Orthopaedic Knowledge Update 2

Home Study Syllabus

American Academy
of Orthopaedic Surgeons

Acknowledgments

Orthopaedic Knowledge Update 2
Home Study Syllabus

Published by the
American Academy of Orthopaedic Surgeons
222 South Prospect Avenue
Park Ridge, Illinois 60068
January 1987

First Edition

Library of Congress Cataloging in Publication Data
86-72286
ISBN 0-89203-018-6

Audiovisual Consultants
Sherman S. Coleman, MD
Thomas H. Comfort, MD
Ramon B. Gustilo, MD
David G. Murray, MD
Andrew J. Weiland, MD
Bertram Zarins, MD

Consultants
Joseph A. Buckwalter, MD
Joseph R. Cass, MD
J. William Fielding, MD
Murray N. Silverstein, MD

American Academy of Orthopaedic Surgeons
Thomas C. Nelson, Executive Director
Fred V. Featherstone, MD, Deputy Executive Director
Mark W. Wieting, Director, Communications and Publications
Wendy O. Schmidt, Project Coordinator

Contents

Lower Extremity

Contributors

Editorial Board

Robert H. Fitzgerald, Jr., MD, Chairman, Rochester, Minnesota
Sherman S. Coleman, MD, Salt Lake City, Utah
Ramon B. Gustilo, MD, Minneapolis, Minnesota
David G. Murray, MD, Syracuse, New York
Bertram Zarins, MD, Boston, Massachusetts

General Orthopaedics Task Force

Chairman	Joseph M. Lane, MD New York, New York
Health Maintenance	Frederick A. Matsen, MD Carol C. Teitz, MD Seattle, Washington
Congenital Abnormalities	Vernon T. Tolo, MD Baltimore, Maryland
Bone Metabolism	John H. Healey, MD Joseph M. Lane, MD I. K. Bills, MD New York, New York
Arthritis	Victor M. Goldberg, MD Cleveland, Ohio
Musculoskeletal Neoplasms	James R. Neff, MD Kansas City, Kansas Franklin H. Sim, MD Rochester, Minnesota
Infection	R. William Petty, MD Gainesville, Florida
Trauma: Hard Tissue	R. Bruce Heppenstall, MD Philadelphia, Pennsylvania
Trauma: Soft Tissue	William E. Garrett, Jr., MD Durham, North Carolina
Neuromuscular Disorders and Gait	Sheldon R. Simon, MD Columbus, Ohio Jacquelin T. Perry, MD Chicago, Illinois
Circulatory, Respiratory, Hematopoietic, Gastrointestinal, Genitourinary, and Integumentary Systems	James H. Herndon, MD Providence, Rhode Island
Prostheses: Implant Materials and Methods of Fixation	E. Y. S. Chao, PhD Rochester, Minnesota
Soft Tissue Implants	William C. Allen, MD Columbia, Missouri
Microsurgery	James A. Nunley II, MD Durham, North Carolina
Bone Grafts	Gary E. Friedlaender, MD New Haven, Connecticut
Imaging of the Musculoskeletal System	Manuel L. Brown, MD Tom H. Berquist, MD Rochester, Minnesota

Upper Extremity Task Force

Chairmen	Peter C. Amadio, MD Robert H. Cofield, MD Rochester, Minnesota
Pediatric Reconstruction	Leonard K. Ruby, MD Boston, Massachusetts
Shoulder: Trauma	Louis U. Bigliani, MD New York, New York
Shoulder: Reconstruction	Robert H. Cofield, MD Rochester, Minnesota
Elbow and Forearm: Trauma in Adult and Pediatric Patients	Robert N. Hotchkiss, MD Baltimore, Maryland
Elbow and Forearm: Reconstruction	Robert G. Volz, MD Tucson, Arizona Bernard F. Morrey, MD Rochester, Minnesota
Wrist and Hand: Trauma	Peter J. Stern, MD Cincinnati, Ohio
Wrist and Hand: Reconstruction	Peter C. Amadio, MD Rochester, Minnesota

Spine Task Force

Chairman	Dan M. Spengler, MD Nashville, Tennessee
Cervical Spine: Pediatric and Reconstructive Aspects	Stephen J. Lipson, MD Boston, Massachusetts
Cervical Spine and Cord: Trauma	Henry H. Bohlman, MD Cleveland, Ohio
Thoracolumbar Spine: Pediatric Aspects	Neil E. Green, MD Nashville, Tennessee
Thoracolumbar Spine: Trauma	Harold K. Dunn, MD Salt Lake City, Utah
Thoracolumbar Spine: Reconstruction	Paul C. McAffee, MD Baltimore, Maryland
Lumbar Spine	Stanley J. Bigos, MD Seattle, Washington Sam W. Wiesel, MD Washington, D.C. Dan M. Spengler, MD Nashville, Tennessee

Lower Extremity Task Force

Chairmen	Robert Poss, MD Bertram Zarins, MD Boston, Massachusetts
Pelvis, Hip, and Femur: Pediatric Aspects	Raymond T. Morrissey, MD Atlanta, Georgia
Trauma: Pelvis and Acetabulum	Joel M. Matta, MD Phillip O. Merritt, MD Los Angeles, California
Trauma: Hip	Richard F. Kyle, MD Minneapolis, Minnesota
Trauma: Femur	Robert A. Winquist, MD Seattle, Washington
Hip Reconstruction: Total Hip Replacement	Dennis K. Collis, MD Eugene, Oregon
Hip Reconstruction: Non-Implant	Richard F. Santore, MD San Diego, California

Knee and Leg: Pediatric Aspects	J. Andy Sullivan, MD Oklahoma City, Oklahoma
Knee and Leg: Soft Tissue Trauma	Lonnie Paulos, MD Salt Lake City, Utah John P. Drawbert, MD Lexington, Kentucky Thomas D. Rosenberg, MD Salt Lake City, Utah
Knee and Leg: Bone Trauma	Jesse C. DeLee, MD San Antonio, Texas
Knee and Leg: Reconstruction	Richard D. Scott, MD Boston, Massachusetts
Ankle and Foot: Pediatric Aspects	Richard E. Lindseth, MD Indianapolis, Indiana
Ankle and Foot: Trauma	Pierce E. Scranton, MD Seattle, Washington
Ankle and Foot: Reconstruction	Roger A. Mann, MD San Leandro, California

Preface

The proliferation of new journals devoted to various aspects of the musculoskeletal system reflects the increase in activity of clinicians and scientists who are attempting to elucidate the pathophysiology and treatment of disease processes affecting the axial and appendicular skeletal structures. This growth in the literature devoted to the musculoskeletal system places an increasing demand on the orthopaedic surgeon. It is becoming impossible for the individual orthopaedic surgeon to be conversant with all of the rapidly developing new concepts and materials described in the medical literature. It is challenging to maintain a working knowledge of the new literature on just a single subspecialty area of orthopaedic surgery. This volume of *Orthopaedic Knowledge Update* utilizes the expertise of surgeons and scientists with specialized experience in various areas. They have summarized, for each area, the literature published between 1983 and 1986, along with pertinent background information. In addition, annotated bibliographies are provided to permit the reader to select those references that will best serve his or her needs.

Publication of the first volume of *Orthopaedic Knowledge Update* was followed by publication of the *Orthopaedic Self-Assessment Examination* and a referenced answer booklet. This second volume of *Orthopaedic Knowledge Update* has these cognitive features and an associated audiovisual tape which emphasizes some of the technologic advances in the recent past. The audiovisual tape covers six subjects presented by knowledgeable surgeons active in each area.

As a learner-centered educational tool, *Orthopaedic Knowledge Update 1* was a resounding success with the Fellowship of the American Academy of Orthopaedic Surgeons. Orthopaedic residents also found it to be an important tool in their education. The success of the first volume of *Orthopaedic Knowledge Update* is a reflection of the efforts of Marc Asher, M.D., and his vision. The syllabus was designed to present the new information in a logical and flowing fashion. The second syllabus has essentially followed the same format with some minor variations which reflect developing areas of interest. The reader will find, in the General Section, chapters dealing with new imaging techniques, bone grafting, microvascular surgery, soft tissue implants, and soft and hard tissue trauma. In the Upper Extremity Section, the pediatric problems of the shoulder, elbow, forearm, wrist, and hand have been combined into one chapter. In the Spine Section, acute and chronic lumbosacral radiculopathies have been combined with mechanical low back pain to form a single chapter.

Fellows of the Academy who subscribed to the first syllabus were randomly canvassed to determine if major changes should be incorporated into subsequent volumes. Although the Ad Hoc Committee on Home Study envisioned that the second and subsequent volumes of the syllabus would be smaller than the initial volume, the Fellowship strongly recommended the inclusion of additional background material. Thus, in size the second volume is comparable to the first. Considerable effort has been devoted to the inclusion of background material that has not been included in the continuing medical education activities and Instructional Courses of the Academy. As with the first syllabus, the process of writing, editing, and printing has required well over a year. Even though contributors made considerable effort to report material as current as possible, material published within the last 6 to 8 months has not been included.

Orthopaedic Knowledge Update 2: Home Study Syllabus is not intended to be a textbook and does not cover all the important information upon which the practice of orthopaedic surgery is based. Basic orthopaedic information is available in many standard textbooks. It is not a yearbook or a periodical. Finally, it is not a statement of principle or a standard of practice.

The *Orthopaedic Self-Assessment Examination* will appear in the Fall of 1987. The Committee on Examinations and Evaluation has had copies of the manuscripts of the syllabus during each phase of development. A major portion of the self-assessment examination will be derived from the material contained within the syllabus.

The completed syllabus reflects intense effort by numerous individuals who donated their time to ensure that *Orthopaedic Knowledge Update 2* will provide the current and future fellows of the Academy with a volume useful as a reference in the daily practice of orthopaedic surgery as well as a guide for in-depth reviews. The members of the editorial board have performed yeoman service. Their careful review of subject matter and probing questions have helped the section chairmen guide individual contributors to make each chapter accurate and yet include new and controversial material. The Academy Fellowship expresses special thanks to all of these individuals for their efforts.

Along with the editorial board, section chairmen, and individual authors, others have contributed to the production of the home study program materials. Robert C. Benassi of the Mayo Clinic coordinated the illustrations used in the videotape. Thomas C. Nelson, Fred V. Featherstone, M.D., Mark W. Wieting, and Wendy O. Schmidt of the Academy staff assisted in the development and printing of this volume. I would also like to thank Susan M. Krusemark, Sharon L. Bratlien, and Rebecca J. Solberg for their assistance.

Robert H. Fitzgerald, Jr., M.D.
Editor

1
Health Maintenance

Because our patients are asking more questions about diet, types of exercise, and stress reduction, this volume of *Orthopaedic Knowledge Update* begins with a section on exercise and health maintenance to provide some basic information. The topics include effect of exercise on cardiac risk factors, measurement of fitness, metabolic and physiologic effects of training, sex differences in athletic performance, and athletic amenorrhea and osteopenia.

Effect of Exercise on Cardiac Risk Factors

The mortality rate from all cardiovascular diseases has diminished by over 30% in the last 15 years. This dramatic result appears to be related to improvements in life-style and decreases in cardiovascular risk factors such as smoking, high blood pressure, excessive body fat, and increased serum cholesterol, triglycerides, glucose, and uric acid values. Many studies have demonstrated that these risk factors are less common or less severe in subjects with higher levels of physical fitness, whether adolescents or adults. The relationship between fitness and risk factors does not appear to be a simple one. For example, if the effects of age, physique, smoking, alcohol use, and stress are rigorously controlled, the effect of fitness on risk factors is not strong. Probably the most reasonable conclusion is that cardiac risk factors can be decreased by a health-maintenance program consisting of increased fitness, avoidance of smoking, minimization of stress, and optimization of diet.

Lipids

Increased serum total cholesterol concentration is a well-known risk factor for coronary artery disease. Low density lipoprotein-cholesterol (LDL-C) may be associated with coronary heart disease more specifically than total cholesterol. High density lipoprotein-cholesterol (HDL-C) level, especially HDL_2, has an inverse relationship with and is a good predictor of coronary heart disease. In one study, every 10 mg/dl change in HDL level was associated with a 50% change in cardiovascular risk. In another study, a 29-week training program statistically improved the plasma lipid profile by decreasing total cholesterol, increasing HDL-C, and decreasing LDL-C and total triglycerides.

The role of serum triglycerides as a cardiac risk factor is not clear. Triglyceride levels decrease in trained subjects after prolonged endurance exercise. Short-term exercise produces no changes in patients with normal triglyceride levels but does lower the level in those with hypertriglyceridemia. Training-related decreases in triglycerides may be due to increased activity of lipoprotein lipase, an enzyme that degrades triglyceride-rich lipoproteins and limits the rate of transport of fatty acids from triglycerides to peripheral tissues. It is not yet clear whether the training-related increase in activity of lipoprotein lipase is induced by exercise alone or by the changes that occur in relation to altered body composition after exercise.

Few studies have examined exercise and cardiac risk factors in women. Levels of lipoprotein lipase generally are higher in women than in men. Estrogen also increases the level of HDL-C. In addition to these inherent advantages in cardiac risk factors, a consistent dose-response association has been found between fitness and cholesterol levels in women.

In summary, most studies support the benefits of physical activity in decreasing the levels of atherogenic lipids in serum. Whether participation in an intense and prolonged exercise training program will prove to be an important therapeutic modality in the prevention of coronary artery disease by improving lipid profiles remains to be determined.

Measurement of Fitness

Many methods have been used for quantifying physical fitness including asking the subject's opinion, measuring the maximum rate of oxygen consumption ($\dot{V}O_2$ max), measuring the anaerobic threshold, and estimating endurance on a bicycle ergometer or treadmill. Each of these methods measures a different factor, giving rise to variable results from clinical studies. Differences in results arise from differences in the circumstances under which the determinations are made—for example, arm ergometry, leg ergometry, stationary bicycle, or treadmill. The following discussion is limited to anaerobic threshold because the current literature indicates that it may be the best predictor of endurance performance and fitness.

Anaerobic Threshold

This is the level of exercise intensity above which the plasma lactate concentration increases and ventilation increases out of proportion to the oxygen intake. Lactate is produced during anaerobic metabolism when the rate of pyruvate formation from glycolysis exceeds the rate of pyruvate oxidation. An increase in plasma lactate may reflect increased production or decreased metabolism of lactate. Acidosis decreases both plasma and muscle lactate concentrations. Hypoxemia, on the other hand, is associated with respiratory alkalosis which can increase plasma lactate levels.

Lactic acidosis is detrimental in a number of ways. In the muscle it accelerates creatine kinase (CK) breakdown and inhibits glycolysis. In addition, associated decreases in muscle pH interfere with the ability of calcium to trigger a muscle contraction. Systemically, lactic acidosis inhibits lipolysis and accelerates carbohydrate utilization. Glycogen is used up more quickly, increasing plasma carbon dioxide levels. Carbon dioxide is also produced when bicarbonate is used to buffer lactic acid. To dispose of this excess carbon dioxide, ventilation must increase. Because of this association between increased plasma lactate and increased ventilation, the anaerobic threshold can be detected by monitoring ventilation rather than plasma lactate concentration. However, it is uncertain whether the lactate threshold and the ventilation threshold are the same—i.e., do the blood lactate levels and the components of gas exchange reflect the same threshold? The ventilation threshold may be determined graphically as the point at which the relationship between ventilation and oxygen uptake changes from a straight line to a curve (Fig. 1). This measurement may be affected by changes in breathing patterns and tidal volume, variations in ventilatory control mechanisms and sensitivity to carbon dioxide, and slow and fast incremental exercise.

In trained athletes the lactate threshold occurs at a higher $\dot{V}O_2$ max than it does in untrained subjects. Training-associated increase in oxidative capacity in both major muscle fiber types also corresponds with increase in the lactate threshold. Fuel substrates may be a factor: a carbohydrate-rich diet decreases the lactate threshold whereas a carbohydrate-poor diet increases it. Increase in plasma free fatty acids also increases the lactate threshold. However, diet changes produce opposite effects in the ventilation threshold.

In addition to disagreements about how the anaerobic threshold should be measured, there is also some debate as to what the anaerobic threshold represents (Table 1). The theories include: 1) an oxygen debt—i.e., the point at which muscle switches to glycolytic (anaerobic) metabolic pathways; 2) a change in muscle fiber type (recruitment from oxidative to glycolytic fiber types); and 3) a change in the balance of regulatory enzymes in muscle.

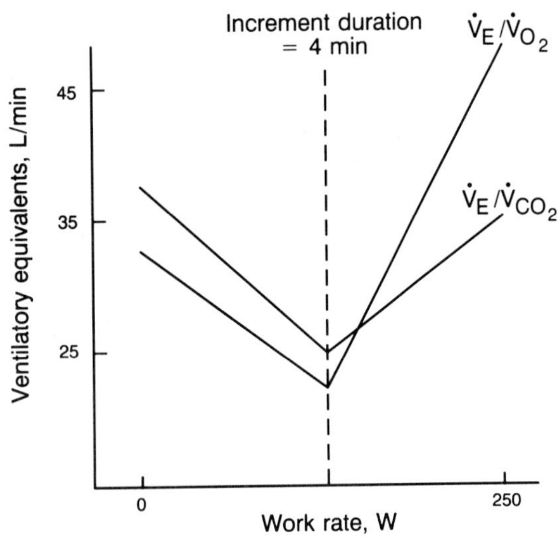

Figure 1

Ventilation threshold. Diagram of changes in ventilatory equivalent for $\dot{V}O_2$ ($\dot{V}_E/\dot{V}O_2$) and for $\dot{V}CO_2$ ($\dot{V}_E/\dot{V}CO_2$). The vertical dashed line denotes the break point in ventilation and gas exchange. The criterion of the systematic increase in $\dot{V}_E/\dot{V}O_2$ without a concomitant increase in $\dot{V}_E/\dot{V}CO_2$ is the most specific gas exchange method for detection of the anaerobic threshold. (From Davis, J.A. Med. Sci. Sports Exerc. 17:6–18, 1985. By permission of the American College of Sports Medicine.)

Table 1. Anaerobic Threshold Controversies

1. What does anaerobic threshold represent?
   - Point at which anaerobic metabolism begins?
   - Changes in muscle (fiber-type) recruitment: shift from slow-twitch to fast-twitch
2. How is it measured?
   - Blood lactate level
     - Amount
       - Absolute increase
       - Relative increase
     - Influential variables
       - pH of serum and muscle
       - Substrate
       - Increased production vs. decreased metabolism
   - Ventilatory threshold ($\dot{V}_E/\dot{V}O_2$)
     - Influential variables
       - Diet
       - Breathing patterns
       - Neural and hormonal sensitivity to CO_2
       - Speed of exercise

All of these controversies do not detract from the apparent usefulness of the anaerobic threshold in predicting endurance performance. Endurance performance is well correlated with the highest oxygen uptake that can be achieved during exercise before a systemic increase in blood lactate concentration occurs. It is also well known that the lactate threshold is higher for endurance-trained subjects than for untrained subjects. Additional correlations between anaerobic threshold and endurance performance include the following.

1. Anaerobic threshold increases approximately 44% with training compared with an increase of 25% in $\dot{V}O_2$ max with training.
2. Anaerobic threshold decreases with age.
3. Anaerobic threshold has the highest correlation ($r = 0.98$) with marathon performance compared with such measurements as relative body fat, $\dot{V}O_2$ max, and percentage of fast-twitch fibers. A few studies have also found that the most successful marathon performers actually run within 5% of their anaerobic threshold.
4. On the basis of the anaerobic threshold, one can predict the highest metabolic rate that can be maintained for long periods of time. This measure may prove to be better than $\dot{V}O_2$ max for assessing exercise intensity and also may be useful as a criterion for disability evaluation.
5. Cessation of training causes decreases not only in $\dot{V}O_2$ max but also in anaerobic threshold.

Hence, the concept of anaerobic threshold is useful because of the high association, predicted theoretically and found experimentally, between endurance exercise tolerance and the onset of lactic acidosis.

In summary, the graphic analysis of ventilation/oxygen consumption ($\dot{V}_E/\dot{V}O_2$) is a favored method for noninvasive detection of the anaerobic threshold. The facts that the ventilation threshold and $\dot{V}O_2$ max vary independently in a population and that endurance training increases the former to a greater extent than the latter support its usefulness as an independent measure of fitness. Potential applications of the anaerobic threshold include: exercise prescription, characterizing and selecting endurance athletes, predicting endurance performance, measuring effects of endurance training, studying effects of drugs on exercise tolerance, and correlating the anaerobic threshold with muscle fiber composition and biochemical properties of skeletal muscle.

Metabolic and Physiologic Effects of Training

Training has a substantial effect on metabolism. For example, a 6-week training program induces a higher rate of lipid utilization, a decreased rate of carbohydrate utilization, a slower lactate increase, and an increased utilization of exogenous glucose. Furthermore, training decreases the sympathoadrenal response to exercise as well as the autonomic recovery from psychosocial stress. This observation may be of particular importance in view of the relationship between stress and coronary artery disease.

Muscle Adaptations

There is a strong association between lactate threshold and ability to perform endurance exercise. The muscle's respiratory capacity is of primary importance in determining the work rate at which blood lactate accumulation begins. Muscle adapts to training by increasing the concentration of mitochondria and by increasing the enzymes for oxidative metabolism, thus increasing the total oxidative potential of the muscle fibers. Muscle also responds to conditioning by an increased capillarization. Thus, increased fitness improves the body's ability to deliver metabolites to the muscle and the muscle's ability to utilize these metabolites.

The proportion of slow-twitch fibers also may play an important role in determining the relative lactate threshold. One study found that the percentage and relative fiber area of slow-twitch fibers were significantly related to the lactate threshold. The ratio of slow-twitch to fast-twitch fibers may exert a genetic influence over the lactate threshold and may control the range in which the relative lactate threshold can shift. This finding supports a current concept that endurance athletes are born rather than made.

Substrate Utilization

During exercise at the same intensity, physically trained individuals derive a much greater percentage of their energy from fatty acid oxidation than do untrained individuals. Increasing lipid oxidation during exercise has been shown to slow the rate of glycolysis and inhibit lactate formation, thereby also influencing the muscle's respiratory capacity. Hence, the beneficial effects of training on endurance performance are not solely incidental to increased $\dot{V}O_2$ max. Changes occur in muscle ultrastructure, capillarization, oxidative capacity, and substrate utilization, all of which may be major determinants of successful, prolonged performance.

Plasma Insulin and Glucose Tolerance

The increased muscle capillarization and increased oxidative enzyme activity in trained muscle also have been used to explain lower plasma insulin levels and improved glucose tolerance in a group of obese women on an aerobic conditioning program for 3 months. These changes in insulin and glucose tolerance were associated with an increased percentage of fast-twitch oxidative fibers and a decrease in fast-twitch glycolytic fibers as well as increased capillarization. From the capillary density around those fibers, 80% of the explained variance of the plasma insulin levels could be predicted. It seems probable that the increased capillarization in muscle constitutes at least one of the factors that facilitate insulin uptake. This increased capillarization is thought to occur prior to changes in enzyme activities and muscle fiber morphology.

The changes in glucose concentration after training also could be predicted by observed changes in enzyme activities. The activities of oxidative enzymes increase while those of glycolytic enzymes decrease. The changes noted are due partly to changes in the autonomic nervous system and depressed pancreatic secretion of insulin and partly to increased peripheral uptake of glucose and insulin in muscle tissue and liver. As proposed by Gollnick and Saltin, the main local adaptation occurring in muscle tissue after training is increased use of fat and decreased carbohydrate consumption. Physical training thus may be an effective means of preventing the development of the carbohydrate metabolism abnormalities that are observed in the obese.

Muscle Strength

Strong muscles commonly are touted as being more resistant to strains and more likely to endure prolonged exercise. However, opinions vary greatly regarding the best techniques for strengthening muscles and for measuring improvements in muscle strength. Strengthening techniques include isometric, isotonic, and isokinetic resistive exercises as well as electrical stimulation of muscle.

One study looked at the relationship between the strength of the human quadriceps and its cross-sectional area. Muscles were trained by using high-resistance, low-repetition, dynamic exercise. Cross-sectional area was determined by ultrasound scanning and measurement of thigh circumference. Strength was determined by measuring maximal voluntary isometric contraction. Measurements of thigh circumference underestimated the amount of quadriceps hypertrophy found on scanning. Moreover, the isometric strength of trained quadriceps increased more than did the cross-sectional area. The authors thought that the strength gains might be due to the improved ability to increase motor unit recruitment in a maximal voluntary contraction. However, others have suggested that type II fibers may be able to generate more force per cross-sectional area than some type I fibers. Hence, preferential hypertrophy of type II fibers would result in greater increase in strength than in muscle cross-sectional area. Biopsies in these subjects, however, showed no evidence of selective hypertrophy of either fiber type. The authors concluded that studies of muscle growth must include a direct measurement of the size of the muscle concerned.

In a recent study on strength changes as a result of electrical stimulation, 58 subjects were divided into three groups: one group trained by using isometric exercise alone; one group did not train and served as a control; and one group underwent daily stimulation of the quadriceps femoris. After 5 weeks, both the isometric exercise group and the electrical stimulation group had statistically significant increases in quadriceps femoris torque compared with the controls. In addition, the electrical stimulation group had a larger strength gain than did the isometric exercise group. However, during exercise, the peak torque of the isometric exercise group was considerably greater than that of the electrical stimulation group. The lower torque observed in the electrical stimulation group suggests that subjects in this group strengthen their quadriceps femoris while experiencing less joint compressive forces than the subjects in the isometric exercise group.

This finding has implications in the rehabilitation of patients after knee arthroplasty. With an appropriate muscle stimulator, transcutaneous electrical stimulation can significantly increase the strength of normal skeletal muscle. In athletes, this may shorten the rehabilitation time required after knee surgery. This therapeutic effect may be achieved by subjecting the joint and surrounding soft tissue to stresses of lesser magnitude than those developed through isometric contractions.

One study examined the effects of adding electromyographic feedback to isometric exercise and found that the combination of biofeedback and isometric exercise brought about greater strength gains than did exercise alone. This finding was explained by possible reorganization of facilitation patterns. These patterns may be responsible for either an increased firing rate or an increased number of motor units recruited. The effect represents motor learning by the subject. More research is needed to refine techniques for measurement of muscle growth and strength and for muscle strengthening.

Sex Differences in Athletic Performance

Sex differences in athletic performance are largely due to variations in body size, body composition, aerobic power, and muscular strength. The differences between any two individuals of the same sex are often greater than those between an average man and average woman. The average man is taller, heavier, and has less body fat than the average woman. Essential body fat is 3% in men and 12% in women. The average woman has 22% to 26% body fat, although trained women may have less than 15% body fat; the average man has 16% body fat. Fat increases the amount of dead weight, so it increases the metabolic cost of weight-bearing activities without increasing the ability to produce energy. Therefore, it decreases performance in some endurance events. Moreover, because of greater body fat, women have relatively less muscle with which to exert a force when strength, power, speed, and endurance are required.

Aerobic Capacity

Men generally have a greater $\dot{V}O_2$ max than women. This difference is in part attributed to less dead weight and the fact that a larger body requires a larger $\dot{V}O_2$ max. Men usually have larger hearts, more hemoglobin, and a larger blood volume than women. Regardless of whether heart size is expressed as absolute volume or relative to body size, the heart in women is only 80% to 90% as large as that in men. Therefore, the stroke volume is smaller in women, but this is compensated for to a degree by an increased heart rate. However, the absolute maximum heart rate is equal in men and women. Therefore, because of the larger heart size and larger stroke volume, the cardiac output (rate times stroke volume) is approximately 30% greater in men than in women. Hemoglobin concentration in men is approximately 2 g/dl greater than it is in women, and men also have a 12% to 25% greater blood volume. The curves of $\dot{V}O_2$ max in men and women overlap (Fig. 2). However, because $\dot{V}O_2$ max is determined in part by cardiac output, blood volume, hemoglobin, and dead weight, the average woman obviously has a decreased oxygen-carrying capacity and therefore a lower $\dot{V}O_2$ max than the average man.

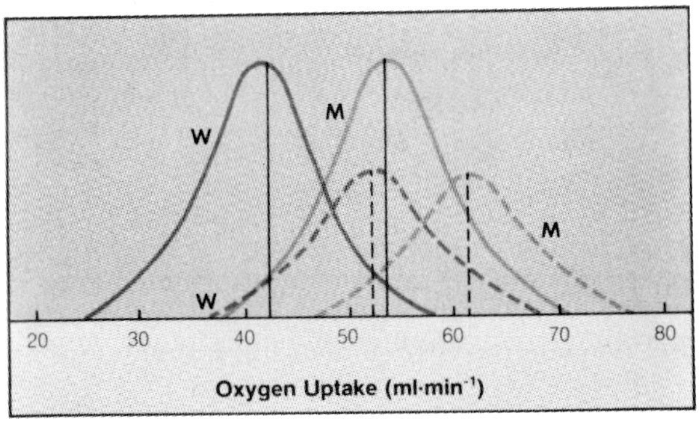

Figure 2

Frequency distribution of aerobic power ($\dot{V}O_2$ max) in men (*M*) and women (*W*). Broken lines represent oxygen uptakes of trained distance runners. (From Wells, C.L., and Plowman, S.A. Physician Sportsmedicine 11:52–63, August 1983. By permission of McGraw-Hill.)

Muscular Strength

Men typically have greater muscular strength than women do. This difference may be behavioral or it may be due to greater size, greater lean body mass, and more muscle fibers. Upper body strength in women is reported to be 56% of that in men, trunk strength about 64%, and lower body strength about 72%. However, if the muscle strength is compared relative to lean body mass, upper extremity strength, as measured by the ability to do biceps curls, in women increases to 76% of that in men, bench press strength increases to 83%, and leg press strength increases to 106%. When strength is examined relative to the cross-sectional area of muscle, it is equal in men and women. Women respond the same as men to exercise and training. In one study, 10 healthy women with a mean age of 30 years underwent arm and leg ergometer tests to measure $\dot{V}O_2$ max during submaximal and maximal exercise. The ratio of upper extremity to lower extremity $\dot{V}O_2$ max was found to be comparable in men and women. Hence, although the absolute $\dot{V}O_2$ max is lower in women than men, their aerobic capacity for arm work is not disproportionately inferior to that of men.

Susceptibility to Injuries

Exercise-related injuries are similar in men and women. Women "midshipmen" have been followed since they were first admitted to the United States Naval Academy at Annapolis. Initially, they had 10% more overuse injuries than the male recruits. In a recent study with a 7-year follow-up, the incidence of overuse injuries is 1.5% higher in women than in men. Women midshipmen have the same number of serious injuries as men and have also been found to be more susceptible to injuries in basketball and gymnastics than their male counterparts. However, women are now able to do more pull-ups than in previous tests. In addition, criteria for passing physical tests are continually revised upward as fitness levels of entering women improve. Because these women continue to improve in fitness level more rapidly than do the male midshipmen peers, the author concluded that the disparities in performance in many cases should be attributed to societal conditions rather than physiologic differences. If the performance requirements ever become the same, women will have to work harder than men to achieve the same standards because of the physiologic differences.

Osteopenia and Athletic Amenorrhea

Exercise and Bone Mineral Content

Approximately one-fourth of women over age 60 have osteoporosis. In postmenopausal women with previously documented osteopenia, regular exercise has been found to increase the mineral content in the vertebral bodies, in contrast to a continuing loss of bone in nonexercising controls. Despite this beneficial effect of exercise on bone mineral content, recent studies have shown that young, premenopausal women who are amenorrheic lose cancellous bone at rates similar to those in postmenopausal women despite, and perhaps due to, intense exercise.

In a well-controlled study in which amenorrheic and eumenorrheic athletes were matched for nutritional levels, percentage body fat, age at menarche, and years of sport participation, the amenorrheic athletes had significantly less vertebral mineral than did the eumenorrheic group. However, there was no difference in the mineral density of the radius. The amenorrheic athletes ran significantly more miles per week and had significantly lower mean estradiol concentrations, progesterone peaks, and prolactin levels than the eumenorrheic athletes. It is not known whether the vertebral bone loss noted in amenorrheic athletes is due to total body mineral loss or to "movement" of the mineral from a relatively nonstressed area to a highly stressed area—for example, from the spine to the legs in a runner. In addition, the effect of mineral loss has not yet been shown to be clinically crucial, at least in the young amenorrheic athlete—i.e., no one has yet found any increased incidence of fracture or stress fracture in premenopausal amenorrheic women compared with eumenorrheic women.

Athletic Oligomenorrhea and Amenorrhea

In the past 5 years, descriptive studies have shown a relatively high incidence of menstrual cycle irregularity in athletes. In a summary of the available literature, the prevalence of oligomenorrhea or amenorrhea was 5% of the general population, 20% of exercising women, and about 50% of women in competitive athletics. It is more prevalent in runners than in swimmers and cyclists, but when all studies are combined, there appears to be no correlation with the weekly mileage, the pace, or the number of years of training. One study showed a trend toward fewer menstrual cycles in runners with low body weight and high mileage; however, less than one-fourth of the runners with disrupted cycles had both low weight and high mileage.

The incidence of oligomenorrhea or amenorrhea is also increased in women who weigh less than 52 kg (115 pounds) and in those who have lost more than 4.5 kg (10 pounds). However, the mechanism for this increased incidence has not been elucidated. Prior menstrual irregularity is commonly found in women who become amenorrheic when exercising. Although athletic oligomenorrhea or amenorrhea initially was thought to be due solely to excessively low body fat levels, subsequent studies have shown that amenorrhea may be caused by many interacting factors including hormonal alterations that accompany exercise and training, stress, caloric expenditure, and loss of body fat.

One of the problems common to many of the studies is documenting that the amenorrheic women are anovulatory. Amenorrhea can represent luteal phase deficiency, euestrogenic anovulation, or hypoestrogenic amenorrhea. In many cases the women are ovulating but not menstruating. In other cases they are menstruating but not ovulating. Even in women with apparently regular menses, one-third will have normal luteal function, one-third will demonstrate luteal phase inadequacy, and one-third will be anovulatory. The central issue is whether the ovaries are functioning to produce estrogen. It is the relative estrogen loss that may be responsible for the recent findings of decreased mineral in the vertebrae of young amenorrheic women.

The accumulated evidence strongly implicates intensive regular training as the direct cause of exercise-induced amenorrhea. It is not understood how chronic exercise stimulates changes in the menstrual cycle but it is known that profound increases can occur in the availability of sex hormones during exercise. Such alterations have been attributed to reduced degradation or enhanced secretion. In addition, other effects may be due to a change in the free fraction of the circulating hormonal pool.

During training, alterations in hormones include acute increases in estradiol, prostaglandins, prolactin, and testosterone. The latter two return to normal within 1 to 2 hours after the cessation of exercise. Some investigators have also found increases in ACTH, opioids, melatonin, and cortisol. In addition, testosterone and cortisol levels have been found to increase just prior to initiation of exercise, possibly due to psychologic stimuli. The roles of follicle-stimulating hormone (FSH) and luteinizing hormone (LH) are particularly critical. A deficiency in either of these gonadotropic hormones or the necessary follicular enzymes will impair estradiol production and consequent maturation of the follicle.

The sensitivity of the hypothalamus-pituitary axis may differ in trained and untrained women. One study of trained runners showed normal FSH and LH secretion from the pituitary gland in response to a stimulation test. However, other authors have found both impaired and augmented LH release in marathon runners. The exercise-stimulated increases in prolactin seen in trained subjects have not been observed in untrained subjects. Chronically short luteal phases secondary to low midluteal phase progesterone levels also have been found in some women who regularly engage in high-mileage exercise. These findings are reversible when exercise intensity is reduced. A decreased rate of metabolic clearance of estradiol has also been correlated with exercise intensity. In addition, chronic exercise can affect the concentrations of the primary plasma receptor for estradiol and testosterone—namely, testosterone-estradiol binding globulin. How the repetitive transient hormone alterations relate to long-term changes in female athletes and how hormonal differences between amenorrheic and eumenorrheic athletes account for the differences in menstrual patterns remain unproven.

Athletes with oligomenorrhea or amenorrhea should be

evaluated. Pregnancy must be ruled out either by history and physical examination or by laboratory test. One should then obtain FSH, LH, prolactin, TSH, T4, and T3 levels. In addition, a progestin challenge test can be done to determine if menstruation can be induced, implying euestrogenic endometrium. Exercise-induced amenorrhea should be a diagnosis of exclusion. An extensive discussion of the treatment of this condition is beyond the scope of this chapter; however, if ovulatory menses return, normal fertility can be expected. Current therapeutic approaches are directed toward reestablishing the menstrual cycle with sequential hormone replacement. Additional research needs to be done in this area in order to develop specific guidelines and prognoses for the amenorrheic athlete.

Motor Vehicle Accident Injury Prevention

Installation of safety belts in all automobiles and light trucks became mandatory in 1966. They have proved to be the most effective safety device available for motorists because they prevent the "second collision" of the occupant with the inside of the vehicle. Usage rates are less than 15% in states without usage laws but can be increased to 40% to 90% with public education and enforcement of mandatory use laws such as those now in effect in more than 20 states.

Protective packaging, both active and passive, can decrease or prevent altogether the majority of serious and fatal injuries to head and spine, chest and abdomen, and extremities. Air bags stored in the steering wheel and lower dashboard are passive restraints for those unwilling to buckle up, a population with a significantly higher accident rate than safety belt users have. Air bags inflate in 0.03 second. Due to improved load distribution, they provide protection superior to that from safety belts in head-on impacts, although there is less roll-over protection because air bags deflate in 0.3 second to prevent rebound. Passive static restraints include rounded-contour, high-energy-absorbing dashboards and energy-absorbing steering wheels and columns. These protect the torso and extremities in head-on collisions. Windshield glass with a plastic, nonlacerative inner surface is designed to act as a net for the head. Some vehicle seat cushions use the buttocks as an energy input target by having an upward-sloping forward shield beneath the seat cushion padding. Two-thirds of the body can be controlled by using the knees and buttocks as such targets against the lower dashboard and seat cushion.

Sports Medicine Injury Prevention and Bracing

Injury Prevention

Sports regulatory bodies have made strides toward eliminating biomechanically inadequate protective devices, establishing standards, and understanding the relationship of footwear to turf and surface fixation. Injurious effects of rigid protective equipment (e.g., football helmets) remain a problem. Vital and vulnerable areas such as the head, eyes, neck, kidneys, genitals, and teeth must be protected from sticks (e.g., in hockey and lacrosse) and from high-velocity, low-mass hazards (e.g., in baseball and racquet sports) by means of helmets, face masks, eye protection, and mouthguards (mandatory in football).

Bracing

The prophylactic value of taping susceptible joints is well established but not of practical use at all levels. The value of braces is not clearly supported by biomechanical and clinical data. There are two basic types of prophylactic knee braces: lateral bars with single-axis, dual-axis, or polycentric hinges; and plastic shells that encircle the thigh and calf and have polycentric hinges. Biomechanical data suggest that prophylactic braces do not provide increased stiffness to valgus loads. A study using the KT-1000 knee arthrometer showed that anterior tibial displacement was unaffected by prophylactic braces. Short-term clinical data on prophylactic knee bracing for football are contradictory. Several studies showed a trend toward a decreased incidence of serious medial ligament injuries, but others showed no changes in incidence and no studies showed reduction of anterior cruciate ligament or meniscus injuries.

Rehabilitative Knee Braces These have some or all of the following features: single- or dual-axis or polycentric hinges, hinge brace arms (either offset or not), underwraps for edema control, thigh and calf enclosures (Velfoam, medial and lateral plastic shells, circumferential plastic shells), straps (that encircle brace components, thigh, and calf), shoe inserts, and exercise and augmentation control springs and straps. One study of four rehabilitative brace types controlling static anterior, valgus, and rotational forces in cadaver limbs, but without control of tightness of brace application, failed to show that such braces restore normal stability. The brace with medial and lateral plastic shells and offset hinges performed best. Largely anecdotal reports of good results must be set against a study that showed that rehabilitative knee braces allow knee extension of 15° to 20° past hinge stop settings.

Functional Knee Braces There are two construction types and designs, featuring hinge posts with or without shells to encompass thigh and calf. No biomedical conclusions are possible because only preliminary and fragmentary data are available; clinical studies have shown that functional knee braces subjectively decrease giving-way episodes in some patients. Greatest benefits have been achieved in those wearers with lesser degrees of ligamentous laxity. No statement can be made as to the effect of functional knee braces on ligament defects other than those of the anterior cruciate ligament.

Conclusion

Bracing remains a topic replete with anecdotal comments and unsubstantiated claims regarding effectiveness. In addition to biomechanical and epidemiologic research, efforts need to be made to curtail unnecessary use in light of the scant evidence on the efficacy of knee bracing.

Annotated Bibliography

Effect of Exercise on Cardiac Risk Factors

Brown, T.F.; Myles, W.S.; and Allen, C.L.: The relationship between aerobic fitness and certain cardiovascular risk factors. Aviat. Space Environ. Med. 54:543–547, 1983.

In 2,500 servicemen, improved fitness was associated with decreased values for cardiac risk factors in young (<40 years old) as well as older men.

Gibbons, L.W.; Blair, S.N.; Cooper, K.H.; and Smith, M.: Association between coronary heart disease risk factors and physical fitness in healthy adult women. Circulation 67:977–983, 1983.

In 1,700 women, the authors found a consistent dose-response association between fitness and HDL cholesterol (HDL-C) level, triglycerides, total cholesterol/HDL-C ratios, blood pressure, and cigarette smoking. The study is one of the few that has looked at fitness and risk factors in women.

Goldberg, L., and Elliot, D.L.: The effect of physical activity on lipid and lipoprotein levels. Med. Clin. North Am. 69:41–55, January 1985.

The authors provide an excellent summary of information on this topic to date.

Hagberg, J.M.; Goldring, D.; Ehsani, A.A.; Heath, G.W.; Hernandez, A.; Schechtman, K.; and Holloszy, J.O.: Effect of exercise training on the blood pressure and hemodynamic features of hypertensive adolescents. Am. J. Cardiol. 52:763–768, 1983.

Six months of exercise training can lower systolic and diastolic blood pressure significantly in hypertensive adolescents.

Heath, G.W.; Ehsani, A.A.; Hagberg, J.M.; Hinderliter, J.M.; and Goldberg, A.P.: Exercise training improves lipoprotein lipid profiles in patients with coronary artery disease. Am. Heart J. 105:889–895, 1983.

In 10 men with coronary artery disease who trained for 6 months, increased maximal work capacity was associated with statistically significant improvements in plasma levels of total cholesterol, HDL-C, LDL-C, and total triglycerides. Changes were maximal in patients with low $\dot{V}O_2$ max, high LDL-C, and low HDL-C initially.

Kannel, W.B.; Doyle, J.T.; Ostfeld, A.M.; Jenkins, C.D.; Kuller, L.; Podell, R.N.; and Stamler, J. (Atherosclerosis Study Group): Optimal resources for primary prevention of atherosclerotic diseases. Circulation 70:155A-205A, 1984.

Since 1968, there has been an annual decrease of 3% in cardiovascular disease mortality which appears to be due to improvements in life-style and modification of cardiovascular risk factors. The authors recommend avoiding a diet excessive in calories, total fat, saturated fat, cholesterol, and salt. They also recommend avoidance of a sedentary pattern of living, weight gain, and cigarette smoking.

Paffenbarger, R.S., Jr.; Hyde, R.T.; Wing, A.L.; and Hsieh, C.-C.: Physical activity, all-cause mortality, and longevity of college alumni. N. Engl. J. Med. 314:605–613, 1986.

This article clearly demonstrates the advantages of a general exercise program for prolonging life. Men performing 2,000 kcal of exercise per week had 25% to 33% lower mortality rates. At highest risk were women who were smokers, had hypertension, and led a sedentary life.

Sedgwick, A.W.; Davidson, A.H.; Taplin, R.E.; and Thomas, D.W.: Relationships between physical fitness and risk factors for coronary heart disease in men and women. Aust. N.Z. J. Med. 14:208–214, 1984.

When the effects of age, physique, smoking, alcohol use, and stress were controlled, the relationships of fitness to blood pressure, serum cholesterol, and serum triglycerides were seen as weak trends of minor clinical importance.

Stamler, J., and Stamler, R.: Intervention for the prevention and control of hypertension and atherosclerotic diseases: United States and international experience. Am. J. Med. 76:13–36, February 27, 1984.

Cigarette smoking is one of the established major risk factors for coronary heart disease. Unequivocal proof has been provided for the important role of smoking in the cause of premature severe atherosclerotic disease and its clinical sequelae. Hypertension is a major risk factor that can be lessened by appropriate treatment. From 1969 to 1981 the mortality rates from all cardiovascular diseases have diminished 33%.

Measurement of Fitness

Davis, J.A.: Anaerobic threshold: Review of the concept and directions for future research. Med. Sci. Sports Exerc. 17:6–18, 1985.

An excellent review of the concept of anaerobic threshold, including controversies and directions for future research. Controversy exists regarding postulated mechanisms for the anaerobic threshold and techniques for measuring the threshold.

Hammond, H.K., and Froelicher, V.F.: Exercise testing for cardiorespiratory fitness. Sports Med. 1:234–239, 1984.

Maximal oxygen consumption measurements do not predict athletic performance.

Ready, A.E., and Quinney, H.A.: Alterations in anaerobic threshold as the result of endurance training and detraining. Med. Sci. Sports Exerc. 14:292–296, 1982.

Twenty-one males achieved significant increases in $\dot{V}O_2$ max and anaerobic threshold during a 9-week training period. Loss of absolute $\dot{V}O_2$ max and a decline in anaerobic threshold both were significant at 6 weeks after the cessation of training.

Tanaka, K.; Matsuura, Y.; Matsuzaka, A.; Hirakoba, K.; Kumagai, S.; Sun, S.O.; and Asano, K.: A longitudinal assessment of anaerobic threshold and distance-running performance. Med. Sci. Sports Exerc. 16:278–282, 1984.

Anaerobic threshold, $\dot{V}O_2$ max, and distance running performances were measured on 21 well-trained male runners. Improved performance was significantly correlated with improvement in $\dot{V}O_2$ at anaerobic threshold but not with changes in $\dot{V}O_2$ max.

Metabolic and Physiologic Effects of Training

Gollnick, P.D.; Hermansen, L.; and Saltin, B.: The muscle biopsy: Still a research tool. Physician Sportsmedicine 8:50–55, January 1980.

Muscle adapts to training by increasing its content of mitochondria and by increasing the enzymes for oxidative metabolism, thus increasing the total oxidative potential of the muscle fibers. Muscle also responds to conditioning by increasing its capillary bed. Thus, increased fitness improves the body's ability to deliver metabolites to the muscle and the muscle's ability to utilize these metabolites.

Hargreaves, M.; Costill, D.L.; Coggan, A.; Fink, W.J.; and Nishibata, I.: Effect of carbohydrate feedings on muscle glycogen utilization and exercise performance. Med. Sci. Sports Exerc. 16:219–222, 1984.

Ten men were studied during 4 hours of cycling. The authors concluded that repeated feedings of solid carbohydrate maintain blood glucose levels, reduce muscle glycogen depletion during prolonged exercise, and enhance sprint performance at the end of such activity.

Krotkiewski, M.; Bylund-Fallenius, A.-C.; Holm, J.; Björntorp, P.; Grimby, G.; and Mandroukas, K.: Relationship between muscle morphology and metabolism in obese women: The effects of long-term physical training. Eur. J. Clin. Invest. 13:5–12, 1983.

Twenty obese women subjected to a physical training program for 3 months changed neither body weight nor body fat. However, lowered plasma insulin levels and improved glucose tolerance were found and were explained by increased muscle capillary bed and increased oxidative enzyme activity.

Krzentowski, G.; Pirnay, F.; Luyckx, A.S.; Lacroix, M.; Mosora, F.; and Lefebvre, P.J.: Effect of physical training on utilization of a glucose load given orally during exercise. Am. J. Physiol. 246:E412–E417, 1984.

A 6-week training program induced a higher rate of lipid utilization, a decreased rate of carbohydrate utilization, a decreased lactate rise, a significant decrease in the sympatho-adrenal response to exercise, and increased utilization of exogenous glucose.

Laughman, R.K.; Youdas, J.W.; Garrett, T.R.; and Chao, E.Y.S.: Strength changes in the normal quadriceps femoris muscle as a result of electrical stimulation. Phys. Ther. 63:494–499, 1983.

Fifty-eight subjects were randomly assigned to one of three groups. After 5 weeks, both the electrical stimulation and isometric exercise groups had statistically significant increases in torque of the quadriceps of the thigh compared with the nonexercised controls.

Lucca, J.A., and Recchiuti, S.J.: Effect of electromyographic biofeedback on an isometric strengthening program. Phys. Ther. 63:200–203, 1983.

Thirty subjects were randomly assigned to one of three groups. After a 19–day training period, significantly greater gains in peak torque were found in the biofeedback-isometric exercise group compared with those in the isometric exercise group or the control group.

Young, A.; Stokes, M.; Round, J.M.; and Edwards, R.H.T.: The effect of high-resistance training on the strength and cross-sectional area of the human quadriceps. Eur. J. Clin. Invest. 13:411–417, 1983.

Increases in isometric strength of a muscle exceed those predicted from increase in cross-sectional area.

Sex Difference in Athletic Performance

Cox, J.S., and Lenz, H.W.: Women midshipmen in sports. Am. J. Sports Med. 12:241–243, 1984.

Seven-year follow-up on Naval Academy women midshipmen revealed more overuse injuries initially. Criteria for passing physical tests are continually revised upward as fitness levels of entering women improve.

Vander, L.B.; Franklin, B.A.; Wrisley, D.; and Rubenfire, M.: Cardiorespiratory responses to arm and leg ergometry in women. Physician Sportsmedicine 12:101–106, May 1984.

The ratio of $\dot{V}O_2$ max values in upper and lower extremities in women was found to be comparable with previously measured values for men. Although absolute $\dot{V}O_2$ during arm and leg ergometry is lower in women than in men, their aerobic capacity for arm work is not disproportionately inferior to men's.

Wells, C.L., and Plowman, S.A.: Sexual differences in athletic performance: Biological or behavioral? Physician Sportsmedicine 11:52–63, August 1983.

A review of the literature on sex differences including body composition, aerobic power (including $\dot{V}O_2$, heart size, cardiac output, and hemoglobin), and strength.

Athletic Amenorrhea and Osteopenia

Drinkwater, B.L.; Nilson, K.; Chesnut, C.H., III; Bremner, W.J.; Shainholtz, S.; and Southworth, M.B.: Bone mineral content of amenorrheic and eumenorrheic athletes. N. Engl. J. Med. 311:277–281, 1984.

The authors tested, and proved false, the assumption that activity might exert a protective effect against bone loss in amenorrheic athletes.

Krølner, B.; Toft, B.; Nielsen, S.P.; and Tøndevold, E.: Physical exercise as prophylaxis against involutional vertebral bone loss: A controlled trial. Clin. Sci. 64:541–546, 1983.

Thirty-one women with previous Colles' fracture of the forearm were allocated to either a physical exercise group or a control group. Lumbar spine bone mineral content of the exercise group increased significantly compared with loss of bone in the control group.

Shangold, M.M.: Causes, evaluation, and management of athletic oligo-/amenorrhea. Med. Clin. North Am. 69:83–95, January 1985.

This article discusses the many interacting factors that may contribute to the development of athletic amenorrhea. The author provides a practical approach for evaluating oligomenorrhea and amenorrheic athletes and recommends several options for treating these patients.

Motor Vehicle Accident Injury Prevention

International Symposium on Occupant Restraint. Arlington Heights, Illinois, American Association for Automotive Medicine, 1981.

This book is a collection of 23 papers on safety belt systems, automatic restraint systems, and child restraints. Design performance, effectiveness, and the societal impacts of safety belt usage laws and the cause of accidents are presented.

Bracing for Prevention of Injury in Sports

American Academy of Orthopaedic Surgeons: Athletic Training and Sports Medicine. First edition. Chicago, 1984.

This manual, prepared by the Sports Medicine Committee of AAOS, is designed for trainers, coaches, and team physicians who are responsible for the health, environment, and physical well-being of athletes in sports competition.

AAOS Sports Medicine Committee: Knee Braces: Seminar Report. Chicago, American Academy of Orthopaedic Surgeons, 1985.

This report summarizes evaluations, by teams of knowledgeable orthopaedists and bioengineers, of objective data available in 1984 regarding the design and effectiveness of prophylactic, rehabilitative, and functional knee braces.

2

Congenital Abnormalities

Congenital abnormalities of the skeleton occur in many settings. Some defects, such as congenital constriction bands, may be isolated to a single region; others may be more generalized, involving various areas of orthopaedic concern in a pattern that may change with time as the child matures. The congenital problems of a single part or a single event are dealt with in other sections. This chapter addresses conditions that are present at birth, that often include several orthopaedic abnormalities, and that frequently are less common than isolated abnormalities.

Skeletal Dysplasias

The number of syndromes reported to be of genetic importance continues to increase. Various classifications have been proposed to allow systematic study of these dysmorphic individuals, but the principal classification of which orthopaedists should be aware is the International Nomenclature of Constitutional Diseases of Bone, published from Paris in 1976. Although specific defects have been demonstrated by electron microscopy and enzyme chemistry for some of these dysplasias, the initial diagnosis generally is made clinically on the basis of recognizable features and abnormalities.

It is best if the diagnosis can be established during infancy, so that the child's family can be given advice regarding expectations for this child and also regarding their chances of having a similarly afflicted child subsequently. Centers that provide multidisciplinary services for patients with skeletal dysplasias are the best sources of care for these patients because of the rarity of the condition and the lack of adequate experience among general orthopaedists. Whereas once all short-stature patients were classified as having either achondroplasia or Morquio's syndrome, much more specificity is required now for appropriate care. Amniocentesis, ultrasonography, and other new techniques may permit diagnosis *in utero*.

Achondroplasia

This is the most common of the short-limbed dysplasias and can readily be diagnosed clinically at birth. Features at birth include a prominent forehead, depression of the nasal bridge, thoracolumbar kyphosis, hypotonia, and short limbs with a normal length of trunk. The diagnosis can be confirmed by radiographic findings of narrowed interpediculate distances in the lumbar spine, vertebral wedging (T-12 or L-1), and short iliac wings with a small sciatic notch.

The underlying cause of achondroplasia has not been fully delineated, but the limb growth disturbance is likely due to abnormal endochondral ossification resulting from an incompletely developed hypertrophic zone in the growth plate. The growth plates in the ilia are normal, and trunk growth is not affected. In the forearm and in the leg, growth of the radius and tibia is affected more than growth of the ulna and fibula, leading to angular limb deformities in these regions.

In many of these children, some motor milestone delay is common. However, the principal orthopaedic care needed is for the spine and the lower extremities. In the spine, one may find stenosis at the level of the foramen magnum or the cervical region, but the most common problems are thoracolumbar kyphosis and lumbar spinal stenosis.

Thoracolumbar kyphosis is generally noted when the child sits upright. Although the kyphosis resolves over the first few years of life in about 90% of the children, bracing is needed if the kyphosis persists. Initially asymptomatic, a progressive kyphosis will lead to spinal cord compression and lower extremity neurologic deficits in adolescence or young adulthood (third decade), at which time the treatment required is usually both anterior and posterior fusion (Fig. 1). Even if a significant kyphosis is not present, in adults spinal stenosis will frequently develop from the narrowed lumbar spinal canal, in combination with hypertrophic degenerative changes at the facet joints. Myelography, through an upper cervical puncture to avoid causing neurologic deficits, should be done to assess possible spinal cord compression and the level of compression. If lumbar spinal stenosis is present without thoracolumbar kyphosis, laminectomy from the lower thoracic spine to the sacrum is performed without fusion.

The most common lower extremity problem is genu varum, due mainly to the relative overgrowth of the fibula but also due to some degree to the joint laxity present. Osteotomy of the tibia alone is generally insufficient and a preferable approach may include a shortening osteotomy of the fibula or an epiphyseodesis of the proximal fibula.

About 10% of patients with achondroplasia have significant respiratory problems. The causes include an abnormal thoracic cage configuration with rib flaring, upper airway obstruction due to skull shape, or upper cervical or foramen magnum cord compression. Careful preoperative assessment and postoperative monitoring (intensive care unit) of the pulmonary function in these patients is needed.

Pseudoachondroplasia

These patients also are short-limbed but this dysplasia may be differentiated from achondroplasia by the normal face and skull and the absence of lumbar spine interpediculate narrowing. The diagnosis is confirmed by radiographs of the epiphyses, metaphyses, and vertebrae—all of which differ from the findings of achondroplasia. Ultrastructural abnormalities include the presence of unique inclusions in the cisternae of the endoplasmic reticulum and the presence of abnormal proteoglycans, probably related to the protein core or to the enzymes that allow formation of the glycosaminoglycan chains.

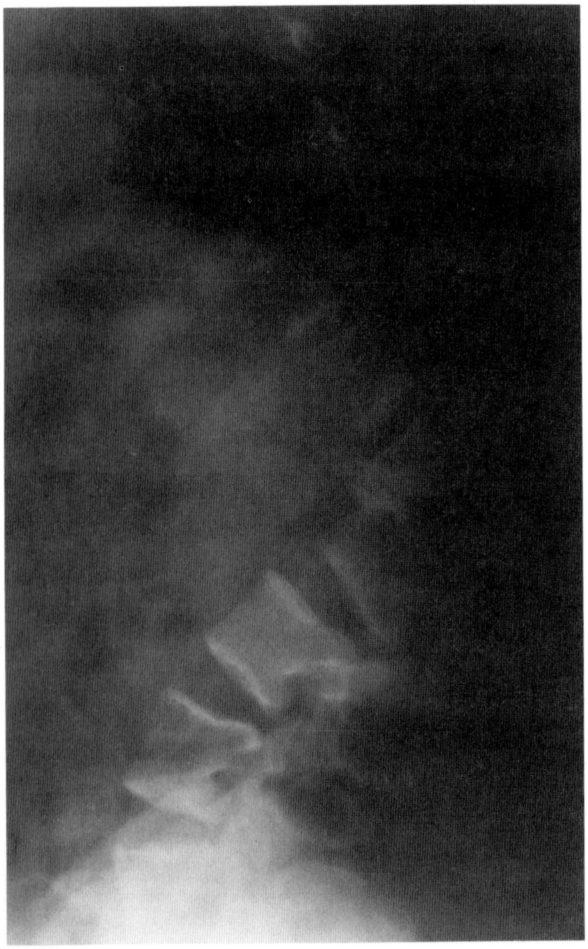

Figure 1

In achondroplasia, thoracolumbar kyphosis is common. Although the kyphosis may resolve, if the deformity is progressive, as in this case, anterior and posterior spinal fusion is needed. If progressive and untreated, this kyphosis will lead to spinal cord compression symptoms in adolescence or early adulthood.

As growth proceeds, the central portion of the physis grows at a slower rate than does the remainder. This may lead to joint incongruity and malalignment, for which osteotomy is useful. Arthrography of the hip and the knee is needed before the needed correction and realignment are planned. In the spine, a progressive kyphosis may develop, although without the clear-cut vertebral body wedging seen in the thoracolumbar area in achondroplasia. If spinal surgery is needed, spinal instrumentation may be safely used to achieve correction.

Diastrophic Dysplasia

With both short limbs and a short trunk, these patients have misshapen ears from cartilage abnormalities, a "hitchhiker" thumb, severe clubfeet, and, frequently, a severe kyphoscoliosis. The underlying cause appears to be a structural alteration of the type II collagen molecule in the physeal area; the proteoglycans appear to be normal.

The clubfeet in diastrophic dysplasia are extremely rigid and cannot be corrected nonoperatively. A wide release at the hindfoot and ankle is required to achieve a plantigrade foot position. Marked flexion positions of the hips and knees frequently require realignment osteotomies. Although about 70% of these patients have some degree of scoliosis, only half of these require treatment. The most severe deformity generally is a rigid, sharply angular kyphosis and scoliosis at the mid-thoracic area. If significant scoliosis and kyphosis is going to be present, it usually is obvious by age 4 or 5 years. Surgical treatment is necessary for progressive curves. Cervical kyphosis is often present in early childhood but generally resolves with increasing age.

Spondylo-Epiphyseal Dysplasia Congenita

These patients have a short-trunk form of dwarfism, and they walk with their shoulders hyperextended and their abdomen protuberant. This syndrome is inherited in an autosomal dominant manner. At birth, these infants may be thought to have achondroplasia because some frontal bossing is present. As with achondroplastic children, hypotonia may be present early, but walking is usual by age 2 years. The body proportions may change over the first 5 years of life, with a gradual decline in the growth of the trunk.

The main orthopaedic manifestations of spondylo-epiphyseal dysplasia are in the spine and hips. The most serious is the atlantoaxial instability that is found in a high percentage of patients and is responsible for myelopathy in up to a third of the patients in reported series. If delayed motor development or recurrent respiratory problems are present, a cervical myelopathy should be suspected as the cause. Occipitocervical fusion, with halo-cast immobilization, is then necessary. The other spinal problems encountered are scoliosis and exaggerated lumbar lordosis. If fusion for scoliosis is necessary, posterior instrumentation can be used safely.

In the lower extremities, the principal problem is coxa vara which frequently produces a waddling gait. Progressive subluxation often occurs if untreated. Arthrography of the hip should precede valgus osteotomy, to permit accurate placement of the femoral head because femoral head ossification is delayed.

Morquio's Syndrome

This syndrome, diagnosed on the basis of corneal opacities and the urinary secretion of keratan sulfate, causes short-trunk dwarfism and is inherited in an autosomal recessive manner. These children are normally proportioned at birth, but short stature starts becoming evident at 2 or 3 years of age. Pectus carinatum or sternal gibbus becomes increasingly apparent after this age, and genu valgum progresses quickly. Despite these problems, the most serious abnormality in Morquio's syndrome is the atlantoaxial instability that commonly is present and is due to a combination of odontoid aplasia and ligamentous laxity.

The myelopathy from this instability is manifested by a gradual decrease in walking activity at age 5 or 6, often ascribed to the knock-knees but actually due to the cervical cord compression. Unchecked, this myelopathy leads to lower limb paralysis, incontinence, and respiratory failure.

Occipitocervical fusion at an early stage will prevent the neurologic dysfunction. If cervical fusion is performed, bone for the graft is best obtained from the proximal tibial metaphysis because in patients with Morquio's syndrome the iliac crest is a very poor source of graft bone.

Because the genu valgum deformity often is severe and may inhibit ambulation, realignment osteotomies are useful at age 8 to 10. Patients with Morquio's syndrome generally have attained their final height by this age, and delay of osteotomy until then usually prevents the need for repeat surgery.

Other Dysplasias

Ultrastructural abnormalities have been discovered recently in several other syndromes, each quite rare. In Kniest syndrome, there appears to be an abnormality of cartilage proteoglycan metabolism. In fibrochondrogenesis, organization of type II collagen is abnormal, and in pyknodysostosis there is an intracellular accumulation of lipid.

All patients with short-stature syndromes require radiographic evaluation of the spine and lower extremities to assess possible problems. As a group, in the spine the most common problems are upper cervical spine instability and thoracolumbar kyphosis; the lower extremities require assessment for angular deformity of the long bones and developing incongruity of the joints resulting from abnormal cartilage growth and maturation.

Connective Tissue Disorders

Marfan's Syndrome

This syndrome probably is diagnosed too often, and terms such as "marfanoid" are used too often to describe tall, thin patients. In fact, the use of the term "marfanoid" probably is inappropriate.

To make the diagnosis of Marfan's syndrome itself, it is necessary to meet at least two, and preferably three or four, of the major diagnostic criteria: 1) positive family history; 2) cardiac involvement, usually mitral valve or aortic abnormalities, diagnosed by echocardiography; 3) inferior lens dislocation; and 4) musculoskeletal features including scoliosis, arachnodactyly, dolichomelia, pectus excavatum, and joint laxity. Although the underlying cause of this autosomal dominant condition remains unknown, abnormalities in the production of the α_1 chain of collagen have been demonstrated in some patients.

Orthopaedic problems in Marfan's syndrome are mainly in the lower extremities and trunk. Pectus excavatum is common and is often associated with scoliosis. Although mild scoliosis is common, progressive curves occur only in 10% to 20%. Treatment of scoliosis in Marfan's syndrome is similar to that of idiopathic scoliosis, but the thoracic lordosis that is a characteristic feature of Marfan's syndrome makes brace treatment (Fig. 2 *A*) less likely to be successful. Scoliosis treatment often begins before age 10. Attempts to use estrogen-progesterone treatment to induce early puberty and limit growth, in the hope of making scoliosis treatment easier, have not met expectations.

Joint laxity is present to variable degrees in all Marfan's syndrome patients. The long, thin foot in these patients makes shoe-fitting difficult, and this is further complicated by calcaneovalgus hindfoot position and laxity of ankle support. The majority of the children with Marfan's syndrome can be managed with regular shoes, with or without orthotics, and few require triple arthrodesis (Fig. 2 *B*). The patellofemoral joint also is frequently symptomatic and may subluxate. Because the collagen is abnormal in Mar-

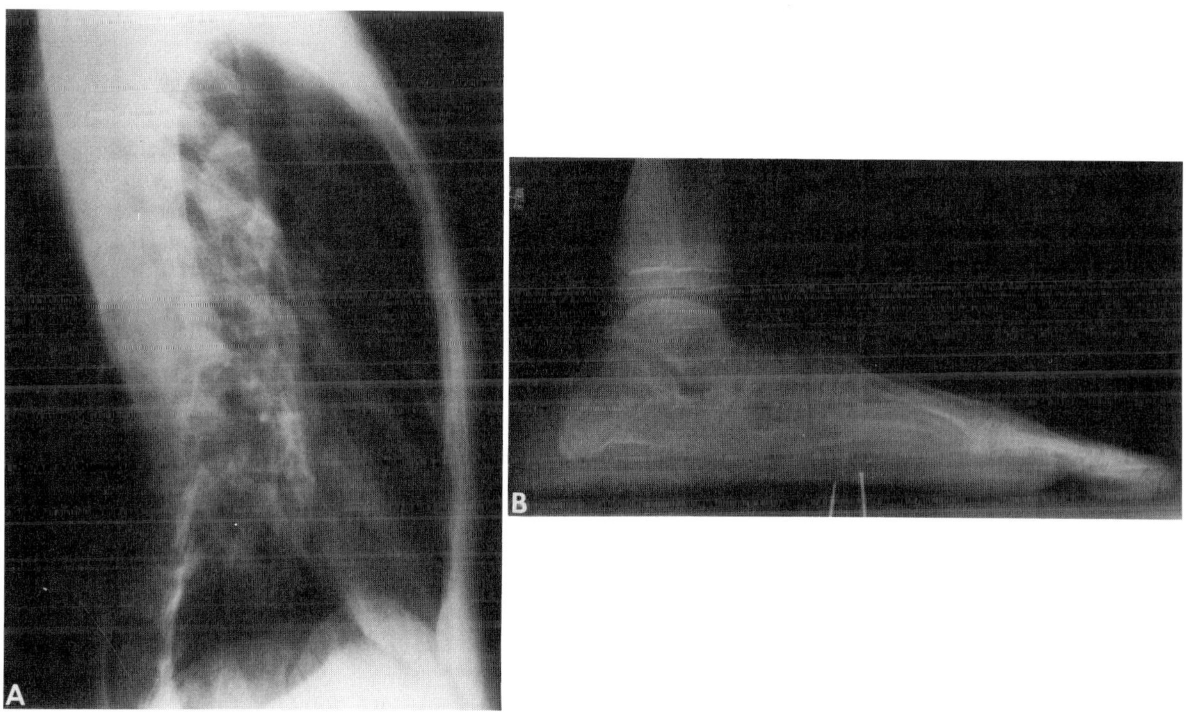

Figure 2

A, In Marfan's syndrome, thoracic lordosis is almost always present to some degree, making the brace treatment of scoliosis less successful. *B,* Most patients with Marfan's syndrome have narrow, flat feet, making shoe-fitting difficult, but they rarely benefit from triple arthrodesis.

fan's syndrome patients, management of patellar problems should be directed to muscular exercises initially, with soft-tissue reconstruction reserved for later, if attempted at all. Protrusio acetabuli is often present to varying degrees, at times leading to symptomatic degenerative joint disease in adult life. If early protrusio is detected in childhood, operative closure of the triradiate cartilage can prevent further protrusio development.

Ehlers-Danlos Syndrome

This syndrome has multiple clinical forms (nine types have been described to date). Lysyl hydroxylase deficiency is present in type VI and defects of collagen synthesis have been demonstrated in types IV and VII, but the exact causes of the other types have not yet been found.

Types II and III are the most common and the least disabling of the various forms of Ehlers-Danlos syndrome; joint hypermobility, some skin laxity, and a tendency to bruise easily are the usual findings. In a patient who presents with recurrent sprains or dislocations or simply with joint laxity, the skin should be carefully inspected. Scars from previous lacerations or operations have a characteristic thin, spread appearance, classically described as resembling cigarette paper. Inheritance of these types is autosomal dominant.

The management of joint instability may be frustrating to both patient and orthopaedist because some degree of instability generally is present in several joints. Symptomatic shoulder instability is usually multidirectional and very careful evaluation is needed because a simple anterior soft tissue repair rarely is successful. As a general principle, strengthening of all muscles controlling the symptomatic joint should be the initial treatment of choice to relieve symptoms in patients with Ehlers-Danlos syndrome. A customized physical exercise program will allow many of these patients to participate in various sports. Soft tissue transfers to enhance joint stability are very likely to stretch out with time because of the underlying abnormality in the collagen. Arthrodesis is a predictable means of stabilizing an unstable symptomatic joint not controlled by muscle training or orthoses.

Osteogenesis Imperfecta

There is a great deal of genetic hetereogeneity among patients with osteogenesis imperfecta, a condition characterized by fragile, easily fractured bones, abnormal tooth development, hearing deficit, and short stature. Numerous classifications are available, the most often cited being congenita versus tarda. The Sillence classification of four types incorporates genetic, clinical, morphologic, and biochemical features but may not allow definite classification at birth or early in infancy.

Children born with the most severe form of osteogenesis imperfecta have multiple fractures of broad, crumpled long bones and ribs at birth and have a softened skull (caput membranaceum) (Fig. 3). More than 90% of these infants die early. If these children survive, they will not become ambulatory. Over 90% of infants who have fractures at birth but have long bones and ribs of normal shape and length will survive; respiratory complications are the cause of death in those who die. Many of these patients eventually become wheelchair dependent, but some remain ambulatory to some degree. Many require multiple osteotomies and intramedullary rod placement. It is unusual for either of these two groups with fractures obvious at birth to have a family history of osteogenesis imperfecta.

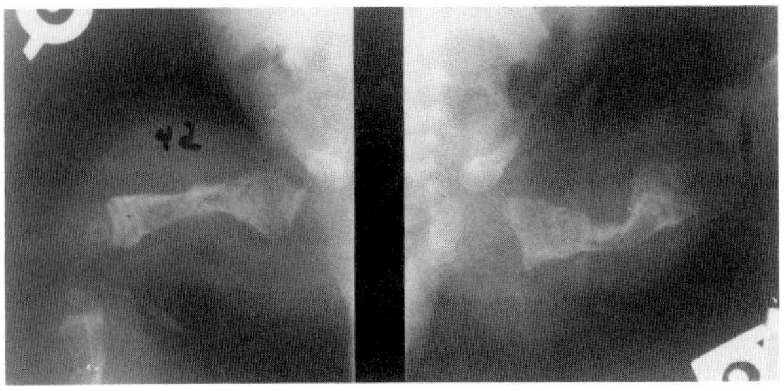

Figure 3

Infants with severe osteogenesis imperfecta have broad, crumpled bones with multiple fractures at birth; they have less than a 10% chance of survival and, if they survive, will not be able to walk.

Patients with fractures that occur after birth but not at the time of delivery frequently have a family history of osteogenesis imperfecta, with dominant inheritance being the most common. If fractures occur before walking begins, about one-third of the children will become wheelchair dependent. If fractures do not occur until after walking begins, almost all will remain ambulatory. Patients in both of these categories frequently need bracing and osteotomies.

Although the presence of blue sclerae is described as a classic feature of osteogenesis imperfecta, some children have normal sclerae and others may not develop blue sclerae until a few years after birth. If there is more than one fracture in an infant with normal-shaped bones and white sclerae, it may be difficult to differentiate between osteogenesis imperfecta and child abuse, but a proper diagnosis should be reached if a family history is looked for and the fracture pattern is studied. In patients who have been given the diagnosis of osteogenesis imperfecta, audiologic examination is important because many have hearing defects from middle and inner ear abnormalities. Abnormal tooth development (dentinogenesis imperfecta) is also common and dental care is needed as soon as teeth appear.

In osteogenesis imperfecta the fractures heal promptly. If bowing is present in the lower extremity long bones, light-weight plastic orthoses—at times, circumferential molded types—should be used to allow weight bearing and bone strengthening. Bone bowing may be present in any long bone. If bowing is sufficient to lead to recurrent fracture by tension-side failure on the convexity of the bow, multiple osteotomy is indicated for realignment. Fixation is best accomplished with a telescoping intramedullary rod inserted through the bone ends and designed to pass across the physis. In the lower extremity, all bowed bones should be straightened concurrently to decrease the time of immobilization postoperatively. Postosteotomy bracing is effective in preventing the recurrence of bowing in many patients.

Spinal deformity commonly is present in osteogenesis imperfecta, and more than half of the more severely involved patients develop scoliosis. The usual bracing methods for scoliosis are less effective in osteogenesis imperfecta because the lateral rib pressure, intended to straighten the spine in the brace, often causes secondary rib deformities and fails to control the scoliosis. Posterior spinal instrumentation methods can be used as in idiopathic scoliosis, but hook reinforcement with methyl methacrylate should be considered in the nonambulatory osteogenesis imperfecta patient.

Comment

Ehlers-Danlos syndrome, Marfan's syndrome, homocystinuria, osteogenesis imperfecta, and other connective tissue disorders probably will be found to have subtle biochemical differences. For the collagen molecule to assemble correctly, it is necessary to have the correct amino acid distribution along its surface, to have correct molecular length, and to have the three chains in a rigid triple-helix conformation. It is already known that a mutation altering one region of the type I procollagen will cause a disease affecting skin, tendons, and ligaments; a similar mutation in another part of the same molecule will cause a disease mainly involving the bone. Other similar examples will continue to be found. No systemic treatment is currently available for any of these connective tissue disorders. Their similarities and the potential overlap of these disorders should be recognized by orthopaedists as they treat the clinical manifestations.

Chromosomal Abnormalities

Down's Syndrome

This is the best-known of the chromosomal abnormalities and is generally due to trisomy 21, although a form may be associated with translocation in this same chromosomal subgroup. Mental retardation is present and developmental milestones are delayed, but unassisted ambulation should be expected in these children. Some degree of short stature is common.

The orthopaedic abnormalities in Down's syndrome result from the generalized ligamentous laxity present in this condition. The most serious, atlantoaxial instability, is present in about 20% of patients with Down's syndrome but is asymptomatic in the majority. All patients with this syndrome should have lateral flexion and extension cervical spine radiographs to assess the stability of C-1/C-2. Generally, those children with less than 6 mm of space between the odontoid and the posterior margin of the anterior atlas ring are asymptomatic and simply require regular neurologic and radiographic reassessment. These asymptomatic children with instability should not participate in contact sports, diving, certain gymnastic activities, or other physical activity liable to injure the cervical spine. In addition to screening for this instability in these children who participate in the Special Olympics, periodic reassessment is important, even in those children found earlier to have atlantoaxial stability, because instability may develop in later childhood.

In almost all patients with 7 mm or more of atlantoaxial instability, neurologic compromise is present and atlantoaxial posterior fusion should be done (Fig. 4). In patients in whom neurologic deficits have already developed, recovery of neurologic function is not consistent after fusion. Because these patients frequently have a broad-based, slow gait as a part of this syndrome, the diagnosis of neurologic defects may be delayed unless one suspects this problem.

The major joints affected by the ligamentous instability are in the lower extremity, especially the hip and knee. The patella is usually hypermobile, and recurrent patellar dislocation may lead to frequent falling episodes, with the knee giving way. Muscle-strengthening exercises are difficult for these children to do, because of their mental retardation, so surgical patellar realignment may be needed. However, there is a substantial incidence of redisplacement postoperatively due to the ligamentous laxity. Voluntary, painless dislocation of the hip may be seen in this syndrome, and if this persists through late childhood into adolescence, acetabular dysplasia is often seen (Fig. 5). Salter or Chiari osteotomy has been reported to be successful in these patients, but some residual subluxation is common. Pes planus is generally present but seldom requires treatment.

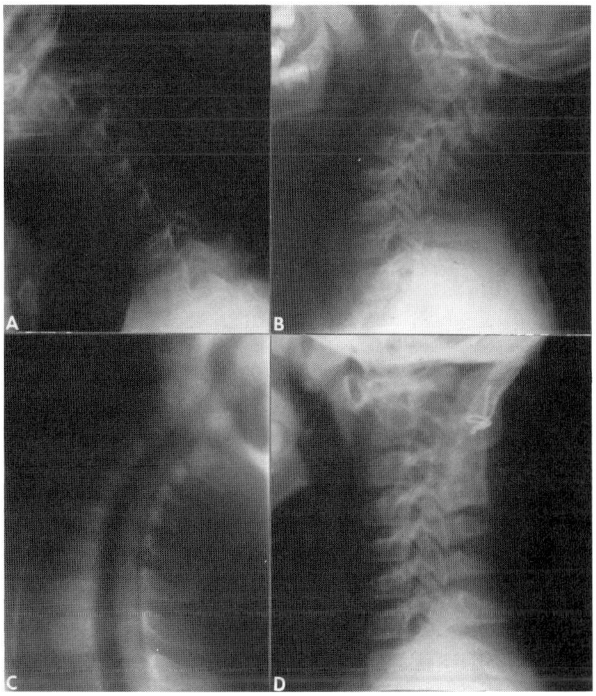

Figure 4

About 20% of children with Down's syndrome have atlantoaxial instability, as in this 7-year-old boy. *A* and *B*, Flexion and extension cervical spine radiographs show the instability (associated with neurologic symptoms in this case). *C*, Air myelogram demonstrates spinal canal stenosis at the atlas level. *D*, Occipitocervical fusion and atlas laminectomy relieved the spinal cord compression.

In patients with Down's syndrome, careful cardiac evaluation is mandatory prior to orthopaedic surgery. The substantial anesthetic risks, especially in the presence of Eisenmenger's complex (a large ventricular septal defect with a reversed shunt) which often is associated with Down's syndrome, must be carefully balanced against the expected benefits in these children.

Turner's and Noonan's Syndromes

Turner's syndrome (karyotype 45,XO) is characterized by short stature, webbed neck, absence of secondary sexual characteristics, and occasional scoliosis. The orthopaedist may be consulted regarding the neck, which is normal radiographically and is rarely symptomatic. Noonan's syndrome has the same phenotype features as Turner's syndrome but is found only in males (XY). Patients with either

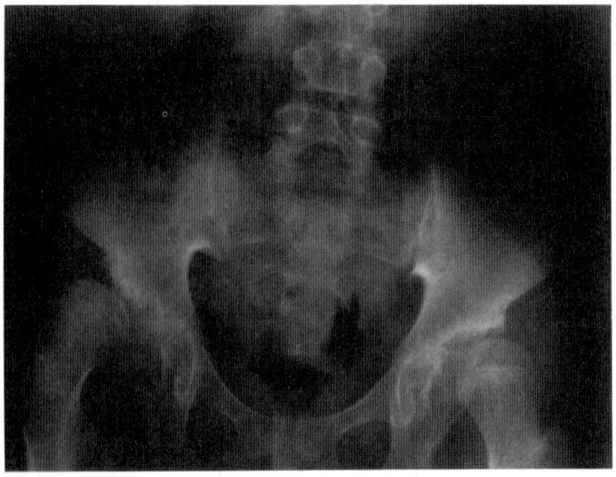

Figure 5

Ligamentous laxity in Down's syndrome may lead to hip dislocations. If these persist, acetabular dysplasia, as shown here, will result. Pelvic osteotomy may be useful to provide hip stability in these children.

of these syndromes have a significantly higher risk of malignant hyperthermia during anesthesia, so dantrolene is often administered preoperatively if orthopaedic surgery, such as spinal instrumentation and fusion, is advised.

Other chromosomal abnormalities may cause orthopaedic problems as a significant feature, such as congenital vertical talus in trisomy 18, and orthopaedic care must be tailored to the individual child, depending on the other syndrome features including the mental status and the expected length of survival.

Neuromuscular Conditions

Duchenne's Muscular Dystrophy

This uniformly fatal muscle disease is inherited in a sex-linked recessive mode and affects only boys. Symmetric pelvic muscle weakness is commonly seen first, with pseudohypertrophy of the calf muscles appearing soon after. Upper extremity involvement usually appears 3 to 5 years after the lower extremity manifestations. Death occurs before age 20 years, from cardiopulmonary failure. Diagnosis at the earliest possible stage is important in order to advise the family regarding the risks of future children having this fatal disease.

The orthopaedic care is focused primarily on trying to keep these boys ambulatory as long as possible and correcting deformities to allow them to function more easily. The common lower extremity problems encountered are ankle equinus and foot equinovarus deformities and hip flexion and abduction contractures. Before these deformities become fixed, physical therapy and the use of lightweight plastic orthoses can prolong the time during which these patients remain ambulatory. The use of a knee-ankle-foot orthosis should be instituted as soon as the child ceases to walk independently and needs some external support. If contractures that prevent this brace application are present, surgical treatment is indicated. Heel-cord lengthening is most often needed, as well as other releases including posterior tibialis tenotomy, iliotibial band release, and hip flexor release. Immediate reambulation and therapy postoperatively, in casts or braces, is needed.

The most useful preoperative predictors of success in maintaining ambulation with this treatment program are 1) residual muscle strength, 2) vital capacity, 3) daily urinary excretion of creatinine, and 4) motivation of the patient. With these criteria, one can predict the success of increasing the time of walking before the child becomes wheelchair dependent.

Once a child with Duchenne's dystrophy becomes confined to a wheelchair, there is an increase in lower extremity joint contractures and a very high incidence of scoliosis. Bracing for scoliosis is usually ineffective in preventing continued progression of the curvature, and the bracing may have a detrimental effect on pulmonary function.

If the scoliosis progresses to 30° or 40°, posterior spinal instrumentation and fusion is recommended to enhance sitting, to prevent further pulmonary effects from the increasing curve, and to improve the ability of the patient to use his hands. Segmental spinal instrumentation and fusion, requiring no external brace or support, is the surgical procedure of choice. It is estimated that these patients will lose approximately 4% of their vital capacity for each additional 10° of thoracic scoliosis. Because, as a part of the natural history of muscular dystrophy, 4% of vital capacity is lost annually from muscle weakness, it appears that early surgical treatment of scoliosis will slow the onset of pulmonary failure.

Charcot-Marie-Tooth Disease

There are two, and perhaps more, different types of Charcot-Marie-Tooth disease, a demyelinating neuropathy. Inheritance is by an autosomal dominant mode in both. In the hypertrophic type, nerve biopsy shows increased fibrosis, and both sensory and motor nerve conduction velocities are low on neurometric examination (conduction usually is <30 m/sec). Symptoms and signs of muscle weakness begin in childhood; more than half of those afflicted show some changes by age 10. In the second type, termed the "neuronal form," onset tends to be later and nerve conduction is normal or only slightly slowed. The eventual clinical picture is similar in both groups.

By far the most common orthopaedic problem in Charcot-Marie-Tooth disease is pes cavus. The initial change resulting from this neuropathy probably is weakness of the foot intrinsic muscles. Peroneal weakness follows, frequently with some weakness of the anterior tibialis as well. The posterior tibialis and triceps surae are generally spared. Plantar releases and ankle-foot orthoses may be adequate treatment in some cases but, because the cavus deformity often becomes more rigid, triple arthrodesis usually is needed to stabilize the foot. Because of the peroneal weakness, it is commonly necessary to transfer the posterior tibialis through the interosseous membrane to balance the foot after the hindfoot has been stabilized. Associated symptomatic toe deformities also may require surgical treatment.

Arthrogryposis Multiplex Congenita

A wide variety of neurogenic and myopathic diseases have the clinical features described as arthrogryposis. These features can result from any lesion that affects the final neuromuscular pathway in the process of limb formation *in utero*. The congenital contractures characteristic of this group of diseases may be caused by lesions in the anterior horn cells, the peripheral nerves, the motor end plates, or the extremity muscles or they may be part of a wide variety of syndromes or chromosomal abnormalities. Arthrogryposis occurs in about 1 per 3,000 births.

When multiple congenital contractures are found at birth, a thorough work-up is needed to determine the cause in that child. This evaluation should include a neurologic examination, neurometric studies, serum enzyme tests, and a muscle biopsy, although this biopsy is best not performed until age 3 or 4 months because interpretation is difficult at earlier ages. If an underlying cause can be determined, genetic counseling of the family regarding risks of having additional similarly affected children is essential. If no specific cause can be determined, the risk of having another child with arthrogryposis is estimated to be about 5%. Real-time ultrasonography can be useful for diagnosing multiple congenital contractures *in utero.*

The multiple joint contractures may cause birth fractures in up to 25% of these patients, mainly involving the femoral shafts and the physes. Contractures are generally symmetric, most commonly involving both upper and lower extremities. In the lower extremity, clubfoot, hip dislocation, and knee flexion deformities are the most common; in the upper extremity, shoulder internal rotation, elbow extension, and wrist flexion contractures are usual. Frequently, absence or marked weakness of muscle adjacent to the contracted joints is seen.

In the first year or two of life, stretching exercises and judicious splinting often lead to some improvement in joint motion, although this motion gain frequently may be lost as the child grows. Associated with most joint contractures are thickened, fibrous joint capsules, making surgical release often necessary and not uncommonly requiring repeat surgery as the child grows. Posteromedial release, with or without talectomy, is most useful for the clubfoot deformity. Hamstring releases, combined with posterior capsulotomy, are used initially for the knee flexion deformity, although in the older child extension osteotomy of the distal femur can be used to improve knee extension (Fig. 6). Bilateral hip dislocation in the severely involved child is generally left unreduced, but a unilateral hip dislocation should be reduced, usually surgically, because otherwise later development of pelvic obliquity and scoliosis of the hip is possible.

The goal of these surgical procedures is to allow ambulation training. To achieve functional ambulation, it is necessary to have 1) hip extension power and range (or the ability to use crutches to substitute for this), 2) knee extension range and power or a knee-ankle-foot orthosis to substitute, and 3) plantigrade feet. Without these abilities, functional ambulation is unlikely and, for these children, sitting and wheelchair skills should be emphasized.

Upper extremity orthopaedic surgery is seldom done before age 4 years. Of greatest importance is to allow hand positioning to enable eating and toileting independently, with other hand functions being of secondary importance. Derotational humeral osteotomy is most useful to improve shoulder position. Triceps-plasty (anterior triceps transfer) to provide elbow flexion may be useful but requires careful preoperative assessment of the patient's needs. Procedures to straighten the flexed-wrist deformity may help hand function, although carefully defined goals must be established because the child may have adapted and have better function with the wrist flexed. Hand surgery to restore mobility is seldom useful.

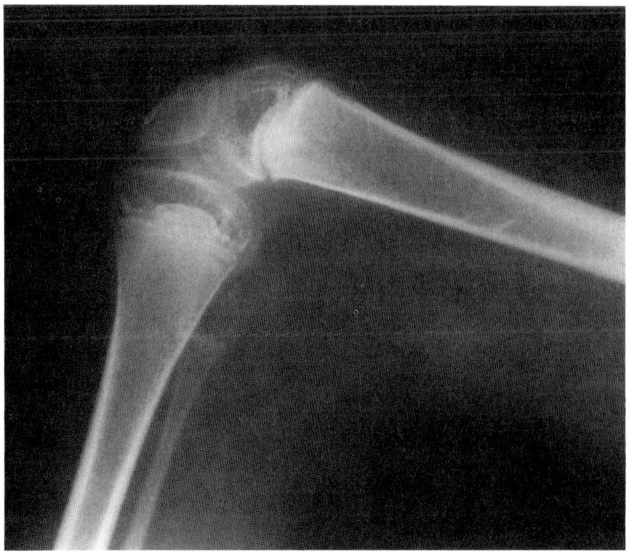

Figure 6

In arthrogryposis multiplex congenita, joint contractures are common, and the contracted side of the joint capsule is thickened and fibrotic. In this example, surgical treatment of this contracture consisted of posterior capsulotomy and hamstring release, with possible extension femoral osteotomy reserved for a later time.

Children with arthrogryposis are best managed in centers that have multiple disciplines available, including neurologists, orthopaedists, geneticists, therapists, and facilities for parental education and support.

Miscellaneous

Sickle Cell Disease

Probably the most important of the hemoglobinopathies, sickle cell disease (with hemoglobin SS) is found in about 1% of North American blacks; sickle cell trait (hemoglobin SA) is present in 7% of blacks in this country. In this disease, erythrocytes periodically form into a sickle shape, leading to the so-called sickle crisis; this usually begins at about 2 or 3 years of age. These crises lead to infarction of affected areas, usually secondary to capillary stasis induced by the sickle-shaped cells. Abdominal organs may be affected, and bone involvement is common.

The initial orthopaedic manifestation of sickle cell disease often is dactylitis, causing swelling of the hand or foot in a young child and leading to the typical radiographic findings of new periosteal bone formation in the metacarpals and metatarsals. The dactylitis resolves without permanent sequelae.

The most difficult orthopaedic dilemma in sickle cell disease is differentiation between a bone infarct and early osteomyelitis. In both, marked extremity pain and fever are common. The erythrocyte sedimentation rate is less useful here because the abnormal cells make interpretation difficult. Bone scans cannot reliably differentiate between infarcts and infection. Therefore, for a febrile patient with bone pain, blood cultures are needed and local aspiration of the affected area with subsequent Gram stain and culture is often useful. *Salmonella* species, probably from small intestinal infarcts, frequently are the causative bacteria, but *Staphylococcus aureus* is also commonly found to cause the osteomyelitis.

If cultures of blood or local aspirate are positive or if clinical findings point to bone infection, the osteomyelitis should be surgically drained and appropriate systemic antibiotic therapy should be instituted. If surgery is to be performed, adequate oxygenation during anesthesia is needed to prevent sickling. Preferably, tourniquets are not used during surgery. Exchange blood transfusions are a useful preoperative precaution to decrease risks of anesthesia.

Another common orthopaedic feature of sickle cell disease is the development of osteonecrosis of the femoral head in late adolescence or early adulthood. Nonoperative treatment (partial weight bearing with crutches and range-of-motion exercises) has been successful in some teenage patients, leading to gradual resolution of the avascular necrosis, but this is rarely successful in adults with sickle cell disease. In these patients, total hip arthroplasty is generally the treatment of choice, even if the patients are in their third decade, because these patients often are thin and somewhat chronically ill and thus are not placing excessive stress on their hip replacements. Preoperative preparation for anesthesia, as noted above, is necessary prior to joint replacement.

Thrombocytopenia-Absent Radius Syndrome

This rare, probably autosomal recessive, syndrome combines hematologic and orthopaedic abnormalities. At birth, the infant has hypomegakaryocytic thrombocytopenia, often requiring multiple platelet transfusions to prevent fatal bleeding. The most common orthopaedic feature is bilateral aplasia of the radii, generally presenting as a radial clubhand. Initial orthopaedic management involves splinting this hand to prevent further flexion contracture, with surgical centralization of the hand on the distal ulna and hematologic stabilization, provided that the elbow flexion range is adequate. A second, frequently associated, orthopaedic problem is dysplasia of the knee joint, which may involve absence of the patella, menisci, or cruciate ligaments. For these problems, treatment must be individualized. If surgical procedures are contemplated in patients with this syndrome, preoperative assessment of platelet function is mandatory.

Hemihypertrophy

This relatively uncommon condition may be diagnosed in infancy when one leg is noted to be longer than the other. Confusion with congenital hip dysplasia is common because of inequality of knee height when the infant is examined with knees and hips flexed. Radiography confirms the increased length of the bones of both the upper and lower extremities on one half of the body as well as increased width of these bones if carefully measured. The principal orthopaedic problem requiring treatment is the leg-length discrepancy. This must be followed regularly with scanograms and plots on appropriate growth prediction charts to determine the best time for possible surgical treatment. The most common orthopaedic procedure required is epiphyseodesis of the distal femur and proximal tibia at the proper time. As a nonorthopaedic consideration in patients with hemihypertrophy, there is an increased risk of Wilms' tumor in early childhood.

Annotated Bibliography

General

Jones, K.L., and Robinson, L.K.: An approach to the child with structural defects. J. Pediatr. Orthop. 3:238–244, 1983.

A systematic method is described for reaching a specific diagnosis of the underlying condition or syndrome present in infants with defects at birth.

Skeletal Dysplasia

Kopits, S.E.: Orthopedic complications of dwarfism. Clin. Orthop. 114:153–179, 1976.

A thorough review of the pertinent aspects of orthopaedic problems most commonly encountered in the assessment and treatment of patients with short-stature syndromes.

Pedrini-Mille, A.; Maynard, J.A.; and Pedrini, V.A.: Pseudoachondroplasia: Biochemical and histochemical studies of cartilage. J. Bone Joint Surg. 66A:1408–1414, 1984.

Pseudoachondroplasia was found to be a generalized cartilage disorder involving proteoglycan abnormalities, a totally different cause from that previously described for achondroplasia in which proteoglycans appear normal.

Pedrini-Mille, A., and Pedrini, V.: Proteoglycans and glycosaminoglycans of human achondroplastic cartilage. J. Bone Joint Surg. 64A:39–46, 1982.

This study defines the defect in achondroplasia as most likely an abnormality in chondrocyte proliferation and in the formation of a fully developed zone of hypertrophy in the physis.

Stanescu, V.; Stanescu, R.; and Maroteaux, P.: Pathogenic mechanisms in osteochondrodysplasias. J. Bone Joint Surg. 66A:817–836, 1984.

This thorough study of the histochemical, immunohistochemical, ultrastructural, and microchemical aspects of the cartilage growth plate in 68 patients with different forms of human short-stature syndromes describes the basic defect found in many of these disorders.

Connective Tissue Disease

Albright, J.A., and Millar, E.A.: Osteogenesis imperfecta (editorial). Clin. Orthop. 159:2, 1981.

This editorial comment on a series of articles relating to osteogenesis imperfecta summarizes both nonoperative and surgical management of this disorder as well as explaining more fully Sillence's classification.

McKusick, V.A.: Heritable Disorders of Connective Tissue. Fourth edition. St. Louis, C.V. Mosby Company, 1972.

Although published 15 years ago, this textbook still continues to provide much of the basic clinical information on a wide variety of connective tissue disorders.

Prockop, D.J.: Osteogenesis imperfecta: Phenotypic heterogeneity, protein suicide, short and long collagen. Am. J. Hum. Genet. 36:499–505, 1984.

This review of the basic collagen defects in osteogenesis imperfecta and other connective tissue diseases emphasizes how only a small change in the collagen molecule can cause a large variation in clinical manifestations of these disorders.

Shapiro, F.: Consequences of an osteogenesis imperfecta diagnosis for survival and ambulation. J. Pediatr. Orthop. 5:456–462, 1985.

Eighty-five patients with osteogenesis imperfecta were reviewed to determine what effect the bone appearance at birth and the time of initial fracture had on survival and subsequent ambulation potential.

Chromosomal Abnormalities

Pueschel, S.M.; Herndon, J.H.; Gelch, M.M.; Senft, K.E.; Scola, F.H.; and Goldberg, M.J.: Symptomatic atlantoaxial subluxation in persons with Down syndrome. J. Pediatr. Orthop. 4:682–688, 1984.

In a prospective study of 236 patients with Down's syndrome, 40 had atlantoaxial instability radiographically but only 7 were symptomatic. Details of the symptomatic patients and recommendations for cervical spine assessment and care in Down's syndrome are presented.

Neuromuscular Conditions

Duchenne's Muscular Dystrophy

Kurz, L.T.; Mubarak, S.J.; Schultz, P.; Park, S.M.; and Leach, J.: Correlation of scoliosis and pulmonary function in Duchenne muscular dystrophy. J. Pediatr. Orthop. 3:347–353, 1983.

In a longitudinal study of 25 patients with Duchenne's muscular dystrophy, the authors demonstrated that the vital capacity diminished approximately 4% annually as a result of the muscle disease. An additional 4% decrease was found for each 10° increase in scoliosis, so early posterior spinal instrumentation and fusion was advocated for the scoliosis.

Moser, H.: Duchenne muscular dystrophy: Pathogenetic aspects and genetic prevention. Hum. Genet. 66:17–40, 1984.

This exhaustive review, with several hundred references, presents what is known currently about the pathogenesis and genetics of Duchenne's dystrophy. No orthopaedic management is discussed.

Vignos, P.J., Jr.; Wagner, M.B.; Kaplan, J.S.; and Spencer, G.E., Jr.: Predicting the success of reambulation in patients with Duchenne muscular dystrophy. J. Bone Joint Surg. 65A:719–728, 1983.

In a statistically based evaluation of 50 patients with Duchenne's dystrophy, the authors derived the biochemical and clinical factors that were important to predict most accurately which patients would likely regain walking skills when treated by surgery and bracing.

Charcot-Marie-Tooth Disease

Bouché, P.; Gherardi, R.; Cathala, H.P.; Lhermitte, F.; and Castaigne, P.: Peroneal muscular atrophy. Part 1. Clinical and electrophysiological study. J. Neurol. Sci. 61:389–399, 1983.

In a review of 144 patients with Charcot-Marie-Tooth disease, the two main groups—hypertrophic and neuronal—are characterized by nerve conduction tests, clinical findings, and genetic features.

Jahss, M.H.: Evaluation of the cavus foot for orthopedic treatment. Clin. Orthop. 181:52–63, 1983.

This author provides a thorough review of his approach to pes cavus and the foot deformities associated with this, particularly as pes cavus relates to Charcot-Marie-Tooth disease.

Shapiro, F., and Bresnan, M.J.: Orthopaedic management of childhood neuromuscular disease. Part II: Peripheral neuropathies, Friedreich's ataxia, and arthrogryposis multiplex congenita. J. Bone Joint Surg. 64A:949–953, 1982.

General orthopaedic care principles are reviewed for several common neuromuscular diseases.

Arthrogryposis Multiplex Congenita

Hoffer, M.M.; Swank, S.; Eastman, F.; Clark, D.; and Teitge, R.: Ambulation in severe arthrogryposis. J. Pediatr. Orthop. 3:293–296, 1983.

Requirements for functional ambulation were determined by a review of 36 patients severely affected with arthrogryposis.

Thompson, G.H.: Arthrogryposis multiplex congenita (editorial). Clin. Orthop. 194:2–3, 1985.

This symposium includes all aspects of the current knowledge of arthrogryposis, including etiology, neuropathology, genetic considerations and classifications, and orthopaedic surgical management.

Miscellaneous

Sickle Cell Disease

Mallouh, A., and Talab, Y.: Bone and joint infection in patients with sickle cell disease. J. Pediatr. Orthop. 5:158–162, 1985.

Although osteomyelitis in sickle cell disease seems to be decreasing in the United States, *Salmonella* osteomyelitis is still common elsewhere. Methods of diagnosis and treatment are reviewed.

Thrombocytopenia-Absent Radius Syndrome

Schoenecker, P.L.; Cohn, A.K.; Sedgwick, W.G.; Manske, P.R.; Salafsky, I.; and Millar, E.A.: Dysplasia of the knee associated with the syndrome of thrombocytopenia and absent radius. J. Bone Joint Surg. 66A:421–427, 1984.

Twenty-one patients with thrombocytopenia-absent radius syndrome were found to have associated intra-articular dysplasia of their knee joints, usually causing varus and a flexion or torsional deformity.

3

Bone Metabolism

This chapter covers the aspects of cell biology, physiology, and endocrinology that govern bone and calcium metabolism. Knowledge of the normal situation permits understanding of disorders that affect the quality and quantity of bone. It also permits the derivation of appropriate methods of therapeutic intervention. Recent advances in the diagnosis and treatment of osteoporosis and Paget's disease now permit stabilization of these disorders. More important, prevention of osteoporosis should start during adolescence, with emphasis on appropriate calcium nutrition and sufficient exercise.

Cellular Control of Bone Metabolism

Bone Cells

The cells that control the metabolism of bone respond to mechanical, electrical, and chemical signals. The response may be specific or nonspecific. In general, specific responses are governed by hormones acting through cell receptors. Nonspecific responses may be mediated by chemical changes but do not occur through specific receptors. Therefore, hormones act in a specific way while mechanical and electrical stimuli and various chemical agents probably act in a nonspecific way.

There are three cell types in bone. Osteoblasts are the bone-forming cells. They line the endosteal surface of bone and actively lay down new bone matrix. When bone is in a static state the cells thin out and are called "lining cells." Osteocytes are osteoblasts that have become encompassed by bone matrix. They function to maintain calcium homeostasis but have a limited role in bone formation and resorption. Osteoclasts are the active agents in bone resorption. They are responsible for the remodeling of bone and form the leading edge of the "cutting cone." Osteoclasts are usually multinucleated but singly nucleated cells may stain histochemically as do the standard osteoclasts.

Extracellular Environment

The extracellular environment around bone maintains a chemical gradient. This bone fluid compartment maintains a stable envelope of ion concentrations that permits normal bone maintenance and the orderly transfer of mineral between the extracellular fluid and the compartment in the bone.

Osteoblasts and Osteocytes

The origin of osteoblasts is controversial. There seem to be two available cell lines from the bone marrow—differentiated (committed) osteoprogenitor cells from mesenchymal or stromal cell lines, and inducible, pluripotential osteoprogenitor cells from hematopoietic stem cells (1 per 2,000,000 hematopoietic cells).

All bone surfaces are continuous and are lined by cells with small intercellular gaps between the cells and their cytoplasmic processes. The endosteal surface is connected to the Volkmann canals of the haversian systems via canaliculi. The cellular layer protects the bone from the extracellular fluid space at large. The small intercellular gaps in the matrix line are metabolically isolated in a thin organic layer of proteoglycan and collagen.

The cellular membrane has a typical trilaminar appearance when viewed by electron microscopy. The inner surface is electronegative and contains large numbers of phosphatidylserine molecules. Thus, as in matrix vesicles, the membrane has a high affinity of binding for cations such as calcium. This membrane configuration is important in calcification. In the case of extracellular vesicle membrane, phosphatases are present that concentrate inorganic phosphates and the membrane localizes free calcium, the substrates necessary to produce hydroxyapatite crystals.

Electrical potentials develop in bone. The majority of piezoelectric and mechanical potentials can develop in dehydrated and demineralized bone. This implicates the bone collagen as primarily responsible for the production of the potentials. The mineral and matrix may be involved in electrical potential formation. These potentials must act through a cellular mechanism. Furthermore, the cells may modulate the electrochemical signals. Some authorities postulate that electrical potentials act by stimulating the release of endogenous prostaglandins and the actions proceed through cyclic AMP as a second intracellular messenger.

Osteoblasts and osteocytes have receptors. Parathyroid hormone and calcitonin are peptide hormones with separate membrane receptors. Physical alterations occur in the cell membrane and trigger intracellular changes in cyclic AMP and cyclic GMP. Steroid hormones such as glucocorticoids have intranuclear receptors. Other sterols such as 1,25-dihydroxyvitamin D probably function by binding to a protein in the cytosol; they are then transported into the nucleus and interact with DNA. Questions remain as to the breakdown and handling of intranuclear vitamin D metabolites. No receptors have yet been identified for estrogen in osteoblasts or osteocytes. Nevertheless, such receptors are abundant in bone marrow, and local effects by second messengers may be present.

Osteoclasts

Osteoclast progenitor cells are derived from the hematopoietic tissue. They resemble cells of the monocyte/macrophage cell line. Among the data that support this hypothesis is the observation that the disordered osteoclast function in osteopetrosis can be corrected by bone marrow transplantation. Monocytes and osteoclasts have similarities in their membranes. The life span of osteoclasts is uncertain but recent evidence suggests that it may be as short as 7 days. Osteoclasts can arise on bone surfaces directly or as blood-borne constituents. Most osteoclasts are formed by the coalescence of monocytes and appear as multinucleated giant cells. Both the typical giant cells and the singly nucleated osteoclasts resorb bone. Osteoclasts reside in Howship's lacunae (resorptive cavities) on bone surfaces. Resorbing surfaces are complexes of convoluted plasma membrane that forms a ruffled border. The microenvironment between the ruffles is thought to be acidic and may foster bone resorption. Between the ruffled borders on the resorbing bone surface is a clear zone. Here, collagen fibrils and vacuoles that digest mineral crystals are found. In the extracellular space, bone matrix is digested by hydrolytic enzymes and collagenase. Parathyroid hormone (PTH) and osteoclast-activating factor (OAF) directly stimulate formation of the ruffled border and are present in amounts proportional to the amount of bone resorption taking place.

Bone Biomechanics

The skeleton serves as mineral reserve, hematopoietic repository, and structural support. The structural elements have important biomechanical properties. Bone is a composite material consisting of type I collagen (providing tensile strength) and hydroxyapatite mineral (providing compressive strength). It is anisotropic in structure and consistency. Histologic and microradiographic analyses have shown that it has well-defined areas of nonmineralized osteoid, partially mineralized osteoid, and fully mineralized osteoid. Nonmineralized osteoid usually constitutes 1% to 2% of the total bone volume. Although all mature bone is essentially lamellar, the cortex is relatively compact with a high volume-to-surface ratio. Interspaced within the cortex are haversian canals, each with a central blood vessel. Circumferential rings around the vessel form each osteon. "Cutting cones" of osteoclasts can be identified removing old cortical bone that will be replaced with a new osteonal system ("remodeling").

Trabecular bone is also largely lamellar but it has a high surface-to-volume ratio. Rather than remodeling by "tunneling resorption" within the trabeculae, there is remodeling on the surface. Osteoclasts initially carve out Howship's lacunae. Within these lacunae, osteoblastic bone formation occurs secondarily.

The material properties of bone are governed by the microdensity of the material. In a homogeneous material, the compressive strength is proportional to the square of the density. When not homogeneous, a material's weakest point is the area of least density. This emphasizes the importance of the structural distribution of the bone mass.

Bone geometry determines bone strength. The tensile strength of a solid rod is the same as that of a tube with the same cross-sectional area of material. However, the tube has a greater moment of inertia and is significantly stronger than the rod when withstanding bending or torsional stresses. Consequently, the farther the material is distributed away from the center of the object, the stronger is the structural strength of that material in torsion and bending. An example of this principle is seen in the femoral diaphysis of an aging individual. As one grows older the outer periosteal diameter increases and the inner endosteal diameter increases. This shifts the bone mass further from the epicenter of the bone. Theoretically, these changes in bone geometry have the potential to maximize skeletal strength for any given amount of bone mass and could partially compensate for the decreased bone mass that accompanies aging. Furthermore, although this process has been demonstrated to occur in males, there are reported data that suggest that in sedentary postmenopausal women the skeleton does not widen with aging. In addition, certain parts of the skeleton such as the femoral neck may be deficient in periosteum and cannot compensate for loss of endosteal bone mass. These observations partially explain the increased frequency of fracture of the femoral neck in elderly women.

Two concepts govern structural properties: modeling and remodeling. In modeling, general appositional growth occurs on the surface of the loaded bone at the greatest distance from the epicenter of the bone. It does not follow the "metabolic bone unit" concept of resorption followed by formation. Modeling is illustrated clinically by periosteal bone formation in stressed bones. It is also seen after aseptic necrosis—the dead trabeculae provide a lattice upon which new appositional bone growth occurs. Lastly, it is clearly illustrated in the external fracture callus where bone formation occurs unilaterally, without preliminary bone resorption.

Remodeling involves an initial process of removing bone from within. This is illustrated by the cutting cone osteoclastic resorption of cortical bone or Howship's lacunar indentations into trabecular bone. In both instances, the bone is temporarily weakened during the remodeling process before it is partially restrengthened by new bone formation. Furthermore, the initial mineralization is incomplete, so the new bone is weaker. The compressive strength of the new metabolic bone unit is significantly decreased compared to the preexisting highly mineralized bone. Lastly, the production of porosities and subsequent reossification during the remodeling process produces a multicomponent bone rather than a single unit of reinforced collagen and mineral. This remodeled bone differs from reinforced concrete produced entirely at one time. It is similar to the process of boring holes into preexisting concrete and producing microfractures and weaknesses. Plugging up the hole with new concrete will never produce its original strength. Osteonal bone and remodeled bone are initially significantly weaker than the cortical bone they replaced. The body recognizes skeletal stress, perhaps by a piezoelectric feedback, and will only remodel the least-stressed bone. Bone cells respond according to "Wolff's law" and deposit bone appositionally in an effort to increase the structural strength of loaded areas.

The implications of modeling and remodeling are clear in terms of osteoporosis. Bone that has undergone significant remodeling and porosity has a markedly weakened microstructure. Conversely, modeled bone maintains an intact microstructure without faults or stress risers while augmenting lamellar bone mass by appositional growth.

Normal metabolic circumstances avoid rapid bone turnover or production of excess osteoid, protecting bone's mechanical structure. Enhanced remodeling can produce microweaknesses. Patients with hyperparathyroidism, hyperthyroidism, or even Paget's disease with its enhanced bone mass all have hypermetabolic remodeling states and are noted for their high incidence of stress fractures. Efforts to strengthen bone by promoting the remodeling process are less likely to succeed than efforts that augment bone by direct appositional modeling.

Bone consists of both cortical and trabecular bone. There are different structural roles for each of these two types of bone. Areas in which large impact stresses are applied from multiple directions do best with the trabecular bone pattern. Cortical bone's primary function is protection against torque and bending loads. Cortical bone forms slowly, and its dimensions develop in response to a long history of specific recurring stresses. The vertebral body consists of a cortical outer shell and a large trabecular interior bone volume. Removing the cortex of the vertebral body lessens the compressive strength by only 7%. Consequently, 93% of the compressive strength of the vertebral body is maintained by the trabecular bone. This also has been noted in the subchondral area of the femur and the proximal tibia. The femoral neck has little trabecular bone and depends on cortical bone for its integrity; it fails mainly in torque and bending modes, for which trabecular bone has little protective role.

Bones rich in trabecular bone are affected first by osteoporosis because of their high surface-to-volume ratio. Cortical bone is slower to dissolve, because of its low surface-to-volume ratio.

Bone Metabolism

Calcium homeostasis is a complex process. All calcium intake is from the diet. Calcium absorption varies with the perceived systemic calcium requirements and is under complex hormonal regulation. Approximately 20% of dietary calcium is absorbed; the remainder is either not absorbable or not absorbed and is excreted in the stool. Under net neutral conditions, urinary excretion of calcium balances the amount of calcium absorbed. Absorption from the gut and excretion in the urine average 150 to 200 mg of calcium per day in normal homeostasis.

The precise calcium requirements remain unknown. It is estimated that, in Western countries, 900 mg of calcium per day is required to maintain calcium balance in 95% of the population. Significant variations exist between individuals, however. Children require significantly more calcium during growth but the minimum amount is not known. Pregnant women, lactating women, adolescents, and postmenopausal women have the greatest calcium requirements—1,500, 2,000, 1,300, and 1,500 mg/day, respectively. Unfortunately, the average American diet provides only 450 mg of calcium per day. Recent data show that adolescents consume only 430 mg of calcium per day. This severe calcium deficiency during growth may adversely affect the peak of bone mass that is obtained at maturity.

In the average adult man, calcium makes up 1,050 g of the total weight. Only 1% of this is located outside the bones. More than 50% of the circulating calcium is bound to plasma proteins (the majority, to albumin). The amount of ionized, free calcium is critical to the maintenance of membrane electrical potential, blood coagulation, and most functions of the living organism. The ionized calcium concentration is maintained within very narrow limits, and bone mineral is sacrificed whenever necessary to increase the ionized calcium level back to a physiologic range.

Bones represent a potential reservoir for calcium and phosphate. Two different methods for the movement of calcium between the bone and body fluids are known. The first method is osteoclastic resorption and osteoblastic bone formation—i.e., the system by which bone is remodeled. This is a relatively slow process. Although the entire skeleton is theoretically available and the system has a huge capacity for supplying calcium, it is unable to respond to short-term calcium demand. Parathyroid hormone is one of the factors controlling the process. Long-term stimulation by parathyroid hormone increases both the number and the activity of osteoclasts. Nevertheless, parathyroid hormone receptors have not been identified in osteoclasts.

The other process is both rapid and reversible. It has the ability to respond to the minute-by-minute demand for calcium. The cells lining the bone surface are responsible for maintaining the plasma calcium concentration. Osteocytes and osteoblasts respond rapidly (within 5 minutes) to parathyroid hormone injection by changing their shape and intracellular organelle content (Golgi apparatus and endoplasmic reticulum). There is evidence that the perilacunar material surrounding osteocytes is a primary source of calcium on a short-term basis. It is this material that parathyroid hormone causes to be transferred rapidly into the body fluid compartment from the bone surface. Calcitonin also may be important in the postprandial storing of calcium in these areas.

Vitamin D also seems to be essential in promoting bone mineralization and in the short-term storing of calcium supplies, but its role is undefined. 1,25-Dihydroxyvitamin D potentiates the activity of parathyroid hormone in its bone resorptive function and activates calcium-binding protein in the gut. 25-Hydroxyvitamin D, or another analogue, may play a role in bone mineralization.

Calcium is absorbed mainly in the duodenum and jejunum. In the duodenum, its absorption is an active transport process. In the jejunum, it is absorbed by facilitated diffusion. Most calcium is taken up in the jejunum because of the greater length of this portion of the bowel and the slower speed of transport in it that provides more time for absorption. The normal intestine has a huge reserve capacity for absorbing calcium.

The presence of 1,25-dihydroxyvitamin D, a metabolite of vitamin D, is necessary for calcium absorption and can greatly enhance the ability of the gut to absorb calcium. This accelerated passage across the gut wall is caused by increases of the surface area available in the gut and the synthesis of proteins involved in transporting calcium. The presence of parathyroid hormone is unnecessary for this direct effect of vitamin D.

The kidney is capable of resorbing only 98% of the calcium filtered in the glomerulus. Less than 200 mg of calcium is usually present in a 24-hour urine collection (normal, <2 mg/kg per day). Calcium resorption is similar to sodium resorption in that it occurs throughout the nephron. Parathyroid hormone closely controls the amount of calcium excreted; administration of small amounts significantly increases the amount of calcium resorbed. Interestingly, parathyroid hormone seems to decrease resorption in the proximal tubule and increase it in the distal tubule.

1,25-Dihydroxyvitamin D_3 increases calcium resorption in the kidney in states of hypocalcemia or low parathyroid hormone level and during total body fluid volume expansion. The results in early studies that showed that vitamin D increased urinary excretion of calcium were primarily from increased intestinal absorption of calcium, which increased the amount of calcium filtered by the kidneys.

Phosphate metabolism is less well understood. It is now

known that 1,25-dihydroxyvitamin D stimulates active phosphate absorption across the gut wall. Phosphate is secreted in the renal tubules, and this process is augmented by increased parathyroid hormone level. Ample phosphate is contained in the standard Western diet, and phosphate deficiency is rare.

Vitamin D

Metabolic Pathway

Vitamin D is unique among vitamins in that it can be manufactured in the human body. It is formed in skin when 7-dehydrocholesterol is exposed to ultraviolet light. Approximately 1 hour of sunlight supplies the daily requirement in a white person; heavily pigmented individuals may require more exposure. This endogenous form of vitamin D is cholecalciferol or vitamin D_3. The other major source of vitamin D is the diet; this form is ergocalciferol or vitamin D_2. The two forms have slightly different structures but act the same. Both are stored in tissues, especially in adipose tissue and muscle. The only significant natural source of vitamin D is cod liver oil. This has led to the supplementation of vitamin D in milk in the United States.

In the liver, vitamin D is converted to 25-hydroxycholecalciferol [25-(OH)D] by either of two vitamin D 25-hydroxylases. The enzyme that is active at normal physiologic levels of vitamin D is located in the microsomes. The other 25-hydroxylase is found in the mitochondria of hepatic cells and is active only at high levels (pharmacologic doses). 25-Hydroxyvitamin D [25-(OH)D] is the major circulating form of vitamin D. It is transported by and bound to an α-globulin.

The next step in the metabolism of vitamin D is the 1-hydroxylation of 25-(OH)D to form the active form, 1,25-$(OH)_2D$. This reaction is catalyzed in the mitochondria of kidney cells. The only other tissue in which this enzyme has been found is the placenta. The production of 1,25-$(OH)_2D$ is under very close control. Parathyroid hormone, phosphate, ionized calcium level, and the amount of 1,25-$(OH)_2D$ itself all regulate 1-hydroxylase activity.

1,25-$(OH)_2D$ meets the criteria for a hormone. Its structure is similar to that of other steroid hormones, and it interacts with target tissues in a similar fashion. 1,25-$(OH)_2D$ diffuses across the cytoplasmic membrane and becomes bound to a cellular protein which helps transport it into the nucleus where it enhances the production of specific mRNA and, subsequently, protein production.

Target Organs

The major target tissues of 1,25-$(OH)_2D$ are bone, intestine, parathyroid gland, and kidney. In the kidney, it increases proximal tubular reabsorption of phosphate and, perhaps, calcium. It also increases 24-hydroxylase activity which produces another metabolite, 24,25-$(OH)_2D$, and decreases 1-hydroxylase activity, thereby acting as a feedback inhibitor of its own formation.

The major role of 1,25-$(OH)_2D$ is in the promotion and mobilization of calcium from bone. It acts by two mechanisms: 1) as a permissive agent, with parathyroid hormone actually causing the mineral resorption, and 2) by promoting differentiation and recruitment of osteoclasts. It also plays a role in bone mineralization, although this may be in the form of another metabolite such as 25-(OH)D or 24,25-$(OH)_2D$.

There is some evidence that 1,25-$(OH)_2D$ has a negative feedback effect on the production of parathyroid hormone because this hormone is known to stimulate 1,25-$(OH)_2D$ production. This point is unproven.

In the intestine, 1,25-$(OH)_2D$ promotes calcium and phosphate absorption. It does this by increasing the active absorption of calcium in the bowel, probably by stimulating the production of a calcium-binding protein.

High levels of 1,25-$(OH)_2D$ induce hydroxylation of 25-(OH)D at the 24 position, in several tissues besides the kidney. 24,25-$(OH)_2D$ may be involved in bone mineralization.

Several degradation products of vitamin D have been found. No known physiologic effect has been demonstrated, however.

Calcium-Binding Proteins

Many calcium-binding proteins have been identified in the calcified bone matrix, including phosphoproteins, γ-carboxyglutamic acid-containing proteins (Gla-proteins), and osteonectin. The phosphoproteins attract calcium by virtue of acidic phosphate groups, often attached to serine. The Gla-proteins attract calcium by virtue of carboxyl groups on glutamic acid residues. Osteonectin was recently described as a binding protein between the collagen of bone matrix and associated hydroxyapatite mineral.

Phosphoproteins are believed to be localized within the "holes" between collagen fibrils. Their phosphate groups attract calcium to this area and may be responsible for the nucleation phenomenon required to initiate mineralization.

The Gla-proteins that have been most studied are vitamin K-dependent clotting factors (factors II, VII, IX, and X) and Gla-protein residues of both prothrombin and factor Xa phospholipid.

Osteocalcin, a Gla-protein, has been isolated recently from bone. It is the most common noncollagenous protein in bone, and it constitutes between 10% and 20% of all noncollagen protein matrix and 1% to 2% of total bone protein. Osteocalcin is synthesized by the bone cells and undergoes the same vitamin K-dependent post-translational modification as prothrombin. The amount of osteocalcin in bone is such that less than 1 per 1,000 calcium ions is bound to it, but the onset of mineralization of bone does coincide temporally and spatially with the formation of osteocalcin. Indeed, there is a linear relationship between osteocalcin content and increasing density of bone.

Animals given warfarin, which blocks Gla-protein production, have a decreased amount of osteocalcin in their bones but no other significant changes in bone structure. Furthermore, the Gla-proteins have been shown to inhibit apatite mineral deposition *in vitro,* suggesting that they are not necessary for initiation of mineralization in bone. Given their high affinity for the calcium of hydroxyapatite, the Gla-proteins may accumulate in bone, at least to some extent, simply because of an affinity for apatite. Although the role of Gla-proteins in bone metabolism is unknown, they may function as local inductive agents as well as systemic hormone-like substances. Gla-proteins have been shown to be elevated in the serum of patients with Paget's disease, primary hyperparathyroidism, renal osteodystrophy, or osteoporosis.

Most of the Gla-protein is excreted in nonmetabolized form in the urine. Approximately 25% of urinary Gla-protein comes from mineralized tissues and associated osteocalcin. Perhaps it will be possible to use urinary Gla-protein excretion as an indicator for bone mineral turnover or even to monitor a patient's anticoagulation and vitamin K status. Serum osteocalcin level has been reported to correlate highly with the bone formation rate as determined by histomorphometry of iliac crest bone.

Many other noncollagenous matrix proteins have been isolated, including bone morphogenetic protein and the putative bone coupling factor. These proteins may be exposed by osteoclastic bone resorption. Their levels may be measured in the serum. They may act both locally and systemically to promote bone formation. Via these inductive substances, bone formation is coupled to bone resorption.

Endocrine Effects

Parathyroid Hormone

Parathyroid hormone, in association with 1,25-$(OH)_2D$, controls the concentration of calcium in body fluids. Its three major target organs are intestine, kidneys, and bone. Two areas of major new discoveries are the peripheral metabolism of parathyroid hormone and its intracellular production. Normally, the hormone is produced in, and secreted exclusively from, the parathyroid gland in humans. Intracellularly, it has two precursors. Preproparathyroid hormone is a 115-amino acid peptide produced directly from mRNA. Its half-life is less than 1 minute, and in the rough endoplasmic reticulum it is cleaved to prohormone which contains 90 amino acids. In the Golgi apparatus, it is cleaved to the major secretion product, parathyroid hormone itself, which contains 84 amino acids. The Golgi apparatus also packages the hormone into vesicles for secretion.

Secretion of parathyroid hormone is a very tightly regulated, but sensitive, system. A change in the ionized calcium concentration as small as 0.1 mg/dl will stimulate release of hormone. The second-messenger system of adenyl cyclase and cyclic AMP regulates that secretion. An increase in calcium flux inhibits cyclic AMP formation and decreases the amount of parathyroid hormone secreted. Hormone release is stimulated by hypocalcemia, prostaglandin E secretion, and β-adrenergic agonists. Interestingly, propranolol has the ability to block parathyroid hormone release; some studies indicate that the parathyroid gland probably has specific β_2-receptors.

At least three immunologically identifiable forms of parathyroid hormone are in the peripheral circulation. One is the intact 84-amino acid molecule that is secreted from the parathyroid gland. The other two forms result from the proteolytic cleavage of it in the liver. The carboxy-terminal part is large and is the predominant circulating form. It is not biologically active and is cleared by the kidney. The amino-terminal fragment is smaller, has a short half-life, and has many of the same actions as the whole molecule. This fragment is taken up almost completely by bone. The complete 84-amino acid molecule is much less active in bone than its amino-terminal peptide. Consequently, immunologic assay results for intact amino-terminal and carboxy-terminal parathyroid hormone have different clinical interpretations and do not correlate consistently with biologic effect.

The action of parathyroid hormone or its amino-terminal peptide on target tissues is related to activation of membrane-bound adenyl cyclase to produce intracellular cyclic AMP. The intracellular events taking place after this step are unclear, but the typical activation of protein kinases and increases in intracellular cytoplasmic calcium are believed to occur. These kinases then further alter cellular metabolism.

Calcitonin

The exact physiologic role of calcitonin is controversial. The theory that it is a vestigial or nonfunctioning hormone in humans probably is incorrect. It does have significant calcium- and phosphate-lowering actions at physiologic doses in humans.

Calcitonin is produced and secreted mainly by the C cells (parafollicular cells) in the thyroid gland. These cells originate in the embryonic neural crest tissue. Small amounts of calcitonin also are present in thymus, pituitary, gut, liver, and cerebrospinal fluid; the significance of this is unclear.

Biosynthesis of calcitonin is similar to that of other exported peptides. First synthesized in a large precursor form, it subsequently undergoes proteolytic cleavage at least twice to reach the final structure of 32 amino acids and a molecular mass of 3,500 daltons. Calcitonin molecules isolated from many sources (pig, cow, rat, etc.) all have the same length, 32 amino acids. Salmon calcitonin, which is available as a drug, differs from human calcitonin at 16 different amino acid positions. This alteration is large enough to cause it to be immunogenic. Interestingly, it is several times more potent for patients than is human calcitonin.

Secretion of calcitonin is controlled by serum calcium levels. Hypercalcemia stimulates secretion, and low calcium levels suppress its release. Several other divalent cations will influence secretion but only at superphysiologic levels and are probably not important *in vivo*. β_2-Adrenergic receptors are believed to exist that stimulate calcitonin release, an effect that can be blocked by propranolol. Pharmacologic doses of the intestinal hormones gastrin, cholecystokinin, and cerulein stimulate its release. This raises the interesting possibility that calcitonin is involved in some way with gastrointestinal function.

Breakdown of calcitonin occurs almost totally in the kidney where it is filtered, resorbed, and then degraded. The half-life is approximately 10 minutes in a patient with normal renal function but increases significantly with renal failure. The best assays available for analysis of calcitonin are radioimmunologic techniques, but all existing assays have difficulty measuring very low levels. In addition, they are not selective for the biologically active hormone but often react also with breakdown products or other similar proteins.

Calcitonin exerts its effect by binding to specific membrane receptors and activating adenyl cyclase which increases intracellular cyclic AMP. Further information about its intracellular effects is unknown.

The major target tissues of calcitonin seem to be bone, kidney, and the gastrointestinal tract. In the bone, its major defined action is the inhibition of osteoclastic bone resorption. Osteoclasts lose their ruffled borders and clear zones within 15 minutes in response to calcitonin. It has been proposed that calcitonin plays an important role in the rapid storage of calcium in the perilacunar space after meals. In the kidney, specific receptors are known to exist for calcitonin. It decreases tubular reabsorption of both calcium and phosphate. In the gut, pharmacologic doses of calcitonin increase secretion of Na^+, K^+, Cl^-, and water and decrease acid secretion.

Calcitonin deficiency causes no known disorder of metabolism. Although calcitonin has no important physiologic role, it is likely that it is involved in the long-term maintenance of calcium homeostasis and skeletal mass.

Calcitonin does have several pharmacologic uses: treating Paget's disease, preventing disuse osteoporosis, and rapid lowering of serum calcium in severe hypercalcemic states.

Estrogens and Corticosteroids

Both males and females experience age-related bone loss, particularly from cortical bone. The rate of trabecular bone loss increases in the first few years after menopause. This rate is correlated with decreasing amounts of endogenous estrogens at menopause. Several studies have shown that estrogen replacement in the postmenopausal years blocks or significantly decreases the loss of bone. Furthermore, a decrease in fracture rates in the appendicular skeleton has been well documented in patients receiving estrogen replacement. When used alone, 0.625 mg of Premarin per day is the lowest effective dose for retarding bone loss. When combined with calcium supplementation, 0.3 mg may be equally effective.

Patients who undergo bilateral oophorectomy before menopause also respond to estrogen therapy. This group is especially at risk for developing osteoporosis because a greater proportion of their lives is spent with low estrogen levels. Discontinuation of estrogen therapy can result in a greatly accelerated rate of bone loss in these patients. To obtain maximal benefit from therapy, estrogen should be started shortly after menopause. This significantly delays the precipitous bone loss and keeps bone mass above the postulated fracture threshold throughout the patient's life. If estrogen therapy is not started within the first 5 to 10 years after menopause, it is of limited benefit.

Two other symptoms of low estrogen level, hot flashes and genitourinary problems, are adequately treated with the low doses of estrogen given to prevent osteoporosis. Estrogen contained in topical creams used to treat atrophic vaginitis is absorbed into the circulation. It is not known what effect this type of estrogen therapy has on the probability of endometrial cancer developing, but the occurrence of this carcinoma is believed to be approximately 8 times higher in women on continuous estrogen therapy. The risk is reduced to 1.5 to 2 times normal when estrogens are used cyclically (21 days/month) and may revert to control level when estrogens are used in conjunction with progestins 10 days per month. Nevertheless, it is recommended that any woman on estrogen therapy should be followed closely with serial Pap smears and an annual endometrial biopsy.

Additional complications of estrogen therapy include an increased risk of cerebrovascular accident, thrombosis, and uterine bleeding. In one study, 13% of patients on supplemental estrogen therapy required hysterectomy. Several reports have indicated that in patients receiving estrogen therapy the incidence of breast cancer varies from 0.6 to 1.7 times normal.

The mechanisms by which decreasing levels of estrogen cause bone loss and estrogen therapy prevents bone loss are unknown. No receptors for estrogens have been demonstrated in osteoblasts. This has led some to believe that the action of estrogen on bone is indirect. Many think that the estrogen effect is mediated by calcitonin. Although baseline calcitonin levels appear to be normal in postmenopausal osteoporotic women, it has been postulated that osteoporotics generate an inadequate calcitonin release in response to dietary calcium loads. The calcium then is not adequately handled, and insufficient calcitonin is present to blunt the effects of parathyroid hormone on bone resorption. However, conflicting reports have recently appeared, so the mechanism of estrogen action remains controversial. Estrogen-progestin therapy may be the safest form of therapy. It should be recommended to patients at high risk for osteoporosis—i.e., patients who experience premature menopause or who have several risk factors such as slender build, a strong family history of osteoporosis, low dietary calcium consumption, significant alcohol intake, or exposure to medications that predispose to osteoporosis.

Corticosteroids may cause bone loss directly by inhibiting calcium absorption across the gut or increasing renal calcium excretion, and indirectly by stimulating secondary hyperparathyroidism. Their principal effects are to decrease production of the intestinal calcium-binding proteins required for calcium absorption. They also decrease bone formation. Severe net bone loss can be produced with doses of only 10 mg of prednisone per day. Alternate-day treatment programs may have less potential to affect bone mass.

Thyroid Hormones

The thyroid gland produces two hormones, thyroxine (T4) and 3,5,3′-triiodothyronine (T3). Both are bound extensively to proteins in the plasma. The major binding proteins in order of decreasing binding affinity are: T4-binding globulin, T4-binding prealbumin, and albumin. T4 is bound approximately 10 times more tightly to these proteins than is T3.

T4 is the major secretory product of the thyroid, which is the only source of T4 in the body. Approximately 80% of T3 is formed from T4 in nonthyroid tissue. The two major organs that convert T4 to T3 by 5′-monodeiodination are the liver and kidney. Although there is less T3 in the circulation, it is 3 to 4 times more active biologically than is T4. Cell function is controlled by T3 that binds to nonhistone nuclear receptors. These complexes then regulate the synthesis of specific proteins by altering the rate of mRNA production. The amount of T4 secreted by the thyroid depends on the level of thyrotropin (also known as thyroid-stimulating hormone; TSH) present. TSH, in turn, is released in response to thyrotropin-releasing hormone (TRH). T4 and T3 have negative feedback loops regulating the formation and release of TSH and TRH.

Patients with hyperthyroidism may develop osteoporotic bone disease. Bone resorption and bone formation take place at stimulated rates, but resorption appears to occur at a slightly faster rate than formation. The radiographic findings may be indistinguishable from those of senile osteoporosis. High normal physiologic levels of thyroid hormones, particularly when given pharmacologically, may affect bone metabolism disproportionately. Consequently, chronic thyroid supplementation may contribute to osteoporosis. TRH stimulation tests including measurement of TSH levels can be helpful in identifying patients receiving excessive thyroid supplementation.

Osteopenia

Osteoporosis

It is estimated that approximately 15% of white women over age 65 years have significant osteoporosis. Up to 30% of these patients will sustain a fracture related to osteoporosis by age 75 years. The short-term, direct cost of the treatment of hip fractures due to osteoporosis was estimated to be more than 3 billion dollars in 1983. Thus, this condition has national significance. Typical fractures related to osteoporosis are located frequently in the proximal humerus, lower forearm, hip, spine, and pelvis.

The amount of bone loss associated with aging has been the subject of numerous research projects. From age 30 until menopause, compact bone is lost at a rate of 3% per decade. After menopause until age 60, bone is lost at 9% to 10% per decade. After age 60, the rate of loss decreases to 3% per decade. The rate of loss of trabecular bone does not appear to differ between the sexes. It progresses at a steady rate of 6% to 8% per decade, starting in mid-adulthood.

The typical patient with osteoporosis is a slender, sedentary, white woman of northern European descent who smokes and has breast-fed several children. Also, her diet is usually deficient in calcium and vitamin D, and she has little exposure to the sun. Blacks or obese women rarely have osteoporosis (obese women are believed to be protected from osteoporosis by virtue of their greater bone mass). Large stores of fat are important in the peripheral conversion of androgens to estrogen, so obese postmenopausal women have higher estrogen levels and this may protect their bone from the rapid postmenopause bone loss. Women with low weight-to-height ratios are particularly at risk for osteoporosis. Because blacks usually have a normal or high weight-to-height ratio, they rarely become osteoporotic; however, those blacks with low weight-to-height ratios have hip fracture rates similar to those in white women.

The differential diagnosis of osteopenic conditions is extensive. The diagnosis of idiopathic or postmenopausal osteoporosis is one of exclusion. Hyperparathyroidism, hyperthyroidism, bone marrow dyscrasias or malignancies, osteomalacia, and other abnormalities must be ruled out. Appropriate laboratory tests should be performed to eliminate these diagnoses. In addition, the general metabolic profile of the patient should be obtained, including calcium balance data, creatinine clearance, urinary hydroxyproline excretion, blood urea nitrogen, and serum phosphorus level. Photon absorptiometry is very helpful in quantitating the degree of osteoporosis. Dual-photon absorptiometry of the spine is helpful in diagnosis and in following treatment. Single-photon absorptiometry of the radius is precise, but there is wide overlap between normals and osteoporotics. Finally, specially calibrated "quantitative" computed tomography scans of the lumbar spine may be the best way to assess trabecular bone. The techniques of noninvasive bone measurement may vary in their levels of radiation exposure, costs, and availability. It is not yet certain which technique has the most value.

Trans-iliac bone biopsy is a reliable diagnostic aid, especially for identifying osteomalacia, if the bone has been labeled previously with tetracycline. Biopsies have established the heterogeneity of the causes that produce osteoporosis and may be helpful in guiding appropriate therapy.

The cause of postmenopausal osteoporosis has not been clearly delineated. The rates of bone resorption and bone formation become uncoupled. This may be due to relative parathyroid hormone excess. Decreased levels of circulating estrogens are often implicated, but there is no evidence showing that estrogen receptors exist in bone cells. Nevertheless, estrogen blocks the bone loss of postmenopausal osteoporosis. Other studies have shown a blunted response of calcitonin secretion to calcium challenge in elderly women. This deficiency may play a role in osteoporosis. A significant number (50% to 60%) of women with osteoporosis are lactase deficient and have a diet very low in calcium. Decreased calcium intake probably also contributes to the pathogenesis of osteoporosis. Reduced physical activity also contributes to osteoporosis; immobilization or weightlessness may cause a rapid loss of bone, as much as 1% per week. Appropriate exercise and weight bearing are necessary to maintain the skeleton and prevent bone loss.

Heparin-induced osteoporosis is a rare cause of spinal fractures. It typically occurs in women who are taking heparin for antepartum thrombophlebitis. The cause is unknown, but it can be avoided if not more than 10,000 units is given daily and therapy is not continued past 120 days. Adequate calcium supplementation also may be helpful.

Treatment

Several different treatments for postmenopausal osteoporosis have been studied. The efficacy of each treatment was judged by the reduction in the vertebral fracture rates that occurred. Calcium supplementation decreased the fracture rate by 50%. Supplementation with fluoride or estrogen further reduced the fracture rate by 50%. The combination of calcium, fluoride, and estrogen reduced the fracture rate to 10% of the original rate. Ironically, higher fracture rates were seen in all groups when patients received 50,000 units of vitamin D per week.

Other studies have specifically evaluated the efficacy of sodium fluoride. Sixty percent of patients treated with fluoride had radiographic evidence of increased vertebral bone mass. Eighty percent of patients increased their trabecular bone volumes by an average of 18% per year as measured by double biopsy. The fracture rates were reduced significantly after 1 year of treatment. Common side effects of fluoride treatment include gastrointestinal upset and arthralgias. The Food and Drug Administration has not yet approved sodium fluoride therapy; the results of ongoing double-blind studies and evaluation of long-term effects are needed.

It is interesting to note that large doses of vitamin D do not substantially alter the fracture rate with any of the above-mentioned treatment regimens. It does appear that a physiologic amount of vitamin D must be available for bone formation to occur normally. A summation of available data suggests that supplementation with calcium or estrogen will halt or decrease bone loss. Calcitonin is perhaps the most effective way to stop bone loss. However, its effectiveness in increasing total bone mass is limited. Furthermore, as a polypeptide, it is only available in an injectible form at the present time.

Sodium fluoride stabilizes the hydroxyapatite crystal and stimulates osteoblastic bone formation. It is this latter function that accounts for its principal effect. Although the newly synthesized bone is slightly irregular (increased osteocytes, increased lacunar size, perilacunar basophilia, and irregularity of collagen weave), overall bone strength is increased. When given in the absence of calcium supplementation, fluoride therapy leads to increased osteoid content and actual bone brittleness. Occasional indigestion and arthralgias are temporary and usually respond to nonoperative treatment; nonsteroidal anti-inflammatory drugs or calcitonin is usually effective. Symptoms resolve when the medication is discontinued.

Generally, postmenopausal women should receive initial treatment with calcium carbonate (1,500 mg of elemental calcium per day) and vitamin D (400 to 800 units per day). Estrogen therapy (0.65 mg of Premarin per day for 3 weeks per month and 10 mg of Provera per day for approximately 10 days) is only used for women who have a premature menopause, are experiencing rapid bone loss as seen by bone biopsy, and are within the first 6 years or so of menopause. Recently, the NIH Consensus on Osteoporosis suggested combined estrogen/progesterone therapy for all women under age 60 if there were no contraindications (e.g., thrombophlebitis or breast cancer). Calcitonin therapy can be substituted in women at high risk for breast or endometrial cancer. Estrogen therapy is terminated after 5 to 10 years.

Sodium fluoride (1 mg/kg per day) is only given to women with documented osteopenia and only after some calcium/vitamin D pretreatment to correct any osteomalacia or excess osteoid. Sodium fluoride is continued with calcium and vitamin D for at least 2 years or until the bone scan and radiographs show no new fractures for 2 years. On the average, most patients receive combined therapy for 3 years. Thereafter, calcium and physiologic doses of vitamin D are continued indefinitely.

Exercise is an important but poorly understood factor in the treatment of osteoporosis. Vigorous training programs have been shown to build bone mass, but these techniques usually are inappropriate for elderly osteoporotics. A program of increasing walking provides the weight bearing and "impact loading" required to maintain bone mass and is well tolerated by the patients. Thoracic extension exercises should be added to the standard lumbar-flexion back-exercise programs used by these women.

It is useful to consider osteoporosis as the end result of two factors: 1) the peak bone mass achieved, and 2) the rate at which that bone is lost. Any factor that diminishes peak bone mass or accelerates bone loss can produce osteoporosis. Osteoporosis thus is a clinically and histologically heterogeneous disorder. Treatment should be individualized to match the contributing factors in each patient.

Osteomalacia

As does its equivalent in children, rickets, osteomalacia has a multitude of causes. These causes can be grouped into the classic deficiency of dietary or endogenous vitamin D, intestinal malabsorption disorders, acquired or hereditary renal disorders, and a "miscellaneous" group. To obtain the correct diagnosis, all of these causes must be considered in an appropriate work-up.

The clinical diagnosis of osteomalacia is often difficult. Patients usually have nonspecific complaints (such as muscle weakness or just diffuse aches and pains, symptoms common in older patients). Frequently, the diagnosis is not made until the disorder is far advanced with evidence of kyphosis or significant decrease in trunk height. Multiple stress fractures may also occur.

Radiographic evidence of osteomalacia often is not specific and can mimic other disorders. The presence of pseudofractures or Looser's transformation zones is good evidence that some degree of osteomalacia is present (Looser's zones are radiolucent areas of bone that are the result of multiple microstress fractures that heal by the formation of osteomalacic bone). Other radiographic signs of osteomalacia include biconcave vertebral bodies and the "trefoil" pelvis. The process of osteomalacia is far advanced when these findings are present.

In many patients trans-iliac bone biopsy is necessary to confirm the diagnosis of osteomalacia. The histologic hallmark of osteomalacia is an increase in width and extent of the osteoid seams. Associated changes include decreased rate of mineral apposition as determined by tetracycline labeling and decrease in surface of the mineralization front. Osteoblasts on the bone surface do not appear to be actively stimulated and show a low, flattened profile.

Osteomalacia appears gradually over a period of several years. Its development depends on the quality and quantity of initial bone stock and the severity of the underlying disorder.

Classic osteomalacia is caused by a decrease in the vitamin D content in the diet. These patients are easily identified because of their unusual dietary habits—e.g., strict vegetarianism or a diet extremely low in fat. Typically, classic osteomalacia occurs in patients who are elderly. It has been proposed that the "mild malabsorption of the elderly" predisposes these patients to bone disease. This disorder is easily treated with small amounts of vitamin D.

Gluten-sensitive enteropathy is a common cause of osteomalacia due to a malabsorption syndrome. It is believed that the disease is present at birth, but it is not uncommon for patients to present as adults with osteomalacia due to gluten sensitivity. Treatment consists of a gluten-free diet (mainly a diet free of wheat and rye) and, initially, low doses of vitamin D.

Changes in gastrointestinal physiology secondary to abnormalities such as dumping syndrome, blind loops, or Crohn's disease may cause steatorrhea and malabsorption. Changes secondary to surgery (60% of Billroth I procedures after 10 years) may alter vitamin D metabolism and calcium homeostasis enough to produce osteomalacia. A more common result, however, is osteoporosis.

Vitamin D metabolites are known to undergo enterohepatic circulation. Thus, a biliary fistula may deplete vitamin D and lead to osteomalacia. Bile salts are important in the process of vitamin D absorption in the bowel, and any disorder of the biliary system or liver may affect vitamin D uptake by the intestine.

There are several known hereditary renal causes of rickets. Patients with these disorders (such as sex-linked dominant hypophosphatemic rickets) often will develop normally if the diagnosis is made early in life. Treatment with phosphate and 1,25-$(OH)_2D$ can maintain normal growth; this usually is discontinued after a mature skeleton is achieved. It may need to be used again as these patients age.

Albright originally described the disorder termed "distal renal tubular acidosis" in 1948. It has a dominant mode of inheritance with a variable penetrance. When patients present, they usually show at least one of the three major complications of the disorder: renal stones, hypophosphatemic paralysis, and osteomalacia. High doses of vitamin D and sodium bicarbonate usually are necessary. It has been suggested that vitamin D deficiency and subsequent osteomalacia occur because of damage done to the renal tubular cells by calcium deposited within the kidney. The tubular cells slowly regain their function of vitamin D metabolism as the disorder is brought under control with bicarbonate. The most common cause of bone loss in chronic renal failure is hyperparathyroidism (due to low serum calcium levels). Osteomalacia frequently is also a concomitant of renal osteodystrophy and usually cannot be explained by a decreased calcium · phosphate product in serum. (The calcium · phosphate product usually is high in chronic renal failure because serum phosphate is high.) Recently, it has been shown that aluminum, either as a contaminant of dialysis baths or by excessive ingestion of aluminum-containing phosphate binders, will concentrate at the calcification front and prevent mineralization. Excessive osteoid then accumulates. There also may be a direct toxic effect on osteoblasts. Finally, aluminum inhibits mineralization directly *in vitro.* Aluminum toxicity produces various bone abnormalities that are manifested clinically as diffuse bone pain. There may be associated toxic effects on the brain; indeed, the so-called dialysis encephalopathy may be related to aluminum disease.

Anticonvulsant osteomalacia occurs in patients on long-term phenytoin (Dilantin) therapy. Patients who are immobile are especially at risk for this form of osteomalacia. Any of the anticonvulsant drugs that induce hepatic enzyme formation in the endoplasmic reticulum (P-450 hydroxylase) can cause the disorder. It is believed that the increased levels of enzymes compete with 25-hydroxylase in metabolizing vitamin D and subsequently produce metabolites of vitamin D that are inactive. Therapy consists of moderate doses of vitamin D. Osteoporosis is also common in the phenytoin-treated patients.

Mild forms of hyperosteoidosis are common in osteopenia (30% of patients). Bone biopsy and morphometric analysis of undecalcified specimens may be the only ways to recognize the subtle forms of osteomalacia. Defective bone mineralization appears to be an independent variable in the successful healing of femoral neck fractures. Therefore, many recommend trans-iliac bone biopsy for all patients with osteopenia who are to undergo operative repair of hip fractures.

Increased Osteodensity

Paget's Disease of Bone

Paget's disease of bone has been found throughout the world but may be more common in the United Kingdom than elsewhere. It is uncommon in Scandinavia, Africa, the Middle East, and the Far East. In the United States, its incidence is roughly 3% in the population more than 40 years old. Geographic clustering has been reported. No genetic link has been found, and there is no associated HLA antigen. A viral cause has been postulated. Intranuclear inclusion bodies have been found in the osteoclasts from pagetic bone of 41 consecutive patients with Paget's disease; control patients without the disease did not have these bodies. The presentation is consistent with that seen in slow virus infections. Measles virus, the cause of subacute sclerosing panencephalitis (SSPE), may be responsible. Interestingly, Sir James Paget was the first to propose that the disease was an inflammatory disorder of uncertain infectious origin. Mirra described a giant cell tumor occurring in bone that was also involved by Paget's disease. Intranuclear inclusion bodies similar to those seen in Paget's disease were demonstrated in the nuclei of the giant cells in the tumor. Bone sarcomas and giant cell tumors have been described in pagetic bone.

Histologically, the initial event in Paget's disease is bone lysis by overly active osteoclasts. This creates the radiolucent areas seen on radiographs in the early phase of the disease. Later, osteoblasts become more active and start to form new bone rapidly. This causes the sclerotic areas present on radiographs. Some believe that the osteoblasts are not abnormal cells but are only responding to the massive resorption of bone in a manner that allows calcium homeostasis to exist in the organism. No inclusion bodies have ever been found in the osteoblasts or osteocytes of pagetic bone.

The local rate of bone turnover is markedly increased in pagetic bone—as high as 20 times normal in some studies using radioactive calcium. This hypermetabolic state causes increased amounts of alkaline phosphatase to appear in the serum and an increased amount of hydroxyproline to be excreted in the urine. Alkaline phosphatase activity correlates with the osteoblastic activity and, therefore, with bone production. Most of the hydroxyproline in the body is contained in collagen, and type I collagen makes up most of the organic matrix of bone. Hydroxyproline clearance is an indicator of bone resorption and osteoclastic activity. Recently, a large peptide containing hydroxyproline was isolated from the urine. Metabolically, patients with Paget's disease typically have normal serum calcium, phosphate, and parathyroid hormone levels. Calcium clearance by the kidneys is not elevated. These are indications that the osteoclastic resorption is closely coupled to osteoblastic bone formation, even though the overall rates are greatly increased.

Paget's disease often is discovered as an incidental finding on radiographs. In patients who become symptomatic, bone pain and deformity are common complaints. Eighty-three percent of patients with this disease have some rheumatologic complaint. Back pain is the most common finding; usually some component of osteoarthritis is also present. Ninety-eight percent of patients with Paget's disease have other problems unrelated to the Paget's disease. This finding emphasizes the importance of looking for alternative sources of pain in patients with Paget's disease.

For treatment, three classes of drugs are available: calcitonin, mithramycin, and the diphosphonates. Each of these drugs acts to decrease osteoclastic resorption of bone. As resorption decreases, so does osteoblastic activity. Typically, hydroxyproline clearance decreases first, and later alkaline phosphatase levels fall. The goal is 50% reduction of the elevated values.

Calcitonin is effective initially in almost all patients. It acts by decreasing both osteoclastic activity and the absolute number of osteoclasts present. "Resistance" to calcitonin therapy develops in a significant number of patients. This resistance is not necessarily due to the development of antibodies to calcitonin. Approximately 60% of patients given salmon calcitonin develop antibodies. To demonstrate antibody-mediated resistance, it is necessary to return the disease to pretreatment levels by discontinuation of therapy and then obtain remission of the disorder with another calcitonin such as human calcitonin.

Mithramycin action is believed to act by binding of the drug to DNA and thereby selectively inhibiting the synthesis of specific RNA sequences. Side effects include hemorrhage, hepatotoxicity, and nephrotoxicity, especially at high dosages. It is primarily utilized to treat impending Paget's paraplegia.

The only diphosphonate available in the United States is diphosphonate disodium etidronate (EHDP) which functions as an analogue of pyrophosphate. This drug takes several weeks before its effect becomes apparent. There may be initial increase in bone pain associated with increased radiographic lucencies. In vitro, the diphosphonates also inhibit the formation of hydroxyapatite crystals. The interference with mineralization is believed to be minimal at doses of 5 mg/kg. The defective mineralization can cause severe osteomalacia. High doses, 20 mg/kg, commonly cause osteomalacia and are no more effective than low doses.

Paget's disease requires treatment when the disorder affects weight-bearing bones or hearing, produces spinal impingement, or is associated with fractures. Pretreatment of patients is recommended before joint replacement is undertaken. Treatment usually is 50 units of calcitonin subcutaneously three times per week for 6 months. Diphosphonate at 5 mg/kg per day may be used sequentially or concurrently.

Osteopetrosis

There are two distinct forms of this rare genetically transmitted disorder: a juvenile or "malignant" form, and the more common adult or "benign" form. An intermediate form has recently been reported.

The juvenile form is also known as "infantile," "precocious," or "congenital" osteopetrosis. The mode of transmission is autosomal recessive. It is characterized by anemia, hepatosplenomegaly, thrombocytopenia, cranial nerve palsies, and usually death at an early age. Radiographic studies show radiodense bone with obliteration of the medullary canal and widening of the metaphysis but no gross alteration in the secondary growth zones other than the increased radiodensity. Histologically, cores of calcified cartilage are seen surrounded by new bone, and an increased number of osteoclasts are present. All knowledge about this disorder is consistent with the conclusion that the skeletal lesions are caused primarily by a markedly decreased rate of cartilage and bone resorption. There is no evidence that there is any alteration in the rate of cartilage or bone formation.

Studies of tissue from humans with the disorder and from several animal models strongly implicate altered osteoclastic activity as the cause. Ultrastructural studies have shown that the number of osteoclasts in bone is increased but that they lack the characteristic ruffled border and clear zone of normal osteoclasts resorbing bone. The cells are responsive to parathyroid hormone but they are not able to form the ruffled border and clear zone. Tissue collagenase, which is important for resorption, cannot be detected in osteopetrotic bone.

Recently, several patients with juvenile osteopetrosis have been cured by bone marrow transplantation. Postoperatively, there was progressive resolution of the osteopetrotic deformities with return to normal blood cell counts, decreased radiodensity of bone, and increased medullary cavity size. These patients were in negative calcium balance as the excess bone was mobilized. These patients need to undergo vigorous hydration to allow the excess calcium to be excreted in the urine. Bone marrow biopsy of one patient showed that the osteoclasts were actively resorbing bone and indicated that their origin was the bone marrow donor.

Patients with osteopetrosis have also been shown to have deficient killer cell function and impaired thymic secretory activity. This has caused some researchers to believe that juvenile osteopetrosis is a more complex disorder than simply a dysfunction of osteoclasts. After bone marrow transplantation, both of the above alterations return to normal levels. It is now postulated that these alterations are caused by the decrease in hematopoietic activity associated with obliteration of the bone marrow cavity.

The adult type of osteopetrosis is also known as "tarda osteopetrosis." It is inherited via an autosomal dominant pattern and does not alter the life expectancy of the affected individual. It is usually an incidental finding on a radiograph taken for another reason. The radiographic findings are increased bone density but little or no disturbance of skeletal remodeling. Occasionally, these patients have bone pain, excessive fracturing, or cranial nerve palsies. Osteoclasts are found in increased number on bone biopsy, and the amount of bone present is increased with some remaining calcified cartilage present. Defective osteoclastic function is believed to be the cause, but the osteoclasts have retained enough function so that severe skeletal deformity does not occur.

Biochemical Mediators of Tissue Repair and Regeneration

Repair and regeneration of traumatized tissues may eventually involve any of a number of highly complex and poorly understood processes including hemostasis, inflammation, fibrogenesis, angiogenesis, neurogenesis, chondrogenesis, and osteogenesis. Histologic and gross biochemical descriptions of the sequential events that ultimately result in repair or regeneration have been available for some time. With these descriptions have been assumptions that biochemical or biophysical signals orchestrate these highly reproducible sequences. Recently, a number of substances that can mediate these changes have been identified and isolated. This section reviews the current understanding of these various substances.

Events of Wound Healing

Repair and regeneration of tissues are normal responses to injury. The biologic phenomena that ultimately lead to tissue repair and regeneration can be artificially divided into four phases for discussion: hemostasis, inflammation, organogenesis (modeling), and remodeling.

Hemostasis. The hemostatic mechanism appears to influence wound healing on at least three levels. First, it establishes hemostasis itself. Second, it initiates and partially mediates the inflammatory response. Third, it initiates organogenesis. The events of hemostasis can be divided into two phases—primary hemostasis (the formation of the platelet plug), and secondary hemostasis (blood clotting).

In response to injury, platelets adhere both to exposed elements of connective tissues (e.g., collagen) and to one another. The former phenomenon is called "platelet adhesion" and the latter, "platelet aggregation." During these events, the platelets secrete numerous substances that are either synthesized at this time or released from platelet storage granules (platelet release reaction). Examples are prostaglandins and thromboxanes for the former and serotonin and ADP for the latter. These substances can induce other platelets to aggregate, thus amplifying the response. The resultant hemostatic plug provides the primary arrest of bleeding. This phase of hemostasis occurs in the first 5 minutes after injury. In addition to its role in primary hemostasis, the platelet plug also provides a nidus for blood coagulation—i.e., it forms a protective and catalytic surface on which the reactions leading to thrombin formation can be initiated and sustained.

Tissue injury and primary hemostasis result in activation of both the intrinsic and extrinsic coagulation cascades. These pathways are amplification mechanisms for the generation of thrombin which in turn will convert large amounts of fibrinogen to fibrin. The polymerization of fibrin will initially act as a net for the entrapment of blood elements, forming the secondary hemostatic plug—a blood clot. This network will later provide a scaffolding for the initial conduction of vascular and connective tissue elements. The clotting mechanism is initiated in the first 5 minutes after injury and has its maximal effect within the first 10 to 15 minutes, although it may continue at a lower level of activity until wound stability has been established.

Inflammation. Inflammation occurs, with variable intensity, in response to all tissue injury. It appears to play at least two important roles in wound healing: wound debridement, and initiation of organogenesis. The inflammatory response can be divided into three phases—activation, amplification, and debridement.

Activation occurs within minutes after injury and is mediated by the products of tissue damage and hemostasis. Examples of these products include collagen, Hageman factor, and kallikrein.

Once the response is activated it is amplified via various biochemical and cellular mechanisms to yield the cardinal signs of inflammation: calor, rubor, tumor, and dolor. On a tissue level, these signs are caused by vasodilation, increased vascular permeability, edema, and hypersensitivity of nerve endings. During this amplification phase, which peaks between 48 and 72 hours after injury, the injured tissues are infiltrated first by neutrophils and then by macrophages.

The amplification process is mediated by multiple biochemical substances that are generated during the events of hemostasis or inflammation. Examples of the former are prostaglandins, thromboxanes, hydroxy fatty acids, and serotonin. Examples of the latter include kallikrein, bradykinin, components of the complement cascade, leukotrienes, and interleukin 1.

Debridement requires immunologic, phagocytic, and biochemical activities. It involves degradation of contaminants or devitalized tissues on at least three levels: bacterial, cellular, and matrix. Bacterial debridement, which probably occurs to some extent in all wounds, is mediated by neutrophils and the immunologic system and is augmented by multiple biochemical pathways. A detailed description of these phenomena is beyond the scope of this discussion.

Cellular debridement is mediated by phagocytic cells, mainly activated macrophages, and is also augmented by multiple biochemical pathways. Cellular phagocytosis is augmented by components of the complement cascade and by various components of the immunologic system. Cellular degradation also occurs as a result of enzymatic digestion. These enzymes are proteolytic in nature and are secreted by platelets, neutrophils, and activated macrophages.

Matrix debridement is mediated by both phagocytic cells and biochemical degradation. As with cellular debridement, the principal mediator is the activated macrophage. Biochemical degradation of the extracellular matrix is also mediated by proteolytic enzymes; especially important in this regard is collagenase.

The activated macrophage is a facultative anaerobe and, as such, is ideally suited for the acidic, anoxic environment of the early wound. The early wound contains the secondary hemostatic plug, modified by factor XIII-mediated binding of fibronectin to fibrin. This fibrin-fibronectin scaffolding facilitates macrophage activation, migration, and phagocytosis. Macrophages are the predominant cell of the wound from about the third to the fifth day. They are the key cell in the inflammatory response, and wound healing does not progress normally in their absence. In addition to their central role in debridement, these cells appear to provide nutrients to the other cells of the wound by degrading macromolecules to amino acids and simple sugars. They also appear to be the source of several growth factors that initiate organogenesis.

Organogenesis. Organogenesis or tissue modeling takes many forms in wound healing, depending on the nature of the injured tissues. It usually involves fibrogenesis, angiogenesis, and neurogenesis and can involve chondrogenesis and osteogenesis.

All types of organogenesis appear to progress through a series of cellular responses including conduction (migration), proliferation, induction (differentiation), and differentiated function. The various types of organogenesis are mutually supportive and inseparable. Moreover, the various types of organogenesis occur sequentially, each adding to or modifying the product of its predecessor. The resultant three-dimensional composite of tissue types serves as a temporary stabilizer of the wound and provides the stock for remodeling.

The earliest form of organogenesis seen in wound healing can be termed "primitive fibrogenesis." Mesenchymal stem cells from adjacent tissues migrate into the wound. They find there the fibrin-fibronectin scaffolding further modified by macrophage-mediated cellular and matrix debridement. These stem cells proliferate and differentiate into cells that some call "myofibroblasts." The myofibroblasts express their differentiated function by generating a new wound scaffolding composed of fibronectin, types I and III collagen, and proteoglycan. This new scaffolding is the predominant tissue in most wounds from days 5 through 10.

Angiogenesis follows primitive fibrogenesis in short order. These two phenomena seem to be coupled in that early fibroblastic proliferation and differentiated function occur directly subjacent to proliferating capillaries, and endothelial cells are seen to proliferate and differentiate into capillaries only in areas where the primitive fibrogenesis scaffolding is in place. These phenomena can result in the reestablishment of wound perfusion in 7 to 14 days if reasonable wound stability has been achieved.

More mesenchymal stem cells migrate to the wound with the ingrowth of the vasculature. These cells then proliferate, differentiate, and express differentiated function in response to various local signals. These signals tell the cells when to divide, what matrix to make, and how to orient in three-dimensional space. Thus, local signals may direct these stem cells to become fibroblasts and generate fibrous tissue or to become chondroblasts and generate cartilaginous tissue or to become osteoblasts and generate osseous tissue. The nature of these signals will be discussed in detail below. Although dependent on wound size and stability, the various forms of organogenesis will usually occur between days 7 and 21.

Remodeling. The tissue composite generated by the organogenesis phase of wound healing provides the stock for tissue remodeling. This process involves both the degradation of existing wound tissue and the generation of new tissue. The new tissue is of similar composition but with a different and biomechanically more efficient orientation. This phase occurs over a prolonged period of time, from 21 days after wounding to 1 year or more. The mediators of these phenomena are not well described and are probably biophysical in nature.

Types of Growth Factors

There are several types of growth factors that orchestrate the sequential phases of repair and regeneration. These factors can be broadly categorized as chemotactic factors, competence factors, progression factors, inductive factors, transforming factors, or permissive factors.

General Characteristics. Growth factors are widely diversified in terms of biochemical composition. Some are small peptides; others are large glycoproteins; and still others are lipids. Despite this diversity, most growth factors have several biologic properties in common.

First, these factors are not biologically available in normal tissue. They are present either in latent form (e.g., sequestered in storage granules) or in an inactive precursor form. When needed, they become available either by secretion or by biochemical modification.

Second, there tends to be multiple, redundant pathways for the generation of these factors or for the generation of other factors with similar biologic activity. Thus, nature has provided multiple back-up systems to ensure that wound healing is achieved.

Third, these factors are generated as part of amplification systems. Activation of small amounts of initiators results in the generation of large amounts of biochemical effectors via biochemical or cellular cascades.

Last, these growth factors and their biologic effects are limited by feedback loops.

Chemotactic Factors. These factors attract cells to the wound at various phases of healing. They tend to be cell-specific—i.e., each factor attracts a specific cell type—and as a result they mediate dramatic shifts in the cell population of the wound.

1. *Prostaglandins.* Numerous prostaglandins are generated by damaged tissues and aggregating platelets in the wound, mainly PGE_2 and $PGF_{2\alpha}$. These acidic, oxygenated lipids are synthesized from arachidonic acid that has been released from membrane phospholipids. They attract neutrophils to the wound.

2. *Prostanoids.* This group includes the thromboxanes and prostacyclin. Thromboxanes are generated mainly by aggregating platelets; prostacyclin is generated mainly by damaged tissues. They are acidic oxygenation products of arachidonic acid and they too attract neutrophils to the wound.

3. *Eicosanoids.* Hydroxy fatty acids, lipoxins, and leukotrienes are examples of these arachidonic acid metabolites. They are generated by damaged tissues, aggregating platelets, and neutrophils. They attract neutrophils and macrophages to the wound.

4. *Complement.* The components of the complement cascade are proteins that are synthesized in the liver. These components are activated in a cascade generated by proteolytic modification. Several activated intermediates in this cascade, particularly the C5a component, attract neutrophils and macrophages to the wound.

5. *Platelet-derived growth factor* (PDGF). This peptide is stored in platelet granules. It is released by platelets as they aggregate. PDGF attracts macrophages and fibroblasts to the wound.

6. *Angiokine-I* (AK-I). This factor is thought to be a protein elaborated by activated macrophages. It attracts proliferating endothelial cells to the wound.

Competence Factors. With the exception of a few constantly dividing cell types, most cells are in the so-called resting (G_0) phase of the cell cycle. A prerequisite for proliferation of these resting cells is the acquisition of "competence." This refers to some poorly understood change in the cell's receptiveness to various mitogens. This change is induced by competence factors. Once a resting cell has been changed, it is competent to enter the G_1 phase of the cell and subsequently divide, if stimulated to do so by an appropriate progression factor (see below). The following are examples of competence factors.

1. *Platelet-derived growth factor* (PDGF). This peptide also has chemotactic activity (described above). It induces competence in numerous cells of mesenchymal origin.

2. *Prostaglandin* $F_{2\alpha}$. This substance has also been described above and has both chemotactic and competence activity.

3. *Fibroblast growth factor* (FGF). This peptide is present in wound fluid and may be generated by activated macrophages. It induces competence in numerous cells of mesenchymal origin.

Progression Factors. Once competent, cells in the G_0 phase will respond to so-called progression factors, enter the cell cycle, and divide. Thus, proliferation requires the sequential influence of two types of mitogens, competence factors and progression factors. During this proliferative phase of organogenesis, differentiation and differentiated function tend to be suppressed. Accordingly, competence and progression factors are often found to inhibit differentiated function. The following are examples of progression factors.

1. *Epidermal growth factor (EGF)*. This peptide is found in wound fluid but its cell of origin is unknown. It stimulates numerous types of competent mesenchymal cells to proliferate, and it inhibits differentiated function.

2. *Interleukin 1*. This peptide is generated by activated macrophages in the wound. It stimulates the proliferation of myofibroblasts and fibroblasts.

3. *Somatomedin A*. This insulin-like peptide is a circulating systemic factor and is a normal constituent of blood plasma. It is generated in the liver. It stimulates the proliferation of competent cells.

4. *Somatomedin C (insulin-like growth factor I, IGF-I)*. This peptide is structurally related to insulin and is a systemic factor generated in the liver. It stimulates the proliferation of numerous types of competent mesenchymal cells.

5. *Insulin-like growth factor II (IGF-II) (multiplication-stimulating activity, MSA)*. This is another systemic peptide related to insulin and generated in the liver. It too stimulates proliferation of competent mesenchymal cells.

Inductive Factors. These factors stimulate differentiation and differentiated function. Additionally, some of these factors appear to stimulate the proliferation of cells that have undergone differentiation. They all tend to be local factors, either generated by the cells mediating wound healing or present in the matrix of the injured tissue itself. The following are examples of inductive factors.

1. *Angiokine-II (AK-II)*. This poorly characterized activity stimulates the local proliferation of vascular endothelial cells.

2. *Angiokine-III (AK-III)*. This poorly characterized activity stimulates differentiated function in proliferating vascular endothelial cells (e.g., tubularization).

3. *Nerve growth factor (NGF)*. This protein is elaborated by fibroblasts in the wound. It stimulates differentiation of medulloblasts into neurons and glial cells.

4. *Cartilage-derived factor (CDF)*. This peptide has been found to be present in both cartilage and bone. It stimulates chondroblast proliferation and the elaboration of cartilaginous matrix.

5. *Bone morphogenetic protein (BMP)*. This highly studied peptide is present in bone. It induces the differentiation of precursor cells into osteoblasts.

6. *Bone-derived growth factors I & II (BDGF I & II)*. These activities are present in bone. They appear to stimulate proliferation of osteoprogenitor cells and the elaboration of osteoid.

Transforming Factors. These factors appear to cause dedifferentiation and proliferation. They are characterized experimentally by their ability to cause cells to lose their sensitivity to contact inhibition and to acquire anchorage independence—i.e., they can proliferate in culture without first adhering to some surface. Their role in wound healing and neoplasia is unclear at the present time. The following are examples of these factors.

1. *Transforming growth factor I (TGF-I)*. This membrane protein appears to be the receptor for EGF (see above). It stimulates proliferation and transformation as described above. As might be expected, its activity appears to be dependent on EGF.

2. *Transforming growth factor II (TGF-II)*. This peptide is present in platelets and appears to regulate the production of TGF-I. Its activity therefore is dependent on both TGF-I and EGF.

Permissive Factors. These factors allow cells to respond to other growth factors in an appropriate way—i.e., they make the cells responsive to stimulation by growth factor. Most of these factors are components of the extracellular matrix and as such are specific to a given tissue. A single growth factor—e.g., an inductive factor—may induce a mesenchymal stem cell to differentiate into completely different cell types depending on the type of permissive factor that is present. The following are examples of these factors.

1. *Fibronectin*. This protein of matrix and cell membrane is generated by many cell types including platelets, myofibroblasts, and fibroblasts. It specifically binds to several fibrillar proteins of the wound, including fibrin, type III collagen, and type I collagen. When associated with fibrin or collagen, it allows activated macrophages to respond to chemotactic factors and move into the wound, it allows myofibroblasts to respond to inductive factors and elaborate type III collagen, and it allows proliferating endothelial cells to respond to inductive factors and grow into the wound. When associated with type III collagen, it allows fibroblasts to respond to inductive factors and elaborate type I collagen and it allows proliferating endothelial cells to express differentiated function in response to inductive factors.

2. *Osteonectin*. This noncollagenous protein of the bone matrix appears to be the hard tissue equivalent of fibronectin and, as such, may interact with osteoprogenitor cells to allow them to be responsive to inductive factors.

Summary

It is now clear that the sequential phases of wound healing are mediated by a highly complex and diverse group of substances that can be loosely categorized as growth factors. New knowledge in this area will surely bring new and exciting approaches to many clinical problems. New information is already implicating these factors in many disease states—most importantly, in neoplastic states. Moreover, once isolated, these substances may be put to use as therapeutic agents. Research has already started to demonstrate their value in several areas of interest to the orthopaedist. These include stimulation of biologic fixation of prosthetic implants, bone graft incorporation in segmental and allographic transplantation, and vascular ingrowth in osteonecrotic states.

Annotated Bibliography

Bone

Bone Cells

Bonucci, E.: New knowledge on the origin, function and fate of osteoclasts. Clin. Orthop. 158:252–269, 1981.

The osteoclast originates within the monocyte/macrophage system and is brought to the bone surface via the bloodstream.

Messer, H.H.: Bone cell membranes. Clin. Orthop. 166:256–276, 1982.

A review of the bone cell membrane and the effects of hormonal, chemical, and electrical stimuli on cell function.

Owen, M.: The origin of bone cells in the postnatal organism. Arthritis Rheum 23:1073–1079, 1980.

Succinct synopsis of modern concepts of osteogenesis and differentiation between the origins of osteoblasts and osteoclasts. A comprehensive bibliography is included.

Bone Biophysics

Goodship, A.E.; Lanyon, L.E.; and McFie, H.: Functional adaptation of bone to increased stress: An experimental study. J. Bone Joint Surg. 61A:539–546, 1979.

An original discussion of the roles of modeling and remodeling of bone in relation to stress.

Pollack, S.R.: Bioelectrical properties of bone: Endogenous electrical signals. Orthop. Clin. North Am. 15:3–14, January 1984.

A concise description of the nature and significance of electrical phenomena in bone.

Bone Formation

Brighton, C.T.; Friedenberg, Z.B.; Black, J.; Esterhai, J.L., Jr.; Mitchell, J.E.; and Montique, F., Jr.: Electrically induced osteogenesis: Relationship between charge, current density, and the amount of bone formed: Introduction of a new cathode concept. Clin. Orthop. 161:122–132, 1981.

An analysis of the various factors affecting bone osteogenesis by electricity.

Harakas, N.K.: Demineralized bone-matrix-induced osteogenesis. Clin. Orthop. 188:239–251, 1984.

Consideration of the biologic basis of bone induction and a good explanation of the different results reported by individual investigators. An excellent bibliography.

Raisz, L.G., and Kream, B.E.: Regulation of bone formation. N. Engl. J. Med. 309:29–35, 1983.

A comprehensive review of the biologic determinants of bone formation.

Mineral Metabolism

Calcium and Phosphorus

Nordin, B.E.C.; Horsman, A.; Marshall, D.H.; Simpson, M.; and Waterhouse, G.M.: Calcium requirement and calcium therapy. Clin. Orthop. 140:216–239, 1979.

Calcium homeostasis in normal and osteoporotic patients is outlined.

Spencer, H.; Kramer, L.; Lesniak, M.; De Bartolo, M.; Norris, C.; and Osis, D.: Calcium requirements in humans: Report of original data and a review. Clin. Orthop. 184:270–280, 1984.

Detailed original work on the calcium intake necessary to achieve positive calcium balance.

Vitamin D/Osteomalacia

Chesney, R.W.: Current clinical applications of vitamin D metabolite research. Clin. Orthop. 161:285–314, 1981.

An understandable review of vitamin D metabolism, providing a good basis for clinical applications.

Kanis, J.A.: Vitamin D metabolism and its clinical application. J. Bone Joint Surg. 64B:542–560, 1982.

A clear, comprehensive review with clinically relevant recommendations for most of the known osteomalacic syndromes.

Renal Osteodystrophy

Malluche, H.H.; Smith, A.J.; Abreo, K.; and Faugere, M.-C.: The use of deferoxamine in the management of aluminum accumulation in bone in patients with renal failure. N. Engl. J. Med. 311:140–144, 1984.

The importance of diagnosing aluminum-related bone disease is emphasized by the successful treatment that is now possible for this condition.

Ward, M.K.; Feest, T.G.; Ellis, H.A.; Parkinson, I.S.; Kerr, D.N.S.; Herrington, J.A.; and Goode, G.L.: Osteomalacic dialysis osteodystrophy: Evidence for a water-borne aetiological agent, probably aluminum. Lancet 1:841–845, 1978.

Osteomalacia in hemodialysis patients correlates with the concentration of aluminum in the dialysate.

Calcium-Binding Proteins

Delmas, P.D.; Wahner, H.W.; Mann, K.G.; and Riggs, B.L.: Assessment of bone turnover in postmenopausal osteoporosis by measurement of serum bone Gla-protein. J. Lab. Clin. Med. 102:470–476, 1983.

Serum bone Gla-protein content correlates with bone formation rates.

Gallop, P.M.; Lian, J.B.; and Hauschka, P.V.: Carboxylated calcium-binding proteins and vitamin K. N. Engl. J. Med. 302:1460–1466, 1980.

The distribution, function, and vitamin K-dependence of calcium-binding proteins are discussed.

Termine, J.D.; Kleinman, H.K.; Whitson, S.W.; Conn, K.M.; McGarvey, M.L.; and Martin, G.R.: Osteonectin, a bone-specific protein linking mineral to collagen. Cell 26:99–105, 1981.

An original contribution detailing the ability of this protein to localize calcium ions and nucleate mineralization of bone.

Endocrine Effects

Martin, T.J.: Drug and hormone effects on calcium release from bone. Pharmacol. Ther. 21:209–228, 1983.

A review of the hormonal basis of calcium release and homeostasis.

Parathyroid Hormone

Habener, J.F.: Regulation of parathyroid hormone secretion and biosynthesis. Annu. Rev. Physiol. 43:211–223, 1981.

This article discusses parathyroid hormone synthesis and metabolism.

Martin, K.J.; Hruska, K.A.; Freitag, J.J.; Klahr, S.; and

Slatopolsky, E.: The peripheral metabolism of parathyroid hormone. N. Engl. J. Med. 301:1092–1098, 1979.

The clinical significance of various fragments of parathyroid hormone is discussed.

Calcitonin

Austin, L.A., and Heath, H., III: Calcitonin: Physiology and pathophysiology. N. Engl. J. Med. 304:269–278, 1981.

A review of recent information about calcitonin physiology and its therapeutic effects.

Gruber, H.E.; Ivey, J.L.; Baylink, D.J.; Matthews, M.; Nelp, W.B.; Sisom, K.; and Chesnut, C.H., III: Long-term calcitonin therapy in postmenopausal osteoporosis. Metabolism 33:295–303, 1984.

Calcitonin may slow bone loss but has limited effect in building new bone.

Tiegs, R.D.; Body, J.J.; Wahner, H.W.; Barta, J.; Riggs, B.L.; and Heath, H., III: Calcitonin secretion in postmenopausal osteoporosis. N. Engl. J. Med. 312:1097–1100, 1985.

Deficiency in calcitonin level (response) is unlikely to be important in postmenopausal osteoporosis.

Estrogen

Bush, T.L.; Cowan, L.D.; Barrett-Connor, E.; Criqui, M.H.; Karon, J.M.; Wallace, R.B.; Tyroler, H.A.; and Rifkind, B.M.: Estrogen use and all-cause mortality: Preliminary results from the Lipid Research Clinics Program Follow-Up Study. J.A.M.A. 249:903–906, 1983.

Estrogen-treated women live longer.

Wilson, P.W.; Garrison, R.J.; and Castelli, W.P.: Postmenopausal estrogen use, cigarette smoking, and cardiovascular morbidity in women over 50. The Framingham Study. N. Engl. J. Med. 313:1038–1043, 1985.

The use of estrogens may increase the risk of cardiovascular disease in postmenopausal women.

Worley, R.J.: Age, estrogen, and bone density. Clin. Obstet. Gynecol. 24:203–218, March 1981.

Estrogens decrease bone loss and fracture rate in postmenopausal women.

Osteopenia

Osteoporosis

Diddle, A.W., and Smith, I.Q.: Postmenopausal osteoporosis: The role of estrogens. South. Med. J. 77:868–871, 1984.

The benefits of estrogen therapy are discussed, and recommendations for the necessary follow-up examinations are given.

Lane, J.M.; Healey, J.H.; Schwartz, E.; Vigorita, V.J.; Schneider, R.; Einhorn, T.A.; Suda, M.; and Robbins, W.C.: Treatment of osteoporosis with sodium fluoride and calcium: Effects on vertebral fracture incidence and bone histomorphometry. Orthop. Clin. North Am. 15:729–745, October 1984.

Bone mass was significantly improved and the spinal fracture rate was reduced in a series of doubly biopsied osteoporotic women who received daily doses of sodium fluoride (1 mg/kg), calcium (1,500 mg), and vitamin D (400 IU) per day.

Lane, J.M., and Vigorita, V.J.: Osteoporosis. J. Bone Joint Surg. 65A:274–278, 1983.

This review covers the pathophysiology, diagnosis, and treatment of osteoporosis.

Riggs, B.L.; Seeman, E.; Hodgson, S.F.; Taves, D.R.; and O'Fallon, W.M.: Effect of the fluoride/calcium regimen on vertebral fracture occurrence in postmenopausal osteoporosis: Comparison with conventional therapy. N. Engl. J. Med. 306:446–450, 1982.

Vertebral fractures are preventable by treatment with calcium, sodium fluoride, and estrogen.

Schneider, R.: Radiologic methods of evaluating generalized osteopenia. Orthop. Clin. North Am. 15:631–651, October 1984.

This article describes the techniques, uses, and misuses of noninvasive bone mass measurements.

Increased Osteodensity

Paget's Disease

Merkow, R.L., and Lane, J.M.: Current concepts of Paget's disease of bone. Orthop. Clin. North Am. 15:747–764, October 1984.

A good recent review of Paget's disease is presented. It includes a good discussion of various orthopaedic aspects such as hip replacement and the treatment of secondary sarcomas in Paget's disease of bone.

Twenty-Fifth Rheumatism Review: Paget's disease. Arthritis Rheum. 26:281–283, 1983.

This article reviews the etiology, pathogenesis, presentation, and treatment of Paget's disease. A good discussion of mithramycin, calcitonin, and diphosphonate therapy is included. This is part of a larger symposium on Paget's disease.

Osteopetrosis

Marks, S.C., Jr.: Congenital osteopetrotic mutations as probes of the origin, structure, and function of osteoclasts. Clin. Orthop. 189:239–263, 1984.

The heterogeneous types of osteopetrosis are described. Included is a detailed discussion of the way that marrow transplantation has helped to elucidate the origin of osteoclasts.

Sorell, M.; Kapoor, N.; Kirkpatrick, D.; Rosen, J.F.; Chaganti, R.S.K.; Lopez, C.; Dupont, B.; Pollack, M.S.; Terrin, B.N.; Harris, M.B.; Vine, D.; Rose, J.S.; Goossen, C.; Lane, J.; Good, R.A.; and O'Reilly, R.J.: Marrow transplantation for juvenile osteopetrosis. Am. J. Med. 70:1280–1287, 1981.

The clinical success of marrow transplantation in reversing osteopetrosis is documented in this article.

Bone Biopsy

Whyte, M.P.; Bergfeld, M.A.; Murphy, W.A.; Avioli, L.V.; and Teitelbaum, S.L.: Postmenopausal osteoporosis: A heterogeneous disorder as assessed by histomorphometric analysis of iliac crest bone from untreated patients. Am. J. Med. 72:193–202, 1982.

Iliac bone biopsies and histomorphometry demonstrate the qualitative and quantitative differences in metabolic bone diseases.

Events of Wound Healing

Hunt, T.K.: Physiology of wound healing. *In* Surgical Physiology, edited by J.F. Burke, pp. 1–13. Philadelphia, W.B. Saunders Company, 1983.

A good review of wound healing with particular attention to the systemic changes that accompany wounding.

Peacock, E.E., Jr.: Wound healing. *In* The Scientific Management of Surgical Patients, edited by R.M. Peters,

E.E. Peacock, Jr., and J.R. Benfield, pp. 27–63. Boston, Little, Brown & Company, 1983.

One of many excellent descriptions of the normal sequence of events in wound healing.

Growth Factors

Canalis, E.: Effect of growth factors on bone cell replication and differentiation. Clin. Orthop. 193:246–263, 1985.

Extensive review of many of the growth factors with special emphasis on their effects on bone metabolism and fracture healing.

Castor, C.W., and Cabral, A.R.: Growth factors in human disease: The realities, pitfalls, and promise. Sem. Arthritis Rheum. 15:33–44, 1985.

Reviews growth factors and discusses their possible involvement in disease.

Gospodarowicz, D., and Tauber, J.-P.: Growth factors and the extracellular matrix. Endocr. Rev. 1:201–227, 1980.

Reviews growth factors with special emphasis on the interactions among cells, their matrix, and growth factors.

Granström, E.: The arachidonic acid cascade: The prostaglandins, thromboxanes and leukotrienes. Inflammation Suppl. 8:15–25, 1984.

An excellent review of the various arachidonic acid metabolites and their activities.

4 Arthritis

Subjects in this section include new concepts of normal joint physiology integrated with recent advances in the pathophysiology of osteoarthritis and the inflammatory arthropathies. New nonoperative and operative treatments of these disorders will be discussed.

Normal Joint Physiology

Articular cartilage is an avascular, aneural, and alymphatic tissue composed of chondrocytes enmeshed in a superhydrated (66%–79% water) matrix of proteoglycans and collagen.

Chondrocytes

These cells are metabolically active and produce and maintain the intercellular matrix. They are unique in being isolated from each other although highly responsive to their environment. Cells from the superficial zone (zone I) are usually oval and elongated with few intracytoplasmic filaments. Chondrocytes from the deeper zones (zones II and III) are more rounded and contain more mitochondria, rough endoplasmic reticulum, and Golgi complex, indicative of a more metabolically active cell. When chondrocytes are grown in high-density cultures and exposed to intermittent compressive forces, they respond by significantly increasing proteoglycan synthesis as shown by increased [^{35}S]sulfate incorporation. Also, the ability of proteoglycans to aggregate is enhanced and the coherence of proteoglycans with other matrix components is improved. This increase in sulfated glycosaminoglycans provides a higher water-binding capacity which will improve resistance to compressive forces. Chondrocytes also respond to cartilage-derived growth factors by increasing hyaluronate synthesis, which seems to induce changes in cell shape consistent with decreased adhesion to the surrounding matrix and increased cellular motility.

Within the chondrocytes are bodies known as lysosomes in which enzymes are stored; these are important in the maintenance of normal joint function as well as in degenerative processes. Acid phosphatase and β glucuronidase have been shown to be present in normal cartilage. A heat-stable hyaluronidase has recently been identified in normal articular cartilage by a viscometric technique. Cathepsins and neutral proteoglycanase also have been identified, but only indirect evidence suggests that a neutral collagenase is present in normal cartilage.

Matrix

The synthetic products of the chondrocyte are *collagen,* a unique triple-helix molecule with specific phenotypes; *proteoglycan,* an anionic macromolecule present in aggregates clustered on a hyaluronic acid backbone, and *water,* trapped within the collagen-proteoglycan complex by hydrostatic forces.

The fibrillar network of cartilage is largely composed of type II collagen. However, type I is present in the superficial layers, and other minor collagens with disulfide bonds have been identified recently in the pericellular areas. The three-dimensional network that is formed provides the tissue with an inextensible volume. There is a slow but measurable turnover of adult articular collagen. The sequence of events in the synthesis of collagen has been reviewed previously; however, it appears that the process is under the control of one gene, although the specific genetic code sequence is as yet unknown. Collagen undergoes changes with normal aging, such as increased thermal stability, decreased solubility, increased mechanical stiffness, and a tendency toward a brown discoloration. Some evidence also suggests a generalized decrease in collagen synthesis with aging.

Proteoglycan exists in the form of aggregates composed of monomers, hyaluronic acid, and link proteins, which, because of their high concentration, exert a swelling pressure that maintains the fibrillar network in its extended form. The monomer contains a hyaluronate binding region of constant size and composition and a peripheral chondroitin sulfate region of variable length. The latter region appears to decrease with aging; the binding region and the intervening keratan sulfate-rich region increase in proportion with aging. The factors that control these age changes are largely unknown, although immunologic epitopes change with age and the chemical structure of keratan sulfate is different in cartilage from older individuals. The three-dimensional structure and aggregation of proteoglycan is important for the normal functioning of joints. A recently identified dermatan sulfate proteoglycan appears to have a unique relationship with collagen and increases in concentration in the surface layers of aged articular cartilage.

The load-bearing function of articular cartilage depends on the interaction between the hydrated proteoglycan gel and the collagenous network. This latter network, although somewhat randomly distributed, shows a preferred radial orientation in the middle and deep zones of articular cartilage and tangential at the surface. Hydrated proteoglycans are essentially absent in the superficial zones but are present in increased concentrations in the deeper zones. The compressive response of normal articular cartilage results in deformation throughout the entire depth of the cartilage. Collagen fibers compact without forming a band structure, and the radial texture usually seen by transmission electron microscopy is lost. By contrast, when proteoglycans are disrupted by treating cartilage with hyaluronidase, compression produces a repeating sequence of obliquely layered parallel bands. This buckling and flattening of the collagenous network results in the loss of normal compressive strength. This clearly shows the highly dependent interaction of matrix molecules for normal articular cartilage function.

Synovium and Synovial Fluid

Synovium, a highly vascularized connective tissue, is devoid of a classic basement membrane. In addition to the type A phagocytic cells and type B secretory cells, there are undifferentiated cells that may act as a source of reparative cells after injury or degenerative processes. The synovial fluid is a dialysate of plasma with the addition of hyaluronic acid secreted by the synthesizing cells of the synovium. The synovium also secretes glycoproteins and other macromolecules which are important in joint lubrication and nutrition.

Glycoproteins appear to be the major lubricant in synovial fluid. Lubricin (a purified glycoprotein) at concentrations as low as 30 μg/ml has lubricating properties similar to those of whole synovial fluid. This glycoprotein gives bovine synovial fluid its boundary lubricating function. The concentrations of hyaluronic acid, sialic acid, and other proteins have no relationship to the lubricating ability of human synovial fluid.

Biomechanical Considerations

Articular cartilage must withstand high loads (2 to 7 times body weight) during normal function. The biphasic model, which considers hyaline cartilage as an interacting mixture of a porous permeable elastic solid (proteoglycan interacting with collagen) and the interstitial fluid, describes the relationship between the mechanical function of cartilage and its biologic structure. Pure shear, when no fluid flow is generated, measures the contribution of the matrix while compressive creep and stress relaxation behavior determine the effects of fluid flow. Collagen determines the tensile and shear stiffness of cartilage as well as imparting strength.

The interaction of water, proteoglycans, and the resulting Donnan osmotic pressure gives cartilage its property of withstanding compression. If the water content of cartilage increases, the compressive modulus decreases and permeability increases. By contrast, if the proteoglycan increases, the modulus increases and the permeability decreases.

One of the major determinants of joint forces is muscle force. The analysis of this contribution is an indeterminate problem. To resolve this, an optimization method is used in which variables are reduced by grouping functionally similar muscles. However, individual muscle efforts must be considered, so that a more even distribution of stresses will be reflected in the final solution. This technique may be used to resolve joint forces more correctly across the humero-ulnar joint during activities such as strenuous weight lifting (calculated at 2 times body weight).

Summary

The complex structures that make up the diarthrodial or synovial joint have distinct anatomic, biochemical, and physiologic characteristics. Articular cartilage is not an inert structure. It responds to its environment by maintaining its cellular and matrix components. Cartilage may be capable of partial reconstitution under certain conditions, although an imbalance of reparative and degradative functions usually results in degeneration. Chondrocytes synthesize matrix components including collagen, proteoglycan, and hyaluronic acid. It is the aggregation of hyaluronic acid molecules that binds water and is entrapped in a network of collagen. This complex matrix structure gives articular cartilage its unique biomechanical property of withstanding large compressive loads for prolonged periods. The synovium and synovial fluid provide the major source of nutrients and lubrication fluid to maintain the normal functional state of the joint. A derangement in any of these highly integrated structures may result in degenerative disease.

Osteoarthritis

This is the most common form of articular cartilage degeneration. The etiopathogenesis is still obscure, but it is not a disease of inevitable occurrence with aging. Osteoarthritis is usually described as primary (idiopathic) or secondary. The central theme in the evolution of osteoarthritis involves material failure, failure of normal chondrocyte response, and extracartilaginous factors. Recent experimental data and clinical observations suggest that each may play a role at various times in the natural course of the disease. Figure 1 summarizes the interplay of these factors.

Experimental Osteoarthritis

The progressive destruction of cartilage seen in the later stages of osteoarthritis appears to have multiple causes. The etiopathogenesis of the early lesions is not well understood. In dogs, unique histologic patterns are seen in different parts of the knee joint after sectioning of the anterior cruciate ligament. Vertical clefts are uniquely present in tibial cartilage; tangential elongated splits are seen in the medial femoral condylar cartilage. This latter lesion is associated with necrosis of the superficial cells. Decreased microhardness and increased water content with unchanged fixed charge density precede these fibrillation changes. The early increased thickness of the femoral articular cartilage is most likely due to both a slight increase in tissue hydration and a real increase in matrix synthesis associated with cell replication in the middle and deep zones.

Conflicting biochemical observations have been obtained with experimental animal models that simulate human osteoarthritis and with *in vitro* cell culture techniques. Increased synthesis of proteoglycan and collagen has been reported. After induction of experimental osteoarthritis by transection of the canine anterior cruciate ligament, the *in vivo* uptake of [^{35}S]sulfate indicative of proteoglycan synthesis by the articular cartilage and menisci was 1.5 to 10 times higher than in control tissue. The medial meniscus and the tibial plateau beneath the meniscus were more stimulated than other areas, suggesting that local mechanical factors were involved. This increase in synthetic activity was confirmed *in vitro* and by ^{35}S autoradiography at 7 to 21 days postoperatively.

The glycosaminoglycan content in the menisci of beagles was decreased early after sectioning of the anterior cruciate ligament; however, by 3 to 18 months it had returned to normal. This was in contrast to the articular cartilage which progressively lost glycosaminoglycans, suggesting that the meniscus may have some capacity to regenerate after this type of joint injury. Early in experimental osteoarthritis,

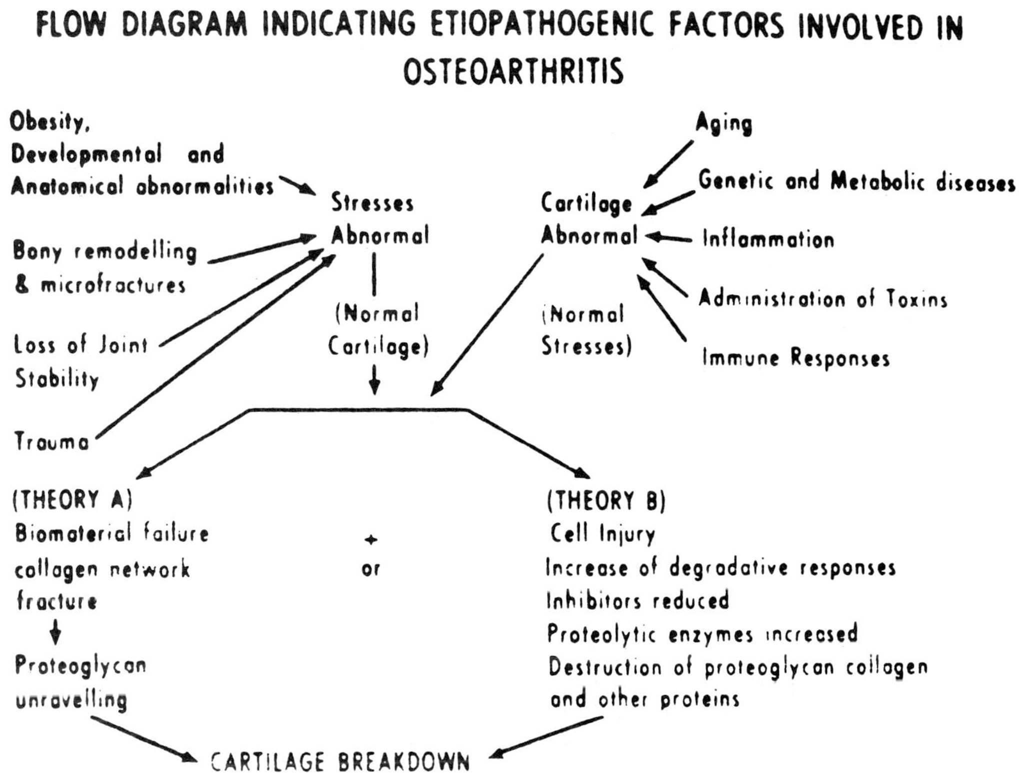

Figure 1

Diagram of etiopathogenic factors involved in osteoarthritis.

the collagen network shows evidence of breakdown and stiffening as assessed by swelling properties and mechanical indentation of experimental femoral condylar cartilage. These changes are seen without the presence of erosions. The proteoglycan aggregates are smaller, and the subunit species increase in amount at about the same time in this experimental model. At longer observation in this laxity model, some regenerative changes due to cell proliferation and increased matrix synthesis are seen.

Proteolytic enzymes active at neutral pH may be responsible for the breakdown of cartilage matrix. Collagenolytic enzyme activity is significantly increased in osteoarthritic cartilage and synovium. The increased activity of the cartilage did not correlate with the synovial collagenolytic activity. The degree of synovial inflammation correlated directly with the cartilage collagenolytic activity. Prednisone inhibited the enzyme activity in cartilage but not in synovium. It appears that stimulating factors rather than collagenolytic enzymes diffuse from the synovium and mediate cartilage breakdown.

Synovial cells disaggregated from osteoarthritic synovium have the capacity *in vitro* of secreting factors that induce the dendritic cells of the tissue to release collagenase and prostaglandin E_2. One of these factors is catabolin which appears to be identical to macrophage interleukin 1. Interleukin 1 may induce the release, from synovial cells and chondrocytes, of factors that break down matrix faster than it can be replaced. Chondrocyte proliferation and vascular and cellular ingrowth from subchondral bone result in remodeling of the joint and osteophyte formation. Growth factors derived from cartilage or bone may modulate uncommitted mesenchymal cells to become chondrocytes in an attempt to heal the degenerative articular cartilage.

Human Osteoarthritis

Articular cartilage from osteoarthritic femoral heads demonstrated overlapping histopathologic patterns from the fibrillated or discolored surfaces, whereas cartilage from osteophytic areas was distinct. *In vitro* incorporation of [^{35}S]sulfate in two peaks of radioactivity on Sepharose CL-2B column chromatography was seen with each of these three tissue types. The average proteoglycan monomer predominated from discolored, fibrillated, and osteophytic cartilages in peak I. The hydrodynamic size of the synthetic proteoglycan monomer was the same for discolored, fibrillated, and osteophytic samples. The proteoglycan monomer isolated from peak II showed similar percentages in the discolored and fibrillated tissue, whereas the proteoglycan monomer content was reduced significantly in the osteophytic tissue. In addition, the endogenous proteoglycans extracted from each cartilage area were generally of a smaller hydrodynamic size than newly synthesized proteoglycan monomer. The glycosaminoglycans were predominantly chondroitin 6-sulfate. These findings indicate that discolored and fibrillated cartilage tissue types from defined topographic areas of human osteoarthritic femoral heads have neither unique histopathologic nor synthetic or endogenous proteoglycan characteristics. By contrast, osteophytic cartilage appeared more distinct histopathologically than either discolored or fibrillated osteoarthritic cartilage but synthesized proteoglycan monomer with hydrodynamic size similar to that of the other cartilage tissue types.

When grown as a *suspension culture* in the presence of [^{35}S]sulfate, osteoarthritic chondrocytes isolated from osteoarthritic femoral heads incorporated isotope at a rate 3 to 4 times greater than normal chondrocytes did. The rate of incorporation was increased with moderate histologic gradings (grades 4–8) whereas chondrocytes isolated from mild grades (grades 0–3) or more advanced stages (grades 9–13) of the disease showed decreased levels of incorporation compared to normal. A strong correlation was seen between increasing histopathologic score and decreasing size of proteoglycan monomer.

Osteoarthritis articular cartilage *organ cultures* demonstrate a 13-fold increase in the rate of incorporation of radioactive sulfate; there is a small but statistically significant increase in incorporation of amino sugars and amino acid into the purified proteoglycan subunit compared to normal cartilage. Additionally, hyaluronate is synthesized more rapidly in the osteoarthritic cartilage compared to normal and more rapidly than the proteoglycan subunit. There is a metabolic heterogeneity in cartilage from osteoarthritic joints which raises the question as to the nature of the hyaluronate being synthesized; *in vivo* aggregating ability of osteoarthritic articular cartilage is poorer than that of normal cartilage.

In one study, cartilage from human knees with osteoarthritis was sampled from three sites on the tibial plateau—the center of the osteoarthritis lesion, the edge of the lesion, and a remote site—and graded histologically. Collagenolytic activity was highest in the center of the lesions, declining to 2.4% in remote sites and 1.4% in controls. Moderately severe disease (grades 6–9) had the highest collagenolytic activity. Half of the metal-dependent collagenolytic activity was in the latent form (activated by aminophenol/mercuric acetate). This increased enzyme activity provides a mechanism for the loss of collagen in osteoarthritis which may be additive to mechanical wear.

Osteoarthritic human articular cartilage contains significant titers of collagen antibody most of the time. Similar results are seen with meniscal extracts. These collagen antibodies may play a pathogenic role in osteoarthritis by interacting directly with the chondrocyte and inducing functional alterations that lead to cell death.

Articular cartilage from osteoarthritic knees that was intact by visual inspection demonstrated no apparent chemical abnormalities compared with normal controls in regard to water content, swelling capacity, fixed-charge density, and content of extractable proteoglycans. When the cartilage surface was not intact, the biochemical changes correlated linearly with the degree of fibrillation. Surface fibrillated specimens had a higher water content in the surface layer but no change in the content or rate of glycosaminoglycan synthesis. Superficial slices demonstrated swelling in solution. Additionally, the extracted proteoglycans showed the same capacity to aggregate as did proteoglycan from the intact cartilage of normal joints. Deeply fibrillated cartilage showed a significant loss of glycosaminoglycans as well as a decreased rate of synthesis of proteoglycans, with increased hydration and ability to swell. The histologic features suggested that the cellular changes in osteoarthritic cartilage occur only after serious damage to the collagen network and a significant depletion of proteoglycans from the matrix.

Differential interference contrast microscopy demonstrated that degenerative tissue from osteoarthritic human femoral heads had a distinct radial fibrous structure in the middle and deep zones compared with normal cartilage which exhibited a "ground glass" type of amorphous structure largely free of a fibrous texture. These fibrous structures appeared as discrete islands or as large zones between cell clusters. The fibrous arrays exhibited a wave-like structure. At a microcompressive stress of only 35 g/mm^2, the aligned fibrous structure in the middle zone collapsed to create a wave pattern immediately adjacent to the relatively undeformed normal-appearing matrix. Propagation of a radial tear through the middle and deep layers of degenerative cartilage required loads significantly less than those in normal tissue. This radial notch deformed entire lacunae, so that occasionally they were released from their surrounding matrix. No direct advancement of a transverse rupture was possible in normal articular cartilage, and any rupture initiated was always associated with an immediate radial deflection down into the deeper zone or up toward the articular surface. Transverse notch propagation in degenerative cartilage was possible only through prominent radial arrays of fibers and in regions of matrix exhibiting no obvious radial texture. The loads required to propagate the transverse notch were always less than those required to initiate the primary radial notch in the degenerative matrix. These differences between osteoarthritic and normal cartilage emphasize a fundamental structural breakdown in the load-bearing function of the tissue.

Summary

Table 1 summarizes the generally accepted biochemical and metabolic changes seen in osteoarthritis. It is important to understand that this common disease is truly complex and most likely may have many different initiating events but common ultimate pathways. Briefly, whether cartilage begins as entirely normal or abnormal as a result of a specific insult, either a material failure of the collagen network occurs or chondrocyte damage with an increase of enzymatic activity and concomitant reduction of inhibitors ensues. The sequence that follows appears to be an

Table 1. Summary of Biochemical Changes in Human and Experimental Osteoarthritis

	Early	Late
DNA content (cell count)	Incr.	Decr.
Water content	Incr. (retention incr.)	Incr.
Proteoglycan concentration	Decr. (synthesis incr.)	Decr. (synthesis decr.)
Collagen	Relative concentration and type unchanged (synthesis incr.)	Decr.
Degradative enzymes		
Cathepsin D	Incr.	Incr.
Acid phosphatase	Incr.	Incr.
Neutral proteoglycanase	Incr.	Incr.
Collagenase	Incr.	Incr.

unravelling of proteoglycans with destruction of the complex interaction of collagen and proteoglycan. These events lead to cartilage breakdown and the pathologic osteoarthritis state. Ultimately, from an understanding of the pathophysiology of osteoarthritis, specific therapeutic modalities may be developed to prevent progression of the disease.

Etiology of Rheumatoid Arthritis

Immunohistologic analysis of diseased synovium from patients with rheumatoid arthritis has demonstrated a variety of abnormalities that parallel various stages of a cell-mediated or delayed type immune response. Many of the infiltrating mononuclear cells in synovium are T cells. It appears that synovial sites are rich in HLA-DR-bearing cells, both in the lining layer and in the nodular aggregates of lymphocytes. These T cells proliferate and secrete lymphokines into their environment, which initiate and augment the inflammatory response. Additionally, the lymphokines stimulate macrophages to increase phagocytic activity and to secrete biologically active mediators of inflammation. These monokines also contribute to the recruitment and activation of inflammatory cells. Additionally, lymphokines can stimulate macrophages to release enzymatic mediators such as plasminogen and collagenase which further contribute to the tissue damage and vascular effects associated with a synovitis.

The most effective therapies appear to affect either mononuclear cell function or the rates of production or deletion of these cells. T-helper cells which infiltrate the synovium are able to exchange information and stimulate B cells which, in the process of polyclonal proliferation, produce antibodies. These antibodies are of a specific IgG subtype and appear directed to connective tissue components. Furthermore, immune complexes are important in sustaining the inflammatory response in the synovium.

Radioimmunoassay studies of extracts from articular cartilage specimens from 16 patients with rheumatoid arthritis demonstrated 37 times more IgM and 13 times more IgG than in normal cartilage extracts. IgM rheumatoid factor was found in 13 of 16 rheumatoid patients but in none of 6 normal controls. IgG rheumatoid factor was detected in four of seven seropositive rheumatoid articular cartilage specimens. More than 60% of the rheumatoid cartilage extracts were positive for native and denatured anti-collagen-II antibodies. These findings suggest that rheumatoid cartilage contains autoantibodies that play an important role in cartilage damage.

The destructive processes of rheumatoid arthritis well may be the expression of a genetically controlled host immune response to a stimulus such as an infectious agent or products derived from an infectious agent, constituents of synovial or connective tissue, or a combination of these. The recent demonstration that a spirochete is the etiologic agent of Lyme disease, a condition that resembles rheumatoid arthritis, suggests that infectious agents must still be considered as possible etiopathologic mediators of the inflammatory process in rheumatoid arthritis.

It appears that the principal immunogenetic association in rheumatoid arthritis is the HLA-Dw4 locus determined by the mixed lymphocyte reaction or its related HLA-DR-4 allotype on lymphocytes. Although there is a strong association with rheumatoid arthritis, it is not as strong a relationship as seen with the HLA-B27 locus with ankylosing spondylitis. For example, control subjects in a large study had a frequency of the HLA-Dw4 locus of 25%, compared with a frequency of 52% in patients with seropositive rheumatoid arthritis. There was no relationship with seronegative rheumatoid arthritis, which suggests that this may in fact be a different disease. Generally, the patient with more severe classic type rheumatoid arthritis has the DR-4 locus more than 80% of the time. RANA, a rheumatoid arthritis nuclear antigen, is induced in lymphoblastoid cell lines infected with the Epstein-Barr virus. A higher percentage of patients with severe seropositive rheumatoid arthritis have antibodies to RANA in their serum compared with nonrheumatoid patients. However, anti-RANA is not specific to the disease; it occurs in a significant number of young persons with infectious mononucleosis.

Of the cells found in synovial fluid from patients with rheumatoid arthritis, 90% are neutrophils. These neutrophils ingest (by endocytosis), *in vitro* and *in vivo,* the immune complexes and complement components that are present in rheumatoid arthritis. Subsequent release of neutrophilic lysosomal enzymes and other mediators of inflammation accounts in part for the rheumatoid synovitis. These mediators also provoke tissue injury and the generation of reactive oxygen species which may enhance the inflammatory response. Neutrophils also produce arachidonic analogs such as leukotriene B_4. This acts as a potent calcium ionophore which activates additional neutrophils.

Specific histochemical and ultrastructural evaluation of the cartilage-pannus junction demonstrated macrophages and fibroblasts as the majority cell types in 25 of 49 rheumatoid joints. Additionally, mast cells, polymorphonuclear leukocytes, dendritic cells, or plasma cells were also present. Small blood vessels occasionally were observed at this junction, but they rarely penetrated the cartilage matrix. No lymphocytes were observed close to the cartilage, but these cells were conspicuous in the pannus tissue remote from the junction.

The presence of macrophages as a predominant cell type and the presence of collagenase markers within the cell and subsequent collagenolysis of the eroded bone matrix suggest that these cells may be responsible for a major portion of the bone erosion. Also, osteoclasts with ruffled borders containing free bone crystals which are in close contact with the bone appear to be stimulated by the rheumatoid synovium. Periarticular bone resorption appears to depend upon the interaction of both macrophage and osteoclast. An additional source of collagenase is the dendritic cells from synovia which secrete this enzyme as well as prostaglandins. These cells later are induced to produce more of these mediators by monokines secreted by macrophages.

Macrophages and neutrophils secrete lysosomal enzymes such as neutral proteases, cathepsin G, and elastase which are capable of degrading proteoglycan and have been detected in the superficial layers of articular cartilage from patients with rheumatoid arthritis. In addition, proteoglycan synthesis in cultured chondrocytes is inhibited as a result of their interaction with these neutrophilic enzymes. Although enzymatic markers have been found at the pannus-cartilage junction, two important enzyme inhibitors, α_2-macroglobulin and α_1-antitrypsin, have been demonstrated at this interface. These enzyme inhibitors were found in synovial cells of the deeper layer of pannus. Additionally, inhibitor markers were found in the vicinity of superficial chondrocytes. The fact that synovial tissue and possibly chondrocytes may produce inhibitors of enzymatic mediators may have important implications with regard to protective mechanisms within joints affected by rheumatoid arthritis.

Summary

Although the etiology of rheumatoid arthritis remains obscure, certain concepts of a reasonable sequence of events have evolved. The destructive processes appear to be a genetically controlled host immune response to some stimulus—e.g., infectious agents or constituents of connective tissue. The HLA-Dw4 locus is more frequently associated with severe seropositive rheumatoid arthritis. The immune response most closely resembles a delayed type immune reaction with T cells predominating. The destructive cascade includes lymphokines and other immune mediators of inflammation which are directed toward connective tissue components. Newer therapeutic modalities that have been successful in ameliorating the manifestations of rheumatoid arthritis have been based on knowledge of these pathophysiologic events.

Other Inflammatory Arthropathies

Juvenile Rheumatoid Arthritis

Three major types of juvenile rheumatoid arthritis have been identified on the basis of the predominant clinical manifestations that occur within the first 6 months of the disease: systemic, polyarticular, and pauciarticular. Table 2 summarizes the differential features of these clinical entities.

Immune complexes containing both the 19S IgM and IgG have been isolated from serum and synovial fluid from patients with juvenile rheumatoid arthritis. These patients were negative for rheumatoid factor, indicating the ineffectiveness of this serologic test for diagnostic confirmation. HLA typing of 200 patients with juvenile types of arthritis demonstrated interesting findings: 1. Boys with onset after 9 years of age were predominantly B27 positive; CW-1 and CW-2 also were increased. 2. Children with polyarthritis and rheumatoid factor showed an increase in the incidence of the DR-4 locus. 3. Patients with systemic onset juvenile rheumatoid arthritis had an association with DR-2. 4. Pauciarticular disease with or without iritis was associated with a 2 times greater incidence of A2, DR-5, and DR-w8 loci. 5. Patients with polyarticular onset and without rheumatoid factor also showed a strong association with DR-5 and DR-w8 but not with A2. 6. None of the groups showed an increase in Bw35. 7. A group of patients with monoarticular onset and subsequent conversion to polyarticular disease did not show an association with the HLA antigens tested. These findings may increase our diagnostic abilities and help to identify markers of specific subsets of this disease.

High-dose aspirin therapy is usually sufficient to control fever and to reduce joint inflammation in the majority of patients. Some patients with polyarthritis may require the addition of gold or other remissive agents. Asymptomatic ocular involvement is a common complication in the pauciarticular type of juvenile rheumatoid arthritis and therefore requires frequent ophthalmologic examination and usually corticosteroid therapy; management should be optimistic because a majority of the patients do well, usually entering remission after 1 or 2 years.

Ankylosing Spondylitis

There is evidence of heterogeneity in the clinical presentation of patients with ankylosing spondylitis. There are different subgroups of patients who demonstrate the HLA-B27 antigen but do not develop ankylosed spines. However, it appears that one-gene cross-tolerance is a viable etiologic hypothesis and that the genetically determined clinical patterns are triggered by different environmental clues, as yet undetermined. Patients with acute anterior uveitis who are HLA-B27 positive with only minor musculoskeletal complaints may represent only a monosymptomatic ankylosing spondylitis syndrome. Many of these patients ultimately develop sacroiliitis or other manifestations of ankylosing spondylitis. However, it is unnecessary to require radiographic evidence of bilateral sacroiliitis as the central feature for making the diagnosis of this disease.

Gout

Monosodium urate crystals have been shown to activate numerous cellular and humoral inflammatory mediator systems *in vitro.* The products of urate-neutrophil interactions are lysosomal proteases, crystal chemotactic factor, prostaglandins, leukotriene B_4, and oxygen radicals. Urate crystals also activate synoviocytes, mononuclear phagocytes, platelets, the classic complement pathway, and the Hageman factor contact system. The therapeutic agents that inhibit acute gouty inflammation inhibit phagocytosis. Colchicine suppresses the production of crystal chemotactic factor by neutrophils without affecting phagocytic de-

Table 2. Clinical Features of Juvenile Rheumatoid Arthritis

Type	Incidence, %	RF and ANA*	Sex	Joints, no.	Systemic symptoms
Pauciarticular	30	Usually negative	F > M	<4	Usually none except iridocyclitis in 20%
Polyarticular	50	Both can be positive, 15–20%	F > M	>4 About 35% have chronic joint problems	Can present with rash, iridocyclitis; differential diagnosis, rheumatic fever
Systemic (febrile form)	20	Unusual for either to be positive but can occur	F = M	Multiple; warm & swollen; cervical spine involvement	Usually present with fever, rash, high leukocyte count, & liver/spleen enlargement

*RF, rheumatoid factor; ANA; antinuclear antibody.

granulation. Indomethacin and phenylbutazone diminish phagocytosis of crystals *in vitro* and also act via inhibition of the cyclooxygenase-dependent generation of arachidonate metabolites from cells interacting with urate crystals.

The problem of the absence of inflammation, even in the presence of urate crystals, remains unsolved. However, recent evidence suggests that there is an inhibitory function of polypeptides *in vitro* to inhibit inflammatory response to urate crystals. The binding of these plasma glycoproteins to urate crystals appears to be a direct response and depends on a chemical interaction. The sequence begins with protein coating of urate crystals, which is permissive at first for neutrophil responses but later suppresses the urate-neutrophil interaction. This later event occurs when low density lipoproteins are present and are adsorbed to crystals. Recent electron microscopy studies demonstrate an abundant amorphous coat on urate crystals in asymptomatic gouty patients. This effect of low density lipoproteins on the crystal-neutrophil interaction may be important in other responses of connective tissue cells to inflammatory mediators.

Chondrocalcinosis

Chondrocalcinosis is a multifactorial syndrome in which several metabolic and physicochemical factors interact to produce calcium pyrophosphate dihydrate crystals. The possible mechanisms associated with deposition of these crystals are an inherited form in which there usually is decreased action of inhibitors of crystallization, aging with possibly disturbed pyrophosphate metabolism, and physical damage to chondrocytes. Additionally, with aging, nucleating agents may be released or decreased inhibitory activity could result with increased cartilage permeation of calcium and pyrophosphate. Joint diseases such as osteoarthritis or ochronosis may produce an environment that promotes transformation to more insoluble forms. Metabolic disorders such as hyperparathyroidism, hypothyroidism, and hemachromatosis result in increased extracellular concentrations of calcium or pyrophosphate, or both, due to increased adenylate cyclase activity as well as metabolic changes in cartilage. Other associations with hypertension, renal insufficiency, Paget's disease, and diabetes have been suggested and may be related to metabolic alterations in cartilage or age-related changes. It is important to note that crystal deposition can occur in the elderly in the absence of inflammation. Figure 2 demonstrates the amplification-loop hypothesis which predisposes to crystal deposition and the acceleration of joint damage by mechanical or inflammatory pathways.

The recent clinical use of intra-articular injection of yttrium-90 as a colloidal silicate in cases of chronic pyrophosphate arthropathy provided significant amelioration of the disease, thereby suggesting a synovial mediation of the inflammatory component. However, pyrophosphate arthropathy is complex and there is great diversity in the clinical syndromes associated with intra-articular deposition of calcium pyrophosphate dihydrate crystals.

Summary

Many of the nonrheumatoid inflammatory spondyloarthropathies appear to be genetically controlled and the result of mechanisms triggered by environmental stimuli. Examples of this are the high incidence of the HLA-B27 locus with ankylosing spondylitis and the relationship of the DR-4 locus with polyarthritis and rheumatoid factor in children. The crystal arthropathies (gout and chondrocalcinosis) appear to manifest their symptoms as a result of macrophage ingestion of urate or calcium pyrophosphate dihydrate crystals and subsequent release of inflammatory mediators. Less frequently encountered crystalline arthropathies such as hydroxyapatite deposition disease appear to manifest this symptom through a similar mechanism.

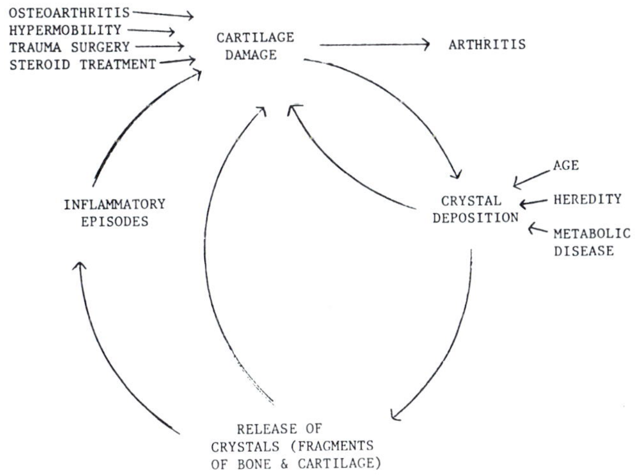

Figure 2

Diagram of the amplification-loop hypothesis which predisposes to crystal deposition.

Infectious Arthritis

In synovial membranes sequentially sampled from animals with experimentally induced bacterial arthritis, bacteria are detectable throughout the superficial synovium within 2 hours after the inoculum is introduced. Within 48 hours, a significant polymorphonuclear leukocyte infiltration of the synovium occurs with concomitant vascular congestion and proliferation of lining cells. If the host's defenses are adequate, the initial joint infection will be eradicated and only transient arthralgias will result. By 1 week after the infection, a chronic proliferation of synovial lining cells occurs with mononuclear cell infiltration and the development of microabscesses. The inflammation in septic arthritis is due not only to the products elaborated by the viable microorganisms but also to the immune response generated by the host. The subsequent destruction of cartilage and bone results from the release of proteolytic enzymes from leukocytes as well as necrosis by direct pressure and lack of nutrition. Host-microbe interactions are important in understanding why bacterial arthritis develops in some patients whereas most bacteremias are self-limited. The risk factors include defects in phagocytic functions with complement deficiencies, impaired host defense mechanisms (as in cancer or chronic use of immunosuppressive drugs or glucocorticosteroids), and direct penetration as well as joint damage secondary to arthritis or prosthetic joint surgery.

The destructive processes are due to the direct attack by microorganisms and also in part to interaction between the immune components of the host and fragments of the microorganism. An excellent example of this is the events leading to Lyme arthritis, the result of a tick-borne spirochete infection. The initial inflammation is the response of acute host defense mechanisms to direct infection by the microorganism. However, joint inflammation with chronic arthritis may result and is secondary to the formation of immune complexes and cryoglobulins in the synovial fluid. It is apparent that the chronicity of the inflammation is a result of the chronic immune response by the host. Penicillin has been an effective therapeutic agent, either at the onset of the disease or in the later stages.

The most common non-gonococcal bacterial arthritis in adults continues to be caused by *Staphylococcus aureus* or *Streptococcus* sp. However, disseminated gonococcal infection is still the most common cause of bacterial arthritis seen in major urban medical centers. The initial presentation of disseminated gonococcal infection is a polyarthritis in 50% of patients; however, small skin papules on the trunk or extremities are very common. Pathologic examination indicates that these are an area of erythema and microinfarction of the skin. It is the hematogenous phase that is associated with the migratory polyarthritis. The diagnosis of septic arthritis or gonococcal arthritis is based on demonstration of microorganisms in the synovial fluid by culture or by Gram stain. Although many other tests are available, these are the only definitive diagnostic tests. The following findings are highly suggestive of a bacterial arthritis: positive culture and Gram stain, leukocyte count markedly greater than 100,000/μl, low glucose concentration in synovial fluid compared with blood, and positive cultures of blood and material from other sites of infection. Helpful, but not definitive, findings are peripheral blood leukocytosis, increased erythrocyte sedimentation rate, positive scans, and appropriate responses to antibiotics. Recent evidence suggests that increased lactate in synovial fluid may help in the diagnosis of infectious arthritis although a modest increase can be seen in noninfectious inflammatory arthropathy such as rheumatoid arthritis.

There is a direct correlation between outcome and the duration of symptoms before diagnosis and treatment. When treatment was instituted within the first 3 to 4 days, more than 95% of the patients recovered completely; when treatment was delayed 1 week or longer, the majority of patients generally had a poor outcome.

Treatment of Arthritis

Nonsurgical

Fifty-three knees in 44 patients with severe rheumatoid arthritis were treated by intra-articular instillation of dysprosium-165 coupled with ferric hydroxide macroaggregate. There was only a 0.3% leakage of the injected dose, which corresponds to a total body dose of 0.4 rad, the equivalent of a battery of low back radiographs. Eighty percent of the treated knees demonstrated clinical improvement, with reduction of the effusion for as long as 1 year after treatment. There was no correlation between the clinical improvement and radiographic evidence of cartilage and bone destruction. However, there was a direct correlation between the pretreatment radiographic stage and the response to treatment; patients in stages I and II had an excellent response after 1 year of follow-up. There was also a correlation between clinical improvement and the results of technetium-99m flow scintigraphy. Scintigraphic improvement was based qualitatively on a decrease of more than 10% in the index ratio of uptake in the treated knee relative to the untreated knee. Radiochemical synovectomy appears to be an effective means of decreasing inflammation, effusion, and pain in patients with rheumatoid arthritis. Although the long-term results cannot be predicted, it appears that radiation synovectomy is most effective in the early stage of the disease, before extensive destruction of cartilage and bone.

The goal of therapy in rheumatoid arthritis is to prevent disability. Although anti-inflammatory drugs such as nonsteroidal compounds are effective in suppressing the proliferative component of the disease, they are ineffective in modifying the underlying immunologic abnormalities. Gold and D-penicillamine specifically act by suppressing the early factors of the immune response. These include antigen processing by macrophages and T lymphocytes, which is so important in the disease cascade. Glucocorticoids appear to function by inhibiting synthesis of proteases and prostaglandins by synovial cells, although multiple other effects on cell function may result in toxicity rather than effectiveness in therapy. Retinoid compounds may be useful in that they inhibit collagenase production by rheumatoid synovial cells without interfering with connective tissue components and therefore may retard the development and potency of the proliferative synovitis of rheumatoid arthritis.

Auranofin, an orally active gold compound, was equally as effective as parenteral gold therapy in a majority of studies when clinical symptoms of recurrent effusion, cartilage destruction, and erosive changes were evaluated. Adverse reactions and withdrawal rates were 2 to 3 times greater with parenteral gold therapy than with auranofin. The nature of the side effects from the two treatments was noticeably different—lower bowel symptoms prevalent with auranofin and mucocutaneous lesions present with parenteral gold. Neither demonstrated significant laboratory index changes, although proteinuria was the usual reason for withdrawal of either drug.

Considerable evidence suggests that T lymphocytes are critical in provoking synovial inflammation in rheumatoid arthritis. Because of this background, lymphocyte depletion (lymphapheresis) has been reported to be temporarily effective in patients with severe rheumatoid arthritis. Blood mononuclear cells were less responsive to mitogens *in vitro* after therapeutic trials of this technique. Lymphoplasmapheresis (plasma exchange in combination with lymphapheresis) was associated with both clinical improvement in rheumatoid arthritis and enhanced response to mitogen. Two trials to test the feasibility of total lymphoid irradiation were associated with some evidence of clinical improvement in patients who were refractory to standard therapeutic approaches. Although there were objective indications of a biologic response to irradiation in these studies, controlled trials were not performed to define the anti-inflammatory effect and its ultimate effect on the natural course of rheumatoid arthritis.

Monoclonal anti-T-cell antibody, used previously to evaluate T-cell subpopulations in rheumatoid arthritis, recently has been used in immunosuppressive therapy for patients with unremitting rheumatoid arthritis.

Endogenous mechanisms that appear to regulate cellular immunity may be useful avenues for treatment. An example of this is the C3a component of the complement cascade, which can inhibit lymphokine production by cultured human blood mononuclear cells. The isolation of this component and the development of a synthetic octapeptide that retains its inhibitory properties remain possibilities for use in treatment. Animal experiments indicate that the use of antigen-specific immunosuppressive techniques, such as anti-idiotypic and suppressive factor pathways, may inhibit clinically relevant effector cells in rheumatoid arthritis. Thymic hormones such as thymopoietin are being evaluated for treatment of severe rheumatoid arthritis, and early results are encouraging.

Nonsteroidal anti-inflammatory drugs are the mainstay of drug therapy in osteoarthritis. Although aspirin is the most cost-effective at a dosage of 3.9 g/day, few patients can tolerate such high doses, and, in one study, 40% of patients treated with aspirin developed gastric erosions and 17% had gastric ulcers. Allergic reactions and renal dysfunction also are seen. The newer nonsteroidal anti-inflammatory drugs such as Piroxicam, Naproxen, and Sulindac provide reasonable pain relief and some degree of anti-inflammatory action. Unfortunately, they still cause gastrointestinal side effects, and noncompliance has been estimated at between 25% and 50% in large series of patients. The mode of action of these drugs is through suppression of prostaglandin synthesis; however, some experimental studies suggest that some of these drugs may accelerate cartilage destruction. Aspirin has been shown to hasten cartilage degeneration in the knees of immobilized dogs.

The one class of drugs that is capable of reversing the degenerative process is known as chondroprotective. Arteparon (a glycosaminoglycan polysulfate) and Rumalon (a glycosaminoglycan sulfate peptide and pentosan polysulfate) are drugs in this class. Arteparon has been shown in some experimental studies to inhibit enzymatic degradation of cartilage. Rumalon appears to have a stimulatory effect on proteoglycan synthesis. The former compound has been shown to protect against progressive articular cartilage damage in experimentally induced osteoarthritis. A few clinical studies utilizing both Rumalon and Arteparon in open, noncontrolled circumstances have suggested that both of these compounds have some ameliorating effect.

Summary Newer modalities of nonoperative treatment of rheumatoid arthritis are radiation synovectomy with dysprosium-165, specific remissive agents (e.g., gold, D-penicillamine), modalities that deplete the T lymphocytes (e.g., lymphapheresis), and immunosuppressive agents (e.g., monoclonal anti-T-cell antibody). Nonsteroidal anti-inflammatory drugs which usually act through suppression of prostaglandin synthesis are the mainstay of drug treatment in osteoarthritis. Experimental drugs known as chondroprotective agents (e.g., Arteparon) have potential in reversing the degenerative process in osteoarthritis.

Surgical

In the treatment of osteoarthritis, osteotomies redirect the articular surface so that those portions of cartilage that are relatively well preserved are transposed to articular regions subject to greatest loads. Secondary deformities are corrected to achieve more physiologic load distribution. Pressures are decreased within the joint, and physiologic conditions are restored so that articular cartilage can respond to forces in a more normal fashion. Additionally, there are biologic effects of juxta-articular osteotomy. The venous drainage is restored and, simultaneously, the increased intraosseous pressure seen in osteoarthritis is reduced. The intraosseous oxygen pressure is increased, which reflects return of the intraosseous blood supply to normal. There appears to be amelioration of the resting pain which may persist for years. Evidence suggests that pain-conducting fibers are interrupted, which may have a direct influence on venous drainage of the joint. These biologic effects of osteotomy may be as important as the purely mechanical ones.

Arthroscopic debridement has become a widespread modality of operative intervention in early osteoarthritis. Considerable laboratory data indicate that, in the best circumstances, articular cartilage repairs with fibrocartilage which ultimately degenerates. However, some preliminary studies in rabbits suggest that, if subjected to constant passive motion, full-thickness hyaline cartilage defects heal with a functional hyaline cartilage; its stability is still unknown. It would appear, therefore, that a functional articular cartilage does not form after arthroscopic debridement or abrasion chondroplasty. In one study of 275 arthroscopic debridements followed for 13 months to 7 years, results were good in 76% and fair or poor in 24%. The good results must be attributed to the removal of mechanical irritants such as crystals, unstable cartilage lesions, or loose bodies. The use of continuous fluid irrigation helps to remove many of these degradative products free within the joint, which are known to perpetuate the degenerative processes. The poorer outcomes were seen in patients with extensive degenerative changes associated with angular deformities. Also, the more active patients tend to worsen with longer follow-up. Although these appear to be impressive results, they should be viewed with caution because the follow-up is short.

Thirty six knee joints with rheumatoid synovitis were evaluated, 2 to 39 months after surgical synovectomy, by arthroscopic techniques that included synovial biopsy and synovial fluid collection. Histologic evidence of synovitis at the time of synovectomy was confirmed in these knees. Regenerated synovial tissue was less permeable to serum proteins and contained lower activities of lysosomal enzymes. The joint fluid contained a decreased number of leukocytes; however, the lysosomal enzyme activity was only slightly lowered and there was no change in the amount of components C3 and C4 of the complement pathway. Of the enzyme activity assayed in the synovial fluid, acid protease cathepsin-D had the greatest decrease. Subjective scores of the joint symptoms improved in almost all cases but with little correlation with objective findings of enzymatic activity or histologic evidence of inflammation.

In 47 cases of wrist synovectomy with resection of the distal ulna performed for severe rheumatoid arthritis, followed for a mean of 33 months, pain relief was complete in 31 and moderate in 8. Pain was unchanged in eight. Five patients had recurrent synovitis and progression of the disease. The range of motion in both supination and pronation and volar flexion and dorsiflexion was significantly improved as was the subjective assessment of function. Radiographic findings of loss of cartilage space and erosions were not modified and progressed in 41 of these cases. Therefore, it appears that, when conservative medical treatment has been utilized for a minimum of 6 months without successful results, wrist synovectomy and distal ulnar resection is an appropriate therapeutic approach.

Eighty-six percent of patients with rheumatoid arthritis were clinically improved after total hip arthroplasty at a mean follow-up of 7 years after the operation. Incidence of mechanical loosening was inversely related to the functional activities of the patient. Revision of the femoral components was required in 1.6% of the patients; no revision was performed for acetabular loosening. The infection rate was 2.6%, which was almost 2 times that in osteoarthritis patients. Radiographic analysis demonstrated a high incidence of femoral component migration and acetabular component lucent lines which did not correlate with the clinical function of these patients but suggested an inferior ultimate result.

One hundred consecutive knees in 75 patients were followed for a mean of 6.6 years after total knee arthroplasty (total condylar prosthesis) for treatment of either osteoarthritis or osteonecrosis. Of these knees, 64 were rated as excellent, 27 as good, 2 as fair, and 7 as failures. The tibial components demonstrated some evidence of radiolucency in 41% of the cases although, with the exception of two loose components, there were no complete radiolucent lines. The majority of these lucencies were seen in the first postoperative year and there was no further change in more than 80% of the patients. There was no gross evidence of wear of the polyethylene tibial component. Failures were usually a result of errors in surgical technique. This original total condylar prosthesis appears to be useful for reconstruction of the osteoarthritic or osteonecrotic knee with satisfactory long-term results.

The results of 798 total knee arthroplasties for rheumatoid arthritis at one institution, with a minimum of 2 years of follow-up, were evaluated. During recent years there has been an increase in the good and excellent results, from 67% to 92%, and revision rates declined. Failures included revision for loosening in 1.3% of the knees, patellofemoral pain in 1.8%, and infection in 0.4%. In this relatively short follow-up, the failure rate was acceptably low and radiolucent lines indicative of potential later failure appeared to be decreasing with improved technical expertise.

Porous-coated implants provide an effective means for implant fixation by bony tissue ingrowth. *In vivo* tests have demonstrated the need for initial implant stability and close apposition of the prosthesis to bone to achieve bony ingrowth. Animal studies indicate an optimal pore size range of 50 to 400 μm. When these requirements are met in total hip arthroplasty, implants appear to function well (Fig. 3). Twenty-six patients with a porous hip prosthesis were followed for 2 to 5 years after operation. The mean Harris hip rating for these patients improved and was equivalent to that in a simultaneous experience using cemented prostheses. Radiographic evaluation indicated a firmly fixed prosthetic device. Radiopaque lines were seen in a third of the patients, at follow-up of 2 years or more, indicating micromotion. No abnormal bone remodeling was seen, so appropriate stress transfer was present. There was no radiographic evidence of bone resorption due to femoral stress shielding by a high-modulus implant with a porous surface.

Total knee arthroplasty has been performed with an implant with a porous coating in the uncemented mode. At follow-up at least 2 years after implantation, there were no clinical interface failures. Radiographs showed that an intimate contact between bone and prosthesis was maintained.

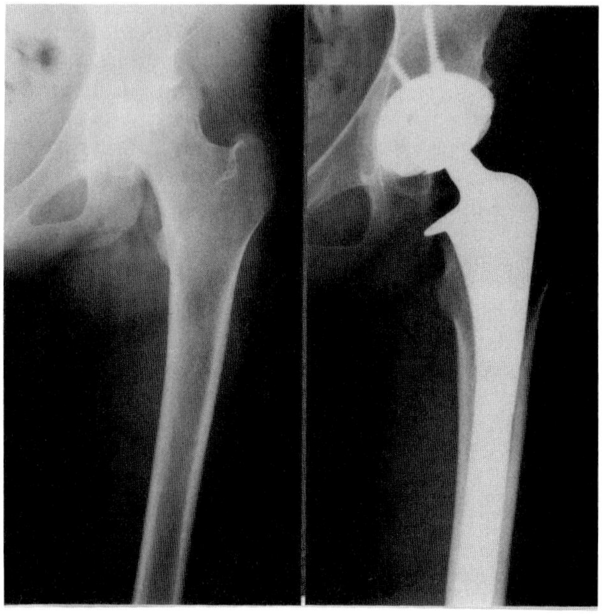

Figure 3

Pre- and postoperative radiographs of the hip in a 47-year-old patient with osteonecrosis, demonstrating the excellent hip reconstruction with an uncemented prosthesis.

Biologic Replacement

Osteochondral autografts of femoral condyles in dogs were frozen at a rate of 2°C per minute and cryoprotected with either glycerol or dimethyl sulfoxide after harvesting; no differences after transplantation were found with either cryoprotective agent. Cartilage survived 10 days of hypothermic storage and tissue culture before transplantation. Allografts were frozen in glycerol with cooling at a rate of 1°C per minute. Although up to 4 months after transplantation there was gross evidence of smooth and shiny cartilage, microscopically there was loss of chondrocytes throughout the cartilage plate and conversion of hyaline cartilage to fibrocartilage. No chronic inflammatory reaction was seen, and the subchondral bone was healed by 4 months. Additionally, bone marrow spaces were filled with normal bone marrow cells from the host.

Fresh osteochondral allografts that had been stored in Ringer's lactate solution at 4°C for 24 hours were transplanted into 100 patients with idiopathic osteoarthritis, post-traumatic arthritis, or osteonecrosis. After a mean follow-up of 3.8 years, successful results were seen in 85% of patients treated because of traumatic injury. However, overall results for patients with osteoarthritis or osteonecrosis were not encouraging. Recovered specimens showed necrotic bone and bone marrow; necrosis appeared to be independent of the length of time that the graft was in place. Articular cartilage showed degenerative changes ranging from fibrillation to complete erosion. In some grafts, pannus formation with resorption of cartilage was also present. There was no histologic evidence of immunologic rejection.

Twenty-five fresh osteochondral allografts were used to treat osteonecrosis of the femoral head with a follow-up of 9 to 63 months after transplantation. The allograft was obtained under sterile conditions and stored at 4°C in Ringer's solution containing antibiotics. The solution was changed every 24 hours under sterile conditions. There was an overall success rate of 68%, and most of the failures were in patients receiving systemic steroid therapy. In non-steroid-treated patients with osteonecrosis, there was an 80% rate of success.

These studies suggest a continued need for studies of alternative methods for treating articular cartilage degeneration.

Annotated Bibliography

Normal Joint Physiology

Armstrong, C.G., and Mow, V.C.: The mechanical properties of articular cartilage. Bull. Hosp. J. Dis. Orthop. Inst. 43:109–117, 1983.

The interaction of two materials—a porous permeable elastic solid and an interstitial fluid—is used as a biphasic model to describe the mechanical behavior of articular cartilage during loading and deformation. Pure shear condition, when no fluid flow is generated, measures the contribution of the matrix; compressive creep and stress relaxation behavior of articular cartilage determine the effects of fluid flow.

Broom, N.D., and Poole, C.A.: Articular cartilage collagen and proteoglycans: Their functional interdependency. Arthritis Rheum. 26:1111–1119, 1983.

The load-bearing properties of articular cartilage depend on an interaction between the hydrated proteoglycan gel and the collagenous network. Treatment of articular cartilage with testicular hyaluronidase dismantles the proteoglycan/hyaluronic acid complex, resulting in a significant loss of compressive strength. Morphologic changes in the unsupported collagenous structure result, with buckling and flattening.

van Kampen, G.P.J.; Veldhuijzen, J.P.; Kuijer, R.; van de Stadt, R.J.; and Schipper, C.A.: Cartilage response to mechanical force in high-density chondrocyte cultures. Arthritis Rheum. 28:419–424, 1985.

Proteoglycan synthesis and deposition is increased, as reflected by incorporation of [^{35}S]sulfate into glycosaminoglycan by high-density cultures of chick epiphyseal chondrocytes *in vitro* when the cells are exposed to intermittent physiologic compression for 24 hours. Additionally, aggregating capacity and coherence with matrix components were improved with intermittent compression force.

Osteoarthritis

General

Moskowitz, R.W.; Howell, D.S.; Goldberg, V.M.; and Mankin, H.J.: Osteoarthritis: Diagnosis and Management. Philadelphia, W.B. Saunders Company, 1984.

This is a comprehensive text that summarizes the knowledge in basic science, diagnosis, and treatment of osteoarthritis.

Experimental

Altman, R.D.; Tenenbaum, J.; Latta, L.; Riskin, W.; Blanco, L.N.; and Howell, D.S.: Biomechanical and biochemical properties of dog cartilage in experimentally induced osteoarthritis. Ann. Rheum. Dis. 43:83–90, 1984.

Breakdown and stiffening of the collagen network occurs in the middle and deep cartilagenous zones of the femoral condyles after sectioning of the anterior cruciate ligaments in the dog. Although cartilage erosions were not seen, proteoglycan aggregates were smaller and subunit species increased in amount in the tibial plateau cartilage.

Hamerman, D., and Klagsbrun, M.: Osteoarthritis: Emerging evidence for cell interactions in the breakdown and remodeling of cartilage. Am. J. Med. 78:495–499, 1985.

Interleukin 1 may be released from synovial membrane cells and induce release of hydrolytic factors—e.g., collagenase and prostaglandin E_2—by other synovial membrane cells and chondrocytes, which would contribute to the degradation of cartilage matrix. Remodelling occurs by chondrocyte proliferation and vascular and cellular ingrowth from subchondral bone, resulting in osteophyte formation. Growth factors derived from cartilage and bone may modulate the entire process.

Pelletier, J.-P.; Martel-Pelletier, J.; Ghandur-Mnaymneh, L.; Howell, D.S.; and Woessner, J.F., Jr.: Role of synovial membrane inflammation in cartilage matrix breakdown in the Pond-Nuki dog model of osteoarthritis. Arthritis Rheum. 28:554–561, 1985.

Collagenolytic activity of cartilage and synovia was significantly increased after anterior cruciate ligament sectioning. The increased activity in cartilage correlated directly with synovial inflammation but not with synovial enzyme content. Prednisone inhibited the increase in enzyme activity.

Sandy, J.D.; Adams, M.E.; Billingham, M.E.J.; Plaas, A.; and Muir, H.: In vivo and in vitro stimulation of chondrocyte biosynthetic activity in early experimental osteoarthritis. Arthritis Rheum. 27:388–397, 1984.

The rate of synthesis of proteoglycans after *in vivo* labeling and *in vitro* incubation with [^{35}S]sulfate was significantly increased in articular cartilage and menisci after sectioning of the anterior cruciate ligament. The increase was due to a general stimulation of chondrocytes in the middle and deep zones of the articular cartilage and throughout the meniscus. The regional response of the cartilage indicates that mechanical factors are acting; stimulation produced by a sham operation suggests that humoral mechanisms also may be involved.

Human

Brocklehurst, R.; Bayliss, M.T.; Maroudas, A.; Coysh, H.L.; Freeman, M.A.R.; Revell, P.A.; and Ali, S.Y.: The composition of normal and osteoarthritic articular cartilage from human knee joints. J. Bone Joint Surg. 66A:95–106, 1984.

No differences in water content, proteoglycan composition and structure, or glycosaminoglycan synthesis rate and cell content were seen between visually intact cartilage from osteoarthritic knees and cartilage from control joints. Deeply fibrillated cartilage had an increased water content and a decreased synthesis rate and content of glycosaminoglycans.

Broom, N.D.: The altered biomechanical state of human

femoral head osteoarthritic articular cartilage. Arthritis Rheum. 27:1028–1039, 1984.

The microcompressive response of osteoarthritic cartilage measured by differential interference contrast microscopy was a collapse of the fibrous structure at a stress of 35 g/mm^2. Propagation of a radial tear through the middle and deep zones of degenerate cartilage involved loads significantly less than those in normal tissue. Transverse notch propagation was possible only in osteoarthritic cartilage. These differences between normal and osteoarthritic cartilage emphasize a fundamental structural breakdown in the load-bearing function of the tissue.

Goldberg, V.M.; Norby, D.P.; Sachs, B.L.; Moskowitz, R.W.; and Malemud, C.J.: Correlation of histopathology and sulfated proteoglycans in human osteoarthritic hip cartilage. J. Orthop. Res. 1:302–312, 1984.

Articular cartilage from fibrillated or discolored cartilage surfaces of femoral heads had neither unique histopathologic nor synthetic or endogenous sulfated proteoglycans specific to that tissue type. Osteophytic tissue incorporated more $^{35}SO_4$ per milligram of tissue protein and showed a distinct histopathologic character, an increased extractability of uronic acid-containing proteoglycan, and a different molecular sieve profile of endogenous proteoglycans.

Pelletier, J.-P.; Martel-Pelletier, J.; Howell, D.S.; Ghandur-Mnaymneh, L.; Enis, J.E.; and Woessner, J.F., Jr.: Collagenase and collagenolytic activity in human osteoarthritic cartilage. Arthritis Rheum. 26:63–68, 1983.

Collagenolytic activity was highest (4.6%) in the center of osteoarthritic lesions, decreasing to 3.7% at the edge and 2.4% at a remote site. The highest enzyme activity was found in the moderately and severely affected groups.

Teshima, R.; Treadwell, B.V.; Trahan, C.A.; and Mankin, H.J.: Comparative rates of proteoglycan synthesis and size of proteoglycans in normal and osteoarthritic chondrocytes. Arthritis Rheum. 26:1225–1230, 1983.

Chondrocytes isolated from cartilage graded histologically as showing moderate osteoarthritis incorporated $^{35}SO_4$ at a rate 3–4 times greater than control cells, but the rate decreased to normal levels with chondrocytes from mild or advanced disease. The proteoglycan synthesized was smaller in size with increasing severity of the osteoarthritis.

Rheumatoid Arthritis: Etiology

Decker, J.L.; Malone, D.G.; Haraoui, B.; Wahl, S.M.; Schrieber, L.; Klippel, J.H.; Steinberg, A.D.; and Wilder, R.L.: Rheumatoid arthritis: Evolving concepts of pathogenesis and treatment. Ann. Intern. Med. 101:810–824, 1984.

Immunohistologic evaluation of rheumatoid synovium demonstrates abnormalities of cell-mediated immune responses. Activated mononuclear cells are the primary mediators that result in tissue destruction. The disease likely is the expression of a genetically controlled host immune response to an undefined agent.

Stastny, P.: Rheumatoid arthritis: Relationship with HLA-D. Am. J. Med. 75:9–15, December 30, 1983.

The HLA-D locus modulates immune responses in rheumatoid arthritis. The Dw4 and DR4 products of this region are associated with the disease in whites, and HLA-DR4 is related to severe rheumatoid factor-positive disease.

Weissmann, G., and Korchak, H.: Rheumatoid arthritis: The role of neutrophil activation. Inflammation 8 Suppl:3–14, 1984.

Neutrophils present in rheumatoid synovial fluid take up immune complexes by endocytosis and then release lysosomal enzymes and other mediators of inflammation. Neutrophils also generate a derivative of arachidonate, leukotriene B_4, that is a potent activator of neutrophils and inducer of local inflammation.

Gout

Terkeltaub, R., and Ginsberg, M.H.: Molecular mechanisms of gouty arthritis: New insights into an old disease. Surv. Synthesis Pathol. Res. 3:386–396, 1984.

Urate-neutrophil interaction produces lysosomal protease, chemotactic factor, prostaglandins, and oxygen radicals. Urate crystals also activate mononuclear phagocytes, synoviocytes, platelets, the classic complement pathway, and the contact system.

Juvenile Rheumatoid Arthritis

Moore, T.L.; Dorner, R.W.; Sheridan, P.W.; and Zuckner, J.: Precipitation of 19S IgM rheumatoid factor-IgG circulating immune complexes in patients with juvenile arthritis by polyethylene glycol and separation by immobilized protein A. Clin. Exp. Immunol. 56:247–252, 1984.

Immune complexes containing 19S IgM and IgG were isolated from sera and synovial fluid from patients with juvenile rheumatoid arthritis, supporting their participation in immune complex formation in this condition. The majority of these patients were rheumatoid factor-negative.

Ankylosing Spondylitis

Kåss, E., and Vinje, O.: Pathogenesis of ankylosing spondylitis and related disorders: Future perspectives. Br. J. Rheumatol. 22 Suppl 2:177–183, 1983.

There is a spectrum of clinical disorders associated with the HLA-B27 locus although a one-gene cross-tolerance theory is strongly supported in ankylosing spondylitis. Genetically determined patterns are triggered by different trigger mechanisms not yet determined.

Chondrocalcinosis

Caswell, A.; Guilland-Cumming, D.F.; Hearn, P.R.; McGuire, M.K.B.; and Russell, R.G.G.: Pathogenesis of chondrocalcinosis and pseudogout. Metabolism of inorganic pyrophosphate and production of calcium pyrophosphate dihydrate crystals. Ann. Rheum. Dis. 42 Suppl:27–37, 1983.

There is great diversity in the clinical syndromes associated with intra-articular deposition of calcium pyrophosphate dihydrate crystal. Crystal deposition commonly occurs in the elderly in the absence of inflammation.

Infectious Arthritis

Goldenberg, D.L., and Reed, J.I.: Bacterial arthritis. N. Engl. J. Med. 312:764–771, 1985.

Within 48 hours, bacterial arthritis produces polymorphonuclear leukocyte infiltration, vascular congestion, and proliferation of synovial lining cells. Cartilage and bone destruction results from proteolytic enzymes released from these leukocytes. Gram stain demonstration of bacteria or recovery of bacteria from the synovial fluid is the only definitive diagnostic test.

Treatment of Arthritis

Nonoperative

Doyle, D.V., and Lanham, J.G.: Routine drug treatment of osteoarthritis. Clin. Rheum. Dis. 10:277–291, August 1984.

Drug therapy in osteoarthritis should consist of a nonsteroidal oral medication that is inexpensive, effective in relieving symptoms, and well tolerated. Chondroprotective agents—e.g., glycosaminoglycan polysulfates (Arteparon) may inhibit enzymatic degradation of cartilage in osteoarthritis.

Harris, E.D., Jr.: Evaluation of pathophysiology and drug effects on rheumatoid arthritis. Am. J. Med. 75:56–61, October 31, 1983.

Nonsteroidal drugs affect mediators of inflammation whereas gold and D-penicillamine affect macrophages and lymphocytes early in the disease cascade. Prednisone inhibits synthesis of proteinases; retinoids may inhibit collagen and proteinase production without affecting normal connective tissue components.

Sledge, C.B.; Atcher, R.W.; Shortkroff, S.; Anderson, R.J.; Bloomer, W.D.; and Hurson, B.J.: Intra-articular radiation synovectomy. Clin. Orthop. 182:37–40, 1984.

Dysprosium-165 coupled to ferric hydroxide macroaggregates has extremely low leakage rates and minimal total body irradiation when injected intra-articularly. Eighty percent of 53 knees with rheumatoid arthritis showed improvement for as long as 1 year after treatment.

Surgery

Engh, C.A.: Hip arthroplasty with a Moore prosthesis with porous coating: A five-year study. Clin. Orthop. 176:52–66, 1983.

Twenty-six porous hip prostheses followed for 2 to 5 years demonstrated results equivalent to those with cemented implants in a comparable high-risk group of patients. No radiographic evidence of bone resorption due to stress shielding was seen.

Insall, J.N.; Hood, R.W.; Flawn, L.B.; and Sullivan, D.J.: The total condylar knee prosthesis in gonarthrosis: A five to nine-year follow-up of the first one hundred consecutive replacements. J. Bone Joint Surg. 65A:619–628, 1983.

Detailed analysis of 100 consecutive total knee replacements for osteoarthritis or necrosis followed for 5 to 9 years demonstrated 91% excellent or good results. Forty-one percent of the tibial components showed radiolucent lines.

Myllylä, T.; Peltonen, L.; Puranen, J.; and Kalevikorhonen, L.: Consequences of synovectomy of the knee joint: Clinical, histopathological, and enzymatic changes and changes in 2 components of complement. Ann. Rheum. Dis. 42:28–35, 1983.

Regenerated synovial tissue after synovectomy, evaluated by arthroscopy, usually demonstrated decreased inflammation, less permeability to serum proteins, and lower activities of lysosomal enzymes.

Tillmann, K.: Pathological aspects of osteoarthritis related to surgery. Inflammation 8 Suppl:57–74, 1984.

Although osteotomies for osteoarthritis have mechanical consequences, they also have a biologic effect based on changes in the circulation to the joint. Pain-conducting nerves may be interrupted, which aids in relieving clinical symptoms.

Biologic Replacement

Malinin, T.I.; Wagner, J.L.; Pita, J.C.; and Lo, H.: Hypothermic storage and cryopreservation of cartilage: An experimental study. Clin. Orthop. 197:15–26, 1985.

Use of osteochondral autografts of femoral condyles that have been frozen at a rate of 2°C/min with either glycerol or dimethyl sulfoxide resulted in normal-appearing cartilage 2½ months after transplantation. Cartilage survived 10 days of hypothermic storage in tissue culture medium. Allografts frozen by standard methods eventually showed loss of chondrocytes and conversion to fibrocartilage.

Meyers, M.H.: Resurfacing of the femoral head with fresh osteochondral allografts: Long-term results. Clin. Orthop. 197:111–114, 1985.

Osteochondral allografts used to reconstruct osteonecrosis of the femoral head prior to osteoarthritis were successful 68% of the time (9 to 63 months after transplantation). When the cause was not steroid related, the success rate was 80%.

5 Musculoskeletal Neoplasms

Although bone and soft tissue neoplasms are uncommon, orthopaedic surgeons are frequently involved in the initial assessment and management of this nonhomogeneous group of tumors. New developments in diagnosis and treatment of such patients are being explored at many institutions in an effort to improve the overall well-being and survival and to diminish treatment-associated morbidity.

Principles of the Biopsy

The biopsy is probably the most important procedure in managing patients with bone and soft tissue tumors. The tissue obtained should accurately reflect the lesion so that pathologic interpretation will lead to a treatment program compatible with the predicted natural history of the neoplasm. Should sampling errors occur or nonrepresentative tissue be submitted, the planning and subsequent management program will be distorted, delaying diagnosis and treatment and possibly being detrimental to the patient.

In managing such patients, considerable effort should be given to the development of a differential diagnosis. In most cases, by using a combination of the historical, physical, and radiographic findings with a thorough knowledge of the natural history of the suspected lesion, one should be able to obtain sufficient tissue for diagnosis without rendering the patient inoperable for possible limb-preservation procedures. If one is unfamiliar with the suspected extension of the lesion and the three-dimensional compartmental anatomy of the extremity, a simple error in incision placement or injudicious exposure of neurovascular structures can render a limb unsuitable for preservation.

It is advisable to discuss the anticipated biopsy with the radiologist and pathologist prior to the procedure. Incision placement should be carefully planned so that the surrounding skin and contaminated soft tissues can be excised *en bloc* with the lesion at the time of definitive surgery.

There are many methods by which tissue and fluid can be obtained for evaluation. Fine-needle aspiration biopsy is appropriate only for those surgeons and pathologists who feel comfortable with this technique. Needles of larger caliber can be used for bone biopsies in special anatomic regions (e.g., vertebral bodies, iliac crest); however, sampling errors become more likely with these techniques. Preferably, a small, appropriately placed open biopsy should be used to obtain several samples of tissue (Fig. 1). Many bone and soft tissue lesions are not homogeneous, and therefore, for accurate diagnosis, several areas of the lesion, including the interface between the lesion and reactive tissue, should be evaluated pathologically.

Many surgeons favor excisional biopsy when the lesion is small (<3 cm) and favorably located and when excision of the lesion and a cuff of surrounding tissue will not result in significant morbidity (e.g., ribs, skin lesions, expendable bones). When a choice is available, however, most oncologic surgeons prefer an incisional technique. If appropriate management of the lesion requires a compartmental resection, then one usually can proceed after biopsy without significantly extending the margins beyond those previously planned. Consequently, the incision should be placed in a manner that permits subsequent wide excision of the tumor.

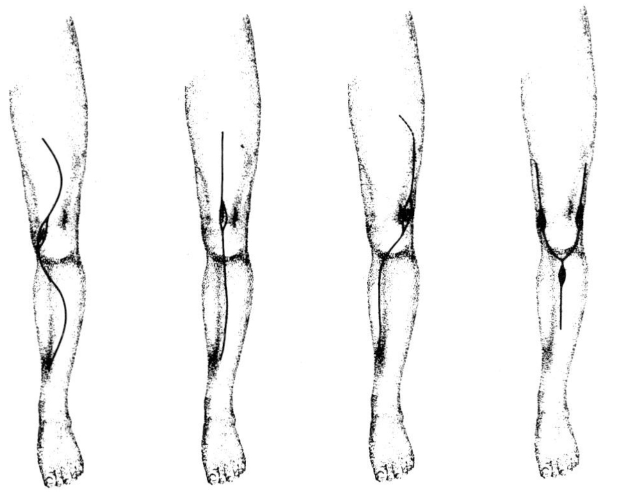

Figure 1

Some of the more common sites for biopsy and the accompanying incisions for resection. Transverse incisions should *not* be used in the extremities.

Postoperative hematoma formation can render a previously resectable lesion unresectable. Techniques that will diminish the likelihood of hematoma formation include the use of a tourniquet (after gravity exsanguination), thrombogenic agents (activated thrombin, Oxycel, Avitene), methyl methacrylate, and hemostatic closure. The tourniquet should be deflated prior to closure in order to secure adequate hemostasis. Presumably, anatomic planes dissected by hematoma should be considered to be contaminated and included in the surgical margins.

Once tissue is obtained for evaluation, proper handling is mandatory. One must be certain that material has been obtained for multiple analyses (e.g., culture, use of different fixatives) to permit full evaluation of the previously entertained diagnosis and to provide sufficient information for differentiating one lesion from another. Tissue for electron microscopy should be obtained and fixed; if not required, it can be disposed of after the diagnosis is secure.

The ever-increasing complexity of the diagnosis and management of patients with bone and soft tissue lesions requires constant update. Even after careful technique has been used in the most ideal situations, errors will be made. However, by constant attention to detail and careful follow-up, many of these errors can be eliminated. A recent multicenter analysis revealed a 2-fold increase in rate of failure to achieve an accurate diagnosis in centers that are not routinely practicing orthopaedic oncology compared to cancer centers.

Primary Tumors

Osteosarcoma

It is estimated that there are approximately 600 to 800 newly diagnosed cases of osteosarcoma in the United States each year (approximately 200/yr in the United Kingdom). Although the common histologic presentation of malignant cells producing osteoid would suggest a homogeneous group of tumors, the morphologic appearance can vary considerably, to include classic osteosarcoma, fibroblastic osteosarcoma, chondrogenic osteosarcoma, telangiectatic osteosarcoma, low-grade central osteosarcoma, and others. In general, low-grade central osteosarcomas and the parosteal and periosteal osteosarcomas are grouped separately because of their favorable prognosis.

Adjuvant Chemotherapy The role of adjuvant chemotherapy in the treatment of patients with osteosarcoma is becoming better defined. In 1972, studies on 1,286 patients given adequate surgical treatment (primary amputations) between 1946 and 1971 revealed 5-year survival of 19.7% with virtually all of the metastases occurring within 2 years postoperatively. It was concluded that, because the majority of patients had amputations or disarticulations for management of their primary tumor, 80% of patients must have had microscopic, subclinical pulmonary metastasis at the time of operation.

On the basis that chemotherapy should be most effective against microscopic disease, clinical trials of adjuvant therapy were initiated in the early 1970s with high-dose methotrexate and leucovorin rescue. Of 12 patients with classic nonmetastatic osteosarcoma, 5 had disease-free survival with 12 years of follow-up. The adjuvant use of doxorubicin as a single agent was tried in another study; 35 (40%) of 88 patients remained free of disease at 5 years. These and other studies demonstrated the efficacy of each agent as an adjuvant in the treatment of osteosarcoma, compared to historical controls. The combined use of high-dose methotrexate with leucovorin rescue and doxorubicin soon followed, with improved disease-free survival suggested. A combination of cisplatin and doxorubicin was tried in 22 patients with osteosarcoma of the extremities; approximately 60% of these patients remain free of disease at 5 years. Currently, it is accepted that adjuvant chemotherapy significantly enhances survival.

The role of adjuvant pulmonary irradiation in patients with osteosarcoma is doubtful. With the development of radiosensitizing agents, however, adjuvant pulmonary radiotherapy may become useful in the future.

Originally, disarticulation or resection of the entire involved bone was recommended for adequate surgical management of extremity lesions because of the intramedullary origin of the tumor and the 25% incidence of documented intramedullary "skip" metastasis. Later studies reviewing the local recurrence rates for patients having transmedullary amputations for primary management alone revealed local recurrences in approximately 5% to 10% of patients, suggesting that the incidence of skip lesions was less than originally believed or that some of the microscopic skips are eliminated by adjuvant chemotherapy. Soon, the standard surgical management was transmedullary amputation 5 to 10 cm from the intramedullary extent of the lesion as defined by bone scan, computed tomography, or magnetic resonance imaging.

Once it became apparent that one could manipulate tumor growth with preoperative (neoadjuvant) chemotherapy, sufficient preoperative time could be gained to construct a custom prosthesis, setting the stage for limb-sparing surgery. Various techniques have been used, including allograft reconstruction, custom prosthesis, arthrodesis, and rotation-plasty. Comparison of patients undergoing preoperative chemotherapy with those undergoing immediate amputation followed by adjuvant chemotherapy showed those patients who waited for construction of a prosthesis appeared to have a longer relapse-free survival than those undergoing immediate amputation and postoperative chemotherapy. Thus, the concept of neoadjuvant chemotherapy was established for the management of patients with osteosarcoma.

Patient Evaluation Clinical staging prior to biopsy is extraordinarily important. Plain films of the chest and lesion along with polytomography and three-phase bone scan represents a minimal evaluation. Computed tomography of the chest and lesion with and without contrast may be used to evaluate the lung for pulmonary metastasis and to gain information on the vascularity of the primary lesion. A gallium scan may be of use if neoadjuvant chemotherapy is being considered. It has been suggested that diminished gallium scan activity after preoperative chemotherapy correlates well with tumor necrosis. Magnetic resonance imaging is also helpful in evaluating the intraosseous and extraosseous extents of the lesion and in detecting skip lesions (best seen on coronal or sagittal reconstructions). Preoperative conventional or digital subtraction angiography may be helpful in determining the extraosseous extent of the lesion in that the unmineralized portion of the tumor may appear isodense with surrounding muscle tissue on computed tomography. Magnetic resonance imaging may better show the edema in the reactive zone about the tumor.

Correlating the above studies will most often delineate the three-dimensional location of the lesion in preparation for biopsy. Needle aspiration may provide sufficient tissue for diagnosis; however, most often a small, judicious, longitudinal incision is required. The incision should be placed in such a way to enable an *en bloc* resection if limb preservation is anticipated, with care not to expose or contaminate any vital structures. Transverse incisions should *not* be used. Absolute hemostasis must be achieved prior to closure and in general the incision should not be drained.

Treatment Various treatment programs are under evaluation at present. Depending on the study, most current protocols utilize some form of systemic or intra-arterial neoadjuvant chemotherapy with or without low-dose rapid fraction radiation therapy. Depending upon the type of reconstruction to be used, local resection of the primary lesion usually follows in 6 to 10 weeks. If the tumor has responded favorably as evidenced by diminished local pain, improved flexion contracture, diminished uptake on gallium scan, mineralization of the previously unmineralized soft tissue portion of the tumor on computed tomography, and retention of a normal tissue plane between vital structures and the tumor, limb preservation may be elected. If, however, the lesion enlarges with subsequent involvement of the vessels, ablative surgery may be required. Once the operative wounds have healed (usually in 3 weeks), adjuvant chemotherapy is initiated and maintained for approximately 40 weeks, depending upon the particular study.

Surgical Treatment After *en bloc* resection of lesions about the knee, the joint can be reconstructed by custom prosthesis, arthrodesis, and rotation-plasty. Resection-arthrodesis is utilized exclusively by some surgeons for lesions about the knee; others choose to use arthrodesis when the primary lesion produces a large extraosseous mass projecting into the quadriceps mechanism (stage II-B) adjacent to the knee joint. The usual operative treatment of such a lesion would require an extra-articular resection including the quadriceps mechanism, with the transmedullary margin 7 cm distant to the closest extent of the lesion and a subadventitial dissection of the vessels. For the unusually rare intraosseous lesions (stage II-A) or when the primary bulk of the lesion does not project anteriorly, some surgeons prefer to reconstruct the extremity by using a custom articulated prosthesis where the prosthesis can be protected with the intact or reconstructed quadriceps mechanism. Soft tissue coverage can be enhanced by gastrocnemius transfer (medial or lateral head or both).

Figures 2, 3, and 4 show three alternative methods of resection-arthrodesis for management of stage II-B osteosarcoma of the distal femur. All patients had extra-articular resections, and significant portions of the quadriceps mechanism were resected with the specimen.

Lesions arising in the proximal humeral metaphysis or the scapula can be managed by prosthetic replacement, allograft replacement, humeral-scapula arthrodesis with fibula graft, or a Tikhoff-Linberg type procedure.

In general, primary amputation is considered for patients presenting with pathologic fracture, very young patients (<9 years old) in whom leg length inequality would be considerable, and patients with stage II-B lesions arising below the knee or below the elbow. However, selected patients with favorable lesions arising below the knee or elbow may be candidates for limb-sparing procedures. Also, some pathologic fractures have been shown to unite while the patient is on intensive neoadjuvant chemotherapy. Several centers have utilized rotation-plasty or expandable custom prostheses in selected young patients with tumors about the knee.

Chemotherapy After the publication of an extensive retrospective study suggesting a change in the natural history of osteosarcoma, the role of adjuvant chemotherapy was in doubt. Patients treated by surgery alone after 1969 appeared to have improved relapse-free survival compared to those treated prior to 1969. Subsequently, a randomized controlled trial was initiated in which patients received surgical treatment with low-dose adjuvant chemotherapy or surgical treatment alone. The results indicated no improvement in disease-free survival for patients receiving low-dose adjuvant chemotherapy. In patients managed by surgical treatment alone, disease-free survival rate was 44%.

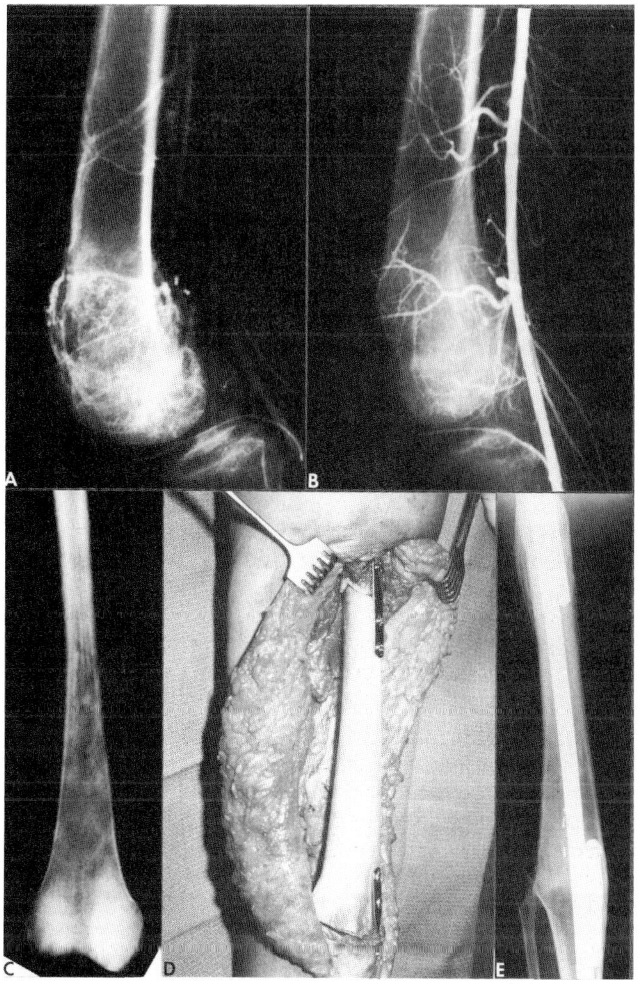

Figure 2

A, Late arterial phase lateral angiogram, showing vascular destructive lesion involving metaphysis of distal right femur in skeletally mature 12-year-old girl later proved to have nonmetastatic "classic" osteosarcoma (in 1977). *B*, Preoperative lateral angiogram of distal femur after completion of two courses of neoadjuvant high-dose methotrexate therapy; flexion contracture and pain were less severe and marked reduction in the neovascularity is apparent without deviation of the major vessels. *C*, Anteroposterior radiograph of deep-frozen allograft, performed to be certain that appropriate size and side were obtained prior to operative procedure. The plan was to remove the condyles and use the allograft as a nonarticulating intercalary graft reconstructed over a custom-fluted intramedullary nail. *D*, Intraoperative photograph, showing intercalary allograft in place with two small plates to stabilize the reconstruction. Autogenous iliac crest graft was then used to augment both proximal and distal host-graft junctions. *E*, Anteroposterior radiograph at 3 years postoperatively, showing solid incorporation of both the proximal and distal host-graft junctions (junctions healed within 6 months postoperatively while patient was on intensive postoperative adjuvant chemotherapy). The patient remains fully ambulatory and brace-free at 9 years postoperatively without evidence of metastatic disease or destruction of the intercalary allograft.

To examine the role of adjuvant chemotherapy in osteosarcoma of the extremity, a multi-institutional osteosarcoma study was initiated. Between June 1982 and May 1984, 18 patients were randomized to adjuvant chemotherapy and 19 to observation (3 of the 19 patients randomized to observation received chemotherapy outside of

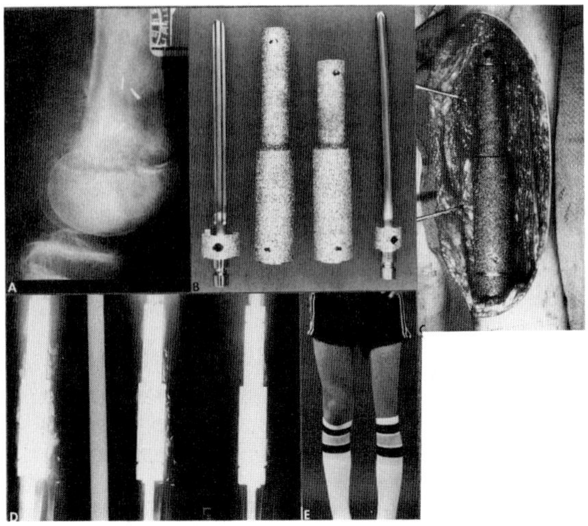

Figure 3

A, Lateral radiograph of distal femur of 12-year-old boy who had pain and associated limp in his left leg for 2 months. Film shows a destructive lesion with neoplastic bone production. Computed tomography revealed intra- and extraosseous stage II-B lesion; however, vessels were free of tumor involvement. Open biopsy confirmed osteosarcoma. *B*, Patient was treated with multi-drug neoadjuvant chemotherapy while a custom titanium fiber-metal implant was constructed. Two fiber-metal spacers were made, to offer a selection of reconstruction lengths. The implant was designed to be assembled through the resection incision with retrograde introduction of the curved 12-mm femoral nail and antegrade insertion of the straight 12-mm tibial nail. Locking screws provide for control of rotation and distraction. *C*, Lateral photograph, showing implant in place with the peroneal nerve and vessels posteriorly. Reconstruction was intentionally 2.5 cm longer to compensate for anticipated growth of the opposite extremity. Autogenous iliac crest graft was placed over the fiber-metal. *D*, Sequential anteroposterior radiographs of the intercalary reconstruction (immediately postoperative, 6 months, and 18 months), showing maturation of the autogenous iliac crest graft. *E*, Anteroposterior photograph, showing clinical result at 18 months. Metastatic disease developed later and the patient died of his disease.

the study). Only 5 of the 19 patients randomized to observation remain disease-free but 13 of the 18 patients randomized to adjuvant chemotherapy remain free of disease. By life-table analysis, this difference in disease-free survival is highly significant ($P = 0.0015$). Of the 70 patients who refused randomization, 51 patients elected adjuvant chemotherapy and 19 elected observation. Of the 19 electing observation, 15 relapsed; only 8 of the 49 patients electing adjuvant chemotherapy (2 patients could not be evaluated) relapsed. These data strongly suggest that the natural history of osteosarcoma remains unchanged. The administration of adjuvant chemotherapy appears to have a significant impact on the disease-free survival for patients with nonmetastatic osteosarcoma of the extremities. The overall survival of both groups, however, remains to be reported.

Pathologic Analysis of Resected Specimen Efficacy of neoadjuvant chemotherapy can be monitored by careful pathologic evaluation of the resected surgical specimen. Depending upon the system used, necrosis ranging from 60% to 90% is common. That this information has prognostic significance was shown in a recently reported European study that confirmed that patients with unfavorable pathologic responses to preoperative chemotherapy experienced a 49% disease-free survival whereas those with a favorable pathologic response experienced an 87% disease-free survival ($P < 0.005$).

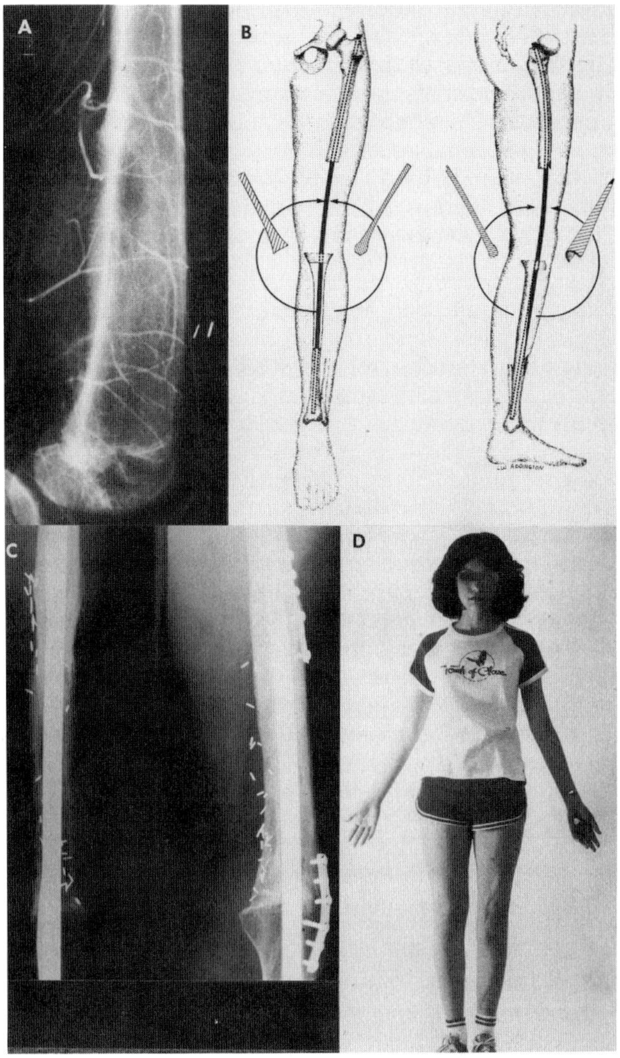

Figure 4

A, Lateral arteriogram after completion of preoperative neoadjuvant chemotherapy for stage II-B nonmetastatic fibroblastic osteosarcoma, revealing hypovascular destructive lesion in distal femoral metaphysis in 14-year-old girl. Computed tomography showed a fatty plane preserved between the lesion and the vessels. *B*, Technique of resection-arthrodesis of the knee with a custom-fluted intramedullary rod and large autogenous cortical grafts to reconstruct the distal femoral defect after tumor-free margins were confirmed intraoperatively. *C*, Grafts at 30 months postoperatively, showing maturation. Graft junctions were supplemented with autogenous iliac crest graft at operation; both were united radiographically at 6 months (patient on intensive adjuvant chemotherapy). *D*, Photograph at 3 years postoperatively, showing clinical result. The patient remains free of disease, clinically and radiographically, at 6 years postoperatively.

To evaluate if patients undergoing limb-sparing procedures did as well as patients with other types of procedures, a multi-institutional retrospective study was begun in July

1975. Evaluation of 227 patients with osteosarcoma of the distal femur has now been completed. In the 73 patients who had limb-sparing procedures there were 8 with local recurrences. Nine of 115 patients undergoing an above-knee amputation had local recurrence; none of 39 patients with hip disarticulations experienced local recurrence. One-third of patients with limb-sparing procedures required at least one additional surgical procedure, and one-fourth eventually required amputation. The Kaplan-Meier estimates for the three surgical groups, however, revealed no significant difference in continuous disease-free survival or ultimate survival for each group (Mantel-Cox test, $P = 0.8$) after a median follow-up of 5.5 years. The continuous disease-free survival for the entire group at 5 years was 42%; overall survival was 55%. They concluded that limb-sparing procedures for osteosarcoma of the distal end of the femur did not compromise either disease-free or overall survival.

A recent multidisciplinary consensus conference evaluating the role of limb-sparing procedures in over 2,000 patients with primary bone and soft tissue sarcomas established the safety and efficacy of limb-preservation procedures as an alternative to amputation in carefully selected patients. Currently, to be a candidate for a limb-salvage procedure, a patient must have a free neurovascular bundle and the potential for reasonable soft tissue coverage.

Management of Patients With Nonresectable Osteosarcoma These patients, usually with the spine or pelvis affected or who refuse surgical resection, remain a problem. The use of intra-arterial radiosensitizers combined with hypofractionated irradiation and chemotherapy for primary treatment has been reported, and early results are encouraging. Significant soft tissue effects were experienced, however.

Ewing's Sarcoma

Ewing first separated this round cell sarcoma from osteosarcoma in 1921. The cell of origin remains obscure. However, investigators recently have identified type VIII collagen secreted from a human Ewing's sarcoma cell line, strongly suggesting an endothelial origin.

The radiographic appearance may resemble that of eosinophilic granuloma and osteomyelitis. It commonly is more metaphyseal-diaphyseal, making the radiographic diagnosis difficult. When the lesion arises in the digits of the hands or feet, the radiographic appearance tends to be more aneurysmal. The primary lesion commonly is associated with a large soft tissue mass that often can be demonstrated by gallium scan, computed tomography, and especially magnetic resonance imaging. Computed tomography remains the standard for evaluating the lung for metastatic disease.

Fever and leukocytosis associated with an increased erythrocyte sedimentation rate at the time of presentation presumably are responses to tumor necrosis and represent a poor prognosis. Any patient presenting with the typical clinical picture of osteomyelitis should be suspected of having Ewing's sarcoma, and representative tissue for routine histopathology, cytology, culture and sensitivity testing, and electron microscopy should be obtained at the time of biopsy.

The biopsy tract should be small and placed longitudinally in such a position that an *en bloc* excision of the lesion could be performed if local excision is indicated later. Absolute hemostasis should be obtained prior to closure to prevent contamination of normal tissue planes, which would render the patient unsuitable for local excision or require unnecessary extension of the radiotherapy ports.

Treatment The primary treatment of Ewing's sarcoma remains chemotherapy and radiation therapy. Most modern protocols include induction chemotherapy followed by irradiation of the primary lesion followed by maintenance chemotherapy for approximately 1 year. Provision for surgical resection of expendable bones after induction chemotherapy is encouraged.

The primary objective of either radiation or surgical therapy in nonmetastatic Ewing's sarcoma is optimal local control. The true local recurrence rate after radiation therapy varies from 12% to 21%. As more patients survive their disease, local recurrence becomes more significant and undoubtedly adversely affects the overall outcome. When local recurrence occurs as the first manifestation of progression of disease, the prognosis is similar to that in patients presenting with metastatic disease.

The role of limited surgical treatment to include the primary excision of expendable bones was established in a large intergroup Ewing's sarcoma study initiated in 1972. Of the 302 patients who could be evaluated, 81 had either partial or complete resections of their primary lesions. Forty patients with complete resections of the primary lesion had improved survival compared with those without resection ($P = 0.03$). The difference between the treatment groups in terms of time to relapse was not statistically significant, however. One center reported that the only survivors of scapular Ewing's sarcoma had undergone surgical resection; none of the patients receiving chemotherapy and irradiation alone were cured. Similarly, the patients with pelvic Ewing's sarcoma who underwent wide excision had a 2-fold greater survival than those in the chemotherapy-irradiation group. These trends in conjunction with the experience at other institutions strongly support the use of limited surgery in the management of the primary tumor in nonmetastatic Ewing's sarcoma of bone.

At present it is recommended that excisional biopsy be utilized for the initial management of small primary lesions of the rib. If residual tumor remains, either resection of the entire rib can be performed or radiation therapy can be administered after induction chemotherapy. It is recommended that expendable bones such as the clavicle, body of the scapula, ribs, wing of the ilium, proximal fibula, and rays of the hands and feet be resected after induction chemotherapy, whenever possible. In many instances, resection with adequate margins may provide satisfactory local control, thereby eliminating the need for and secondary effects of radiation therapy. Amputation or disarticulation may be elected to manage pathologic fractures or extensive destructive lesions of the weight-bearing bones (where pathologic fracture is highly probable) or when a significant limb length inequality could be anticipated (patients less than age 8).

The late development of secondary malignancy in patients surviving Ewing's sarcoma has become of increasing concern among oncologists. The oncogenic effects of radiation therapy and chemotherapy, used alone or in combination, are well recognized. Three of the 302 patients who could be evaluated in the intergroup study had secondary osteosarcomas within the radiation treatment portals and died. Four of 24 patients who had primary Ewing's sarcoma arising within the pelvis and who survived 5 years had secondary malignancies and died; 3 of these 4 received both chemotherapy and radiation therapy. A pediatric cooperative oncology group is conducting a study utilizing induction chemotherapy (12 weeks) followed by either limited surgery or tailored-port radiation therapy in an effort to decrease therapy-associated late effects.

Chondrosarcoma

The histologic appearance varies. The lesions are classified into primary chondrosarcoma, secondary chondrosarcoma, dedifferentiated chondrosarcoma, and clear cell variety. Some tumors may arise *de novo* in extraskeletal tissues, producing an extraskeletal soft tissue variety; in general, these cells do not produce bone and can be distinguished from their benign counterpart by the increased cellularity and pleomorphic appearance.

Primary chondrosarcoma usually arises in adults and presents in older patients compared with secondary chondrosarcoma. The clinical course is generally slow and protracted except for the high-grade lesions which grow rapidly and produce tissue nearly unrecognizable as cartilage. Because most chondrosarcomas do not develop an extensive vascular network and tend to grow by local enlargement and lobulation, surgical excision is required for adequate treatment of this radioresistant and chemotherapy-resistant tumor (Fig. 5). Chemotherapy and radiation therapy can be used for palliation but in the dedifferentiated chondrosarcoma they can be therapeutic.

Treatment The case histories and histopathologic slides of 280 patients managed between 1909 and 1975 at one large treatment center have been retrospectively reviewed. Mesenchymal and clear cell varieties were excluded. One hundred thirty previously untreated patients with localized disease underwent curative procedures and were studied separately. The survival for the 130 patients who had curative procedures was 79% at 5 years, 66% at 10 years, 56% at 15 years, and 47% at 20 years. Women tended to have a better overall prognosis. Among the 69 patients with lesions less than 10 cm in diameter, the 10-year survival rate was 75%; among the 58 with lesions greater than 10 cm, the 10-year survival rate was 57%.

In general, those patients who had local recurrence did less well than those who did not (43% at 10 years, compared to 79%). Also, those patients with histologically higher grade lesions also did less well: 10-year survival was 77% with grade 1, 59% with grade 2, and 36% with grade 3. The younger patient with a smaller lesion of low grade that can be adequately resected has the best overall chance for survival (Fig. 6).

It is important to recognize that clear cell chondrosarcomas commonly are misdiagnosed radiographically as benign lesions and tend to calcify late. In general, these tumors are frequently undertreated, and multiple local recurrences are common. Initial complete excision of the lesion is the treatment of choice. Reconstruction depends on anatomic location and includes custom prosthesis, arthrodesis, and allograft.

Mesenchymal Chondrosarcoma

First recognized as a separate entity in 1972, this rare lesion is characterized by a bimorphic pattern with clusters of small round cells producing a "hemangiopericytoid" appearance.

Formerly, the usual approach to the management of potentially resectable lesions was compartmental surgery when possible or palliative radiotherapy for nonresectable lesions. At present, chemotherapy patterned after that used

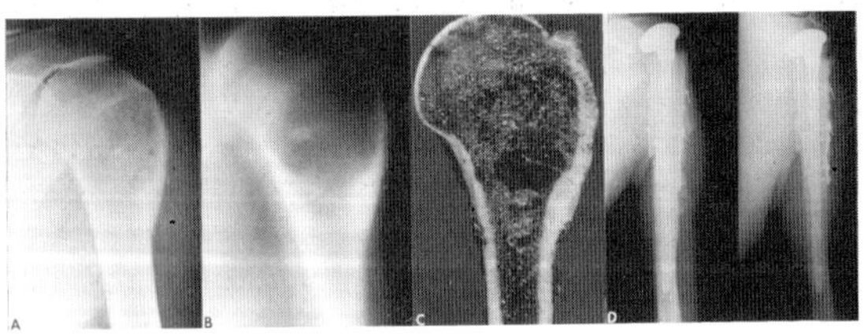

Figure 5

Chondrosarcoma. *A*, Anteroposterior radiograph of left proximal humerus, showing destructive expansile lesion in metaphysis in 38-year-old right-handed male laborer. *B*, Polytomogram shows characteristic calcification of lesion, later proved by biopsy to be grade 1 chondrosarcoma (stage I-A). *C*, Cut specimen, showing area of involvement and biopsy defect. A transarticular resection was performed, sparing the rotator cuff. *D*, Limb and shoulder were reconstructed with a long-stem prosthesis and bilateral proximal fibular grafts. Small portion of the fibular collateral ligament was retained with each graft and reconstructed to the rotator cuff (Left). The patient remains free of disease, clinically and radiographically, at 30 months postoperatively (Right). The patient can actively abduct 45° and lifts objects heavier than 25 kg without pain.

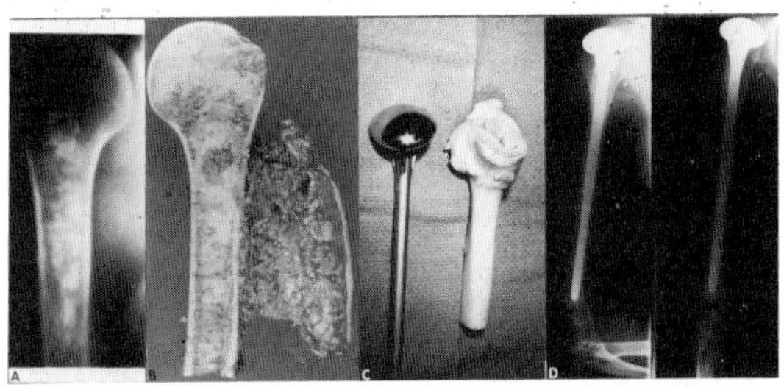

Figure 6

Chondrosarcoma. *A*, Anteroposterior polytomogram of right proximal humerus in 56-year-old right-handed woman who had noted the onset of low-grade pain, worse at night, 8 months prior to evaluation. Note lesion associated with punctate calcifications. The bone scan showed increased activity in the proximal humeral metaphysis, encompassing the proximal 10 cm. A double-contrast arthrogram with intra-articular xylocaine showed no intra-articular involvement (stage I-A) and did not relieve the patient's pain, suggesting an extra-articular source of the pain. *B*, Cut specimen shows the *en bloc* transarticular resection of 17 cm of the proximal humerus after open biopsy confirmed grade 1 chondrosarcoma. The resection included all the continuous tissue associated with the biopsy track. *C*, Preparation of deep-frozen allograft and a long-stem proximal humerus prosthesis. The prosthesis was passed through the allograft, secured by using methyl methacrylate, and then passed into the prepared intramedullary canal. Methyl methacrylate was used to secure the composite reconstruction to the shaft of the humerus, and the rotator cuff was carefully repaired with permanent sutures. *D*, Results 2 years after insertion. Patient has limited abduction and rotation but excellent function of the elbow and hand 4 years postoperatively.

for Ewing's sarcoma and osteosarcoma has produced some promising early results.

At a single large institution, 35 patients with mesenchymal chondrosarcoma have been reviewed. Thirty tumors arose in the skeleton and five occurred in extraskeletal sites. The lesions ranged in size from 4 to 30 cm (mean, 12.5 cm). Five patients with the small round cell variety and eight with the hemangiopericytomatoid variant were managed with combination chemotherapy, surgery, and radiation therapy; median survival was 37.9 months and 28% were alive at 10 years. The use of multimodality therapy for this unusual tumor may provide a maximal therapeutic result.

Giant Cell Tumor of Bone

Giant cell tumor of bone represents approximately 20% of the primary benign tumors of bone. They occur most commonly in patients 20 to 40 years old and develop in the metaphyseal-epiphyseal region of long bones after closure of the epiphyseal plate. More than half occur about the knee; the next most common site is the distal radius followed by the sacrum. Only 3% of giant cell tumors occur in the vertebrae. The malignant giant cell tumor of bone constitutes 5% to 8% of all giant cell tumors of bone. Only five biopsy-proved benign giant cell tumors of bone have been reported in patients prior to epiphyseal plate closure.

Other lesions radiographically confused with giant cell tumors include aneurysmal bone cyst, chondroblastoma, and, most difficult of all, the brown tumor of hyperparathyroidism. If a question arises as to the possibility of hyperparathyroidism, radiographs of the hands and distal clavicle and a serum parathyroid hormone level should be obtained to exclude this possibility.

Histopathologic grading of the tumor has not been successful except for those lesions that have obvious sarcomatous changes. In one attempt to grade 86 giant cell tumors of bone, histologically it was not possible to correlate mitotic count or vascular permeation with local recurrence. Recurrence correlated best with inadequacy of initial treatment. Also, attempts were made to correlate histopathologic features with "aggressive" radiographic characteristics such as cortical destruction; however, the "aggressive lesions" could not be identified on a histologic basis.

Treatment Treatment primarily has been local intralesional curettage with or without bone graft; a few lesions have been excised (marginal resection) because of extensive bone destruction (Fig. 7).

In 222 cases of giant cell tumor reported in 1970, the recurrence rate was 78% in 45 patients treated with curettage alone, 24% in 91 patients treated with curettage and graft, 23% in 44 patients treated with resection alone, 18% in 22 patients treated with resection of the lesion and graft, and 0% in those managed by amputation. Recurrence rate was 60% in patients managed by radiation therapy alone. Intravascular extension did not correlate with subsequent development of pulmonary metastasis. Seeding of the tumor into adjacent tissues was thought to be related to local recurrence in 12 patients. The incidence of seeding did not appear to be related to the site or location of the tumor, and all were grade 1 lesions histologically. Thirteen of the 222 patients had known metastasis—to lung in 11, to the brain in 1, and to lymph node in 1; they were histopathologic grade 1 in two cases, grade 2 in five cases, and grade 3 in six cases.

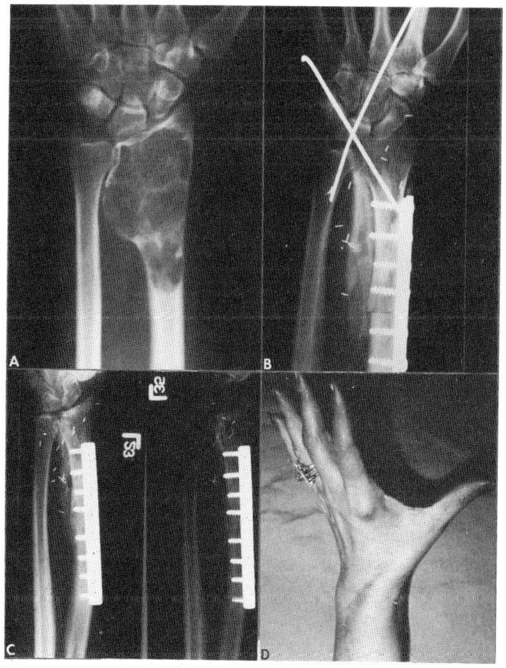

Figure 7

Giant cell tumor of bone. *A*, Anteroposterior radiograph of left wrist of 38-year-old right-handed woman, showing expansile lesion of the distal radius recognized after minor trauma. Needle biopsy revealed grade 1 giant cell tumor of bone. *B*, Anteroposterior radiograph after resection of distal radius, reconstruction by using ipsilateral proximal fibula and capsule, and immediate postoperative fixation with the application of autogenous crest graft. Transfixing pins were removed at 6 weeks. *C*, Oblique radiographs, showing area of reconstruction at 2 years, without evidence of subluxation. The patient lacks 15° of full extension and has 10° limitation of pronation and supination. *D*, Result at 2 years. Function of the wrist, hand, and fingers is excellent. Patient has no pain but avoids heavy lifting and pushing.

Attempts to decrease the incidence of local recurrence and to preserve function have led some authors to use cryosurgery. In a recent study, 12 patients with histopathologically proved giant cell tumor of bone were treated by closed cryotherapy along with curettage and bone grafting; there were two recurrences, one in soft tissue and one in bone. Five of the 12 patients sustained six pathologic fractures. The frequently associated problem of late pathologic fracture remains.

The results of treatment with introduction of bone cement (methyl methacrylate) were recently updated. Two local recurrences occurred (15%) in 14 patients followed for at least 3 years; both of these were managed by recurettage and repeat cementation. Two of the 14 patients have subsequently developed radiographic degenerative changes about the joint. These recent studies emphasize the need for thorough curettage through a large cortical window. The lesions are then subjected to cryosurgery or thermotherapy provided by the heat generated during polymerization of the cement. The former extends the tumor kill 1 to 2 cm but has a significant late fracture rate; the latter extends necrosis 1 to 2 mm but has low morbidity. If the tumor has extensive expansion, particularly with cortical breakthrough, resection is suggested followed by reconstruction with allograft or arthrodesis.

Giant cell tumor is a rare complication of pregnancy. However, because of the high incidence of giant cell tumor among females and the peak occurrence in the third decade of life, pregnant patients occasionally present with a concomitant giant cell tumor of bone. In general, a judicious biopsy should be performed to confirm the diagnosis; termination of the pregnancy is not usually indicated in most patients (Fig. 8).

Malignant Fibrous Histiocytoma of Bone

It is now well recognized that the primary site of malignant fibrous histiocytoma may be bone rather than soft tissue with extension and invasion of adjacent bone. The natural history of the disease has not been well recognized until recently when a summary of the diagnosis and treatment of 90 patients with this lesion of bone, observed between 1940 and 1981, was reported. Forty-eight originally diagnosed cases and 42 retrospectively diagnosed cases were extensively analyzed.

The histopathologic criteria for diagnosis included three basic types of cells: spindle fibroblasts, histiocytes, and malignant-appearing and benign giant cells. Osteoid production was interpreted as an indication of osteosarcoma, and these patients were excluded. The typical fibroblastic, storiform arrangement of cells was the representative underlying component of the tissue.

Two-thirds of the tumors were in males, evenly distributed between the second and sixth decades of life. Radiographically the lesions most commonly arose in the metaphysis of long bones and were equally located eccentrically or centrally. In general (86%), they were destructive lesions with ill-defined margins. Tumor calcification was not observed. Cortical destruction was noted in 85% of lesions, and 20% of patients presented with pathologic fracture. Sixty-seven tumors arose in apparently normal bone and 23 tumors arose in bone associated with preexisting bone abnormalities (Paget's disease in 5, dedifferentiated chondrosarcoma in 5, postirradiation in 3, bone infarcts in 3, multiple osteochondromata in 2, and various other lesions in 5). The most common primary site of origin was the distal femoral metaphysis, followed by the proximal tibial metaphysis and the proximal femur. The most common primary site of origin in a flat bone was the ilium followed by rib and scapula.

Surgical therapy could be evaluated in 68 patients; 46 patients were judged to have had adequate surgical margins and 22 had inadequate margins. Local recurrence occurred in 21 patients overall (31%); the specific frequencies were 64% in those with inadequate margins, 21% after wide amputation, 17% after wide resection, and 6.5% after radical compartmental margins. Local recurrence was found to be similar in patients with stage II-A or II-B lesions (33% vs. 28%).

Metastasis developed in 52 patients: pulmonary in 44, bone in 6, both lung and bone in 1, and regional lymph node involvement in 1.

Twenty patients received adjuvant chemotherapy. Survival rates were highest in those patients managed by adequate surgery plus adjuvant chemotherapy (57% 5-year survival). Adjuvant chemotherapy was not effective in preventing local recurrence when associated with inadequate surgery. All patients with stage I-B lesions were long-term survivors; patients with stage II-A lesions had a trend (not statistically significant) to higher survival rate than those with II-B lesions. Patients with lesions arising in bone with preexisting abnormalities appeared to have a poorer outcome than those with lesions arising in apparently normal bone. Radiotherapy effected clinical cure in only three patients.

Adjuvant chemotherapy has been reported, by other authors, to have had an apparent beneficial effect in a small series. Also, chemotherapy has been used in a neoadjuvant manner, similar to its use in osteosarcoma management, followed by limb preservation and adjuvant chemotherapy (Fig. 9).

From the available literature, it appears that a prudent course of therapy for nonmetastatic stage II-A or II-B lesions would be wide excision or wide amputation followed by adjuvant chemotherapy. Small, favorably located lesions in skeletally mature individuals may be considered for limb-preservation procedures either with or without neoadjuvant chemotherapy.

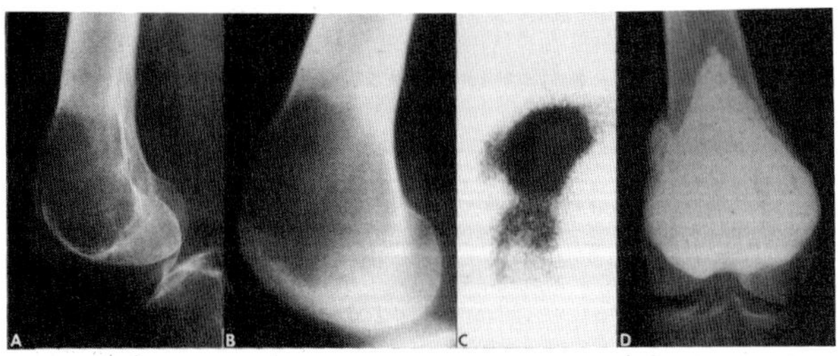

Figure 8

A, Lateral radiograph, showing destructive lesion in metaphyseal-epiphyseal region of distal femur associated with a small anterior pathologic fracture in 26-year-old woman in 6th month of pregnancy. Open biopsy confirmed the diagnosis of grade 2 giant cell tumor of bone. *B*, After delivery of normal infant, polytomograms confirmed destructive nature of lesion (fracture had been allowed to heal with protective splint). Arthrogram revealed no intra-articular involvement. *C*, Lateral view bone scan, showing typical "donut" sign commonly seen in expansile vascular lesions. No other lesions were identified. *D*, Anteroposterior projection of distal femur, showing 2-year follow-up after cementation. Patient has full range of motion and walks without a limp. There has been no evidence of local recurrence.

Chordoma

This unusual tumor constitutes 1% to 4% of malignant bone tumors arising from notochordal remnants in such diverse places as the posterior nasopharynx, spheno-occipital region, intervertebral disks and bodies, and sacrococcygeal region. This lesion arises almost exclusively in the midline, approximately half in the sacrococcygeal region, 35% in the spheno-occipital region, and the remainder in the cervical spine. It is the most common primary bone tumor of the sacrum.

The spheno-occipital lesions occur slightly more often in men in the third through fifth decades of life; the sacrococcygeal lesions are 3 times more common in men and appear in a slightly older population, in the fifth decade. This may be related to the often-discovered large asymptomatic masses in the sacrum whereas lesions of similar size in the cervical region would be incompatible with life. Approximately 10% of chordomas produce hematogenous

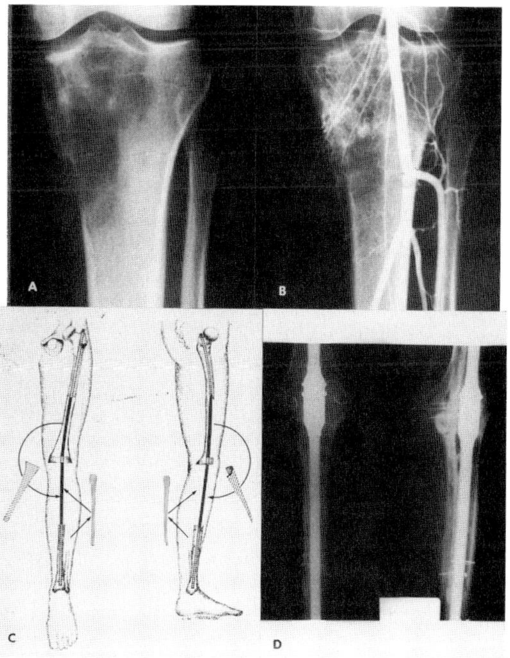

Figure 9

A, Anteroposterior projection showing destructive, malignant fibrous histiocytoma (biopsy-proved) of bone in 51-year-old accountant. Arthrography showed joint not involved, and chest had no evidence of metastatic disease. *B*, Angiogram after two courses of multi-drug neoadjuvant chemotherapy, revealing marked reduction in neovascularity compared to prechemotherapy angiogram. Clinical improvement was evident (marked reduction in size of associated soft tissue mass). *C*, Resection-arthrodesis with femoral turn-down procedure was performed. Reconstruction and skin closure required transfer of gastrocnemius muscle flap and split-thickness skin graft. *D*, Reconstruction at 2 years postoperatively. One year of adjuvant chemotherapy was delivered; both graft junctions healed within 6 months. The segmental intramedullary nail used was unique in that it could be inserted through the resection incision and not violate the buttock tissues. The patient remains free of disease.

metastasis, with some lesions presenting in such unusual locations as the skin.

The presenting symptoms in patients with the spheno-occipital variety include pituitary dysfunction (amenorrhea, loss of libido, weight gain), visual field defects, and, most commonly, diplopia due to an abducens nerve paresis. The mass need not be large, because of the critical location of the lesion.

Initial presenting symptoms with the sacrococcygeal variety are in large part associated with bowel and bladder dysfunction. Constipation is the most common. Motor loss is often a late finding. Because the tumor almost always presents as a presacral mass, it often is a large, bulky mass in contrast to the spheno-occipital variety. A recent study noted the late diagnosis of sacral lesions. In that series, two-thirds of the patients had undergone lumbar spinal surgery prior to the recognition of a sacral tumor.

Pathology The histopathologic subtyping of chordoma appears to be important because lesions with chondroid elements tend to follow a more indolent and protracted course. Nineteen patients with chondroid chordoma had a mean survival of 15.8 years compared with 4.1 years in patients with pure chordoma. Overall, however, the course of both types ultimately includes tumor recurrence or metastasis and death if the tumor is not completely resected.

The microscopic differential diagnosis of chordoma includes chondrosarcoma, ependymoma, and metastatic mucin-producing adenocarcinoma. Reticulin staining, previously reported to be of no value, has recently regained support with the report of *in vitro* studies that demonstrate extracellular reticulin production from chordoma cells. The absence of reticulin production in mucin-producing adenocarcinomas may be useful in excluding these occasionally nearly indistinguishable lesions.

Enzyme histochemical characterization of chordomas has also added another powerful tool to separate pure chordoma from other variants. 5′-Nucleotidase activity has been evaluated in sections from four chordomas. All four tumors showed strong positivity localized in the plasma membrane; fetal notochordal remnants, chondrosarcomas, ependymomas, and chondroid chordomas did not.

Treatment Treatment of the spheno-occipital variety often is not curative because of the adjacent vital structures. However, it is generally agreed that, when feasible, surgical resection is the preferred treatment. When only incomplete resection (tumor spillage or intralesion margins) is possible, the addition of radiation therapy is indicated. A recent paper described lesions involving the cervical vertebrae (two patients) and base of the skull (seven patients) and reported eight of the nine patients free of disease at 10 months to 3 years after treatment with a combination of photon and proton beam techniques. Dose levels as high as 8,040 cGy in 38 fractions were achieved without evidence of radiation morbidity.

In general, surgery remains the primary treatment for sacrococcygeal chordoma. In a recent report on chordomas involving the sacrum, the recurrence rate was 28% in 25 patients with complete surgical resections (marginal to wide margins) and 64% in 25 patients in whom the lesion was entered (intralesion margin) at the time of operation. It has been reported that, as long as the upper half of the first sacral vertebra remains intact, the pelvis will permit adequate stability for near-normal standing and walking. If the S-2 nerve root can be preserved, adequate bowel and bladder function could be expected postoperatively. If only the S-1 root remains, then satisfactory bowel and bladder function can be expected after training. Incomplete resection results in recurrence. Consequently, sufficient resection of the sacrum is required to provide a normal tissue margin, even if bladder and bowel function is compromised.

When complete surgical resection cannot be achieved, the addition of radiation therapy in doses of 6,500 cGy or greater is required to achieve a worthwhile level of palliation.

Secondary and Treatment-Related Sarcomas of Bone

It is now well recognized that chemotherapy and radiation therapy are oncogenic. Although postirradiation sarcoma of bone is well documented, secondary malignancies related to chemotherapeutic agents are less well known.

The occurrence of sarcoma in bone within a radiation therapy portal was first recognized in three patients given such therapy for tuberculous bone disease. Since then, numerous patients have been described with sarcoma arising in preexisting benign lesions and also within normal bone after exposure to ionizing radiation.

The criteria for the diagnosis of postirradiation sarcoma of bone arising from a benign process are as follows.

1. The benign nature of the initially treated lesion must be evident microscopically or radiographically.

2. The secondary sarcoma must have arisen within the radiotherapy portal.

3. A relatively long latent period must have elapsed (5 years) before the clinical appearance of the secondary lesion.

4. All secondary sarcomas must be identified microscopically.

The criteria were modified in 1971 to include malignant tumors without microscopic evidence of osteoid production, such as Ewing's sarcoma, lymphoma of bone, carcinoma of the breast, and Hodgkin's disease.

A report from a large cancer center (where radiation therapy has been used extensively) described 66 patients with documented osteosarcoma arising in bone and soft tissue previously exposed to radiation therapy. In 42 patients, the bone was normal prior to radiation therapy; 24 patients had had radiation therapy for osseous lesions. The overall mean latent period was 10.5 years; it was 8.7 years for those under age 16 years and 13.8 years for adults ($P = 0.02$). The sexes were affected equally, and the majority of lesions arose in the pelvis, hip, or shoulder girdle. No patient received less than 2,000 cGy. Fifty-nine lesions arose in bone and seven were extraskeletal in origin. The cumulative disease-free survival rate was 17% at 5 years.

In an experience reported from another institution, of 78 patients with postirradiation sarcomas, 35 had had previously normal bone and 43 had preexisting osseous lesions. The mean latent period was 14.3 years, and 90% of the microscopically proved lesions were either osteosarcoma or fibrosarcoma. Prompt radical surgery was recommended for extremity lesions; 30% of patients survived 5 years without recurrence. There were no disease-free survivors among patients with tumor arising in the pelvis, shoulder girdle, or vertebrae.

Secondary malignancies arising in conjunction with the use of anticancer agents in animals have also been recognized. The use of cyclophosphamide in animals commonly produces tumors of the urinary bladder, hematopoietic system, and nervous system.

Chemotherapy-induced secondary malignancies in humans have been recently reviewed. The median latent period was 54 months. Cyclophosphamide induced primarily acute leukemias, carcinoma of the urinary bladder, and squamous cell carcinoma of the skin. Leukemia accounted for approximately 90% of the secondary malignancies associated with the use of melphalan.

Current multimodality therapy includes both chemotherapeutic agents and radiation therapy. Factors contributing to increased risk of development of a secondary malignancy are chemotherapy, radiation therapy, and genetic factors. A study of the risk of subsequent malignancies developing in patients surviving Ewing's sarcoma revealed an enhancing effect, not simply an additive one, when radiation therapy was combined with chemotherapy. The development of secondary malignancies in children appears to be accelerated (requiring fewer years) compared to that in adults.

Combined multimodality Ewing's sarcoma protocols now are seeking to decrease the risk of significant late effects (including late-developing malignancies) by using induction chemotherapy to decrease the volume of irradiated tissue and using tailored ports along with resection of expendable bones (eliminating the need for radiation therapy). The true significance of late-developing malignancies will not become evident until both our ability to manage these tumors and patient survival improve.

Soft Tissue Sarcoma

Benign mesenchymal tumors outnumber malignant neoplasms by approximately 100:1. It is estimated that approximately 4,500 new malignant neoplasms arise in soft tissues yearly (approximately 3 times the rate of osteosarcoma). In general, the lesions are classified according to their histogenic similarity to the parent tissue. Often, an extracellular matrix may be produced by the cells that can be identified by routine histopathologic techniques or by more elaborate studies (e.g., histochemistry, electron microscopy, immunoperoxidase).

The biopsy method varies from needle-aspiration cytology to open techniques, depending on the choice of the physician and the pathologist. Many institutions now rely on needle aspiration with the needle track being placed within the anticipated operative field. If the diagnosis can be made from the cytologic study, treatment can proceed; however, if sufficient tissue cannot be obtained, then open biopsy is performed. Although needle aspiration frequently will permit a diagnosis as to histogenesis, often it cannot provide the grade of the lesion. By using simultaneous cytophotometric DNA analysis, some institutions are attempting to correlate the aspiration histopathology data with flow studies to provide both the diagnosis and the grade.

The compartmental growth characteristics of soft tissue sarcomas are now well recognized and accepted (Fig. 10). This is due to the characteristic expansile growth up and down muscle fibers and fascial planes in the path of least resistance. The dense fascial compartment represents an anatomic barrier to tumor growth and is transgressed infrequently. If the tumor does invade adjacent structures outside of the compartment, it frequently does so along vascular perforations through the limiting fascia or when nerves course from one compartment to another (e.g., the ulnar nerve perforating the posterior septum in the arm).

The anatomic location and size of the primary tumor are extremely important. In a recent two-institution study, 66% of 113 patients with soft tissue sarcomas in extremities managed by surgery alone were alive with a follow-up of at least 5 years. At the time of diagnosis, 17 tumors (15%) were less than 5 cm in diameter, 64 (57%) were less than 10 cm in diameter, and 49 (43%) were 10 cm or larger. Thirty-seven tumors (33%) were malignant fibrous histiocytomas, 24 (21%) were liposarcomas, and 15 (13%) were leiomyosarcomas; the remaining 37 (33%) tumors consisted of malignant schwannoma, fibrosarcoma, myxofibrosarcoma, synovial cell sarcoma, and others. Ninety-two (81%) were believed to be high-grade and 21 (19%) were low-grade. Seventeen tumors (15%) originated in the upper extremity and 96 (85%) were in the lower extremity. Seventy-six tumors (67%) were intracompartmental and 37 (33%) were extracompartmental. Nineteen of the extracompartmental tumors originated within an anatomic compartment and had extended to another compartment; the 18 others originated extracompartmentally.

One hundred three patients (91%) were treated by limb-

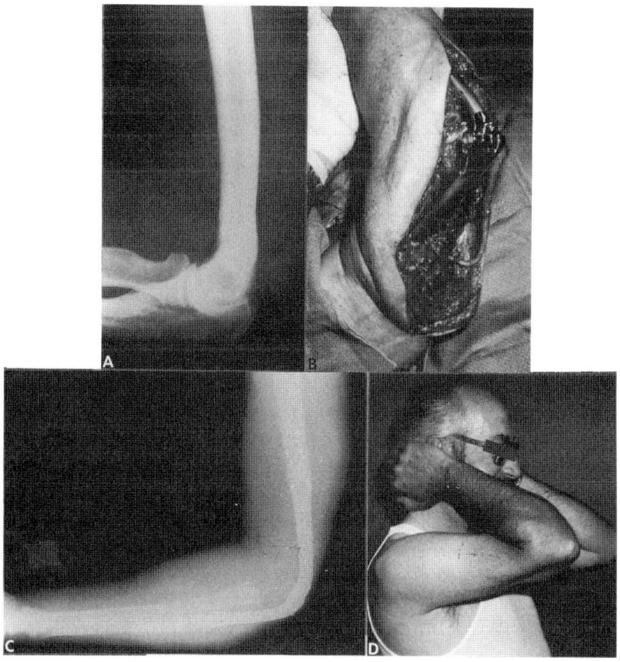

Figure 10

Synovial cell sarcoma. *A,* Lateral radiograph of 51-year-old right-handed farmer who noted development of painless mass over the posterior aspect of his right elbow 3 years prior to this study. The mass was firm and fixed to the shaft of the humerus. An arthrogram revealed involvement of the olecranon fossa. Biopsy revealed the diagnosis. *B,* Extra-articular resection of the elbow to include the distal third of the humerus was performed and reconstructed by using a custom Vitallium elbow prosthesis. The ulnar nerve can be seen to the right of the prosthesis, and the cut end of the proximal radius can be seen to the left. *C,* Lateral radiograph of the extremity taken 2 years after resection reveals no loosening. Triceps function was absent; however, the patient could achieve full extension of the elbow with gravity. *D,* Clinical photograph showing the degree of function of the elbow. The patient's forearm and hand function were essentially normal with full pronation and supination. The prosthesis functioned well until the patient died of pulmonary metastasis 4 years postoperatively.

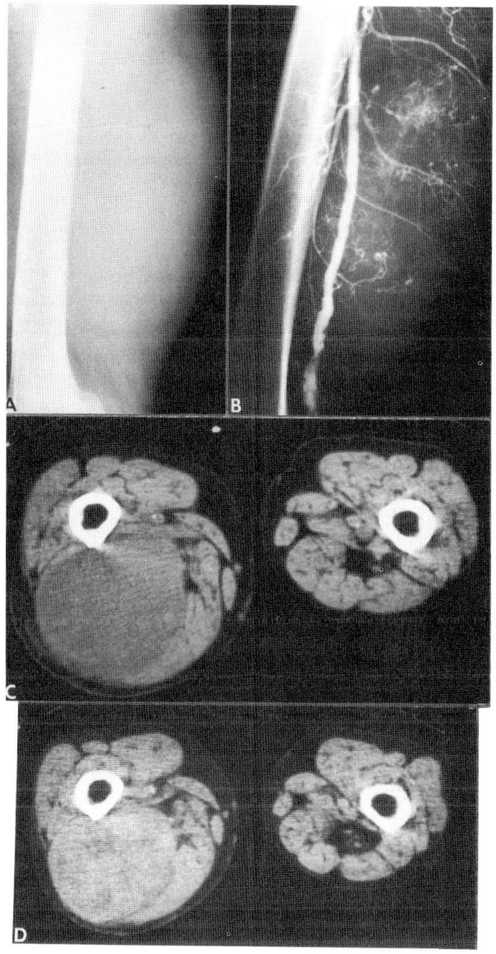

Figure 11

Grade 2 liposarcoma. *A,* Lateral radiograph in 81-year-old man who had noted an enlarging painless mass in the posterior aspect of his right thigh approximately 6 months prior to this study. There was no leg or foot pain. The bone scan showed no evidence of bone involvement. Open biopsy revealed a grade 2 (I-IV) liposarcoma. *B,* Preoperative lateral angiogram suggested a marked reduction in the neovascularity compared to a pre-radiation-therapy angiogram. At local resection, the sciatic nerve was free from the tumor mass. The entire lateral hamstrings were resected from origin to insertion. An additional 2,000 cGy was given to the tumor bed after 3 weeks for wound healing. The patient remains free of disease clinically and radiographically at 5 years after resection. *C,* Prone computed tomography scan through the mass showed the vessels to be free of tumor; however, the status of the sciatic nerve was uncertain. The computed tomogram of the chest revealed no evidence of metastatic disease. A total of 4,500 cGy was delivered preoperatively to the tumor over 5 weeks. *D,* Computed tomogram at 4 weeks after completion of the radiation therapy, showing marked decrease in size of the mass. The patient also experienced increased range of motion of his knee with resolution of local edema.

sparing surgery (3 radical resection, 77 wide resection, and 23 marginal excision) and 10 (9%) had an amputation.

The tumor recurred locally in 23 (22%) of the 103 patients with limb-sparing surgery—16% (12/76) in intracompartmental tumors and 32% (12/37) in extracompartmental tumors. None of the three patients with radical resection had local recurrence. The local recurrence rate was 65% after marginal excision and only 10% after wide excision. The tumor-related survival at 5 years was 66%.

Another institution reported the results in 40 patients with soft tissue sarcomas of the thigh. When wide margins were achieved, with low-grade lesions there were no local recurrences but with high-grade lesions 30% (3/10) recurred locally. No local recurrences were reported when radical margins were achieved. The margin required for local control correlated best with the biologic aggressiveness (grade) of the lesion.

At present, several centers are evaluating the use of neoadjuvant chemotherapy in biologically responsive soft tissue sarcomas (such as malignant fibrous histiocytoma) followed by limb-sparing surgery. Most commonly, however, preoperative radiation therapy (4,500 cGy) is used followed by limited compartmental surgery (Fig. 11). Also, intra-arterial neoadjuvant chemotherapy with or without concomitant radiation therapy is being evaluated as a way to provide maximal local reduction in the size of the mass and to minimize the need for removal of large segments of tissue. The ability to provide adequate local control without endangering survival (local recurrences) by using these protocols is not known at this time.

Carcinoma Metastatic to Bone

Pathogenesis of Metastasis The pathogenesis of metastasis is a dynamic and selective process and only recently has become better understood. The process of metastasis consists of a sequence of interrelated steps, each dependent on the preceding event.

The initial phase of metastasis consists of local invasion of normal stromal cells by the primary tumor cells. Invasion continues by increased local pressure and dissection of tumor cells along the lines of least resistance, release of lytic enzymes, and increased motility of tumor cells. The tumor cells invade local lymphatic or vascular channels where they may remain or may become dislodged and circulate as tumor emboli. During this process, the emboli must survive many potential lethal events (e.g., vascular turbulence, normal immune "killer cells") and it is believed that only a few (less than 0.1%) emboli actually survive to become embedded and adherent to the endothelial cells of a distant preferred capillary bed where the process of invasion continues. The tumor cells extravasate into the surrounding tissue where new capillary networks are developed through the influence of tumor angiogenesis factor and a new colony of commonly biologically heterogeneous cells proliferates.

Mechanisms of Bone Destruction Hypercalcemia is a commonly associated metabolic complication of cancer and its most common clinical symptoms are nausea, vomiting, anorexia, lethargy, confusion, stupor, and coma. These symptoms should not be confused with the terminal events of cancer. The hypercalcemia of cancer is most commonly associated with carcinoma of the breast and squamous cell carcinoma of the lung; however, not all tumors of the lung are associated with hypercalcemia (i.e., anaplastic and oat cell tumors). The hypercalcemia observed as a secondary effect is related to the capacity of the tumor to secrete specific hypercalcemia factors.

Bone resorption related to neoplasia results in osteolytic metastatic sites and hypercalcemia. The secondary hypercalcemia may or may not result in clinical symptoms (i.e., rate of destruction); however, the associated bone destruction commonly results in increased morbidity. No single process of altered bone cell metabolism is believed to be responsible for the bone destruction produced.

There are three general categories of tumors, each producing bone destruction by a different means. Hematologic malignancies such as multiple myeloma result in either focal or generalized bone destruction which is produced by activating osteoclasts. Cultured myeloma cells produce a soluble factor that stimulates osteoclasts to resorb bone. This factor may be the same lymphokine that is released by lymphocytes and is designated "osteoclast-activating factor (OAF)." Other hematologic malignancies that produce an osteoclast-activating factor include lymphoma, lymphosarcoma, and Burkitt's lymphoma.

Hypercalcemia in patients with carcinoma of the breast is most commonly seen only after widespread bone metastasis is discovered. It is observed in approximately 30% of patients. As the process of metastasis occurs, the emboli lodge in the sinusoids of the hematopoietically active bone marrow and migrate to the endosteal surfaces. The process of bone destruction with this specific solid tumor probably includes several types of cells—tumor cells, osteoclasts, lymphocytes, and monocytes. The osteoclast is probably the cell primarily responsible for bone destruction in response to stimulation by prostaglandins produced by monocytes and tumor cells and osteoclast-activating factor produced by lymphocytes (i.e., the inflammatory response of the tumor). Tumor cells and monocytes can resorb bone directly. The attraction of tumor cells and monocytes to bone surfaces appears to be related to the chemotactic effects of fragments of type I collagen released during bone remodeling.

Hypercalcemia has been described in another group of patients with solid tumors but without bone metastasis. This syndrome has been described as the humoral hypercalcemia of cancer. Calcium absorption from the gut and concentrations of 1,25-dihydroxyvitamin D are decreased, suggesting that parathyroid hormone is not the responsible mediator. Many patients do have increased urinary excretion of prostaglandin E-M (the primary urinary metabolite of prostaglandins E), implicating prostaglandin E as a causative factor for bone resorption. Numerous studies now suggest that the prostaglandin production is insufficient to explain the hypercalcemia seen in humans.

Tumors produce a family of polypeptides known as transforming growth factor (TGF). These substances primarily have two significant properties: they stimulate cell growth and replication, and they confer the transformed phenotype to the transformed cell. Study of these growth factors may lead to a better understanding of the mechanisms of bone destruction in solid tumors without metastasis. Because all tumor cells secrete transforming growth factor but only a few tumors are associated with hypercalcemia, it is suggested that probably several transforming growth factors stimulate bone resorption.

Survival Survival after pathologic fracture varies according to the type of the primary tumor. Patients with carcinoma of the lung rarely survive more than 1 year and often do not survive for 6 months, whereas patients with carcinoma of the thyroid commonly survive 5 years or longer. In general, as a group, approximately 50% of patients sustaining a pathologic fracture will survive more than 6 months and approximately 30% will survive 1 year. As our ability to manage the primary tumor through the use of chemotherapy, radiation therapy, and surgery improves, a corresponding increase in post-fracture survival time will require improved surgical methods and development of improved implants for better management of these patients.

Treatment The most common site for pathologic fracture associated with metastatic disease is within the distribution of hematopoietic marrow in the adult skeleton. The spine, ribs, and proximal femur are most common. Of these fractures, those affecting the femur are the most common and are managed by surgical intervention. Fractures in the non-weight-bearing portion of the skeleton, such as the humerus, may or may not be managed by surgical means, depending upon the location of the fracture and the condition of the patient. Functional cast bracing can lead to union in the majority of patients but re-fracture is frequent.

Prevention of pathologic fracture is preferred, through frequent follow-up examinations, including appropriate radiographs and bone scans. Early chemotherapeutic management or radiation therapy can prevent pathologic fracture; however, once sufficient bone destruction has occurred, consideration must be given to prophylactic internal fixation.

General guidelines have been developed for prophylactic internal fixation. Painful destructive lesions in long bones—2.5 cm in diameter or areas of destruction occupying more than 50% of the circumference of the cortex—have been shown to fracture with minimal trauma. Also, painless lesions occupying more than 50% of the cortical surface fail with minimal trauma. Patients with these defects in long bones should be considered for prophylactic internal fixation. The predictability of failure of the involved bone is sufficiently great to warrant the risks and hazards of surgical intervention, provided that reasonable survival is anticipated.

The use of poly(methyl methacrylate) has improved the overall management of pathologic fractures. The material can be used to fill large areas of destruction in bone to achieve better transmission and dispersal of loads across the areas of reconstruction and to augment fixation of surgical implants. The material is not significantly altered by high-dose irradiation, thereby making it an ideal filler material for reconstruction. If large quantities of poly(methyl methacrylate) are under pressure, patients may develop a pseudo-fat emboli syndrome with a decrease in PA_{O_2}. Volumetric expansion and respiratory support are necessary.

Consideration should be given to preoperative radiation therapy, especially in patients with bone metastasis due to carcinoma of the kidney and thyroid. These metastatic lesions are frequently vascular, and significant blood loss should be expected. Rapid fraction preoperative radiation therapy in some instances can significantly decrease blood loss and postoperative morbidity.

The treatment of patients with pathologic fractures has progressed significantly over the past 15 years with the addition of better supportive and occasionally curative chemotherapy, radiation therapy, and surgery. A significant improvement has been the use of better biomaterials, implant design, and construction. The use of poly(methyl methacrylate) has afforded better fixation and stress distribution for previously inoperable fractures. The philosophy of early management of impending fractures through improved follow-up has decreased the morbidity commonly associated with the management of these patients.

Limb-Preserving Surgery in the Management of Bone Tumors

Management of patients with musculoskeletal neoplasms continues to be one of the most challenging areas in oncology. In recent years there have been great advances, including better understanding of the histologic criteria for diagnosis, better clinical staging procedures, and use of adjuvant treatments. All of these developments have contributed to our ability to perform more limb-sparing resections for neoplasms. Until recently, excision with a wide margin was reserved for aggressive benign or low-grade malignant tumors. In the past decade, successful use of adjuvant chemotherapy coupled with improved reconstructive techniques has stimulated increased interest in limb-saving procedures for high-grade malignant lesions as well.

For a limb-sparing procedure to be a viable alternative in the management of patients, it must meet two criteria. First, and most important, is local control of the tumor. This requires that the recurrence rate must be comparable to that with ablative surgery. Second, the resection must be compatible with maintenance of a functional status that is an improvement over the status after amputation and fitting of a prosthetic device.

Preoperative Assessment

When a patient presents with a bone sarcoma, thorough evaluation is necessary prior to deciding on limb salvage. Advances in preoperative investigative measures, particularly computed tomography and magnetic resonance imaging, have enhanced the ability to determine the exact extent of tumor involvement. This information is critical in choosing between amputation and limb-saving resection. Ideally, the tumor should involve only a short segment of the affected bone without extensive intramedullary involvement. Although cortical destruction with soft tissue extension (stage II-B) is present with most high-grade sarcomas, it is preferred that the soft tissue extension be small and located away from neurovascular structures. Generally, for the patient with a large lesion and soft tissue extension involving the neurovascular structures, amputation is selected.

Proper selection of patients with high-grade sarcomas for limb-saving resection is essential. The important factors are age and functional status of the patient, nature and grade of the lesion, extent of osseous destruction, and extent of soft tissue involvement. For the most part the reconstructive techniques used after the bone resection are applicable to patients whose epiphyses have closed. For children who are still growing, amputation is probably the most realistic surgical procedure; however, use of expandable or "growing" prostheses may extend the indications for limb salvage into younger age groups. In addition, excellent functional results are being obtained with the rotation-plasty procedure.

In the selection of the reconstructive method, there are various aspects to be considered. Many of these are purely medical, such as the patient's age, height, weight, general medical condition, expected survival, and intelligence. Other factors to be considered are the patient's socioeconomic status, education, training, and motivation. Finally, the patient's expectations are often the deciding factor and may require preoperative patient education and preparation.

The surgeon has preferences based on experience and training, and these may or may not provide the patient with a wide variety of options. In addition, the surgical facility may not have access to the necessary reconstructive armamentarium. However, such facilities do exist, and such procedures are best not performed by the surgeon who does only occasional tumor cases.

General Aspects of Surgical Techniques for Resection and Reconstruction

The success of limb-sparing procedures depends on achieving local control of the tumor and restoring useful function. Wide local excision of the lesion and the subsequent skeletal reconstruction are surgically demanding and should be performed according to well-established principles of oncologic surgery. The biopsy wound must be carefully planned and accurately placed so that it can be completely circumvented at the time of definitive resection. Contamination of multiple compartments by a poorly planned biopsy incision or by a hematoma after the biopsy may preclude a successful limb-sparing procedure.

The reconstruction after massive resection is a complex surgical problem that can be managed by various techniques, depending on location of the tumor. The simplest application of total resection without amputation may be used when the lesion is located in a totally or partially expendable bone that does not need replacement, such as a scapula, clavicle, or end of a fibula. It is important to evaluate these limb-sparing procedures separately for each area.

Knee

One of the most frequently encountered regions where a limb-sparing procedure may be feasible is the knee joint. Safe local control of a tumor with an appropriate surgical margin results in a large osseous or soft tissue defect. In this situation the reconstructive goal is to preserve as much function as possible but often this is a difficult surgical problem with no single answer. Various solutions to this problem have been described. Salvage of a mobile joint may be attempted by using either an allograft or a custom-made prosthetic replacement. Segmental reconstruction to achieve a knee arthrodesis can be performed with a local autogenous bone graft (either vascularized or nonvascularized), an intercalary allograft, a custom-made fiber-metal implant, or a combination of these.

Resection Resection of lesions of the proximal tibia or distal femur is carried out with the patient in a supine position. Preoperative assessment will determine whether the resection should be intra-articular or extra-articular. If an adequate margin can be achieved with an intra-articular resection, this is preferred because of the better functional result. However, large extracompartmental lesions involving the knee necessitate an extra-articular resection. A long, medial parapatellar incision reflecting the patella laterally is customary, but another approach may be dictated by location of the biopsy incision. The peroneal nerve is carefully protected laterally, as are the posterior neurovascular structures. For tibial lesions, the patellar tendon is detached and reflected upward. It also may be necessary to resect the proximal fibula with the specimen. An adequate *en bloc* resection requires removal of the distal femur or proximal tibia with its surrounding capsule, ligaments, and muscles. With lesions in the distal femur, this resection involves removal of a large portion of the vastus lateralis, vastus medialis, and vastus intermedius; the rectus femoris is preserved to provide extensor power. With a proximal tibial resection, a portion of the surrounding anterior tibial muscle group and the popliteus are sacrificed. If the patellar tendon has been detached, after the resection it is reattached with a staple.

Reconstruction ***Segmental Total Knee Arthroplasty*** The use of a custom-made segmental prosthesis in total knee replacement is effective in restoring skeletal continuity of either the distal femur or the proximal tibia while maintaining the function of the knee joint (Fig. 12). If the resection includes sacrificing the surrounding soft tissues, joint capsule, ligaments, and dynamic muscular stabilizers, the resulting lack of stability frequently requires a fully constrained type of implant for total knee replacement. Recently, improvements in the implant design of the fully constrained prostheses have resulted in adoption of the Kinematic rotating hinge. In addition, porous surface coating is incorporated in the segmental portion of the implant to enhance extracortical biologic fixation. It is hoped that these biomechanical improvements will be reflected in future clinical results.

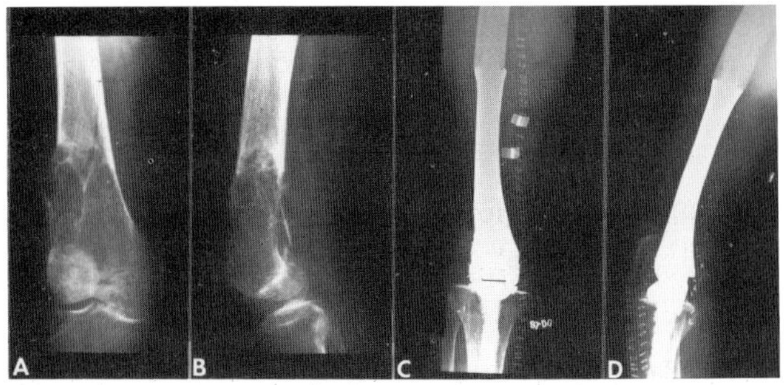

Figure 12

A and *B*, Anteroposterior and lateral views of left distal femur, showing extensive lytic destructive lesion. Open biopsy revealed a fibrosarcoma. *C* and *D*, Anteroposterior and lateral views of right distal femur after resection and custom total knee arthroplasty.

Prosthetic reconstruction has inherent advantages, particularly the maintenance of motion and immediate functional restoration. One would consider arthroplasty in patients who meet the following criteria: older age, high-grade malignant lesion, femoral lesion or intra-articular resection, limited life expectancy, and not suited for other reconstructive options. The early results have been satisfactory, but long-term survival of the prosthesis is an area of concern that limits widespread acceptance. Recent advances in implant design and the use of bone ingrowth materials to provide biologic fixation should improve the long-term results. The postoperative use of chemotherapy has encouraged the use of a prosthesis because one does not have to rely on bone graft incorporation. In one series of 41 custom knee prostheses, good or excellent results were reported in the majority, with preservation of motion (90%) and absence of pain (76%); however, 41% had significant complications including the necessity for revision in nine patients. The survival curve demonstrated the probability of failure of a custom arthroplasty to be 35% at 5 years and 42% at 8 years.

Osteochondral Allograft Increased emphasis has been placed on biologic reconstructive alternatives because of concerns involving the durability of prosthetic materials. This concern is increasing now because more patients with life-threatening sarcomas are expected to survive longer with the improvements in medical and surgical management. Many continue to prefer allograft replacement, but it is limited by availability and the complication and failure rates are still high, so it remains experimental. One would consider an osteoarticular allograft reconstruction for the young patient with an ideal weight who has a benign or low-grade malignant lesion and is unwilling to accept an arthrodesis. However, this biologic replacement should become increasingly useful (Fig. 13). Chemotherapy is always a concern when an allograft reconstruction is contemplated. There are data to suggest that chemotherapy and radiation therapy retard allograft "survival" but this does not contraindicate their use. For the most part, allograft reconstruction is better for aggressive benign tumors.

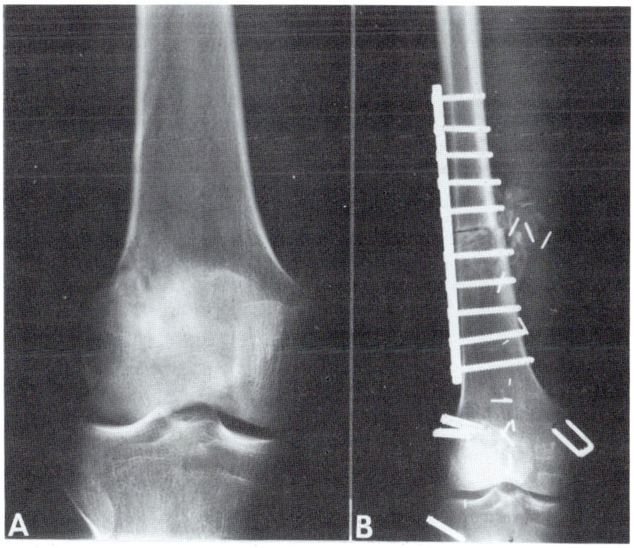

Figure 13

Anteroposterior radiographs of distal femur. *A,* Stage II-A osteosarcoma. *B,* After resection and allograft replacement. (B from Sim, F.H.; Bowman, W.E., Jr.; Wilkins, R.M.; and Chao, E.Y.S.: Limb salvage in primary malignant bone tumors. Orthopedics 8:574–581, 1985. By permission of Slack.)

Resection Arthrodesis One of the preferred methods of restoring skeletal continuity after resection of a lesion of the knee, particularly in a young and active patient, is segmental arthrodesis (Fig. 14). Although being unable to bend the knee is a functional handicap and an inconvenience to the patient, a segmental arthrodesis provides a stable, pain-free, weight-bearing extremity that will last the patient throughout life with the least restriction in strenuous walking and recreational activities. Indications for arthrodesis to restore skeletal continuity after resection of a lesion at the knee include: young age, active patient, and benign or aggressive benign lesion. With this technique, as with others, one can expect a significant rate of complications. Even though the patient is not able to bend the knee, 75% of the patients rate their result as good or excellent subjectively. These results reflect good patient selection and preoperative emotional preparation and acceptance of this procedure.

Various methods are available for achieving a segmental arthrodesis. Most popular is a hemicylindric sliding graft from the ipsilateral tibia or femur, augmented with a fibular graft. Considerable experience has been reported with this technique. Excellent results also have been achieved with an intercalary allograft segment (Fig. 15). Moreover, a vascularized fibular graft has advantages when a long segmental defect is to be reconstructed (Fig. 16). A vascularized free fibular graft may be combined with the femoral turn-down or tibial turn-up procedure. Preliminary experience with a fiber-metal prosthesis indicates great potential in achieving stability, with the prosthesis serving as a scaffold into which bone grafts grow and completely replace the osseous structure of the segmentally resected area to achieve extracortical fusion (Fig. 17). This technique has the advantage that the ipsilateral tibia or femur is not compromised and the technique is not technically demanding. Development of this custom implant into a modular system will lead to better utilization; however, this technique should remain experimental inasmuch as its advantages over other methods are not clear because of limited clinical experience.

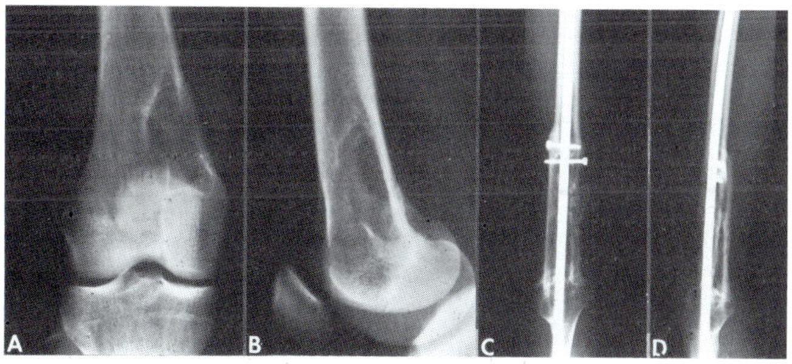

Figure 14

A and *B,* Anteroposterior and lateral radiographs, showing lytic destructive lesion in right distal femur. Open biopsy revealed malignant fibrous histiocytoma. *C* and *D,* Anteroposterior and lateral radiographs of distal femur after resection of tumor and segmental arthrodesis.

Proximal Femur

Currently, a great deal of interest has been shown in limb-saving resection involving the proximal femur because of the large functional loss associated with an amputation at this level.

Resection Resection of proximal femoral lesions is carried out with the patient in the lateral position, to give wide exposure. The femoral neurovascular structures are isolated anteriorly, and the sciatic nerve is isolated and protected posteriorly. The length of the proximal femoral resection depends on the extent of the osseous lesion as determined by preoperative bone scan and computed tomography. The lesion is removed with its surrounding muscles which usually include the psoas, adductor longus, adductor brevis, gluteus medius, and gluteus minimus and occasionally a large portion of the gluteus maximus.

Reconstruction Previous reconstructive techniques to restore skeletal continuity after wide excision of osseous hip lesions were plagued with prolonged morbidity and catastrophic complications such as infections, nonunion, fracture, and disintegration. Use of a fibula to salvage a mobile joint is doomed to failure because of the large weight-bearing stresses. Arthrodesis with a shortened extremity has also been used. However, development of proximal femoral replacement prostheses has opened new horizons for rehabilitation of these patients (Fig. 18). These have been effective in restoring the integrity of the proximal femur and preserving hip joint function. When the acetabulum can be spared, particularly in younger patients, a bipolar design can be used.

Allograft replacement of the proximal femur has few advocates. However, results of using an allograft as a sleeve around a prosthesis (bioimplant) have been encouraging. Generally, the allograft segment heals to the host bone and has the advantage of providing an osseous site for reattachment of the remaining functional muscles.

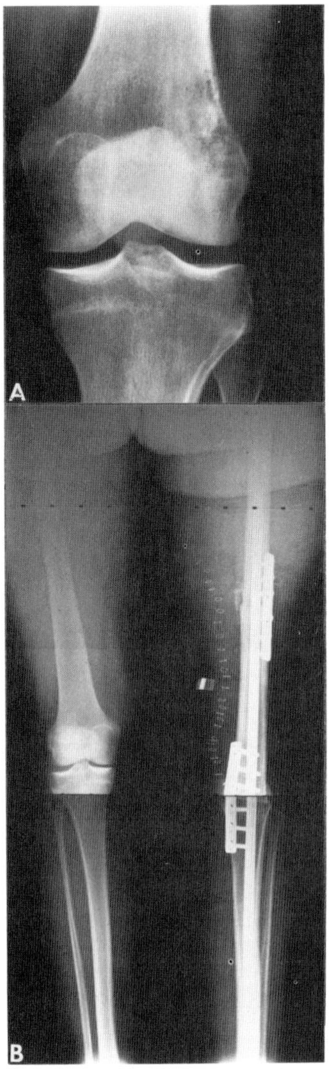

Figure 15

A, Anteroposterior radiograph of distal left femur, showing osteosarcoma. *B,* After reconstruction with an intercalary allograft segment. (From Sim, F.H.; Beauchamp, C.P.; and Chao, E.Y.S.: Reconstruction of musculoskeletal defects about the knee for tumor. Clin. Orthop. [in press]. By permission of J.B. Lippincott Company.)

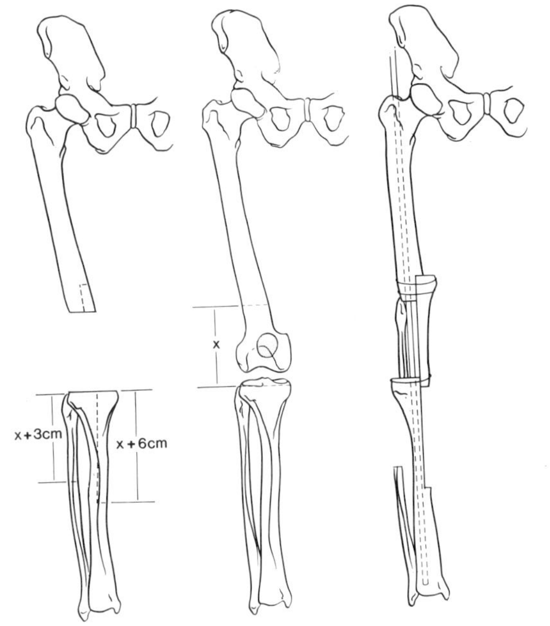

Figure 16

Diagrams of technique of resection arthrodesis with sliding tibial hemicylindric graft. (From Sim, F.H.; Beauchamp, C.P.; and Chao, E.Y.S.: Reconstruction of musculoskeletal defects about the knee for tumor. Clin. Orthop. [in press]. By permission of J.B. Lippincott Company.)

Pelvis

Primary malignant bone tumors of the pelvis present the most challenging problems in the field of oncology. These lesions generally carry a worse prognosis than more distal tumors. Moreover, hemipelvectomy, which has been the standard surgical treatment, is a debilitating and disfiguring procedure with a high incidence of postoperative morbidity. As a result, there is a great deal of interest in limb salvage for these lesions. In many cases, the surgical margin is similar to what might be achieved with an amputation.

Resection Resection of a lesion of the pelvis is performed with the patient positioned as for a hemipelvectomy. Extensive exposure provides access to both intrapelvic and extrapelvic structures. The incision begins at the posteroinferior iliac spine, follows the iliac crest and inguinal ligament, and then turns distally toward the anterolateral aspect of the thigh. If more exposure is needed, the incision may curve laterally and posteriorly at the junction of the proximal and middle thirds of the thigh. Furthermore, if the ischiopubic region needs to be exposed, a supplemental incision may be used along the remaining portion of the inguinal ligament. Large flaps are then developed, and the sciatic nerve and femoral neurovascular structures are identified and protected. The technique of resection will vary with location of the tumor in the pelvis.

Resections are classified into three groups, which is very helpful in planning the appropriate reconstruction. Type I resection involves the iliosacral or posterior region; when the surrounding gluteal musculature is resected, this becomes a type IA resection. Resection of the acetabulum is classified as type II. Preoperative staging must determine whether extra-articular resection is necessary; when this is performed the resection is classified as type IIA. Resection involving the ischiopubic region is classified as type III. Some large lesions occupy more than one region. The technical difficulty of the resection is increased when the tumor involves the sacroiliac joint or the acetabulum. In the posterior pelvis, a hemilaminectomy usually is required for adequate resection.

Reconstruction After resection, the method of reconstruction varies with the anatomic location of the lesion. After a type I resection involving the sacroiliac region, patients often do well with no reconstruction; however, it is generally preferred to close the defect and approximate the remaining pelvis to the sacrum by hinging the symphysis

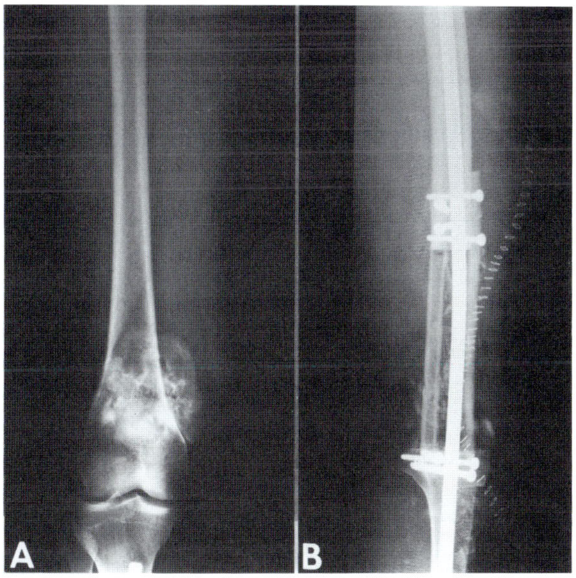

Figure 17

A, Anteroposterior radiograph of distal femur, showing large osteosarcoma. *B,* Reconstruction of distal femur with segmental arthrodesis using vascularized fibular grafts after resection of osteosarcoma. (From Sim, F.H.; Ivins, J.C.; Taylor, W.F.; Chao, E.Y.S.: Limb sparing surgery for osteosarcoma. Mayo Clinic experience. Cancer Treat. Symp. 3:139–154, 1985.)

pubis (Fig. 19). Fixation can be achieved with wires or screws and augmented with autogenous bone grafts. After a type IA resection, this type of reconstruction is necessary to restore function. Care must be taken to allow adequate room for the sciatic nerve to exit from the pelvis; this usually requires enlarging the inferior portion of the pelvis at this site.

A major problem of reconstruction develops when the lesion involves the acetabular region. If only a portion of the acetabulum is removed, the acetabulum may be reconstructed with autogenous bone grafts. However, when lesions involve the entire acetabulum and a total acetabular resection is necessary (type II), it is generally pre-

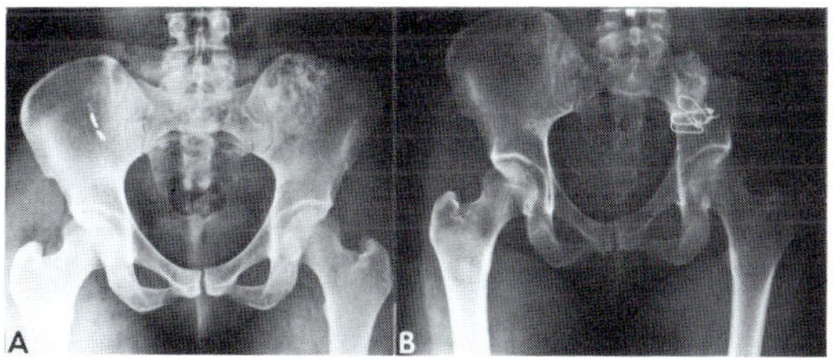

Figure 19

Anteroposterior radiographs of pelvis. *A,* Chondrosarcoma involving left sacroiliac region. *B,* After resection of chondrosarcoma and fusion of remaining ilium to the sacrum.

ferred to fuse the proximal femur to the remaining ilium (Fig. 20). If inadequate ilium remains after the resection (combined types I and II), the proximal femur may be stabilized against the ischium. When a lesion requires resection of the entire hemipelvis, the femur is usually left flail.

After resection of a lesion in the anterior pelvis (type III), usually reconstruction is not necessary unless a portion of the acetabulum has been resected.

Shoulder

Limb ablation for tumors about the shoulder is more devastating than its counterpart in the lower extremity. Prosthetic devices to compensate for shoulder disarticulation or forequarter amputation are cumbersome and do not allow independent function. Most patients prefer not to use them. This is particularly true if the dominant extremity is involved. If, while adhering to the general principles of oncologic surgery, one can resect the tumor involving the shoulder girdle without compromising the distal aspect of the extremity, the functional results will be infinitely better than can be achieved with any of the prosthetic devices now available.

Resection Resection of a lesion involving the shoulder girdle is carried out with the patient in the semi-sitting or lateral position. For resection to be successful, preoperative assessment must determine that there is a sufficient margin

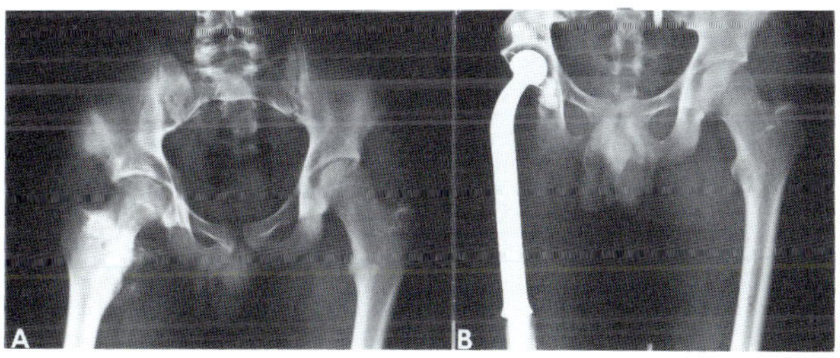

Figure 18

A, Anteroposterior radiograph of femur. *B,* After resection and proximal femoral replacement arthroplasty. (From Sim, F.H.; Bowman, W.E., Jr.; Wilkins, R.M.; and Chao, E.Y.S.: Limb salvage in primary malignant bone tumors. Orthopedics 8:574–581, 1985. By permission of Slack.)

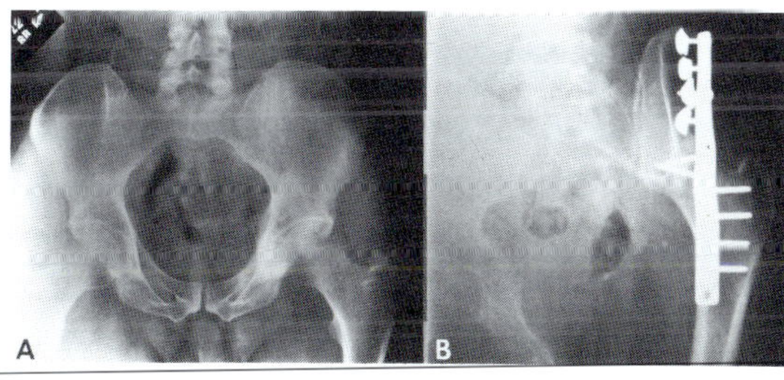

Figure 20

Anteroposterior radiographs of left hip. *A,* Chondrosarcoma involving the periacetabular region. *B,* After periacetabular resection and femoral iliac arthrodesis. (From Sim, F.H.; Bowman, W.E., Jr.; and Chao, E.Y.S.: Limb salvage and reconstructive techniques. *In* Diagnosis and Treatment of Bone Tumors: A Team Approach, edited by F.H. Sim, pp. 75–104. New Jersey, Slack, 1983. By permission of Mayo Foundation.)

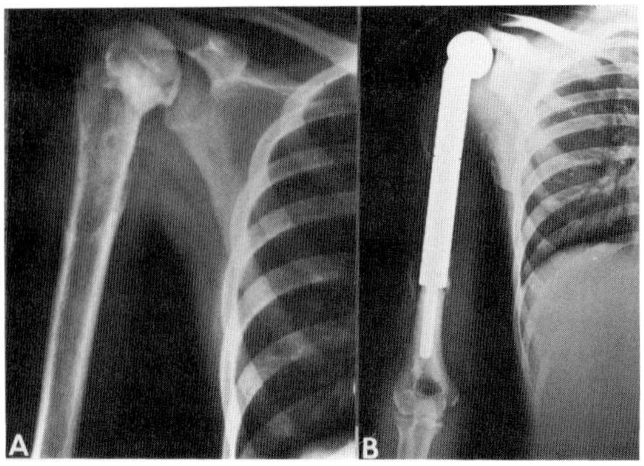

Figure 21

A, Proximal humerus, showing extensive destruction by an osteosarcoma. *B*, After resection and custom prosthetic replacement of the upper humerus.

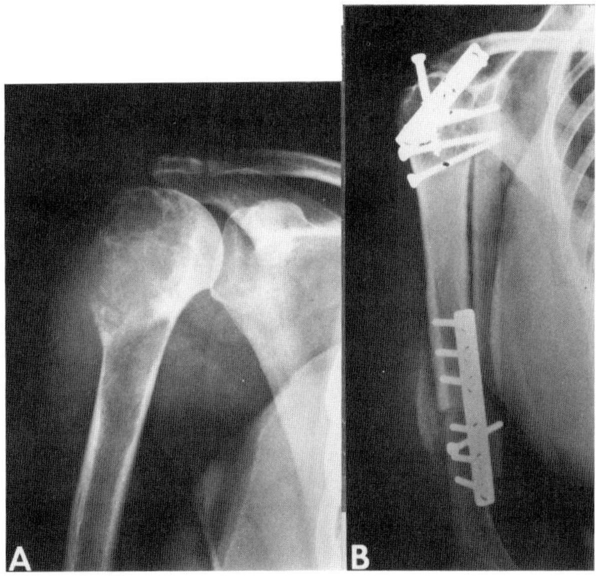

Figure 22

A, Right proximal humerus and shoulder, showing destruction by large chondrosarcoma. *B*, After removal of tumor and resection arthrodesis.

of normal tissue not involving the neurovascular structures. Most commonly the Tikhoff-Lindberg incision is used unless the biopsy site was poorly positioned and another incision is required. Large flaps are developed and, if indicated, the clavicle is resected to allow exposure of the neurovascular structures. With high-grade lesions, the resection generally involves removal of the rotator cuff as well as the overlying deltoid muscle and sacrificing the axillary nerve.

Reconstruction Resection of various osseous components of the shoulder girdle creates defects in function, mobility, and strength that correlate with the relative significance and contribution to the integrative function of the shoulder. Partial excision of the clavicle, including the acromioclavicular joint, creates minimal disability. A full range of motion is possible with a slight decrease in strength in abduction and forward flexion on resistance. Partial scapulectomy is still compatible with good powerful shoulder mobility because the articulations of the shoulder axis are maintained and much of the periarticular soft tissue is preserved. However, total scapulectomy requires removal and interruption of both shoulder articulations and excision of the soft tissues that stabilize and move the proximal humerus. In this instance, the active shoulder mobility is dramatically decreased and is not within functional limits.

When the proximal humerus together with the scapula and clavicle are resected (Tikhoff-Lindberg interscapulothoracic resection), the shoulder joint is left flail. Modification of this procedure includes use of an intramedullary nail or prosthesis to anchor the remaining segment of the humerus to the anterior chest wall or clavicle. The tendinous portions of the anterior and posterior musculature and remnants of the rotator cuff, latissimus dorsi, teres major, and pectoralis major are advanced under tension and sutured into the prosthesis, the chest wall, or themselves. Patients with this type of reconstruction after a Tikhoff-Lindberg resection have improved elbow mobility and strength. Use of a prosthesis in these instances also allows retention of length and bulk in the proximal aspect of the extremity and results in an improved cosmetic appearance.

Resection of the proximal humerus leaves a defect that may be reconstructed in various ways, and one of various bone grafting techniques may be utilized. However appealing the use of autogenous tissue, it has not enjoyed the success that one might expect. Delayed union, nonunion, resorption, and fatigue fractures are common problems and contribute to the lack of success with singular fibular replacements. Dual fibular grafts are more suitable to the stresses in the area. With recent advances in microsurgical techniques, a vascularized fibular placement may be an alternative.

Allografts may be useful with benign or low-grade malignant lesions. This biologic spacer provides a structure to which soft tissue can be reattached. Moreover, combining the allograft with a prosthesis (bioimplant) to provide improved strength and an articulating surface is becoming more popular. There is considerable experience with the proximal humeral placement endoprosthesis (Fig. 21). The purpose of the prosthesis in these cases is to act as a spacer that will provide a stable fulcrum through which the distal aspect of the extremity can function. To this end, use of a proximal humerus prosthesis has been successful. Most patients continue to enjoy full mobility and use of the elbow, wrist, and hand.

Although resection arthrodesis of the shoulder is difficult and arduous and healing time is prolonged, it is the only procedure that is compatible with restoration of function, mobility, and strength at the shoulder after wide local excision for tumors. It is generally preferred to use this extensive procedure when there is a good chance for a cure and to use prosthetic replacement for patients with high-risk life-threatening sarcomas. When the patient is thought to have survived the sarcoma, more extensive reconstruction with a resection arthrodesis can be carried out if necessary. Various techniques can be used to achieve the arthrodesis. One method uses dual nonvascularized fibular grafts with internal fixation provided by a custom plate. A more recent technique utilizes an intercalary allograft, to provide immediate stability and fixation, combined with a vascularized fibular graft for its biologic healing potential (Fig. 22). Although resection arthrodesis of the shoulder is an extensive surgical procedure, the functional results justify its use.

Comment

The use of these limb-sparing procedures in patients with bone tumors remains a highly selective process. For limb salvage to represent a viable alternative in the management of primary bone tumors, the outcome must compare favorably with that after the standard oncologic surgical practice of amputation. It therefore must afford the potential for improvement in function achieved with prosthetic devices while not jeopardizing the patient's life by increasing the potential for recurrent disease. The latter is by far the more important consideration. It is becoming increasingly clear that limb salvage offers a successful alternative to mutilating and often crippling amputation. In comparing the different techniques of reconstruction that are available after tumor resection, many clinical and functional factors must be considered. Experience indicates that, for each location, there are various reconstructive procedures that promise utility and functional restoration but the procedure selected should be tailored to the needs of the patient. The musculoskeletal oncologic surgeon must have the versatility to choose among surgical options to treat this challenging problem.

Annotated Bibliography

The Biopsy

Mankin, H.J.; Lange, T.A.; and Spanier, S.S.: The hazards of biopsy in patients with malignant primary bone and soft-tissue tumors. J. Bone Joint Surg. 64A:1121–1127, 1982.

This retrospective study performed by the Musculoskeletal Tumor Society reviewed information on 329 patients with lesions of bone and soft tissue. Results in 143 patients biopsied by referring institutions and 171 patients biopsied in treating centers are compared. Biopsy-related problems occurred 3 to 5 times more frequently when biopsies were performed at referring institutions.

Simon, M.A.: Biopsy of musculoskeletal tumors. J. Bone Joint Surg. 64A:1253–1257, 1982.

The criteria for evaluating and biopsying patients with musculoskeletal tumors are described. Current concepts in staging patients with musculoskeletal neoplasms are also discussed.

Osteosarcoma

Goorin, A.M.; Abelson, H.T.; and Frei, E., III: Osteosarcoma: Fifteen years later. N. Engl. J. Med. 313:1637–1643, 1985.

The past 15 years of experience with osteosarcoma are reviewed (99 references).

Link, M.; Goorin, A.; Miser, A.; Green, A.; Pratt, C.; Belasco, J.; Pritchard, J.; Baker, A.; Kirkpatrick, J.; Ayala, A.; Shuster, J.; Abelson, H.; Simone, J.; and Vietti, T.: The role of adjuvant chemotherapy in the treatment of osteosarcoma (OS) of the extremity: Preliminary results of the Multi-Institutional Osteosarcoma Study (MIOS) (abstract). Proc. Annu. Meet. Am. Soc. Clin. Oncol. 4:237, 1985.

This reports the results of a prospective study of patients treated with a six-drug adjuvant therapy regimen or with surgery alone. The 2-year actuarial disease-free survival was 18% for patients with surgery alone and 56% for those in the chemotherapy group.

Martinez, A.; Goffinet, D.R.; Donaldson, S.S.; Bagshaw, M.A.; and Kaplan, H.S.: Intra-arterial infusion of radiosensitizer (BUdR) combined with hypofractionated irradiation and chemotherapy for primary treatment of osteogenic sarcoma. Int. J. Radiat. Oncol. Biol. Phys. 11:123–128, 1985.

The use of intra-arterial radiosensitizers combined with hypofractional irradiation and chemotherapy is discussed. These innovative techniques may be of use in the future in patients with nonresectable osteosarcoma.

National Institutes of Health, Consensus Development Panel: Limb-sparing treatment of adult soft-tissue sarcomas and osteosarcomas. J.A.M.A. 254:1791–1794, 1985.

The results of the Consensus Conference on Limb-Sparing Treatment of Adult Soft-Tissue and Osteosarcomas, held December 3–5, 1984, are reviewed. The conference considered the results in over 2,000 patients with high-grade sarcomas and concluded that limb-sparing treatment programs are clearly established and have been shown to be appropriate and feasible options.

Winkler, K.; Beron, G.; Kotz, R.; Salzer-Kuntschik, M.; Beck, J.; Beck, W.; Brandeis, W.; Ebell, W.; Erttmann, R.; Göbel, U.; Havers, W.; Henze, G.; Hinderfeld, L.; Höcker, P.; Jobke, A.; Jürgens, H.; Kabisch, H.; Preusser, P.; Prindull, G.; Ramach, W.; Ritter, J.; Sekera, J.; Treuner, J.; Wüst, G.; and Landbeck, G.: Neoadjuvant chemotherapy for osteogenic sarcoma: Results of a Cooperative German/Austrian study. J. Clin. Oncol. 2:617–624, 1984.

The preliminary results of a study by the German Society of Pediatric Oncology (COSS-80) are reported. The median survival at 19.5 months was 73% for 116 patients. These results suggest a beneficial effect from systemic chemotherapy performed in a multi-institutional setting.

Ewing's Sarcoma

Bacci, G.; Picci, P.; Gherlinzoni, F.; Capanna, R.; Calderoni, P.; Putti, C.; Mancini, A.; and Campanacci, M.: Localized Ewing's sarcoma of bone: Ten years' experience at the Istituto Ortopedico Rizzoli in 124 cases treated with multimodal therapy. Eur. J. Cancer Clin. Oncol. 21:163–173, 1985.

The results of multimodality treatment of 124 patients with Ewing's sarcoma are reported. At a median follow-up of 65 months, 48% were disease-free. Those patients with nonpelvic primary lesions managed by four-drug chemotherapy and surgery had the best overall result.

Evans, R.G.; Nesbit, M.; Askin, F.; Burgert, E.O., Jr.; Cangir, A.; Foulkes, M.; Gehan, E.; Gilula, L.; Kissane, J.; Makley, J.; Neff, J.; Perez, C.; Pritchard, D.J.; Tefft, M.; Thomas, P.; and Vietti, T.: Local recurrence, rate and sites of metastases, and time to relapse as a function of treatment regimen, size of primary and surgical history in 62 patients presenting with non-metastatic Ewing's sarcoma of the pelvic bones. Int. J. Radiat. Oncol. Biol. Phys. 11:129–136, 1985.

This paper reports the experience with 62 patients with nonmetastatic Ewing's sarcoma of the pelvis (IESS-I). The overall poor prognosis of pelvic primary lesions is discussed and the multifactorial analysis is described.

Hayes, F.A.; Thompson, E.I.; Hustu, H.O.; Kumar, M.; Coburn, T.; and Webber, B.: The response of Ewing's sarcoma to sequential cyclophosphamide and Adriamycin induction therapy. J. Clin. Oncol. 1:45–51, 1983.

The results in 19 patients managed at St. Jude Children's Research Hospital by using cyclophosphamide and doxorubicin induction therapy are reviewed. The roles of cytoreduction chemotherapy, limited surgery, and reduced radiation therapy portals are discussed.

Lewis, R.J.; Marcove, R.C.; and Rosen, G.: Ewing's sarcoma: Functional effects of radiation therapy. J. Bone Joint Surg. 59A:325–331, 1977.

The long-term morbidity was assessed in 55 patients who had Ewing's sarcoma and survived at least 2 years. The authors recommended that patients with upper extremity lesions be managed by radiation therapy; selected cases (younger patients and some older patients with lesions in the lower extremity) generally were best treated by primary amputation.

Springfield, D.S., and Pagliarulo, C.: Fractures of long bones previously treated for Ewing's sarcoma. J. Bone Joint Surg. 67A:477–481, 1985.

The authors describe the results in 28 patients with Ewing's sarcoma followed for a minimum of 2 years. Nine patients had primary lesions in the ulna, radius, tibia, and fibula, and none had late pathologic fracture. Of the remaining patients, eight had pathologic fractures. Those patients managed by early internal fixation and bone grafting appeared to have the best overall functional result.

Thomas, P.R.M.; Perez, C.A.; Neff, J.R.; Nesbit, M.E.; and Evans, R.G.: The management of Ewing's sarcoma: Role of radiotherapy in local tumor control. Cancer Treat. Rep. 68:703–710, 1984.

The role of radiation therapy in the management of Ewing's sarcoma is reviewed. Radiotherapy and surgery are compared as modalities for local control.

Chondrosarcoma

Bjornsson, J.; Unni, K.K.; Dahlin, D.C.; Beabout, J.W.; and Sim, F.H.: Clear cell chondrosarcoma of bone: Observations in 47 cases. Am. J. Surg. Pathol. 8:223–230, 1984.

The authors reviewed their experience in the management of 47 patients with clear cell chondrosarcoma. The lesion is more common in males (2.6:1) and has a propensity to develop in long bones. *En bloc* excision with a cuff of normal tissue appears to be the treatment of choice.

Kreicbergs, A.; Boquist, L.; Borssén, B.; and Larsson, S.-E.: Prognostic factors in chondrosarcoma: A comparative study of cellular DNA content and clinicopathologic features. Cancer 50:577–583, 1982.

A retrospective analysis of 45 surgically treated chondrosarcomas with respect to the prognostic significance of cellular DNA content and different clinicopathologic factors is described. The results indicated that ploidy probably is the best predictor of the clinical course in chondrosarcoma.

Pritchard, D.J.; Lunke, R.J.; Taylor, W.F.; Dahlin, D.C.; and Medley, B.E.: Chondrosarcoma: A clinicopathologic and statistical analysis. Cancer 45:149–157, 1980.

The authors report a clinicopathologic study of 280 patients with chondrosarcoma of the spine, limb girdle, and limbs. Size of the primary tumor and histopathologic grade were the most significant prognostic factors.

Mesenchymal Chondrosarcoma

Bertoni, F.; Picci, P.; Bacchini, P.; Capanna, R.; Innao, V.; Bacci, G.; and Campanacci, M.: Mesenchymal chondrosarcoma of bone and soft tissues. Cancer 52:533–541, 1983.

The clinicopathologic features of seven patients with mesenchymal chondrosarcoma are reported. Five tumors were in bone and two were in soft tissue. Six patients were treated surgically and had no local recurrence. No patient survived more than 4 years.

Huvos, A.G.; Rosen, G.; Dabska, M.; and Marcove, R.C.: Mesenchymal chondrosarcoma: A clinicopathologic analysis of 35 patients with emphasis on treatment. Cancer 51:1230–1237, 1983.

Thirty-five patients with mesenchymal chondrosarcoma (30 in the skeleton) were evaluated. The authors report that the "hemangiopericytoid" variant responds well to radiation therapy and chemotherapy, suggesting a role for these modalities in the treatment program.

Giant Cell Tumor of Bone

Goldenberg, R.R.; Campbell, C.J.; and Bonfiglio, M.: Giant-cell tumor of bone: An analysis of two hundred and eighteen cases. J. Bone Joint Surg. 52A:619–663, 1970.

An analysis of 218 cases of giant cell tumor of bone, including the clinical presentation, radiographic description, and treatment, is reported. This thorough analysis still is one of the most complete discussions of this unusual entity available.

Jacobs, P.A., and Clemency, R.E., Jr.: The closed cryosurgical treatment of giant cell tumor. Clin. Orthop. 192:149–158, 1985.

Twelve patients managed by closed cryotherapy, curettage, and bone grafting were reviewed retrospectively. The treatment techniques are outlined. Five patients had six postoperative pathologic fractures; however, only two lesions recurred.

Johnston, G.A.; Simon, M.A.; and Azizi, F.: Giant cell tumors of bone in pregnancy: Report of two cases. J. Reprod. Med. 24:43–45, 1980.

Two patients with biopsy-proved giant cell tumor of bone associated with pregnancy were reviewed. In general, the results of follow-up suggest that termination of pregnancy was not indicated.

Persson, B.M.; Ekelund, L.; Lövdahl, R.; and Gunterberg, B.: Favourable results of acrylic cementation for giant cell tumors. Acta Orthop. Scand. 55:209–214, 1984.

The clinical results in 14 patients with giant cell tumor of bone treated with curettage and cementation are reviewed. Two of 14 tumors recurred, and both were treated with cementation. Joint function was normal in 11 patients and only 2 had radiographic changes of degenerative osteoarthritis.

Malignant Fibrous Histiocytoma

Capanna, R.; Bertoni, F.; Bacchini, P.; Bacci, G.;

Guerra, A.; and Campanacci, M.: Malignant fibrous histiocytoma of bone: The experience at the Rizzoli Institute: Report of 90 cases. Cancer 54:177–187, 1984.

Ninety patients with malignant fibrous histiocytoma of bone were observed at the Rizzoli Institute between 1940 and 1981. Sixty-eight with nonmetastatic disease had surgical therapy; 20 also received chemotherapy. Use of adjuvant chemotherapy improved survival but was not effective in preventing local recurrence in patients with inadequate surgery.

den Heeten, G.J.; Koops, H.S.; Kamps, W.A.; Oosterhuis, J.W.; Sleijfer, D.T.; and Oldhoff, J.: Treatment of malignant fibrous histiocytoma of bone: A plea for primary chemotherapy. Cancer 56:37–40, 1985.

The authors report their results of treatment of seven patients with malignant fibrous histiocytoma of bone. Two patients had either no or partial treatment with chemotherapy after surgery, and both died (7 and 51 months after diagnosis). The five remaining patients completed chemotherapy; three patients received neoadjuvant chemotherapy. All five patients were alive with a mean follow-up of 45 months, suggesting a definite role for chemotherapy.

McCarthy, E.F.; Matsuno, T.; and Dorfman, H.D.: Malignant fibrous histiocytoma of bone: A study of 35 cases. Hum. Pathol. 10:57–70, 1979.

Thirty-five cases of primary malignant fibrous histiocytoma of bone are reviewed. Twenty-one patients had a minimum of 3 years of follow-up; 9 patients were free of disease, 2 were alive with disease, and 10 were dead. In four patients, the lesions were multicentric and in four they were associated with bone infarcts.

Chordoma

Bottles, K., and Beckstead, J.H.: Enzyme histochemical characterization of chordomas. Am. J. Surg. Pathol. 8:443–447, 1984.

Four cases of chordoma were characterized by enzyme histochemistry. All chordomas exhibited strong 5′-nucleotidase positivity, providing a marker to differentiate chordoma from other neoplasms of similar appearance.

Kaiser, T.E.; Pritchard, D.J.; and Unni, K.K.: Clinicopathologic study of sacrococcygeal chordoma. Cancer 53:2574–2578, 1984.

Sixty-three patients underwent surgical therapy for sacral chordoma at the Mayo Clinic between 1952 and 1979. Local recurrence occurred in only 28% of 25 patients treated with adequate surgical margins; recurrence rate was 64% in 25 patients in whom the tumor was entered at the time of surgery. The authors concluded that aggressive surgery is indicated.

Mindell, E.R.: Chordoma. J. Bone Joint Surg. 63A:501–505, 1981.

The author describes and discusses the present concepts of diagnosis and management of patients with chordoma.

Rich, T.A.; Schiller, A.; Suit, H.D.; and Mankin, H.J.: Clinical and pathologic review of 48 cases of chordoma. Cancer 56:182–187, 1985.

The results of treatment of 48 patients with the diagnosis of chordoma at the Massachusetts General Hospital are reviewed. The results of surgical therapy, radiation therapy, and combination therapy are discussed. The 5-year actuarial survival rate was 76% for patients treated surgically and 50% for those given radiation therapy.

Secondary and Treatment-Related Sarcomas of Bone

Huvos, A.G.; Woodard, H.Q.; Cahan, W.G.; Higinbotham, N.L.; Steward, F.W.; Butler, A.; and Bretsky, S.S.: Postradiation osteogenic sarcoma of bone and soft tissues: A clinicopathologic study of 66 patients. Cancer 55:1244–1255, 1985.

Sixty-six patients with secondary radiation-induced osteosarcoma are reviewed. Postirradiation osteogenic sarcomas most commonly arose in bones about the shoulder and pelvic region. The 5-year cumulative disease-free survival rate was 17%.

Meadows, A.T.; Strong, L.C.; Li, F.P.; D'Angio, G.J.; Schweisguth, O.; Freeman, A.I.; Jenkin, R.D.T.; Morris-Jones, P.; and Nesbit, M.E.: Bone sarcoma as a second malignant neoplasm in children: Influence of radiation and genetic predisposition. Cancer 46:2603–2606, 1980.

Forty of 188 patients who had secondary chondrosarcoma or osteosarcoma are analyzed. All had neoplasms previously managed during childhood. A greater susceptibility was found in 23 which appeared to hasten the onset of secondary malignancies.

Schmähl, D.; Habs, M.; Lorenz, M.; and Wagner, I.: Occurrence of second tumors in man after anticancer drug treatment. Cancer Treat. Rev. 9:167–194, 1982.

The authors discuss reported cases of secondary treatment-related malignancies in which sufficient data were available to permit review of dosage and latent period. This detailed report correlates total drug dosage with diagnosis and latent period.

Weatherby, R.P.; Dahlin, D.C.; and Ivins, J.C.: Postradiation sarcoma of bone: Review of 78 Mayo Clinic cases. Mayo Clin. Proc. 56:294–306, 1981.

Seventy-eight patients developing postirradiation sarcomas in irradiated bones are extensively reviewed. Analysis of the clinical presentation, pathology, and treatment indicates that prompt radical surgery is the treatment of choice when possible.

Soft Tissue Sarcoma

Eilber, F.R.; Eckhardt, J.; and Morton, D.L.: Advances in the treatment of sarcomas of the extremity: Current status of limb salvage. Cancer 54:2695–2701, 1984.

The current status of multimodality treatment of extremity lesions is reviewed. The role of neoadjuvant chemotherapy is outlined along with the routes of administration.

Rydholm, A.: Management of patients with soft tissue tumors: Strategy developed at a regional oncology center. Acta Orthop. Scand. [Suppl.] 203:3–76, 1983.

This extensive review of the management of patients with soft tissue sarcomas constitutes the majority of up-to-date opinions on current surgical therapy of patients with soft tissue tumors.

Carcinoma Metastatic to Bone

Fidler, I.J., and Hart, I.R.: Biological diversity in metastatic neoplasms: Origins and implications. Science 217:998–1003, 1982.

This excellent, well-referenced, review article describes the pathogenesis of the process of metastasis.

Fidler, M.: Prophylactic internal fixation of secondary neoplastic deposits in long bones. Br. Med. J. 1:341–343, 1973.

The author retrospectively reviewed 19 patients in whom metastasis to bone was managed. Those lesions associated with pain and larger than 2.5 cm in diameter were commonly associated with spontaneous pathologic fracture. The author recommends prophylactic fixation of these lesions.

Mundy, G.R.; Ibbotson, K.J.; D'Souza, S.M.; Simpson, E.L.; Jacobs, J.W.; and Martin, T.J.: The hypercalcemia of cancer: Clinical implications and pathogenic mechanisms. N. Engl. J. Med. 310:1718–1727, 1984.

The authors review the present knowledge regarding the hypercalcemia of cancer. The subject is developed from clinical presentation and mechanisms of action to treatment. There are 114 references.

Limb Salvage

General

Jaffe, N.; Watts, H.; Fellows, K.E.; and Vawter, G.: Local en bloc resection for limb preservation. Cancer Treat. Rep. 62:217–223, 1978.

Preoperative chemotherapy combined with local *en bloc* resection allows limb preservation without recurrence. The chemotherapy used included high-dose methotrexate, vincristine, and citrovorum factor.

Johnston, J.O.: Local resection in primary malignant bone tumors. Clin. Orthop. 153:73–80, 1980.

A general overview of the indications and technical considerations for resection about the hip and knee.

Mankin, H.J.; Doppelt, S.H.; Sullivan, T.R.; and Tomford, W.W.: Osteoarticular and intercalary allograft transplantation in the management of malignant tumors of bone. Cancer 50:613–630, 1982.

One hundred six patients were treated with wide resection and allograft replacement. In the 45 with adequate follow-up, 74% had successful transplants, 13% had infections, 10% required bracing, and 10% had pathologic fractures.

Nilsonne, U.: Limb-preserving radical surgery for malignant bone tumors. Clin. Orthop. 191:21–26, 1984.

The well-planned, adequately staged, *en bloc* resection of a malignant tumor need not compromise a patient's survival or increase the risk of local recurrence and can be functionally superior to amputation.

Parrish, F.F.: Treatment of bone tumors by total excision and replacement with massive autologous and homologous grafts. J. Bone Joint Surg. 48A:968–990, 1966.

An Instructional Course Lecture that thoroughly reviews the indications for *en bloc* resection and describes the various surgical techniques for osteochondral allografting around the knee, distal forearm, and proximal humerus.

Wilson, P.D., and Lance, E.M.: Surgical reconstruction of the skeleton following segmental resection for bone tumors. J. Bone Joint Surg. 47A:1629–1656, 1965.

An Instructional Course Lecture that gives an in-depth consideration of the reconstruction necessary after tumor resection. Various methods for reconstruction of upper and lower limbs are reviewed.

Knee

Campanacci, M., and Costa, P.: Total resection of distal femur or proximal tibia for bone tumours: Autogenous bone grafts and arthrodesis in twenty-six cases. J. Bone Joint Surg. 61B:455–463, 1979.

Twenty-six patients underwent *en bloc* resection of tumors about the knee, and the defects were reconstructed with an intramedullary rod and autogenous bone to achieve arthrodesis. Ninety-two percent achieved union; 20% had infection.

Enneking, W.F., and Shirley, P.D.: Resection-arthrodesis for malignant and potentially malignant lesions about the knee using an intramedullary rod and local bone grafts. J. Bone Joint Surg. 59A:223–236, 1977.

Twenty patients with aggressive tumors about the knee were treated by local resection and arthrodesis with an intramedullary rod and autogenous segmental cortical grafts from the same limb. Normal activity was resumed by 1 year.

Sim, F.H., and Chao, E.Y.S.: Prosthetic replacement of the knee and a large segment of the femur or tibia. J. Bone Joint Surg. 61A:887–892, 1979.

Total replacement of the knee and a long segment of the femur or tibia (75–150 mm) in 13 patients provided a stable extremity, excellent relief of pain, and a useful range of motion.

Hip

Dobbs, H.S.; Scales, J.T.; Wilson, J.N.; Kemp, H.B.S.; Burrows, H.J.; and Sneath, R.S.: Endoprosthetic replacement of the proximal femur and acetabulum: A survival analysis. J. Bone Joint Surg. 63B:219–224, 1981.

Eighty-one patients underwent reconstruction with an endoprosthesis after proximal femoral resection. Sixty-three percent of the prostheses survived 10 years. The survival of patients with chondrosarcoma and osteoclastoma compared favorably with survival after amputation or excision of the tumor.

Sim, F.H., and Chao, E.Y.S.: Segmental prosthetic replacement of the hip and knee. *In* Tumor Prostheses for Bone and Joint Reconstruction: The Design and Application, edited by E.Y.-S. Chao and J.C. Ivins, pp. 247–266. New York, Thieme-Stratton, 1983.

Segmental total joint replacement was successful in providing joint functional recovery of the hip in 55 patients. The length of the replacement varied from 80 to 250 mm. Good functional results were obtained.

Pelvis

Enneking, W.F., and Dunham, W.K.: Resection and reconstruction for primary neoplasms involving the innominate bone. J. Bone Joint Surg. 60A:731–746, 1978.

Oncologically adequate procedures were performed in two-thirds of the cases. In the remaining cases, the adequacy of the procedure was compromised by poor biopsies, occult microextensions, and surgical error. Recurrence rate after inadequate procedures was 100%; it was 4% after adequate procedures. Three types of pelvic procedures were performed: resection of the iliac wing, periacetabular resection, and resection of the pubis.

Steel, H.H.: Partial or complete resection of the hemipelvis: An alternative to hindquarter amputation for periacetabular chondrosarcoma of the pelvis. J. Bone Joint Surg. 60A:719–730, 1978.

After excision of the hemipelvis with preservation of the lower extremity, five patients with periacetabular chondrosarcoma were able to walk with no support or with minimal lateral support (follow-up, 3 to 6 years).

6
Infection

The microbiology of musculoskeletal infections is increasingly associated with the isolation of methacillin-resistant staphylococci, especially *Staphylococcus epidermidis.* Although the short-term use of perioperative antibiotics and the use of unidirectional airflow operating rooms have decreased the incidence of postoperative wound sepsis, sepsis continues to complicate musculoskeletal surgery. This topic and newer techniques in the diagnosis and surgical treatment of osteomyelitis, biofilms, the role of poly(methyl methacrylate), and nutrition in postoperative sepsis are covered in this chapter.

Microbiology

The bacteria most frequently causing infections of the musculoskeletal system associated with surgery and trauma in adults and hematogenous infections in children still are the staphylococci. When perioperative antibiotic coverage is administered for clean operative procedures, *Staphylococcus epidermidis* is the most frequent organism causing infection, especially when implants are placed. *S. aureus* commonly causes such infections as well but is more common in infections associated with trauma. Gram-negative bacilli also are commonly associated with infections after trauma. In children, *S. aureus* is the most common causative organism of both osteomyelitis and septic arthritis, but infections caused by *Pseudomonas aeruginosa, Haemophilus influenzae,* and streptococcal organisms are not unusual in this age group.

Before optimal treatment can be given, it is essential to isolate the causative bacteria and to determine which antimicrobial agents are most effective against them. Patterns of antibiotic resistance continue to change; reliance on expected antibiotic effectiveness against a given organism will result in an increased incidence of treatment failure. Increasing numbers of *S. epidermidis* are resistant to methicillin; some routine laboratory techniques will suggest that these organisms are sensitive to cephalosporins but none of them should be considered sensitive. Some gram-negative bacilli that are resistant to second- and third-generation cephalosporins are becoming apparent. *Bacteroides* species other than *B. fragilis* and clostridia other than *Clostridium perfringens* that are resistant to penicillin are being found with increasing frequency. Some routine laboratory techniques will not detect true resistance patterns, and in these circumstances it is essential to utilize macrotube broth dilution techniques for 24 or, preferably, 48 hours of growth; in some instances disk diffusion and agar diffusion techniques will be effective.

Antimicrobial Agents

Perioperative Use in Clean Orthopaedic Cases

During the past 15 years, evidence has accumulated to demonstrate the effectiveness of perioperative use of antimicrobial agents to decrease the incidence of infection in operations involving total joint replacement or internal fixation of hip fractures. For clean cases, in most institutions the first-generation cephalosporins remain the most effective prophylactic agents because of their effectiveness against staphylococci and against many gram-negative bacilli.

An evaluation of antimicrobial concentrations in blood, muscle, and hematoma in patients undergoing operation for femoral fractures has demonstrated that cefazolin reached concentration levels 2 times higher than those of either cefamandole or cefoxitin in the tissues evaluated. In the same study, all three agents penetrated hematoma adequately without correlation with the duration of time from injury to administration of the agent. In a study evaluating cefamandole and cephalothin in the treatment of experimental staphylococcal osteomyelitis, cefamandole had an increased concentration in bone but also had increased inactivation by β-lactamase. Animals treated with cephalothin had a better clinical course, with significantly more weight gain and less severe infection than those treated with cefamandole. This improved course with cephalothin probably can be explained on the basis of the increased stability of this agent despite the high level of β-lactamase associated with a high level of *S. aureus* contamination. Of the first-generation cephalosporins, cefazolin is the preferred agent because of its higher peak serum value, longer half-life, and lower cost.

A recent well-controlled study demonstrated that the infection rate in patients undergoing amputation of the lower extremity for ischemia was decreased by using cefoxitin, beginning 30 minutes before operation and continuing for 24 hours. In the patients who received placebo, there were eight clostridial infections and three of these patients died. There were no clostridial infections and no deaths in the patients who received cefoxitin.

For prophylactic use to prevent infection in clean operative cases, the antimicrobial agent should be administered just prior to operation and for 24 to 48 hours postoperatively. There are no controlled studies to demonstrate the effectiveness of shorter duration of administration, although it may be that shorter administration would be as effective. Continuation of administration for a long period of time not only is unnecessary but, in fact, may be harmful because of increased incidence of toxicity from the agent, increased incidence of infection due to changes in bacterial flora, and general increase in bacteria with resistance to the antimicrobial agent. In addition to the orthopaedic operative procedures for which prophylactic antimicrobial therapy has been shown to decrease infection rate, it may be reasonable to consider using it in patients undergoing other procedures of long duration involving implants or extensive bone and joint exposure. The risks of prophylactic antimicrobial use may outweigh the benefits in patients undergoing procedures of short duration, particularly those involving only soft tissue.

Complications of Antimicrobial Administration

Hypersensitivity reaction is the most common complication of the penicillin and cephalosporin agents; there is significant cross sensitivity between the penicillins and the cephalosporins. If it is important to use an agent to which the patient reports a sensitivity, skin testing should be performed to verify the history. Patients can be desensitized as is done with other allergenic materials. Ototoxicity and renal toxicity remain the major complications associated with the aminoglycosides. These complications can be greatly decreased by establishing dosage regimens based on peak and trough serum levels measured once or twice a week and serum creatinine measured every other day. One of the first indications of renal toxicity is an increasing serum trough level; if this occurs the dosage should be decreased or the time interval between doses should be increased, or both. Careful clinical history and examination should be repeated frequently to determine if the patient is developing any signs of vestibular or hearing dysfunction. In those patients in whom toxicity is suspected, audiograms may be helpful. Significant bleeding problems have been associated with both carbenicillin and moxalactam; similar complications have occurred less frequently with many other antimicrobial agents. Patients receiving these agents must be observed for this complication.

Pseudomembranous colitis was originally reported to be associated with administration of clindamycin but since then it has been found with many different antimicrobial agents including cephalosporins. Any patient who is receiving moderate- to long-term administration of an antimicrobial agent and develops significant diarrhea should be checked by culture for *Clostridium difficile.* A serum titer method for the detection of *C. difficile* infections has been adapted for clinical use. The appropriate treatment for infection with this organism includes intravenous administration of fluids as supportive therapy and oral administration of vancomycin. If the involvement is severe, proctoscopic examination may be helpful to determine if steroids should be administered.

Changing Patterns of Resistance to Antimicrobial Agents

There has been an increasing incidence of methicillin-resistant *S. epidermidis;* these organisms are not sensitive to cephalosporins. Appropriate laboratory studies are necessary to determine their sensitivity patterns; vancomycin is still an effective drug for almost all the staphylococci resistant to methicillin and cephalosporins. *Corynebacterium* spp. occasionally cause musculoskeletal infection; *Corynebacterium* spp. with multiple resistance patterns have been isolated but not commonly in musculoskeletal infections. These organisms are sensitive to vancomycin. Increasing numbers of gram-negative bacilli are developing resistance to the second- and third-generation cephalosporins. In addition, there may be antagonism between the second- and third-generation cephalosporins and other β-lactam agents (penicillins and cephalosporins). Among anaerobic organisms, most penicillin-resistant *Bacteroides* spp. and *Clostridium* spp. remain susceptible to clindamycin; if these organisms are resistant to clindamycin, the agents most likely to be effective are chloramphenicol and metronidazole. Some enterococcal group D streptococci have become β-lactamase producers and are highly resistant to the aminoglycosides. Infections with these organisms are difficult to treat; it is hoped that agents effective against these enterococci will be developed.

Route of Administration

Most patients with osteomyelitis or septic arthritis will require intravenous administration of the antimicrobial agent. In the past this has required long-term hospitalization but during the past few years there has been increasing use of home intravenous therapy programs. Recent reports indicate the successful use of the Hickman or Broviac catheter for long-term intravenous therapy at home (Fig. 1). The major disadvantage of these catheters is that an operation is required for their placement but their advantages include long-term durability and decreased incidence of pneumothorax, thrombosis, breakage, and septic complications. In addition, the patients can administer their own medication.

In the past, infections of the musculoskeletal system caused by fungi such as *Blastomyces dermatitidis* have required treatment with amphotericin B. Amphotericin B still is an effective agent but has relatively high toxicity and requires intravenous administration. Recent reports indicate that ketoconazole, an orally administered agent, may become an effective alternative to amphotericin B for some fungal infections.

Oral administration of antimicrobial agents to children with musculoskeletal infections has proved to be effective.

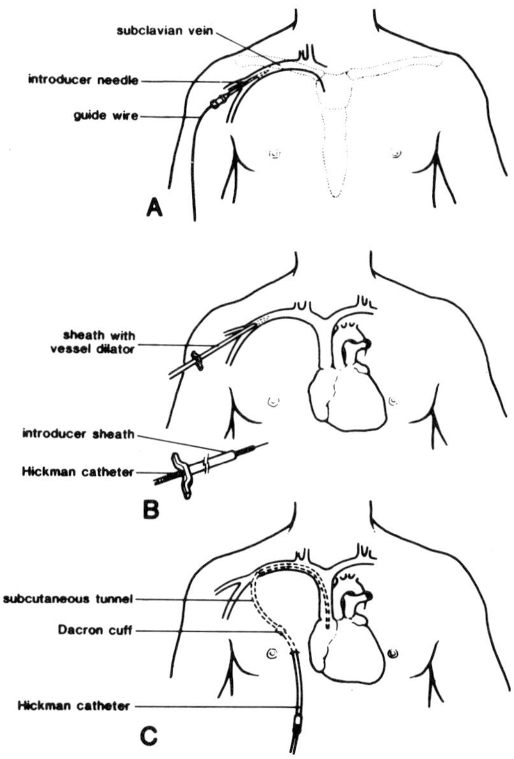

Figure 1

Use of the Hickman catheter. *A*, Introducer needle is placed into the subclavian vein. The guide wire is passed through the needle into the vein; then the needle is removed and the guide wire is left in place. *B*, Vessel dilator and introducer sheath are passed over the guide wire and into the vein. The guide wire and vessel dilator are removed. The Hickman catheter is passed through the introducer sheath into the vein. *C*, Sheath is removed with the catheter in place. The catheter is passed through a long subcutaneous tunnel and out through the skin of the chest wall.

If treatment failures are to be avoided, rigid criteria must be applied: 1) there must be an adequate clinical response to parenteral therapy, 2) the causative bacteria must be isolated and found sensitive to an agent that can be absorbed after oral administration, 3) the patient must be able to tolerate the chosen agent, 4) adequate serum bactericidal activity (peak titer >1:8 with trough titer >1:2) must be demonstrated with oral administration of the agent, and 5) patient compliance must be ensured (this often requires continued hospitalization).

Operating Room Environment

Since the advent of total joint replacement, there has been considerable controversy regarding the effectiveness of unidirectional airflow systems and body exhaust suits for the prevention of infection. A recent prospective study in Great Britain established the effectiveness of these units for total hip and total knee replacements. Unfortunately, there are no studies to prove the effectiveness of the systems for other total joint replacements or other orthopaedic procedures. It has been established that, if a unidirectional airflow system is used without body exhaust apparatus, appropriate surgical suite organization and discipline are essential to avoid a detrimental effect from the use of these units. One study revealed an increased infection rate after total knee arthroplasty with the use of the unidirectional airflow system without body exhaust apparatus, probably because of interposition of surgical team members between the air source and the operative wound. If unidirectional airflow systems are used without body exhaust apparatus, the area between the air source and the operative site must be kept clear at all times (Fig. 2). Although the effectiveness of the unidirectional airflow system has been established clearly only for total hip or knee arthroplasty, it seems reasonable to encourage its use for other procedures of long duration and involving implantation of large foreign bodies.

It has been demonstrated that conversation in the area of the operation may be a major source of bacterial contamination. This source of contamination can be significantly reduced by utilizing an effective mask placed under an appropriate overlapping hood (Fig. 3).

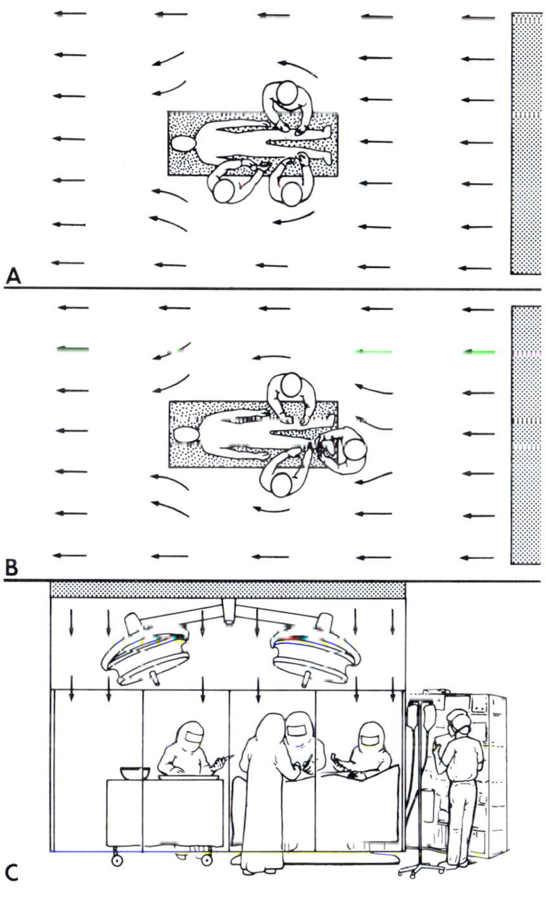

Figure 2

Ultraclean air-handling systems. *A*, With horizontal flow system, there must be no obstruction between air source and operative wound. *B*, If operating room personnel come between air source and operative wound, infection rate may be increased to more than if no special air-handling system were used. *C*, Vertical system combined with body exhaust apparatus provides excellent operative environment. Use of body exhaust systems with either horizontal or vertical system frees the surgical team from concern about coming between air source and operative wound.

Osteomyelitis

Diagnosis

Osteomyelitis is best diagnosed by appropriate bacterial culture techniques and histologic examination. In many instances, it is helpful to detect an infectious process prior to an invasive procedure to permit better planning of the treatment for the patient. Both the accuracy and the specificity of radioactive isotope imaging techniques have improved in the evaluation of musculoskeletal infections. The three most useful imaging agents are technetium-99m, gallium-67, and indium-111. For technetium-99m imaging, the radioisotope is administered as the phosphate and the patient is scanned in two phases. The early phase is within the first 10 to 15 minutes, when the majority of the radioisotope is in equilibrium in the extracellular compartment and there is increased accumulation in areas of increased blood flow, such as that associated with cellulitis. In the late phase, 2 to 4 hours after injection, 30% to 40% of the radioisotope has been excreted in the urine and the

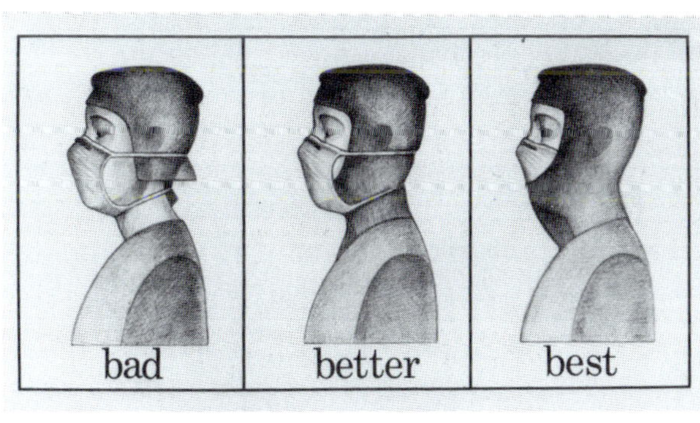

Figure 3

When bottom and sides of face mask are covered by a hood, bacterial fallout during conversation is minimized. (From Letts, R.M., and Doermer, E. J. Bone Joint Surg. 65A:357–362, 1983. By permission of the journal.)

remainder is retained within the skeleton in both the organic matrix and the mineral phase. This retention has been interpreted as an indication of the amount of activity within bone. Gallium-67 imaging involves injection of the radioisotope and scanning over a period of 1 to 3 days. Increased uptake of the isotope in areas of infection can be explained by three mechanisms: direct bacterial uptake, protein-bound tissue uptake, and direct leukocyte uptake. Imaging with indium-111 requires collection of 80 to 90 ml of venous blood, separation of the leukocytes in it, and labeling them with indium-111 *in vitro;* the laboratory procedure requires approximately 3 hours. Patients then are given their own indium-111-labeled leukocytes intravenously and are scanned at 18 to 24 hours afterward.

Technetium-99m imaging is very sensitive and is the technique of choice for acute hematogenous osteomyelitis. In an extensive study in children, the injection of technetium-99m phosphate (at 215 μCi/m^2 of body surface) was followed by immediate blood pool scanning and then delayed scanning approximately 2 hours later. A diffuse initial increased uptake followed by focal uptake in the skeleton was interpreted as a positive image. Some positive images showed specific unlabeled ("cold") areas in the skeleton on the delayed image. The images were correctly interpreted as revealing osteomyelitis in 55 of 62 patients who had osteomyelitis, and appropriate negative determinations were made in 74 of 79 patients. All soft tissue infections were identified correctly by this technique, and among 37 positive studies for septic arthritis, 8 were falsely positive. Other studies have shown less accuracy and specificity in neonates, but this study revealed no difference in accuracy and sensitivity for patients in this age group. In the entire group of 280 children evaluated, sensitivity of the technetium-99m image was 89%, the specificity was 94%, and the overall accuracy was 92%.

Although technetium-99m imaging is sensitive for chronic musculoskeletal septic processes, large numbers of false-positive results are reported because many of these infections occur after surgery or trauma. To improve the results in chronic infectious processes, the sequential technetium/gallium imaging technique was developed. This involves a sequence of a delayed technetium image and a 48- or 72-hour gallium image. The results are considered positive for infection if the gallium and technetium images are noncongruous or are congruous but the gallium uptake is greater than that of technetium. The overall accuracy reported with this technique varies from 65% to 80%.

The accuracy of the indium-labeled leukocyte imaging technique has been compared with sequential technetium/gallium images in the same group of patients suspected of having low-grade chronic musculoskeletal infection. Indium-labeled leukocyte imaging had an accuracy of 83%; the accuracy of sequential technetium/gallium imaging was 57%. When a prosthesis was in place, the indium image

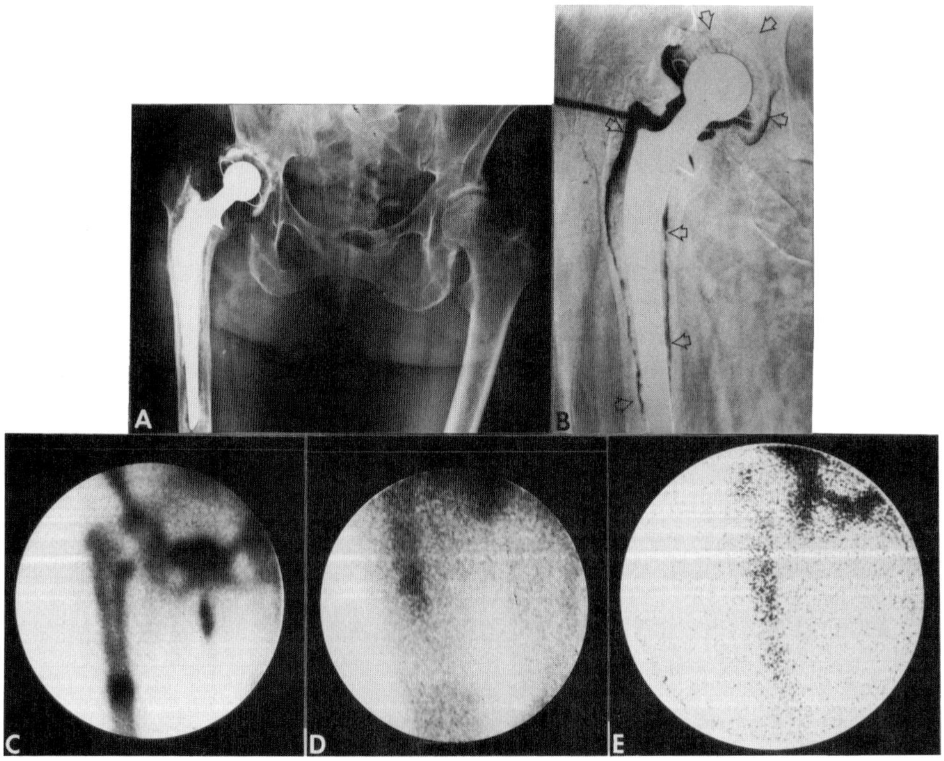

Figure 4

A, Radiograph, showing evidence of prosthetic loosening after right total hip arthroplasty. *B,* Subtraction arthrogram of right hip is not diagnostic of infection, although loosening is evident. *C,* Technetium-99m image demonstrates increased uptake at tip of femoral stem, medial part of calcar, and greater trochanter. *D,* Gallium-67 uptake is increased at distal tip of femoral stem. Uptake is less intense than that of technetium and thus was interpreted as negative for infection. *E,* Accumulation of indium-labeled leukocytes about femoral stem is positive for infection. (From Merkel, K.D.; Brown, M.L.; Dewanjee, M.K.; and Fitzgerald, R.H., Jr. J. Bone Joint Surg. 67A:465–476, 1985. By permission of the journal.)

was 94% accurate and the technetium/gallium image was 75% accurate. In addition, it was noted that interpretation of the indium images was made with more confidence and accuracy compared with the sequential technetium/gallium images (Fig. 4). The indium-111 technique has a major disadvantage in the demanding quality control required for reproducible and accurate results but it has an advantage over the technetium/gallium technique in being completed within 24 hours and having lower cost. Radionuclide imaging is usually not necessary for diagnosis of septic arthritis. The incidence of false-negatives with technetium imaging in septic arthritis is high. If a radionuclide image is necessary to help in the diagnosis of septic arthritis, a sequential technetium/gallium image probably would be helpful.

Causes

Anaerobic Bacteria The most common anaerobic coccus associated with osteomyelitis is *Peptococcus magnus; Bacteroides* is the most common genus of gram-negative anaerobic bacteria causing osteomyelitis. In one large series of patients with osteomyelitis, anaerobic organisms were cultured from the infected site of 22%; 9 infections were solely by anaerobes and 31 were by a mixture of anaerobic and aerobic organisms. The 5-year treatment success rate was lower in those patients with anaerobic involvement, 48%, than in the overall group. The infections caused solely by pure anaerobic organisms had more successful results than mixed infections. It is important to utilize appropriate anaerobic culture techniques when evaluating difficult infections.

Tuberculosis In a controlled trial comparing debridement and anterior spinal fusion with standard chemotherapy and ambulatory treatment in the management of tuberculosis of the spine, it was found that there was earlier bony fusion, a slight decrease in loss of vertebral height, and slightly less kyphosis in those patients treated surgically. However, the results were excellent in both groups when evaluated at both 5 and 10 years after treatment.

Drug Abuse *P. aeruginosa* is commonly associated with bone and joint infections in patients who have a history of drug abuse. The vast majority of infections in this group of patients have involved the spine and pelvis, with occasional involvement of the shoulder, knee, hip, and tibia. In general, the patients are not severely toxic but have an increased erythrocyte sedimentation rate, >30 mm in 1 hour. Symptom duration has been reported to range from 1 day to 1 year before presentation. Only 5 of 35 radiographs of the involved part were positive at the time of initial presentation; all 30 technetium bone images were positive. All patients were treated with an aminoglycoside and carbenicillin for 4 to 6 weeks; none had surgical debridement. The treatment was apparently successful in all patients except four who had septic arthritis (three in the knee and one in the hip). These patients required synovectomy and debridement combined with antimicrobial therapy before the infections cleared.

In an additional study, seven patients had culture-proved osteomyelitis of the pubis—five due to *P. aeruginosa,* one due to *S. aureus,* and one due to *Escherichia coli.* Six of these seven patients were parenteral drug abusers and one had undergone operation for urinary incontinence. All were treated successfully with antimicrobial agents without surgical debridement. This condition must be differentiated from the benign condition, osteitis pubis; the differentiating features include history of drug abuse, increased erythrocyte sedimentation rate, presence of sequestrum, and a positive culture of material obtained by needle or open biopsy.

Therapy

Surgical Since the introduction of local muscle flap procedures for the treatment of osteomyelitis, there have been numerous advances in this area including use of free tissue transfers for treatment of chronic osteomyelitis. With either local or vascularized flaps, thorough soft tissue and bone debridement and antimicrobial treatment, often combined with an additional debridement or period of pack changes, frequently will be successful in the treatment of chronic osteomyelitis. In a series of 42 patients, 93% were treated successfully with these combined techniques. However, 22 of the patients required additional surgical treatment for associated nonunion or other problems before a successful clinical result was obtained. The most common infecting organism in this series was *P. aeruginosa.* A 93% success rate in curing osteomyelitis in patients with such organisms is a substantial improvement over techniques not utilizing flap coverage.

Local flap transfers that have been developed for difficult problems include the vastus lateralis, rectus femoris, or rectus abdominis flap for treatment of persistent infections about the hip including those occurring after removal of failed total hip arthroplasty. Transfer of the vastus lateralis and rectus femoris flaps has not caused lower extremity dysfunction, and in small series the success rate in clearing the infection has been high. Use of the rectus abdominis flap has also been reported to be successful. These procedures should be considered true salvage procedures; the bone resection required for successful flaps may prevent reimplantation of a total hip arthroplasty in the future (Fig. 5).

Vascularized bone grafts may be useful in refractory cases of chronic osteomyelitis in long bones. Treatment of refractory infected forearm nonunions by this technique has been successful (Fig. 6).

Pin track osteomyelitis sometimes occurs after use of traction or external fixation pins (Fig. 7). Pins placed entirely within one bone cortex are more likely to cause persistent pin track infection. Treatment includes debridement and appropriate antimicrobials. Cancellous bone grafting may be helpful in resistant cases.

Hyperbaric Oxygen Therapy Studies in animals indicate improved outcome in the treatment of gas gangrene, and possibly chronic osteomyelitis, when hyperbaric oxygen treatment is combined with other accepted methods of treatment. Major side effects of hyperbaric oxygen therapy include cerebral oxygen toxicity with grand mal seizures, barotrauma to the middle ear or sinuses, and confinement anxiety. These complications can be virtually eliminated by appropriate pretreatment evaluation and orientation and the use of properly selected medications. It is known that increased oxygen tension (80 mm Hg or more) inhibits production of toxins by *C. perfringens.* In hyperbaric oxygen therapy at a pressure of 2 atmospheres, oxygen tension is raised to 250 mm Hg; at 3 atmospheres, it reaches

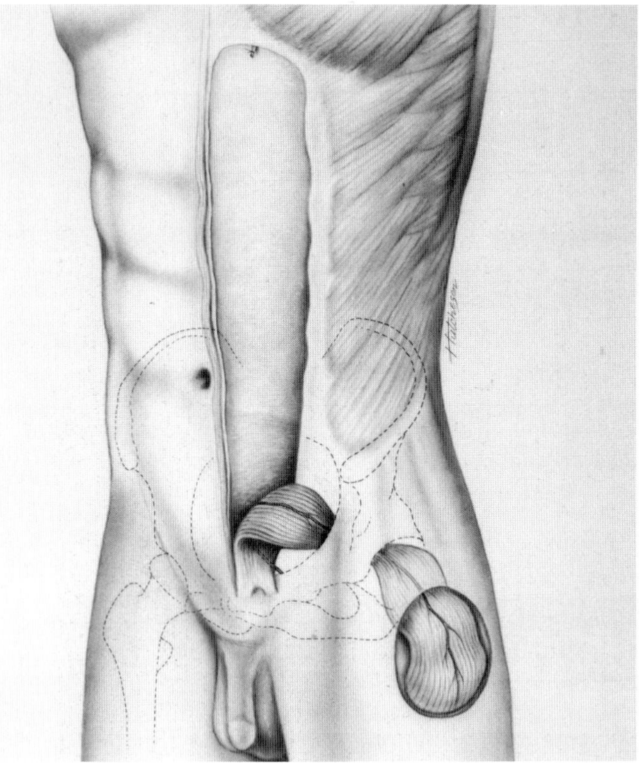

Figure 5

Rectus abdominis mobilized on inferior pedicle and passed through acetabulum to hip wound.

450 mm Hg. The alpha toxin of *C. perfringens* that has already been produced is stable but other toxins such as the theta toxin are inactivated. Increased oxygen tension also counteracts the hypoxic environment that is usually present in tissues in which clostridial infection develops. A reversal of the hypoxia allows formation of peroxides which inactivate and kill clostridial organisms.

Surgery remains a vitally important feature of treatment of infections caused by gas-forming organisms. Removal of devitalized tissue decreases catalase production, which is of benefit because catalase inactivates the peroxides that inhibit and kill the bacteria. A recent study demonstrated that gas gangrene is not limited to patients who have experienced trauma; in a large series of patients, 35% of the cases occurred after clean surgical procedures and 16% occurred spontaneously. In the same series, in which the patients were treated with antimicrobial agents, surgical debridement, and hyperbaric oxygen, the survival rate was 81%. Poor prognosis for survival was associated with spontaneous occurrence, presentation more than 30 hours after onset of symptoms, shock at the time of presentation, and intercurrent disease such as diabetes or neoplasia. Although it has been demonstrated that hyperbaric oxygen may be a useful adjunctive treatment of clostridial infection and may be helpful in the treatment of osteomyelitis, we must await controlled trials to determine its true effectiveness and indications.

Toxic Shock Syndrome

Toxic shock syndrome usually has been associated with the use of absorbable vaginal tampons but is being seen with increasing frequency postoperatively in both males and females. Usually, a high temperature develops in the early postoperative period and, if the condition is not recognized and treated, hypotension, nausea, vomiting, and diarrhea ensue and other organ systems may become involved. If the condition is not recognized, the mortality rate will be increased; the overall mortality rate of toxic shock syndrome is 7% to 10%. In patients who have toxic shock syndrome after operation, the wound usually has a benign appearance. When a high, unexplained fever develops postoperatively, an exudate or aspirate from the wound should be cultured; if staphylococci are found, open wound debridement and treatment with antimicrobial agents should be undertaken immediately.

Septic Arthritis

There is general agreement that septic arthritis of the hip joint should be treated by immediate open drainage and appropriate antimicrobial agents. However, there is considerable controversy concerning the surgical treatment of septic arthritis in most other joints. Some series suggest improved results after open surgical drainage of all joints with septic processes; other reports suggest excellent results under some circumstances with repeated joint aspiration. In an experimental animal model, septic arthritis was induced in the knee joint with *S. aureus;* 24 hours later, when the animals had pain and limped, some were treated by arthrotomy and saline lavage and others were treated by daily aspiration (all animals were given penicillin). Animals treated by repeated aspiration had diffuse erosion and widespread degeneration of the articular cartilage, and there was marked and extensive fibrillar change. Animals that had open arthrotomy had only minor articular cartilage changes with rare focal areas of degeneration and minimal erosion and fibrillar changes; in these animals the chondrocytes appeared normal (Fig. 8). Open synovectomy and debridement may alter catabolin production which may be important in the destruction of glycosaminoglycans of the articular cartilage. Arthroscopic drainage and debridement have been utilized in the treatment of septic arthritis; this appears to be a reasonable method of achieving the advantages of open debridement with fewer of its disadvantages but to date there are no controlled studies demonstrating whether it is more or less effective than either repeated aspiration or open debridement.

Infected Total Joint Arthroplasty

Although the infection rate after total joint replacement arthroplasty is low, the consequences of such infections remain a major problem in orthopaedic surgery. Use of special air-handling systems and body exhaust suits, perioperative treatment with antimicrobial agents, and meticulous surgical technique are responsible for the low incidence of infection after these procedures. Hematogenous infection of such replacement arthroplasty obviously occurs, but our knowledge of the pathogenesis of these infections is limited. There are no data supporting the use

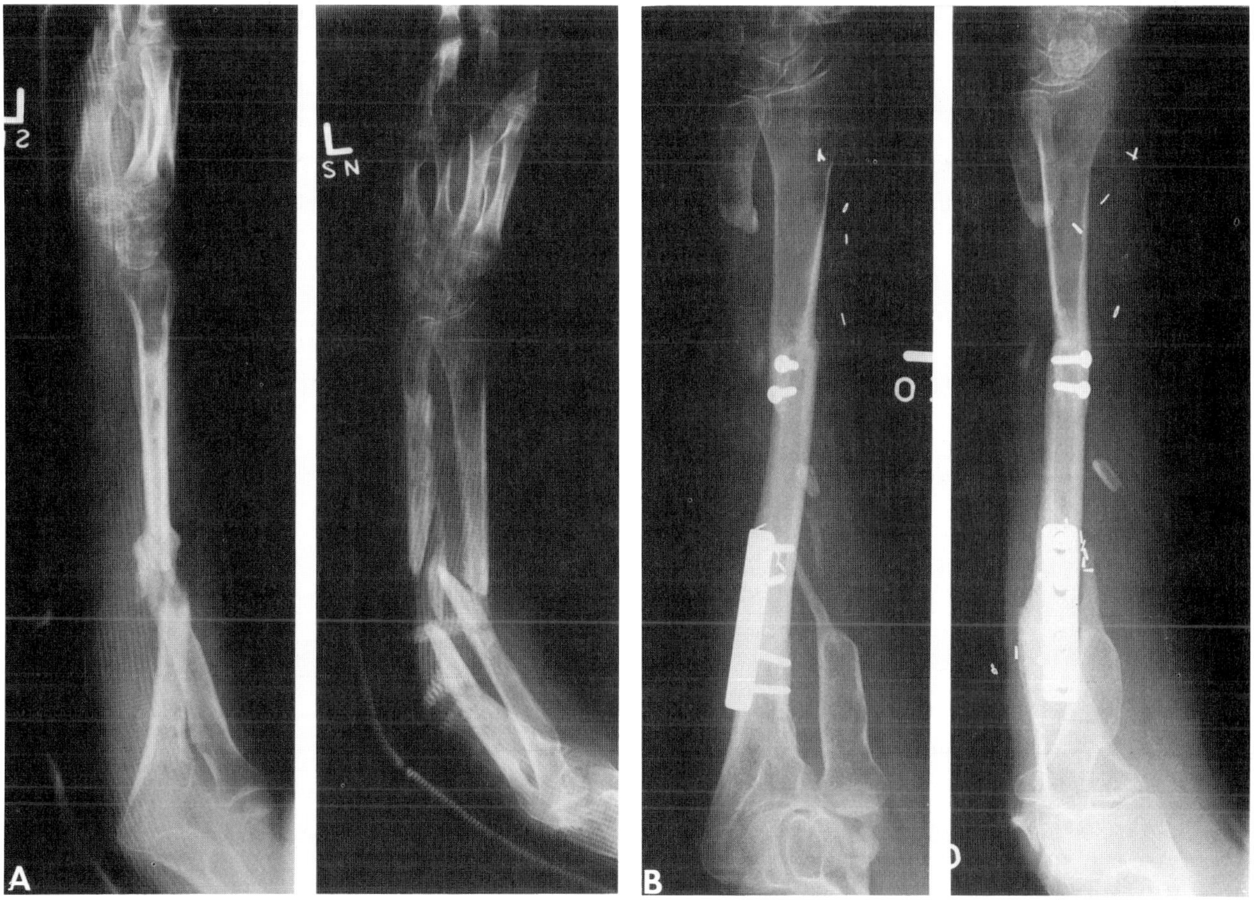

Figure 6

A, Anteroposterior and lateral radiographs, showing sequestrum, angulation, and nonunion of the forearm. *B*, Proximal and distal union of the ulnar and radial junctions is evident at 5 months after vascularized fibular bone graft to achieve function by conversion to a one-bone forearm. (From Dell, P.C., and Sheppard, J.E. J. Hand Surg. [Am.] 9:653–658, 1984. By permission of the American Society for Surgery of the Hand.)

of antimicrobial coverage for procedures such as dental work and urinary tract manipulation; it seems prudent to continue to recommend such coverage for these procedures as well as their vigorous use for treating diagnosed infections until we have more knowledge about the complications. Although some investigators, primarily surgeons in Europe, have reported high success rates with one-stage reimplantation for infected total joint replacement, the consensus of surgeons in the United States is that, if reimplantation of total joint arthroplasty components is contemplated, success rates will be higher if these procedures are performed in stages. However, under special circumstances involving strong indications for limiting the approach to a single surgical procedure and in infections caused by organisms of low virulence with high sensitivity to antimicrobial agents, a one-stage reimplantation may be used. Infections caused by gram-negative organisms such as *P. aeruginosa* are less likely to be successfully treated by reimplantation of arthroplasty components in either one stage or two stages; if reimplantation is elected, a two-stage procedure is better.

Although most work related to infection associated with total joint arthroplasty has involved the hip, recent studies suggest that some patients with infected total knee arthroplasty may be treated successfully by methods similar to those used for the hip. Acute infections in the knee may be treated by debridement without removal of arthroplasty components; chronic infections are best treated by complete debridement including components and bone cement, followed by reimplantation at a later stage. When arthrodesis is selected as the treatment of choice for infected total knee replacement, the knee should have complete debridement followed by external fixation with biplanar application of the external fixation pins. Some difficult treatment problems may be solved by initial clearing of the infection followed by arthrodesis fixed by a long intramedullary rod.

The results of treatment of infected total hip arthroplasty by resection arthroplasty have been poor in large numbers of patients; a recent report indicates results not as poor as those suggested previously although the criteria for a satisfactory result were somewhat lax (Harris hip score > 65) in that study. An additional finding was that those patients who had resection of proximal femoral bone along the intertrochanteric line with prominences removed from the periacetabular area seem to have better results than those who did not have such resection. Results also indicated

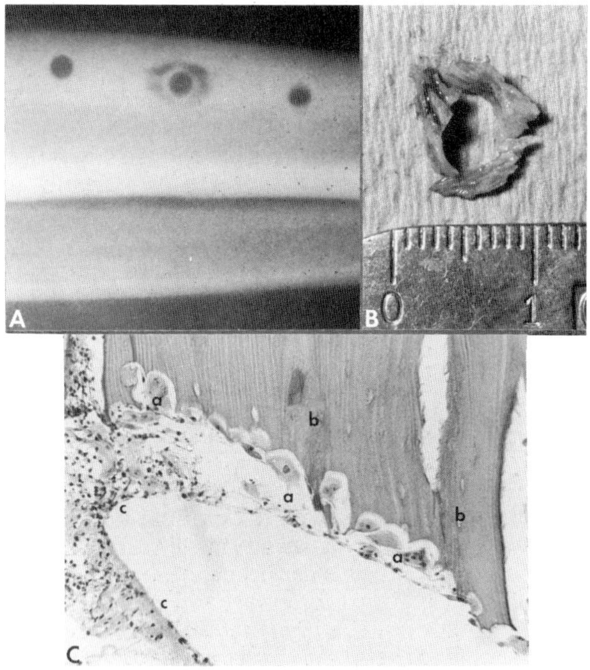

Figure 7

A, Classic ring sequestrum involving the middle pin hole of an external fixation apparatus. *B*, Typical small ring sequestrum with fragmentation. *C*, Histologic section, showing row of mononuclear and multinuclear osteoclasts (*a*) and eroding necrotic bone (*b*) of the ring sequestrum. Granulation tissue is also seen (*c*).

that completeness of cement removal made little difference in whether or not the patients achieved dry wounds. However, if reimplantation of total arthroplasty components is planned in the future, it is essential that all cement be debrided.

Influence of Implant on Infection

It has been found in recent experimental studies that all biomaterials commonly used for total joint arthroplasty increase the incidence of infection with *S. aureus*. However, the infection incidence for *E. coli* and *S. epidermidis* was not increased with most biomaterials but was increased markedly with the use of poly(methyl methacrylate). Incorporation of an antimicrobial agent in the poly(methyl methacrylate) reversed this increased incidence of infection to an incidence lower than the incidence when no implant was used. Both systemic antimicrobial therapy and irrigation of the operative site with antimicrobial solution produced a trend toward lower incidence of infection but neither was nearly as effective as use of poly(methyl methacrylate) bone cement. Two separate experiments have established that poly(methyl methacrylate) containing an aminoglycoside antimicrobial agent is effective in preventing infection in wounds contaminated with *S. aureus* and other bacteria.

Adherence of microorganisms to various objects has been studied for many years. Recent studies indicate that this mechanism may be an important factor in sepsis associated with orthopaedic and other implants. Adherence is enhanced by a polysaccharide biofilm which appears to protect the bacteria from host defense mechanisms and antimicrobial agents. In addition, this film makes culture of organisms difficult; even when special techniques were used, organisms could not be cultured successfully but were demonstrated by electron microscopy (Fig. 9). These experiments may lead to a further decrease in the incidence of and improved treatment for infections associated with total joint arthroplasty.

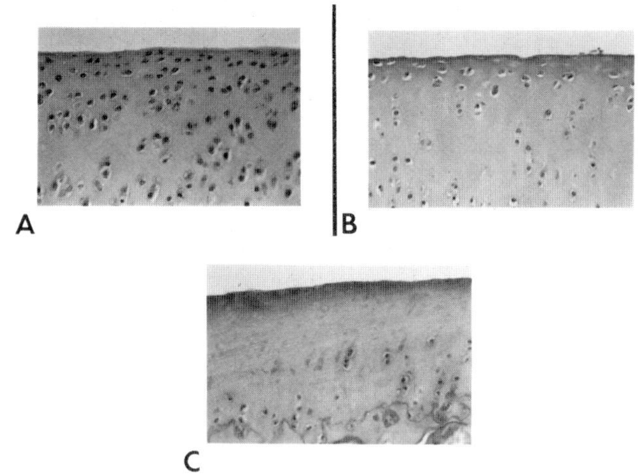

Figure 8

A, In uninfected rabbits, the articular cartilage is normal. *B*, Section at 5 days after arthrotomy and irrigation for treatment of infection shows minimal decrease in number of chondrocytes in the most superficial layer of articular cartilage; otherwise, the cartilage appears normal. *C*, Section at 5 days after aspiration shows necrosis of superficial areas of articular cartilage with areas of acellularity and cloning of chondrocytes. There is diffuse fibular degeneration.

Synthetic sutures have been found to be superior to natural suture material in resistance to infection. The synthetic monofilament and braided absorbable sutures are most resistant to infection, followed by braided nonabsorbable sutures. Use of natural suture materials should be avoided in wounds potentially susceptible to infection. Monofilament synthetic sutures and polyglycolic acid sutures are best for use in the presence of bacterial contamination.

Importance of Nutritional Status in Prevention of Infection

In 1930 it was first recognized in orthopaedic patients that negative nitrogen balance, weight loss, and tissue wasting developed in patients with fractured femurs. In the past 2 decades, it has been demonstrated that complications can be decreased markedly by maintaining appropriate nutritional status. In orthopaedics, as in other areas of medicine, the gross signs and symptoms of malnutrition—such as marked weight loss, pitting edema, and intercostal or interosseous wasting—have been recognized. More subtle indicators of malnutrition have not been widely reported, and the consequences of malnutrition have not been widely recognized.

The basal energy expenditure of a normal 70-kg man at rest is approximately 1,800 kilocalories/day. A patient with a major fracture has a 20% to 25% increase in energy expenditure; a patient with multiple trauma or infection has

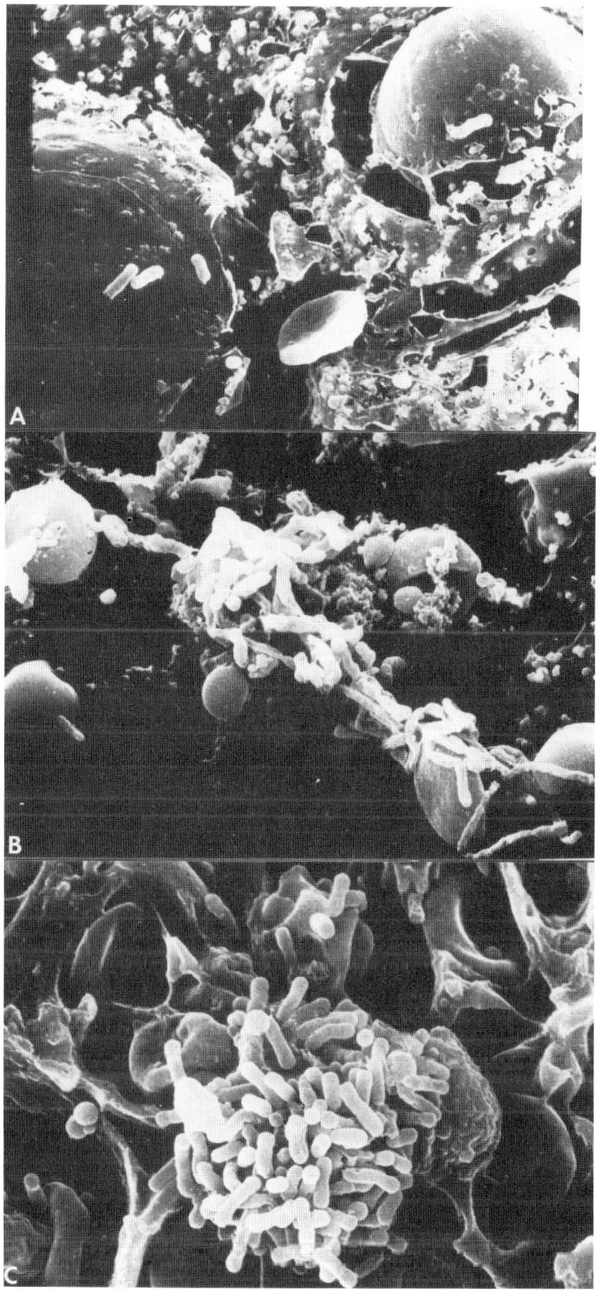

Figure 9

A, Scanning electron micrograph of intramedullary methyl methacrylate from infected and loosened total hip prosthesis, showing rod-shaped bacteria in association with, and often partly buried in, extensive biofilm on surface of this biomaterial. *P. aeruginosa* was isolated from this specimen. *B,* Biofilm is incompletely formed in this area and individual adherent bacterial microcolonies can be discerned. *C,* Surface of bone from infected total hip joint, showing development of discrete adherent microcolonies in which bacteria of a single morphotype are partly surrounded by amorphous condensed material. (From Gristina, A.G., and Costerton, J.W. J. Bone Joint Surg. 67A:264–273, 1985. By permission of the journal.)

an increase of 30% to 55%. Liver and skeletal muscle glycogen stores, which are about 300 g (1,200 kilocalories), can be depleted in 12 hours or less during severe stress. Utilization of body fat stores may not spare visceral and skeletal muscle protein because fat is not a readily available energy source during severe stress.

Failure of a delayed cutaneous response to skin antigen testing and low total lymphocyte counts are indicators of decreased immune competence and are often associated with malnutrition that is not readily recognized. In an excellent review of 129 orthopaedic patients who were carefully evaluated by easily performed tests of nutritional status, it was found that 42% had some degree of clinical or subclinical malnutrition. Patients undergoing elective total hip replacement had the lowest incidence of malnutrition (29%) and those with multiple trauma and femoral fractures had the highest (59%). Trauma, including major surgery, was demonstrated to cause further nutritional deficit. The infection rate was significantly higher in patients with malnutrition than in those who had normal nutrition. A protocol for evaluation and treatment of nutrition problems in orthopaedic patients has been developed (Fig. 10). Although clinical trials are necessary to evaluate specific treatment programs, use of such a protocol can be expected to provide significant benefit to orthopaedic patients at this time.

Acquired Immune Deficiency Syndrome

What has now become known as the acquired immune deficiency syndrome (AIDS) epidemic began in the United States in 1978. Since that time, extensive research has generated significant knowledge about this disease but treatment has remained primarily supportive. Several populations have been described to be at increased risk of infection; these include homosexual men, intravenous drug

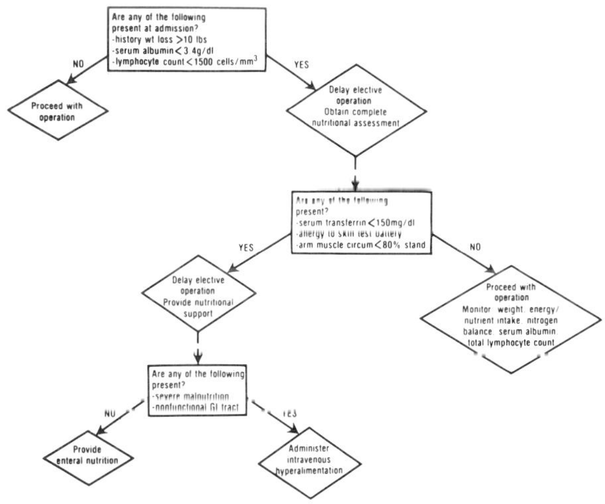

Figure 10

Flow chart depicting a rational screening approach to identify patients who are nutritionally at risk, utilizing tests that are readily available in most clinical situations. (From Jensen, J.E.; Jensen, T.G.; Smith, T.K.; Johnston, D.A.; and Dudrick, S.J. J. Bone Joint Surg. 64A:1263–1272, 1982. By permission of the journal.)

abusers, and recipients of transfusions of blood products. In addition, infection has been passed between heterosexual partners, to children born of mothers with AIDS or in high-risk groups, and by needle puncture.

Human T-cell lymphotrophic virus, type III/lymphadenopathy-associated virus (HTLV-III/LAV) transmission appears to occur by blood-borne means and intimate sexual contact. The virus has been isolated from saliva, but to date there is no evidence of direct transmission by this fluid. Infection with the HTLV-III/LAV is not synonymous with AIDS, and many have been found to carry the virus but are asymptomatic. Individuals with hemophilia should be considered to be in the high-risk group for both carrying the virus and having AIDS. Many of these patients have significant disorders of the musculoskeletal system that require treatment by orthopaedic surgeons. In addition, others who are infected with the virus or have AIDS may present with significant musculoskeletal disorders requiring treatment.

In addition to other musculoskeletal disorders, these patients may have infection of the musculoskeletal system. In patients with normal immune competence, these are problems that are often difficult to treat; treatment of patients with AIDS who have musculoskeletal infection will require close cooperation between the orthopaedic surgeon and the internal medicine specialist or other specialists.

Guidelines issued for care of these patients include precautions similar to those utilized for patients with hepatitis B infection (Table 1). Orthopaedic surgeons treating these patients should adhere strictly to these precautions. Recent research indicates that, even over an extended period of time, close nonsexual contact with patients with AIDS represents a minimal risk of infection with HTLV-III/LAV.

Table 1. Precautions for Preventing Acquisition of HTLV-III/LAV Infection in Health-Care Workers

1. Sharp items (needles, scalpel blades, and other sharp instruments) should be considered potentially infective and handled with extraordinary care to prevent accidental injury. Disposable syringes, needles, scalpel blades, and other sharp items should be placed into puncture-resistant containers located as close as possible to the area in which they are used. Needles should not be recapped, bent, broken, removed from syringes, or otherwise manipulated by hand.
2. When the possibility of exposure to blood or other body fluids exists, the minimal protection requires gloves. Gowns, masks, and eye-coverings may be necessary when performing procedures involving more extensive contact with blood or other potentially infected body fluids—e.g., dental or endoscopic procedures, postmortem examinations, and surgical procedures. Hands should be washed immediately if they become contaminated with body fluids.
3. To minimize the need for mouth-to-mouth resuscitation, mouthpieces, resuscitation bags, or other ventilation devices should be readily available if needed for resuscitation.
4. Pregnant health-care workers are not known to be at greater risk of contracting HTLV-III/LAV infection but, if the health-care worker does become infected during pregnancy, the infant is at increased risk of infection resulting from perinatal exposure.

Annotated Bibliography

Antimicrobial Agents

Berman, A.T., and Johnson, M.D., III: The use of the Hickman catheter in orthopaedic infections: Brief note. J. Bone Joint Surg. 67A:650–651, 1985.

The authors report an excellent experience with the Hickman catheter for long-term intravenous use in the hospital and at home. The complication rate was low and patient compliance was high because of the ease of drug administration.

Jones, S.; DiPiro, J.T.; Nix, D.E.; and Bhatti, N.A.: Cephalosporins for prophylaxis in operative repair of femoral fractures: Levels in serum, muscle, and hematoma. J. Bone Joint Surg. 67A:921–924, 1985.

These investigators found that higher levels of antimicrobial agents were obtained with cefazolin than with either cefamandole or cefoxitin, both in serum and in fracture hematoma. Antimicrobial penetration of the hematoma did not correlate with the time interval between fracture and drug administration.

Mader, J.T., and Wilson, K.J.: Comparative evaluation of cefamandole and cephalothin in the treatment of experimental *Staphylococcus aureus* osteomyelitis in rabbits. J. Bone Joint Surg. 65A:507–513, 1983.

Cefamandole was shown to reach higher concentration in bone than did cephalothin. However, cefamandole had increased inactivation by β-lactamase, and the clinical course of the animals was improved more by cephalothin than by cefamandole, probably because of cephalothin's greater resistance to β-lactamase inactivation.

Moore, R.M., and Green, N.E.: Blastomycosis of bone: A report of six cases. J. Bone Joint Surg. 64A:1097–1101, 1982.

Patients had good response to intravenous administration of amphotericin B and oral administration of ketaconazole. Ketaconazole had the advantage of oral administration and probably has less potential for serious toxicity.

Scoles, P.V., and Aronoff, S.C.: Antimicrobial therapy of childhood skeletal infections. J. Bone Joint Surg. 66A:1487–1492, 1984.

Positive bacterial identification and appropriate sensitivity studies are essential in selecting antimicrobials for treatment of childhood musculoskeletal infections. When appropriate criteria are met, some children may be treated by oral therapy for most of the duration of their therapy.

Sonne-Holm, S.; Boeckstyns, M.; Menck, H.; Sinding, A.; Leicht, P.; Dichmann, O.; Prag, J.B.; Baekgaard, N.; Ostri, P.; and Gøtrik, J.K.: Prophylactic antibiotics in amputation of the lower extremity for ischemia: A placebo-controlled randomized trial of cefoxitin. J. Bone Joint Surg. 67A:800–803, 1985.

Administration of cefoxitin decreased the infection rate after amputation for lower limb ischemia. There were no clostridial infections and no deaths in those patients treated with antimicrobial agent; of those who had no such treatment, eight had clostridial infection and three died.

Operating Room Environment

Letts, R.M., and Doermer, E.: Conversation in the operating theater as a cause of airborne bacterial contamination. J. Bone Joint Surg. 65A:357–362, 1983.

In a study using human albumin spheres as a tracer, the investigators determined that conversation is important in spreading bacteria in the area of the wound. Their studies demonstrated that the best protection, other than aspirator suits, was a mask of appropriate size and quality with a hood placed such that the hood overlapped the mask.

Osteomyelitis

del Busto, R.; Quinn, E.L.; Fisher, E.J.; and Madhavan, T.: Osteomyelitis of the pubis: Report of seven cases. J.A.M.A. 248:1498–1500, 1982.

A group of patients who had true osteomyelitis of the pubis are described; most were drug abusers. This condition must be differentiated from a benign condition, osteitis pubis; differentiating features include sequestrum formation, bone destruction, and positive cultures.

Dell, P.C., and Sheppard, J.E.: Vascularized bone grafts in the treatment of infected forearm nonunions. J. Hand Surg. [Am.] 9:653–658, 1984.

Four patients with persistent infected forearm nonunions were treated with vascularized fibula transfer. Each patient had a pain-free stable forearm without evidence of infection. This technique may be helpful in those patients in whom conventional techniques have failed.

Fitzgerald, R.H., Jr.; Ruttle, P.E.; Arnold, P.G.; Kelly, P.J.; and Irons, G.B.: Local muscle flaps in the treatment of chronic osteomyelitis. J. Bone Joint Surg. 67A:175–185, 1985.

Thirty-nine of 42 patients with osteomyelitis had successful eradication of their infection after adequate debridement, antimicrobial therapy, and local muscle flap transfer. Most patients required additional surgery to achieve union or for other reasons.

Green, S.A., and Ripley, M.J.: Chronic osteomyelitis in pin tracks. J. Bone Joint Surg. 66A:1092–1098, 1984.

Most persistent pin track infections are caused by *Staphylococcus aureus* and occur in bones in which pins have been inserted entirely within one cortex. Treatment by debridement, open packing, and appropriate antimicrobials, with cancellous bone grafting in persistent cases, usually is successful.

Hall, B.B.; Fitzgerald, R.H., Jr.; and Rosenblatt, J.E.: Anaerobic osteomyelitis. J. Bone Joint Surg. 65A:30–35, 1983.

Most cases of osteomyelitis due to anaerobic organisms are mixed infections with aerobic organisms. Infections caused solely by anaerobic organisms had a better prognosis than did mixed infections. The prognosis in anaerobic osteomyelitis is poor compared to osteomyelitis caused by aerobic organisms.

Hart, G.B.; Lamb, R.C.; and Strauss, M.B.: Gas gangrene. J. Trauma 23:991–1000, 1983.

In patients with gas gangrene, survival was high when hyperbaric oxygen therapy was used in addition to antimicrobial agents and surgical therapy. The occurrence of both postoperative and spontaneous gas gangrene is emphasized.

Howie, D.W.; Savage, J.P.; Wilson, T.G.; and Paterson, D.: The technetium phosphate bone scan in the diagnosis of osteomyelitis in childhood. J. Bone Joint Surg. 65A:431–437, 1983.

The use of technetium bone scans was very helpful diagnostically in children with hematogenous osteomyelitis. It also correctly identified all soft tissue infections in the children evaluated. Accuracy was less for septic arthritis.

Medical Research Council Working Party on Tuberculosis of the Spine: A 10-year assessment of a controlled trial comparing debridement and anterior spinal fusion in the management of tuberculosis of the spine in patients on standard chemotherapy in Hong Kong. J. Bone Joint Surg. 64B:393–398, 1982.

Long-term results were equally favorable with standard chemotherapy and ambulatory status of the patients compared with anterior spinal fusion. The only advantage of spinal fusion was a slight decrease in vertebral height loss and slightly less kyphosis.

Merkel, K.D.; Brown, M.L.; Dewanjee, M.K.; and Fitzgerald, R.H., Jr.: Comparison of indium-labeled-leukocyte imaging with sequential technetium-gallium scanning in the diagnosis of low-grade musculoskeletal sepsis: A prospective study. J. Bone Joint Surg. 67A:465–476, 1985.

Indium-labeled-leukocyte imaging was more accurate than sequential technetium/gallium scanning in the diagnosis of low-grade musculoskeletal sepsis. The indium-labeled-leukocyte technique also was more accurate when a prosthesis was in place. Interpretations were made with more confidence and accuracy with the indium technique.

Miskew, D.B.W.; Lorenz, M.A.; Pearson, R.L.; and Pankovich, A.M.: *Pseudomonas aeruginosa* bone and joint infection in drug abusers. J. Bone Joint Surg. 65A:829–832, 1983.

Technetium scanning was very helpful in early localization of osteomyelitis in these patients. Patients with osteomyelitis were successfully treated with antimicrobials without surgical debridement. Those patients with septic arthritis required surgical debridement in addition to antimicrobial therapy.

Weiland, A.J.; Moore, J.R.; and Daniel, R.K.: The efficacy of free tissue transfer in the treatment of osteomyelitis. J. Bone Joint Surg. 66A:181–193, 1984.

Advantages of free tissue transfer in the treatment of chronic osteomyelitis include addition of a permanent blood supply to the region, avoidance of further recipient tissue compromise, and provision for radical debridement. Most free tissue transfers survive, but not all result in successful treatment.

Toxic Shock Syndrome

Irvine, G.W.; Kling, T.F., Jr.; and Hensinger, R.N.: Postoperative toxic shock syndrome following osteoplasty of the hip: A case report. J. Bone Joint Surg. 66A:955–958, 1984.

The authors describe the clinical course of a 13-year-old girl who had fatal toxic shock syndrome after osteoplasty of the hip. Early signs included persistent high temperature and malaise.

Infected Total Joint Arthroplasty

Canner, G.C.; Steinberg, M.E.; Heppenstall, R.B.; and Balderston, R.: The infected hip after total hip arthroplasty. J. Bone Joint Surg. 66A:1393–1399, 1984.

Patients with true Girdlestone arthroplasty had better results for both pain relief and function than those who did not have proximal femoral resection along the intertrochanteric line and removal of prominences from the acetabular area.

Influence of Implants on Infection

Chu, C.-C., and Williams, D.F.: Effects of physical configuration and chemical structure of suture materials on bacterial adhesion: A possible link to wound infection. Am. J. Surg. 147:197–204, 1984.

Chemical nature and coating material appear to be major factors in determining bacterial attachment to suture material.

Of the absorbable sutures, polydioxanone (PDS) had the lowest bacterial adherence rate.

Fitzgerald, R.H., Jr.: Experimental osteomyelitis: Description of a canine model and the role of depot administration of antibiotics in the prevention and treatment of sepsis. J. Bone Joint Surg. 65A:371–380, 1983.

Poly(methyl methacrylate) with *Staphylococcus aureus* consistently produced osteomyelitis in experimental animals. Addition of gentamicin to the polymer prevented the occurrence of osteomyelitis but was not effective for the treatment of established *Staphylococcus aureus* osteomyelitis.

Gristina, A.G., and Costerton, J.W.: Bacterial adherence to biomaterials and tissue: The significance of its role in clinical sepsis. J. Bone Joint Surg. 67A:264–273, 1985.

Microbial adherence to implants is enhanced by the polysaccharide biofilm; this film may protect bacteria from both antimicrobial agents and host defense, partially explaining the difficulty of treating infection associated with implants. These protected bacteria may be very difficult to culture.

Petty, W.; Spanier, S.; Shuster, J.J.; and Silverthorne, C.: The influence of skeletal implants on incidence of infection: Experiments in a canine model. J. Bone Joint Surg. 67A:1236–1244, 1985.

Incidence of infection due to *Staphylococcus aureus* increased when cobalt-chrome, stainless steel, polyethylene, and bone cement were placed. The highest incidence of infection was associated with bone cement; bone cement was the only implant material associated with an increased incidence of infection with *Staphylococcus epidermidis* and *Escherichia coli.*

Sharp, W.V.; Belden, T.A.; King, P.H.; and Teague, P.C.: Suture resistance to infection. Surgery 91:61–63, 1982.

Synthetic sutures are more resistant to infection than are natural sutures. Monofilament sutures and polyglycolic acid sutures may be used in the presence of bacterial contamination.

Nutrition

Jensen, J.E.; Jensen, T.G.; Smith, T.K.; Johnston, D.A.; and Dudrick, S.J.: Nutrition in orthopaedic surgery. J. Bone Joint Surg. 64A:1263–1272, 1982.

The lowest incidence of nutritional depletion was identified in patients undergoing total hip replacement (29%), followed by an elective surgical group (35%) and patients with multiple trauma and femoral fractures (59%).

Acquired Immune Deficiency Syndrome

Centers for Disease Control: Recommendations for preventing transmission of infection with human T-lymphotropic virus type III/lymphadenopathy-associated virus in the workplace. MMWR 34 no. 45:682–695, 1985.

The highest risk for health-care workers in regard to acquiring HTLV-III/LAV infection in the workplace would involve parenteral exposure to a needle or other sharp instrument contaminated with blood of an infected patient. Appropriate precautions should be taken to avoid such exposure, and exposure to body fluids of patients infected with HTLV-III/LAV should be avoided.

Friedland, G.H.; Saltzman, B.R.; Rogers, M.F.; Kahl, P.A.; Lesser, M.L.; Mayers, M.M.; and Klein, R.S.: Lack of transmission of HTLV-III/LAV infection to household contacts of patients with AIDS or AIDS-related complex with oral candidiasis. N. Engl. J. Med. 314:344–349, 1986.

This report indicates that household contacts who are not sexual partners of, or born to, patients with AIDS are at minimal or no risk of infection with HTLV-III/LAV.

7 Trauma: Hard Tissue

Epidemiology

An alarming increase in incidence of fractures of the proximal femur has been reported in both the foreign and the English-language literature. In the United Kingdom, these patients occupy approximately 20% of all orthopaedic beds. Overall, the incidence of this fracture has doubled over the past 28 years, and the increase has occurred at all ages and in both sexes. The increased incidence is greater than the increase in the proportion of elderly in the population. For example, the 80- to 84-year-old group demonstrated a 280% increase; frank osteomalacia was present in 10% to 20%. This increased incidence of hip fractures has been attributed to improved care facilities and more allied health workers for the elderly.

Several studies from Sweden have raised concern about the increased incidence. In Gothenburg, the female-to-male ratio was 3.4:1 for cervical fractures and 2.2:1 for trochanteric fractures. Only 2.7% occurred in patients less than 50 years of age. From 1965 to 1983, the rate increased 109%.

Cervical fractures predominated in the lower age groups. However, there was a higher incidence of trochanteric fractures than of cervical fractures in the elderly. It was predicted that the rate of fracture will double in 16 years in men and in 30 years in women. In Malmö, Sweden, the cumulative risk of hip fracture in a person living to age 90 is 45% in women and 24% in men.

In Uppsala, the incidence of hip fractures increased from 43 per 10,000 in 1965 to 65 per 10,000 in 1980. In the 85-year-old group, femoral neck fractures were over 3 times more common and trochanteric fractures were more than 4 times more common in 1980 than in 1965. In 1965, fractures of the femoral neck were almost 2 times more common than trochanteric fractures but in 1980 the incidences were almost equal.

In Malmö, a 6-fold increase in hip fractures was documented over the last 30 years. Men had a greater increase than women, and the greatest increase occurred in the very elderly.

In Finland, hip fracture accounted for 9% of all surgical hospital days in 1980. The number of femoral neck fractures was predicted to double from 1968 to 1985. As in other series, men under 50 had a greater incidence of femoral neck fracture than women, but this trend reversed after age 50 years. In 1980, the female-to-male ratio was 3:1 for femoral neck fractures and 2:1 for trochanteric fractures.

In the United States, the risk of hip fracture doubles every 6 years after age 50 years. White women have a 1.5 to 4 times greater incidence than black women after age 40 and an approximately 2 times greater incidence than white men after age 50 years. There does not appear to be a difference in incidence between black women and black men. This finding has been explained by the fact that whites have a decreased bone mass compared to blacks. The significance of the problem is evident by the fact that more than 200,000 hip fractures occur in the United States per year. This is compounded by the fact that the case fatality rates 1 year after fracture are as high as 50%.

Osteoporosis has been a predisposing condition for this problem. Alcohol consumption, particularly by men, has been a leading cause of osteoporosis in all age groups. In women, postmenopausal conditions account for the vast majority of cases of osteoporosis. A combination of vitamin D and calcium supplementation may be of benefit in decreasing the progression of the disease (see Chapter 3).

Smoking has been identified as a cause of osteoporosis in both sexes. Inactivity is an obvious factor. Osteomalacia accounts for a significant percentage of these problems. Prior gastric resection predisposes to malabsorption and decreased bone mass.

Some medications may have an adverse effect on bone mass. Tranquilizers have a marked effect on bone mass. Steroids have been demonstrated to decrease bone mass.

The orthopaedic surgeon still sees patients who are on long-term phenytoin (Dilantin) therapy for seizure disorders but have not had vitamin D and calcium supplementation. Unfortunately, the fact that phenytoin therapy leads to osteomalacia has received little attention in the neurology literature.

A program of gentle exercise is of paramount importance in decreasing the progression of osteoporosis, which will eventually decrease the incidence of hip fractures in the elderly.

Unfortunately, whether the noted increased incidence of hip fractures is due to one or more new risk factors or reflects an increase in prevalence or severity of existing factors is unknown at present.

Stress Fractures

The incidence of stress fractures (339 fractures in 295 trainees) was evaluated at an Army hospital in the United States. From this and other studies, four factors have been identified. Sex was a predisposing factor in that women had a greater incidence than men—3.41% and 0.9%, respectively. Second, race was a definite factor, with whites having a higher incidence than blacks. The white women were at the greatest risk, with an incidence of 11.8%. Third, age was a predisposing factor, with an increased incidence in stress fractures with advancing age. Fourth, stress fractures may result from underlying osteopenic metabolic bone disease—most notably rickets, osteomalacia, hyperparathyroidism, or osteoporosis. Additionally, stress fractures occur with Paget's disease, osteopetrosis, and pyknodysostosis. Of interest was the fact that the metatarsal bone was affected most often in these trainees, with an incidence of 28.3%. Other fracture incidences were 25.1% in the calcaneus and 15.6% in the medial tibial plateau.

In clinical practice, a difficult management problem is posed by the runner who has pain in the tibial region that limits activity. It is important to rule out the presence of a stress fracture. If there is no evidence of a definite stress fracture on regular radiographs, it frequently is useful to obtain a technetium bone scan which will reveal an altered level of activity if there is a stress fracture present. Restriction of the running activities will usually resolve the problem. However, these fractures do not always heal with limited activity, and frank nonunion may ensue.

Metabolism

Calcium metabolism in humans is regulated by multiple factors including parathyroid hormone (PTH), calcitonin (CT), and vitamin D metabolites. Bone tissue is a major target organ for these hormones (see Chapter 3). Growth hormone, thyroid hormone, anabolic agents, and vitamin D have been found to have beneficial effects on the process of fracture repair. On the other hand, steroids have been noted to have a negative effect. Callus formation is a very active process that consumes local calcium. Because calcium homeostasis is regulated by PTH, CT, and vitamin D metabolites, it is important to understand their function in fracture repair. Recently, studies in dogs and in humans have investigated the function of these molecules in normal fracture healing.

In the dog, a bridging callus is usually present at a fracture site by 3 to 4 weeks. Callus is apparent clinically and radiographically by 3 weeks. Hypocalcemia and reciprocal hyperphosphatemia develop 24 hours after the fracture in the dog model. Serum magnesium level fluctuates similar to that of calcium, but the changes are less obvious. These changes represent an immediate, nonspecific post-traumatic reaction (acute-phase reaction) to the injury. An interesting finding was the immediate increase in alkaline phosphatase level (this enzyme is produced by osteoblasts). It is thought that alkaline phosphatase activates osteoblastic bone formation, particularly calcification.

During fracture healing, there is an increase in serum levels of CT, 24,25-dihydroxyvitamin D [24,25-$(OH)_2$-D], and PTH. Serum 25-hydroxyvitamin D [25-(OH)-D] levels decrease consistently. It has been noted previously that PTH, CT, and 25-(OH)-D levels in dogs are similar to those in humans. CT is a calcium-preserving hormone and an antagonist to most of the actions of parathyroid hormone (see Chapter 3). It inhibits bone resorption by direct inhibition of the osteoclast. In the dog model, serum CT levels increase during the bone healing process, which confirms observations in humans. This supports the reports that suggest an important positive role for CT in bone repair.

In the kidney, two active end-metabolites of vitamin D are formed—namely, 1,25-$(OH)_2$-D and 24,25-$(OH)_2$-D. These metabolites are formed from the common precursor 25-(OH)-D. 1,25-$(OH)_2$-D is the principal factor governing calcium and phosphorus absorption from the gastrointestinal tract and regulates calcium and phosphorus concentrations in the extracellular fluid (see Chapter 3). Some investigators suggest that 24,25-$(OH)_2$-D may act directly on bone cells. However, all investigators agree that it is in part an inactive metabolite of vitamin D. In the dog model, serum levels of 24,25-$(OH)_2$-D are increased during fracture healing. The conversion of the precursor to 24,25-$(OH)_2$-D explains the persistently low concentrations of 25-(OH)-D during the fracture healing period. Obviously, vitamin D is a prerequisite for normal fracture healing. An increase in serum levels of PTH during regular fracture healing is explained by the body's effort to mobilize calcium and increase its availability for callus calcification.

Patients with fractures were also studied for PTH, CT, and vitamin D metabolites during regular healing. The plasma calcium level on the day of fracture was significantly decreased compared with a group of healthy volunteers of similar age and sex. Serum CT level on the day of fracture was significantly increased and it continued to increase during the healing period. A significant increase was noted in the plasma level of 24,25-$(OH)_2$-D on the day of fracture, and this continued to increase up to 6 weeks later. No significant changes were found in serum PTH levels on the day of fracture or during the healing process. The results suggest a possible physiologic active role for CT. The changes in 24,25-$(OH)_2$-D in fracture healing in humans may reflect inactive byproducts of vitamin D metabolism or a product that has a specific function. Further studies will be necessary to define its role.

Steroid Effects

The administration of high doses of cortical glucocorticoids has been associated with osteoporosis and pathologic fractures. However, the majority of these studies were in patients who had active rheumatoid arthritis or renal disease. It is difficult to separate the effect of steroid administration from that of immobilization of the joints (these patients have chronic joint inflammation). Corticosteroid administration affects bone in a characteristic distribution, with predominant loss of trabecular bone density in the axial skeleton such as the ribs and vertebrae. These areas are known to have a high content of trabecular bone with a rapid turnover rate. This is in contrast to the less dramatic changes in bone density and less frequent fractures that occur in the appendicular skeleton, where cortical bone predominates.

The effects of long-term steroid therapy in asthmatic patients were studied. An association between corticosteroid administration and pathologic fractures of the vertebrae and ribs was evident. Patients who had these fractures had received steroids in large doses for prolonged periods. The diminished trabecular bone mass in the forearm of patients receiving long-term treatment was consistent with the tendency to fracture in vertebrae and ribs which contain high proportions of trabecular bone. The data confirmed the usefulness of the ratio of cortical to trabecular mass; this ratio was constant regardless of age and sensitivity to the preferential effect of steroid on trabecular bone.

Only one study has demonstrated a rough but statistically significant relationship between duration of steroid therapy and selective loss of trabecular mass in patients with various steroid-treated disorders, primarily rheumatoid arthritis. It is also known that rheumatoid arthritis itself may lead to osteoporosis and therefore may have a detrimental effect in addition to that of steroid administration. If long-term steroid therapy is required for asthma or other medical conditions, then the orthopaedist will be required to treat the significant bone loss that results as well as to manage the fractures.

Bioelectricity

The biophysical properties of bone have received a great deal of recent attention. Electrical impulses have never demonstrated an ability to hasten normal fracture healing. It is true that the application of electrical current or electrical fields to a fresh fracture may hasten early phases of healing, but the end result is a fracture that heals in the same overall time interval. In other words, there is no decrease in the time required for a fracture to heal with the use of electricity.

The situation is entirely different with nonunions. Electricity in its various forms has been used as a treatment modality for management of delayed union and nonunion. In selected fractures it has been as successful as conventional surgical methods of treatment. Electricity may be applied to bone in three different forms.

Direct Current

Direct current may be applied to bone in two different manners.

1. A semi-invasive method involves insertion of Teflon-coated stainless steel cathodes percutaneously into a nonunion site and connecting them to a power pack. The stainless steel cathodes are programmed to deliver current at 20 μA to the nonunion site. Four cathodes are generally utilized for this method.
2. A completely invasive system has been developed for the application of direct current to bone. The system involves implantation of a cathode directly at the fracture site, connecting it to a battery covered by an inert coating, and burying the entire apparatus in the tissue.

Both of these systems have shown an ability to heal nonunions, with the success rate varying from 70% to 90%, depending on the bone involved.

Inductive Coupling

This involves application of a coil or a pair of coils on a common axis, termed "Helmholtz aiding." The coil or coils are positioned externally in a manner such that the coil's axis passes through the limb near the site to be stimulated. Time-varying current at 10 to 100 V is passed through the coils, producing a time-varying magnetic field, generally between 0.1 and 20 gauss, within the limb. This field produces a secondary time-varying potential field, resulting in local voltage gradients of 1 to 10 mV/cm and associated local currents in the tissue between the coils. The fields and the resulting currents diminish rapidly as distance from the coils increases. The power requirements are large and, in the past, this unit required the use of household current as a power source. Recently, a portable system has been developed. The success rate with this system has been similar to that with the direct current systems.

Capacitive Coupling

Several new studies have been published in regard to this new technique of electrical stimulation. Electrodes are placed externally, on the opposite sides of a limb portion containing the tissue that is to be stimulated. Although high potential gradient static fields have been utilized, lower gradient dynamic fields are much more common.

The power requirements of this system are modest and provided by a simple 9-V battery which is changed daily. In a preliminary study, 22 well-established nonunions in 20 patients were treated with a capacitively coupled electrical signal that was applied noninvasively through stainless steel capacitor plates on the skin surface over the approximate site of the nonunion.

Seventeen (77%) of the nonunions achieved solid osseous union after an average of 22.5 weeks of treatment with capacitive coupling. It was concluded that, because capacitive coupling is noninvasive, involves portable equipment, allows full weight-bearing on the lower extremity in a cast, is easy to apply, and does not require precise localization of the capacitor plates, it has distinct advantages over other methods of treating nonunion with electricity.

This system has also been utilized to study disuse osteoporosis and normal fracture healing. Disuse osteoporosis in the rat tibia was reversed in a sciatic denervation model.

The fact that an appropriate electrical signal was able to reverse osteoporosis in an animal model that was heretofore considered irreversible points out the effectiveness of electrically induced osteogenesis and the importance of continued investigation of capacitive coupling in the treatment of osteoporosis.

Annotated Bibliography

Epidemiology

Boyce, W.J., and Vessey, M.P.: Rising incidence of fracture of the proximal femur. Lancet 1:150–151, 1985.

The incidence of fractures was recorded prospectively in 1983 and compared with rates in the same population 27 years previously. The incidence was found to have doubled in both sexes, and the increase was apparent at all ages. The increases in the age-specific incidence must be due to changes in the cause of the fracture.

Farmer, M.E.; White, L.R.; Brody, J.A.; and Bailey, K.R.: Race and sex differences in hip fracture incidence. Am. J. Public Health 74:1374–1380, 1984.

Incidence rates for hip fractures in the United States were estimated from the National Hospital Discharge Survey for the years 1974–1979. Risk approximately doubles every 5 years after age 50. Age-specific rates by 5-year age groups were compared among the four race/sex groups. White women were at twice the risk for hip fracture compared with black women and at 2.7 times the risk for hip fracture compared with white men. No significant differences were observed between black women and black men.

Johnell, O.; Nilsson, B.; Obrant, K.; and Sernbo, I.: Age and sex patterns of hip fracture: Changes in 30 years. Acta Orthop. Scand. 55:290–292, 1984.

There was a continuous increase in hip fractures over the 30 years. The trend was most obvious in the oldest age groups and in men.

Lüthje, P.: Fractures of the proximal femur in Finland in 1980. Ann. Chir. Gynaecol. 72:282–286, 1983.

In 1980, 2,449 patients with femoral neck fracture and 1,096 with trochanteric fracture were treated in Finland. The female-to-male ratio was 3:1; the femoral neck-to-trochanteric fracture ratio was 2:1. Age-specific incidence was higher for women than for men in both groups. The number of femoral neck fractures will have doubled between 1968 and 1985.

Schmidt Brudvig, T.J.; Gudger, T.D.; and Obermeyer, L.: Stress fractures in 295 trainees: A one-year study of incidence as related to age, sex, and race. Milit. Med. 148:666–667, 1983.

A study of 339 stress fractures in 295 military trainees suggests that sex, race, and age all have significant influence in the development of stress fractures in the military training population.

Wallace, W.A.: The increasing incidence of fractures of the proximal femur: An orthopaedic epidemic. Lancet 1:1413–1414, 1983.

Analysis of hospital admissions in Nottingham reveals a disproportionate increase in fractures of the proximal femur in women over age 75 years, from 8/1,000 per year in 1971 to 16/1,000 per year in 1981. Work is urgently required to establish prophylactic treatment for this group of patients.

Zain Elabdien, B.S.; Olerud, S.; Karlström, G.; and Smedby, B.: Rising incidence of hip fracture in Uppsala, 1965–1980. Acta Orthop. Scand. 55:284–289, 1984.

For every 5-year interval, the number of hip fractures increased by 21–25%. The study demonstrated that the incidence of hip fractures has increased particularly in the older age groups. If the age-specific incidence continues to rise in the older age groups, the frequency of hip fractures will be doubled within 20 years.

Zetterberg, C.; Elmerson, S.; and Andersson, G.B.J.: Epidemiology of hip fractures in Göteborg, Sweden, 1940–1983. Clin. Orthop. 191:43–52, 1984.

A dramatic progressive increase in the incidence of cervical and trochanteric fractures of the proximal end of the femur was observed in Gothenburg from 1940 to 1983. Only 20% of the 109% rate increase can be explained by age factors in the population. It is probable that the fracture incidence will double in 16 years in men and in 30 years in women.

Metabolism

Adinoff, A.D., and Hollister, J.R.: Steroid-induced fractures and bone loss in patients with asthma. N. Engl. J. Med. 309:265–268, 1983.

Long-term steroid therapy in asthmatic patients appears to be associated with decreased trabecular bone density and increased prevalence of rib and vertebral fractures.

Bagnoli, F.; Bruchi, S.; Sardelli, S.; Vispi, L.; Buonocore, G.; Franchi, F.; and Bracci, R.: Calcitonin and parathyroid hormone in newborn infants with fracture of the clavicle. Calcif. Tissue Int. 36:357–360, 1984.

The results indicate that fracture of the clavicle is a significant and peculiar factor in stimulating calcitonin secretion. Serum calcium levels appear to be controlled by calcitonin rather than autoregulating the secretion of it.

Meller, Y.; Kestenbaum, R.S.; Mozes, M.; Mozes, G.; Yagil, R.; and Shany, S.: Mineral and endocrine metabolism during fracture healing in dogs. Clin. Orthop. 187:289–295, 1984.

The data demonstrate the changes in levels of calcium-regulating hormones in response to bone injury. This suggests that calcitonin and 24,25-$(OH)_2$-D can be associated with the process of callus formation.

Meller, Y.; Shainkin-Kestenbaum, R.; Shany, S.; Zuilli, I.; Yankowitz, N.; Giat, J.; Konforti, A.; and Torok, G.: Parathyroid hormone, calcitonin, and vitamin D metabolites during normal fracture healing in humans: A preliminary report. Clin. Orthop. 183:238–245, 1984.

No significant changes were found in serum PTH and plasma 25-OH-D_3 levels on the day of fracture or during the healing process. The results suggest a possible physiologic active role for calcitonin and 24,25-$(OH)_2$-D_3 in fracture healing in humans.

Bioelectricity

Black, J.: Tissue response to exogenous electromagnetic signals. Orthop. Clin. North Am. 15:15–31, January 1984.

Studies in animals have clearly established that various forms of electrical stimulation positively affect the course of fracture healing. The situation with regard to stimulation of regeneration and to prevention and treatment of osteoporosis is less clear, reflecting the early stages of research on these phenomena. However, early indications suggest that the underlying conditions will also be shown to be subject to electrical control in animals. The human application will be based in part on the progress of studies in animals.

Brighton, C.T.: The semi-invasive method of treating nonunion with direct current. Orthop. Clin. North Am. 15:33–45, January 1984.

The results of treating 467 nonunions with direct current over the preceding 12 years was presented. A dose-response curve of 10–20 μA was established. When treated adequately with constant direct current, a typical nonunion with a gap not greater than half the diameter of the bone and not containing a synovial pseudarthrosis will heal at a rate equal to that after bone graft surgery.

Brighton, C.T.; Hozack, W.J.; Brager, M.D.; Windsor, R.E.; Pollack, S.R.; Vreslovic, E.J.; and Kotwick, J.E.: Fracture healing in the rabbit fibula when subjected to various capacitively coupled electrical fields. J. Orthop. Res. 3:331–340, 1985.

The results show that there is a dose-response curve for capacitive coupling in fracture healing and that a 220-mV 250-μA 60-kHz applied electrical signal (0.33 V·cm internal electrical field) is the most effective for fracture stimulation in this model.

Brighton, C.T.; Nichols, C.E., III; and Arangio, G.A.: Amelioration of oxygen-induced osteoporosis in the in vitro fetal rat tibia with a capacitively coupled electrical field. J. Orthop. Res. 3:311–320, 1985.

It was concluded that an appropriate capacitively coupled electrical field can inhibit oxygen-induced osteoporosis in an *in vitro* mammalian long bone model. The signal was a 60-kHz sine wave with a 10-V peak-to-peak output; current density and field in a culture dish were calculated to be 5.2 $\mu A/cm^2$ and 0.32 mV/cm, respectively.

Brighton, C.T., and Pollack, S.R.: Treatment of recalcitrant non-union with a capacitively coupled electrical field: A preliminary report. J. Bone Joint Surg. 67A:577–585, 1985.

Twenty-two well-established nonunions in 20 patients were treated with a capacitively coupled electrical signal (sine wave at 60 kHz; 5 V peak-to-peak) that was applied noninvasively through stainless steel capacitor plates on the skin overlying the approximate site of the nonunion. The total overall results were 77% solid union at an average of 22.5 weeks of treatment.

Brighton, C.T.; Tadduni, G.T.; and Pollack, S.R.: Treatment of sciatic denervation disuse osteoporosis in the rat tibia with capacitively coupled electrical stimulation: Dose response and duty cycle. J. Bone Joint Surg. 67A:1022–1028, 1985.

The authors conclude that a capacitively coupled electrical signal, delivered through gel-coated electrodes, can largely reverse an established disuse osteoporosis due to neurectomy in rat tibia. Only a 100% duty-cycle signal was effective in reversing the loss of bone mass in the neurectomized tibia.

Downes, E.M., and Watson, J.: Development of the iron-cored electromagnet for the treatment of non-union and delayed union. J. Bone Joint Surg. 66B:754–759, 1984.

An iron-cored electromagnet was developed as a stimulator of bone union. In 80 patients treated for various forms of failed union over an 8-year period, a 70% success rate was achieved.

Marcer, M.; Musatti, G.; and Bassett, C.A.L.: Results of pulsed electromagnetic fields (PEMFs) in ununited fractures after external skeletal fixation. Clin. Orthop. 190:260–265, 1984.

External skeletal fixation *in situ* and pulse electromagnetic fields were used to treat 147 patients with nonunions who had a mean of 3.3 operative procedures. The overall success rate was 73%. The humerus had a lower success rate, as with other techniques.

Rodriguez Fuentes, A.E.; Marcondes de Souza, J.P.; Valeri, V.; and Mascarenhas, S.: Experimental model of electric stimulation of pseudarthrosis healing. Clin. Orthop. 183:267–275, 1984.

Direct-current electrical stimulation was evaluated in induced pseudarthrosis in the radius of adult dogs. Statistically significant data demonstrate activation of endochondral ossification and bone union by electrical stimulation.

Wahlström, O.: Stimulation of fracture healing with electromagnetic fields of extremely low frequency (EMF of ELF). Clin. Orthop. 186:293–301, 1984.

A randomized controlled study of the treatment of Colles' fractures with and without a low-frequency electromagnetic field was performed. The clinical relevance of the results is not known for certain, but one interpretation of the data is that this stimulation improves or accelerates the early phase of fracture healing. Further studies are required.

8

Trauma: Soft Tissue

This chapter covers aspects of repair of soft tissue with an emphasis on muscle, tendons, ligaments, articular cartilage, meniscal tissues, and nerves. More information on ligament injury and repairs specific to the knee is provided elsewhere.

Muscle Injury

Injury to muscle tissue can be conveniently considered as *direct* or *indirect*. Direct injury is the result of a laceration or a direct blow to the muscle; indirect injury is the result of a strain or muscle damage caused by excessive stretch, muscle contraction, or both.

Direct

Laceration Few clinical and research studies have dealt with the recovery of muscle after laceration and repair. (This paucity of information is in sharp contrast to the data available for recovery of nerve or connective tissues.) Muscle tissue can be sutured if the connective tissues or tendons around the muscle provide enough strength for suture repair. The fate of the muscle might then depend on the nature of the recovery process. Muscle tissue might regenerate across the laceration and restore the muscle to its previous appearance, as has been shown for some very thin muscles. Alternatively, the muscle might heal with a dense connective tissue scar and no regeneration of muscle across the gap. The recovery of muscle function then would depend on the separate fates of the two segments created by the laceration.

It appears that for larger muscles the recovery process is the latter alternative—healing with a dense scar at the laceration site. In one study the portion of the muscle containing the motor point remained physiologically active, whereas the portion of the muscle separated from the motor point and from intramuscular innervation became fibrotic with many histologic features of denervated muscle. The portion isolated from the motor point healed and was able to transmit tension and shortening generated in the innervated portion.

The extent of physiologic recovery is dependent on the architectural arrangement of the muscle fibers (Fig. 1). In general, the ability of muscle to produce tension is proportional to the cross-sectional area of muscle fibers, and the ability to shorten is relative to the length of the muscle fibers. In a penniform muscle as shown in Figure 1, only the muscle segment containing the nerve supply continues to function. Because only half of the muscle fibers are in this segment, only half of the tension of the whole muscle can be generated. The intact fibers are their full original length and therefore shortening near the normal amount is possible if light loads are used to test shortening ability. The distal segment becomes fibrotic and is able to transmit the tension generated in the proximal innervated segment. The distal segment remains viable if its blood supply is not destroyed but cannot function as active muscle if isolated from its nerve supply.

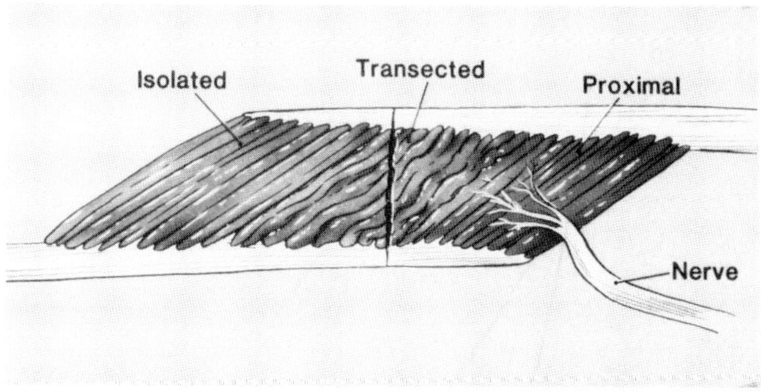

Figure 1

Diagram of lacerated muscle. Oblique orientation of muscle fibers is shown. The laceration leaves fibers intact proximally and distally but divides the central fibers. The segment distal to the laceration becomes isolated from its nerve supply by the scar. (From Garrett, W.E., Jr.; Seaber, A.V.; Boswick, J.; Urbaniak, J.R.; and Goldner, J.L. J. Hand Surg. [Am.] 9:683–692, 1984. By permission of the American Society for Surgery of the Hand.)

Blunt Trauma Unlike laceration, blunt trauma produces muscle injury without disrupting the muscle belly. Blunt trauma has long been known to affect the deeper muscles in proximity to bone. The potential for myositis ossificans is also recognized. Standardized crush injuries have been studied experimentally. Controlled blunt trauma causes disruption of the muscle fibers in a manner somewhat similar to laceration as discussed above. There is an initial intense inflammatory reaction with eventual clearing of the necrotic muscle and formation of a dense connective tissue scar. Continuity of the muscle fibers is disrupted in the area of the blunt trauma.

In one study in sheep, the quadriceps femoris overlying the femur was bluntly injured. The force was applied to the soft tissue directly anteriorly but, interestingly, only the muscle tissue adjacent to the bone—i.e., the vastus intermedius—was damaged severely. One may consider that the pressure was transmitted through the fluid compartment and only where the pressure could not be transmitted through the bone did damage occur. Although not obviously damaged by the initial injury, the underlying femur reacted to the injury with predictable periosteal hyperplasia and new bone formation. Heterotopic bone formed within the reactive scar tissue in 17% of the legs of the injured sheep (Fig. 2). The heterotopic bone formed within the scar tissue and appeared to result from metaplastic ossification.

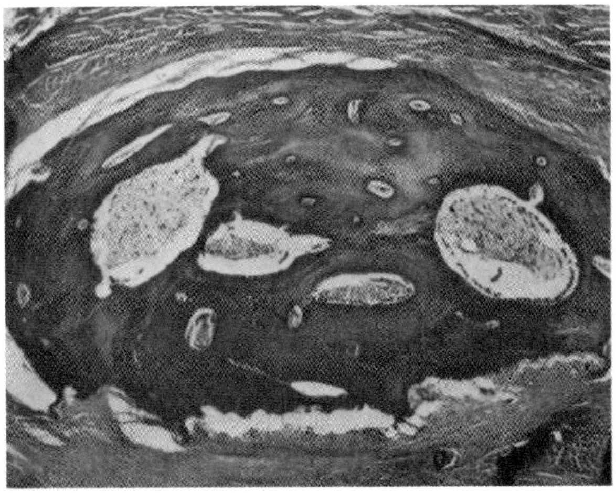

Figure 2

Ectopic bone in thigh of sheep killed 3 months after blunt trauma. (From Walton, M., and Rothwell, A.G. Clin. Orthop. 176:273–281, 1983. By permission of the J.B. Lippincott Company.)

In a separate study, blunt trauma was produced in the gastrocnemius of rats. Again, collagen scar proliferated in the defect. The muscle from younger animals demonstrated a more rapid and intensive reparative process than muscle from older animals.

Indirect

Skeletal muscle trauma occurs more frequently as an indirect injury or strain in which no direct blow or external contact is made with the muscle tissue. Epidemiologic studies show muscle strains to be among the most frequent injuries sustained in athletics. The high incidence of strain injuries of the back in occupational situations has also been documented in detail. These injuries are more prevalent with heavy labor and are a large and costly problem for the national economy.

Studies of strain injuries in the extremities have stressed the frequency of these injuries in two-joint muscles which are subjected to simultaneous stretch at two joints under certain conditions. Frequently injured are the hamstring muscles, rectus femoris, and gastrocnemius. Muscles at risk for strain injury often contain a high percentage of type II fibers. These fibers are capable of faster speeds of contraction, higher forces, and poorer endurance than the type I fibers. The fiber type distribution in a muscle is related to its physiologic use and it is likely that muscles whose use requires fast and powerful contractions are both higher in percentage of type II fibers and more susceptible to injury.

There is general agreement that strain injuries are very likely to recur. Perhaps poor rehabilitation practices influence the reinjury rate. There is also general agreement that the stronger a muscle group, the less likely is injury. It is difficult to test many of the concepts of injury prevention. Muscle imbalance and joint inflexibility have often been considered to predispose to indirect muscle injury. However, a prospective blind study has revealed that muscle imbalance documented by an isokinetic dynamometer did not predispose to injury. Similarly, ligamentous laxity has not been shown conclusively to be a predictor of injury.

One of the problems relative to investigating strain injuries to muscle is the lack of good structural and pathologic studies demonstrating the nature, location, and recovery of muscle following strain injuries.

Delayed Muscle Soreness and Injury

Attention has been focused in the past few years on the nature of the soreness and pain felt 24 to 72 hours after heavy exercise. Exercise requiring higher intensity and higher force production is more likely to cause soreness than is exercise at lower intensity levels and requiring more endurance. This soreness has also been associated with a muscular weakness that is transient as shown in the classic studies by Hough over 80 years ago. Recently, the changes in structure and strength after high-intensity exercise have been investigated. Muscle biopsy in athletes with delayed muscle soreness showed changes in the sarcomere structure, particularly in the Z-band and particularly in type II fibers. These changes were apparent by electron microscopy.

Particular reference has also been made by several investigators to the concurrence of muscle soreness and *eccentric* muscle contraction. Eccentric muscle contraction refers to muscle activation associated with lengthening or stretching of the muscle rather than shortening of it. Muscle activation and concomitant shortening is termed "concentric contraction." For example, in jumping, the quadriceps femoris undergoes concentric contraction involving muscle activation and shortening to supply the force to extend the knee. In landing from the jump, the quadriceps again is activated but it is being stretched (an eccentric contraction) as it absorbs kinetic energy and prevents falling. Repetitive stresses in the eccentric mode are associated with a higher rate of delayed muscle soreness. For example, if one leg is used to jump a certain height repetitively and the other leg is used to land from the height, the leg used for landing is more likely to exhibit delayed soreness.

A transient weakness accompanies delayed muscle soreness. Recent studies have demonstrated additional weakness after eccentric muscle contraction (25% to 50% weaker) and this weakness was evident even when the muscles were directly stimulated by electrical currents. However, the muscle has been shown to recover from the weakness and there are no data showing long-term detrimental effects on performance after delayed muscle soreness.

With the increase in popularity of jogging and high-endurance exercise such as marathon running, questions have been raised regarding potential injury to muscle. Several studies have shown transient increases in serum enzymes such as creatine kinase which are thought to represent muscle injury. The beneficial cardiovascular aspects of endurance training have been demonstrated frequently and clearly. The literature to date does not describe permanent injury to muscle after long-duration aerobic exercise such as marathon running. The available studies of serum enzyme changes and structural changes show strong evidence of a reparative process as well as an injury process and there are no conclusive studies showing ultimate detrimental effects on muscle. In fact, it is apparent that many of the beneficial cardiovascular effects are not due to changes in the cardiovascular system *per se* but to beneficial changes in the aerobic capacity of the skeletal muscle.

Tendon Injury

Controversies about the basic biologic events in tendon injury and repair have received considerable attention in the recent and current literature. Much of the controversy is about the cellular source of tendon healing. Previously it was thought that most of the healing that occurred in a lacerated tendon was due to the new blood supply and fibroblasts brought by the scar formation and adhesions formed between the tendon and the surrounding tissues. Recent studies have emphasized the intrinsic ability of tendons to heal without adhesions to surrounding tissue. Knowledge of the source of healing certainly must have a large influence on initial treatment and postoperative management of tendon injuries. If scar tissue and extrinsic blood supply are necessary for tendon healing, then immobilization might be necessary to allow temporary adhesions. If healing is possible due to intrinsic ability of the tendon or the synovial fluid, then motion might be begun early in order to decrease adhesions and allow maximal return of range of motion.

Recent studies emphasize that synovial diffusion accounts for a large portion of the nutrition of normal tendons. All tendons have a measurable blood flow but differences in perfusion and diffusion suggest that most of the normal tendon nutrition comes from diffusion from surrounding tissues. Blood supply within tendons comes primarily from the region of the muscle tissue and from the paratenon. In the hand flexor tendons, additional blood supply comes from the vincula.

In spite of the importance of the surrounding tissue in the nutrition of tendons, it has been demonstrated that severed flexor tendons can repair without any extrinsic blood supply brought by scar tissue or adhesions to the tendon. When flexor tendons were severed, repaired, and then transferred to the synovial cavity of the knee joint, the superficial layers were able to heal and bridge the suture gap without adhesions to the surrounding synovium. The fibroblasts responsible for healing the tendon injury were from the tendon and possibly the synovium; the macrophages present in the gap were primarily contributed by the surrounding synovium.

Lacerated tendons from rabbits were transferred to a tissue culture medium after laceration and demonstrated intrinsic ability to heal in the absence of extrinsic blood supply or synovial diffusion. Within the tissue culture medium, the tendon healing process included both phagocytosis of cellular debris and new collagen synthesis. The former occurred from cells derived from the epitenon and the latter, from endotenon-derived cells.

At present there is a great deal of evidence to show that tendon repair can occur from intrinsic capabilities, either through cells within or covering the tendon or from the synovial fluid. It is quite likely that extrinsic factors are also active in tendon healing in the clinical situation.

Controlled Motion in Tendon Healing

The intrinsic ability of tendons to heal has increased interest in the use of motion during the healing period. Motion might deprive the tendon of extrinsic blood supply through adhesions, but it also might enhance ultimate recovery of range of motion. Controlled passive motion has a beneficial effect on flexor tendon healing in dogs. When the tendons were immobilized, the bulk of the repair came from the digital sheath rather than from the epitenon. Mobilized tendons healed more quickly with earlier restoration of a smooth tendon surface (Fig. 3). Later studies have shown revascularization across a repaired flexor tendon by

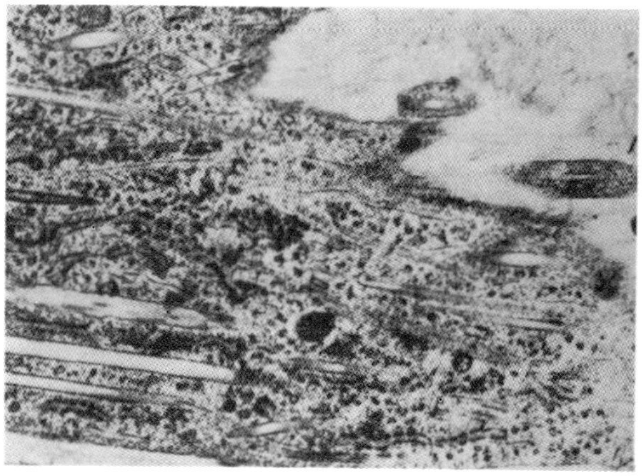

Figure 3

Scanning electron micrograph of tendon after repair with early controlled passive motion postoperatively. The repair surface is smooth and without adhesions. The sutures remain visible. (From Gelberman, R.H.; Vande Berg, J.S.; Lundborg, G.N.; and Akeson, W.H. J. Bone Joint Surg. 65A:70–80, 1983. By permission of the journal.)

2 weeks with gaps healing by cellular proliferation from the epitenon and endotenon.

There are hopes that controlled early motion or continuous passive motion might allow healing of tendons, particularly digital flexor tendons, without excessive scar formation and motion limitation. There now appears to be good scientific evidence that intrinsic healing is not only possible but may also be superior. One risk of early motion is tendon rupture if the tension generated by the motion exceeds the strength of the tendon at the repair site.

Biomechanics of Tendon Healing

Classic studies of tendon healing show a gradual return of strength in repaired tendon. However, collagen content does not appear to increase significantly after 5 to 6 weeks. The increases in strength that occur long after 5 to 6 weeks therefore are likely to be due to remodeling and reorganization of the collagen rather than to an absolute increase in collagen. More recent studies using bone-tendon-muscle-tendon-bone preparations and modern testing apparatus have confirmed the classic studies. Maximum load increased slowly and was less than half of normal at 4 weeks. Cellularity in the repaired tissue decreased and collagen fiber orientation became more mature as healing progressed. In the early healing phase there appears to be an increase in the amounts of glycoproteins such as fibronectin (fibronectin is a glycoprotein thought to be responsible for linking cell surfaces to connective tissue frameworks). Type III collagen is also increased in the early phase of healing.

Ligament Injury

Basic understanding of the biomechanics of ligament injury and of the biology of ligament healing has increased substantially in recent years. Much of the interest has been generated by an increased awareness of the poor outcome expected from healing of an untreated injury to the anterior cruciate ligament. The anterior cruciate ligament will be discussed later in the section on the lower extremity. This review will consider new knowledge regarding ligaments other than in the knee joint and general information about ligaments.

The ligaments of the ankle joint have been investigated in much detail in the past few years. Previous literature was ambiguous regarding which ankle ligaments must be injured to produce instability or clinical signs. Several recent studies point out the importance of the anterior talofibular (ATF) ligament. Sectioning of just this ligament alone produced measurable laxity in response to anterior, inversion, and rotation forces; the laxity was more pronounced for anterior and rotational forces than for inversion forces. Testing of the ankle under physiologic joint loading conditions also demonstrated that stability in response to inversion stress was provided by articular surface contact rather than by ligaments. These studies together point out the nature of *rotary* instability of the ankle due to ATF ligament deficiency rather than to a simple inversion instability. The ATF ligament fibers are directed in an appropriate plane to resist internal rotation of the talus on the tibia (or external rotation of the tibia on the talus).

Results of biomechanical studies and radiographic stress tests are in agreement. Anterior displacement of the talus is primarily a function of the status of the ATF ligament with little or no additional motion when the calcaneofibular ligament also is excised. However, inversion stress tests show much more instability when both ligaments are injured than when either ligament alone is injured.

The strength of the human ankle ligaments and autogenous reconstructive grafts has been reported. The ATF ligament showed surprisingly high strain-to-failure and low load-to-failure values, explaining its propensity for injury. Several of the frequently used autogenous grafts were also tested. All of the tendon grafts showed significantly greater strength than the ATF and significantly greater stiffness (Table 1). This may explain the general success of reconstructive ankle procedures in terms of restoring stability and the frequent increase in stiffness after these procedures.

In many respects the recent progress in the understanding of ligamentous instability of the ankle is similar to the previous evolution in understanding of the ligamentous instability of the knee. Injury to the ATF ligament can cause a rotary instability, but secondary restraints lessen other instabilities such as inversion. The ligament function is dependent on the position of the ankle and the application of force, as in the knee. Finally, consideration of the strengths of the tissues used to reconstruct the ankle ligaments helps to explain the surgical results. In the knee the relative weakness of the autogenous substitutes made it clear why many of the grafts previously used were insufficient. The relative strength of the ankle substitute grafts explains why the reconstructive procedures usually are able to restore stability.

Cartilage Injury

Articular Cartilage Injury

With the increasing use of arthroscopy and the search for new techniques by which arthroscopic surgical procedures may be beneficial, there has been renewed interest in the response of hyaline cartilage to injury. A review of the basic biologic processes associated with the healing of lesions in articular cartilage has given the orthopaedic surgeon a better scientific basis for evaluating whether these procedures may in fact be useful. Laceration or trauma to hyaline cartilage that does not extend to underlying bone can remain for years without healing or necessarily progressing. A partial-thickness shaving of articular cartilage similarly shows no appreciable healing or restoration of articular cartilage. This can be explained by the lack of a vascular supply in articular cartilage. Clot formation and reorganization are necessary to restore tissue continuity.

Lacerations that are deeper and penetrate the vascular region of the underlying bone react in a different manner. Initial bleeding causes hematoma formation which progresses to fibroblastic repair tissue and ultimately differentiates into a tissue resembling cartilage. Under different conditions the scar is more likely to resemble fibrocartilage or hyaline cartilage. The lesions do not appear to be repaired completely but do show ability to heal. The ability to repair decreases as the size of the defect increases. These data suggest that partial-thickness cartilage shaving is unlikely to result in any significant cartilage repair. Perforation of the subchondral bone does bring the potential for some tissue regeneration with fibrocartilage. There is no good evidence that a large area of cartilage loss can be induced to regenerate by multiple perforations of the subchondral bone.

It has been shown that full-thickness articular cartilage defects into the subchondral bone of rabbits heal differently, depending on the motion of the joint in the postoperative period. Light microscopy was used to evaluate the results. Healing with a tissue resembling hyaline cartilage occurred in a small percentage of animals treated by immobilization or intermittent active motion. In adult animals treated postoperatively by continuous passive motion, healing occurred in 44% of the defects (Fig. 4). These lesions were small (1 mm in diameter) and were created in normal (not osteoarthritic) cartilage, but the clinical promise is evident.

Table 1. Biomechanical Data

	Anterior talofibular ligament	Calcaneofibular ligament	Peroneus brevis	Split peroneus brevis	Extensor, 4th toe
Specimens, no.	12	16	4	5	6
Max. load, newtons	138.9 ± 23.5	345.7 ± 55.2	258.2 ± 63.5	258.8 ± 110.6	130.1 ± 20.9
Max. strain	0.53 ± 0.06	0.38 ± 0.03	0.10 ± 0.03	0.08 ± 0.02	0.09 ± 0.01
Velocity of deflection, cm/sec	101 ± 7	106 ± 4	54 ± 19	82 ± 24	71 ± 6

From Attarian, D.E.; McCrackin, H.J.; Devito, D.P.; McElhaney, J.H.; and Garrett, W.E., Jr. Am. J. Sports Med. 13:377-381, 1985. By permission of the American Orthopaedic Society for Sports Medicine.

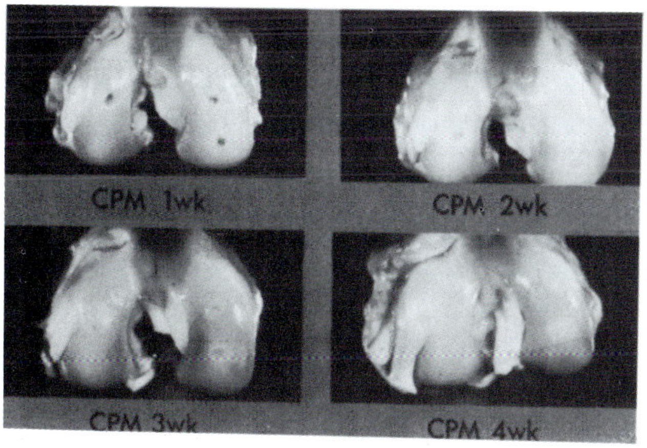

Figure 4

Gross appearance of rabbit femoral condyles after creation of articular cartilage defects and treatment with continuous passive motion (*CPM*) for various periods of time. Note the progression of healing and the resemblance to normal cartilage. (From Salter, R.B.; Simmonds, D.F.; Malcolm, B.W.; Rumble, E.J.; MacMichael, D.; and Clements, N.D. J. Bone Joint Surg. 62A:1232–1251, 1980. By permission of the journal.)

The effect of blunt trauma on cartilage has been reinvestigated recently. Blunt trauma does not create cartilage laceration or subchondral fracture, unlike the mechanisms of trauma mentioned above. Controlled loads applied to canine patellofemoral joints caused reproducible histologic changes, particularly in the zone of calcified cartilage. Increased cellularity and vascular invasion were evident in this zone. Biochemical changes were also prominent, with an increase in water content and an increased proteoglycan content as measured by hexuronic acid content. Although proteoglycan content increased, there was less association of collagen with the proteoglycan. These changes are similar to the chronic changes in articular cartilage with osteoarthritis. This is an interesting finding and may reveal an association between blunt joint trauma and the changes in chondromalacia.

Meniscal Injury

For many years, standard orthopaedic treatment of torn menisci was complete surgical excision. In the 1970s there were reports of successful repairs of peripheral tears of menisci in association with collateral ligament disruptions. In recent years there has been new emphasis on the ability of menisci to heal. Above, the discussion regarding healing of articular cartilage stressed that superficial cartilage lesions not penetrating to a vascular supply were unlikely to heal. This principle also holds for meniscal fibrocartilage. A tear in the avascular central portion of the meniscus creates no bleeding, no clot, no subsequent fibrous reorganization, and no scar formation. However, a tear near the peripheral meniscocapsular junction may involve the vascularized portion of the meniscus and may heal if sutured and immobilized properly. Several clinical series demonstrate a good response of peripheral meniscus tears after suture fixation in stable knees or knees made stable by surgical repair or reconstruction of the deficient ligaments.

Experimental support also exists for the concept of meniscal healing. The peripheral 25% of the meniscus contains blood vessels that originate in the capsular and synovial tissues. Lacerations of meniscus in the avascular portion do not heal. Lacerations extending into the vascularized portion of meniscus heal with fibrovascular scar (Fig. 5). If lesions in the avascular region can be connected to the peripheral vascular tissue, they can heal with scar formation made possible by the connection which acts as a vascular access channel.

Nerve Injury

Advances in basic and clinical knowledge about nerve injury and repair have not been as frequent as advances in other tissues of interest to orthopaedic surgeons. Nerve transection and repair disrupts the nerve axons distal to the laceration and results in their death and eventual wallerian degeneration. If this alone were the limiting factor in nerve recovery, one might expect a nerve crush injury with death of the distal axons to recover similarly to a laceration and repair. However, nerve crush injuries (or axonotmesis) recover much better than lacerations do. The disruption of the connective tissue framework and the malalignment of the approximated nerve endings appears to be one of the biggest obstacles to predictable and successful nerve repair.

New attention has been addressed to the old technique of direct muscular neurotization. This technique does not restore motor nerve continuity but instead inserts the proximal stump of a transected motor nerve directly into the muscle belly. This technique has been effective in restoring some function in animal models, although the function may not be equal to that from the functional recovery of repaired nerves. However, in some clinical situations, direct nerve repair may not be possible (e.g., due to avulsion of the distal nerve) and direct implantation of the proximal stump into the muscle belly may be warranted. Clinical

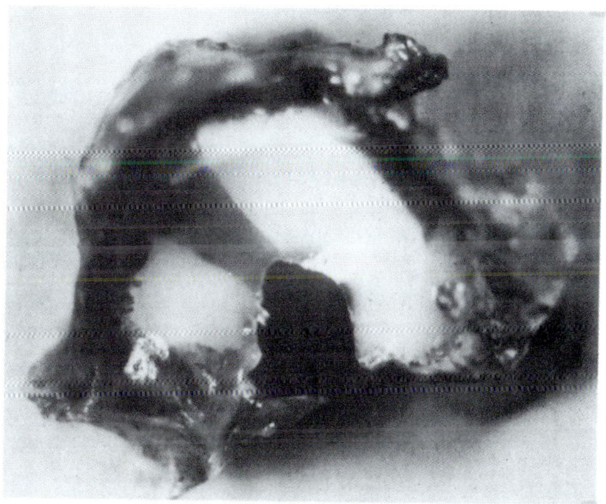

Figure 5

Meniscus perfused with India ink 10 weeks after complete transection. The radial incision reached to the peripheral vascular region. Fibrovascular scar has filled the lesion and resumed the normal contour of the meniscus. (From Arnoczky, S.P., and Warren, R.F. Am. J. Sports Med. 11:131–141, 1983. By permission of the American Orthopaedic Society for Sports Medicine.)

studies, particularly from Italy, have demonstrated the usefulness of this technique of nerve reconstruction in the limited indications for which it is warranted.

A new approach to the repair of peripheral nerve lacerations is worthy of note. An extremely careful and sophisticated approach has been developed to place nerves back into proper alignment without necessarily causing distal cell death. The approach involves suturing nerves not to each other but to a rubber mechanical platform that will distribute the tension and allow better alignment and less scar tissue at the repair site. The nerves are frozen carefully, cut with a vibrating blade, and soaked in a solution resembling intracellular fluid and containing nonspecific enzyme inhibitors to prevent some intracellular destructive changes (Fig. 6). With all of these technical improvements, the functional recovery of lacerated nerves was clearly superior to nerve repaired by conventional microsurgical technique. These techniques were developed in the rat model using the sciatic nerve. No data are available for primates.

Wound Healing

The cellular and biochemical events involved in the wound healing process have received much attention in recent years. Better understanding of these phenomena may allow clinical manipulation of wound healing and delayed healing problems. Many of the advances found by studying wound healing in skin and subcutaneous tissue are also applicable to other soft tissues such as ligament, tendon, and cartilage as well as to the healing of bone.

The products of coagulation are increasingly regarded as active participants in the healing process. Platelets and products of platelets are specifically involved. Platelets bind to collagen and release various products. Prostaglandin release is mediated by platelets. These arachidonic acid derivatives are among the primary mediators of the inflammatory response. Various products of the prostaglandin pathway induce vasodilation and edema (prostacyclin), platelet contraction and vasoconstriction (thromboxane), and leukocyte chemotaxis (leukotrienes). The balance among these products is very much involved in the cellular events of wound healing.

Platelets also secrete a specific growth factor that causes proliferation of fibroblasts and the production of collagen. Growth factors appear to be present also in epidermis, cartilage, fibroblasts, and other tissues. These growth factors stimulate the cells involved in the reparative process. They appear to have an effect separate from that of inflammation and produce new tissue growth, not invasion by inflammatory cells.

Central in the initial clotting sequence is the presence of fibrin and fibronectin. The initial granulation scaffold appears to be composed largely of the fibrin polymer and fibronectin. Fibronectin, a very large glycoprotein, is gaining increasing recognition for its importance in the extracellular matrix of tissues and in the adhesion of cells to the connective tissue matrix (Fig. 7). Fibronectin binds to fibrin and also to fibroblasts or regenerating cells. In this manner the fibronectin may act as a chemotactic factor for fibroblasts or epidermal cells and as a mediator of selective cell adhesion. In addition to the fibronectin in the clot matrix, an additional form of fibronectin exists bound to cell membranes. For example, cell surface fibronectin of platelets is involved in the initial adhesion of platelets to collagen.

The inflammatory cells present in a wound are now realized to be highly involved in the healing process and not simply with the inflammatory process. The initial cells seen in wound healing are polymorphonuclear leukocytes. The neutrophils have a central role in prostaglandin synthesis and mediate the factors listed above. After several days, the wound is populated more by monocytes or monocytes transformed to macrophages. These cells ingest and remove cell debris and dead tissue. Macrophages also produce growth factors and are involved in proliferation of

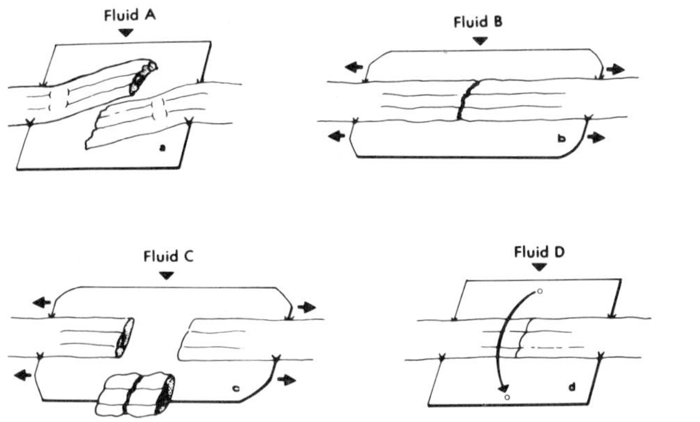

Figure 6

Four phases of nerve reconnection by the technique of de Medinaceli. In fluid A (resembling extracellular fluid), the nerve is sutured to a rubber support away from the severed ends. Then the nerve is cooled to 10°C and soaked in fluid B (resembling intracellular fluid) and the rubber is stretched until the nerve ends come into contact. The nerve ends are then carefully frozen and the lacerated ends are trimmed with a vibrating blade. The nerve ends are reapproximated after tension on the rubber support is released and the cut ends are in close proximity. (From de Medinaceli, L.; Freed, W.J.; and Wyatt, R.J. Exp. Neurol. 81:488–496, 1983. By permission of Academic Press.)

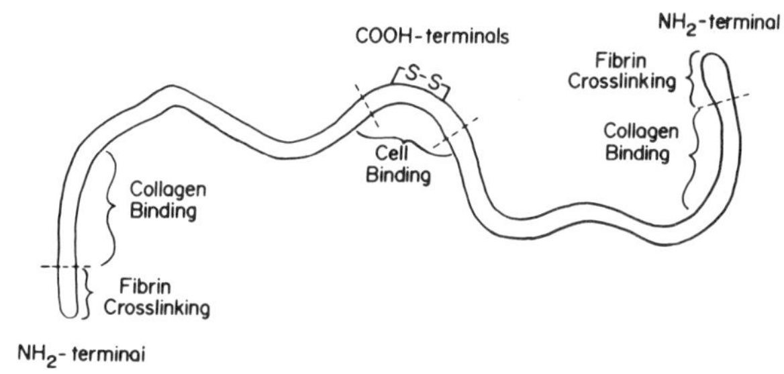

Figure 7

Model of the fibronectin molecule. The major plasmin cleavage sites are indicated by dotted lines, but the multiple cleavage sites that produce the family of high molecular weight peptides are not accounted for precisely. The molecule is drawn to scale; its dimensions are 160 nm long by 2 nm thick. (From Erickson, H.P.; Carrell, N.; and McDonagh, J.: Fibronectin molecule visualized in electron microscopy: A long, thin, flexible strand. J. Cell Biol. 91:673–678, 1981. By permission of the Rockefeller University Press.)

fibroblasts and vascular ingrowth. A deficiency of serum monocytes can interfere with normal healing.

The fibroblast is the cell eventually responsible for new collagen production and the formation of extracellular scar tissue. An additional related cell is the myofibroblast which has the collagen-producing ability of the fibroblast and an intercellular network of contractile proteins which may help with wound contraction. These cells exist in the granulation tissue and are capable of attaching to the extracellular matrix by fibronectin. Active force generated in the myofibroblasts and connection of myofibroblasts to the connective tissue matrix may be responsible for much of the early wound strength, before adequate deposition and alignment of the extracellular collagen.

The eventual strength of the healed wound is restored by collagen. The collagen is arrayed in longitudinal fibers, and tissue strength is proportional to the mean fiber diameter. Initially, collagen synthesis is quite high with predominantly type I collagen; a good proportion of type III collagen is present, at least initially. The ultimate tensile strength of the wound appears to be related to the arrangement and crosslinking of collagen as well as to the absolute amount of collagen. Much of the later increase in tensile strength is associated not with an increase in the amount of collagen but with alignment along lines of tension.

Obviously, there are many factors involved in soft tissue and wound healing. The clotting factors, including platelets and the fibrin network, not only achieve hemostasis but also act in transformation of the clot to reparative tissue. Prostaglandin products help to mediate the inflammatory response. Specific growth factors stimulate new cell production and angiogenesis. Fibroblasts and myofibroblasts connected with the connective tissue framework of fibrin and fibronectin provide initial wound strength. Finally, collagen production and alignment provide final strength. More knowledge of the specific cellular and biochemical events may greatly influence our treatment of soft tissue injury in the future.

Annotated Bibliography

Muscle Injury

Direct

Garrett, W.E., Jr.; Seaber, A.V.; Boswick, J.; Urbaniak, J.R.; and Goldner, J.L.: Recovery of skeletal muscle after laceration and repair. J. Hand Surg. [Am.] 9:683–692, 1984.

Complete and partial transverse lacerations were created in rabbit muscle distal to the motor point. Good function was present in the segment containing the motor point; the distal segment became fibrotic and transmitted tension although it did not shorten. The return of function was related to muscle geometry.

Walton, M., and Rothwell, A.G.: Reactions of thigh tissues of sheep to blunt trauma. Clin. Orthop. 176:273–281, 1983.

A standardized crush injury was created in the anterior thigh muscles of sheep. Acute inflammation followed by extensive scarring was noted in the muscles directly overlying the bone. Heterotopic bone formation was sometimes seen arising by intramembranous ossification within the scar tissue.

Indirect

Garrett, W.E., Jr.; Califf, J.C.; and Bassett, F.H., III: Histochemical correlates of hamstring injuries. Am. J. Sports Med. 12:98–103, 1984.

The authors examined the hamstring muscles because of the frequency of strain injury in athletic and occupational medicine. A relatively high percentage of type II (fast-twitch) muscle fibers was found in these muscles. These are subjected to stretch at two joints, are used as decelerators after contracting eccentrically, and have the ability to contract forcefully and rapidly. These facts are probably correlated with their propensity to injury.

Klein, B.P.; Jensen, R.C.; and Sanderson, L.M.: Assessment of workers' compensation claims for back strains/sprains. J. Occup. Med. 26:443–448, 1984.

The authors examine data from the Bureau of Labor Statistics Supplementary Data System to evaluate the incidence of back strains/sprains in U.S. industrial employees. These data showed that strains/sprains accounted for almost 90% of back injuries with an average direct cost of more than $3,500 per incident and over $1 billion total cost.

Delayed Muscle Soreness

Davies, C.T.M., and White, M.J.: Muscle weakness following eccentric work in man. Pflugers Arch. 392:168–171, 1981.

The separate effects of positive (concentric) and negative (eccentric) work were examined by having subjects box-step using one leg to climb the box and the other leg to absorb the energy of the fall. The loss of strength and soreness were much more pronounced in the leg working eccentrically.

Tendon

Gelberman, R.H.; Vande Berg, J.S.; Lundborg, G.N.; and Akeson, W.H.: Flexor tendon healing and restoration of the gliding surface: An ultrastructural study in dogs. J. Bone Joint Surg. 65A:70–80, 1983.

Healing in canine flexor tendons was examined. Immobilized tendons relied more on connective tissue ingrown from the digital sheath whereas mobilized tendons healed more by cells derived from the epitenon.

Hooper, G.; Davies, R.; and Tothill, P.: Blood flow and clearance in tendons: Studies with dogs. J. Bone Joint Surg. 66B:441–443, 1984.

Blood flow in intact tendons in dogs was measured with labeled microspheres and compared with clearance of a diffusible radionuclide. Clearance was greater than flow, suggesting that diffusion was an important source of nutrition in intact tendons.

Manske, P.R.; Gelberman, R.H.; Vande Berg, J.S.; and Lesker, P.A.: Intrinsic flexor-tendon repair: A morphological study *in vitro*. J. Bone Joint Surg. 66A:385–396, 1984.

Rabbit flexor tendons received a 90% mid-section laceration and then were excised and placed in a tissue culture medium (without blood supply or synovium). In the absence of extrinsic cell sources derived from the epitenon and endotenon, the tendon demonstrated capacity for repair.

Ligament

Attarian, D.E.; McCrackin, H.J.; Devito, D.P.; McElhaney, J.H.; and Garrett, W.E., Jr.: A biomechanical study of human lateral ankle ligaments and autogenous reconstructive grafts. Am. J. Sports Med. 13:377–381, 1985.

The biomechanical characteristics of human ankle ligaments and autogenous structures used for ankle reconstruction were tested. The anterior talofibular ligament was surprisingly weak. All commonly used reconstructive tissues were considerably stronger and less elastic.

Johnson, E.E., and Markolf, K.L.: The contribution of the anterior talofibular ligament to ankle laxity. J. Bone Joint Surg. 65A:81–88, 1983.

Using fresh-frozen cadaver ankles, the authors demonstrated that sectioning the anterior talofibular ligament caused increased laxity in anterior, inversion, and rotational directions. Anterior laxity was more pronounced in dorsiflexion, and inversion laxity was more pronounced in plantar flexion.

Stormont, D.M.; Morrey, B.F.; An, K.-N.; and Cass, J.R.: Stability of the loaded ankle: Relation between articular restraint and primary and secondary static restraints. Am. J. Sports Med. 13:295–300, 1985.

This study added physiologic loading to the ankle joint to determine the stabilizing effect of the ligaments. Loading of the articular surface was responsible for all of the stability of inversion-eversion and 30% of the stability in rotation.

Cartilage

Articular

Donohue, J.M.; Buss, D.; Oegema, T.R., Jr.; and Thompson, R.C., Jr.: The effects of indirect blunt trauma on adult canine articular cartilage. J. Bone Joint Surg. 65A:948–957, 1983.

A controlled blunt impact was applied to canine patellofemoral joints. Pathologic changes were found in all specimens, with the zone of calcified cartilage being altered most consistently. This may be a model for articular cartilage injury without fracture.

Mankin, H.J.: The response of articular cartilage to mechanical injury. J. Bone Joint Surg. 64A:460–466, 1982.

This excellent review of articular cartilage injury examines healing in cartilage after a superficial laceration, a deep penetrating injury, and blunt impact. The intrinsic potential for healing of articular cartilage is discussed.

Salter, R.B.; Simmonds, D.F.; Malcolm, B.W.; Rumble, E.J.; MacMichael, D.; and Clements, N.D.: The biological effect of continuous passive motion on the healing of full-thickness defects in articular cartilage. J. Bone Joint Surg. 62A:1232–1251, 1980.

Small articular cartilage defects were created in rabbit femoral condyles, and healing was assessed after treatment by immobilization, intermittent active motion, or continuous passive motion. Results, as measured by light microscopic analysis, were far superior in animals treated by continuous passive motion.

Meniscal

Arnoczky, S.P., and Warren, R.F.: The microvasculature of the meniscus and its response to injury: An experimental study in the dog. Am. J. Sports Med. 11:131–141, 1983.

Lesions were created in normal canine menisci. Complete transection in a radial direction cut through the vascular periphery and resulted in healing. Longitudinal incisions did not heal unless they were connected to the peripheral vascular supply by a vascular access channel.

Nerve

de Medinaceli, L.; Freed, W.J.; and Wyatt, R.J.: Peripheral nerve reconnection: Improvement of long-term functional effects under simulated clinical conditions in the rat. Exp. Neurol. 81:488–496, 1983.

Peripheral nerve injuries were reconnected by a novel combination of techniques including freezing the nerves, soaking them in fluids resembling intracellular fluid, cutting with a vibrating knife, and suturing the nerves not to themselves but to a rubber support structure. The results were much improved over those of conventional microsurgery.

Orgel, M.G.: Experimental studies with clinical application to peripheral nerve injury: A review of the past decade. Clin. Orthop. 163:98–106, 1982.

This article reviews new approaches to peripheral nerve injury and concludes that technologic advances have reached their peak. New attention must be concentrated on avoiding excess scar and in providing better orientation of regrowing cells.

Wound Healing

Carrico, T.J.; Mehrhof, A.I., Jr.; and Cohen, I.K.: Biology of wound healing. Surg. Clin. North Am. 64:721–733, August 1984.

The authors give a good background on the biologic processes in tissue repair. The inflammatory processes, collagen metabolism, and wound contraction literature are reviewed.

Forrest, L.: Current concepts in soft connective tissue wound healing. Br. J. Surg. 70:133–140, 1983.

This article is an excellent review of the cellular and biochemical events in soft tissue repair. The myofibroblast-fibronectin network is discussed clearly. The increase in wound strength and changes in collagen type and content are well presented.

Knighton, D.R.; Hunt, T.K.; Thakral, K.K.; and Goodson, W.H., III: Role of platelets and fibrin in the healing sequence: An in vivo study of angiogenesis and collagen synthesis. Ann. Surg. 196:379–387, 1982.

The initiation and early events in wound healing are evaluated. The important roles of fibrin and growth factors released by platelets are stressed.

9

Neuromuscular Disorders and Gait

The process called "walking" is a repeated cycle of limb motions, controlled by selective muscle action, that carries the body forward while also maintaining optimal upright stability. Included are actions directed toward absorption of the shock of floor impact and conservation of energy. Except for knee flexion in swing, most joint function depends on small but critical 15° to 20° arcs. A 10° deviation can be obstructive. This narrow margin between normal and abnormal function makes the diagnosis of gait deviations difficult. To overcome these limitations, objective instrumented systems for evaluating gait disorders have been developed. Their value in identifying functional problems and determining the effectiveness of treatment is becoming more and more evident. Because walking is such a complex interaction of joint motions and muscle actions, a summary of the critical events is provided as background for the survey of the recent literature.

Normal and Abnormal Gait

During each stride (cycle) the limb moves through eight unique synergistic motion patterns (phases of gait) to accomplish three basic tasks: weight acceptance; single limb support; and limb advancement (Table 1). As these tasks are accomplished the ankle and knee use four positions and the hip two. A posture that is appropriate in one gait phase would signify dysfunction at another point in the cycle because the functional need has changed. As a result, timing often is as significant as posture. The relative significance of one joint's motion compared to the other varies among the gait phases. This is another factor that makes observational gait analysis difficult.

Each joint has its own normal pattern of motion and muscle control. During stance, the stimulus is forward fall of body weight. As a result, muscle action is eccentric (i.e., restraining a lengthening force). In swing, joint function is directed to clearing the floor, advancing the limb, and preparing for the next stance period. Muscle action is concentric.

Ankle

The mode of foot/ankle mobility and muscular control is the most significant determinant of both limb stability and body progression.

Initial floor contact with the heel establishes the heel rocker which will be used to preserve progression and initiate shock absorption during the limb's loading response. After heel contact, the ankle undergoes rapid plantar flexion. Vigorous deceleration of the tibialis anterior (assisted by the extensor hallucis longus) provides a controlled heel rocker. Two purposes are served: part of the impact shock is absorbed directly, and the tibia is advanced to preserve progression and accelerate knee flexion for further shock absorption.

Controlled dorsiflexion to 10° (midstance) and subsequent heel rise (terminal stance) throughout the single limb support period are the main sources of body progression. Active deceleration of the tibial advance is a critical component of knee stability. Reversal of ankle motion toward dorsiflexion immediately follows floor contact by the forefoot. The stimulus is forward momentum of the body weight. Deceleration of this motion by soleus and gastrocnemius activity provides a controlled ankle rocker. The

Table 1. Functional Elements of Walking

Task	Phase	Action	Joint involved
1. Weight acceptance	Initial contact	Start stance	ASC*
	Loading response	Roll onto foot	Ankle
		Shock absorption	Knee
		Limb stability	Knee
		Trunk stability	Hip
2. Single limb support	Midstance	Roll over foot	Ankle
		Limb stability	Ankle
			Knee
	Terminal stance	Roll beyond foot	Ankle
		Limb stability	Ankle
3. Limb advancement	Preswing	Preparatory flexion	Knee
	Initial swing	Limb advancement	Hip
		Toe clearance	Knee
	Midswing	Limb advancement	Hip
		Toe clearance	Ankle
	Terminal swing	Limb deceleration	Hip
		Limb extension	Knee

*Ankle-subtalar complex.

muscles yield as they hold to allow the tibia, and thus the body, to move forward. The restraining force, however, is sufficient to make the rate of tibial advance slower than that of the femur. This allows the knee to extend. Body weight moves across the length of the foot, reaching the metatarsal head area as the ankle attains 10° dorsiflexion. Increased (strong) gastrocnemius and soleus action stabilizes the ankle and allows the heel to rise.

The forefoot becomes the final progressional rocker. During this action the ankle moves into slight plantar flexion (5°) just before the forwardly aligned body weight drops onto the other foot. The limb then unloads; the muscles of the gastrocnemius/soleus group promptly relax. Hence, the functions of these muscles are to decelerate tibial advance for knee stability and to stabilize the ankle for a forefoot rocker. Push-off is not their role. The large arc of plantar flexion that occurs in preswing is functionally insignificant because the limb is virtually unloaded; it contributes to clearance but not to balance. Strength demands on the gastrocnemius/soleus musculature increase as the stride is lengthened.

Dorsiflexion to neutral in swing is the final event. It is responsible for toe clearance in midswing.

Three types of pathologic circumstance prevent effective ankle motion: 1) plantar flexion contracture, 2) weakness of plantar flexion muscles, and 3) weakness of dorsiflexion muscles.

Plantar flexion contracture is functionally significant when the ankle cannot attain a 5° dorsiflexed posture by the end of midstance. This angle is necessary for body weight to advance onto the forefoot. Dorsiflexion to 0° is not enough; this keeps body weight in the area of the ankle joint. A 15° plantar flexion contracture is not uncommon. Insensitivity to this posture stems from the fact that it is a natural event—it is the resting posture of the ankle and is a normal occurrence during the loading response. Contractures form as an incidental element of immobilization. Spontaneous positioning of the ankle will be in 15° of plantar flexion if specific efforts are not taken to avoid it. Inability to achieve dorsiflexion blocks the body's efforts to move forward over the supporting foot. Stride length and gait velocity are decreased. The knee may be strained into hyperextension. Forefoot pressure is prolonged and the intensity is increased, leading to pain and skin damage. Substitution of early heel-off (occurring in middle rather than terminal stance) improves progression but continues to strain the forefoot and knee.

Gastrocnemius/soleus insufficiency introduces tibial instability with a corresponding increase in quadriceps demand. Lacking the ability to restrain a dorsiflexion torque, body weight is kept close to the heel throughout the single limb support period. Stride length is shortened. Endurance is reduced. Heel rise is delayed until the limb is unloaded. This is a very disabling situation that is difficult to recognize. The signs are persistent heel contact with excessive dorsiflexion at the end of single stance, persistent knee flexion in midstance, and lack of knee flexion during weight acceptance. All of these signs are subtle, and instrumented gait analysis may be needed to make the diagnosis. Because several motion patterns are possible, dynamic electromyography (EMG) also is indicated.

Clinical definition of gastrocnemius/soleus weakness is obscure. Manual testing is convenient but does not reproduce the force used in a single heel rise. Hence, this examination is woefully inadequate. Grade 5 strength supine is no better than grade 2 standing. The lesser perimalleolar plantar flexors (the peroneus group, tibialis posterior, and toe flexors) can meet the challenge of manual testing but not the standing demand. Repetitive, single limb heel rise (full range at least 18 times is normal) and instrumented force testing are the only valid measures.

Tibialis anterior weakness causes the familiar footdrop. This is the most frequently treated yet least significant gait error involving the ankle. Functional significance is low because there are so many ways to adjust for it (slightly increased hip flexion and contralateral vaulting, circumduction). Orthotic assistance at the onset of disability is indicated. Only the more severely disabled patients who lack an alternate means of lifting the foot continue to use the orthosis, however.

Knee

Three essential actions occur at the knee: flexion to decrease the impact of floor contact, extension for weight-bearing stability, and flexion for toe clearance in swing.

Weight acceptance is accomplished by knee flexion of about 15°. This provides valuable shock absorption but it also introduces postural instability. Two mechanisms are involved. Body weight is behind the foot at the time of initial contact, and the heel rocker rolls the tibia forward. Both events place the body vector line behind the knee. Quadriceps activity preserves limb stability. When the flexion is limited to 15° the functional demand is well tolerated. Peak stance-phase knee flexion occurs just at the onset of single limb support. Throughout midstance the knee progressively extends over the stable tibia. As the body weight line reaches and then moves ahead of the knee axis in late midstance, the quadriceps relax, and knee extension stability depends entirely on tibial control at the ankle.

Knee flexion for swing begins in the terminal double support period (preswing). Approximately 40° is attained passively as body weight rolls beyond the metatarsal heads, and distal stability is lost. Only if the rate of knee flexion is excessive is there any restraining muscle action. Knee flexion is increased in initial swing (60°) for toe clearance. Momentum from hip flexion and slight local knee flexion action (biceps femoris, short head) are the sources.

The final knee action is progressive knee extension to neutral in preparation for the next weight-bearing period. This begins passively in midswing and then is completed by quadriceps activity in terminal swing.

Assessment of knee position is complicated by the fact that two bony landmarks are eccentric to the joint axes they are supposed to indicate. The greater trochanter prominence is 3 cm behind the center of the femoral head, and the apex of the lateral malleolus is 1 cm behind the ankle axis. Use of these anatomic landmarks without corrections for their eccentric alignment can indicate 15° knee flexion when that joint is seen to be fully extended on the radiograph.

There are three significant gait errors. Each relates to the key function listed above.

1. Inadequate knee flexion during the loading response generally is not listed but it deprives the patient of valuable shock absorption. The primary cause is quadriceps weakness. Patients substitute by using premature ankle plantar flexion to prevent the normal heel rocker. A second substitution is increased hip extensor muscle action. Slight

forward lean of the trunk provides proximal stability so the hip extensors can relatively draw the femur back.

2. Persistent knee flexion during single limb support increases the duration of quadriceps demand. If knee position exceeds 15°, it also increases the supporting force needed. Both situations lead to premature fatigue. A flexion contracture or persistent hamstring muscle action are well-recognized causes. Weak gastrocnemius/soleus musculature must be added to this list. Walking on a flexed knee increases energy costs because the extensor muscle must remain active.

3. Insufficient knee flexion in initial swing causes a toe drag unless the patient substitutes. Possible substitutions include lateral trunk lean, circumduction, and vaulting by the other foot. All of these alternate mechanisms increase the energy cost of walking.

Hip

Sagittal plane motion is simple. Starting from 45° of flexion, the hip progressively extends during stance. In swing there is rapid reversal into flexion for limb advancement. Demands on the extensor musculature are brief, lasting only during the weight acceptance period. The dominant control is by the single joint muscles (gluteus maximus and adductor magnus). Relaxation of the hamstrings avoids excessive knee flexion. At the end of stance, the hip is drawn toward hyperextension, with iliacus activity being the restraining force. Limb advancement in early swing is accomplished by a mixture of low flexor muscle activities.

Hip control in the coronal plane is more demanding. Gluteus medius activity starts with the onset of stance and persists through most of the single limb support period. The upper gluteus maximus also functions as an abductor. In addition, the hip is subjected to rotational forces as the trunk moves from behind to ahead of the supporting limb.

The significant functional errors are insufficient hip extension range and inadequacy of hip extensor, abductor, or flexion musculature. Flexion contractures commonly are accommodated by increased lumbar lordosis. In time, lumbosacral pain may be an additional complication. Patients who lack this range must lean forward. This introduces the need for a cane or crutch. Backward lean of the trunk (or lordosis) also is the postural substitution for hip extensor weakness. The two causes may be differentiated by timing: an extensor weakness requires accommodation at initial contact whereas demands of a flexion contracture may wait until mid or terminal stance. Hip abductor weakness leads to coronal plane instability. The immediate reaction is a drop of the contralateral side of the pelvis. Upright balance is maintained by a lateral trunk lean toward the supporting limb. Insufficiency of hip flexor strength leads to a loss of limb advancement unless the person can substitute by a contralateral lean or increased pelvic motion.

Instrumentation Systems

At present, five types of instrumentation systems are applicable to clinical use: motion analysis, dynamic EMG, force plates, footswitch stride analysis, and measurement of energy costs. Automated motion systems are replacing photography by being more rapid and more comprehensive; at least five systems now are available. Dynamic EMG provides a direct means of identifying inappropriate muscle action. This is an invaluable aid in determining the appropriate surgical plan for improving the gait of persons disabled by cerebral palsy, head trauma, stroke, etc. Use of this technique to identify compensatory muscle action in other types of impairment also is increasing. Definition of stride characteristics by use of footswitches or other methods classifies the patient's ability to walk. It is an excellent means of measuring the functional effectiveness of treatment. Energy cost determination identifies the physiologic strain of a gait disorder. To replace the inconvenience of direct oxygen measurement, calculations of mechanical work are being explored. However, the excessive muscular effort that may be used to minimize a limp cannot be realized by summation of segment displacement. Consequently, the ratio between the two sets of data is low even though the correlations are good.

Recent Findings by Instrumented Gait Analysis

Experimental evaluation of clinicians' observations demonstrated that they could perceive only 22% of the deviations. Step length and step time proved particularly difficult to assess. Also, just a change in the angle of the lower limb during the step cycle visually transformed a walk into a running pattern. This finding implied that gait disorders involving increased flexion of the lower extremities might erroneously be judged insignificant.

A second limitation of clinical examination was identified by dynamic EMG verification of manual muscle testing. In assessing the response of the muscles crossing the ankle, the manual tests suffered from lack of selectivity when maximal effort was exerted. The test based on standing with the knee flexed and extended did not differentiate between the soleus and the gastrocnemius. The flexor hallucis longus was more active during the tibialis posterior test than when the great toe flexion was resisted. In addition, all the tests at maximal effort showed multiple muscle involvement. This would cloud the clinical interpretations of when a pathologic condition had altered the strength of the target muscle.

Sports

Race walking recently has become popular as a means of reducing the incidence of injury from running. Its speed, averaging 12.5 km/hr, distinguishes it from customary fast walking (8.7 km/hr) and makes it comparable to running. Dynamic EMG showed increases in both amplitude and duration of muscular activity that were similar in magnitude to the muscular effort of running and exceeded that of fast walking. The pattern of limb motion was different, however.

Elderly Persons

A comparison of stride characteristics of young to middle-aged subjects (ages 20–50 yr) and elderly subjects (ages 65–85 yr) showed that step length and stride time did not differ significantly between the groups, but the elderly had much higher stride widths and double support times. Step length and stride time are thought to be determined predominantly by the gait-patterning mechanism. Stride width and double support time may be determined predominantly by the balance-control mechanism. Although overall the elderly had the capacity to walk at the same speeds as the younger subjects, comfortable walking on average seemed to be 78% of maximal speed in elderly women and 70% in men. One implication of this is that timing of automobile traffic signals at intersections is not compatible with the functional capacity of older persons.

Increased variability in gait should not be regarded as a normal concomitant of old age. A specific cause may be found in about half of patients examined. Myelopathy from cervical spine disease and multiple sensory disorders should be sought. Normal-pressure hydrocephalus is another possibility in patients with seemingly idiopathic senile gait disorders. Such patients often have ventricular enlargement by computed tomography, compared with age-matched controls.

Arthritis

Patients with unilateral hip disease 5 years after total hip arthroplasty appear to have an accelerated decline in function unassociated with pain. Revision rates for mechanical failure by 10 years was 58% for the elderly and 66% for fast walkers. Rheumatoid patients studied prior to and after total knee replacement were found to have significant poorer function than those who had degenerative disease of the knee. In a group of elderly patients undergoing standard knee replacement arthroplasty for isolated degenerative arthritis of one knee, most of the measurements of gait returned to normal levels by 2 years. Compared with the normal subjects, these patients spent approximately 30% more time in double limb stance and had prolonged gait cycle times.

An association between degenerative joint disease and decline in proprioception is suggested to be a possible cause of this. If it exists, loss of proprioception and the resulting abnormal gait patterns may place increased stress on components and contribute to loosening. There is some evidence that joint position sense decreases with aging in controls and further significant decreases occur with joint disease; however, no further worsening has been noted as a result of total knee arthroplasty. Another factor pertinent to performance is the fact that most patients do not have arthritis of a single joint. In the majority of patients, normal gait and function are not typically achieved after total knee replacement; velocity and stride length move toward more normal values postoperatively but do not fully attain this functional level.

Myelodysplasia

In comparison to normal children, children with myelodysplasia walked slower and consumed more oxygen per distance traveled but had a similar rate of oxygen consumption per time. A swing-through gait pattern was 33% more energy-efficient than a four-point gait pattern for these children, and wheelchair propulsion produced velocities and energy efficiencies similar to those in normal children walking. The combination of hip flexion deformity, pelvic obliquity, and scoliosis is likely to preclude walking. This also is true for a severe degree of any one of these factors. Oxygen consumption and velocity in myelodysplastic children are related to the level of the lesion and the strength of hip and knee extension. Patients with myelomeningocele vary in their ability to use an orthosis having reciprocal control hip flexion and extension. The hip device is most successful if strong hip flexors are present, although ambulation is possible for some with no active hip musculature.

Patients with weak or no plantar flexor activity were not able to counteract dorsiflexion moments at the ankle. They delayed the forward progression of the center of pressure to avoid the unstable collapse of the foot into dorsiflexion. A shorter step length and earlier heel strike resulted. If a flat shoe is worn, an ankle-foot orthosis with the anterior stop set at 5° of plantar flexion may be more effective in restoring the values to normal than an ankle-foot orthosis with the anterior stop set at 5° of dorsiflexion but this does not consistently achieve normal values. However, most people wear shoes with a heel height that (for their foot size) represents the equivalent of 5° of plantar flexion. Hence, the orthosis must accommodate this. Evidence has accumulated that transfer of the tibialis anterior to the heel cord to act either dynamically or statically is ineffective for children with myelomeningocele. It does not develop the desired phasic contraction during the stance phase of walking, and bracing requirements at the ankle are unaffected by the procedure.

Muscular Dystrophy

The velocity of fast walking seems to be a simple and useful index for characterizing disease progression in Duchenne muscular dystrophy. A decline in the fast walking rate begins between ages 4 and 6 years and can amount to about 30% of normal. This measure of disease progression seems to follow a unique course in each subject. By the age of 10, the specific decay rate can be characterized mathematically.

Cerebral Palsy

The benefits of using computerized gait analysis to plan and evaluate operations introduces objectivity into the documentation of outcome. The gait measurements of such patients can be used to determine a gait typology. This differs from and complements the present diagnostic classification system of quadriplegic, diplegic, or hemiplegic and may yield better predictors of treatment outcome. Such a typology seems most related to the degree of functional spasticity present in each extremity in addition to the number of extremities involved. Stride length, gait velocity, and range of motion are related to the severity of physical handicap. Those patients classified as functionally moderately spastic may be considered to have only moderate impairment of neurologic function. In these children, surgical treatment seems to have a more variable gait result. Mildly handicapped children are capable of varying the components of their walking pattern to a larger extent than those more severely affected but at the same time do not have the same degree of automatic motor control as nonhandicapped children have.

Hamstring lengthening has been found to decrease mild knee flexion contracture. When performed distally, this procedure rarely causes recurvatum. It can also reduce hip flexion contractures and has little effect on lumbar lordosis. Hindfoot valgus, especially early, is due to muscle imbalance. The deformity has been found to be decreased by peroneal lengthening if performed early. Split transfer of the tibialis posterior tendon to the peroneus brevis has been shown to provide good correction of equinovarus without causing calcaneal deformity.

Stroke

Key quantitative variables of motor recovery in hemiplegic gait appeared to be walking speed and symmetry of the swing phase. Patients with a greater degree of motor recovery walked faster and more symmetrically than those with less motor recovery. None of the other temporal variables of gait showed a significant relationship with the stage of motor recovery. Tension produced by the ankle plantar flexor group in the stance phase of gait was mainly due to an increase in gastrocnemius and soleus activity.

Recent evidence suggests that, during slow gait in spastic adults (and children with cerebral palsy), clonus is generated by a peripheral mechanism of self-excitation rather than by a central spinal pacemaker. The exaggerated monosynaptic reflexes, however, may represent only a small part of leg extensor activation during gait, and tension development does not depend on these reflexes. In many spastic patients the abnormally high tension development in the gastrocnemius/soleus may be due to passive muscle stretch. With a mild equinus deformity it has been found that approximately one-fifth of the total internal moment was contributed by the passive resistance of the surrounding structures. This may be considered a pseudostretch reflex behavior due to their mechanical properties. In hemiplegic patients this may be identified by the delayed EMG responses and the decreased strength of the spastic leg.

Scoliosis

Harrington instrumentation to correct scoliosis can decrease lordosis to a level that may impair walking. Patients accommodate by exaggerated hip and knee flexion in quiet standing. During walking, the compensation is inadequate terminal swing knee extension with excessive knee flexion and ankle dorsiflexion during stance.

Foot

Patients can be treated with free muscle flaps covered with thick split-thickness skin grafts for extensive defects of the foot at or below the medial and lateral malleoli. Detailed gait analysis of these patients has confirmed the foot's weight-bearing capabilities and shown that cutaneous sensibility may not be necessary for success. Mitchell osteotomies of the first metatarsal are known to be satisfying procedures. Excessive first metatarsal shortening, dorsiflexion of the osteotomy, and failure to correct the intermetatarsal angle to 10° or less correlate with poorer results. Gait analysis demonstrates that these patients did not have normal foot mechanics postoperatively.

Bone Tumors

The gait of patients treated by *en bloc* resection and local internal prosthetic replacement for osteosarcoma about the knee was compared with that of patients undergoing equivalent amputation. Their free-walking velocity, oxygen consumption per distance traveled, and percentage of maximal aerobic capacity used during walking demonstrated a lower energy cost during gait. A tibial rotation-plasty for osteosarcoma of the distal end of the femur may be a worthwhile alternative to above-knee amputation. EMG of gait showed that the rotated calf muscles assumed the function of extensors of the prosthetic knee to a substantial degree and, despite some abnormalities, the children walked at speeds comparable to those of normal children.

Orthotic Devices

Maximal reduction of forefoot loads was achieved in a short-leg walking cast or an ankle boot with a posteriorly placed flat rubber heel. Use of a centrally placed rocker heel led to increased forefoot loads, especially with placement under the first metatarsal head. The height of the cast and configuration of the sole of the cast shoe seemed to have little effect on the observed patterns of force distribution.

Orthotics were found to be valuable adjuncts for the treatment of arthritic patients who had ankle and hindfoot pain and deformity. A significant increase in velocity and single limb support time occurred with shoes, and a further significant increase was gained with an orthosis. The improvement seemed to be associated with a decrease in ankle and hindfoot pain after use of the orthosis.

Orthotic devices usually prescribed for ambulatory treatment of Legg-Calvé-Perthes disease did not meet the severe kinematic requirements necessary for a comfortable gait. Improved kinematic characteristics were obtained by the use of six joints placed symmetrically at two levels of the brace. However, comfort is only one feature to consider in the treatment of Legg-Calvé-Perthes disease with orthoses. Gait analysis of these patients with and without various abduction orthoses has shown that the three-dimensional containment of the hip is reproducibly altered by various devices. Specifically, the Atlanta brace increased posterior coverage and slightly improved lateral coverage, whereas Petrie casts improved lateral and anterior coverage at the expense of posterior containment.

The molded polypropylene orthosis offers many advantages in the treatment of foot and ankle problems in cerebral palsy. Numerous balancing, stance phase, and swing phase difficulties have been treated with an ankle-foot orthosis with appropriate molding to correct each specific problem. Gait analysis has confirmed the merits of these orthoses. The manner of improvement appeared to be mechanical. Any decrease in muscle tone appeared secondary to the improved mechanisms. In a similar fashion, inhibitive casting may be useful temporary adjunct for management of both foot deformity and associated proximal hypertonicity in hemiplegic and able-bodied subjects.

Progressive trimming of a rigidly designed polypropylene ankle-foot orthosis makes it more flexible and comparable in function to the commercially available Engen and Teufel orthoses. Gait analysis showed that the more flexible orthoses did not provide as good a terminal stance roll-off as the rigid orthosis that encloses the malleoli, but they did provide an adequate amount of toe clearance during swing.

In the United Kingdom, about 85% of patients with below- or above-knee amputations are fitted with uniaxial feet. In contrast, in the United States about 80% are fitted with SACH feet. An experimental prosthesis permits the interchange of the ankle-foot component while keeping the rest of the components the same. Although patients showed a preference for the foot that they were accustomed to, gait analysis indicated differences in the function between the two prosthetic feet that could be significant. A neutral alignment of below-knee prostheses minimized asymmetry of gait at the hips and knees. The indices of symmetry showed that alignment changes in the prosthetic foot disrupted gait to a greater extent than did other alignment variations. Asymmetry of hip flexion-extension motion was more sensitive to alignment changes than were other asymmetries. For above-knee amputees, comparison of constant-friction and hydraulic swing-control prosthetic knee joints showed that the latter provided more versatility. The amputees had a wider range of walking speeds, improved equality in the duration of successive swing and stance phases, and greater uniformity of forward progression of the prosthetic limb when walking with the hydraulic knee. Abnormalities persisted with both types of prostheses.

Functional Electrical Stimulation

Increasingly, efforts are being made to restore function to spastic, paralyzed muscles through the use of functional electrical stimulation (FES). Direct electrical stimulation to a muscle has been found to decrease hypertonicity. FES of an agonist also was associated with a concomitant inhibition of the antagonist in the healthy individual. The mechanisms for its direct effectiveness on the spastic muscle are not well understood. Nevertheless, in various studies it has been found that about half of randomly selected patients with spinal cord injury who have knee joint spasticity might benefit from FES. FES-restrengthened muscles of paraplegic patients have been used for simple FES-assisted standing.

Use of FES to provide paraplegic patients who have complete lesions of the spinal cord the ability to rise from sitting to standing, to maintain a standing position, and to walk with a reciprocal gait has had some success. Four channels of electrical stimulation seemed to be sufficient for synthesis of a simple reciprocal gait pattern in these patients. During the double stance phase, knee extensor muscles of both knees were stimulated. The phase of the contralateral lower extremity was accomplished by stimulating the synergistic flexor muscle by external contact. Three types of contact were used: two hand switches used by the therapist, switches built into the handles of the walking frame (or crutches) used by the patient, and computer control. Stainless steel electrodes activated by timers have been placed in the quadriceps and hip flexors, extensors, and abductors as needed for modeling FES. Early evidence suggested that patients had improved function but still desired some supervision in walking. A 10-fold increase in knee torque was noted in some, thereby providing nearly normal strength. Further improvements will require the development of an implantable, multichannel, programmable microprocessor-controlled stimulator, a multiple computer program to organize various functions (step, start, train, etc.), and appropriate sensors to warn against hazards (obstacles, change in terrain, etc.).

Annotated Bibliography

Brinkmann, J.R., and Perry, J.: Rate and range of knee motion during ambulation in healthy and arthritic subjects. Phys. Ther. 65:1055–1060, 1985.

This study determined that the normal swing phase knee range of 60° is accomplished at 340°/sec while subjects walked at their average velocity of 180 m/min. In contrast, patients with knee disability secondary to rheumatoid arthritis averaged a 15° active range imposed on a 21° flexion contracture; their rate of motion was 25% of normal. After total knee arthroplasty (mean interval, 16 months) the range of knee flexion was doubled and the rate of motion increased to 58% of normal. Osteoarthritis patients displayed a preoperative knee flexion range of 33° which was accomplished at approximately half the normal rate. Postoperatively, there was only a mild increase in the range (to 40°) but the rate of motion improved to 70% of normal.

Cohen, L.; Morgan, J.; Babbs, R., Jr.; Karrison, T.G.; and Giacomoni, M.: Fast walking velocity in health and Duchenne muscular dystrophy: A statistical analysis. Arch. Phys. Med. Rehabil. 65:573–578, 1984.

Fast walking velocity was measured in 180 males and 155 females (ages 3.5 to 24 years) and serially over periods of 18 to 132 months in 15 patients with Duchenne muscular dystrophy. A decline in the fast walking rate began between ages 4 and 6. This measure of disease progression followed a unique course in each subject and could be mathematically characterized by a unique decay rate and a unique walking velocity [age 10 years]. The measurement of fast walking velocity has proved to be a simple and useful index for characterizing disease progression in Duchenne muscular dystrophy.

Gabell, A., and Nayak, U.S.L.: The effect of age on variability in gait. J. Gerontol. 39:662–666, 1984.

The intercycle variability in gait of two temporal parameters (stride time and double support time) and the step-to-step variability of two spatial parameters were assessed in two groups of subjects—aged 21 to 47, and aged 66 to 84. Step length and stride time did not differ significantly between the two groups, but stride width and double support time were much higher for the elderly group. Step length and stride time are thought to be determined predominantly by the gait-patterning mechanism. Stride width and double support time may be determined predominantly by balance-control mechanisms. Increased variability in gait should not be regarded as a normal concomitant of old age.

Gage, J.R.; Fabian, D.; Hicks, R.; and Tashman, S.: Pre- and postoperative gait analysis in patients with spastic diplegia: A preliminary report. J. Pediatr. Orthop. 4:715–725, 1984.

The benefits of using computerized gait analysis to plan and to evaluate operations were assessed by studying the data from children with spastic diplegia to examine the changes in estimated external work of walking, stride length, walking velocity, and joint rotations preoperatively and postoperatively. Computerized gait analysis has enabled us to be more objective in the evaluation and documentation of outcome.

Goh, J.C.H.; Solomonidis, S.E.; Spence, W.D.; and Paul, J.P.: Biomechanical evaluation of SACH and uniaxial feet. Prosthet. Orthot. Int. 8:147–154, 1984.

In the United Kingdom, about 85% of below- and above-knee amputees are fitted with uniaxial feet, whereas in the United States about 80% are fitted with SACH feet. An experimental prosthesis permitted the interchange of the ankle-foot component while keeping the rest of the components the same. In general, patients showed a preference for the foot that they were accustomed to, and kinematic and kinetic analysis showed differences in the function between the two prosthetic feet.

Gronley, J.K., and Perry, J.: Gait analysis techniques: Rancho Los Amigos Hospital Gait Laboratory. Phys. Ther. 64:1831–1838, 1984.

In this description of the Rancho Los Amigos Hospital Gait Laboratory activities, use of dynamic electromyography for clinical decisions relevant to the spastic patient is emphasized. Differentiation in activity of adjacent muscles by wire electrodes is illustrated with two examples: rectus femoris versus the vasti; and biceps femoris long head versus short head. Both of these examples are functionally significant in treating a patient with a stiff-legged gait (adult stroke and head trauma patients as well as cerebral palsy children). Other techniques described are electrogoniometer motion analysis, footswitch stride analysis, energy cost, and visible vector determinations from the forceplate. Staffing also is described.

Hannah, R.E.; Morrison, J.B.; and Chapman, A.E.: Prostheses alignment: Effect on gait of persons with below-knee amputations. Arch. Phys. Med. Rehabil. 65:159–162, 1984.

This study investigated the effect, on gait, of changing prosthetic alignment for five patients with amputations. Symmetry was measured at different prosthesis alignment settings and used to assess the possibility of aligning below-knee prostheses on the basis of symmetry of lower limb motion. Optimal or neutral alignment of below-knee prostheses, as selected by clinically experienced personnel, tended to minimize asymmetry of gait at the hips and knees for persons with below-knee amputations. The indices of symmetry showed that alignment changes to the prosthetic foot disrupt gait to a greater extent than do other alignment changes. An index was selected that showed sensitivity to changes in gait caused by changes in prosthesis alignment for below-knee amputations.

Janda, J.P.S.; Skinner, S.R.; and Barto, P.S.: Posterior transfer of tibialis anterior in low-level myelodysplasia. Dev. Med. Child. Neurol. 26:100–103, 1984.

A clinical and electromyographic evaluation was performed on six children with myelomeningocele who previously had undergone bilateral transfer of the tibialis anterior to the heel cord. Electromyographic studies indicated that the transferred muscle usually did not develop the desired phasic contraction during the stance phase of walking. Bracing requirements at the ankle were unaffected by the procedure. The authors concluded that this transfer is undesirable for children with myelomeningocele.

Keenan, M.A., Creighton, J., Garland, D.E., and Moore, T.: Surgical correction of spastic equinovarus deformity in the adult head trauma patient. Foot Ankle 5:35–41, 1984.

The results of 59 surgical procedures in 54 adults with traumatic head injury for correction of spastic equinovarus deformity of the foot by using the split anterior tibial tendon were reviewed. The patterns of lower extremity muscle activity preoperatively by dynamic electromyography showed no significant difference from those in the hemiplegic stroke population—namely, spastic calf muscles with overactive toe flexors and anterior tibial muscle. The split anterior tibial tendon transfer was found to be a safe and effective procedure for the head trauma patient because it corrects the equinovarus deformity, allowing for improved shoe wear and wheelchair positioning in the nonambulatory individual and improved ambulation with decreased brace wear in the more functional patient.

Laughman, R.K.; Stauffer, R.N.; Ilstrup, D.M.; and Chao, E.Y.S.: Functional evaluation of total knee replacement. J. Orthop. Res. 2:307–313, 1984.

An automated method of laboratory assessment that permits the objective evaluation of knee joint function is described. Biomechanical parameters were statistically selected, weighted, and combined to develop a Performance Index. Patients were studied prior to total knee replacement. Patients with rheumatoid arthritis were found to have significantly poorer function than those with degenerative disease. The newer generation of prostheses were found to produce better functional results. A patellar resurfacing component produced improved knee function.

Lehmann, J.F.; Condon, S.M.; de Lateur, B.J.; and Smith, J.C.: Ankle-foot orthoses: Effect on gait abnormalities in tibial nerve paralysis. Arch. Phys. Med. Rehabil. 66:212–218, 1985.

Ambulation with a tibial nerve block was performed with and without the assistance of an ankle-foot orthosis with a rigid anterior stop adjusted to either 5° of plantar flexion or 5° of dorsiflexion. The gait abnormalities resulting from tibial nerve paralysis include delayed advancement of the center of pressure, delayed ipsilateral heel-off and early contralateral heel-strike, decreased step length, decreased ankle dorsiflexion moment, and increased knee flexion moment. This study provides quantitative information on the degree to which these abnormalities were corrected by appropriately adjusted ankle-foot orthoses. The orthosis with the anterior stop set at 5° of plantar flexion was more effective in restoring the values to normal than the one with the anterior stop set at 5° of dorsiflexion but still did not consistently achieve the normal values.

Lehmann, J.F.; Esselman, P.C.; Ko, M.J.; Smith, J.C., deLateur, B.J.; and Dralle, A.J.: Plastic ankle-foot orthoses: Evaluation of function. Arch. Phys. Med. Rehabil. 64:402–407, 1983.

Five polypropylene ankle-foot orthoses were evaluated as to the amount of plantar flexion-dorsiflexion resistance that was provided when worn by hemiplegic and able-bodied subjects. Progressive trimming of the Seattle design polypropylene orthosis made it more flexible and comparable in function to commercially available orthoses. The latter orthoses did not provide a push-off substitute as well as the Seattle design orthosis which enclosed the malleoli, but they did provide an adequate amount of toe clearance during swing.

Lerner-Frankiel, M.B.; Vargas, S.; Brown, M.B.; Krusell, L.; and Schoneberger, W.: Functional community ambulation: What are your criteria? Clin. Management 6:12–15, 1986.

Representative areas of the community were measured to determine the distance disabled persons would need to walk (supermarkets, large drug stores, offices, crosswalks). These values were related to the velocity and endurance capabilities of 10 patients (hemiplegic and amputees) judged to be independent community walkers. It was found that supermarkets and large drug stores required walking 150–600 m and the office areas demanded 30–160 m. All patients identified could accomplish the shorter distance but only half would be able to manage shopping in the large stores.

Locke, M.; Perry, J.; Campbell, J.; and Thomas, L.: Ankle and subtalar motion during gait in arthritic patients. Phys. Ther. 64:504–509, 1984.

The purposes of this study were 1) to document ankle and subtalar motion during gait in 20 healthy subjects and in 25 patients with rheumatoid arthritis (RA) and 2) to determine stride characteristics with and without the use of an extended University of California Biomechanics Laboratory orthosis in RA patients with painful ankle and hindfoot deformity. A significant increase in velocity and single limb support time occurred with shoes and a further significant increase occurred with the orthosis in association with a decrease in ankle and hindfoot pain after using the orthosis. This study demonstrates the value of an orthosis for the treatment of RA patients with ankle and hindfoot pain and deformity.

Marsolais, E.B., and Kobetic, R.: Functional walking in paralyzed patients by means of electrical stimulation. Clin. Orthop. 175:30–36, 1983.

Stainless steel wire electrodes activated by timers were placed in the quadriceps and hip flexors, extensors, and abductors as needed. Muscle force and foot contact evaluations were done by using the Cybex and walkway at the Cleveland Veterans Administration Gait Laboratory. After implantation of electrodes, all three patients had improved function but still desired some supervision in walking. A 10-fold increase in knee torque was noted in one patient, thereby providing him with nearly normal strength. This shows the feasibility of functional neuromuscular stimulation gait augmentation in a previously nonwalking patient outside the laboratory.

May, J.W., Jr.; Halls, M.J.; and Simon, S.R.: Free microvascular muscle flaps with skin graft reconstruction of extensive defects of the foot: A clinical and gait analysis study. Plast. Reconstr. Surg. 75:627–639, 1985.

Patients at the Massachusetts General Hospital have been treated with free muscle flaps covered with thick split-thickness skin grafts for extensive defects of the foot at or below the medial and lateral malleoli. Detailed gait analysis of these patients has confirmed its weight-bearing capabilities and has shown that cutaneous sensibility may not be necessary for its success.

Merkel, K.D.; Katoh, Y.; Johnson, E.W., Jr.; and Chao, E.Y.S.: Mitchell osteotomy for hallux valgus: Long-term follow-up and gait analysis. Foot Ankle 3:189–196, 1983.

This study of Mitchell first-metatarsal osteotomies performed on 69 patients with an average follow-up of 7 years found that more than 86% of the patients were completely satisfied and that the procedure was equally effective in all age groups. Gait analysis demonstrated that these patients do not have normal foot mechanics postoperatively. Excessive first metatarsal shortening, dorsiflexion of the osteotomy, and failure to correct the intermetatarsal angle to 10° or less correlated with poorer results. This study demonstrates a relationship between metatarsal shortening and osteotomy plantar flexion.

Mills, V.M.: Electromyographic results of inhibitory splinting. Phys. Ther. 64:190–193, 1984.

The purpose of this study was to compare the integrated electromyographic activity of spastic muscles in brain-damaged patients before and during splint application. Eight patients with spasticity that produced limb posturing were systematically monitored for electromyographic activity during 2-hour intervals without and then with a splint. A paired *t* test showed increase in the position of the limb into extension in the splinted condition. No significant reduction in integrated electromyographic activity occurred during the splinted condition compared with the nonsplinted condition. Therefore, splinting can effectively control postural defects caused by spastic limb posturing without significant changes in muscle tone.

Murray, M.P.; Guten, G.N.; Mollinger, L.A.; and Gardner, G.M.: Kinematic and electromyographic patterns of Olympic race walkers. Am. J. Sports Med. 11:68–74, 1983.

The performance of two Olympic race walkers was studied during free-speed, fast, and race walking. The race walkers achieved an average speed of 12.5 km/hr compared with the 8.7 km/hr average speed by normal men of the same age during fast walking. All of the muscles monitored in the race walkers showed an increase in the amplitude of electromyographic activity during race walking compared with fast walking. Several suggestions for prevention of injuries associated with race walking are made.

Murray, M.P.; Jacobs, P.A.; Gore, D.R.; Gardner, G.M.; and Mollinger, L.A.: Functional performance after tibial rotationplasty. J. Bone Joint Surg. 67A:392–399, 1985.

Two children who had had a tibial rotation-plasty for osteosarcoma of the distal end of the femur were studied by gait analysis. Both had marked loss of strength in the plantar flexors on the side of the prosthesis. Electromyographic recordings showed that the rotated calf muscles had assumed the function of extensors of the prosthetic knee to a substantial degree. Despite some abnormalities, the children walked at speeds that were comparable to those of normal children. Functionally, it is a worthwhile alternative to above-the-knee amputation.

Murray, M.P.; Mollinger, L.A.; Sepic, S.B.; Gardner, G.M.; and Linder, M.T.: Gait patterns in above-knee amputee patients: Hydraulic swing control vs constant-friction knee components. Arch. Phys. Med. Rehabil. 64:339–345, 1983.

Multiple displacement patterns, stride dimensions, and temporal components during slow, free-speed, and fast walking were compared in the same seven above-knee amputees using prostheses with constant-friction knee components and using hydraulic swing-control knee components. With hydraulic-type prostheses, the amputees showed a wider range of walking speeds, improvement in the equality of the durations of successive swing and stance phases, and greater uniformity of forward progression of the prosthetic limb during walking. Abnormalities persisted with both types of prostheses.

Otis, J.C.; Lane, J.M.; and Kroll, M.A.: TI energy cost during gait in osteosarcoma patients after resection and knee replacement and after above-the-knee amputation. J. Bone Joint Surg. 67A:606–611, 1985.

In a group of patients treated for osteosarcoma about the knee, comparisons of free walking velocity, oxygen consumption per meter traveled, and percentage of maximal aerobic capacity used during walking demonstrated that patients with resection and prosthetic knee replacement had a lower energy cost during gait than equivalent amputees did.

Perrin, T.; Dorr, L.D.; Perry, J.; Gronley, J.; and Hull, D.B.: Functional evaluation of total hip arthroplasty with five- to ten-year follow-up evaluation. Clin. Orthop. 195:252–260, 1985.

Forty-seven patients with unilateral hip disease and total hip arthroplasty had gait analysis during a follow-up period of 5–10 years to correlate the levels of function with mechanical loosening. Patients followed longer than 5 years appeared to have an accelerated decline in function unassociated with pain. Revision rate for mechanical failure by 10 years is 58% for age and 66% for fast walkers.

Perry, J.: Integrated function of the lower extremity including gait analysis. *In* Adult Orthopaedics, edited by R.L. Cruess and W.R.J. Rennie, pp. 1161–1207. Vol. 2. New York, Churchill Livingstone, 1984.

This chapter reviews the basic elements of lower extremity function as well as the modes of normal and abnormal gait. Values contributing to limb stability are distinguished from those used for progressional mobility. Generic terminology defines the functional analysis format. The impact of the different types of pathology and the characteristic gait deviations are described.

Perry, J.; Ireland, M.L.; Gronley, J.; and Hoffer, M.M.: Predictive value of manual muscle testing and gait analysis in normal ankles by dynamic electromyography. Foot Ankle 6:254–259, April 1986.

By dynamic electromyography the relative intensities of the foot and ankle muscles were identified during the manual muscle tests of grade 5 (normal), 3 (fair), and 1 (trace). The practice of recording four muscles simultaneously demonstrated poor selectivity by the muscle test. The soleus was not differentiated from the gastrocnemius by the flexed knee stance. There was significant muscle action in all the tests. This introduces considerable doubt about the clinical validity of manual testing when muscle strength is abnormal.

Pratt, D.J.: Energy of gait in below-knee casts with different soles. J. Biomed. Eng. 7:63–67, January 1985.

This paper presents guidelines for the use of soles on below-knee walking casts. Volunteer subjects fitted with below-knee casts with three commercial soles and two "homemade" ones were used. Recommendations are included regarding the design of soles to be used in this clinically demanding situation.

Rab, G.T.; Wyatt, M.; Sutherland, D.H.; and Simon, S.R.: A technique for determining femoral head containment during gait. J. Pediatr. Orthop. 5:8–12, 1985.

Kinematic gait analysis was carried out on patients with Legg-Calvé-Perthes disease with and without various abduction orthoses. The three-dimensional containment of the hip is reproducibly altered by various devices; specifically, the Atlanta brace increases posterior coverage and slightly increases lateral coverage, and Petrie casts improve lateral and anterior coverage at the expense of posterior containment.

Saleh, M., and Murdoch, G.: In defence of gait analysis: Observation and measurement in gait assessment. J. Bone Joint Surg. 67B:237–241, 1985.

In a comparison of visual observation and use of a quantitative gait measurement system, visual observation was found to be an unreliable clinical skill. The observers recorded only 22.2% of the predicted gait deviations and were unable to comment on 15.6% of all the required observations. The gait parameters that were difficult to assess visually—step length and step time—are considered to be of value as diagnostic clinical indicators in gait assessment.

Shereff, M.J.; Bregman, A.M.; and Kummer, F.J.: The effect of immobilization devices on the load distribution under the foot. Clin. Orthop. 192:260–267, 1985.

Maximal reduction of forefoot loads was achieved by means of a short-leg walking cast or an ankle boot with a posteriorly placed flat rubber heel. A centrally placed rocker heel led to increased forefoot loads, especially under the first metatarsal head. The height of the cast and configuration of the sole of the cast shoe had little effect on the observed patterns of force distribution.

Simon, S.R.; Trieshmann, H.W.; Burdett, R.G.; Ewald, F.C.; and Sledge, C.B.: Quantitative gait analysis after total knee arthroplasty for monarticular degenerative arthritis. J. Bone Joint Surg 65A:605–613, 1983.

Quantitative gait analysis was used to determine the functional results of total knee arthroplasty in a group of 12 elderly patients with isolated degenerative arthritis of one knee. All patients had had a standard replacement arthroplasty at least 2 years before the study. Most of the measurements of gait had been restored to normal levels. Three patients had external torque across the implants and in the control knee that were comparable in magnitude but varied in relative frequency between the two groups. Compared with the controls, the patients spent approximately 30% more time in double limb stance and had prolonged cycle times.

Skinner, H.B.; Barrack, R.L.; Cook, S.D.; and Haddad, R.J., Jr.: Joint position sense in total knee arthroplasty. J. Orthop. Res. 1:276–283, 1984.

Normal gait and function are not typically achieved after total knee replacement. Irreversible loss of joint proprioceptive function occurs due to the disease process. Loss of proprioception and the resulting abnormal gait patterns may place increased stress on components and contribute to loosening. An association between degenerative joint disease and decline in proprioception is suggested. Strongest correlations were seen in total knee arthroplasty patients when a clinical and proprioceptive score was compared with gait parameters. Results showed statistically significant decreases in joint position sense from young controls to old controls and further significant decreases with joint disease; however, no further worsening was noted as a result of total knee arthroplasty.

Vaughan, C.L.: Biomechanics of running gait. Crit. Rev. Biomed. Eng. 12:1–48, 1984.

In this paper, various biochemical aspects of sprinting, middle- and long-distance running, and jogging are reviewed. The topics covered include the class of running gait (sprinting, jogging, ascending/descending, load carrying, treadmill); electromyography; joints; kinematics (both linear and angular); kinetics (forceplate, joint forces and torques, work/energy/power, air resistance); mathematical techniques and models; orthopaedic aids; various pathologies; different methods of recording motion; and sports footwear and surfaces.

Vodovnik, L.; Bowman, B.R.; and Winchester, P.: Effect of electrical stimulation on spasticity in hemiparetic patients. Int. Rehabil. Med. 6:153–156, 1984.

Cyclic electrical stimulation was given to 10 hemiparetic patients with clinical signs of knee joint spasticity. None of the patients experienced increased spasticity. The decrease in spasticity ranged from none to substantial, with some other beneficial side effects.

Williams, L.O.; Anderson, A.D.; Campbell, J.; Thomas, L.; Feiwell, E.; and Walker, J.M.: Energy cost of walking and of wheelchair propulsion by children with myelodysplasia: Comparison with normal children. Dev. Med. Child. Neurol. 25:617–624, 1983.

The oxygen consumption in 15 myelodysplastic children during walking and propelling a wheelchair was studied. In comparison with normal children, they walked slower and consumed more oxygen per meter but had a similar time rate of oxygen consumption. A swing-through gait pattern was 33% more energy efficient than a four-point gait pattern for these children. Wheelchair propulsion produced velocities and energy efficiencies similar to those in normal children walking. Oxygen consumption and velocity measurements were found to be significantly related to the clinical factors of level of lesion and strength of hip and knee extension.

Wong, M.A.; Simon, S.; and Olshen, R.A.: Statistical analysis of gait patterns of persons with cerebral palsy. Stat. Med. 2:345–354, 1983.

Gait measurements were used to determine a gait typology for patients with cerebral palsy. The procedure identified four subpopulations from the sample data. The typology differs from the present diagnostic system which classifies a cerebral palsy patient as quadriplegic, diplegic, or hemiplegic.

10

Circulatory, Respiratory, Hematopoietic, Gastrointestinal, Genitourinary, and Integumentary Systems

Circulatory System

Hemorrhagic shock is classified as mild, moderate, and severe. In mild shock there is a 20% to 25% decrease in blood volume with a slight tachycardia, mild hypotension, and mild vasoconstriction. In moderate shock the blood loss is 25% to 35%, resulting in a thready pulse, tachycardia, hypotension, marked vasoconstriction, diaphoresis, restlessness, and decreased urine output. In severe shock there is a 35% to 50% loss in blood volume with severe hypotension, tachycardia, vasoconstriction, obtundation, and absence of urine output. Homeostatic responses are initiated that can only be interrupted by exogenous volume restoration in the form of intravenous administration of fluids (Fig. 1). Changes secondary to low flow rate result in decreased oxygen delivery to vital organs and consequently a shift from aerobic to anaerobic metabolism with eventual organ failure. One important change is that eventually there is a period of complete microcirculatory arrest in skeletal muscle, followed by obstruction of many capillaries by leukocytes when reperfusion is started. This results in local variations of hypoxic injury in muscle. Patients who eventually die of shock have severe ischemic myocardial damage as demonstrated by a positive nitro-BT test.

Vigorous ventilatory and circulatory supports are essential in early resuscitation of patients in shock. Blood replacement and crystalloid solution administration are the most important treatments for hypovolemic shock. Lactated Ringer's solution is isotonic, and intravenous administration of it appears to decrease the requirement for whole blood; however, it may contribute to acidosis. Recently, dextran-70 has been shown to decrease the total fluid requirement and maintain urine output and was associated with a lower incidence of adult respiratory distress compared to treatment with Ringer's solution in a group of adult patients in severe shock after pelvic and femoral fractures. The effectiveness of synthetic oxygen-carrying blood replacement products in patients who have sustained blood loss is being evaluated. However, their place in treatment of patients who sustain traumatic or surgical blood loss is yet to be determined. Pneumatic anti-shock trousers are often used in the immediate resuscitation of severely injured patients. Thigh compartment syndrome may result from these trousers unless their pressure is elevated only high enough to restore adequate blood pressure, and the duration of application should be no longer than clinically necessary.

After minimal resuscitation of the patient, the orthopaedist often is faced with treatment of multiple fractures which may be associated with significant hemorrhage. Hemorrhage remains the most common cause of death after pelvic fractures. Methods for control of hemorrhage from these fractures include direct surgical approach for ligation of vessels, ligation of the internal iliac vessels, use of the G-suit, external fixation of the fracture, skeletal trac-

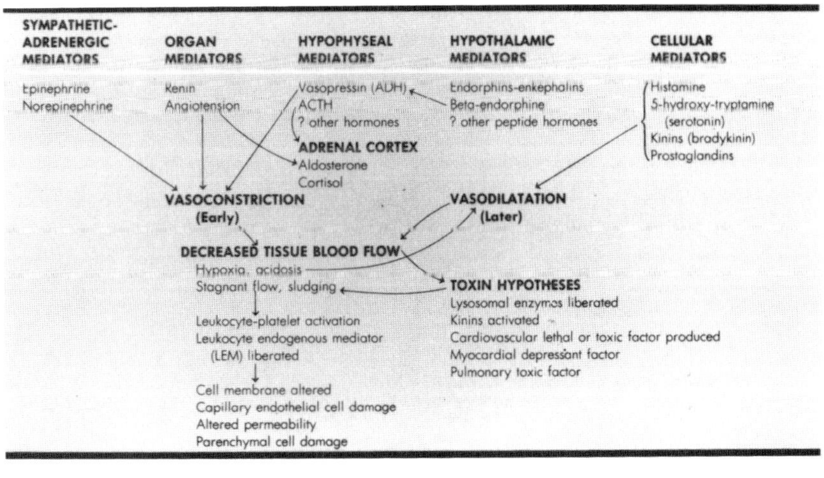

Figure 1

Vasoactive and neuroendocrine mediators in shock. (From Baue, A.E.: Shock and cardiac arrest. *In* Hardy's Textbook of Surgery, edited by J.D. Hardy, pp. 33–65. Philadelphia, J.B. Lippincott Company, 1983. By permission of the publisher.)

tion, massive fluid and blood replacement, and therapeutic embolization of bleeding vessels. Patients who present with pelvic fractures also may have intra-abdominal injury that should receive priority. An injured viscus should be treated surgically. However, the retroperitoneal space should not be opened because it usually is impossible to control the bleeding vessels by direct surgical treatment. The G-suit is effective because of compression and tamponade of the bleeding sites and immobilization of the fractures.

A technique used increasingly in recent years for severe pelvic bleeding after trauma or surgical procedures is diagnostic angiography followed by therapeutic embolization of bleeding sites with an autologous clot or gelatin sponge. Stabilization of the pelvic fracture should be accomplished as soon as possible by external and, possibly later, internal fixation.

Toxic shock has been reported in infants with osteomyelitis and septicemia. It has also been reported in a patient after an elective wrist arthrodesis and in another patient after femoral head osteoplasty, both with secondary *Staphylococcus aureus* wound infections. Although seen predominantly in menstruating women, it occurs in postmenopausal women and men, especially as a postoperative complication. The wound may be benign, but it should be explored in the operating room; high-dose antibiotic therapy and multiorgan system support are necessary. Septic shock continues to be a major clinical problem, and the best means of resuscitation remains uncertain. A combination of antibiotics, 3% colloid solution, and corticosteroids resulted in improved long-term survival in experimental septic shock even when begun after sepsis had started. Irreversible burn shock that persists despite fluid resuscitation remains a significant cause of early mortality in thermally injured children. Because circulating serum factors have been implicated in the pathophysiology of burn shock, exchange transfusion has been tried and reported successful in patients not responding to conventional volume therapy.

Malignant Hyperthermia

This autosomal dominant abnormality of muscle physiology may be triggered by many stimuli, including stress and various anesthetic agents. Patients with this condition are particularly prone to development of musculoskeletal abnormalities including myopathy, recurrent dislocations, scoliosis, and kyphosis. Halothane and succinylcholine most commonly are implicated in stimulation of a hyperthermic reaction. The first signs are rapidly increasing temperature and tachycardia. Sinus tachycardia may lead to ventricular tachycardia, fibrillation, and death. The core body temperature may rise as rapidly as 2°C per 5-minute period and can reach 47°C. The pathogenesis of malignant hyperthermia involves a calcium transport abnormality due to defects in several different cell membranes including the sarcoplasmic reticulum and the mitochondria. This results in recurrent sarcomeric contraction and muscle rigidity, leading to increases in metabolic rate, temperature, CO_2 production, and oxygen use, with resultant cyanosis. Myoglobinuria may occur and lead to renal failure. The mortality rate, which is directly related to the severity of the fever, is high. It has been associated with Duchenne muscular dystrophy, with the use of neuroleptic drugs, and with osteogenesis imperfecta.

Patient Evaluation

Serum levels of creatine kinase may be increased in some patients susceptible to malignant hyperthermia, but this is not a consistently reliable screening test. An accurate family and personal history is the best method. The report of a serious illness or death after stress of any type, including surgery, is a key diagnostic factor. Patients may have large muscle mass with a history of cramping, exercise intolerance in hot weather, and acrocyanosis associated with stress. The phosphorylase ratio has not been shown to identify patients susceptible to malignant hyperthermia, and muscle biopsy with specific *in vitro* muscle fiber testing in specialized laboratories is necessary to establish the diagnosis in suspected individuals.

Management

Careful intraoperative monitoring is important. Any increase in temperature of 1°C or more, even from a subnormal reading, requires investigation. If malignant hyperthermia is suspected intraoperatively, the surgical procedure should be terminated as rapidly as possible, muscle relaxants and anesthetic agents should be discontinued, and the patient should be hyperventilated with oxygen. Dantrolene sodium appears to exert a beneficial action on the sarcoplasmic reticulum by inhibiting calcium release from the sarcotubular system. It should be administered intravenously in an initial dose of 1.5 mg (1–3 mg)/kg of body weight, followed by doses of 1 mg/kg up to a total dose of 10 mg/kg or until a clinical response is seen. Sodium bicarbonate is used to manage acidosis. Mannitol and furosemide may be needed to maintain urine output. Administration of glucose is helpful in decreasing the serum potassium level. Procainamide is an effective treatment for arrhythmias. Cooling of the patient with ice bath or fans is essential. Intravenous use of iced fluids is also helpful. Cooling methods may be discontinued when the patient's temperature falls to 38°C. Patients who recover from malignant hyperthermia will have severe muscle pain and swelling. Most will experience muscle soreness and weakness with any significant activity for many months. Dantrolene sodium at 1 to 1.5 mg/kg given orally 12 and 4 hours before operation may prevent this syndrome.

Anesthesia

Hypotensive anesthesia during major hip and spinal surgery is effective for decreasing intraoperative and total blood loss and for shortening operative time. There is no significant difference in thromboembolism between hypotensive and normotensive anesthesia. In spinal surgery, hypotensive anesthesia significantly reduces intraoperative blood loss, but blood requirement is decreased only in patients under age 18 years, not adults.

To detect spinal cord dysfunction intraoperatively, somatosensory cortical-evoked potential monitoring or a wake-up test, or a combination of the two, is generally used. A balanced anesthesia technique consisting of nitrous oxide, narcotics, and a muscle relaxant is well suited for both techniques. Patients receiving fentanyl instead of morphine do not require postoperative respiratory support.

Regional blocks in the lower extremity have limited use. Sciatic and femoral nerve blocks for the evaluation of knee injuries achieve satisfactory relaxation and analgesia in most patients. Obturator nerve blocks, however, carry an unacceptably high morbidity. Continuous blocks are successful in the brachial plexus for long procedures such as reattachments and for treating reflex sympathetic dystrophy. In the lower extremity, a continuous sciatic nerve block has been helpful in relieving pain in ischemic gangrene of the foot.

Intravenous regional anesthesia is becoming more common for reduction of fractures and major surgery in the upper extremity (and at times in the lower extremity). It may be utilized for procedures distal to the elbow joint in patients who otherwise would require general or regional block anesthesia. Bier's block is superior to fracture site infiltration in terms of patient acceptability and in ease of reduction. Major potential complications associated with this technique include sensitivity to the drug, cardiac and neural reactions, and tourniquet pain. Patients exposed to excessive cortical stimulation after release of the tourniquet may experience light-headedness, agitation, and confusion. On rare occasions, muscle twitching and convulsions follow these symptoms. Rapid deflation of a tourniquet with release of the anesthetic agent may result in cardiac arrest and shock due to depression of respiratory and cardiovascular centers in the medulla oblongata. Patients with severe reactions must be treated with respiratory support, fluid administration, anticonvulsants, and vasopressor agents. Reactions can be decreased or eliminated by delaying release of the tourniquet until 1 hour after drug administration. If release is necessary sooner, it should be done gradually.

Local infiltration at the surgical site (especially back and knee) has been helpful in relieving the patient's postoperative pain and decreasing the amount of narcotics required postoperatively. In patients with femoral neck fracture, a lateral cutaneous nerve block significantly decreased the postoperative pain and opiate requirements.

Osteonecrosis

Death of bone tissue may occur anywhere in the skeleton. When necrosis of bone occurs in limited areas of the diaphysis or metaphysis, the skeleton continues to perform its support function. Unless a radiograph is taken for another reason, these infarcts go unnoticed. A possible, but rare, long-term complication of bone infarction may be transformation to a malignant fibrous tumor. Only when necrotic bone no longer performs its support function, usually adjacent to a joint surface, do symptoms occur.

Cause

The cause of osteonecrosis after a specific episode of trauma is the loss of blood supply for a long enough time to result in cellular death. The cause of nontraumatic osteonecrosis is less clear. Compromise of blood supply to bone tissue may be present, but there may be other factors (Table 1). Steroid administration may be involved in the pathogenesis of osteonecrosis after renal transplantation as well as in other diseases, but it is difficult to correlate the steroid dosage with the occurrence of osteonecrosis. It is most commonly associated with long-term steroid therapy but can occur after short-term high-dose treatment. It can also occur as a complication of cancer chemotherapy that often includes corticosteroids (in some cases it does not).

Older patients who have a low serum phosphorus value, have evidence of significant bone disease, and experience delay in renal function returning to normal after the procedure are more likely to have osteonecrosis after renal transplantation. An additional complication of the procedure found in one large series of patients was a 26% incidence of fractures which involved the pelvis more commonly than the long bones. All fractures healed without complication, usually after closed methods of treatment.

Steroid intake results in an increase in serum cholesterol, fatty metamorphosis of the liver, and occurrence of fat emboli in small vessels. In addition, there is an increase of approximately 25% in the marrow fat cell volume and of 15% in the total volume of the marrow compartment, due to osteoporosis. An increase in cell volume to greater than the marrow compartment space volume may increase pressure and cause damage to the vascular sinusoidal elements.

Similar changes may occur with heavy alcohol intake. Increased vascular pressure and delayed emptying of radiopaque dye from the intraosseous space are found in patients who have osteonecrosis associated with alcohol intake.

The mechanism of development of osteonecrosis in patients presenting with severe pressure changes is probably multifactorial, involving ischemia due to intravascular and extravascular nitrogen bubbles, fibrin thrombi, platelet aggregation, clumping of formed elements of blood (mainly erythrocytes with lipids), and blood flow changes. It is suggested that emboli may not be a cause of osteonecrosis in metabolic disorders but that the bone cells are unhealthy because of metabolic disorders, so that toxic substances, such as alcohol and steroids, may be enough additional insult to cause cell death and eventually result in osteonecrosis.

There are no significant alterations in the biochemical and metabolic features of the cartilage overlying necrotic bone in either traumatic or nontraumatic forms of osteonecrosis. Secondary changes due to mechanical factors and similar to those in osteoarthritis eventually occur in the cartilage.

In patients who present with unilateral symptomatic osteonecrosis, a search for similar skeletal lesions at other sites is warranted (particularly in the contralateral hip) because some forms of treatment are effective only before osteochondral collapse and significant symptoms develop. If a patient is symptomatic and no radiographic changes are noted, a radioactive bone scan or magnetic resonance imaging may be helpful. Tomography may demonstrate the "crescent sign" or transchondral fracture earlier than plain radiographs.

Diagnosis

Biopsy is the definitive method of diagnosis. Venography and pressure studies may be done at the same time to confirm the results. Noninvasive studies include radiographs and quantitative bone scans. However, the diagnosis is difficult, especially in stage I and stage II disease (Table 2). In such cases, the new technology of magnetic resonance imaging is indicating that diagnosis of osteonecrosis of the femoral head may be possible even before changes on the bone scan.

Histologically, initially there is a disappearance of hematopoietic elements and a fat cell necrosis, followed by total necrosis of the marrow and osteocytes. With repair,

Table 1. Conditions Associated With Osteonecrosis (Risk Increases With Number of Conditions)

Alcoholism*	Gaucher's disease*	Pancreatitis†
Arthropathy	Gout	Peripheral vascular disease
Neuropathic	Hemoglobinopathy*	Pregnancy
Carbon tetrachloride poisoning	Hepatitis	Systemic lupus erythematosus†
Chemotherapy	Histiocytosis	Thermal injuries*
Clotting defects	Hypercortisonism*	Burns
Congenital malformation	Hyperlipemia†	Electrical injuries
Convulsive disorders	Hyperuricemia†	Frostbite
Cushing's syndrome*	Irradiation*	Thrombophlebitis
Diabetes†	Leriche's syndrome	Trauma*
Dysbaric phenomena*	Microfractures	Fractures
Endocarditis	Myxedema	Dislocations
Fat embolism†	Obesity	

*Generally accepted contributory factor.
†Commonly reported associated factor.
From Jones, J.P., Jr.: Osteonecrosis. *In* Arthritis and Allied Conditions: A Textbook of Rheumatology, edited by D.J. McCarty, pp. 1356–1373. Tenth edition. Philadelphia, Lea & Febiger, 1985. By permission of the publisher.

new woven bone is laid down on dead trabeculae (Fig. 2). As the dead trabeculae are resorbed, the remaining unstressed woven bone may fracture, leading to collapse and fragmentation and eventually to altered joint configuration.

Treatment

The treatment for osteonecrosis depends on the cause, stage of involvement, symptoms, and location. The most common site of osteonecrosis requiring surgical treatment is the femoral head. Once osteochondral fracture and collapse occur in the femoral head, most patients require major reconstructive surgery. Loosening of the components, however, is very common in young adults and in patients with renal disease (dislocation is 5 to 8 times more common in transplant patients compared to nontransplant patients). Patients with osteonecrosis associated with alcoholism may benefit from decompression of the femoral head and neck by drilling. Patients who have no osteochondral fracture prior to the drilling procedure have no progression of symptoms after decompression in the large majority of patients. Whether this procedure is a significant improvement over conservative therapy and whether it is effective regardless of cause are still unknown.

Patients who have a crescent sign or osteochondral fracture have shown temporary symptomatic improvement but continue to have evidence of progressive destruction on radiographs. Pulsed electromagnetic field treatment is currently under investigation. Osteonecrosis of the femoral condyle may heal if detected early and treated by protection from weight-bearing, appropriate immobilization, or realignment osteotomy. When osteonecrosis develops at the femoral condyle after renal transplantation, the osteonecrotic segment occasionally may heal without sequelae. Those patients progressing to osteochondral fracture and collapse may require realignment osteotomy, removal of loose bodies, arthrodesis, or prosthetic reconstruction.

Table 2. Stages of Osteonecrosis

Stage	Description
I	Radiograph is normal; diagnosis is based on histologic changes of ischemic necrosis; no osteochondral fracture; magnetic resonance imaging and bone scan are positive
II	Radiographic changes are present but may not be typical for ischemic necrosis; no osteochondral fracture
III	Characteristic radiographic changes of ischemic necrosis with wedge-shaped increased density and mottled osteoporosis; subchondral lucent line is visible, and head is no longer spherical
IV	Marked radiographic changes in femoral head with secondary degenerative changes in hip joint

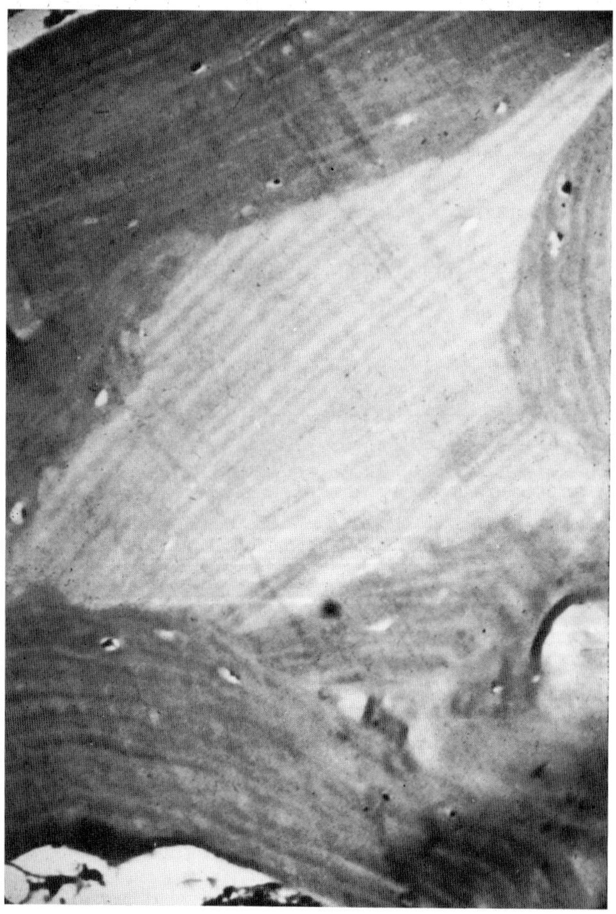

Figure 2

Histologic section, showing osteonecrosis. Note new bone with living cells covering dead bone devoid of osteocytes.

Both post-traumatic and nontraumatic osteonecrosis of the talus may require major surgical reconstruction. Osteonecrosis of the humeral head not associated with a major traumatic episode should be treated with activity limitation to reduce the forces across the shoulder joint and passive or assisted exercises to maintain motion. Healing may occur without surgical intervention. Even with moderate deformity, many patients will continue to function well. Those who have severe symptoms can be treated successfully with prosthetic replacement, usually without resurfacing of the glenoid.

Osteonecrosis *per se* is not painful, and the symptoms are the result of biologic attempts to repair the necrotic bone. Methods that prevent the reparative process in experimental animals may allow continued function of the skeletal support without development of symptoms. Such therapeutic techniques involve chemical fixation of bone to prevent repair or removal of necrotic bone and replacement with plastic. Another procedure still considered experimental is the replacement of the subchondral bone and articular cartilage with human allografts. These techniques are being studied and may have future application in the treatment of osteonecrosis. The close association of metabolic bone disease (osteopenia) and osteonecrosis requires attention.

Respiratory System

Adult Respiratory Distress Syndrome

The adult respiratory distress syndrome (ARDS) is acute respiratory failure due to noncardiogenic pulmonary edema. It is a complex sequela of shock, systemic sepsis, trauma, viral respiratory infections, and many other insults. This disorder is particularly tragic because it often affects healthy young patients. ARDS is common and lethal, affecting an estimated 150,000 persons each year. The mortality rate is 50% despite supportive therapy. The syndrome occurs in approximately 2% of all patients who sustain severe trauma.

The tachypnea, dyspnea, hypoxemia, and decreased compliance are resistant to routine methods of oxygen administration. Patients also exhibit restlessness, anxiety, cough with significant pulmonary secretions, and often an expiratory wheeze. In later stages of the disease, almost complete consolidation in the lung fields may occur.

The cause probably is multifactorial. Fluid overload, lung emboli, aspiration of gastric contents, shock, and particulate matter (such as platelet aggregates and fibrin thrombi) passing through standard blood filters and lodging in the pulmonary capillaries have been suggested as etiologic factors. Sepsis is currently thought to be a major factor. Recent experimental and clinical evidence implicates complement-mediated neutrophil aggregation and stasis in pulmonary capillaries in the genesis of the pulmonary endothelial injury that characterizes early ARDS. Intravascular coagulation, platelet aggregation, and prostaglandins are related to ARDS in a yet undefined way. The neutrophil-mediated injury and the coagulation-mediated injury may amplify each other's effects in ARDS. The end result is alveolar injury, interstitial disarray, and eventual fibrosis.

Early diagnosis is essential for management. Assays for C5a and Di antigen and possibly for other specific markers or mediators of pulmonary endothelial injury may help to identify incipient ARDS before respiratory failure develops. This would allow prospective controlled clinical trials to establish the efficacy of new treatment modalities. A quantitative method for measuring increased pulmonary capillary permeability that uses human serum albumin labeled with radioactive technetium allows early diagnosis of ARDS and accurately differentiates this condition from pneumonia or cardiogenic pulmonary edema.

Mechanical ventilation may be successful treatment, but if the PaO_2 cannot be increased to 70 mm Hg with an FIO_2 of 0.5, positive end-expiratory pressure (PEEP) is necessary. In addition, these patients require adequate blood volume replacement and the use of cardiotonic drugs, if necessary, to maintain cardiac function.

There has been the suggestion that prophylactic mechanical ventilation with PEEP decreases the incidence of ARDS. Early use of PEEP at 8 cm H_2O in high-risk patients has no effect on the incidence of ARDS or other associated complications. Early methylprednisolone therapy is also controversial in pulmonary failure, and recent studies have failed to prove the efficacy of steroids. Also, patients on steroid therapy have an increased risk of infection. Intensive pulmonary care and general supportive care remain the preferred therapy for ARDS.

Fat Embolism Syndrome

Fat embolism syndrome is a clinical symptom complex consisting of tachypnea, tachycardia, fever, mental status change, and petechiae. It occurs much more commonly in young adults than in any other age group and is rare in children. Its incidence correlates positively with the number of long bones fractured, open fractures, and fractures caused by vehicular accidents.

It was believed that fat embolism syndrome was caused by the alteration of pulmonary function brought on directly by fat emboli from the fractured bone. Although fat emboli are found in the lungs of patients who sustain fractures and other major musculoskeletal trauma, there now is evidence that fat emboli are metabolized into free fatty acids which have a toxic action on the lung parenchyma and produce respiratory distress and chemical pneumonitis. The thromboplastin released from damaged tissue is a strong stimulus of platelet aggregation. Thromboplastin causes disseminated intravascular coagulation and a disturbance of the colloidal stability of plasma lipids, allowing the formation of additional intravascular fat particles. Both platelets and erythrocytes adhere to fat particles, producing emboli that consist of fat macroglobules, platelets, and erythrocytes and that lodge in the lungs, resulting in further release of free fatty acids. Finally, hypovolemia and poor oxygenation have an important role in development of the clinical manifestations of fat embolism syndrome.

Embolic marrow fat from the fracture site appears to be the central pathophysiologic agent. It is concentrated in the pulmonary vascular bed where it causes an inflammatory response and serves to activate the clotting cascade, to increase platelet activity, and to initiate the release of vasoactive substances. The lung's final common pathway of response is manifested by capillary leakage, inflammation and edema, and eventual fibrosis.

Great concern has been expressed about the relationship of the fat embolism syndrome to intramedullary fixation of fractured femurs, especially immediately after injury. The fat embolism syndrome rarely occurs after immediate (<24 hours) intramedullary nailing of femoral shaft fractures, but any delay greater than 24 hours is associated with a 5-fold increase in the incidence of ARDS (Fig. 3).

A similar syndrome has been reported after total hip arthroplasty and femoral prosthesis placement with methyl methacrylate. Less commonly, the syndrome may occur after total knee replacement, usually with a long-stem prosthesis (it also has been reported after implantation of a total condylar prosthesis). It is important to plug the distal femur before cementing the femoral component. Reports suggest that leaving the femoral canal unplugged or nonvented can result in high intramedullary pressures, so that fat and marrow elements are forced into the venous drainage. Acute respiratory or cardiac failure shortly after the femoral component has been cemented into place has been reported at a higher incidence in patients being treated for fresh femoral neck fractures or pathologic fractures requiring long-stem prostheses than in patients undergoing total hip replacement for arthritis. Intraoperative monitoring of patients at risk is warranted.

Maintenance of normal blood volume and proper oxygenation are important in preventing the clinical manifestations. Treatment includes blood volume replacement, cardiotonic drugs, and respiratory support. Oxygen (30% to 40%) delivered by mask is adequate in many patients, but some will require positive-pressure breathing. In addition to supportive measures, use of steroids has been recommended. Patients who have a blood alcohol level of less than 0.02 mg/dl are more likely to develop clinical fat embolism syndrome than are patients with higher blood alcohol levels. On this basis, alcohol has been recommended as a treatment for this syndrome, but results are inconclusive. In experimental animal studies, methylprednisolone suppresses many abnormalities that occur during this syndrome. Steroids inhibit platelet aggregation, platelet factor 3 availability, and serotonin release; depress the release of tissue thromboplastin from injured tissues; and produce an increase in lung surfactant content. Atelectasis, inflammation, and alveolar membrane thickening are decreased by methylprednisolone administration. There is also increased cardiac output, increased pulmonary vasodilatation, and decreased pulmonary shunting. Glucose administration partially ameliorates the decrease in PaO_2 after trauma but does not prevent occurrence of the syndrome. Most evidence suggests that patients with clinical fat embolism syndrome should be treated by cardiorespiratory support but, in resistant cases or in the presence of multiple fractures, methylprednisolone treatment may be considered.

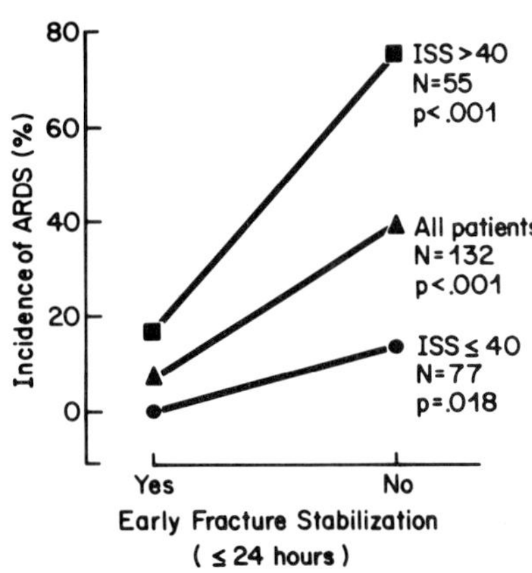

Figure 3

Incidence of ARDS as related to early or late operative stabilization and injury severity (ISS). (From Johnson, K.D.; Cadambi, A.; and Seibert, G.B. J. Trauma 25:375–383, 1985. By permission of Williams & Wilkins.)

Respiratory Function With Spinal Deformity

Respiratory complications after spinal fusion for scoliosis are increased in patients who have nonidiopathic curves, mental retardation, anterior spine fusions, a relative arterial hypoxemia, and an obstructive component in pulmonary function testing and are more than 20 years old.

Pulmonary function is normal on routine testing in young adults with scoliosis with curves of up to 46° although there are some reports of a small tidal volume in scoliotics with a higher respiratory frequency in order to maintain adequate ventilation. In severe thoracic scoliosis with respiratory failure, a restrictive lung pattern, polycythemia, cor pulmonale, and abnormal blood gas values are present. Therapy with supplemental oxygen, digoxin, diuretics, intermittent positive-pressure ventilation four times daily, and tracheostomy may not produce improvement. However, 12 hours of night-time ventilation through a permanent tracheostomy allowed patients to have increased activity approaching a normal life-style. If acute respiratory failure develops, successful management is possible, long-term survival is expected, and pulmonary function will deteriorate at slower than the expected rate.

Pneumothorax

Spontaneous pneumothorax and bullae can be caused by Marfan syndrome. The frequency of spontaneous pneumothorax in patients older than 12 years with Marfan syndrome is 4.4%. Definitive surgical treatment should be performed at the first occurrence of pneumothorax because of the high rate of recurrence after treatment with a chest tube.

Atelectasis

Atelectasis occurs frequently in patients treated with assistive ventilation for respiratory failure due to neuromuscular disease. Infection occurring soon after intubation is often a principal cofactor.

Hematopoietic System

Bleeding Disorders

Hemophilia This genetically inherited group of bleeding disorders is characterized by deficiency or absence of specific coagulation factors, most commonly factor VIII. The degree of deficiency, and thus the degree of coagulation defect, determines the severity of the clinical problem. Patients with a factor VIII level less than 1% of normal have a marked deficiency; at 1% to 5% they have a moderate deficiency, and at 5% to 25% they have a mild deficiency. All have bleeding episodes and possible serious joint, skeletal, and soft tissue sequelae.

The home administration of factor VIII has substantially decreased the need for hospitalization, allows earlier treatment for bleeding, decreases the cost of treatment, and probably improves psychosocial development. For acute hemarthroses it has been shown that higher (40%) doses had no more effect than lower (20%) doses on retransfusion rate or time to complete resolution but did decrease residual loss of motion. Bleeding into the knees, ankles, or elbows commonly presents with pain and swelling. Restriction of motion is seen in all patients with bleeding into the knee and elbow and in most with bleeding into the ankle. When treatment begins within 3 hours after onset of symptoms, there is a direct relationship between the severity of these findings and the time for complete restoration of function. Use of home therapy on a demand schedule has also been shown to maintain normal range of motion in the knee joint in severely affected hemophiliacs with normal joints. However, if even mild disease is present in the joint, the ability to maintain or to improve the joint with such demand therapy appears to be decreased. Severe hemophilic arthropathy generally is correlated with the severity and frequency of bleeding into the joint. Although damage to joints is caused by both mechanical and chemical influences, enzymatic processes appear to be the primary cause of cartilage matrix degradation.

The presence of inhibitors has been a relative contraindication to surgical treatment in hemophiliacs because of potential difficulties in achieving hemostasis. Inhibiting antibodies occur in 4% to 20% of patients with classic hemophilia but are much less common in patients with mild to moderate forms. Administration of large doses of factor VIII daily has resulted in a marked decrease in the level of inhibitors in some patients, allowing surgical treatment. Autoplex, an activated prothrombin-complex concentrate, has been shown to be successful in allowing surgical treatment (elective synovectomy) with control of hemostasis and no evidence of thrombosis or consumption coagulopathy.

Ultrasonography provides a means to establish the diagnosis of bleeding into muscle. It also can be used to evaluate the success of therapy and to follow the patient's course until resolution of the hematoma. Frequent sites of bleeding are the quadriceps, followed by the calf, anterior tibial compartment, adductors, hamstrings, and sartorius. If treatment is delayed more than 2 hours after the onset of symptoms there is a significant prolongation of recovery time after bleeding into the quadriceps. Bleeding into the calf muscles requires less replacement than bleeding into the quadriceps, but recovery time is not prolonged with bleeding treated as late as 3 hours after onset of symptoms. Bleeding within closed compartments may cause neuropathy and muscle contracture. Patients who present with hemophilia and symptoms and signs suggestive of compartment syndrome should have immediate replacement therapy to achieve a factor VIII level adequate for operation. If increased compartment pressure is confirmed, fasciotomy should be performed. Repeated bleeding into muscles may cause an expanding pseudotumor that may be life-threatening. Excision is sometimes necessary.

Iron deposits have been demonstrated throughout the synovium in hemophiliacs. Superficially, a granular material has been shown to be highly iron-saturated ferritin, and ovate bodies in the deeper layers of the synovium are almost pure iron. It appears that the iron-saturated ferritin in the synovial membrane could increase or perpetuate inflammation by promoting lipid peroxidation.

The subchondral cyst appears to begin as a subchondral hematoma beneath the load-bearing surfaces of the joint. As it expands, it destroys local bone and cartilage to become an osteochondral cyst. Because the thickness of the articular cartilage is often maintained over these defects, radiographs do not reflect the extensive destruction seen at operation. The pathogenesis of these cysts can be correlated with the observed changes of condylar flattening and intercondylar notch widening in hemophilic arthropathy.

Patients with hemophilia commonly have fractures as a result of osteoporosis, joint stiffness, and muscle weakness. Most fractures can be treated nonoperatively. Circular casts should not be applied initially. Instead, the fracture should be splinted and the patient given replacement therapy until all bleeding is under control. A factor VIII level of 30% or more should be maintained for 2 to 7 days, depending on the severity of the fracture.

In patients with synovitis and recurrent hemarthroses but preservation of joint (cartilage) space, synovectomy may decrease pain and prevent recurrent bleeding. Release of contractures may result in substantial functional improvement in patients with joint contractures resulting from bleeding into muscle or from compartment syndromes.

Results can be satisfactory without major complications if, during operation and in the immediate postoperative period, factor VIII levels can be maintained between 60% and 120%. The duration of replacement therapy depends on individual wound healing and the postoperative treatment. Radioactive synovectomy with gold (^{198}Au) or rhenium (^{186}Re) is successful in 88% of patients; there is no subsequent increased bleeding into the joint. It has the advantage of little coverage with antihemophilia factor and can be done on an outpatient basis.

Continuous passive motion can aid postoperative rehabilitation in difficult pediatric knee and elbow problems. It reduces hospitalization time, the patients gain greater range of motion, and postoperative manipulation is virtually eliminated.

Other indications for surgical treatment include osteotomy for bony deformity, removal of pseudotumor, total joint arthroplasty in severe arthropathy, and occasionally amputation of a useless or chronically infected extremity. Current medical management programs for established joint disease in hemophiliacs are unsatisfactory. D-Penicillamine may be beneficial in chronic synovitis/arthritis, and ibuprofen significantly decreases pain in hemophiliacs without alterations in platelet function, bleeding times, or coagulation with no increase in bleeding and no change in the amount of concentrate used.

Patients with severe hemophilic arthropathy may be treated successfully with total joint replacement. Caution must be exercised in patients with such arthropathy because they probably have some increased risk of infection due to the frequent necessity for intravenous replacement therapy throughout their expected long life spans.

The frequency of hemarthroses diminishes markedly and the requirement for factor concentrate decreases substantially after total knee replacement. This marked clinical improvement is evident in all patients, but long-term results are not known.

Septic arthritis also occurs in hemophilia, and awareness that infection may be present in an acutely swollen joint should promote aspiration and bacteriologic study. With the increased incidence of AIDS, joint infection may become more common.

Another serious complication in hemophilia is intracranial hemorrhage. The majority of these patients have severe hemophilia, and the hemorrhage may occur spontaneously. The risk of intracranial hemorrhage after head trauma is 13%. After aggressive use of factor replacement within 6 hours after injury, there were no instances of intracranial hemorrhage in one study.

Patients with lesser forms of hemophilia or other coagulation defects may present with musculoskeletal disorders that require surgical treatment. If the coagulation deficiency is unrecognized, catastrophic postoperative bleeding may result. The most effective way to avoid this catastrophe is to obtain an adequate history. Many drugs (such as aspirin and other anti-inflammatory agents) may increase the bleeding tendency by decreasing coagulation efficiency. All patients scheduled to undergo operation should be asked about previous bleeding tendency, particularly in connection with dental extraction or tonsillectomy. If there is any question of coagulation defect based on history, the most appropriate evaluation is assay for specific coagulation factors. If coagulation defects are found, the patient should receive adequate replacement therapy with cryoprecipitate or factor concentrate before and after operation.

Platelet Deficiencies Patients who present with congenital musculoskeletal defects such as radial clubhand commonly have an associated platelet deficiency. A significant advance in their treatment is the transfusion of platelets from tissue-matched donors. If pooled platelets from random donors are used, patients become refractory to treatment after several weeks and may exhibit clinical signs of rejection, including bleeding, fever, chills, and headache. Tissue-matched donor platelets are more effective, and fewer donor packs are required than when random donor platelets are used.

With radial aplasia and thrombocytopenia there may be intra-articular dysplasia of the knee, resulting in genu varum, flexion deformity, and torsional deformity that become evident in the first 2 years of life. Corrective osteotomies are not helpful; the rate of recurrence of deformity is high. Upon completion of growth, the deformity stabilizes. Diagnosis of the syndrome of thrombocytopenia and absent radius is now possible in the prenatal state by ultrasonography. Hypogammaglobulinemia is often associated with this syndrome and may explain the observation of a high incidence of associated infections.

Thrombocytopenia is frequently encountered in patients with lymphoproliferative disorders, systemic lupus erythematosus, and, to a lesser extent, rheumatoid arthritis, pernicious anemia, and autoimmune hemolytic anemia. In a significant proportion of these patients, antibody-mediated immune destruction of platelets can be confirmed by positive platelet antibody tests. Thrombocytopenia is also associated with the use of D-penicillamine, gold, and heparin; it has been reported with hemangioma (Kasabach-Merritt syndrome) and inclusion body myositis.

Thromboembolism

Venous thromboembolic disease is the most prevalent type of complication after operation on or trauma to the lower extremities in adults, and pulmonary embolism is the most common fatal complication. Thrombophlebitis occurs in 40% to 60% of patients over age 40 years not protected by anticoagulants. The incidence is similar after fractures of the femur or tibia. Fewer thrombi occur in the calves of patients who have had tourniquets placed, probably because there is increased systemic fibrinolytic activity after release of the tourniquet. The incidence of thromboembolic disease is much less after spine fusion than after lower extremity surgery. It is more likely in extensive operations that involve longer fusions and increased blood loss. This complication tends to be encountered in the proximal venous system, usually in the left iliac vein which is more vulnerable to stasis when a patient is prone.

Risk factors associated with an increased incidence of venous thrombosis include age, obesity, trauma, myocardial infarction, heart failure, malignant disease, and use of oral contraceptives. Congenital deficiency of antithrombin III and the presence of a lupus anticoagulant are also associated with an increased incidence of venous thrombosis.

Diagnosis Sole reliance on clinical findings such as complaints of pain, swelling, tenderness, Homan's sign, fever, and leukocytosis leads to marked underdiagnosis of thromboembolic disease. Only 5% to 30% of instances of thrombophlebitis will be detected by physical examination alone. Objective testing is mandatory for accurate diagnosis. Measurements of venous hemodynamics by plethysmography and Doppler ultrasonography can detect obstructions to venous blood flow produced by proximal thrombi. These methods are most accurate for thrombi in major veins (thigh) and are less accurate for thrombi in small veins (calf) because of the insignificant difference in outflow. These tests are not as exact as either venography or radioactive fibrinogen scanning. Thermographic techniques have been tested on a small scale and may have future application but currently are limited to experimental use.

Isotope venography and preoperative antithrombin III activity and lipoprotein concentration may be useful in detecting venous thrombosis. Another method under investigation is an assay that measures coagulation and fibrinolysis processes by the products present in the serum. These methods show some promise but will require considerable improvement in technique and documentation before consideration for routine clinical use.

Radioactive fibrinogen (labeled with ^{125}I) is 90% accurate in detecting thrombophlebitis in the calf after total hip replacement. However, because of the presence of fibrin, it is positive in any area scanned close to the site of operation or trauma. Therefore, it is not useful for detecting thrombophlebitis in the thigh after hip surgery or in the calf after knee surgery. It has the advantages of ease of repeatability and causes little patient discomfort.

The diagnostic standard is still radiocontrast venography. It is the most exact evaluation technique, with high accuracy in diagnosis of clots in the femoral and calf veins and approximately 70% reliability for clots in the iliac veins. It has the disadvantages of causing some pain, is difficult to repeat frequently, and may induce thrombophlebitis in 5% of patients and allergic reaction in 0.02%.

Continuous epidural anesthesia has been found to be associated with a significantly lower incidence of thrombophlebitis and pulmonary embolism compared to general anesthesia. Also, patients undergoing total hip replacement under general anesthesia who developed thrombosis had received significantly more blood replacement than did those patients who did not develop thrombosis. No significant difference has been observed between normotensive and hypotensive anesthesia in regard to the incidence of thrombophlebitis.

Arterial embolism to the extremities is a rare but serious

complication. Large emboli occluding the proximal arteries of the lower limb are treated by embolectomy; death or permanent disability occurs in 63% of these patients. Smaller emboli occluding the arterial supply of the upper limb or distal lower limb usually are not fatal but disability is increased if embolectomy is not performed. Use of heparin treatment after catheter embolectomy has decreased mortality, the number of amputations, and the incidence of recurrent emboli.

Prophylaxis Methods recommended for prevention of thromboembolic disease include physical or mechanical measures, use of anticoagulants such as heparin and warfarin, and therapy with antithrombotic drugs.

The ideal treatment would be a highly effective method associated with few or no potential complications. The anticoagulant drugs now available are effective for prophylaxis but their use carries a risk of bleeding complications. Oral warfarin therapy is the approach best documented but is associated with a 10% to 20% incidence of hemorrhagic complications. It has been reported recently that these complications can be significantly decreased by using it only in patients with a partial thromboplastin time of 50 sec or less while on therapy. Dextran in molecular weights of 40,000 to 70,000 is as effective as warfarin in preventing thrombophlebitis after hip surgery. The risk of hemorrhagic complications is similar and it may cause allergic reactions.

Heparin in low doses is effective in thoracic, abdominal, and pelvic surgical procedures but its effectiveness after lower extremity surgery and trauma is controversial. The mechanism of action of low-dose heparin therapy probably is an increased rate at which antithrombin III inhibits activated factor X and thrombin. In a major surgical procedure (such as total hip arthroplasty) or after major trauma, the coagulation system activation may be so intense that thrombin generation exceeds the rate at which it is inhibited, even in the presence of small amounts of heparin. Thrombin generation also releases platelet factor 4 which has antiheparin activity. In a group of patients undergoing total hip replacement who were given 3,500 IU of heparin every 8 hours, the incidence of deep-vein thrombosis diagnosed by venography was 39%. In a similar group who received heparin at doses adjusted to maintain the activated partial thromboplastin time between 31.5 and 35 seconds, the incidence of deep-vein thrombosis was 13%. The frequencies of blood transfusions, decrease in hemoglobin level, and wound hematoma were identical in both groups.

Doses of heparin somewhat higher than those recommended after abdominal procedures have been used for the prevention of thromboembolic disease in the lower extremity. A small device known as a coagulometer was used to assess the state of the coagulation system in one group of patients and, thus, the heparin dose. With this technique, heparin in relatively low dosage was effective in preventing thromboembolic disease after surgery for hip fractures. An additional finding was that most patients were in a state of significant hypercoagulability at 5 to 7 days postoperatively; therefore, heparin therapy was continued well beyond this time. Many low-dose heparin regimens are discontinued at 5 to 7 days or at the time of patient mobilization. Although the incidence of bleeding complications after general surgical procedures with low-dose heparin therapy postoperatively has been minimal or nonexistent, after lower extremity orthopaedic surgical procedures most patients have an increased likelihood of bleeding complications.

A potentially serious complication with use of heparin for antithromboembolism prophylaxis is the paradoxic effect of arterial embolism. Clinically apparent arterial embolisms may occur 7 to 15 days after the start of heparin administration. Heparin induces a thrombocytopenia (platelet count less than 100,000/μl and perhaps as low as 30,000/μl). Most patients who have clinically apparent embolism have premonitory symptoms involving the gastrointestinal tract and musculoskeletal system in the prior 1 to 2 days. The most common embolization site is the aortic bifurcation, but occurrences are possible in other major arteries including the iliac and femoral. The emboli consist of platelet-rich fibrin with a few erythrocytes and may be caused by aggregation of platelets due to prolonged administration of heparin. It has also been suggested that an anti-heparin antibody may become active, leading to platelet aggregation. The mortality rate after major embolism occurring during heparin therapy is 60%. The recommended treatment is immediate surgical removal of the embolus and discontinuation of heparin therapy.

Agents that inhibit the aggregation of platelets include aspirin, sulfinpyrazone, dipyridamole, and hydroxychloroquine. The antithrombotic action of aspirin is related to its inhibition of the prostaglandins, thromboxane (a potent stimulus to platelet aggregation), and prostacyclin (a vasodilator and inhibitor of platelet aggregation synthesized by human endothelial cells). Aspirin blocks the activity of prostaglandin cyclo-oxygenase by irreversible acetylation, thus preventing the formation of active prostaglandins. Thus, aspirin has both a thrombotic and an antithrombotic effect. In low dosage (no more than 600 mg b.i.d.) prostaglandin production in platelets may be affected more than that in endothelial cells, resulting in a net antithrombotic effect. An excessive dose of aspirin (10 times that required for an antithrombotic effect) may reduce effectiveness or even increase thrombosis. In general, low-dose aspirin therapy is useful in decreasing the incidence of both thrombophlebitis and pulmonary embolism. At least one study found a significant difference in effectiveness between males and females: aspirin was prophylactically useful only in males. However, this is controversial because another study did show effectiveness in females, although not as great as that in males. There has been no evidence of increased bleeding complications with aspirin therapy. Except for fractures about the hip, the effectiveness of aspirin has not been evaluated in lower extremity trauma.

Dipyridamole has as its primary effect the blocking of platelet phosphodiesterase and increasing cyclic AMP. Numerous investigations of various combinations of anticoagulant and antithrombotic medications have yielded no evidence that a drug combination is more effective than the use of one agent; and in many instances the use of combination therapy has resulted in increased complications, particularly bleeding.

Physical and mechanical means of preventing thromboembolic disease include early mobilization of patients after operation or trauma, the use of antithromboembolism stockings, and the early initiation of muscle exercises with lower extremity motion. More sophisticated mechanical means include passive motion applied during the operation and use of mechanical compression devices during and after operation to improve venous outflow from the lower extremities. Venography has shown that leg compression decreases the incidence of calf vein thrombosis from 45% to 15% but does not decrease the incidence of thrombosis in the thigh.

Treatment Administration of heparin by continuous intravenous infusion to maintain the activated partial thromboplastin time at 1.5 to 2.5 times normal is continued for approximately 1 week. Oral warfarin therapy is begun, usually at about 3 days after initiation of heparin therapy. This overlap allows the prothrombin time to reach the effective range (1.5 to 2 times normal). Oral anticoagulant therapy is continued for about 4 to 6 months to avoid recurrent episodes of deep-vein thrombosis.

Pulmonary Embolism This occurs in 5% to 19% of patients with deep-vein thrombosis after lower extremity trauma who are unprotected by anticoagulants. Such emboli are fatal in 1% to 2% of patients after total hip replacement and in 5% to 10% of patients after hip fracture. Prophylaxis decreases the incidence and mortality of pulmonary embolism.

Diagnosis is based on findings of dyspnea, chest pain, tachypnea, decreased arterial oxygen tension, and changes in the electrocardiogram (S_1Q_3 pattern of cor pulmonale, axis shift, bundle-branch blocks, and nonspecific ST- and T-wave changes). Each of these changes is nonspecific, but a new appearance in the appropriate clinical setting is highly suggestive of pulmonary embolism. Radionuclide ventilation-perfusion scanning is the most commonly used test for the objective diagnosis of pulmonary embolism. Scans are considered as having low, intermediate, or high probability of pulmonary embolism on the basis of the degree of conformity to a vascular pattern and the degree of ventilation-perfusion mismatch. Ninety percent of patients with high-probability lesions will have pulmonary embolism on angiography; only 5% with low-probability lesions will have pulmonary embolism on angiography. Pulmonary angiography remains the final diagnostic test if questions remain.

Heparinization is the treatment of choice for pulmonary embolism, followed by oral warfarin therapy for 4 to 6 months. For life-threatening massive emboli, open thoracotomy and embolectomy may be necessary. In cases of repeated pulmonary embolism, partial obstruction of the inferior vena cava with an umbrella may be necessary to avoid a fatal embolus.

Gastrointestinal System

Trauma

Patients who sustain severe trauma or undergo major surgery are susceptible to significant gastrointestinal complications, and hemorrhage is the most common serious problem. Patients with gastric hemorrhage postoperatively should be evaluated by endoscopy or angiography or both. Bleeding is usually from a vessel supplied by the left gastric artery and can be controlled in most patients by infusion of vasopressin into this artery. Another effective nonoperative method for control is administration of antacid by a nasogastric tube on an hourly basis to maintain the stomach pH at 7.0. Administration of cimetidine may also be helpful. If antacid is given for prophylaxis in high-risk patients, development of bleeding ulcers is decreased substantially by maintaining the stomach pH at 3.5 or greater. For gastrointestinal hemorrhage in patients who have already had major surgery or suffered severe trauma, operation has a high mortality rate and should be used only as a last resort.

Diagnosing an acute abdominal emergency during spinal shock can be extremely difficult. Loss of sensory, motor, and reflex functions masks the typical signs, and the abdominal examination is unrevealing. During the first month after spinal cord surgery, intra-abdominal lesions were seen in 5% of those who had spinal shock, and patients whose lesions were above the T-5 level were at the greatest risk. Common problems were peptic ulcer disease, pancreatitis, and upper gastrointestinal hemorrhage. Administration of dexamethasone was associated with pancreatitis but gastric ulcers were uncommon. Respiratory distress was associated with peptic ulcer disease. These problems occurred as early as 3 days after injury.

Experimental studies have revealed a marked decrease in rate of emptying of the stomach after trauma; this is related more to the time of the development of severe pain, edema, and shock than to the time of injury. Pentobarbital sedation significantly slows the emptying of stomach contents, both before and after trauma.

Nutrition in Orthopaedics

Patients who have sustained orthopaedic trauma or who have undergone a major orthopaedic operation have increased metabolic requirements. This often is overlooked because the subtler forms of nutritional depletion are not recognized and because of the unavailability of clinical techniques for assessing nutritional status. Healthy patients with a major fracture have a 20% to 25% increase in their energy requirements. This can increase up to 55% in patients with multiple trauma or infection. Fat appears to be relatively unavailable as an energy source during severe stress, so protein is utilized with a consequent loss of visceral protein and skeletal muscle mass. Such protein depletion has been correlated with increased mortality rate, increased surgical failure rate, impaired wound healing, increased rate of wound infection, sepsis and other infections, progressive weakness, and delayed physical rehabilitation.

No single test can identify malnutrition, but the use of a battery of tests can permit early recognition of nutritional depletion (Table 3). Body fat is assessed by measuring the triceps skinfold. Skeletal muscle mass is evaluated by circumference of arm muscle and the creatinine/height index. Visceral protein depletion is estimated by determining the serum albumin and transferrin concentrations and also by loss of immunocompetence as manifested by a decreased reactivity to recall skin antigen testing and total lymphocyte count. Such patients are anergic and are at increased risk for sepsis and death.

In patients undergoing elective orthopaedic surgical procedures or who sustained multiple trauma, significant nutritional depletion of at least a moderate or severe degree has been identified by at least one of the studies listed in Table 3 (Fig. 4). The incidence of nutritional depletion ranged from 29% for arm muscle circumference to 56% for skin antigen testing; the mean was 42%. Patients with multiple trauma and femoral fractures had the highest incidence of nutritional depletion, 59%; the group undergoing elective surgery averaged 35%. Thus, trauma and major surgery may induce a state of malnutrition, and compli-

Table 3. Criteria for Measuring Nutritional Depletion

Index	Moderate depletion	Severe depletion
Triceps skinfold*	65–85	<65
Arm-muscle circumference*	<100	<85
Creatinine:height index*	65–85	<65
Transferrin concentration, mg/dl	150–199	<150
Albumin concentration, g/dl	3.0–3.4	<3.0
Total lymphocyte count, no./mm³	1,000–1,500	<1,000
Skin antigen testing, mm of induration	1–9	None

*Percentage of standard value. From Jensen, J.E.; Jensen, T.G.; Smith, T.K.; Johnston, D.A.; and Dudrick, S.J. J. Bone Joint Surg. 64A:1263–1272, 1982. By permission of the journal.

cations are more frequent in patients who are nutritionally depleted (Table 4). The best single predictor of complications is the arm muscle circumference. Abnormalities in serum albumin and transferrin levels and evidence of anergy indicate an increased risk of complications.

Body weight provides only a gross indication of a patient's overall nutritional status, is often impossible to obtain accurately in orthopaedic patients because of immobility and traction, and can be altered by expansion of extracellular fluid volume in the malnourished state. The routine use of a patient's weight/height relationship should be replaced by the accepted but seldom used measures of protein nutritional status mentioned above.

Genitourinary System

Trauma

Renal failure commonly occurs in crush injuries with traumatic rhabdomyolysis. In patients with extensive crush injuries, immediate induction of an alkaline solute diuresis has prevented azotemia or renal failure in most cases. Renal failure in such cases is associated with a high mortality rate.

Rhabdomyolysis and associated myoglobinuric acute renal failure have been reported after oral administration of phenmetrazine hydrochloride or amoxapine, methadone intoxication in legionnaires' disease, muscle weakness in alcoholics with type II fiber atrophy and decreased muscle phosphorylase levels, intravenous vasopressin infusion, toxic shock syndrome, and prolonged seizure activity. Abnormal sonograms and "hot kidneys" during bone scintigraphy have been helpful in diagnosis.

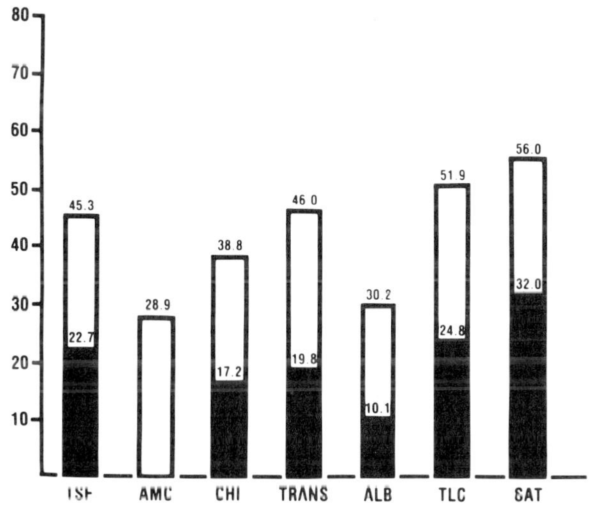

Figure 4

Total incidence of nutritional depletion (*open bars,* moderate; *solid bars,* severe) ranged from 28.9% of the population for arm muscle circumference to 56% for skin antigen testing. TSF, triceps skinfold; AMC, arm muscle circumference; CHI, creatinine/height index; TRANS, serum transferrin concentration; ALB, serum albumin concentration; TLC, total lymphocyte count; and SAT, skin antigen testing. (From Jensen, J.E.; Jensen, T.G.; Smith, T.K.; Johnston, D.A.; and Dudrick, S.J. J. Bone Joint Surg. 64A:1263–1272, 1982. By permission of the journal.)

Drug Toxicity

Acute renal failure has been associated with the use of various drugs including some of the antirheumatics, gold, zomepirac, and high doses of dicloxacillin (in prophylaxis for joint replacement surgery). Ibuprofen can significantly decrease glomerular filtration rate, renal plasma flow, and sodium clearance. These changes are fully reversible within 1 week after withdrawal of the drug. Renal failure has also been associated with polymyositis and Wilson's disease.

Advances in management of acute renal failure include the use of daily dialysis, lower heparin doses, single-needle dialysis, bicarbonate-based dialysis fluid, artificial kidneys with biocompatible membranes, H2 antagonists, and soft Silastic Tenckhoff catheters (if peritoneal dialysis is used).

Infection

Urinary tract infections are the most common nosocomial infections, affecting 5.4% to 8.6% of all hospitalized patients. Use of antibiotics and catheterization are important associated factors. In a large group of men requiring catheterization after total hip arthroplasty, the deep infection rate of the arthroplasty was 6.2%. If a man requires catheterization after total hip arthroplasty, there is a 10% chance that he will require prostatectomy which, in one series, had a mortality rate of 8.6%. Men who complain of urinary tract symptoms should have urologic evaluation and treatment prior to total joint replacement.

In approximately one-third of the patients who have an indwelling urethral catheter, high-level bacteriuria or candiduria (>10^5 colony-forming units/ml) develops. Also important is that in 37% of the patients who have low-level bacteriuria or candiduria (<10^5 organisms/ml) the bacterial counts progressed to more than 10^5/ml in 96% of the cases. The urinary tract of catheterized patients therefore is highly susceptible to infection once small numbers of microorganisms gain access, and even counts below 10^5/ml may be clinically important.

Table 4. Effect of Nutritional Depletion on Incidence of Postoperative Complications

Complications	Total N	Total D	Elective surgery N	Elective surgery D	Total hip replacement N	Total hip replacement D	Trauma N	Trauma D	Femoral fractures N	Femoral fractures D
Mechanical	0	2	0	2	0	1	0	0	0	0
Pulmonary	5	30	3	8	1	3	2	22	2	10
Wound	4	27	2	10	1	1	0	17	0	4
Sepsis	2	20	0	0	0	0	2	20	2	9
Urinary	0	7	0	4	0	1	0	3	0	1
Cardiovascular	0	3	0	2	0	2	0	1	0	0
Death	0	3	0	0	0	0	0	3	0	1
Miscellaneous	0	7	0	4	0	2	0	3	0	0
Total	11	99	5	30	2	10	4	69	4	25

Complications, no.*

*N, normal nutritional status; D, nutritional depletion.
From Jensen, J.E.; Jensen, T.G.; Smith, T.K.; Johnston, D.A.; and Dudrick, S.J. J. Bone Joint Surg. 64A:1263-1272, 1982. By permission of the journal.

When a patient presents with urinary tract infections, elective surgery should be delayed until the infection is cleared, particularly those procedures involving implantation of orthopaedic devices. Traditional treatment for urinary tract infections is the administration of antibiotics, based on appropriate sensitivity studies, for 10 to 14 days. Recent evidence suggests that, in women with no evidence of urinary tract abnormalities, urinary tract infections can be cleared with a 3-day treatment as effectively as with the 10-day course. Preliminary investigation also suggests that even shorter courses of antibiotic therapy may be equally as effective.

Among men on geriatric wards the prevalence of bacteriuria is 33% and the incidence of infections is 45% per year. With single-dose therapy, 15 patients were cured, 11 were not, and the majority (40 patients) relapsed. When treated to eradication of the bacteriuria and later reevaluated, all but one patient had relapsed, suggesting that if joint replacement would be required in this group of patients the urinary tract infection could be cured with proper therapy in preparation for the surgical event, but the patients remain at risk for future bacteriuria and possible joint sepsis. Urinary tract infections also have been found in women with the spastic striated external sphincter syndrome and in men with rheumatoid factor-negative arthritis, especially ankylosing spondylitis or Reiter's syndrome (57% of these men had a urologic infection). In Reiter's syndrome the common infections are balantitis and urethritis; in ankylosing spondylitis, prostatitis is most common.

Integument

Wounds

Open fractures have been classified as type I, II, or III depending on the severity of the soft tissue injury. Infection rates markedly increase with type III wounds, varying from 10% to 50%. Other complications with type III injuries include delayed union, nonunion, and amputation. Factors that predispose to these complications include 1) massive soft tissue damage and loss, 2) severe wound contamination, 3) impaired vascularity, and 4) fracture instability. To improve the classification and to predict prognosis more accurately, type III wounds are divided into three subtypes in order of worsening prognosis:

1. Type IIIA: Adequate soft tissue coverage of a fractured bone despite extensive soft tissue laceration or flaps, or high-energy trauma irrespective of the size of the wound.
2. Type IIIB: Extensive soft tissue loss with periosteal stripping and bone exposure; this is usually associated with massive contamination.
3. Type IIIC: Open fracture associated with arterial injury requiring repair.

Amputation rates are approximately 10% in type IIIA, 16% in type IIIB, and 42% in type IIIC; infection rates are approximately 4%, 52%, and 42%, respectively.

Soft tissue coverage for exposed bone is an old concept but is still controversial in regard to type of coverage and timing of coverage. Aggressive wound management with early fracture coverage by a muscle flap, myocutaneous, or free flap technique significantly shortens healing time and decreases the incidences of nonunion and infection and the costs of hospitalization and rehabilitation.

Skin Ulcers

In the elderly, and more commonly in women over age 70, pressure sores develop during hospitalization for hip fracture. Most patients have more than one sore; common sites are the sacrum, heels, and buttocks. The mortality rate among patients with pressure sores is reported to be as high as 27%, and their mean length of hospitalization far exceeds that of other patients. Prevention of pressure sores demands the help of the whole orthopaedic team, not just the nursing staff. Use of the Clinitron bed has been helpful in prevention and treatment.

Annotated Bibliography

Circulatory System

Bass, R.R.; Allison, E.J., Jr.; Reines, H.D.; Yeager, J.C.; and Pryor, W.H., Jr.: Thigh compartment syndrome without lower extremity trauma following application of pneumatic antishock trousers. Ann. Emerg. Med. 12:382–384, 1983.

Patients with prolonged application (>120 minutes) of pneumatic anti-shock trousers should be closely monitored for the development of compartment syndromes.

Bradford, D.S.; Szalapski, E.W., Jr.; Sutherland, D.E.R.; Simmons, R.L.; and Najarian, J.S.: Osteonecrosis in the transplant recipient. Surg. Gynecol. Obstet. 159:328–334, 1984.

The incidence of severe osteonecrosis was highest among recipients of cadaver kidneys. All experienced dramatic relief of their pain and improved function with total hip replacement. Dislocation was the most common complication.

Britt, B.A.; Scott, E.; Frodis, W.; Clements, M.-J.; and Endrenyi, L.: Dantrolene: *In vitro* studies in malignant hyperthermia susceptible (MHS) and normal skeletal muscle. Can. Anaesth. Soc. J. 31:130–154, 1984.

Dantrolene acts on the sarcoplasmic reticulum to prevent the release of calcium. Therefore, it is effective only when given prior to total loss of calcium from the sarcoplasmic reticulum.

Elmstedt, E., and Svahn, T.: Skeletal complications following renal transplantation. Acta Orthop. Scand. 52:279–286, 1981.

Overall incidence of osteonecrosis in renal transplantation patients is 11%. Fractures are also common (26%). All fractures healed without complication.

Ficat, P., and Grijalvo, P.: Résultats à long terme du forage-biopsie pour les ostéonécroses de la tête fémorale aux stades I et II. A propos de 133 cas revus après un délai moyen de 9 ans 6 mois (abstract). Rev. Chir. Orthop. 70:253–255, 1984.

At a median follow-up of 9.5 years, clinical results were good or very good in 89% of cases treated by core decompression.

Ficat, R.P., and Arlet, J.: Ischemia and Necroses of Bone. Baltimore, Williams & Wilkins, 1980.

A thorough review of osteonecrosis with discussion of diagnosis and management.

Fletcher, J.E., and Rosenberg, H.: *In vitro* interaction between halothane and succinylcholine in human skeletal muscle. Implications for malignant hyperthermia and masseter muscle rigidity. Anesthesiology 63:190–194, 1985.

Succinylcholine induced significant contractures in all preparations first exposed to halothane. In contrast, halothane added in the presence of succinylcholine did not induce contractures to the same extent.

Glimcher, M.J., and Kenzora, J.E.: The biology of osteonecrosis of the human femoral head and its clinical implications: I. Tissue biology. II. The pathological changes in the femoral head as an organ and in the hip joint. III. Discussion of the etiology and genesis of the pathological sequelae; Comments on treatment. Clin. Orthop. 138:284–309; 139:283–312; 140:273–312, 1979.

Osteonecrosis probably has multiple causes. A new approach to treatment involves prevention of the repair process because it appears that the symptoms relate to the presence of this process.

Henao, F., and Aldrete, J.S.: Retroperitoneal hematomas of traumatic origin. Surg. Gynecol. Obstet. 161:106–116, 1985.

Traumatic retroperitoneal hematomas should not be opened unless it is necessary to exclude associated injuries. When they are opened, continued bleeding is associated with a high mortality rate.

Jardon, O.M.; Wingard, D.W.; Barak, A.J.; and Connolly, J.F.: Malignant hyperthermia. A potentially fatal syndrome in orthopaedic patients. J. Bone Joint Surg. 61A:1064–1070, 1979.

The most important factor in recognizing the potential of malignant hyperthermia is a positive family history of sudden death or a medical history of serious illness after stress of any type. Dantrolene sodium is effective in preventing development of this syndrome.

Jones, S.F., and White, A.: Analgesia following femoral neck surgery. Lateral cutaneous nerve block as an alternative to narcotics in the elderly. Anaesthesia 40:682–685, 1985.

Lateral cutaneous nerve blocks greatly increased the time to the first dose of opiate after fixation of femoral neck fractures.

Lawhon, S.M.; Kahn, A., III; Crawford, A.H.; and Brinker, M.S.: Controlled hypotensive anesthesia during spinal surgery: A retrospective study. Spine 9:450–453, 1984.

Intraoperative and postoperative blood loss were significantly reduced in children. In adults, only intraoperative blood loss was significantly reduced.

Modig, J.: Advantages of dextran 70 over Ringer acetate solution in shock treatment and in prevention of adult respiratory distress syndrome. A randomized study in man after traumatic-haemorrhagic shock. Resuscitation 10:219–226, 1983.

Dextran-70 seems to have an advantage over Ringer's lactate solution both in shortening the shock period and in reducing the frequency of adult respiratory distress syndrome.

Pathak, K.S.; Brown, R.H.; Nash, C.L., Jr.; and Cascorbi, H.F.: Continuous opioid infusion for scoliosis fusion surgery. Anesth. Analg. 62:841–845, 1983.

Continuous infusion of narcotic produced stable suppression of somatosensory cortical-evoked potentials, making it easier to interpret during surgery. Wake-up tests were smooth and repeatable.

Poplawski, Z.J.; Wiley, A.M.; and Murray, J.F.: Posttraumatic dystrophy of the extremities: A clinical review and trial of treatment. J. Bone Joint Surg. 65A:642–655, 1983.

Treatment consisted of one or more intravenous injections of lidocaine and corticosteroid followed by physical therapy. The most important factor predicting success was an interval of less than 6 months between onset of symptoms and treatment.

Rovner, R.A.; Baird, R.A.; and Malerich, M.M.: Fatal toxic shock syndrome as a complication of orthopaedic surgery: A case report. J. Bone Joint Surg. 66A:952–954, 1984.

The surgeon must be aware that a benign-appearing wound does not preclude the presence of nonsuppurative *Staphylococcus aureus* infection that is capable of producing the toxin responsible for toxic shock syndrome.

Stock, J.R.; Athanasoulis, C.A.; Harris, W.H.; Waltman,

A.C.; Novelline, R.A.; and Greenfield, A.J.: Transcatheter embolization for the control of wound hemorrhage following hip surgery. J. Bone Joint Surg. 62A:1000–1003, 1980.

Techniques similar to those used for bleeding after pelvic fractures are used for continued hemorrhage after hip surgery. Autologous clot or surgical gelatin is effective in stopping hemorrhage.

Stratta, R.J.; Saffle, J.R.; Kravitz, M.; Ninnemann, J.L.; and Warden, G.D.: Exchange transfusion therapy in pediatric burn shock. Circ. Shock 12:203–212, 1984.

Exchange transfusion therapy facilitates resuscitation from burn shock in children who do not respond to conventional volume therapy.

Sugioka, Y.; Katsuki, I.; and Hotokebuchi, T.: Transtrochanteric rotational osteotomy of the femoral head for the treatment of osteonecrosis: Follow-up statistics. Clin. Orthop. 169:115–126, 1982.

Excellent results were obtained in 98 (77%) of 128 hips followed 2 to 9 years postoperatively. Results are related to extent of head avascularity.

Respiratory System

Anderson, P.R.; Puno, M.R.; Lovell, S.L.; and Swayze, C.R.: Postoperative respiratory complications in non-idiopathic scoliosis. Acta Anaesthesiol. Scand. 29:186–192, 1985.

Postoperative pulmonary complications are higher with non-idiopathic curves than with idiopathic scoliosis.

Gossling, H.R., and Pellegrini, V.D., Jr.: Fat embolism syndrome: A review of the pathophysiology and physiological basis of treatment. Clin. Orthop. 165:68–82, 1982.

Fat embolism syndrome is an infrequent complication of fractures, in contrast to subclinical fat embolization which occurs after nearly all long bone fractures.

Hoeppner, V.H.; Cockcroft, D.W.; Dosman, J.A.; and Cotton, D.J.: Nighttime ventilation improves respiratory failure in secondary kyphoscoliosis. Am. Rev. Respir. Dis. 129:240–243, 1984.

Nighttime ventilation may be an effective alternative for long-term treatment of cardiorespiratory failure caused by secondary kyphoscoliosis.

Johnson, K.D.; Cadambi, A.; and Seibert, G.B.: Incidence of adult respiratory distress syndrome in patients with multiple musculoskeletal injuries: Effect of early operative stabilization of fractures. J. Trauma 25:375–383, 1985.

There is a significant increase in the incidence of adult respiratory distress syndrome associated with a delay in operative stabilization of major fractures in patients with multiple orthopaedic injuries.

Rinaldo, J.E., and Rogers, R.M.: Adult respiratory-distress syndrome: Changing concepts of lung injury and repair. N. Engl. J. Med. 306:900–909, 1982.

Specific therapy aimed at the pathophysiologic sequences that destroy pulmonary architecture in adult respiratory distress syndrome will be necessary to improve outcome dramatically.

Weigelt, J.A.; Norcross, J.F.; Borman, K.R.; and Snyder, W.H., III: Early steroid therapy for respiratory failure. Arch. Surg. 120:536–540, 1985.

Steroids failed to improve pulmonary function and were associated with an increased infection rate.

Hematopoietic System

Bleeding Disorders

Aronstam, A.; Browne, R.S.; Wassef, M.; and Hamad, Z.: The clinical features of early bleeding into the muscles of the lower limb in severe haemophiliacs. J. Bone Joint Surg. 65B:19–23, 1983.

Eighty percent of bleeding into muscle in hemophiliacs occurs in the quadriceps and calf muscles. Recovery after quadriceps bleeding took longer compared with calf bleeding.

Boardman, K.P., and English, P.: Fractures and dislocations in hemophilia. Clin. Orthop. 148:221–232, 1980.

Most fractures can be treated closed, but full cast should not be applied until the danger of continued hemorrhage is past. Open reduction and internal fixation can be performed with adequate replacement therapy.

Brettler, D.B.; Forsberg, A.D.; O'Connell, F.D.; Cederbaum, A.I.; Chaitman, A.K.; and Levine, P.H.: A long-term study of hemophilic arthropathy of the knee joint on a program of Factor VIII replacement given at time of each hemarthrosis. Am. J. Hematol. 18:13–18, 1985.

In severe hemophilia, demand therapy prevents progression of arthropathy in normal joints but, if affected at the initiation of the program, the knee joints may go on to progressive arthropathy and restriction of motion.

Fernandez-Palazzi, F.; de Bosch, N.B.; and de Vargas, A.F.: Radioactive synovectomy in haemophilic haemarthrosis. Follow-up of fifty cases. Scand. J. Haematol. [Suppl.] 40:291–300, 1984.

Synovectomy with gold or rhenium gives excellent control of recurrent hemarthroses. It is simple and inexpensive and can be an outpatient procedure.

Greene, W.B.: Use of continuous passive slow motion in the postoperative rehabilitation of difficult pediatric knee and elbow problems. J. Pediatr. Orthop. 3:419–423, 1983.

Continuous passive motion after surgery enhances the rehabilitation process, resulting in improved joint mobility and eliminating the need for postoperative manipulation.

Hegde, U.M.; Williams, K.; Devereux, S.; Bowes, A.; Powell, D.; and Fisher, D.: Platelet associated IgG and immune thrombocytopenia in lymphoproliferative and autoimmune disorders. Clin. Lab. Haematol. 5:9–15, 1983.

Patients with lymphoproliferative disorders, rheumatoid arthritis, and other problems have significant antibody-mediated destruction of platelets.

Small, M.; Steven, M.M.; Freeman, P.A.; Lowe, G.D.O.; Belch, J.J.F.; Forbes, C.D.; and Prentice, C.R.M.: Total knee arthroplasty in haemophilic arthritis. J. Bone Joint Surg. 65B:163–165, 1983.

Total knee replacement led to marked clinical improvement in all patients with hemophilia. Pain lessened, frequently hemarthroses diminished, and requirements for factor consequently decreased substantially.

Thromboembolism

Aaron, R.K., and Ciombor, D.: Venous thromboembolism in the orthopedic patient. Surg. Clin. North Am. 63:529–537, June 1983.

Thromboembolism, the most common complication in orthopaedic surgery, is difficult to diagnose clinically. Patients at risk should be treated prophylactically to avoid clots and possible fatal pulmonary emboli.

DeLee, J.C., and Rockwood, C.A., Jr.: The use of aspirin

in thromboembolic disease. J. Bone Joint Surg. 62A: 149–152, 1980.

Aspirin in low doses (600 to 1,200 mg/day) is effective in reducing thromboembolic disease in men over age 40 after total hip arthroplasty.

Dorr, L.D.; Sakimura, I.; and Mohler, J.G.: Pulmonary emboli followed total hip arthroplasty: Incidence study. J. Bone Joint Surg. 61A:1083–1087, 1979.

Pulmonary embolism, diagnosed by the development of new perfusion defects without associated ventilatory defects and confirmed by pulmonary angiography, occurs in 6% of patients undergoing minor orthopaedic surgery. Pa_{O_2} may not be a good indicator of pulmonary embolism after major hip surgery.

Harris, W.H.; McKusick, K.; Athanasoulis, C.A.; Waltman, A.C.; and Strauss, H.W.: Detection of pulmonary emboli after total hip replacement using serial $C^{15}O_2$ pulmonary scans. J. Bone Joint Surg. 66A:1388–1393, 1984.

O-labeled carbon dioxide ($C^{15}O_2$) may provide an excellent means of detection of silent emboli and an improved method of evaluating the efficacy of prophylactic agents.

Leyvraz, P.F.; Richard, J.; Bachmann, F.; Van Melle, G.; Treyvaud, J.-M.; Livio, J.-J.; and Candardjis, G.: Adjusted versus fixed-dose subcutaneous heparin in the prevention of deep-vein thrombosis after total hip replacement. N. Engl. J. Med. 309:954–958, 1983.

Adjusted low-dose heparin prophylaxis appears to be a safe and efficacious method to reduce the frequency of deep-vein thrombosis in patients undergoing total hip replacement.

Modig, J.; Borg, T.; Karlström, G.; Maripuu, E.; and Sahlstedt, B.: Thromboembolism after total hip replacement: Role of epidural and general anesthesia. Anesth. Analg. 62:174–180, 1983.

Deep-vein thrombophlebitis and pulmonary embolism occur less frequently in patients under continuous epidural anesthesia compared with general anesthesia for total hip replacement.

Stulberg, B.N.; Insall, J.N.; Williams, G.W.; and Ghelman, B.: Deep-vein thrombosis following total knee replacement: An analysis of six hundred and thirty eight arthroplasties. J. Bone Joint Surg. 66A:194–201, 1984.

Untreated patients had an 84% incidence of thrombophlebitis whereas treated patients had an incidence of 57% after total knee replacement. No one prophylactic regimen was more effective than another.

Gastrointestinal System

Berlly, M.H., and Wilmot, C.B.: Acute abdominal emergencies during the first four weeks after spinal cord injury. Arch. Phys. Med. Rehabil. 65:687–690, 1984.

Patients with spinal cord injuries, especially those with lesions above T-5, are at risk for upper gastrointestinal bleeding, peptic ulcer disease, and pancreatitis.

Hubbard, C.N., and Richardson, E.G.: Pseudo-obstruction of the colon: A postoperative complication in orthopaedic patients. J. Bone Joint Surg. 65A:226–229, 1983.

Cecal dilation can develop rapidly to dangerous proportions. Early recognition by physical examination and abdominal radiographs with early nasogastric suction, intravenous fluid therapy, and frequent turning of the patient are essential to avoid operative intervention or possible perforation and sepsis.

Jensen, J.E.; Jensen, T.G.; Smith, T.K.; Johnston, D.A.; and Dudrick, S.J.: Nutrition in orthopaedic surgery. J. Bone Joint Surg. 64A:1263–1272, 1982.

Over 42% of patients undergoing orthopaedic surgical procedures were found to be clinically or subclinically malnourished. Patients with multiple trauma had the highest incidence of nutritional depletion (59%), followed by patients undergoing elective surgical procedures (35%) and patients undergoing total hip replacement (29%).

Munns, S.W.; Morrissy, R.T.; Golladay, E.S.; and McKenzie, C.M.: Hyperalimentation for superior mesenteric-artery (cast) syndrome following correction of spinal deformity. J. Bone Joint Surg. 66A:1175–1177, 1984.

This paper describes the use of hyperalimentation.

Genitourinary System

Cierny, G., III; Byrd, H.S.; and Jones, R.E.: Primary *versus* delayed soft tissue coverage for severe open tibial fractures: A comparison of results. Clin. Orthop. 178:54–63, 1983.

Early wound healing by use of various tissue transfers significantly improves end results of open severe tibial fractures with respect to union, tissue loss from infection, healing time, and costs of hospitalization and rehabilitation.

Cinotti, G.A.: Clinical assessment of the renal toxicity of antirheumatic drugs. Arch. Toxicol. [Suppl.] 7:338–349, 1984.

Antirheumatic drugs may cause a significant although generally reversible reduction of glomerular filtration rate, renal plasma flow, sodium clearance, and hyperkalemia in a wide range of extrarenal and renal disease states. Chronic drug ingestion has been associated with analgesic nephropathy.

Fair, W.R.; Crane, D.B.; Peterson, L.J.; Dahmer, C.; Tague, B.; and Amos, W.: Three-day treatment of urinary tract infections. J. Urol. 123:717–721, 1980.

In women without genitourinary abnormalities, a 3-day course of antibiotics is as effective in the treatment of urinary tract infections as a 10-day course.

Gustilo, R.B.; Mendoza, R.M.; and Williams, D.N.: Problems in the management of Type III (severe) open fractures: A new classification of Type III open fractures. J. Trauma 24:742–746, 1984.

The current designation of type III open fractures is too inclusive. Three subtypes, in order of worsening prognosis, have been identified.

Gwathmey, F.W., and House, J.H.: Clinical manifestations of congenital insensitivity of the hand and classification of syndromes. J. Hand Surg. [Am.] 9:863–869, 1984.

Common findings include ulceration, infections, fractures, stiffness of fingers, self-mutilation, and traumatic amputation. Reconstructive surgery is not indicated and amputation may be necessary.

May, J.W., Jr.; Gallico, G.G., III; and Lukash, F.N.: Microvascular transfer of free tissue for closure of bone wounds of the distal lower extremity. N. Engl. J. Med. 306:253–257, 1982.

Free flap coverage is possible to close difficult wounds of the distal leg, enhancing bone healing and decreasing osteomyelitis.

McGuire, E.J.; Woodside, J.R.; and Borden, T.A.: Upper urinary tract deterioration in patients with myelodysplasia and detrusor hypertonia: A followup study. J. Urol. 129:823–826, 1983.

Upper tract deterioration after many years of normality demonstrates that these patients require prolonged and careful urologic and radiographic follow-up.

Nicolle, L.E.; Bjornson, J.; Harding, G.K.M.; and MacDonell, J.A.: Bacteriuria in elderly institutionalized men. N. Engl. J. Med. 309:1420–1425, 1983.

Asymptomatic bacteriuria is common in elderly institutionalized men. Forty-five percent have urinary tract infections that can be successfully treated, but almost all recur after cessation of treatment.

Stark, R.P., and Maki, D.G.: Bacteriuria in the catheterized patient: What quantitative level of bacteriuria is relevant? N. Engl. J. Med. 311:560–564, 1984.

The urinary tract of catheterized patients is highly susceptible to infection once small numbers of microorganisms gain access.

Versluysen, M.: Pressure sores in elderly patients: The epidemiology related to hip operations. J. Bone Joint Surg. 67B:10–13, 1985.

Pressure sores are common in elderly women with hip fractures. Mortality in these patients was 27%. Hospital stay was increased. Prevention requires everyone's help, requiring more skill and attention than the nurse alone can offer.

Weiland, A.J.; Moore, J.R.; and Hotchkiss, R.N.: Soft tissue procedures for reconstruction of tibial shaft fractures. Clin. Orthop. 178:42–53, 1983.

Various soft tissue procedures including free flaps provide a new and successful solution to different open fractures of the leg.

Wroblewski, B.M., and del Sel, H.J.: Urethral instrumentation and deep sepsis in total hip replacement. Clin. Orthop. 146:209–212, 1980.

The incidence of deep sepsis and mortality is significantly increased in patients who undergo total hip replacement and require catheterization or prostatectomy.

11

Prostheses: Implant Materials and Methods of Fixation

Introduction

In orthopaedic surgery, implant devices are classified as "functional" rather than "aesthetic" because they must provide active or passive function to sustain physiologic and biomechanical activities in the body. Therefore, implant materials must be strong and inert, and fixation of implant to bone and soft tissue must be durable under different internal and external loads. The three major categories of orthopaedic implants are 1) bone and joint replacement prostheses, 2) artificial tendons and ligaments, and 3) bone fracture fixation devices. Artificial tendons and ligaments generally require incorporation with host tissue to bear load for prolonged periods; their functional and material requirements are markedly different from those of bone and joint replacement prostheses. Fracture fixation devices are only intended to endure short periods of *in vivo* service, until bone fractures unite; thus, their performance criteria are less stringent. This review concentrates mainly on bone and joint replacement implants.

Three classes of material have been used in joint prosthetic designs: metallic alloys, bioceramics, and polymers. These materials can be fabricated in both solid and porous forms for specific applications. Although the biocompatibility of each material is established, their unique functional characteristics and specific roles in implant design differ. Some knowledge about these materials is essential for orthopaedic surgeons when selecting devices for clinical application.

The underlying skeletal and joint structures of the body bear functional loads of substantial magnitude. This predicates the need for strong, durable implant devices and methods of fixation to bone. Three basic forms of implant fixation have been used: 1) mechanical fixation through interference fit; 2) interlocking with grouting material (bone cement—i.e., poly[methyl methacrylate]); and 3) biologic fixation through tissue ingrowth.

Each fixation method has advantages and disadvantages, but none is free of short-term and long-term problems. Short-term problems include infection, dislocation, fracture (of the implant or bone), and loosening. The long-term problems involve wear of the articulating surface, material degradation, systemic reaction to implant material, and bone remodeling or resorption due to physiologic load alteration. Long-term problems could also include loosening and fracture of the implant, which are usually manifestations of biologic responses, and material fatigue and degradation, which will take longer to manifest their effects. However, the definitions of "short-term" and "long-term" are relatively vague because these problems also depend on other factors. On the basis of current clinical follow-up results and advances in implant material selection and prosthetic design, it is postulated that duration for 10 years will be selected as the separation point between short-term and long-term performance of orthopaedic prosthetic devices for bone and joint replacement.

It is important to establish such a benchmark for implant evaluation. However, this criterion should not be used as a standard at the present time in selecting an implant fixation method because a large number of patients have had successful clinical results well beyond 10 years after bone and joint replacement with any of the three types of implant fixation. It is more important to identify the proper indication and optimal implant material and design configuration for each fixation method. When this is accomplished, orthopaedic surgeons will have choices from which to select the device and the surgical procedure that are best for a patient. This is the ultimate goal of medical scientists and bioengineers engaged in research and development related to implant design and fixation.

Metallic Implants

Because development of an acceptable implant material is always a long and costly process, current metallic materials are still limited to surgical grade 316L stainless steel, Co-Cr-Mo alloys, and Ti-6Al-4V. Although other rare and inert metals such as tantalum and niobium have been tried, their inferior mechanical properties, which affect their ability to withstand severe *in vivo* loading, have limited their popularity. Co-Ni-Cr alloy (MP35N) has superior mechanical strength compared to Co-Cr-Mo but its high content of Ni presents potential problems in corrosion resistance and tissue compatibility. For the same reasons, stainless steel is not recommended for porous coating construction because a high Ni content increases the potential for corrosion when the surface area of the prosthesis is substantially increased.

To compare different metals in implant design, a few fundamental definitions regarding material mechanical properties must be reviewed. On a typical stress-strain curve in a uniaxial loading test of a material specimen, the slope of the elastic range (tan ξ) is defined as Young's modulus (Fig. 1). The strain at yielding stress (elastic limit) is defined as elastic strain. The maximum stress before fracture is called ultimate strength, and the corresponding strain is ductility. The total area beneath the stress-strain curve (strain energy) is called toughness of the material. If the material is loaded beyond its elastic limit, it will experience plastic deformation. These basic mechanical properties are important considerations in implant design because sufficient material strength as well as compliance (modulus) with bone must be sought; all related biologic and implant materials vary widely in these key properties (Figs. 2 and 3).

Although small, the incidence of metal implant fracture has stimulated the development and adoption of so-called

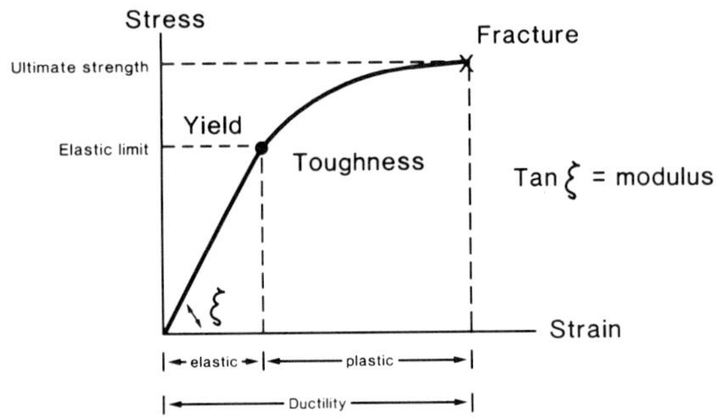

Figure 1

Definitions of important material properties in orthopaedic implants. Stress is defined as the force per unit area; and strain is the elongation per unit length (normal strain).

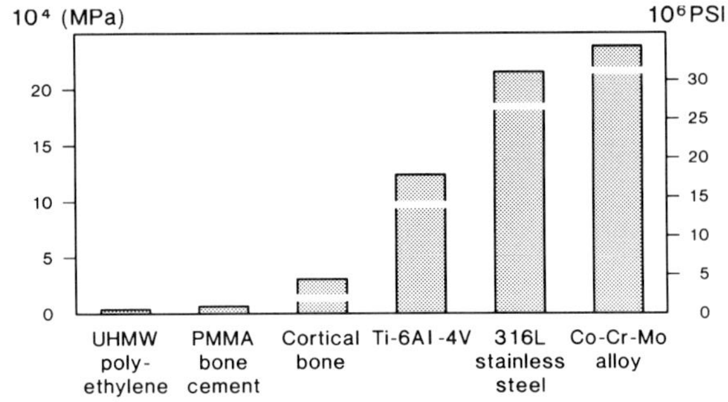

Figure 2

Elastic moduli (Young's modulus) of different implant materials and of cortical bone. The broken section of each data column represents the standard variation of the value reported. Data consolidated from the literature to show typical ranges of expected values. UHMW, ultrahigh molecular weight; PMMA, poly(methyl methacrylate).

supermetals. Basically, these metals are similar in metallic composition but a special forging process (compression under high pressure) and casting of fine metallic powders are used to increase their fatigue strength. These processes also tend to decrease the grain size and thus minimize material defects. Forged Co-Cr-Mo and Ti alloys as well as MP35N are now being introduced for implant design. Implants made of such supermetals are stronger but also cost more. The forging process cannot be easily adopted for prosthetic devices of complex geometry. At the present time, none of the porous-coated implants can be made by this process because of the effects of the sintering temperatures required in creating the porous coatings.

Although the common implant metals have lower strength, this factor can be compensated for through proper design because the geometry of an implant can significantly change the distribution of stress in a prosthetic system. The stresses in the bone, stem, and interface material (bone cement) of prostheses with the same geometry will be influenced primarily by the modulus of the prosthetic material (Fig. 4). On the other hand, implant performance can be augmented by changing the cross-sectional shape of prostheses made of the same materials. Therefore, use of supermetals for bone and joint prostheses may be indicated only in special situations. The performance of implants should be evaluated based on the stiffness property of the stem/cement/bone composite under axial loading (axial stiffness [*EA*]), bending (bending stiffness [*EI*]), and torsion (torsional stiffness [*GJ*]), in which *E* is the material's Young's modulus, *A* is the cross-sectional area of the implant, *I* is the area moment of inertia, *J* is the polar area moment, and *G* is the shear modulus.

Ceramic Implants

Ceramics represent a broad class of materials that contain metallic and nonmetallic elements bonded ionically in a highly oxidized state. In general, this class of materials has a high modulus and low ductility, is extremely inert, has high compressive strength but low tensile strength, and has inferior crack resistance characteristics. However, certain elements, such as zirconium, can produce ceramic material (ZrO_2) of high tensile strength and relatively low modulus that permit machining. There are two classes of ceramic material—biostable (inert) and bioactive (degradable). The biodegradable material is also called bioglass. The most common biostable ceramic is Al_2O_3 with high purity. It comes in two forms, single-crystal formations and multi-

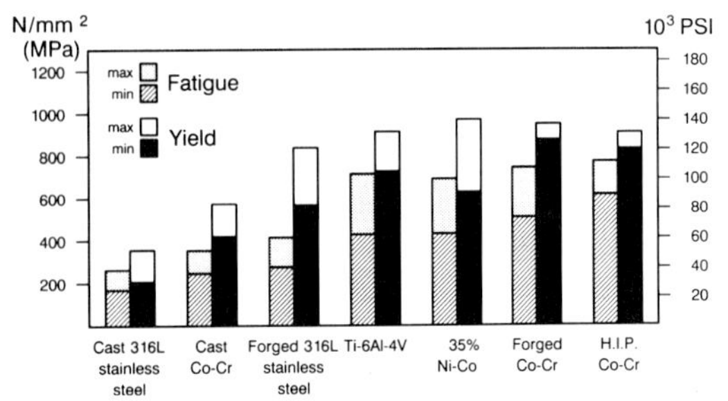

Figure 3

Yield and fatigue strengths of different metallic implant materials, including some of the supermetals. The fatigue strength is normally assumed to be 50% of the ultimate strength of the material. The stippled or open section on top of each data column represents the standard deviation of the values reported.

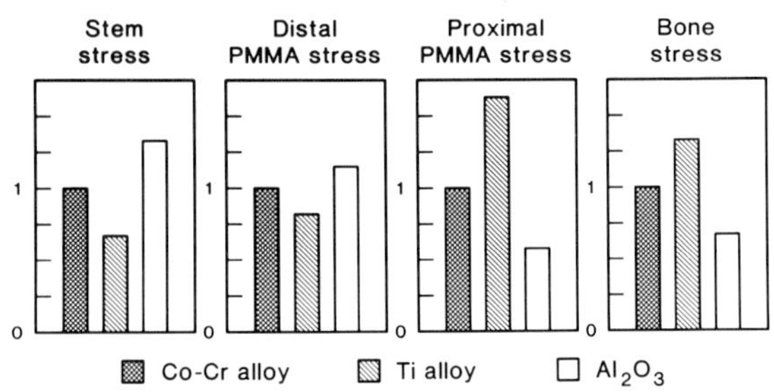

Figure 4

Effect of prosthetic stem material modulus on implant system stress distribution in cemented total hip replacement arthroplasty. The Co-Cr-Mo alloy was used as the reference for comparison. The modulus of Al_2O_3 is higher than that of Co-Cr alloy, and both are substantially higher than the modulus of Ti alloy (see Figure 5).

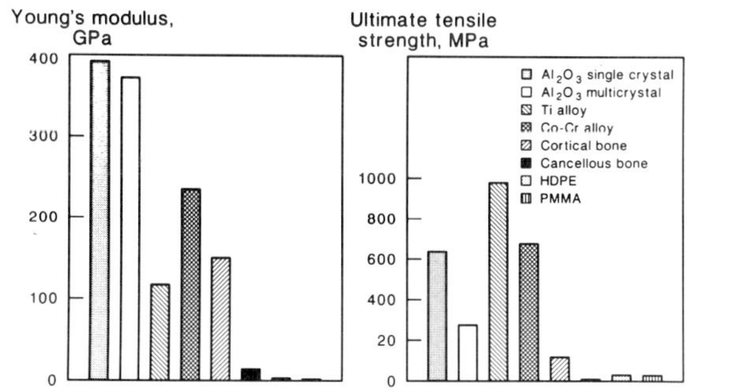

Figure 5

Key mechanical properties of different implant materials and bone. 1 MPa = 1 N/mm²; 1 GPa = 10^3 MPa.

crystal formations, with different mechanical properties (Fig. 5).

The most exciting property of ceramic material is its conduciveness to tissue bonding due to its high surface wettability characteristics as reflected by high surface tension (energy) (Fig. 6). With this property, there is also less friction and wear. The *in vitro* wear rate of ceramic on ceramic has been the lowest among all artificial articulating joint surface designs. Ceramic on polyethylene wear resistance was also found to be superior to that of metal on polyethylene. The small grain size in ceramic material allows an ultrasmooth surface finish. Corrosion resistance and high tissue compatibility are additional advantages of this material which make it a candidate for orthopaedic implant designs. The controllable degradation of bioglass allows the possibility of resorptive implant devices which can serve as structural scaffolds to allow tissue incorporation while maintaining initial strength during the early postoperative implantation period. The raw materials available for this class of ceramic implants are unlimited, but manufacturing costs are still high.

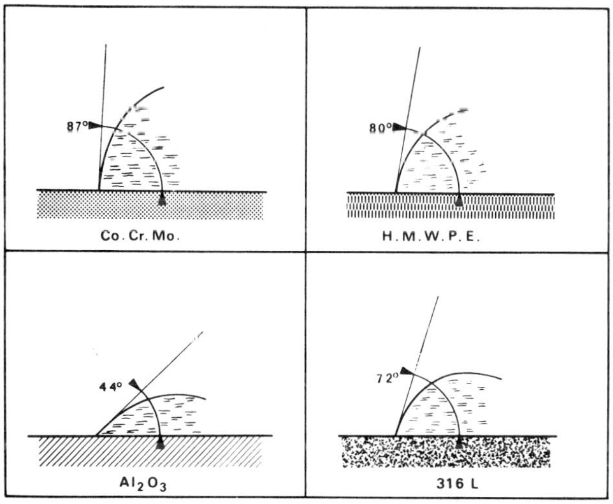

Figure 6

Surface wetting characteristics of four implant materials. Alumina or bioceramic (Al_2O_3) has the best wetting coefficient, reflected by the small fluid contact angle, which influences cell adhesion and lubrication properties.

Bioceramic material also has a number of weaknesses that make it less suitable for orthopaedic applications and may explain why it has not been popular in the United States. Its brittle nature and low resistance to crack propagation have prevented its use in high-tensile-stress environments. It has a high modulus compared to bone, which can create adverse effects such as bone fracture because of its high, noncompliant elastic modulus (Fig. 5). Ceramic material may also lose some of its initial mechanical strength as a result of *in vivo* degradation. Its ability to bond to metal is poor, and, at the present time, fabrication costs are relatively high.

These potential weaknesses could be circumvented by proper implant design using geometry to compensate for material properties. Thus, bioceramics are used for hip joint socket and femoral head in total hip prostheses. An alumina-to-alumina (Al_2O_3) articulation is avoided to minimize impact crack initiation problems. Instead, ceramic-to-HDP (ultrahigh-molecular-weight polyethylene) articulating surfaces are being used. Single-crystal Al_2O_3 is used for finger joint designs but remains linked only to HDP components. Finally, the high inertness and low frictional wear characteristics of ceramics could make them attractive for coating metallic implants. As a class of prosthetic implant material, ceramics should not be discounted in orthopaedic applications because they have certain potential advantages over metals.

Polymer Implants

The most popular polymer used for bone and joint implants is ultrahigh-molecular-weight polyethylene (HDP). Thus far, polyethylene has been the best mating material for articulating with either metal or ceramic. This material is classified as thermoplastic, and its mechanical properties will change with temperature. Although *in vivo* degradation and aging of HDP have not been firmly established, high-dose radiation can alter its physical behavior. Cold flow (plastic deformation) and surface wear have been factors of concern because HDP particles may stimulate biologic reaction at the prosthesis-bone or cement-bone interface. Due to the inherent weakness in most polymeric materials against tension and shear, HDP prosthetic components must be carefully designed to avoid such weaknesses.

Metal backing has been demonstrated to minimize plastic deformation of HDP, thus minimizing loosening problems. However, metal backing will decrease the effective thickness of HDP, thus making plastic deformation and wear more worrisome in long-term *in vivo* applications. Carbon fiber reinforcement has been utilized to improve the mechanical properties of this material. Although creep (increasing deformation with time under constant load) and tensile strength could be improved with such reinforcement, resistance to surface wear and fracture crack propagation may be decreased (Fig. 7). Loose carbon fibers were found in surrounding tissues. Consequently, the advantages of carbon fiber reinforcement of HDP may not be as beneficial as originally anticipated.

Other types of polymer and copolymer, such as Teflon (polytetrafluoroethylene [PTFE]), polyester (polyethylene tetraphthalate), and polyacetal (Delrin), have been tried and abandoned because of their high wear rates and the

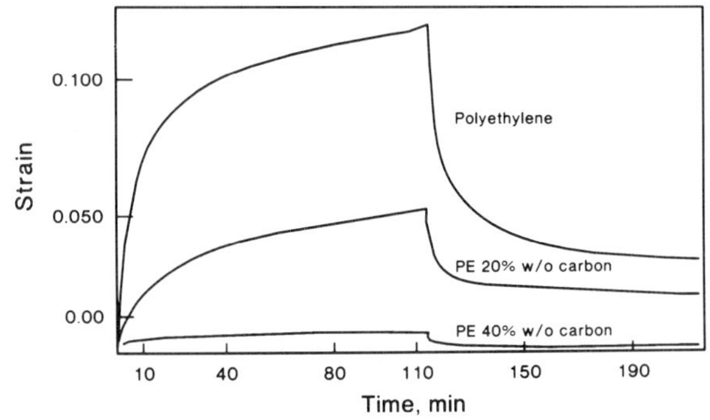

Figure 7

Effect of carbon fiber reinforcement on creep property of HDP. Creep is defined as change in strain with time under constant stress. (From Sclippa, E., and Piekarski, K.: Carbon fiber reinforced polyethylene for possible orthopedic uses. J. Biomed. Mater. Res. 7:59–70, 1973. By permission of John Wiley & Sons.)

adverse biologic reactions to wear particles. Therefore, HDP still remains a polymer of choice in joint prosthesis design, but it may require further improvement.

Silicone rubber is another class of plastics that has been widely used for interpositional spacers in joints. This class of material is intrinsically weak and can evoke a high incidence of mechanical failure. Nylon fiber reinforcement has been tried but produced little improvement. In addition, foreign body giant cell synovitis and focal bony destruction were found to be associated with silicone fragments from the prosthetic implant. Under repeated compressive and shearing loads, this type of polymer may not withstand severe mechanical insult when used as a prosthetic material for joint implant design.

Implant Fixation

Interference Fit

Mechanical fixation of prosthetic components through interference or press fit does not provide intimate interface locking or permanent bonding with bone. Generally, a layer of fibrous tissue will form at the interface as a result of initial microscopic movement. If prosthetic stability is maintained, the fibrous tissue may become bone and thus provide better apposition and load sharing for the implant. If the layer remains fibrous, it will act as a shock absorber and improve the quality of the implant-bone interface. However, if prosthetic stability is not maintained, interface motion may increase and stimulate bone resorption and remodeling that can lead to gross loosening.

Irregularities on the surface of the prosthetic stem in the form of notches, grooves, fenestrations, or screw threads often are sites of stress concentration. Stems usually contain zones of high stress, and these stress raisers can weaken the stem and cause fracture. Materials of different elastic modulus, ranging from ceramics to HDP, have been implanted by using this form of prosthesis fixation. Use of a material of high modulus that is grossly noncompliant to bone can accelerate bone resorption and remodeling unless interdigitation through tissue ingrowth is incorporated in the prosthetic design. Even in such situations, bone fracture due to mismatching of modulus can occur. In low-modulus material, such as HDP, the weak link in the fixation system will be the plastic material. If HDP is designed in the form of a plug or stem, tensile fatigue fracture may occur under high cyclic loading. Metallic reinforcement must be considered.

In a retrospective study of a large series of hip endoprostheses with both cemented and noncemented mechanical fixation of similar stem designs, the loosening rate was significantly higher in the noncemented group at different lengths of follow-up. Because prosthesis loosening is affected by many factors, such as disease, age, activity level, body weight, and joint loading, mechanical fixation without cement or porous ingrowth could be successful when associated conditions are favorable.

Recently, smooth prosthetic surfaces have been coated with inert materials such as ceramics or carbon in attempts to enhance direct tissue bonding. The benefits of this practice need to be demonstrated. The adhesive strength of such coatings must be strong to prevent film breakdown.

Grouting Material (Bone Cement)

Self-curing acrylic cement or poly(methyl methacrylate) (PMMA) has been used successfully for many years to stabilize prosthetic implants based on the mechanical interlocking principle. PMMA contains polymer in powder form and a liquid monomer which are handmixed. The time period from initiation of mixing until the mixture achieves a doughy state (PMMA mixture does not stick to surgical glove material) is defined as "dough time"; the entire time period required for the bone cement to set is called "setting time." The difference between these two time periods is defined as "working time," during which the cement must be applied and the implant inserted. During the final stage when the cement "sets," its temperature rises to nearly 80°C.

Both dough time and setting time vary slightly from one type of cement to another and can be altered by environmental conditions. To increase the working time of bone cement, the most effective method is to decrease the ambient temperature around the cement. Although these physical properties are important in the application of PMMA, its implant fixation performance depends mainly on the basic mechanical characteristics and surgical techniques used during cementing and implant insertion.

Mechanical Properties of PMMA Compared to cortical bone, PMMA is relatively weak in nearly all mechanical properties: compressive strength, 60%; tensile strength, 25%; shear strength, 60%; fatigue strength, 47%; and stiffness, 10%. Its low tensile strength must be compensated for by implant design and fixation technique to avoid fracture failure. Its low modulus appears to be a unique advantage in that it allows a gradual transfer of stress to bone.

Mixing additives with PMMA significantly changes its mechanical properties. Antibiotics decrease its tensile and fatigue strengths. When 10% $BaSO_4$ is added, the decrease of all mechanical parameters is minimal. Adding carbon fibers to the cement mixture effectively increases its elastic modulus, tensile strength, and fatigue life, but its intrusion property is significantly decreased, which will cause difficulty in surgical application.

The porosity of bone cement can be significant, depending on the mixing and insertion techniques used. Blood and gas inclusions further increase PMMA porosity, which significantly decreases its fatigue strength. High temperature and the lapse of time during the cement-setting stage can cause bone necrosis. Lowering ambient temperatures and using proper cement thickness can effectively decrease this adverse effect. The viscosities of PMMA from different commercial sources are different. For optimal bone intrusion by cement, PMMA viscosity should be less than 100 $N \cdot s/m^2$. Finally, dimensional changes in PMMA during curing are negligible (less than 1%).

Potential Problems of Cement Fixation In spite of the demonstrated successes, cemented implant failure still occurs, mainly in the form of aseptic loosening. Such failure has been postulated to be caused by mechanisms that are biomechanical or biologic in origin. It is still unclear whether these two loosening mechanisms act individually or together. One factor may stimulate the other and vice versa, thus forming a vicious cycle that finally leads to implant loosening. In any event, the physical properties of the cement, the cement's response to a tissue environment, the distribution of stress in the bone-cement-implant system, and the surgical technique all must play key roles in the loosening problem. Therefore, it is important to review the potential problems associated with cement and its use for fixing implants.

Inherent Mechanical Weakness Due to the low tensile and fatigue strengths of cement, fracture of the cement layer in certain critical regions of the implant is possible. Such breakage will entirely alter stress conditions in the prosthetic system, which can cause implant loosening or even implant fracture. High porosity, particularly with blood and gas inclusions, will further decrease the strength of cement. A relatively high viscosity in certain cements can obstruct intrusion of the cement into bony spaces and decrease interlocking fixation.

The thickness of the cement layer also affects optimal stress transmission in the implant system. When cement is overly thick, curing temperatures are high and create a hazard to the surrounding tissues. With cements of current mechanical properties, thicknesses of 3 to 5 mm were found to be more desirable. Naturally, these analyses were based on idealized surgical technique and uniform thickness without voids. In reality, less than ideal application of the cement will magnify its mechanical weakness.

Defects in Cement Application Technique During mixing and insertion of the cement, porosity and voids can appear both within the cement and at the interface. A lack of pressure on the surface of the bone or in the cortical canal makes it impossible to achieve an effective interlock between the bone and the cement layer. In addition, nonuniform cement thickness and large interface gaps defeat the purpose of the mechanical interlocking principle for implant fixation.

Systemic Biologic Reaction Cement-bone interface loosening has been postulated as the result of soft tissue membrane formation. This membrane can be infiltrated with macrophages with high acid phosphatase activity. The host bone can appear to be resorbed. If new bone formation is absent and motion continues at the interface, mechanical loosening is inevitable. Granuloma and reactive foreign body giant cells have been observed in loosened implant interfaces with massive osteolysis. However, it remains obscure whether the cement fragmentation found at the interface was the cause or the effect of such systemic changes. Other potential biologic and physiologic problems are related to monomer toxicity which may cause hypotension during total joint replacement procedures. No definitive data are available to refute or support such hypotheses on the systemic effects of bone cement. Additional studies should be performed and careful precautions must be taken to ensure safety during PMMA application.

Stress-Related Bone Remodeling Intramedullary implant fixation, with or without cement, appears to be unphysiologic in reproducing normal bone stress distribution. Consequently, stress-induced bone remodeling, according to Wolff's law, must be considered. Bone stresses are sensitive to the mechanical property of the stem, which can be significantly augmented by the thickness of the cement. The negative aspect of bone remodeling is stress-shielding resorption. This has been a relatively rare finding except when a massive stem is involved. In most cases in which positive bone remodeling was observed, the cortex at the tip of the cemented stem became hypertrophied in response to the high bone stress in this region. However, in the midsection of the bone, the stresses are low, which may be a factor that contributes to osteolysis in this region.

Improvements in PMMA Properties and Application Techniques Many attempts have been made to improve the mechanical properties of PMMA and its surgical application technique in the past 10 years. The results of these efforts are responsible for the much improved clinical outcome of cemented prosthetic implants in terms of decreased aseptic loosening. Further development and investigation are still required to be able to predict accurately the longevity of cement fixation in younger patients. The following are the main areas of advancement related to PMMA.

Development of New Bone Cement Several low-viscosity bone cements have been introduced for clinical use, which may improve interdigitation with bone to achieve micro interlocking. Other physical properties have also improved, but basic mechanical strengths have remained practically unchanged. There is a need for new cements that have low viscosity and low modulus but also provide high tensile and fatigue strengths. A new class of copolymer, butyl methacrylate in a methyl methacrylate matrix, appears promising and should be investigated.

Improvement in Cement Mixing and Application Techniques Better bone bed preparation by using the water-pick technique and distal plugging of the cortical canal have provided a better bone-cement interface interlocking property. Cement pressurization with special instruments and the application of cement with a syringe deep in the medullary cavity also appear to be highly beneficial. Cement mixing under centrifugation or in a vacuum has been demonstrated to increase fatigue strength and decrease porosity.

Application of Optimal Design Concept Important parameters of stem modulus and cement thickness have been identified by using stress analysis techniques to optimize the mechanical performance of current cements. Better stems can be designed that exhibit ideal stress-sharing characteristics in the stem-cement-bone system to minimize potential adverse effects. Through such analyses, stem and cement stresses can be maintained at a safe level while bone stress is maximized to prevent osseous resorption.

Positive bone remodeling may be achieved to prolong fixation strength. It is possible that many of the potential problems in cement application can be successfully resolved by using the new implant design concept, provided that meticulous surgical technique and special instruments are utilized.

Porous Ingrowth

The concept of "biologic fixation" through tissue ingrowth into voids on a porous-surfaced implant has become attractive because of residual problems with both the interference-fit fixation method and use of PMMA bone cement. Extended experimental studies in animals have demonstrated the validity of this concept. In addition, the basic requirements have been identified to establish porous ingrowth as a method for implant fixation. These requirements include:

(1) physical dimension and geometry of pore structure,
(2) base materials to be used for porous layer and solid substrate and their bonding strengths,
(3) mechanical property of the implant and its initial stability requirements,
(4) corrosion and biocompatibility of porous material,
(5) manufacturing process and quality control, and
(6) type and extent of tissue ingrowth and possible methods of enhancement.

Although not all these requirements are met by current experimental prostheses, initial clinical results are very promising. There is no doubt that this method should be pursued enthusiastically but carefully so that its clinical results will be equal to or better than those with other implant fixation techniques. The task may be difficult because cement fixation has a long and good track record.

Type of Porous Material and Structure The base materials used to coat prosthetic surfaces are the established implant materials—namely, porous metals, porous ceramics, and porous polymers. Because porous ceramics and porous polymers are still in the experimental stage, this review will concentrate on the more popular and extensively studied porous metals.

Fiber-Metal Composite This type of material is composed of thin stainless steel, titanium, or Co-Cr-Mo wires cut and kinked by using meshing gears and pressed in die punches to form the specific shape for the porous coating. The porous layer is bonded on the solid substrate through a sintering process (high-temperature diffusion to provide a metallurgic bond) in an inert gas environment or in a vacuum. The porosity ranges from 40% to 50%, with a mean pore size of 270 μm and good interconnectivity. It has been shown in animal experiments that such porous material allowed successful tissue and bone ingrowth with high interface shear strength. Titanium and Co-Cr-Mo are resistant to corrosion, even in the thin wire state, but stainless steel wire is more susceptible to metal ion release and corrosion in the *in vivo* environment. Currently, the Galante-Harris hip and Miller-Galante knee with titanium fiber-metal as the porous surface coating are under clinical trial.

Void Metal Composite Both Co-Cr-Mo and Ti-6Al-4V alloys have been used as base materials. The investment casting technique is used by mixing magnesium microspheres with the base alloy. Under high temperature, the magnesium vaporizes, leaving pores on the surface of the base alloy which form the porous surface. Pore diameters range from 275 to 460 μm. The various fabrication techniques produce different void depths and pore connectivities. Although the porous surface is integrated with the metal base, information on the mechanical and metallurgic properties of such materials has been insufficient. The Judet hip prosthesis is an example of this class of porous surface preparation.

Sintered Micro and Macro Beads Co-Cr-Mo and Ti are the two materials that have been processed in this manner. Metal powder or macro beads (420 to 595 μm) are compacted on a solid substrate by gravity within a ceramic mold, and sintering is achieved at the submelting temperature of the base metal. Porosities range from 30% for the fine powder to 44% for larger beads. Pore diameters vary from 100 to 400 μm. The ultimate tensile strength and modulus depend on the size of the particles used in the process. The corrosion resistance of the Co-Cr-Mo alloy has been quite satisfactory. The AML (Austin-Moore long stem) hip prosthesis and the PCA (porous coated anatomic) total knee and total hip are examples of such implants currently being used clinically.

Potential Problems With Porous Implants In nearly all animal experiments, porous ingrowth fixation has been uniformly confirmed under various loading conditions and with various implant designs. The most important factor affecting the quality of bone ingrowth is implant stability. Because animal experiments are short-term, insufficient information is available to assess the long-term performance of this fixation method under more severe loading and environmental conditions. Similarly, although extremely promising, the available clinical results are based on short follow-up and a relatively small patient population. Consequently, a number of potential problems related to porous implant applications must be recognized and investigated to improve the long-term efficacy of biologic fixation.

Fabrication and Quality Control of Porous Coating Current fabrication techniques for the various types of porous implants are still quite complex and thus increase the cost of the final product. Finished prostheses cannot be inspected for possible flaws that may have occurred during sintering without using destructive testing methods. Inadequate bonding of the porous surface and solid substrate can cause the metal fibers or beads to loosen. More reliable and simplified methods of quality control should be developed. Efficient, consistent, and cost-effective manufacturing processes must be developed to produce implants that are affordable.

Initial Implant Fixation and Long-Term Bone Remodeling Multiple sizes of implants can be fabricated, but there are occasions when a perfect fit cannot be achieved to meet the initial stability requirement. Under such circumstances, alternative means of implant fixation must be considered. In addition, intramedullary fixation through bone ingrowth may not be the ideal form of fixation because it tends to shield stress at the shoulder region of the prosthesis, which could cause bone resorption. Extracortical bone bridging fixation over the porous-coated implant may be more physiologic because stress will be transferred from the bone to the implant and back to the bone. In this case, the stem does not need to be porous-coated and the initial fixation stability can be achieved through press fit or cement.

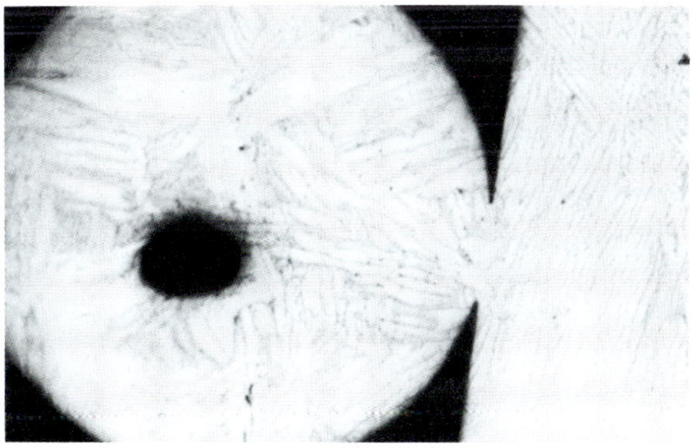

Figure 8

Microstructural changes of the Ti-6Al-4V alloy substrate (at right) and the pure titanium beads in the porous surface sintering process. The substrate has a lamellar microstructure which is completely different from its original equiaxis, α-β morphology. Co-Cr alloy will undergo a similar process, with the substrate grain growing in size and porosity as a result of sintering. (From Cook, S.D.; Georgette, F.S.; Skinner, H.B.; and Haddad, R.J., Jr.: Fatigue properties of carbon- and porous-coated Ti-6Al-4V alloy. J. Biomed. Mater. Res. 18:497–512, 1984. By permission of John Wiley & Sons.)

However, this implant design is limited to segmental bone and joint replacements where the prosthesis contains a porous-coated straight segment that juxtaposes with the bone cortex.

Histochemical investigations of the various mechanisms of tissue ingrowth for biologic fixation are needed because osseous integration depends not only on interface stability but also on the chemistry and composition of the surface of the implant. Animal studies should also be carried out to observe bone remodeling adjacent to the porous coating. If significant bone resorption occurs, the stem could become overstressed and liable to fatigue fracture.

Metal Substrate Weakening Due to Sintering High-temperature sintering tends to weaken the solid substrate and may cause prosthetic fracture. Co-Cr-Mo or titanium alloys undergo a grain growth near the surface that produces abnormal microstructural changes during the sintering process (Fig. 8). This effect may become significant in a solid metal substrate that is in the form of a plate, such as the metal-backed tibial tray in a total knee prosthesis. These metallurgic changes can decrease the fatigue strength of the implant (Table 1). In Ti fiber-metal, the sintering process can create notches on the surface of the solid substrate (Fig. 9). These notches can become sites of stress concentration which tend to decrease fatigue strength significantly (Table 2). Therefore, a better sintering technique must be developed. On the other hand, improved implant design should be utilized to minimize such problems. Porous coating on the stem decreases the effective diameter of the solid substrate and can predispose it to fatigue fracture. When possible, a porous layer should be avoided at critical stress regions on the prosthetic surface.

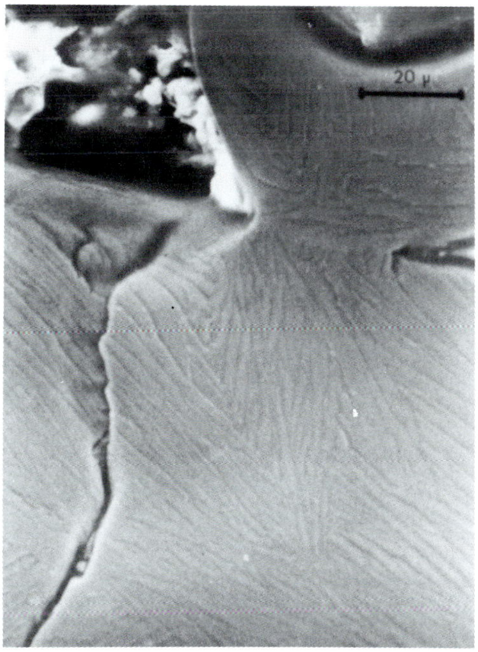

Figure 9

Notch effect during fatigue loading that caused fracture cracks adjacent to the titanium fiber-metal bonding to the Ti-6Al-4V substrate, resulting from the sintering process. Scale bar = 20 μm. (From Yue, S; Pilliar, R.M; and Weatherly, C.G.: The fatigue strength of porous-coated Ti-6%Al-4%V implant alloy. J. Biomed. Mater. Res. 18:1043–1058, 1984. By permission of John Wiley & Sons.)

Metal Ion Release and Surface Corrosion Due to the larger surface area of porous materials, there may be an increased rate of corrosion and ion release. Significantly high levels of Co and Cr ions have been detected in experimental animals. Ti ion release was also found in both short- and long-term animal experiments. These results may serve as early warnings to justify continuing investigation of the effects of porous coating on systemic changes in surrounding tissues. Small metal particles can be found in adjacent tissues in experimental animal models after only short-term implantation of porous-coated prostheses (Fig. 10).

Table 1. Fatigue Strength of Co-Cr-Mo Alloy: Effect of Sintering Process*

Process	Fatigue strength psi	Fatigue strength MPa
Forged	90	600
Cast	35	250
Sintered	25	150
Sintered with controlled coating	30	200

*Data from Pilliar, R.M. Clin. Orthop. 176:42–51, 1983.

Table 2. Fatigue Strength of Ti-6Al-4V: Effect of Sintering Process*

Process	Fatigue strength psi	Fatigue strength MPa
Wrought	95	650
Heat-exposed	85	600
Sintered	30	200
Sintered and aged	55	375

*Data from Pilliar, R.M. Clin. Orthop. 176:42–51, 1983.

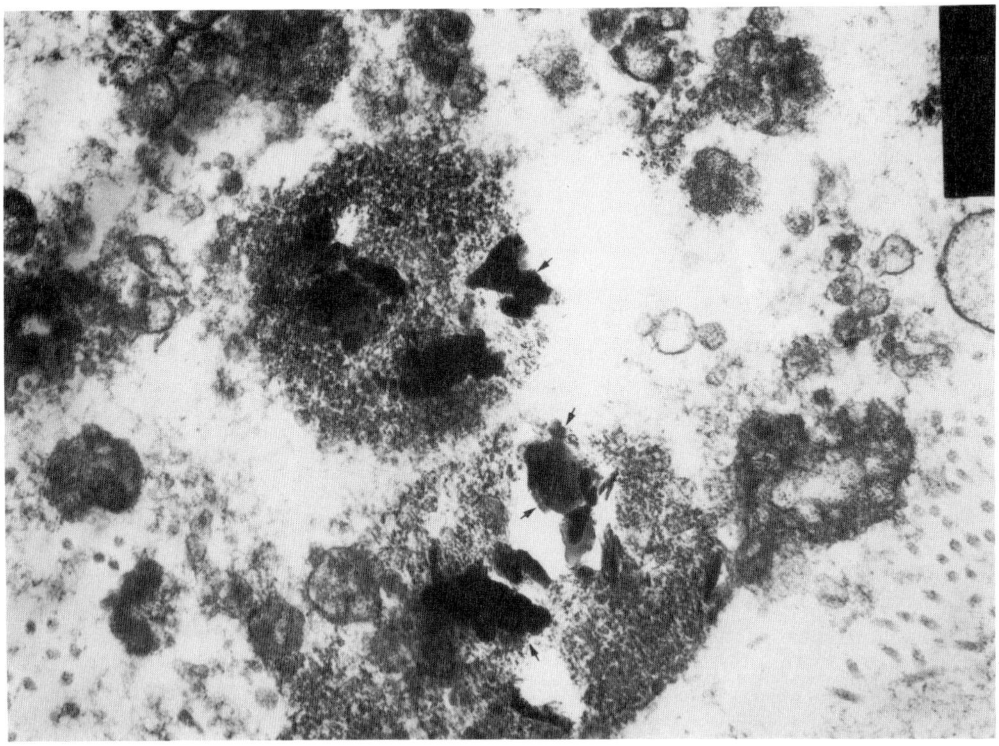

Figure 10
Electron microprobe analysis of tissue sample (X33,000) adjacent to a titanium fiber-metal segmental bone prosthesis in canine mid-femur at 3 months after implantation. Titanium ions (*small arrows*) were also identified by energy spectrum analysis.

Implant Removal This paradoxic problem is real and must be considered in implant design. Using a modular system with extracortical biologic fixation and press-fitting or cementing the solid stem could minimize this problem. Animal experiments must be conducted to validate the concept of extracortical fixation with initial cement fixation and to avoid the possible adverse effects of bone resorption due to stress shielding. Unfortunately, such a composite fixation concept cannot be used at certain anatomic regions.

Summary

Existing metallic implant materials appear to be safe and effective. The adverse mechanical properties associated with each type of alloy can be compensated for by prosthetic design. The supermetals, with their much improved fatigue performance, are desirable but their high cost must be considered in implant design and application. Young and physically active patients with high body weight are ideal candidates to receive prosthetic devices made of high-strength metal to minimize the long-term fatigue failure problem. The technology for incorporating porous coatings on high-strength metals needs to be developed to be able to utilize the unique advantages that these metals can provide. The choice of implant and its material composition should be based on clinical judgment.

Bioceramics have limited advantages, but their superior wear characteristics and tissue compatibility must be considered in joint replacement prosthetic design when high tensile strength is not required. The more critical factor in using ceramic material for implant design is modulus mismatching with bone. However, design alterations and modular structure compositions can combine the advantages of different materials to optimize implant performance *in vivo.* New ceramic materials are being developed that can have mechanical properties closer to those of metal and bone. Resorptive bioglass still remains an intriguing class of implant materials to be explored for orthopaedic implant application. Coating metals with ceramic material to increase their biologic inertness is an attractive idea and should be pursued.

HDP has been the hallmark material for providing an ideal articulating surface for low-friction arthroplasty. However, its low resistance to plastic deformation and tensile crack failure require further improvement. HDP wear particles may cause adverse biologic reactions at the prosthesis-bone interface and must be carefully investigated. New polymers with improved mechanical and biologic responses are needed in the field of orthopaedic implant development. However, silicone rubber and its derivatives seem to be undesirable because of their residual lack of mechanical strength and high degree of tissue reaction. New polymers with high flexibility are needed for interpositioning joint spacers in certain reconstructive procedures.

Fixation based on interference fit without cement may be less appealing in view of inferior clinical results compared to cement fixation. The prosthetic surface irregularities required to achieve implant stability may cause long-term fatigue weakness. However, in certain anatomic regions, this method of implant fixation may be effective under low-load conditions.

Cement fixation has the longest and best record for implant fixation. In addition, many improvements have been made, both in PMMA properties and in surgical techniques of application. It is safe to predict that future results will be even better. Acrylic cement is a rather forgiving material and will compensate for poor bone quality and surgical errors. However, long-term loosening and unknown biologic reactions must not be discounted when implants are to be used in young persons with many years of active functional life remaining. It is safe to predict that a higher percentage of implant fixations in orthopaedic patients will rely on PMMA. A combined mode of implant fixation that uses bone cement to achieve initial prosthetic stability and porous ingrowth to provide long-term incorporation of the implant to bone would be the ideal solution. This concept is under extensive investigation in the segmental bone and joint replacement field which utilizes the concept of extracortical bone bridging over porous-coated prosthetic segments.

Biologic fixation through bone ingrowth into the porous surface of an implant appears to be logical and promising. Although numerous types of material and porous forms have been tried, final selections are limited to only a few that have demonstrated good results. Efforts should be directed toward perfecting these materials rather than toward exploring other alternatives. Although there are a number of potential problems involved with porous implants, these problems may be resolved with today's technology. Extensive clinical trials are needed in large medical centers. Enthusiasm for porous implants should be carefully balanced with consideration of their many unknown characteristics.

Annotated Bibliography

Ahmed, A.M.; Raab, S.; and Miller, J.E.: Metal/cement interface strength in cemented stem fixation. J. Orthop. Res. 2:105–118, 1984.

The strength of interfaces with the cancellous bone surrounding the cement mantle was significantly less than the strength of those with cortical bone. A marked degradation of strength of SS316LVM-cement interfaces was found with saline immersion; after 60 days of immersion, the interface strength was only 10–20% of the value for bulk cement. Interfaces formed with metals precoated with a thin film of poly(methyl methacrylate) had greater strength than interfaces formed with uncoated metals. The strength of precoated SS316LVM-cement interfaces formed with all three brands of cement did not change after saline immersion for 60 days.

Askew, M.J.; Steege, J.W.; Lewis, J.L.; Ranieri, J.R.; and Wixson, R.L.: Effect of cement pressure and bone strength on polymethylmethacrylate fixation. J. Orthop. Res. 1:412–420, 1984.

The effects of the quality of the bone and of the cement pressurization magnitude and duration on the fixation achieved with poly(methyl methacrylate) bone cement were studied *in vitro*. Pressure magnitude is the most influential of the factors considered in the cement penetration behavior and in the development of failure load capacity. Bone strength decreases as cement penetration increases, reflecting an increase in the porosity and a decrease in the area fraction. The strength of the fixation achievable for any bone is limited by the intrinsic strength of the bone. For the most effective fixation, an optimal depth of cement penetration is 4 mm and an optimal bone area fraction is 0.20.

Berman, A.T.; Reid, J.S.; Yanicko, D.R., Jr.; Sih, G.C.; and Zimmerman, M.R.: Thermally induced bone necrosis in rabbits: Relation to implant failure in humans. Clin. Orthop. 186:284–292, 1984.

Exposure of bone to high temperatures has become common, especially with the increasing use of poly(methyl methacrylate) bone cement. In rabbit tibia, bone necrosis was consistently seen in histologic sections at scald temperatures ≥70°C. These results led to the suggestion that joint replacement systems in human bone, with this bone cement, be designed to limit intraoperative temperature maxima 70°C.

Bourne, R.B.; Oh, I.; and Harris, W.H.: Femoral cement pressurization during total hip arthroplasty: The role of different femoral stems with reference to stem size and shape. Clin. Orthop. 183:12–16, 1984.

Aseptic loosening is the most common cause of femoral component failure after total hip arthroplasty. Improvements have been made in cementing technique. The results of this study favor the use of the largest femoral component stem, preferably one with a rounded rectangular cross section, that will fit comfortably in a given femoral canal and still allow a surrounding cement envelope such that bone cement pressurization will be enhanced with implant introduction.

Brown, S.A., and Bargar, W.L.: The influence of temperature and specimen size on the flexural properties of PMMA bone cement. J. Biomed. Mater. Res. 18:523–536, 1984.

A three-stage investigation was undertaken to examine the influence of specimen size and polymerization environment on the flexural properties of poly(methyl methacrylate). These experiments demonstrated that molding thin 1.6–mm specimens resulted in increases of 14% in stress and 30% in strain to failure compared with 3.2–mm specimens. Thicker cement samples reached higher temperatures, and cement samples polymerized at lower temperatures (21°C versus 37°C) had 12% greater stress and 105% greater strain to failure.

Cook, S.D.; Georgette, F.S.; Skinner, H.B.; and Haddad, R.J., Jr.: Fatigue properties of carbon- and porous-coated Ti-6Al-4V alloy. J. Biomed. Mater. Res. 18:497–512, 1984.

This study investigated the effects that both a porous Ti-6Al-4V alloy coating and a ULTI carbon coating have on the fatigue properties of a Ti-6Al-4V alloy substrate system. The results of this study revealed endurance limits for Ti-6Al-4V alloy, tested with a rotating beam system, of 617 MN/m^2 (uncoated as-received), 624 MN/m^2 (ULTI carbon-coated), 377 MN/m^2 (sinter heat treated), 220 MN/m^2 (notched), and 138 MN/m^2 (porous-coated) (MN/m^2 = 1 Pa). The low endurance limit of the porous-coated material is due to the transition from the as-received equiaxed microstructure to a lamellar microstructure upon sintering and to the notch effect created by the porous coating.

Doi, K.; Kuwata, N.; and Kawai, S.: Alumina ceramic finger implants: A preliminary biomaterial and clinical evaluation. J. Hand Surg. [Am.] 9:740–749, 1984.

A hinge-type prosthesis composed of alumina ceramics and high-density polyethylene is described. Follow-up results (12 to 31 months) have been most encouraging, with satisfactory functional recovery and no fracture or dislocation of the implants.

Engh, C.A.: Hip arthroplasty with a Moore prosthesis with porous coating: A five-year study. Clin. Orthop. 176:52–66, 1983.

The 5-year clinical experience with Moore hip prostheses with a porous coating has been encouraging. The results have been equivalent to those of a simultaneous experience using cemented prostheses. The tissue ingrowth has produced stress transfers sufficiently uniform to provide roentgenographic signs of healthy bone modeling. With 4-year follow-up radiographs now available in 10 patients, there has been no evidence of bone resorption due to femoral stress shielding by the relatively high-modulus implant with a porous surface.

Freeman, M.A.R.; Samuelson, K.M.; and Bertin, K.C.: Freeman-Samuelson total arthroplasty of the knee. Clin. Orthop. 192:46–58, 1985.

Experience with cementless fixation over the last 6 years indicates that the technique offers greater opportunities for bone conservation. However, in the senior author's view, it is not a technique that should be generally used as yet. It is hoped that investigations of this problem will take place in a restrained, scientific way rather than in response to the dictates of fashion and commerce.

Harris, W.H.: Advances in total hip arthroplasty: The metal-backed acetabular component. Clin. Orthop. 183:4–11, 1984.

Detailed, long-term studies of cemented total hip arthroplasties clearly show that failure of fixation of the acetabular component is a major problem, with an increasing incidence and an unusual complexity. Long-term follow-up studies of 51 patients who underwent total hip arthroplasty performed by the author during the period 1971 to 1975 and using metal-backed acetabular components confirm the improved fixation that results from the use of this design. Both the analytic data of stress distribution and the clinical follow-up studies strongly support the use of metal-backed acetabular components in cemented total hip arthroplasty.

Hierton, C.; Blomgren, G.; and Lindgren, U.: Factors associated with early loosening of cemented total hip prostheses. Acta Orthop. Scand. 54:168–173, 1983.

Patient data and radiographs from a series of 237 consecutive total hip replacements were evaluated by means of a computer program in an attempt to study factors correlated with early loosening. The authors found that the loosening rate was significantly influenced by several factors, emphasized the importance of thorough technique, and suggested that total hip replacement should be performed by specialized surgeons.

Huiskes, R., and Nunamaker, D.: Local stresses and bone adaption around orthopedic implants. Calcif. Tissue Int. 36 Suppl 1:110–117, 1984.

Mechanical stresses, caused by joint loading, play a key role in the adaption of interface bone and in the loosening process. The results indicate that loosening and bone resorption are associated with high peak stresses at the interface in the immediate postoperative stage. In addition, there appeared to be similarity between the local stress patterns and the bone morphology at the interface if resorption did not occur. Finally, it was found that implants of high local stiffness generate lower peak stresses in bone compared with low-stiffness implants.

Hungerford, D.S., and Krackow, K.A.: Total joint arthroplasty of the knee. Clin. Orthop. 192:23–33, 1985.

The vast majority of total knee components can be mechanically fixed rigidly without the addition of methyl methacrylate. In general, clinical examinations (up to 4 years) suggested that results in the cementless group were as good as results in the cemented group.

Kusleika, R., and Stupp, S.I.: Mechanical strength of poly(methyl methacrylate) cement-human bone interfaces. J. Biomed. Mater. Res. 17:441–458, 1983.

A device was constructed to test the strength of the interface between poly(methyl methacrylate)-based bone cement and human cancellous bone under pure tension. On the basis of experimental findings, better stress-dissipating qualities and higher tensile strength are suggested as two important necessary improvements of bone cements based on poly(methyl methacrylate).

Lewis, J.L.; Askew, M.J.; Wixson, R.L.; Kramer, G.M.; and Tarr, R.R.: The influence of prosthetic stem stiffness and of a calcar collar on stresses in the proximal end of the femur with a cemented femoral component. J. Bone Joint Surg. 66A:280–286, 1984.

Three-dimensional finite-element models of the proximal end of the femur were used to examine the influence of stem material, stem geometry, and use of a calcar collar on the stresses in and around implanted total hip-replacement femoral components. A slender titanium-alloy stem with a collar allows creation of calcar stresses of approximately 80% of the anticipated normal levels. Proximal cement stresses were increased by the use of titanium-alloy stems but were decreased to low levels by a functioning collar. The goal of the designer of a prosthesis is to decrease cement and cement interface stresses around the femoral stem and to create stress distributions in the bone that will prevent resorption.

Linder, L.; Lindberg, L.; and Carlsson, Å.: Aseptic loosening of hip prostheses: A histologic and enzyme histochemical study. Clin. Orthop. 175:93–104, 1983.

Twenty-one total hip arthroplasties were revised because of aseptic loosening. The bone and soft tissue membrane bordering the cement in a total of 37 biopsies from the acetabulum and femur were studied histologically and by enzyme histochemistry. The soft tissue membrane was infiltrated with macrophages and had high acid phosphatase activity. The host bone seemed to have been resorbed by a soft tissue front moving outward from the cement. Reactive new bone formation began at the bone-soft tissue border and appeared to constrain the resorptive process. Articular wear seemed to play no part in initiating the loosening process. The role of bone cement in this respect is obscure because there were no obvious local signs of cytotoxicity. These observations support the theory of mechanical instability as the primary cause of the tissue reaction.

Morscher, E.W.: Cementless total hip arthroplasty. Clin. Orthop. 181:76–91, 1983.

The differences between prostheses fixed with and without cement are mainly in the design and nature of the surface implant. Clinical experience with noncemented hip endoprostheses to date is promising, although the observation time for most models is short.

Oh, I.; Bourne, R.B.; and Harris, W.H.: The femoral cement compactor: An improvement in cementing technique in total hip replacement. J. Bone Joint Surg. 65A:1335–1338, 1983.

Even with new cementing techniques, cement pressurization is low in the most proximal area of the femoral canal. To correct this problem, the femoral cement compactor was devised. This device increased the pressurization of bone cement in the proximal area of the femur by 71% and increased the duration of the pressurization 4-fold compared with the results achieved by finger-packing methods.

Pilliar, R.M.: Powder metal-made orthopedic implants with porous surface for fixation by tissue ingrowth. Clin. Orthop. 176:42–51, 1983.

Orthopaedic implants made of metal powder and having a porous coating provide an effective means for implant fixation by tissue ingrowth. Additionally, the use of metal alloy powders for forming porous surfaces offers the advantage of uniform coatings on complex shapes. This animal study indicated an optimal pore size of 50–400 μm. However, sintered Co-Cr-Mo could cause a 30% reduction of fatigue strength of the solid substrate, due mainly to abnormal grain growth at the diffusion temperature required.

Rampoldi, A.: Mittelmeier's ceramic hip prosthesis. Ital. J. Orthop. Traumatol. 10:305–311, September 1984.

The results are reported for 59 noncemented ceramic hip prostheses; 29 had a follow-up of 1 to 3 years. The results of this limited series, albeit with a comparatively short follow-up, are sufficiently encouraging to recommend the use of this prosthesis when the indications are correct.

Schreiber, A.; Jacob, H.A.; Dietschi, C.; Brandenberg, J.E.; and Züllig, R.: Surface replacement hip arthroplasty with the Freeman double cup. Ital. J. Orthop. Traumatol. 9:157–165, 1983.

The authors report their clinical experience with 43 hip arthroplasties using Freeman's double femoral cup. The patients were followed for 3 to 6 years after operation. At that time, only 44% were totally free from pain, and migration of the femoral cup, which was severe and progressive, was observed radiographically in almost half the cases. Biomechanical studies were also performed with photoelastic models and the technique of finite elements. These studies indicated overloading on contact between the edge of the femoral cup and the cortical bone (especially medially) but without any load over the whole of the spongy bone. Consequently, there was bone resorption in the overload zone and osteoporosis in the spongy bone. The femoral cup rapidly became unstable, and this produced progressive migration, thus constituting a vicious cycle.

Shoji, H.; Karube, S.; D'ambrosia, R.D.; Dabezies, E.J.; and Miller, D.R.: Biochemical features of pseudomembrane at the bone-cement interface of loosened total hip prostheses. J. Biomed. Mater. Res. 17:669–678, 1983.

Biochemical and histologic features of pseudomembrane formed at the bone-cement interface of 13 failed total hip replacements were studied. Overall biochemical features in the light of the histologic appearance suggested that pseudomembrane resembles granulation tissue. The bone healing mechanism at the bone-cement interface appears to differ from that of fracture healing.

Spector, M.; Davis, R.J.; Lunceford, E.M.; and Harmon, S.L.: Porous polysulfone coatings for fixation of femoral stems by bony ingrowth. Clin. Orthop. 176:34–41, 1983.

Sixteen porous polysulfone-coated canine femoral stems were inserted into 14 dogs. Bone was formed within at least 30% of the surface pores of the implants. These observations support the concept of coating femoral prostheses with porous material for cement-free stabilization.

Tullous, H.S.; McCaskill, B.L.; Dickey, R.; and Davidson, J.: Total hip arthroplasty with a low-modulus porous-coated femoral component: Progress report. J. Bone Joint Surg. 66A:888–898, 1984.

Fifty-seven patients had 63 total hip replacements performed with a femoral stem carrying a soft, low-modulus, porous coating of Proplast and a conventional acrylic-cemented acetabular component. Seventeen (36%) of the 47 hips were judged to be clinical failures; five of the failures were revised by inserting a new femoral component and fixing it with acrylic cement. The coating had insufficient strength to withstand normal weight-bearing loads. To improve performance, a more stable prosthesis with a stronger porous coating is needed.

Walker, P.S.; Soudry, M.; Ewald, F.C.; and McVickar, H.: Control of cement penetration in total knee arthroplasty. Clin. Orthop. 185:155–164, 1984.

A radiographic study of 45 knees immediately after and at least 2 years after operation showed that the average depth of cement penetration was 1.5–3.0 mm at different locations around the interface and that there was a strong inverse relationship between the development of radiolucency and the initial cement penetration. In laboratory studies of penetration in the upper tibia, penetration was approximately proportional to bone pore diameter and to the square root of the applied pressure and inversely proportional to the time after initial mixing. The suggested ideal depth of cement penetration is 3–4 mm.

Woodman, J.L.; Jacobs, J.J.; Galante, J.O.; and Urban, R.M.: Metal ion release from titanium-based prosthetic segmental replacements of long bones in baboons: A long-term study. J. Orthop. Res. 1:421–430, 1984.

Forty-five baboons that had received titanium-based fiber-metal composite segmental bone replacements were studied along with 13 controls without implants. In the 38 sacrificed baboons with implants, increased titanium levels were noted in the lungs, spleen, adjacent muscle, and regional lymph nodes. Vanadium content was significantly increased in the lungs of some animals; increases in aluminum were noted in adjacent muscle, lung, and regional lymph nodes. In the seven living baboons with implants, a 6-fold increase in urinary titanium level was noted in comparison with seven living controls without implants. Aluminum levels were increased in the serum of the group with implants.

Wroblewski, B.M., and van der Rijt, A.: Intramedullary cancellous bone block to improve femoral stem fixation in Charnley low-friction arthroplasty. J. Bone Joint Surg. 66B:639–644, 1984.

To improve the fixation of the stem in primary Charnley low-friction arthroplasty, the medullary canal was routinely closed off with a cancellous bone block. In a prospective study of 611 consecutive arthroplasties, no radiologic evidence of loosening of the stem was seen in 604 cases. The method is recommended for routine use in primary total hip arthroplasty.

Yue, S.; Pilliar, R.M.; and Weatherly, G.C.: The fatigue strength of porous-coated Ti-6%Al-4%V implant alloy. J. Biomed. Mater. Res. 18:1043–1058, 1984.

The fatigue behavior of Ti-6Al-4V (extra-low interstitial) alloy coated with Ti-6Al-4V powder was investigated in rotating bending fatigue testing. The high-cycle-fatigue strength of porous-coated specimens was substantially less than that of uncoated specimens of the same microstructure. Scanning electron microscopy revealed crack initiation close to particle substrate contact interfaces, and it is concluded that stress intensification due to these interface regions is a major source of weakness with respect to fatigue strength. Sintering resulted in delineation of prior β grain boundaries, and it is suggested that this also contributes to the inferior fatigue strength of porous-coated Ti-6Al-4V.

12
Soft Tissue Implants

Introduction

The majority of the soft tissue implants used in orthopaedic surgery are utilized in reconstruction of the knee. Although they are not exclusively limited to this application, we will discuss their use in this setting. Once they are perfected, much wider application is certainly likely. These materials are not currently available for general use but are undergoing clinical investigation as required by the Food and Drug Administration. For some devices, limited clinical results are available and will be presented; for others, no results are available.

Biomechanical Properties of Human Knee Ligaments

Few statements can be made that are universal to all human ligaments. To date, the few quantitative results described in the literature differ considerably. The knee is one exception; for it, much data exist. Three general types of studies have been performed. The first is ligament stress under nearly physiologic conditions in joints with preserved ligament structures. The next is determination of individual ligament rupture strength on isolated ligaments with bony attachments preserved; this is an established method because most ruptures occur at sites of insertion and seldom are intraligamentary. Finally, isolated ligaments are used to determine specific ligamental properties such as modulus of elasticity, extensibility, and relaxation parameters which must be measured without the influence of anchorage.

With normal range of motion, the force-strain characteristics of the medial and lateral collateral ligaments (MCL and LCL) can be assessed with and without abduction, adduction, or torsional influences (Fig. 1). In the MCL, tension is maximal at full extension. Between 0° and 25° of flexion this force is borne primarily by the dorsal portion. Forces are minimal between 25° and 80° and then greatly increase in the ventral portion until a maximum is reached at full flexion. An abduction moment of 4,000 N · mm increases the tensile forces to about 3 times normal (Fig. 2).

In the LCL, tensile forces gradually decrease with flexion and reach zero at 40° of flexion (Fig. 1). An adduction moment of 4,000 N · mm increases the tensile force to a peak at 70° of flexion and then decreases it to near zero at 135° (Fig. 2). Strains measured during these studies were not proportional to the forces; therefore, strain measurements do not permit quantitative statements about loads on ligaments.

Force-strain diagrams can be generated that allow several determinations (Fig. 3). The maximum of the curve is defined as the rupture strength. The force at the linear limit indicates the load at which stress is reversible without damage to the ligament. Greater forces cause disruption of individual ligament structures without causing total rupture, until the rupture force is reached. The strain at linear

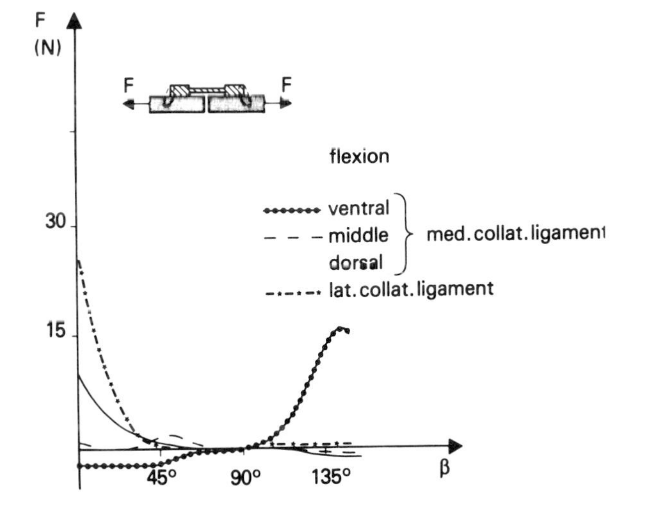

Figure 1

Tensile force as a function of the angle of flexion. (From Claes, L. Aktuel. Probl. Chir. Orthop. 26:10–17, 1983. By permission of Hans Huber Publishers.)

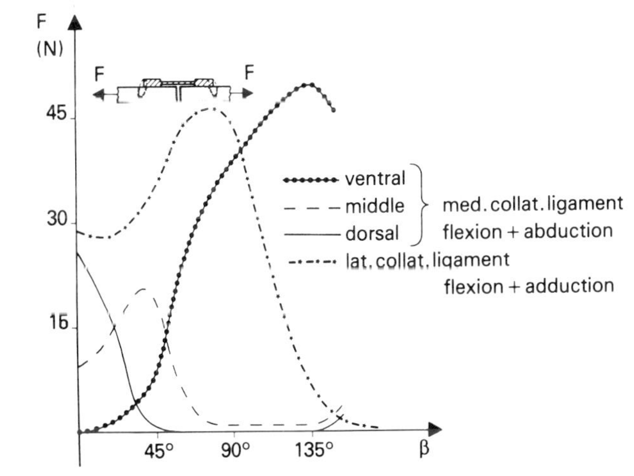

Figure 2

Ligament tensile forces as a function of flexion angle under abduction and adduction moments of 4,000 N · mm. (From Claes, L. Aktuel. Probl. Chir. Orthop. 26:10–17, 1983. By permission of Hans Huber Publishers.)

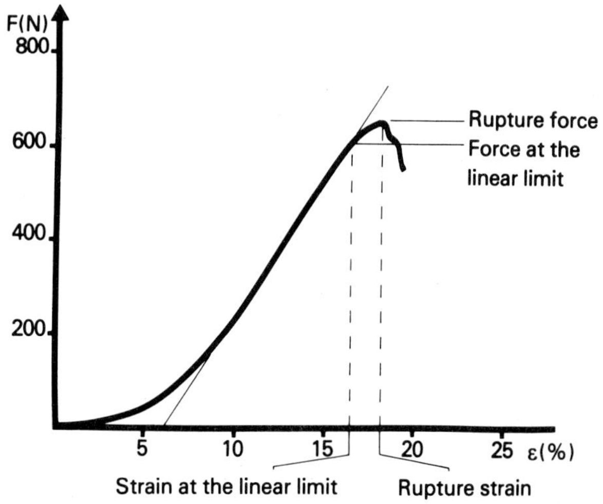

Figure 3

Characteristic force-strain diagram of a test for tensile strength on human knee ligaments. (From Claes, L. Aktuel. Probl. Chir. Orthop. 26:10–17, 1983. By permission of Hans Huber Publishers.)

limit and rupture strain provide a measure of the extensibility of the ligaments.

Stiffness is defined as the quotient of force and absolute strain; it is the slope of the force deformation graph. It characterizes the biomechanical properties in a way similar to calculations of modulus of elasticity but dispenses with calculations of cross-sectional area (Fig. 4).

The rupture forces of the various knee ligaments are shown in Table 1, rupture strains are in Table 2, forces at the linear limit are in Table 3, strains at the linear limit are in Table 4, and stiffnesses are in Table 5. These tables, summarizing the findings by various authors, show that there are distinct differences in the rupture forces of the various ligaments. The highest values are reported for the posterior cruciate ligament (PCL). The weakest ligament of the knee is the LCL. Rupture strains show no distinct differences in relation to ligament type. Stiffness of the cruciate ligaments is approximately twice that of the collateral ligaments although there is no difference between the cruciates. Young ligaments are stronger and stiffer than older ligaments.

Cyclic loading experiments have shown that an increase

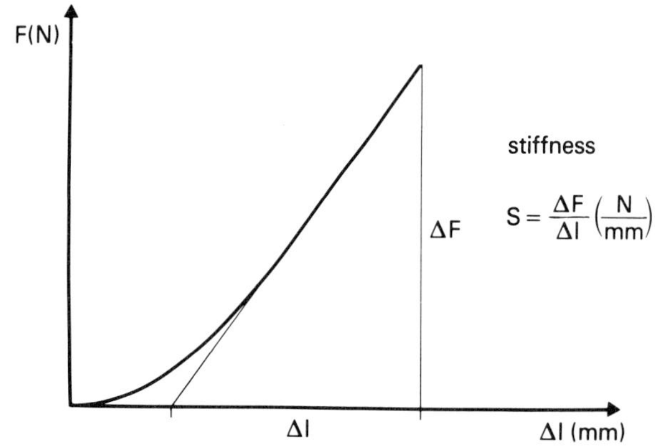

Figure 4

Definition of ligament stiffness. (From Claes, L. Aktuel. Probl. Chir. Orthop. 26:10–17, 1983. By permission of Hans Huber Publishers.)

in load velocity leads to increases in stiffness, modulus of elasticity, and rupture strength and a decrease in strain. These studies indicate that ligaments can store deformation energy under dynamic load and release it in phases of relief. The ligaments thus are in a position to decrease peak loads and absorb impacts to the knee joint.

Stents

Stents are meant to function as internal splint devices while the effects of secondary procedures are gaining strength or, in some cases, are actual permanent replacements for damaged or lost ligaments and tendons.

Proplast Tendon Transfer Stabilizer

The Proplast ligament currently consists of a high-strength core of polyaramid fiber (a high-strength chemically and thermally stable aromatic polyaramid), embedded in fluorinated ethylene/propylene polymer (FEP, a melt processable perfluorocarbon polymer of extreme chemical and thermal inertness) that is coated with the Proplast tissue ingrowth stabilizing material (a porous, low-modulus composite of tetrafluoroethylene polymer [PTFE] and either graphite or aluminum oxide). The actual ligament replacement shown in Figure 5 is the Mark III model, a rectan-

Table 1. Rupture Force*

	Force, N			
	Collateral ligaments		Cruciate ligaments	
	Medial	Lateral	Anterior	Posterior
Kennedy et al.	477±34	—	482±28	940±48
Trent et al.	526	384	633	571
Claes	654.2±151.9	354±139	—	—
Noyes et al.:				
Old	—	—	734±266	—
Young	—	—	1,730±660	—
Tremblay et al.	—	—	530	670
Piziali et al.	—	—	350–620	1,315–1,745
Noyes	—	—	475	927

*From Claes, L. Aktuel. Probl. Chir. Orthop. 26:10–17, 1983. By permission of Hans Huber Publishers.

Table 2. Rupture Strain*

	Strain, %			
	Collateral ligaments		Cruciate ligaments	
	Medial	Lateral	Anterior	Posterior
Kennedy et al.	23.0±24.0	—	30.8±23.0	28.3±19.0
Claes	18.15±3.48	20.89±7.55	—	—
Noyes et al.:				
Young	—	—	44.3±85.0	—
Old	—	—	30.0±10.0	—
Noyes	—	—	30.8	28.3

*From Claes, L. Aktuel. Probl. Chir. Orthop. 26:10–17, 1983. By permission of Hans Huber Publishers.

Table 3. Force at the Linear Limit*

	Force, N			
	Collateral ligaments		Cruciate ligaments	
	Medial	Lateral	Anterior	Posterior
Kennedy et al.	463±32	—	402±28	813±51
Claes	538±165	258±133	—	—
Noyes et al.:				
Young	—	—	1,170±750	—
Old	—	—	622±283	—
Noyes	—	—	396.5	801.0
Tremblay et al.	—	—	470.0	—

*From Claes, L. Aktuel. Probl. Chir. Orthop. 26:10–17, 1983. By permission of Hans Huber Publishers.

gular structure consisting of the polyaramid fabric/FEP polymer composite core throughout its length with the middle third coated with PTFE and entirely hyperflexible. An integral leader is present to facilitate implantation, with preplaced staple holes in the proximal and distal segments that are coated with Proplast II (PTFE and aluminum oxide). This device is a temporary internal splint; it eventually breaks or disintegrates. The Proplast ligament has a projected functional life of 36 months. When used as an anterior cruciate ligament (ACL) replacement, late failure typically occurs suddenly and dramatically, with rupture of the intra-articular portion of the ligament. Most cases required removal of the ligament but, in some cases, knee function continued adequately despite the presence of the ruptured intra-articular prosthesis.

Current use is supplemented with secondary procedures. Those most often performed medially with anterior cruciate stents are semimembranous advancement, posterior medial capsular reefing, MCL advancement, pes plasties, or revisions. On the lateral side, posterior lateral reefing, some form of iliotibial band transfer, biceps advancement, and forward displacement of the bony attachments of the popliteus and fibular collateral ligament with arcuate ligament tightening are performed.

With posterior cruciate stents, multiple adjunct procedures are used, the most common of which are semimembranous transfer and gastrocnemius tendon transfer, posterolateral reefing including repair of the arcuate system, and reconstruction of lateral functional deficits.

The postoperative routine includes use of a long leg cast with a pelvic support belt for 4 weeks, at which time a hinged cast with 30° to 60° limited motion is placed. Total immobilization is for 7 to 8 weeks, followed by routine rehabilitation.

The usual fixation method is by the "over the top" technique of MacIntosh or one of its modifications. A raw bony surface is provided to allow tissue ingrowth. The drill hole placement is crucial to prevent breakage of the stent and allow ingrowth. Figure 6 shows the stents in place for the ACL and PCL. As a salvage for severely injured knees, when the alternative is arthrodesis or total knee replacement, the above-described procedures have produced satisfying results in 80% of the 110 patients reviewed.

Table 4. Strain at the Linear Limit*

	Strain, %			
	Collateral ligaments		Cruciate ligaments	
	Medial	Lateral	Anterior	Posterior
Kennedy et al.	19.6±1.7	—	29.9±2.0	20.7±1.9
Claes	9.0±1.8	10.4±3.5	—	—
Noyes et al.:				
Young	—	—	25.5±8.1	—
Old	—	—	21.9±6.9	—
Noyes	—	—	22.9	20.7
Tremblay et al.	—	—	25.0	30.0

*From Claes, L. Aktuel. Probl. Chir. Orthop. 26:10-17, 1983. By permission of Hans Huber Publishers.

Table 5. Stiffness*

	Stiffness, N/mm			
	Collateral ligaments		Cruciate ligaments	
	Medial	Lateral	Anterior	Posterior
Trent et al.	72	62	141	183
Claes	93.9 ± 20.6	47.4 ± 12.6	—	—
Noyes et al.:				
Old	—	—	129 ± 39	—
Young	—	—	182 ± 56	—

*From Claes, L. Aktuel. Probl. Chir. Orthop. 26:10-17, 1983. By permission of Hans Huber Publishers.

Gore-Tex Prosthetic Ligament

The Gore-Tex prosthetic ligament is a permanent implant intended for repair of chronic instabilities. It is pure PTFE expanded to form a structure consisting of solid nodes of PTFE interconnected by strong, highly oriented PTFE fibrils. It has very high tensile strength, contains 75% air by volume, and has fibrils averaging 60 μm in length. Due to its inertness, it is not subject to biochemical degradation, nor do its mechanical properties degrade with time. The material is sufficiently porous to allow ingrowth from surrounding fibrous and osseous tissue. In its original form, the Gore-Tex ligament was manufactured in a continuous woven strand 16 to 18 cm long that ended in a loop for screw fixation to bone. This configuration has been replaced by a multifilament design constructed of bundles of fibers arranged in a braided fashion in the body of the device to optimize load distribution, with eyelets at each end for fixation.

The biomechanical characteristics of Gore-Tex are excellent, with a mean ultimate strength of 4,830 ± 280 N at a strain rate of 2.6% sec^{-1}. In torsional and bending fatigue tests, minimal elongation takes place over a 50-year equivalence of cyclic tests. The immediate intraoperative fixation strength is 1,824 ± 566 N.

The relative stiffness of the Gore-Tex ligament may result in a slight laxity of the knee when placed in 90° of flexion. However, because maximal loads on the ACL occur with the knee in full extension, this appears to be inconsequential. Tests in sheep have demonstrated good biocompatibility. Histologic studies in dogs have shown ingrowth of osseous and fibrous tissue in bone tunnels and attachment sites. In addition, synovium-like tissue was attached to some portions of the intra-articular segments. As with other ligaments, with Gore-Tex there tends to be fragmentation, wear, and abrasion at the entrance to bony tunnels. This can be minimized by adherence to strict surgical placement of the holes and adequate beveling of their edges.

To date, 130 human ACL reconstructions have been reported with up to 15 months of follow-up; 129 of these have shown improved stability.

As with any permanent implant that does not encourage fibrous ingrowth replacement or is not supplemented with autogenous tissue, late fatigue failure would appear to be a serious concern.

Xenotech

The Xenotech ligament is a bioprosthesis made of bovine tendon treated with glutaraldehyde, a material used in tanning leather. Glutaraldehyde increases the strength of collagen by cross-linking the fibers, thereby making the collagen stronger, nonallergenic, and more flexible. This type of material was first used in humans in the form of glutaraldehyde-treated porcine heart valves for replacing damaged human valves. It was designed to act as a permanent replacement, not a scaffolding or an augmentation device.

Animal studies have shown excellent biocompatibility, with no evidence of rejection phenomena. Histologic evaluations of the implants demonstrated a progressive ingrowth of host tissues into the xenograft. These host tissues grew parallel to the collagen fibers of the graft and consisted of blood vessels and fibroblastic elements. Resorption of the xenograft material is not seen.

As of January 1985, 424 grafts have been placed in humans. Discussion of the preliminary results at the 11th annual meeting of the American Orthopaedic Society for Sports Medicine indicated a 3% infection rate and a 7.6% complication rate. There was no evidence of immune response or adverse tissue reaction. Occasionally, a synovitis

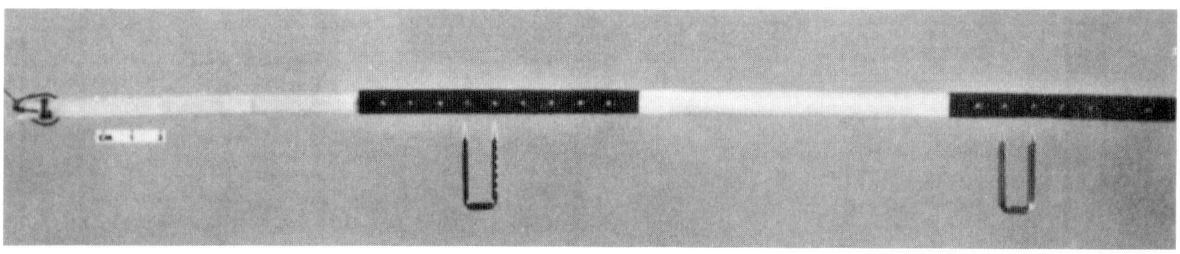

Figure 5

Proplast cruciate ligament implant. (From Homsy, C.A.; Prewitt, J.M., III; and Woods, G.W. Aktuel. Probl. Chir. Orthop. 26:52–57, 1983. By permission of Hans Huber Publishers.)

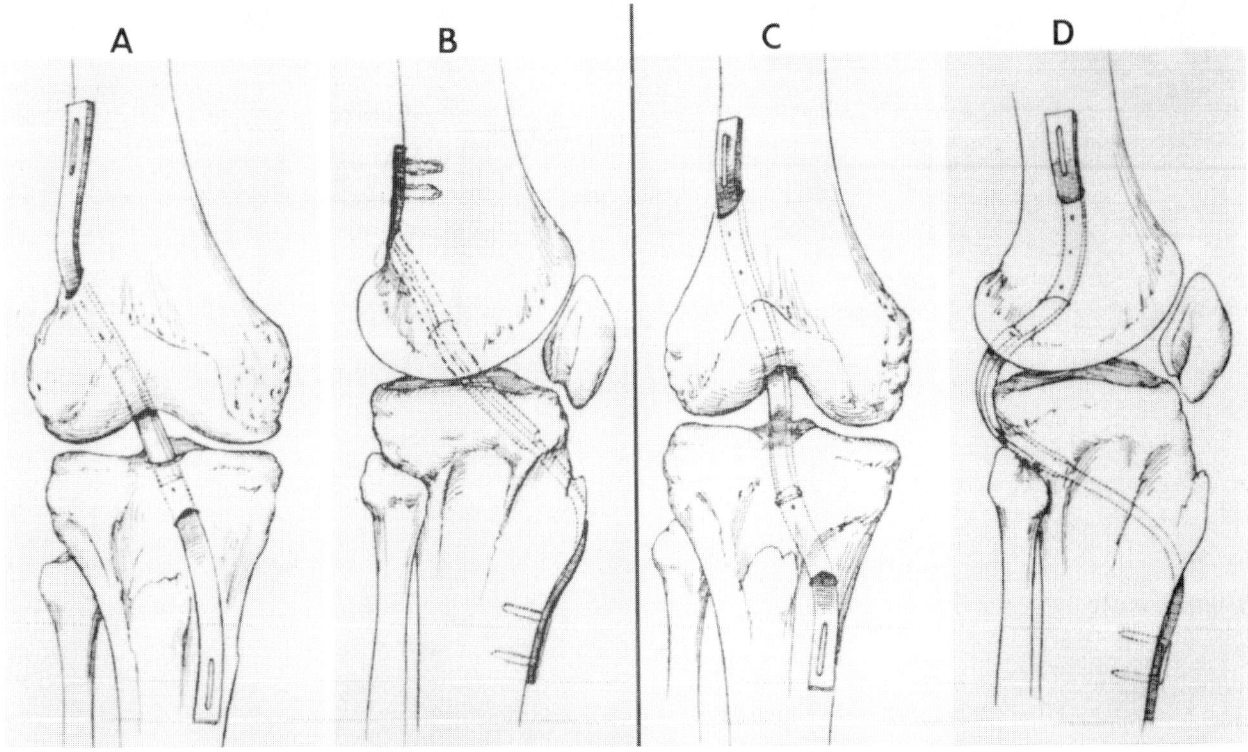

Figure 6
Anterior (*A* and *B*) and posterior (*C* and *D*) cruciate stents. *A* and *C*, Anteroposterior views. *B* and *D*, Lateral views. *A*, Stent in proper position, utilizing tunnel through lateral femoral condyle. *B*, "Over the top" method. (From James, S.L.; Kellam, J.F.; Slocum, D.B.; and Larson, R.L. Aktuel. Probl. Chir. Orthop. 26:116–120, 1983. By permission of Hans Huber Publishers.)

was encountered associated with particulate matter from an abraded graft. This was thought to be a response to a mechanical irritant and consistent with findings in other studies with different prosthetic material. Information is not yet available concerning biomechanical characteristics or implant and fixation techniques.

Polyester

Polyester bands have been used for various applications in medicine for some time and their tissue compatibility has been proven. They are now being used in clinical trials for ligament replacement.

One such replacement is a textile band of braided polyethylene terephthalate, 20 cm long and 10 mm wide, sterilized by gamma irradiation. It has been used to reconstruct knees that have chronic instability of the anteromedial or anterolateral type and have failed prior surgical procedures. A combined cruciate and collateral reconstruction using the "one-ligament" technique is performed. This technique requires a single bony attachment for anterolateral instability and two points for anteromedial instability. Anchorage is achieved by creating a small osteoperiosteal flap with a chisel; the ligament end is placed under this. The flap is then fixed with a small fragment screw or a Kirschner wire. For ACL/MCL repairs, the ligament is routed posteriorly over the lateral femoral condyle subperiosteally into the knee joint. It is then passed through a tibial bone tunnel made in the plateau to the medial tibial condyle, paralleling the usual course of the ACL. Finally, the polyester band is placed in the bed of the MCL extra-articularly and is secured beneath a second bone flap in the medial femoral condyle. ACL/LCL replacements are performed in a similar fashion using a single attachment site. The ligament is routed posteriorly over the lateral femoral condyle subperiosteally into the joint and then into a tibial bone tunnel, this time to the lateral tibial condyle. Subsequently, the band parallels the LCL and both ends of the ligament are anchored beneath the bone flap in the lateral femoral condyle.

Detailed biomechanical property studies are not available for this device; however, limited clinical experience indicates that the results of replacement of ligaments with polyester bands are generally comparable to those achieved with autologous pedunculated or free tissue transplants with regard to band stability and total function. The major concern here is the same as for any replacement that does not result in collagenous replacement of the graft material by ingrowth—i.e., ultimate failure of the device.

Ligament Augmentation Devices

Ligament augmentation devices are intended to function as internal splints to protect autogenous repairs during ischemic and revascularization phases. Most of the different alloplastic materials described in this report could be used in this fashion; however, most trials have utilized Dacron, carbon fiber, or polypropylene. An extensive coverage of carbon fiber follows later, so it will not be discussed here.

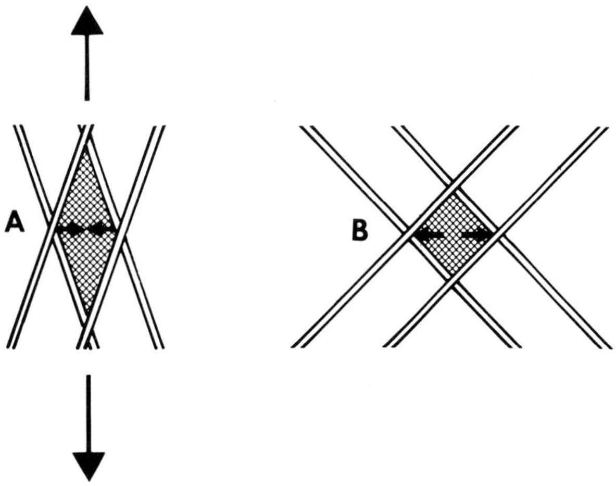

Figure 7

Biomechanical model for demonstration of elastic behavior of ligament replacement with carbon fibers and connective tissue. *A,* Ligament under load. *B,* Ligament after load removed. (From Claes, L., and Neugebauer, R. Aktuel. Probl. Chir. Orthop. 26:58–62, 1983. By permission of Hans Huber Publishers.)

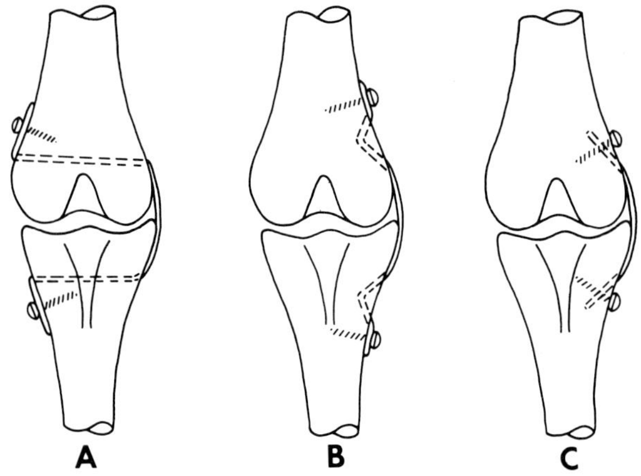

Figure 8

Intraosseous methods of anchorage for replacement of the medial collateral ligament of the knee. *A,* Intracondylar anchorage. *B,* Borehole anchorage medial. *C,* Flake anchorage medial. (From Claes, L., and Neugebauer, R. Aktuel. Probl. Chir. Orthop. 26:58–62, 1983. By permission of Hans Huber Publishers.)

Polypropylene

The Kennedy ligament augmentation device (LAD) is constructed of nine tows (or strands) of high-tenacity (8 g/denier) polypropylene yarn, with each tow containing 180 fibers. These tows are braided into a flat strap-like structure 6 mm wide by 1 mm thick. The ends are heat-sealed to prevent unraveling.

Histologic studies have shown a typical chronic foreign body response at the periphery of the implant. Fibers are often apposed by a cuff of mononuclear or foreign body giant cells surrounded by vascular fibrous tissue. There is no evidence of deep penetration of the graft by fibrous ingrowth; only the outermost two or three fibers show fibroplasia with deposits of collagen.

Biomechanical tests have been encouraging. The tensile strength of ligament is 1,513 ± 14 N, which is equivalent to the strength of young human knee ligaments. With cyclic loading in fatigue tests, the strength decreases only 9% after 500,000 cycles and then remains constant through 1,000,000 cycles. The intraoperative strength of the ligament including anchorage points falls to 364 N, indicating that fixation is the strength-limiting factor.

Dacron

Dacron has a long history of clinical use and an excellent record of biocompatibility. It has had FDA approval for several years for acromioclavicular reconstruction. The current implant consists of four high-strength Dacron tapes enclosed in a loosely woven Dacron velour sleeve designed to promote tissue ingrowth. It is twice as strong and twice as stiff as the normal ACL. *In vitro* testing has shown good fatigue strength, but in animal models it was shown to fray or wear at the entrance or exit from bone tunnels. *In vivo* experiments have documented fibrous tissue ingrowth into both the intra- and extra-articular portions of the device.

Fixation has been by means of staples at the proximal and distal attachments with dependence on later tissue ingrowth for long-term stabilization. One animal study had disappointing results with a high failure rate of the implant. In addition, in those animals in which the implant did not fail, Dacron-augmented central-third patellar reconstructions (modified Jones type) had an ultimate tensile strength of only 75% of that of unaugmented central-third reconstructions in the contralateral limb. The authors' conclusion was that the Dacron implant stress-shielded the autogenous patellar tendon transfer, thereby leading to its resorption.

Histologic studies show fibrous tissue ingrowth into the velour envelope to infiltrate between the filaments of Dacron in the inner core. Augmentation with iliotibial band or central patellar tissue enhances this ingrowth. Some investigators state that autogenous repairs augmented by Dacron have improved immediate stability and strength that increases with time as ingrowth occurs.

Biodegradable Tissue Scaffoldings

Biodegradable scaffoldings provide immediate stability for the joint at the time of operation. Subsequently, they serve as a framework upon which fibrous tissue grows, thus replacing the device. As this infiltration occurs, the artificial ligament is gradually degrading; eventually, the load is transferred to the new ligament. By far, the greatest volume of literature concerning soft tissue implants involves carbon fiber or polylactic acid (PLA)-coated carbon fiber.

Carbon Fiber

Carbon fiber has been studied as an orthopaedic implant since the mid 1970s. It has excellent tissue compatibility. In regard to providing immediate stability and subsequently degrading slowly as collagen and fibrous tissue grow in, carbon fiber has been promising to date.

Except for a few studies that have shown lymph node uptake of carbon particles draining from implant sites, no significant tissue reactions have been found. No significant negative effect of the lymph node uptake has been noted.

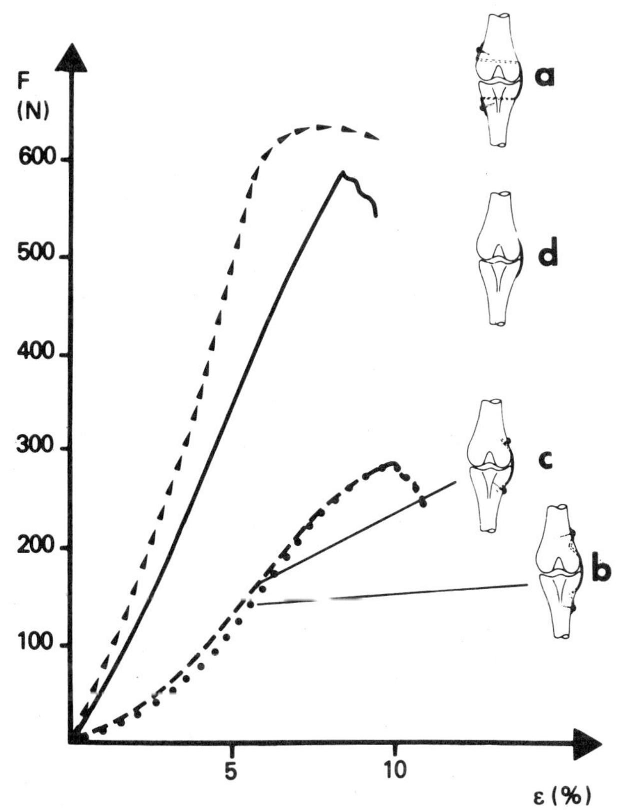

Figure 9

Stress-strain behavior of the replacement of the medial collateral knee ligament in sheep at 12 weeks after operation. Curves: a, intracondylar anchorage; b, bore-hole anchorage medial; c, flake anchorage medial; d, normal medial collateral ligament. (From Claes, L., and Neugebauer, R. Aktuel. Probl. Chir. Orthop. 26:58–62, 1983. By permission of Hans Huber Publishers.)

Biomechanically, carbon fiber has shown very compatible characteristics. The properties of the implanted ligament depend upon its construction. A carbon fiber consists of pure carbon in a graphite structure. The fibril has a diameter of 7 to 8 μm and is thinner than a hair. When loaded to the point of rupture, the fibrils display only elastic deformation; there is no plastic deformation. Fatigue loading does not produce creep. Due to the anisotropic layer structure of the fiber, the shear strength perpendicular to the longitudinal axis of the fiber is poor. This means that high-shear stresses occurring when the fibers are bent over sharp edges can break the carbon fibrils.

Braiding the carbon fibers improves the elastic properties of the implant. A type A ligament made of 32 tows with 3,000 filaments each and a 43° interbraid angle had an average tensile rupture strength of 2,461 ± 238 N. This is roughly 3 times the rupture strength of native knee ligaments. The elasticity of this type A fiber is 0.63% at 300 N. A type H. S. fiber consists of 96,000 fibrils aligned uniaxially. It has a strain of only 0.02% at 300 N. Natural ligaments show a strain of 10% to 20% at this load.

The elasticity of the braided carbon fiber ligament increases after implantation to nearly equal that of the native ligament. This is due to fibrous ingrowth between the braided fibrils that can be compressed and then recoiled (Fig. 7). In addition, the viscoelastic properties of the anchorage site increase the elasticity.

In cadaver knees with mechanical anchorage only and no bioingrowth, tensile tests showed an average breaking force of 434.3 ± 122.0 N. The native MCL of the same knee had a rupture force of 650 ± 154 N. Thus, intraoperative anchorage can be expected to reach 66% to 89% of the strength of the natural ligament. In *in vivo* tests in sheep with the three anchorage techniques in Figure 8, after 12 weeks of implantation the intracondylar anchorage was stronger than the natural ligament (Fig. 9). The extensibility of the implanted ligament after 12 weeks was similar to that of the native ligament (Fig. 9).

To date, 63 knees with chronic ligament laxity have been treated with flexible carbon fiber and reported. Excellent or good results were achieved in 67%, and function improved from that preoperatively in 71%. A lack of correlation between subjective instability and objective physical signs was noted frequently. Combined collateral cruciate repairs and collateral repairs as isolated procedures gave better results than intra-articular (cruciate) reconstructions. Collateral replacements became infiltrated with collagen tissue which takes over the role of a new ligament. Arthroscopic and histologic examinations of biopsy specimens of intra-articular reconstructions showed that infiltration of collagen tissue into the carbon fiber occurred at a slower and less predictable rate. This is presumably due to the rich mesenchymal environment in the extra-articular site that provides precursor cells. The presence of these precursor cells in sufficient number and activity intra-articularly is less certain. There was no clinical or macroscopic evidence of synovitis in the series, but synovial irritation was noted microscopically.

PLA-Coated Carbon Fiber

In an attempt to improve the handling characteristics, decrease the migration of carbon particles, and protect the ligament in intra-articular applications, polylactic acid (PLA) has been used to coat the fiber tows. PLA, a biodegradable polyester, has been widely used as a component of suture material (Vicryl; Ethicon Inc.). It undergoes grad-

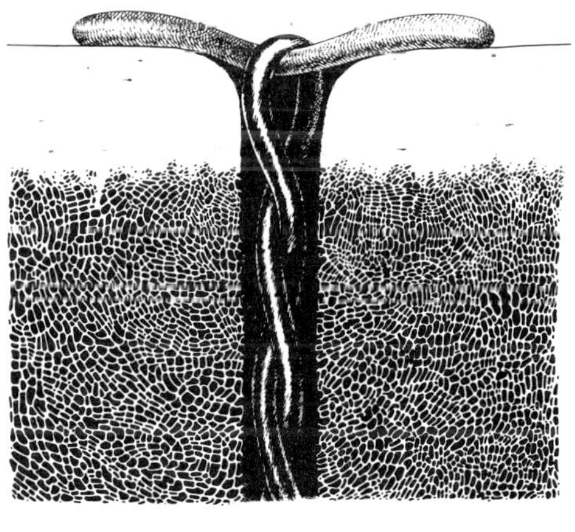

Figure 10

Toggle anchoring a terminal loop of carbon fiber tow. (From Strover, A.E. Aktuel. Probl. Chir. Orthop. 26:127–134, 1983. By permission of Hans Huber Publishers.)

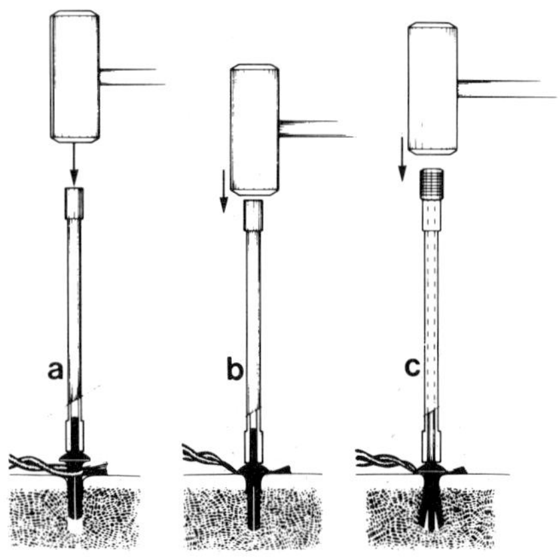

Figure 11

Bollard. *a*, The bollard introduced into a beveled hole. *b*, It is punched down firmly with the mallet and punch tube. *c*, The bollard is expanded by using the bollard punch to advance its central pin. (From Strover, A.E. Aktuel. Probl. Chir. Orthop. 26:127–134, 1983. By permission of Hans Huber Publishers.)

ual hydrolytic de-esterification to lactic acid; then, it is subsequently metabolized to carbon dioxide and water. PLA has been found to be biocompatible and elicits no immune response, probably due to the absence of peptide linkages. A typical tow contains 10,000 fibers, each 6 to 8 μm in diameter; the fibers of the tow are dipped in a dilute solution of PLA in chloroform. As the chloroform evaporates, the PLA is left coating the tow. This process can be used to coat either uniaxial tows or braided implants. Histologic studies in dogs similar to those that showed carbon particle migration in uncoated carbon trials revealed no lymph node uptake of carbon from PLA-coated fibers.

Furthermore, in extra-articular applications, the fibers have shown collagenous ingrowth at the periphery of implants by 2 weeks, infiltration by 4 weeks, and PLA degradation by 8 weeks. The PLA has not delayed ingrowth but seems to protect the ligament implants from fragmentation and particle migration. By 12 months, the new collagen fibers are nearly identical to normal tendon fibers as seen by scanning electron microscopy, with no inflammatory or giant cell reaction. Carbon fibers are still present but are fragmented and contained within the neoligament.

Biomechanical characteristics are similar to those of uncoated fibers both *in vivo* and *in vitro*.

Several clinical trials have recently been reported. One group reported improved stability in 58 of 64 patients undergoing reconstruction with braided type A fibers coated with collagen to improve handling. The intra-articular portion was wrapped with a sheet of dura or fascia lata to protect it from the intra-articular environment and to provide a mesenchymal cell pool. This technique has shown improved bioingrowth.

Another group has reported 82 patients who had an iliotibial band "over-the-top" reconstruction; there was significant improvement in stability, pain, function, and strength with follow-up of 24 months with carbon-PLA-polycaprolactone composites (copolymer carbon fiber).

Two other investigators have reported promising preliminary results in 30 patients undergoing late reconstruction for chronic laxity with a combined ACL lateral complex reconstruction using central-third quadriceps, central-third patellar tendon, and prepatellar tissue, augmented with PLA carbon fiber.

In different composition, these materials are being explored as possible bone plates and intramedullary devices for fracture fixation. In this application, the composite would function as a temporary prosthesis rather than a scaffold; it would be rigid upon implantation but then gradually degrade and avoid the stress-prevention atrophy that results from the currently available metallic devices. Additional advantages include radiolucency, no need for surgical removal, and excellent biocompatibility.

New anchorage techniques are being developed to allow ease of application of these prostheses and firm fixation that permits ingrowth from bone and soft tissues. One such system uses a toggle and a bollard, as shown in Figures 10 and 11, made of carbon fiber composite.

Annotated Bibliography

Biomechanical Properties of Human Ligaments

Claes, L.: Biomechanical properties of human ligaments. Aktuel. Probl. Chir. Orthop. 26:10–17, 1983.

Biomechanical properties of human ligaments are described with the knee as a test model. Literature reports are summarized in tabular form covering rupture force, rupture strain, force at linear limit, stiffness, and viscoelastic properties.

Stents

Bolton, C.W., and Bruchman, W.C.: The GORE-TEX™ expanded polytetrafluoroethylene prosthetic ligament: An *in vitro* and *in vivo* evaluation. Clin. Orthop. 196:202–213, 1985.

New design characteristics and preliminary results in 130 patients with up to 15 months of follow-up are discussed.

Bolton, W., and Bruchman, B.: Mechanical and biological properties of the GORE-TEX expanded polytetrafluoroethylene (PTFE) prosthetic ligament. Aktuel. Probl. Chir. Orthop. 26:40–51, 1983.

The Gore-Tex ligament is evaluated and data on yield strength, creep, elongation recovery time, fatigue life, and modulus of elasticity are provided. Early, limited-protection mobility is possible. Fixation techniques are described; in addition to implant method, these are crucial to satisfactory long-term performance.

Homsy, C.A.; Prewitt, J.M., III; and Woods, G.W.: Proplast knee ligament implants: Design and in vitro testing. Aktuel. Probl. Chir. Orthop. 26:52–57, 1983.

The Proplast ligament is described, including its evolution and design characteristics. No clinical results are presented.

James, S.L.; Kellam, J.F.; Slocum, D.B.; and Larson, R.L.: The Proplast prosthetic ligament stent as a replacement for the cruciate ligaments of the knee. Aktuel. Probl. Chir. Orthop. 26:116–120, 1983.

The Proplast ligament is evaluated and its evolution is described. Operative techniques of knee ligament reconstruction for ACL, PCL, LCL, MCL, and combined ligament injuries are detailed, as well as postoperative management. The conclusion is that this prosthetic ligament is useful for salvage of severely injured knees when the alternative would be arthrodesis or total joint replacement.

McMaster, W.C.: A histologic assessment of canine anterior cruciate substitution with bovine xenograft. Clin. Orthop. 196:196–201, 1985.

The bovine xenograft ACL replacement is discussed; benign host response without cellular evidence of rejection is described. Host tissue ingrowth with blood vessels and fibroblastic elements also occurs.

Mockwitz, J., and Contzen, H.: Alloplastic correction of chronic knee ligament instability with polyethylene terephthalate. Aktuel. Probl. Chir. Orthop. 26:110–115, 1983.

Eleven patients underwent knee ligament reconstruction with polyester bands. The results are comparable to those after autologous tissue transfers. These authors thought polyester reconstruction should be used only if autologous tissue is not available.

Ligament Augmentation Device

Andrish, J.T., and Woods, L.D.: Dacron augmentation in anterior cruciate ligament reconstruction in dogs. Clin. Orthop. 183:298–302, 1984.

Dacron augmentation of a central-third patellar tendon repair of the ACL in dogs is presented. The hypothesized protection during the revascularization phase of healing was not proved. Nearly half of the augmented repairs performed significantly poorer than the central-third-repaired unaugmented contralateral limbs.

McPherson, G.K.; Mendenhall, H.V.; Gibbons, D.F.; Plenk, H.; Rottman, W.; Sanford, J.B.; Kennedy, J.C.; and Roth, J.H.: Experimental mechanical and histologic evaluation of the Kennedy ligament augmentation device. Clin. Orthop. 196:186–195, 1985.

The Kennedy ligament augmentation device is described, including biomechanical characteristics and histologic studies in the goat model.

Park, J.P.; Grana, W.A.; and Chitwood, J.S.: A high-strength Dacron augmentation for cruciate ligament reconstruction: A two-year canine study. Clin. Orthop. 196:175–185, 1985.

One of four Dacron-augmented knee reconstructions was performed in each of 48 adult dogs. Histologic studies are discussed. An over-the-top technique with intra- and extra-articular components using augmented fascia lata was most effective.

Biodegradable Scaffoldings

Alexander, H.; Weiss, A.B.; and Parsons, J.R.: Absorbable polymer-filamentous carbon composites: A new class of tissue scaffolding materials. Aktuel. Probl. Chir. Orthop. 26:78–91, 1983.

A new PLA-coated carbon fiber implant was tested in the dog. Results of biocompatibility and biomechanics studies are reported. Additionally, a series of 30 patients who received PLA-coated carbon fiber replacements is presented and future trends are discussed.

Aragona, J.; Parsons, J.R.; Alexander, H.; and Weiss, A.B.: Medial collateral ligament replacement with a partially absorbable tissue scaffold. Am. J. Sports Med. 11:228–233, 1983.

In an animal model, MCL repair with PLA-coated carbon fiber is shown to be better than ligament healing with scar and no repair.

Claes, L.; Burri, C.; Neugebauer, R.; Wolter, D.; and Rose, P.: The influence of various carbon fibre braiding techniques and methods of fixation on the extensibility of ligament prostheses. Biomaterials 4:134–136, 1983.

The number of carbon fiber tows and the type of braid and braid angle affect the elasticity of alloplastic carbon implants. The best results were found with a fiber made of 32 tows and a braid angle of 43°. The type of fixation contributes more to the elasticity than does the strand itself.

Claes, L., and Neugebauer, R.: Mechanical properties of ligament replacement with carbon fibres. Aktuel. Probl. Chir. Orthop. 26:58–62, 1983.

Assessments of number of tows, braiding technique, and anchorage of the prosthesis are described. The conclusions are that carbon fibers are as strong as stainless steel, small-diameter fibrils allow braiding and increase the flexibility, the resulting ligament is 2 to 3 times stronger than the natural ligament, connective tissue growth between the braided fibers increases elasticity, and intraosseous anchorage increases the rupture strength up to 107% of that of a natural ligament.

Leyshon, R.L.; Channon, G.M.; Jenkins, D.H.R.; and Ráliš, Z.A.: Flexible carbon fibre in late ligamentous reconstruction for instability of the knee. J. Bone Joint Surg. 66B:196–200, 1984.

Sixty-three knees with chronic ligament instability treated with flexible carbon fiber are reviewed. Use as an intra-articular cruciate replacement should be reserved for extremely unstable knees with multiple ligament laxities. In this type of knee, combined collateral and cruciate replacement is valuable in improving knee stability.

Nixon, A.J.; Stashak, T.S.; Smith, F.W.; and Norrdin, R.W.: Comparison of carbon fibre and nylon suture for repair of transected flexor tendons in the horse. Equine Vet. J. 16:93–102, 1984.

For simple flexor tendon lacerations, PLA-coated carbon fiber composites are no better than simple nylon suture repair. Histologic studies of the prosthesis are presented showing fibrous ingrowth.

Strover, A.E.: Technical advances in the reconstruction of knee ligaments using carbon fibre. Aktuel. Probl. Chir. Orthop. 26:127–134, 1983.

Instruments and techniques for carbon fiber reconstruction of the ACL, PCL, MCL, LCL, and combined ligament deficiencies are described as used in 150 patients. No results are presented.

Weiss, A.B.; Blazina, M.E.; Goldstein, A.R., and Alexander, H.: Ligament replacement with an absorbable copolymer carbon fiber scaffold: Early clinical experience. Clin. Orthop. 196:77–85, 1985.

Acute and chronic knee instability in 82 patients was treated with copolymer carbon fiber reconstruction, with 24-month follow-up. The surgical technique of augmenting an over-the-top iliotibial band transfer with carbon fiber is described.

Witvoet, J., and Christel, P.: Treatment of chronic anterior knee instabilities with combined intra- and extra-articular transfer augmented with carbon-PLA fibers. Clin. Orthop. 196:143–153, 1985.

Clinical results in 30 patients are encouraging after PLA-coated carbon fiber reconstruction of chronic knee instability with a combined intra- and extra-articular augmented MacIntosh type technique.

Reviews

Claes, L.; Burri, C.; Neugebauer, R.; Piehler, J.; and Mohr, W.: Animal experiments for comparison of various alloplastic materials in ligament replacements. Aktuel. Probl. Chir. Orthop. 26:101–107, 1983.

This article reviews some of the various materials currently used in ligament replacement including: Teflon, polyester, polyaramid, and carbon fiber in repair of the MCL in sheep. The authors felt that carbon fiber was the most suitable material to date.

Kennedy, J.C.: Application of prosthetics to anterior cruciate ligament reconstruction and repair. Clin. Orthop. 172:125–128, 1983.

A summary article reviewing the use of stents, degrading scaffolding replacement, and ligament augmentation devices. The conclusion was that further clinical testing is necessary prior to widespread use of any of these modalities.

13
Microsurgery

During the 1970s, microsurgery was drawing a great deal of attention from both the lay public and the medical world. As the techniques became more refined and results more predictable, the indications for microsurgical procedures expanded. In the late 1970s and early 1980s, we were bombarded with new "free tissue transfers." However, once surgeons began evaluating their postoperative results critically, the indications for these microsurgical procedures became better delineated. Within the last 3 years, we have seen the application of basic microsurgical techniques to many difficult clinical problems that previously were thought to be hopeless, such as massive soft tissue loss in trauma, osteomyelitis, osteonecrosis of the femoral head, and the failed nerve repair. In nearly every case, this new technology has led to better clinical results in these situations.

Microsurgical Technique

Little progress has been made in refining microsurgical techniques for the repair of small blood vessels or nerves. The ability to repair such structures still seems to be limited to those with a diameter of at least 0.3 mm.

There has been some research into vein grafting techniques. In free tissue transfers, the length of the vascular pedicle frequently will be inadequate for primary anastomosis of the recipient vessels to the normal donor vessels. In these cases it has been the practice of most microsurgeons to use a reversed vein graft. The techniques for obtaining and maintaining patency of these vein grafts had not been investigated extensively. Recently, however, it was demonstrated that, by using subcutaneous and perivenous infiltration of the surrounding tissues with papaverine coupled with atraumatic dissection technique and controlled distention of the vein, one could improve vein graft patency rates. In addition, storage of harvested vein grafts in cold heparinized *blood* containing papaverine produced grafts with improved endothelial preservation, and theoretically this should also improve patency rates. With the combination of these techniques, the surgeon should be able to achieve a much higher patency rate in the very small vein grafts used for microvascular surgery.

Monitoring Techniques

Despite a lack of change in basic microsurgical technique for repairing small blood vessels, great progress has been made in monitoring techniques. Monitoring techniques were developed so that one could ascertain whether or not an anastomosis was patent. In the past, once the skin or muscle was closed over the anastomosis, a free flap or free tissue transfer had been monitored by observing skin color, the temperature of the flap, capillary refill, and bleeding characteristics of the flap after stabbing. All of these were subjective determinants, and one easily could be misled. More recently, laser Doppler velocimetry, transcutaneous oxygen measurements, and tissue pH monitoring have been advocated for monitoring free tissue transfers.

Transcutaneous Oxygen Measurements

The technique of transcutaneous oxygen measurement uses an O_2 sensor which must be firmly attached to the surface of the replanted part or to the free flap. This sensor must be kept at a constant temperature of 42°C to provide reliable data. If the temperature of the sensor is too high, a superficial skin burn will occur beneath the sensor; if the temperature is too low, the data obtained are unreliable. In free tissue transfers, the body Po_2 must be mapped out in the donor area before operation because the values may vary in different anatomic regions of the body. After replantation or free tissue transfer, the Po_2 is monitored constantly.

In addition, every 1 or 2 hours the patient is subjected to an O_2 response test. During this test, for a 5-minute period the patient inhales 100% O_2 delivered at 4 liters/min. If the anastomosis is patent, an increase in Po_2 is detected (Fig. 1). Conversely, absence of an increase in Po_2 *usually* indicates a lack of blood flow. This test can be quite useful if the technique is followed meticulously (the temperature of the probe is critical). This test also requires the

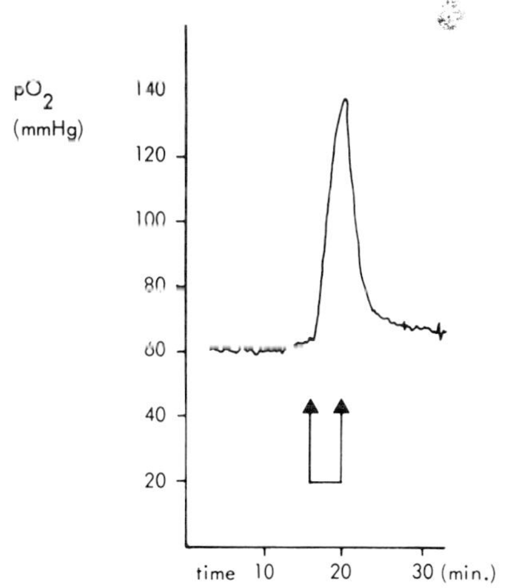

Figure 1

Oxygen response test. (From Smith, A.R.; Sonneveld, G.J.; Kort, W.J.; and van der Meulen, J.C. J. Hand Surg. 8:139–145, 1983. By permission of the American Society for Surgery of the Hand.)

patient's cooperation for the inspiration of 100% oxygen. For this reason, the technique is not completely usable in the comatose or heavily sedated patient.

Tissue pH Measurement

For years it has been known that, with vascular ischemia, there is a rapid decrease in tissue pH. With the availability of continuous pH monitoring systems, originally designed for use in the neonate, it was only natural that this technology be applied to patients undergoing replantation or free tissue transfers. A pH sensor is introduced into the replanted or transplanted part through a 1-mm stab wound and is then held at a depth of 3 mm within the tissue. When *arterial* occlusion occurs, there is a precipitous decrease in pH; with *venous* occlusion, the decrease is much slower (Fig. 2). Some investigators found this monitoring technique useful and reliable in a small series (nine patients) of different free tissue transfers. In their hands, this technique seemed to give earlier warnings of impending problems than did clinical judgment alone.

Laser Doppler Velocimetry

By attaching the laser Doppler, an instrument that emits visible red light through a single optical fiber, to the skin, one can measure the quantity of *moving* erythrocytes in the skin. The device is based on the fact that moving erythrocytes produce a shift in reflected light which can be measured; stationary erythrocytes produce no such shift. At first glance, this would seem to be a useful technique for assessing capillary blood flow in replanted parts. However, it was found that in a clinical setting this device could be fallible and was not an accurate indicator of tissue profusion.

Comment

It appears that these new devices available for monitoring have some usefulness but thus far the ideal device—which would be simple, cheap, reliable, and easy to apply—has not yet been discovered. Table 1 compares various monitoring techniques.

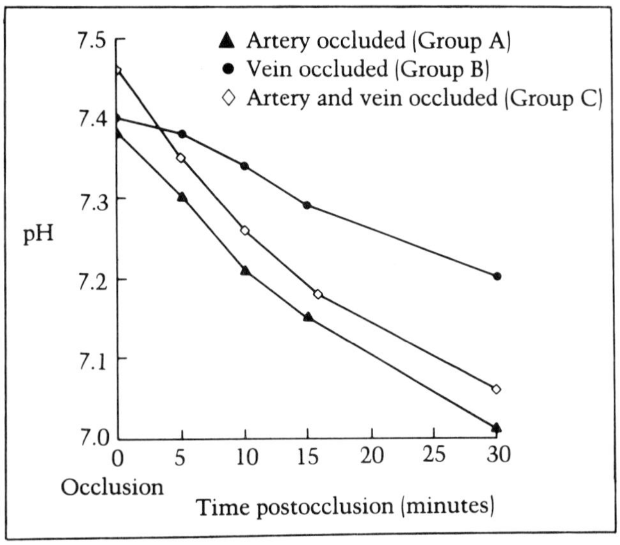

Figure 2

Effect of vascular occlusion on tissue pH. (From Raskin, D.J.; Erk, Y.; Spira, M.; and Melissinos, E.G. Ann. Plast. Surg. 11:331-339, 1983. By permission of Little, Brown and Company.)

Free Flaps

Fasciocutaneous Flaps

One of the most exciting developments in microvascular surgery in the last few years has been the discovery of the fasciocutaneous system for supplying blood to the skin. The blood supply to skin was originally described by Manchot in 1889, yet it was not until 1973 that McGregor called attention to the difference between axial and random pattern flaps. His work led to our present understanding of the direct cutaneous system of blood vessels that supply the skin.

With the work of Ger in 1967, we came to understand the myocutaneous system in which vessels to the skin arise in the muscle and then pass up perpendicularly to the skin, enabling the surgeon to elevate vast quantities of skin on a single blood vessel. This technique requires that one also take the muscle with the skin flap.

In 1981, Poten gave us the third system of blood supply to the skin—the fasciocutaneous system. In the fasciocutaneous system, perforators pass up to the superficial surface of the skin in fascial septae that are located between muscle bellies (Fig. 3). These fascioseptal or fasciocutaneous vessels then fan out at the level of the deep fascia and form a plexus that supplies the overlying skin. In addition, the blood supply to this skin frequently has directionality; this will allow reversal of blood flow while still preserving the skin flap—i.e., the radial arm flap.

Several investigators have studied the fasciocutaneous flaps of the upper arm in great depth. They have demonstrated that these flaps may be unidirectional (as in the medial arm flap where the blood supply is via an end artery) or they may be bidirectional (as in the lateral arm or Chinese forearm flap where the blood supply may enter from either end). The advantages of these new fasciocutaneous flaps over cutaneous or myocutaneous flaps are quite apparent: 1) the skin territory to be raised on a single vessel may be quite large, 2) there is no need to sacrifice a usable muscle as must occur with a myocutaneous flap, 3) the flap is quite thin and one need not even take the overlying skin (as an example, the superficial temporal artery flap which is only fascial) and in fact these fasciocutaneous flaps are especially useful in conjunction with tendon and joint repairs in which gliding is imperative, and 4) many of the fasciocutaneous flaps contain sensory nerves and can thus be innervated (i.e., the lateral arm, dorsalis pedis, and lateral thigh flaps). Although it is not anticipated that the fasciocutaneous flap will supplant the myocutaneous flap in usefulness, these new flaps will surely become adjuncts for the microvascular surgeon.

In the upper extremity, the lateral arm flap has been used quite successfully; the donor defect is minimal. There has also been a great deal of experience gained with the radial arm (Chinese) flap; this is useful but leaves a large donor defect and, preferably, the radial artery should be reconstructed with a vein graft. For the lower extremity, the anatomy and use of the free fasciocutaneous thigh flaps—both medial and lateral—have been described. This is the most common donor area for split-thickness skin grafts

Table 1. Monitoring Techniques

Method	Ease of use	Reliability	Continuous	Cost
Observation (color, capillary refill)	Easy	Good	Yes	Low
Temperature	Easy	Fair	Yes	Low
Laser Doppler	Hard	Poor	Yes	High
Transcutaneous Po_2	Hard	Good	No	High
Tissue pH	Easy	Good	Yes	Low

and may become the most common donor site for a fasciocutaneous free flap. The pedicle to the thigh flap is long and large, and the flap itself encompasses a large skin territory. The recently described posterior calf fasciocutaneous free flap may prove useful but the donor defect is great and the dissection is quite difficult. The ulnar artery forearm free flap has been used for harvesting tendon and bone with skin. Even though this flap may be taken and used without reconstruction of the ulnar artery, it seems to offer no advantages over other flaps and has several disadvantages compared with other current techniques.

To assess the usefulness of innervated free flap, a Japanese group studied seven cases of dorsalis pedis free flaps transferred to the hand with sensory reconstruction done simultaneously. In no case was epicritic sensibility restored to the flap. Thus, one must question the continued search for free flaps that can be transferred as an innervated free tissue transfer.

Myocutaneous Flaps

Just as virtually any area of skin may be transferred by microvascular techniques, so can any muscle be moved. This ability to transfer whole muscles has provided a means for closure of many difficult wounds. The heel, which in the past frequently was covered with an unstable split skin graft, now may be covered by a plantar myocutaneous island pedicle flap, thus eliminating the need for free flaps to this area. Sacral defects due to trauma or developmental anomalies may be covered by gluteus maximus myocutaneous flaps that are rotated into these large defects. The elbow has always been a difficult area in which to obtain skin coverage because of the elbow's poor blood supply and unique bony anatomy. Many have advocated a free flap to obtain skin coverage for the elbow. Recently, however, the external oblique fasciocutaneous flap has provided a good alternative to free tissue transfer in many patients with open elbow joints.

Intrathoracic and extrathoracic chest wounds that are infected or are in irradiated skin portals have always been extremely difficult areas in which to provide skin coverage. This is made more difficult by the fact that latissimus dorsi has usually been sacrificed at the time of initial thoracotomy. There also may have been damage to the pectoralis major at the time of thoracotomy. In these most demanding circumstances, the serratus anterior, rotated as a muscle pedicle, has provided an alternative solution to the management.

For lower extremity reconstruction, especially for proximal-third open tibial fractures, the medial gastrocnemius muscle flap rotated on its vascular pedicle can provide a means of obtaining soft tissue coverage (Fig. 4). This myocutaneous flap can only be used in the proximal third of the tibia because its vascular pedicle is very short. Recently, use of this muscle distally has been extended by releasing the muscle proximally from the femur and extending the skin and soft tissue distally so that a distal advancement of 8 cm is possible. This should enhance the usefulness of this pedicle island flap in difficult fractures of the middle third of the tibia.

The patient with a type III open fracture of the tibia

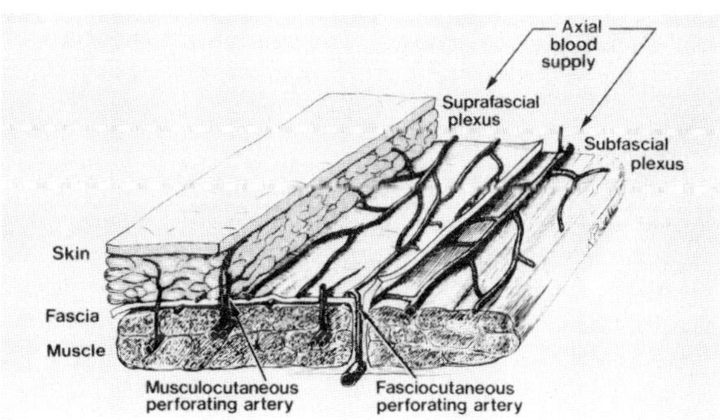

Figure 3

Fasciocutaneous free flap. (From Walton, R.L., and Bunkis, J. Plast. Reconstr. Surg. 74:76–85, 1984. By permission of the American Society of Plastic and Reconstructive Surgeons.)

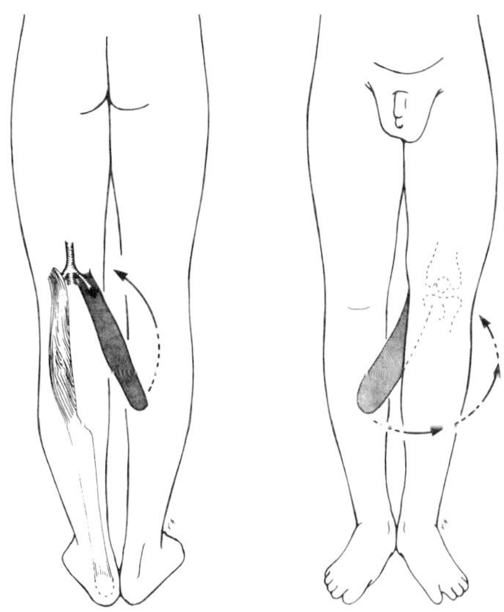

Figure 4

Medial gastrocnemius muscle flap. Muscle blood supply is proximal to popliteal crease; arc of rotation allows coverage for proximal third of tibia. (From Mathes, S.J., and Nahai, F.: Clinical Atlas of Muscle and Musculocutaneous Flaps, p. 146. St. Louis, C.V. Mosby Company, 1979. By permission of the publisher.)

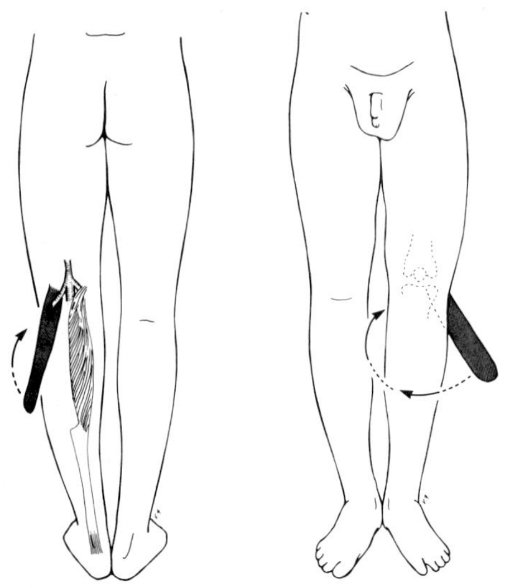

Figure 5

Lateral gastrocnemius muscle flap. Blood supply enters proximally, allowing rotation to front of tibia. (From Mathes, S.J., and Nahai, F.: Clinical Atlas of Muscle and Musculocutaneous Flaps, p. 148. St. Louis, C.V. Mosby Company, 1979. By permission of the publisher.)

presents a challenge not only in terms of bone healing but also in terms of soft tissue coverage. Knowledge of the muscles of the lower leg as well as their intrinsic blood supply is usually all that is necessary to plan a rotational flap (myocutaneous or muscle alone) which, in the majority of cases, will cover defects of the proximal and middle thirds of the tibia. The muscles most useful for this purpose are the medial and lateral gastrocnemius and the soleus—occasionally the flexor digitorum longus will be needed to complete coverage of a distal wound (Figs. 4, 5, and 6). Open fractures of the distal third of the tibia are the most difficult in which to obtain skin coverage because of the paucity of muscles available for rotational flaps; it is this area where the free cutaneous, myocutaneous, fasciocutaneous, or osteocutaneous flaps are of most value; these difficult procedures are best left to those with adequate microvascular surgical experience.

Bone

Debate continues about the timing of skin coverage in the treatment of open fractures. Many advocate immediate coverage of all open fractures to prevent desiccation of bone and its natural consequence—osteomyelitis. Others have proposed delaying closure of all open wounds until the surgeon is sure that there is no infected or necrotic material which will be buried. A review of type III open fractures of the tibia has demonstrated that if wound coverage was achieved within 7 days after injury there was a wound healing problem in only 20% of cases but when coverage was achieved between days 8 and 30 there was an 83% complication rate. In this series, there was also a shortening of the time to union in patients with immediate coverage: 4 months in patients undergoing early coverage and 6.4 months in the late reconstruction group. This paper should convince most orthopaedic surgeons of the advantage of early muscle coverage as an adjunct in the treatment of type III open fractures of the tibia.

Osteomyelitis

Because of encouraging reports on the use of muscle flaps in the treatment of chronic osteomyelitis and the subsequent excellent results obtained with the use of free muscle transfer in treating chronic osteomyelitis, there has been renewed interest in the treatment of this difficult disease. In a recent experience with local muscle pedicle flaps for osteomyelitis in 42 patients, 39 showed no evidence of infection for 2 years or more after operation. However, despite eradication of the infection, 22 patients required further operation to achieve bony union. These results are quite favorable compared with historical data on chronic osteomyelitis.

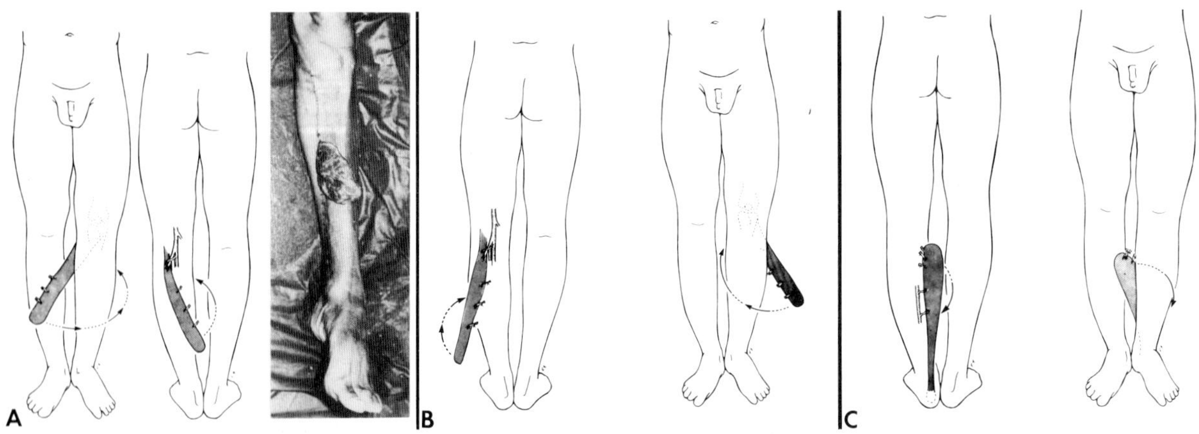

Figure 6

Soleus muscle flap. Dominant vascular pedicle is proximal; with ligation of minor distal pedicles, muscle can be transposed laterally (*A*) or medially (*B*). Less reliable, the major pedicle is ligated and the flap is rotated on minor inferior arteries (*C*). (From Mathes, S.J., and Nahai, F.: Clinical Atlas of Muscle and Musculocutaneous Flaps, p. 162–164. St. Louis, C.V. Mosby Company, 1979. By permission of the publisher.)

Some centers have approached this problem of patients with osteomyelitis not amenable to a local muscle flap by using free muscle or myocutaneous flaps. In general, the more extensive disease process requires soft tissue and full debridement or ablation. In 33 patients in whom a myocutaneous free flap was used after radical debridement for the treatment of osteomyelitis, at a mean follow-up of 41.4 months there was recurrent sepsis in 20%; 80% of the patients had no evidence of recurrent disease although many of them were candidates for amputation prior to the free muscle transfer. Thus it appears that muscle transfer, whether through pedicle graft or free flap, does offer significant help to patients with chronic osteomyelitis.

Free Bone Transfer

The most common donor sites for free osseous transfers in the past have been rib, anterior iliac crest, and fibula. In 1985, the osteo or osteomyocutaneous free flap from the posterior iliac crest was first described. This important new free bone transfer allows the use of an 8 by 13 cm piece of bone from the posterior iliac crest region. The vascular pedicle for this free flap is a posterior branch of the superior gluteal artery. This new flap may prove to be quite useful because it allows a much larger and thicker piece of corticocancellous bone to be transferred than is possible from the anterior iliac crest. The dissection of this posterior iliac flap should prove easier than the dissection for the anterior flap and should eliminate the complications of abdominal hernia that are occasionally seen after anterior iliac crest transfer.

One of the early drawbacks to the use of the vascularized transfer of the fibula was the lack of a good skin island to accompany the bone transfer. This meant that, in severe trauma, soft tissue coverage must precede bone repair. However, this problem seems to have been solved by Chinese workers who have described a 10 by 20 cm skin flap that can be raised with the fibula and also is based on the peroneal artery. This new skin flap requires the sacrifice of a minimal amount of muscle and should greatly enhance use of the free fibula as a single-stage reconstruction in patients who are missing both cortical bone and soft tissue.

Free Nerve Transfer

Free vascularized neural transfer has not been universally accepted, primarily because an adequate donor site has yet to be found. In surgery for complete brachial plexus palsy, use of the ulnar nerve with its ulnar artery may have some advantages over nonvascularized nerve grafts in terms of early healing, but the ulnar nerve would be available only occasionally for free neural transfer. The anatomy and the surgical dissection of a free vascularized sural nerve have been reported. This free tissue transfer is based on the cutaneous perforator vessels from the peroneal artery or the muscular perforating branch of the posterior tibial artery supplying the sural nerve. This free neural transfer has several advantages over other free neural transfers: 1) the sural nerve is quite long and the nerve may be divided and folded upon itself to yield a much larger nerve with two or three cables still based on one vascular bundle; 2) a skin flap may be taken with the nerve so that, by monitoring the skin, one can be sure that the underlying nerve is alive; and 3) the sensory deficit from loss of the sural nerve is minimal and well tolerated by most people. The efficacy of free vascularized nerve grafts has yet to be substantiated clinically. Thus, conventional sural nerve grafting remains the primary way of overcoming a large neural defect.

Free Muscle Transfer

One of the biggest advantages of microsurgery has been the ability to transfer whole muscles on a single neurovascular pedicle. Initially this technique was used only for myocutaneous free flaps when the muscle was transferred only to ensure skin survival. Subsequently, investigators documented the usefulness of a free *functioning* muscle transfer. This technique has proved to be useful for facial paralysis and as a replacement for fibrotic muscles after Volkmann's ischemic contracture. The most commonly used muscles for this purpose are the gracilis and pectoralis major; however, many situations exist in which a smaller muscle with greater excursion would be more useful.

It has also been demonstrated that a fascicular territory exists within a muscle and that the muscle may be divided safely along individual single motor fascicles (Fig. 7). This single motor fascicle within a given muscle has two distinct advantages for the reconstructive surgeon: many times, only a small portion of the muscle need be taken and after the splitting off of only what is needed the remaining body of the muscle is left as a functioning unit; and the entire muscle may be removed but the different fascicular territories in the muscle may be individually innervated by individual motor nerves, which will then allow independent contraction within a single muscle. This technique of individual innervation has been used successfully in replacing the multiple muscles for facial renervation as well as in achieving independent replacement of finger flexor and thumb flexor function in patients with Volkmann's contracture. Certainly, the future of free muscle transfer looks extremely promising with this new technique.

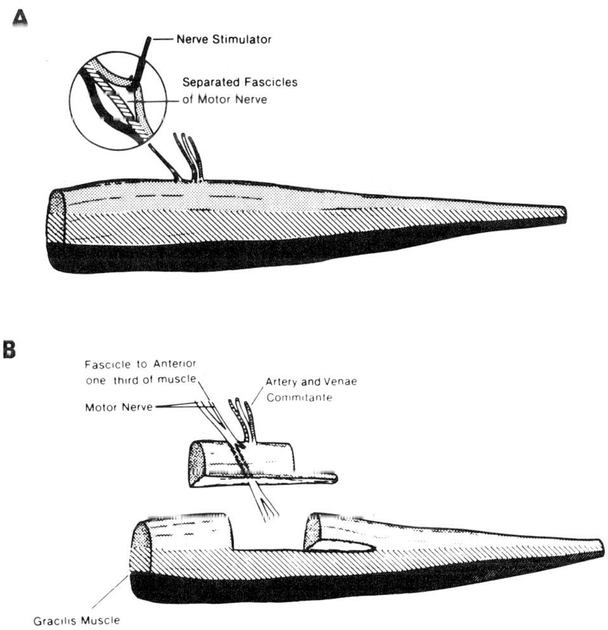

Figure 7

Division of gracilis for small free muscle transfer. *A*, Motor nerve is separated in fascicles, and each fascicle is stimulated to identify its territory of contracting muscle. *B*, Motor territory of a single fascicle for transfer. (From Manktelow, R.T., and Zuker, R.M. Plast. Reconstr. Surg. 73:751–755, 1984. By permission of the American Society of Plastic and Reconstructive Surgeons.)

Annotated Bibliography

Adcock, O.T., Jr.; Adcock, G.L.D.; Wheeler, J.R.; Gregory, R.T.; Snyder, S.O., Jr.; and Gayle, R.G.: Optimal techniques for harvesting and preparation of reversed autogenous vein grafts for use as arterial substitutes: A review. Surgery 96:886–893, 1984.

The technical aspects of vein graft harvesting can make a large difference in postoperative patency rates. Techniques for tissue dissection, types of irrigation and storage solutions used, temperature of the solutions, distention pressure, and pharmacologic agents are described in detail.

Arnold, P.G.; Pairolero, P.C.; and Waldorf, J.C.: The serratus anterior muscle: Intrathoracic and extrathoracic utilization. Plast. Reconstr. Surg. 73:240–248, 1984.

Use of the anterior serratus as a rotational flap to cover infected intrathoracic and extrathoracic chest wounds is described clearly.

Baek, S.-M.: Two new cutaneous free flaps: The medial and lateral thigh flaps. Plast. Reconstr. Surg. 71:354–363, 1983.

This is an anatomic description of the medial thigh flap raised on a direct branch of the superficial femoral artery and the lateral thigh flap based on the third branch of the deep femoral artery. Both allow large free tissue transfers with reliable vascular pedicles.

Baksi, D.P.: Treatment of post-traumatic avascular necrosis of the femoral head by multiple drilling and muscle-pedicle bone grafting: Preliminary report. J. Bone Joint Surg. 65B:268–273, 1983.

When combined with excision and drilling of osteonecrosis of the femoral head, muscle-pedicle bone grafting can be effective in slowing or preventing further collapse of the femoral head in many cases. This technique is also applicable when osteonecrosis is complicated by nonunion.

Chen, Z.-W., and Yan, W.: The study and clinical application of the osteocutaneous flap of fibula. Microsurgery 4:11–16, 1983.

Demonstration of the technique for using the inclusion of skin and subcutaneous tissue when harvesting a free fibular bone graft is described. It allows for the single transfer of 10 by 20 cm areas of skin within the same vascular territory as the free bone transfer alone.

Cheng, H.H.; Rong, G.W.; Yin, T.C.; Wang, H.Y.; and Jiao, Y.C.: Coverage of wounds in the distal lower leg by advancement of an enlarged medial gastrocnemius skin flap. Plast. Reconstr. Surg. 73:671–677, 1984.

By releasing the gastrocnemius both proximally and distally and taking a random portion of skin on the distal end of the flap, this rotational pedicle flap can be extended to allow coverage of the distal leg. By utilizing this mobilization technique, one is able to advance the flap distally 8 cm.

Cierny, G., III; Byrd, H.S.; and Jones, R.E.: Primary *versus* delayed soft tissue coverage for severe open tibial fractures: A comparison of results. Clin. Orthop. 178:54–63, 1983.

A well-controlled comparison between primary and delayed coverage of grade III open tibia fractures demonstrated that fewer complications and quicker union occurred with primary coverage.

Cormack, G.C., and Lamberty, B.G.: Fasciocutaneous vessels in the upper arm: Application to the design of new fasciocutaneous flaps. Plast. Reconstr. Surg. 74:244–250, 1984.

The currently popular lateral arm flap based on the middle collateral artery as a terminal branch of the deep brachial artery is described. Anatomic designs of the flap are discussed; no cases are included.

Cormack, G.C., and Lamberty, B.G.: Fasciocutaneous vessels. Their distribution on the trunk and limbs, and their clinical application in tissue transfer. Anat. Clin. 6:121–131, 1984.

Fasciocutaneous flaps are based on a relatively new anatomic concept: The vessels that supply the skin pass along *fascial* septa between adjacent muscles. The distribution of these fasciocutaneous flaps on the trunk and limbs is described.

Cummings, C.W.; Trachy, R.E.; Richardson, M.A.; and Patterson, H.C.: Prognostication of myocutaneous flap viability using laser Doppler velocimetry and fluorescein microfluorometry. Otolaryngol. Head Neck Surg. 92:559–563, 1984.

Two instruments, microfluorometer and laser Doppler, that complement one another in assessing tissue viability are compared. The former is of greater clinical value for measuring flap perfusion in the period immediately after development of the flap; the latter is more capable of assessing blood flow 24 hours postoperatively.

Doi, K.; Kuwata, N.; Kawakami, F.; Tamaru, K.; and Kawai, S.: The free vascularized sural nerve graft. Microsurgery 5:175–184, 1984.

The anatomy of the blood supply to the sural nerve is demonstrated and the use of this vascularized sural nerve graft in three cases is described.

dos Santos, L.F.: The vascular anatomy and dissection of the free scapular flap. Plast. Reconstr. Surg. 73:599–603, 1984.

The cadaveric dissection that led to the discovery of the cutaneous branch of the circumflex scapular artery and thus to the development of the free scapular flap.

Fisher, J.: External oblique fasciocutaneous flap for elbow coverage. Plast. Reconstr. Surg. 75:51–59, 1985.

This is a good pedicle flap for covering the problem elbow. It is easy to raise, and requires only a Velcro shoulder immobilizer in the postoperative phase.

Fisher, J.; Arnold, P.G.; Waldorf, J.; and Woods, J.E.: The gluteus maximus musculocutaneous V-Y advancement flap for large sacral defects. Ann. Plast. Surg. 11:517–522, 1983.

When utilized bilaterally, this excellent myocutaneous pedicle flap will cover sacral defects 10 to 18 cm in diameter.

Fitzgerald, R.H., Jr.; Ruttle, P.E.; Arnold, P.G.; Kelly, P.J.; and Irons, G.B.: Local muscle flaps in the treatment of chronic osteomyelitis. J. Bone Joint Surg. 67A:175–185, 1985.

Local muscle flaps can be used to treat large defects of soft tissue and bone after adequate debridement of their osteomyelitic regions. This technique was successful in eradicating the infectious process in 93% of the patients studied who were followed for a minimum of 2 years.

Jones, B.M.: Monitors for the cutaneous microcirculation. Plast. Reconstr. Surg. 73:843–850, 1984.

An excellent overview of the monitors that are available both clinically and in the laboratory. Based on this review, it appears that the thermistor is the best technique currently available. An implantable probe probably holds the best hope for the future.

Lovie, M.J.; Duncan, G.M.; and Glasson, D.W.: The ulnar artery forearm free flap. Br. J. Plast. Surg. 37:486–492, 1984.

A new fasciocutaneous free flap based on the ulnar artery has the advantage that it does not contain hair and one can take a portion of the tendons of ulnar flexor muscle of the wrist, the long palmar muscle, and ulnar bone with the flap.

Manktelow, R.T., and Zuker, R.M.: Muscle transplantation by fascicular territory. Plast. Reconstr. Surg. 73:751–755, 1984.

Division of the gracilis into smaller subunits based on a single nerve supply to a separate muscle fascicle is demonstrated. This technique allows for smaller free muscle transfer which is especially useful for fascial reanimation.

Mialhe, C., and Brice, M.: A new compound osteo-myocutaneous free flap: The posterior iliac artery flap. Br. J. Plast. Surg. 38:30–38, 1985.

A new osteomyocutaneous free flap is based on the superficial branch of the superior gluteal artery which harvests the posterior iliac crest and part of the greatest and middle gluteal muscles. A disadvantage of this flap is the short pedicle length; however, large (up to 8 cm) bony defects can be managed with this technique.

Raskin, D.J.; Erk, Y.; Spira, M.; and Melissinos, E.G.: Tissue pH monitoring in microsurgery: A preliminary evaluation of continuous tissue pH monitoring as an indicator of perfusion disturbances in microvascular free flaps. Ann. Plast. Surg. 11:331–339, 1983.

A useful technique for monitoring free flaps is described; the disadvantage is that it requires a stab wound into the flap for insertion of electrodes. It appears that this is a sensitive indicator of the micro blood supply.

Skef, Z.; Ecker, H.A., Jr.; and Graham, W.P., III: Heel coverage by a plantar myocutaneous island pedicle flap. J. Trauma 23:466–472, 1983.

This interesting technique for coverage of the heel uses a myocutaneous island pedicle flap that is innervated. This appears to be a difficult technique with minimal application.

Smith, A.R.; Sonneveld, G.J.; Kort, W.J.; and van der Meulen, J.C.: Clinical application of transcutaneous oxygen measurements in replantation surgery and free tissue transfer. J. Hand Surg. 8:139–145, 1983.

An excellent overview of the applicability of transcutaneous oxygen monitoring in replantation as well as free tissue transfers is provided. The oxygen response curve appears to be the most accurate predictor of flap viability.

Song, Y.G.; Chen, G.Z.; and Song, Y.L.: The free thigh flap: A new free flap concept based on the septocutaneous artery. Br. J. Plast. Surg. 37:149–159, 1984.

The anatomic considerations for this fasciocutaneous free flap are illustrated. This flap is similar to the tensor fascia lata free flap or the lateral thigh flap and offers no distinct advantages.

Takami, H.; Takahashi, S.; and Ando, M.: Use of the dorsalis pedis free flap for reconstruction of the hand. Hand 15:173–178, 1983.

An attempt to restore sensation to the mutilated hand was followed by the transfer of the free flap from the dorsal artery of the foot, with sensation to the flap preserved by utilizing the superficial peroneal nerve. No conclusion can be drawn from this report.

Walton, R.L., and Bunkis, J.: The posterior calf fasciocutaneous free flap. Plast. Reconstr. Surg. 74:76–85, 1984.

This flap removes all of the skin from the popliteal crease to the distal third of the calf; vessels are 1 to 1.5 mm in size and the flap can be well innervated with numerous sensory nerves. Although the flap is useful, the donor-site defect is significant.

Weiland, A.J.; Moore, J.R.; and Daniel, R.K.: The efficacy of free tissue transfer in the treatment of osteomyelitis. J. Bone Joint Surg. 66A:181–193, 1984.

These authors report a 20% recurrent sepsis rate after free tissue transfer for chronic osteomyelitis. Type 3 osteomyelitis is the most difficult to treat with this technique.

Yoshimura, M.; Imura, S.; Shimamura, K.; Yamauchi, S.; and Nomura, S.: Peroneal flap for reconstruction in the extremity: Preliminary report. Plast. Reconstr. Surg. 74:402–409, 1984.

A peroneal free flap that uses the large peroneal artery and vein and multiple fasciocutaneous perforators is described. This can be used either as a rotational flap or as a free flap.

14 Bone Grafts

Terminology

Bone grafts may be classified according to tissue composition (cortical, cancellous), anatomic considerations (site of origin, size, shape), blood supply (nonvascularized, revascularized), preservation method (fresh, frozen, freeze-dried), additional chemical or physical manipulations (demineralization, irradiation), genetics (Table 1), or combinations of these variables. Each aspect can influence biologic, immunologic, and biomechanical properties of the graft which, in turn, may affect clinical efficacy in specific circumstances (Table 2).

Although there is some rationale for designating viable osseous tissues as "grafts" (that are transplanted) and nonviable biologic preparations as "implants" (that are implanted), common usage has tended to lump both categories together as "grafts" with the appropriate descriptive adjectives appended—e.g., fresh revascularized segmental fibular autograft; freeze-dried irradiated cancellous wafer allograft; frozen distal femoral osteochondral allograft.

Biology

The process of bone graft incorporation represents a complex interaction of graft-derived and recipient-site factors. In general, grafts must be invaded by a blood supply that emanates from the host bed and carries with it cells that differentiate into bone resorbing (osteoclast) and bone-forming (osteoblast) populations. Osteoblasts are presumed to arise from stromal precursor cells found in the marrow; osteoclasts are derived from circulating monocytes of hematopoietic stem cell origin. The graft itself serves as a passive template for the influx of vascular and cellular activity (osteoconduction) and also may provide active signals to the host response capable of influencing, if not regulating, the process of incorporation (osteoinduction).

In addition to the local and systemic hormonal control of intact bone turnover (physiologic homeostasis, discussed elsewhere), there is evidence for the role of locally synthesized bone-derived growth factor(s) and matrix-associated bone morphogenetic protein (BMP). BMP is a low molecular weight (17,000–18,000) noncollagenous protein that is able to stimulate DNA synthesis and undifferentiated cell replication but does not appear to influence differentiated osteoblasts directly.

Table 1. Terminology of Genetic Relationships in Transplantation

Current (adjective)	Previous	Definition
Autograft (autogenous)	Autograft	Between sites in the same individual
Isograft (isogeneic) or syngraft (syngeneic)		Between genetically identical individuals
Allograft (allogeneic)	Homograft	Between members of the same species
Xenograft (xenogeneic)	Heterograft	Between different species

The final phase of bone graft incorporation is replacement of preexisting osseous tissue with host-derived osteogenic activity. This new bone eventually falls into the normal sequence of homeostatic remodeling (turnover), a process that responds to physiologic stresses—mechanical or biologic.

The precise mechanisms of graft incorporation and regulation are not completely understood, but the histologic patterns associated with the process have been characterized and found to vary somewhat with different types of graft material as well as with various local and systemic factors that affect the host bed.

Autografts

Nonvascularized Grafts The histologic pattern of repair observed with a nonvascularized bone autograft—that is, osseous tissue transferred without an intact blood supply and without immediate reanastomosis of its vascularity—begins with hematoma formation followed by gradual transformation into a fibrovascular response. These initial events are similar to fracture repair. Except for a small proportion of superficial bone-derived cells that survive by diffusion, the graft undergoes substantial necrosis and this, in turn, causes an inflammatory response within the contiguous fibrovascular stroma. Neovascularization and invasion of the graft by blood vessels arising from the host bed and fibrovascular tissues occur next. Up to this point, cortical and cancellous grafts behave in a similar fashion, but significant differences can be identified qualitatively and quantitatively as the process of incorporation proceeds.

Cortical Cortical grafts revascularize through preexisting haversian canals as well as through the bone periphery, and this vascular invasion requires a preceding wave of osteoclastic activity to remove necrotic cortex and widen vascular channels. Radiographically and mechanically, the graft becomes more porous and weaker. This normal physiologic trend is reversed as an osteoblastic response is established in the areas of prior resorption. Because the process spreads slowly throughout the graft, it has been described as "creeping substitution." As a rule, less than half of the preexisting cortex is replaced, but this is generally sufficient for biologic and biomechanical integrity. Once new bone is laid down, it becomes subject to normal ongoing remodeling.

Cancellous Cancellous bone is revascularized relatively quickly, reflecting the loose distribution of bony mass and intrinsic porosity. Osteoblastic activity ensues, laying down new bone on preexisting nonviable trabeculae. Resorption

Table 2. Summary of Advantages and Disadvantages of Different Types of Grafts

Graft type	Advantages	Disadvantages
Autografts:		
Fresh	Optimal biologic behavior No transfer of disease Histocompatible Best choice when donor site morbidity is acceptable and supply is sufficient	Donor site morbidity Limited availability Sacrifice of normal structures
Revascularized	Little dependence on host bed (e.g., irradiation, chemotherapy) Rapid healing	Technically difficult Limited availability of donor sites Sacrifice of normal structures
Allografts:		
Fresh	No preservation required Articular cartilage viable Particularly suited to joint resurfacing alone	Availability and need may not coincide Little time for proper laboratory tests for sterility or disease Most intense immune response
Frozen	Simple, but expensive long-term Permits cartilage cryopreservation Decreased immunogenicity No change in biomechanical properties Particularly suited to massive osteoarticular and segmental deficits	Requires careful screening of donors Cannot be sterilized secondarily Transit over long distances requires maintenance of freezing temperature Cartilage viability limited
Freeze-dried	Can store indefinitely at room temperature Easy transportation at room temperature Can recover clean and sterilize secondarily Compatible with demineralization Particularly suited to intercalary segmental loss or within cystic defects	Storage and preservation techniques expensive and complicated Structural changes Lengthy and perhaps less-reliable incorporation Incompatible with cartilage cryopreservation
Demineralized	Potent osteoinductor Easy to contour Particularly suited to cystic defects and small or irregular bony gaps or for supplementing stable fusions	Little intrinsic strength Complex processing

follows such that the dead bone is sandwiched between new bone (and results in a radiodense appearance) and is then gradually remodeled away. Cancellous bone is replaced more rapidly and completely than cortical grafts.

Comment The success of nonvascularized bone graft incorporation clearly reflects a satisfactory contribution of cells and blood supply from the host bed, and this is usually recognized clinically as a need for healthy soft tissue coverage of the graft at the time of transplantation. Conversely, various local and systemic factors may detract from the host contribution. For example, systemic chemotherapy that interferes with cell metabolism or replication will also curtail the availability of necessary osteogenic precursor cells at the graft site. Locally, irradiation causes soft tissue fibrosis, obliteration of small blood vessels, and interference with cell replication. Likewise, the inflammatory infiltrate associated with infection can block the cellular and vascular contributions of the recipient bed from effectively reaching the graft.

Vascularized Grafts Grafts transferred on their vascular pedicle or undergoing immediate reanastomosis of their blood supply do not experience cell necrosis or go through the sequence of events described for incorporation of a conventional nonvascularized graft. Instead, they unite to the adjacent skeleton in a fashion analogous to fracture repair (a relatively rapid process), and the bulk of the graft remains viable and continues to remodel. Consequently, there is no necrosis, no substantial unopposed matrix resorption, and no need to replace preexisting bone. This obviates the transient loss of mass and mechanical strength normal to nonvascularized graft incorporation. Similarly, the contributions of the recipient site are minimal, with the exception of the vascular pedicle, and vascular grafts can "survive" the otherwise unnurturing environment posed by radiation-induced changes.

Allografts

The use of allografts avoids potential donor site morbidity and overcomes the limitations in size, shape, and quantity of tissue inherent with use of autogenous sources. These advantages must be weighed against the possible transfer of disease from donor to recipient and the significance of immunologic responses associated with allografts. Immune rejection directed against vascular endothelium and osteogenic cells has precluded the clinical use of revascularized allografts. Attention therefore has focused on nonvascularized allografts and a wide variety of preservation techniques and clinical or physical manipulation of these grafts have been explored.

Freezing and Freeze-Drying The most common and apparently effective methods for bone graft preservation involve freezing or freeze-drying (lyophilization). Both approaches decrease immunogenicity (freeze-drying more so than simple freezing), and allografts preserved in these manners are biologically useful. The sequence of histologic events associated with use of preserved allografts is qualitatively similar to that with autografts, but quantitatively the nature of repair varies with the specific storage technique applied. In canine cortical graft models, approximately 20% of freeze-dried allografts are histologically and radiographically indistinguishable from autografts, 20% are associated with massive resorption and fragmentation, and 60% demonstrate an intermediate course characterized by a slow but successful incorporation that is often associated with delayed union and fracture of the segment. Observations in different animals with preserved cancellous allografts confirm the generally successful but delayed pattern of repair.

Freezing also provides an opportunity to cryopreserve intact articular cartilage. Dimethyl sulfoxide (8% to 10%) or glycerol protects the viability of 40% to 50% of the chondrocytes, and this appears to be sufficient to maintain the specialized matrix. Other recent approaches to cartilage grafting (repair of full-thickness articular defects) include the use of tissue-cultured chondrocytes in the presence of vitamin E and the use of perichondral grafts positioned over full-thickness articular defects. Preliminary results of each technique have been encouraging, but the ability of these grafts to withstand prolonged weight-bearing and normal joint function has not been confirmed.

Demineralized Matrix Preparations The use of demineralized matrix preparations has been explored over the past 20 to 30 years, starting with the pioneering observations by Urist. Bone that is either partially or completely demineralized remains a potent inducer of new bone, but at the sacrifice of structural properties. Certain proteins, including the bone morphogenetic protein (BMP), associated with the osseous matrix survive, and perhaps are even better expressed, after demineralization, and these bone morphogenetic factor(s) either directly stimulate osteogenesis or, more likely, induce or recruit precursors capable of differentiating into osteogenic cell populations. Isolation, purification, and synthesis of BMP have been the subjects of recent work but it remains incomplete.

Synthetic Bone Substitutes

Various synthetic hydroxyapatite and calcium phosphate crystalline (or ceramic) preparations have been manufactured with the intent of duplicating the structure and chemical composition of bone mineral. These implantable materials are biocompatible and, to varying degrees, biodegradable. They clearly permit osteoconduction but probably have no intrinsic inducing properties. Their mechanical properties are generally poor but improve as a composite is formed with the ingrowth of new bone. These materials appear to be efficacious in filling cystic defects or functioning as a biologic spacer, and they may well have application as vehicles or delivery systems for bone inducers such as bone marrow-derived stem cells (precursors) or BMP.

Immunologic Considerations

Like other tissues transplanted across genetic or histocompatibility differences, bone allografts evoke immunologic responses, and their nature and magnitude vary with the manner in which the graft is pretreated and implanted.

The potentially antigenic components of bone include collagen, matrix, and cells. Collagen is a weak sensitizer. Some matrix components such as hyaluronic acid and isolated chondroitin sulfates are nonantigenic, but proteoglycan subunits and link protein elicit immune responses in allogeneic and xenogeneic systems. The diverse cell populations in bone (osteogenic, chondrogenic, fibrous, fatty, neuronal, hematopoietic) are clearly the most potent source of immunogens regardless of the assay approach utilized (histology, skin graft rejection patterns, *in vitro* cytotoxicity). In most animal models the anticipated cell-mediated or humoral antibody responses directed against alloantigens are less intense if the graft is frozen prior to transplantation, and the intensity is decreased even more if the bone is lyophilized or irradiated.

Only a small amount of information is available concerning humans, but it appears to parallel the experience in animals as well as the patterns observed in human recipients of solid organ transplants.

Despite consensus regarding the antigenicity of bone grafts, the animal data are conflicting in regard to correlating the presence of immune responses with the biologic fate of the preserved allografts. Fresh bone allografts do poorly by most criteria, although the occurrence of cell-mediated or humoral responses in animals does not preclude a satisfactory result. Nonetheless, improvements in repair associated with immunosuppression as well as extrapolation from other tissue and organ transplant systems strongly suggest that some degree of adverse biologic behavior is caused as consequences of immunologic responses directed against bone-related antigens. In humans, there is preliminary evidence that certain responses, such as presensitization to DR antigens, may be beneficial to graft survival and biologic function whereas the development of humoral antibody or responses against the class I antigens (ABC loci) appears to be harmful.

Bone-Banking Methods

The objective of bone banking is to provide a mechanism for storing grafts until they are required and ensuring safety and predictably satisfactory biologic and biomechanical behavior. These goals are reflected in the guidelines and standards for bone banking developed by the American Association of Tissue Banks and are briefly summarized here.

Donor selection is accomplished by review of the past and current medical history and appropriate laboratory data to exclude donors who harbor significant and potentially transmissible diseases (infection, malignancy, hepatitis, venereal disease, acquired immune deficiency syndrome [AIDS]), have disorders affecting biomechanical properties of bone (collagen disorders, metabolic bone disease), or provide an opportunity to transfer toxic substances (poisons, radioactivity). It must be emphasized that protection of the recipient from inadvertent transfer of disease is of paramount importance. Serologic tests are available to screen potential donors for hepatitis, venereal disease, and AIDS. It is imperative that these tests be utilized and that the medical record be scrutinized with great care.

Grafts may be removed in a sterile environment with standard operating room technique; these tissues are maintained in sterile packages, usually deep-frozen. Alternatively, tissues recovered clean but nonsterile can be subjected to secondary methods to control contamination including exposure to ethylene oxide, high-dose irradiation, or strong acids (such as hydrochloric acid). These secondarily sterilized grafts are usually freeze-dried for long-term preservation. The AAA technique of Urist combines antigen extraction with chloroform/methanol, demineralization and sterilization with hydrochloric acid, and lyophilization.

The advantages of deep-freezing (usually at −70°C to −80°C) include maintenance of biomechanical properties, relatively inexpensive technology and easy storage, and an opportunity to cryopreserve articular cartilage (with glycerol or dimethyl sulfoxide). Freeze-drying permits storage for indefinite periods at room temperature in evacuated containers, but there is some loss of structural integrity (although this may be unimportant unless grafts are used as major weight-bearing segments). Demineralization appears to enhance osteoinduction, but these grafts have little intrinsic strength (Table 2).

Accurate record keeping is crucial in bone banking.

Clinical Considerations

No single bone graft preparation is ideal for all clinical applications. However, fresh autogenous bone graft must be considered the biologic and biomechanical standard with which alternatives are compared.

Failure of autografts generally can be traced to inadequacies in the host bed that preclude or limit its necessary contributions or to failure to protect the graft mechanically during the incorporation process. It is of particular note that revascularized autografts have performed well in comparison to nonvascularized grafts in host beds compromised by irradiation, loss of soft tissue, and even infection, as well as in circumstances such as congenital pseudarthrosis of the tibia in which a major segmental resection may be required to remove the diseased (abnormal) tissue.

Preserved allografts have been used with substantial success in filling benign cystic defects and in supplementing fracture nonunions and arthrodesis of joints (including scoliosis fusions). Osteochondral grafts, containing articular cartilage and a thin wafer of subchondral bone, have been used to resurface unicompartmental knee joint space destroyed by degenerative disease or osteonecrosis. Similar approaches have been used to graft bone and cartilage defects related to osteonecrosis of the femoral head. Results of these procedures involving reconstruction of joint surfaces with allogeneic tissues have been less predictable than repair of bony defects alone, but they still offer an opportunity to restore function without the sacrifice of additional bone stock as required with synthetic arthroplasties.

Perhaps most exciting has been the use of massive osseous and osteochondral allografts after limb-sparing tumor ablations. It is now clear that adequate wide resections of neoplasms can be accomplished in selected cases without compromise of end results, but restoration of function requires replacement of these massively resected portions of the skeleton. Allografts potentially offer a solution. Segmental or intercalary allografts become incorporated in more than 90% of cases. Osteoarticular grafts (including a cryopreserved articular surface) can be expected to provide good or excellent function in 50% to 70% of patients, and the combined experience in large series using these limb-sparing oncologic procedures, regardless of graft anatomy, approaches 70% to 80%. An additional variation of reconstruction includes the use of allograft for segmental bone stock combined with a metallic arthroplasty for the joint surface, usually involving the hip and most often including a long intramedullary stem. Failures (nonunion, resorption, infection, and graft fracture) of massive osteochondral allografts usually result from the inherent properties of the graft but may reflect a compromised host bed or the local effects of systemic chemotherapy on repair.

Demineralized bone grafts have proved particularly useful in the induction of new bone required for cystic defects, osseous gaps after mid-face surgery, and periodontal disease and in supplementing fusions where stabilization by the graft itself is not crucial. Synthetic mineral substitutes likewise are useful in small defects, and both synthetics and bone allografts are being evaluated as composites with autologous bone marrow or osteoinductive preparations such as BMP.

Annotated Bibliography

Biology

General Considerations and Physiology of Remodeling

Baron, R.; Vignery, A.; and Horowitz, M.: Lymphocytes, macrophages and the regulation of bone remodeling. Bone Mineral Res. 2:175–243, 1984.

A detailed summary of the cellular nature and control of bone remodeling.

Canalis, E.: Effects of growth factors on bone cell replication and differentiation. Clin. Orthop. 193:246–263, 1985.

Describes locally synthesized factors (e.g., bone-derived growth factor) and their influence on cell replication and differentiation as well as their relationships to bone turnover and repair.

Friedlaender, G.E.; Mankin, H.J.; and Sell, K.W., editors: Osteochondral Allografts: Biology, Banking, and Clinical Applications. Boston, Little, Brown and Company, 1983.

Summary of biology, immunology, bone-banking methods, and clinical applications of osteochondral allografts.

Raisz, L.G., and Kream, B.E.: Regulation of bone formation. Part 1. N. Engl. J. Med. 309:29–35, 1983.

Review of normal homeostatic bone remodeling and its regulation.

Osteoinduction and Role of Bone Marrow

Burwell, R.G.: The function of bone marrow in the incorporation of a bone graft. Clin. Orthop. 200:125–141, 1985.

Role of bone marrow precursor cells in bone graft incorporation biology.

Mulliken, J.B.; Kaban, L.B.; and Glowacki, J.: Induced osteogenesis—the biological principle and clinical applications. J. Surg. Res. 37:487–496, 1984.

Description of preliminary animal and clinical data relevant to a demineralized bone preparation.

Muthukumaran, N., and Reddi, A.H.: Bone matrix-induced local bone induction. Clin. Orthop. 200:159–164, 1985.

Description of segmental cellular changes in implants responding to collagenous bone matrix-induced osteogenesis.

Nade, S.; Armstrong, L.; McCartney, E.; and Baggaley, B.: Osteogenesis after bone and bone marrow transplantation: The ability of ceramic materials to sustain osteogenesis from transplanted bone marrow cells: Preliminary studies. Clin. Orthop. 181:255–263, 1983.

Osteogenesis induced by different ceramic materials augmented by bone marrow and implanted in an intramuscular site.

Urist, M.R.; Huo, Y.K.; Brownell, A.G.; Hohl, W.M.; Buyske, J.; Lietze, A.; Tempst, P.; Hunkapiller, M.; and DeLange, R.J.: Purification of bovine bone morphogenetic protein by hydroxyapatite chromatography. Proc. Natl. Acad. Sci. USA 81:371–375, 1984.

Description of purification approach and biochemical characteristics of BMP.

Nonvascularized Grafts

Burchardt, H.: The biology of bone graft repair. Clin. Orthop. 174:28–42, 1983.

Review of the histologic pattern of cortical and cancellous autograft and allograft incorporation.

Heiple, K.G.; Goldberg, V.M.; Powell, A.E.; Bos, G.D.; and Zika, J.M.: Biology of cancellous bone graft repair. *In* Osteochondral Allografts: Biology, Banking, and Clinical Applications, edited by G.E. Friedlaender, H.J. Mankin, and K.W. Sell, pp. 37–49. Boston, Little, Brown and Company, 1983.

Provides a detailed description of histologic aspects of cancellous bone graft incorporation, including autografts and preserved allografts.

Prolo, D.J., and Rodrigo, J.J.: Contemporary bone graft physiology and surgery. Clin. Orthop. 200:322–342, 1985.

Summarizes histologic changes occurring in bone graft incorporation and speculates regarding control mechanisms and role of inductive materials.

Vascularized Grafts

Dell, P.C.; Burchardt, H.; and Glowczewskie, F.P., Jr.: A roentgenographic, biomechanical, and histological evaluation of vascularized and non-vascularized segmental fibular canine autografts. J. Bone Joint Surg. 67A:105–112, 1985.

Describes different mechanisms of graft incorporation associated with vascularized and nonvascularized segmental autografts in dogs.

Shaffer, J.W.; Field, G.A.; Goldberg, V.M.; and Davy, D.T.: Fate of vascularized and nonvascularized autografts. Clin. Orthop. 197:32–43, 1985.

Vascularized canine ulnar autografts repair faster and remain stronger than nonvascularized grafts.

Weiland, A.J.; Phillips, T.W.; and Randolph, M.A.: Bone grafts: A radiologic, histologic, and biomechanical model comparing autografts, allografts, and free vascularized bone grafts. Plast. Reconstr. Surg. 74:368–379, 1984.

Repair with segmented and matchstick autografts, fresh segmental allografts, and vascularized autografts in a femoral segmental defect was evaluated in a dog model. Various criteria were used to assess results.

Synthetic Mineral Preparations

Holmes, R.; Mooney, V.; Bucholz, R.; and Tencer, A.: A coralline hydroxyapatite bone graft substitute: Preliminary report. Clin. Orthop. 188:252–262, 1984.

Describes the structure and nature of hydroxyapatite from naturally occurring coral. This implant encouraged osteoconduction and was associated with very little resorption in dogs. Clinical results in cystic defects were encouraging as well.

Renooij, W.; Hoogendoorn, H.A.; Visser, W.J.; Lentferink, R.H.F.; Schmitz, M.G.J.; Van Ieperen, H.; Oldenburg, S.J.; Janssen, W.M.; Akkermans, L.M.A.; and Wittebol, P.: Bioresorption of ceramic strontium-85–labeled calcium phosphate implants in dog femora: A pilot study to quantitate bioresorption of ceramic implants of hydroxyapatite and tricalcium orthophosphate *in vivo*. Clin. Orthop. 197:272–285, 1985.

Demonstrates biodegradability of tricalcium phosphates but not ceramic hydroxyapatites.

Miscellaneous

Amiel, D.; Coutts, R.D.; Abel, M.; Stewart, W.; Harwood, F.; and Akeson, W.H.: Rib perichondrial grafts for the repair of full-thickness articular-cartilage defects: A morphological and biochemical study in rabbits. J. Bone Joint Surg. 67A:911–920, 1985.

Rabbit rib perichondrium was used to repair full-thickness defects in the femoral condyle. Half the results were associated with production of neocartilage that was histologically and biomechanically similar to hyaline cartilage. Failures were associated with condylar fracture, loss of fixation, or infection.

Burchardt, H.; Glowczewskie, F.P., Jr.; and Enneking, W.F.: The effect of Adriamycin and methotrexate on the repair of segmental cortical autografts in dogs. J. Bone Joint Surg. 65A:103–108, 1983.

Describes the adverse influence of chemotherapy on bone graft incorporation in a canine fibular model.

Immunologic Considerations

Friedlaender, G.E.: Immune responses to osteochondral allografts: Current knowledge and future directions. Clin. Orthop. 174:58–68, 1983.

Summarizes sources of bone and cartilage immunogenicity and decreases in detectable responses by freezing and freeze-drying.

Friedlaender, G.E.; Powell, A.C.; and Thornhill, T.S.: Immunology in orthopaedics. *In* AAOS Instructional Course Lectures. XXXIII:531–547. St. Louis, C.V. Mosby, 1984.

Provides an overview of the immune system and its application to orthopaedic aspects of transplantation, infection, and oncology.

Goldberg, V.M.; Powell, A.; Shaffer, J.W.; Zika, J.; Bos, G.D.; and Heiple, K.G.: Bone grafting: Role of histocompatibility in transplantation. J. Orthop. Res. 3:389–404, 1985.

Major histocompatibility differences were associated with poor repair of cancellous ulnar segments in dogs, but closely matched vascularized allografts did well (as did closely matched nonvascularized allografts).

Bone-Banking Methods

Friedlaender, G.E., and Mankin, H.J.: Bone banking: Current methods and suggested guidelines. *In* AAOS In-

structional Course Lectures. XXX:36–51. St. Louis, C.V. Mosby, 1981.
Describes in detail the guidelines proposed by the American Association of Tissue Banks for banking of musculoskeletal tissues and discusses the background rationale.

Pelker, R.R.; Friedlaender, G.E.; and Markham, T.C.: Biomechanical properties of bone allografts. Clin. Orthop. 174:54–57, 1983.
Strength of bone was unaltered by various freezing temperatures (−20°C to −170°C) but was decreased by freeze-drying or irradiation with 3 Mrad or greater.

Tomford, W.W.; Doppelt, S.H.; Mankin, H.J.; and Friedlaender, G.E.: 1983 bone bank procedures. Clin. Orthop. 174:15–21, 1983.
Bone banking methods and rationale are described.

Tomford, W.W.; Duff, G.P.; and Mankin, H.J.: Experimental freeze-preservation of chondrocytes. Clin. Orthop. 197:11–14, 1985.
Cryopreservation of intact articular surface and isolated chondrocytes resulted in 40% to 50% and 90% viability, respectively.

Clinical Considerations

Aurori, B.F.; Weierman, R.J.; Lowell, H.A.; Nadel, C.I.; and Parsons, J.R.: Pseudarthrosis after spinal fusion for scoliosis: A comparison of autogeneic and allogeneic bone grafts. Clin. Orthop. 199:153–158, 1985.
The incidence of pseudarthrosis was about the same in autograft recipients (4.4%) and in allograft recipients (5.3%).

Mankin, H.J.; Doppelt, S.; and Tomford, W.: Clinical experience with allograft implantation. The first ten years. Clin. Orthop. 174:69–86, 1983.
In 91 patients receiving osteochondral allografts, at 2-year or longer follow-up over 70% had a good or an excellent clinical result. Failures reflected infection, fracture, and nonunion.

Weiland, A.J.; Moore, J.R.; and Daniel, R.K.: Vascularized bone autografts: Experience with 41 cases. Clin. Orthop. 174:87–95, 1983.
A description of the surgical techniques and rationale for free vascularized fibular grafts is provided as well as a summary of clinical cases emphasizing the indications and satisfactory results associated with this approach.

15

Imaging of the Musculoskeletal System

Introduction

The numerous advances in imaging techniques in recent years add to the complexity of choosing the proper technique for a given clinical problem. Newer techniques such as magnetic resonance imaging (MRI), three-dimensional reconstruction of computed tomography (CT) images, and developments in isotope studies will be discussed in this section. These techniques also will be described later in the clinical sections as they apply to specific diagnostic problems.

Magnetic Resonance Imaging

Unlike the images of conventional radiography or CT, those of MRI are created by using a static magnetic field, magnetic gradients, and radiofrequency pulses. Most instruments operate at field strengths between 0.15 and 2.0 tesla (a measure of magnetic field strength). MRI does not require ionizing radiation.

Nuclei with an uneven atomic number (^{1}H, ^{23}Na, ^{31}P, etc.) have spin and charge and act like small magnets. Hydrogen (^{1}H) is currently used for MRI because of its abundance and strong signal. In the body, these nuclei are normally randomly oriented (Fig. 1 *A*). When patients are placed in a static magnetic field, the nuclei tend to align themselves parallel to the magnetic field (Fig. 1 *B*). Applications of radiofrequency pulses induce the nuclei to rotate into the transverse plane (90° to the plane of the magnet) (Fig. 1 *C*), which produces a signal that is detected by the receiver coil. Different information and image features are obtained, depending on the pulse sequences used. The pictures seen on MRI depend on flow, proton density, chemical shift, and two relaxation parameters termed T_1 and T_2. More physiologic information is obtained with MRI than with conventional radiography or CT.

The spin lattice relaxation time (T_1) is the time it takes the nuclei to return to the axis of the magnetic field (Fig. 1 *D*). The spin-spin relaxation time is due to nuclear interactions that result in the return of the transverse magnetization to equilibrium (Fig. 1 *E*). The relaxation times are prolonged in abnormal tissues, which assists in detection of pathology.

The information seen on the images is affected by the pulse sequence. For example, inversion recovery (IR) and partial saturation (PS) sequences are T_1 weighted. With these sequences, pathologic lesions will appear darker than normal tissue. Spin-echo (SE) sequences with a long repetition and echo time are T_2 weighted and abnormal tissue has a high signal intensity (white) (see Figure 20). These sequences provide excellent soft tissue contrast and, combined with the ability to image in the axial, coronal, and sagittal planes, are an excellent technique for detecting and determining the true extent of lesions.

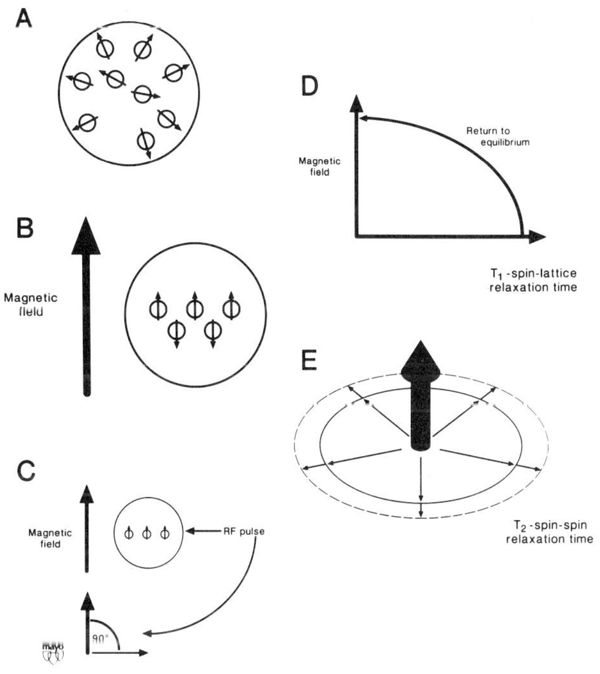

Figure 1

Basic principles of MRI. See text for details. (From Berquist, T.H.: Magnetic resonance (MR) in urology. Urol. Annu. [in press]. By permission of Appleton-Century-Crofts.)

There are no known biologic hazards with MRI. However, the presence of certain ferromagnetic materials in the patient must be considered. Pacemakers are converted to fixed rate by the magnetic field. Many cerebral aneurysm clips are ferromagnetic and may torque on the vessels. Therefore, patients with these implants currently are not examined with MRI. Fortunately, most orthopaedic appliances are not ferromagnetic; these patients can be examined safely and the artifact is usually minimal compared to that on CT.

Images of the normal musculoskeletal anatomy demonstrate high signal (white) intensity with fat, marrow, and neural tissue. Muscle is intermediate in density. Cortical bone, ligaments, tendons, and menisci look black (low signal) and articular cartilage appears gray. There is more water in articular cartilage than in menisci. Normally, flowing blood does not produce a signal. Therefore, vessels also generally appear black. This obviates the need for contrast material (often needed with CT) for definition of vessels and soft tissue lesions.

Computed Tomography

The musculoskeletal applications of CT continue to expand. The value of CT in diagnosis of neoplasms, trauma, infection, and many other lesions is well documented. In the last few years, improved software has permitted new reconstructive techniques that allow images to be formatted in coronal and sagittal planes as well as in three-dimensional reconstruction.

Three-dimensional reconstruction can be accomplished with most conventional CT equipment. The amount of time required to produce three-dimensional images is about the same as needed to generate coronal or sagittal reconstructions.

For best results, very thin (2 mm) slices are obtained with a conventional CT scanner. Thicker slices (4 to 10 mm) have also been used because examination of a large area such as the pelvis by using 2-mm slices can require up to 75 slices. Three-dimensional images can be obtained by using the density thresholds of bone and soft tissues.

Three-dimensional images are useful in characterizing complex fractures of the pelvis and shoulder or in other areas, such as the wrist, foot, or facial bones, where anatomy is complex (Fig. 2). Three-dimensional images are more easily reviewed than the usual multiple axial images provided by conventional CT.

Digital Subtraction Techniques

Digital subtraction provides a means of removing unwanted information from the image. The technique was originally conceived to study vascular structures by using intravenous injection of contrast medium instead of the more invasive arterial approach. Because of problems such as misregistration, cardiac output variables, and lack of small vessel detail, arterial as well as venous routes of administration are now being used. More recently, this technique has been used in conjunction with arthrography.

Subtraction techniques require fairly expensive equipment including an image intensifier and a television system. A digitized computer system allows real-time visualization of the images produced. The advantages of digital subtraction are speed, real-time visualization, permanent disk storage, ease in differentiation of barium-impregnated cement from contrast material, and intravenous contrast for study of arterial and venous structures. The disadvantages are cost, misregistration in moving areas (abdomen), poor detail of small vessels compared to conventional angiography, patient immobilization longer than with conventional subtraction arthrography, less articular detail, and more limited field of view.

In orthopaedic practice, digital subtraction techniques can be used in arthrography (particularly in patients with total joint replacement) and in preoperative evaluation of musculoskeletal neoplasms. The extremities can be easily immobilized, which decreases vascular misregistration problems experienced in the chest and abdomen. To date, this technique has had limited applications in orthopaedic practice because of its high cost and limited availability.

Nuclear Medicine

Several new techniques in nuclear medicine are of potential importance to orthopaedists, including dual-photon absorptiometry for the measurement of spinal and hip bone mineral, use of indium-111-labeled leukocytes for the detection of sites of musculoskeletal infection, and lymphoscintigraphy to map drainage sites from melanoma and other soft tissue tumors. Other techniques that may provide useful information but require further clinical evaluation include use of radiolabeled antibodies for detecting metastatic sites and use of single-photon emission CT (SPECT) for more accurate localization and detection of osseous abnormalities. Radiation exposures for several examinations ordered by orthopaedists are given in Table 1.

Bone Mineral Analysis

The techniques for measuring bone mineral content include single-photon absorptiometry (SPA) of the forearm, dual-photon absorptiometry (DPA) of the lumbar spine and femoral neck, and quantitative CT (QCT) of the lumbar spine and femoral neck.

SPA uses an iodine-125 source to scan the forearm. The results of SPA reflect primarily cortical bone. DPA uses a gadolinium-153 source which produces two primary photon peaks, at approximately 44 and 100 keV. These energies allow DPA to correct for variations of beam length and overlying soft tissues, permitting calculation of total bone mineral in the lumbar spine or hips, structures composed primarily of trabecular bone. QCT allows measurement in the spine or femur; it can be programmed to measure essentially only trabecular bone.

SPA has a precision of approximately 3% and an accuracy of approximately 6%. The major limitation in SPA is that it reflects primarily the cortical bone in long bones and therefore, although it may better reveal overall skeletal status, it is not useful for the trabecular bone in spine and hips—the clinically more critical sites. DPA has a precision of approximately 2% and an accuracy of approximately 4%. Although DPA allows quantitation of spine and hip bone mineral, it reflects an integration of the cortical and trabecular bones in these sites. Problems with DPA occur in measurements at sites of compression fracture, severe osteoarthritis, or extensive calcifications in the aorta which may cause falsely increased values. QCT can be performed in one of two modes: with a single-energy technique which has a precision of approximately 2% but has an accuracy of only 10% to 20% in elderly patients due to significant marrow fat; or with a dual-energy technique which has a precision of approximately 4% and an accuracy of approximately 5%. Radiation exposure is approximately 10 mrad from DPA and 400 to 1,500 mrad from QCT (Table 2).

Although there is controversy in the literature as to whether DPA or QCT is superior for measuring spine and hip bone mineral, there is little controversy over the limited utility of SPA for diagnosing osteoporosis or for predicting fracture risk in the individual patient (Fig. 3).

Indium-111-Labeled Leukocytes

Techniques have been recently introduced that allow the labeling of various cellular components of blood with indium-111 (^{111}In) while preserving their structure and function. There are several methods for labeling leukocytes, all of which begin with a Volex-induced erythrocyte sedimentation to yield leukocyte-rich plasma. The leukocytes can be further separated by centrifugation, or a relatively pure granulocyte preparation can be obtained by layering the leukocyte-rich plasma on two different densities of Ficoll-

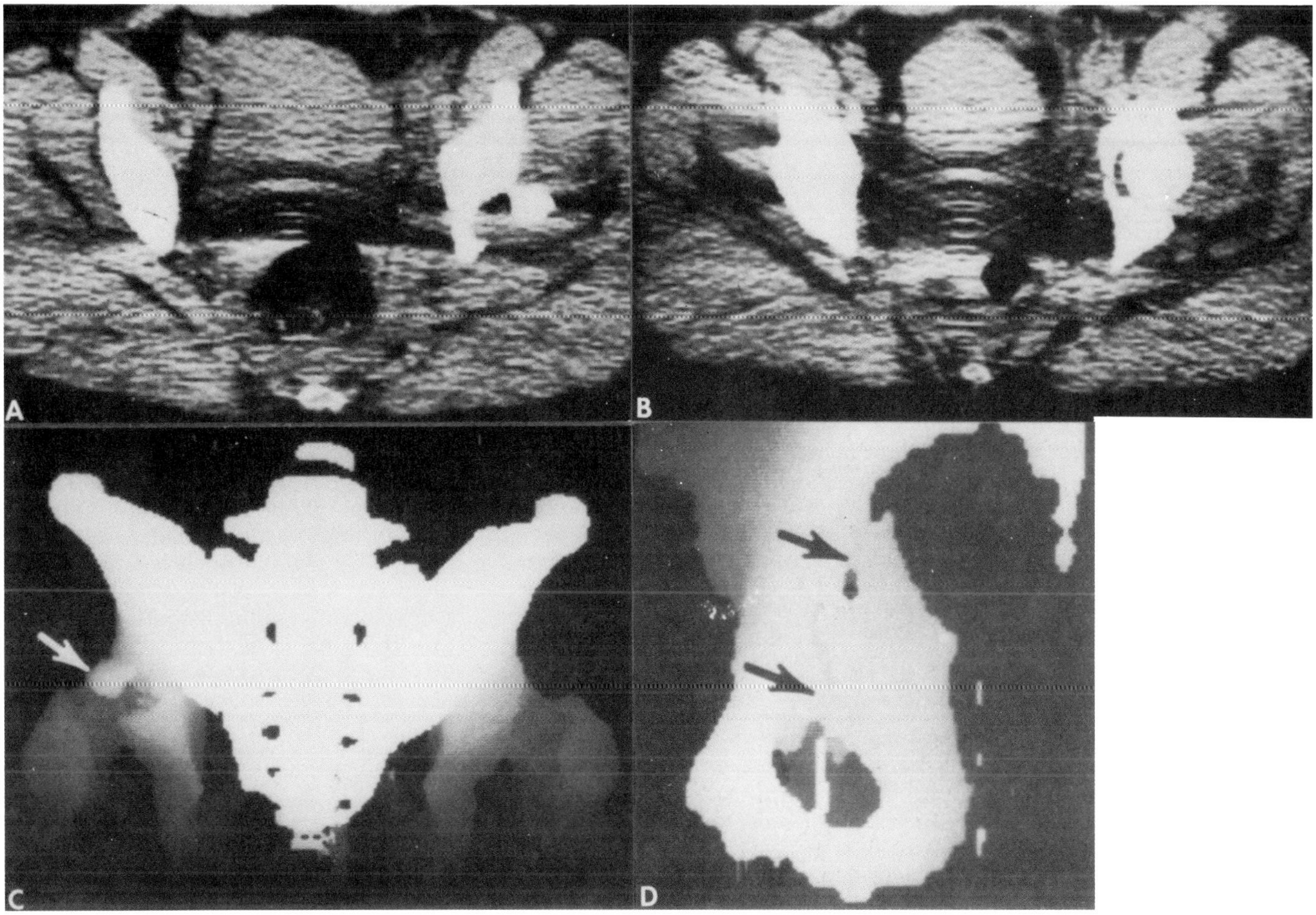

Figure 2

A and *B*, Conventional axial CT images of acetabular fracture through the superior (*A*) and mid acetabulum (*B*). *C* and *D*, Surface reconstruction of the posterior right hemipelvis (*C*) and left hemipelvis (*D*) as viewed from within the pelvis. (From Totty, W.G., and Vannier, M.W. Radiology 150:173–177, 1984. By permission of the Radiological Society of North America.)

Hypaque solution. The resulting leukocyte or pure granulocyte pellet is then incubated with ^{111}In oxine, ^{111}In tropolone, or ^{111}In acetylacetone (only the ^{111}In oxine is currently approved by the Food and Drug Administration) for approximately 10 to 20 minutes at room temperature. The In-labeled complex is lipophilic and allows entry of the label into the cell where it binds to cytoplasmic proteins and other subcellular organelles. The preparation is then

Table 1. Radiation Exposure From Common Orthopaedic X-ray Examinations*

	Dose, rad		
	Skin entrance exposure	Ovaries/testicles	Bone marrow
Chest (PA & Lat.)	0.050	†/†	0.004
Knee (AP & Lat.)	0.035	†/†	†
Hand	0.015	†/†	†
Pelvis (AP)	0.400	0.105/0.038	0.019
Lumbar spine (AP & Lat.)	0.900	0.162/0.004	0.054
CT of pelvis	5.700	4.700/1.700	1.25
Hip fluoroscopy (1 min.)	4.000	1.050/0.400	0.200
	Target organ	**Ovary**	
Bone scan (20 mCi of ^{99m}Tc MDP)	4.000 (bladder)	0.600	0.800
Gallium scan (5 mCi)	4.500 (colon)	1.200	2.900
^{111}In scan (500 μCi)	8.600 (spleen)	0.300	0.300

*Assume one film unless otherwise noted.
†Insignificant (< 0.001 rad).

Table 2. Methods of Bone Mineral Analysis

Method	Site	% Cortical/% trabecular	% Precision/% accuracy	Radiation exposure, mrad	Cost, $
Single-photon absorptiometry	Distal radius	80/20	2-4/2-4	<10	50-125
	Mid radius	95/5			
Dual-photon absorptiometry	Spine	40/60	3-5/2-4	<10	75-200
	Hips	75/25	3-5/?	<10	
Quantitative CT:					
Single energy		0/100	3-8/6-30	400-1,200	200-400
Dual energy*		0/100	5-10/4-6	400-1,200	

*Not widely available yet.

washed to remove unbound ^{111}In and injected back into the patient who provided the cells.

Results with the ^{111}In-labeled leukocyte preparations have been very promising in acute osteomyelitis; some laboratories report good results in chronic osteomyelitis. The differences among the various reports may relate to differences in the indium complex used as well as to whether a mixed leukocyte population or pure granulocytes were used. (See section on infection.)

Radiolabeled Monoclonal Antibodies

Currently, a number of investigators are evaluating the usefulness of radiolabeled (^{131}I, ^{111}In, ^{99m}Tc) antibodies in various malignancies. In principle, the radiolabeled antitumor antibodies could be used for diagnosis and treatment. The early work involved polyclonal antibodies specific for tumor-associated antigens (e.g., carcinoembryonic antigen, α-fetoprotein, human chorionic gonadotropin, melanoma-associated antigen, a kidney antigen, and ferritin); more recently, monoclonal antibodies (derived from mouse hybridomas) against colon, breast, melanoma, and anti-T lymphocyte antigens have been used. Various forms of labeled antibodies including intact IgG and the $F(ab')_2$ and Fab fragments have been used. The problems with radiolabeled antibodies are significant and include slow clearance of nonspecific activity from soft tissue and blood, nonspecific localization of labeled antibody in liver and other normal tissues, difficulty in penetration of the radiolabeled antibody into poorly vascularized tumors, and the cross reactivity of antibody with normal antigen present in organs and tissues. There is also a problem in using a single-species hybridoma because repeat studies are not possible due to the development of human anti-mouse antibody. Attempts are being made at more specific localization by interstitial injection to look for nodal sites of metastasis in early disease.

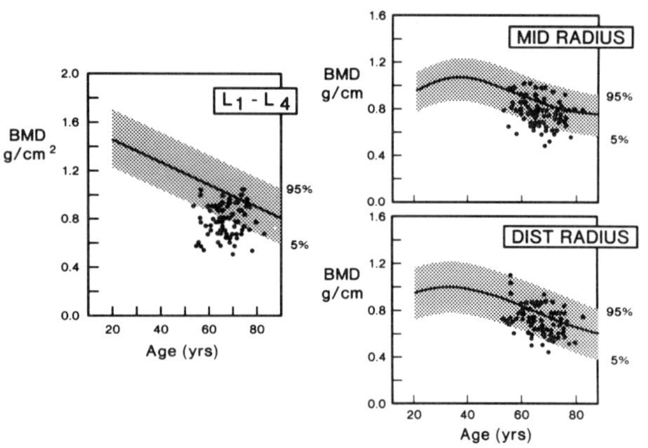

Figure 3

Bone mineral density (BMD) in the lumbar spine measured with DPA (*Left*) and BMD in the mid and distal radius measured with SPA (*Right*) in 76 women with osteoporosis. Stippled areas represent 5th through 95th percentile range for 105 age- and sex-adjusted normal women. Note the incomplete separation of the patient population from the control population. DPA gives the best distinction between patients with osteoporosis and normal subjects. (From Riggs, B.L.; Wahner, H.W.; Dunn, W.L.; Mazess, R.B.; Offord, K.P.; and Melton, L.J., III: Differential changes in bone mineral density of the appendicular and axial skeleton with aging: Relationship to spinal osteoporosis. J. Clin. Invest. 67:328–335, 1981. By permission of the American Society for Clinical Investigation.)

Lymphoscintigraphy

Technetium-labeled colloids can be injected interstitially to determine lymph drainage from a specific primary tumor site. This is useful particularly when radical dissection is being considered for definitive therapy, such as in malignant melanoma. In one series of malignant melanoma patients, the drainage determined by scans was not predicted 72% of the time and resulted in a change in both the location and extent of nodal dissection in half of the patients. The study is easy to perform, involves a minimal radiation exposure, and can be performed in hours. It is important to note that the images do not determine sites of lymph node metastasis but rather indicate only the drainage patterns.

Single-Photon Emission Computed Tomography

SPECT uses standard radionuclides such as ^{99m}Tc diphosphonate. Images are acquired over 360° with a rotating gamma camera, and computerized back-projection produces axial, coronal, and sagittal reconstructions of areas of interest. Work in this area is preliminary but initial reports suggest that it is potentially useful in diagnosis of low back problems, abnormalities in the temporomandibular joint, and osteonecrosis in hips. The procedure is relatively easy to perform and takes an additional half hour of imaging time; it is now widely available.

Thermography

Increase in body temperatures as a result of a disease process is a well-established phenomenon. The body emits infrared radiation with wavelengths in the range of 3 to 75 μm. This radiation can be detected by special photoelectric or photochemical detectors, so variations in the skin temperature can be measured. Theoretically, the increased blood supply to an area of inflammation or neoplasm should cause an increase in temperature in the involved area which could be detected on the thermogram.

Thermography was first used diagnostically in 1956 for detection of breast cancer. The technique requires no ionizing radiation but it has many potential inaccuracies. For example, a cool-down period of 15–30 minutes is required prior to the study to allow skin temperatures to equilibrate. Controlling the temperature of the area to be studied can be difficult.

The use of thermography has remained controversial and most think that the technique adds little to the clinical examination. There are reports of using this technique in following patients with arthropathy and low back pain. In a study of ankylosing spondylitis the technique was not specific and could not detect abnormalities any earlier than routine radiography. The technique is currently not used actively in most centers.

Trauma

Algorithm 1 summarizes the imaging approaches for common injuries.

Spine

Patients suspected to have spine injury should be stabilized until they can be completely evaluated. Routine radiographs are usually sufficient for diagnosis of significant spinal injuries. The extent and mechanism of injury can usually be detected accurately in the majority of cases. In certain situations, conventional tomography or CT also may be required.

Table 3 summarizes the role of imaging techniques in detection of common spinal injuries.

Isotope bone scans play little or no role in the evaluation of acute spinal injuries. Bone scintigraphy, however, has been reported to be helpful in spondylolysis and spondylolisthesis by defining areas where there is increased metabolic activity due to areas of stress or breaks in the pars intra-articularis (Fig. 4). In one study in 19 adult patients with radiographic evidence of spondylolysis or spondylolisthesis, SPECT allowed more accurate localization and was more sensitive than planar bone scintigraphy in identifying sites of painful pars defects. In six patients with spondylolisthesis or spondylolysis and no back pain, the SPECT images were normal.

In another study, there was good correlation between radiographs and the isotope bone scan when there was a stress fracture with irregular lucent lines in an area of sclerosis, but the bone scan often was negative when an ununited fracture with a large lucent defect and well-defined margins was found radiographically. This study concluded that, if no radiographic abnormalities were present at the site of localized pain, scintigraphy should be used to exclude stress injuries not radiographically apparent.

Routine Radiographs Routine radiographs of the cervical spine should include AP, lateral, both obliques, and open-mouth odontoid views. All views can be obtained without moving the patient. Additional views may be useful if the odontoid or AP view is difficult to obtain. These include angled (20°–30° to head and 20°–30° to feet) AP views which aid in evaluating the bodies and lamina. If the odontoid is difficult to visualize, one can double expose a coned-down projection over the AP view on the same film. Pillar views also may be useful in evaluation of the posterior elements (>40% of fractures) but this requires turning the patient's head. Therefore, initial films should be studied carefully first. If no significant injury is noted but symptoms dictate, the pillar views can and should be obtained.

The lateral view allows detection of about 90% of significant injuries to the cervical spine (Table 4). The most important factor is being certain that all seven cervical vertebrae and the first thoracic vertebra are included on the film. This may require a swimmer's view (the safest

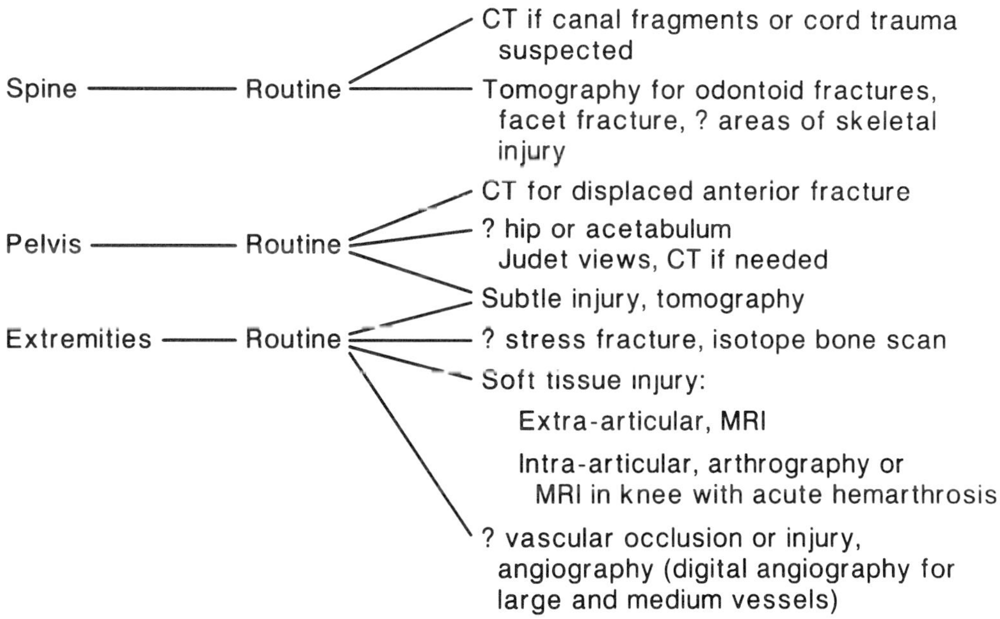

Algorithm 1
Imaging of orthopaedic trauma.

Table 3. Diagnostic Techniques for Evaluation of Spinal Injuries

Injury	Usefulness*				
	Routine radiography	Conventional tomography	CT	MRI	Myelography
Vertebral body fracture	E	E	E	E	NI
Odontoid fracture	F	E	P	E	NI
Neural arch fracture	F	F–E	E	F	NI
Facet fracture	P	E	P	P	NI
Fracture/dislocation	A	E	E	E	NI
Soft tissue injury	P†	P	P	E†	NI
Obstruction or cord compression	F	F	A	E	E
Nerve root avulsion	P	P	P	P	E

*E, excellent; A, adequate; P, poor; NI, not indicated.
†Flexion/extension views often needed.

technique), upper extremity traction (can hyperextend the neck), or tomography to be certain that the lower cervical spine is well seen. Signs of instability should be searched for on the lateral view. These include: 1) widened interspinous distance, 2) vertebral subluxation > 3 mm, 3) compression of the vertebral body by > 25%, 4) narrowed or widened disk space, 5) facet joint widening, and 6) angulation.

For the thoracic and lumbar spine, AP and lateral views are usually adequate for identification of significant fractures. The entire spine, including the cervical portion, should be studied in patients who have had high-velocity trauma or if any abnormality is noted in any of the spine segments. The incidence of multiple distant injuries is approximately 17%.

Conventional and Computed Tomography CT has replaced conventional tomography for evaluation of many complex spinal injuries. Detection of fragments in the spinal canal and evaluation of the cord and epidural space can be readily accomplished. Metrizamide CT may be particularly useful in evaluating subtle changes in the spinal canal. Sagittal reconstruction may be valuable for correlating the area of injury with the adjacent spinal segments.

Conventional tomography is still a valuable tool in the evaluation of spine trauma. Use of a Versitome unit allows one to obtain tomograms in the AP, lateral, oblique, and axial planes without moving the patient. Certain types of injury are less well defined with CT—e.g., odontoid fractures and facet fractures because the fracture is in the plane of the image (Figs. 5 and 6). Tomography of the odontoid is particularly helpful. Up to 20% of type II odontoid fractures cannot be seen on conventional views. Type I fractures can be even more difficult to detect. Both AP and lateral tomograms should be obtained. Oblique tomograms are occasionally required for subtle facet injuries.

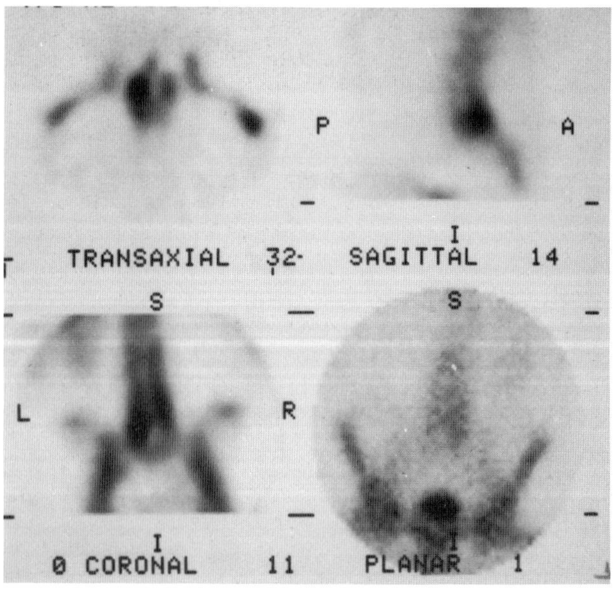

Figure 4

Fifty-year-old man with low back pain. SPECT images demonstrate area of focal increased uptake at left side of L-5 vertebra. Transaxial and coronal images clearly localize this activity to within the pars intra-articularis. It was due to a site of spondylolisthesis.

Motion Studies Evaluation of soft tissue injury may require flexion/extension or lateral bending views. These studies are most commonly used to evaluate patients with suspected instability or to exclude ligament injury in the cervical region. They should be performed fluoroscopically. This will increase safety and accuracy. In the immediate

Table 4. Evaluation of Lateral View of Cervical Spine*

Upper cervical spine (C1-2):
- Distance from anterior ring of C-1 to odontoid
  - Adults, ≤2.5 mm
  - Children, ≤4.5 mm
- Prevertebral soft tissues
  - Airway to anterior inferior margin of C-2
    - Adults, ≤7 mm
    - Children, ≤7 mm

Lower cervical spine (C3-7):
- Soft tissues
  - Airway to anterior margin of C-6
    - Adults, ≤22 mm
    - Children, ≤14 mm
- Alignment
  - Subluxation (<3 mm) may be seen of C-2 on C-3 and of C-3 on C-4 in children up to late teens (rarely into early 20s)
  - Subluxation in adults is abnormal (usually C4-7)
- Disk space
  - Uniform = normal
  - Compressed = flexion injury
  - Widened anteriorly = extension injury
- Interspinous distance
  - Should decrease from C-3 to C-7

*From Berquist, T.H.: The spine. *In* Diagnostic Imaging of the Acutely Injured Patient, edited by T.H. Berquist, pp. 39-67. Baltimore, Urban & Schwarzenberg, 1985. By permission of Mayo Foundation.

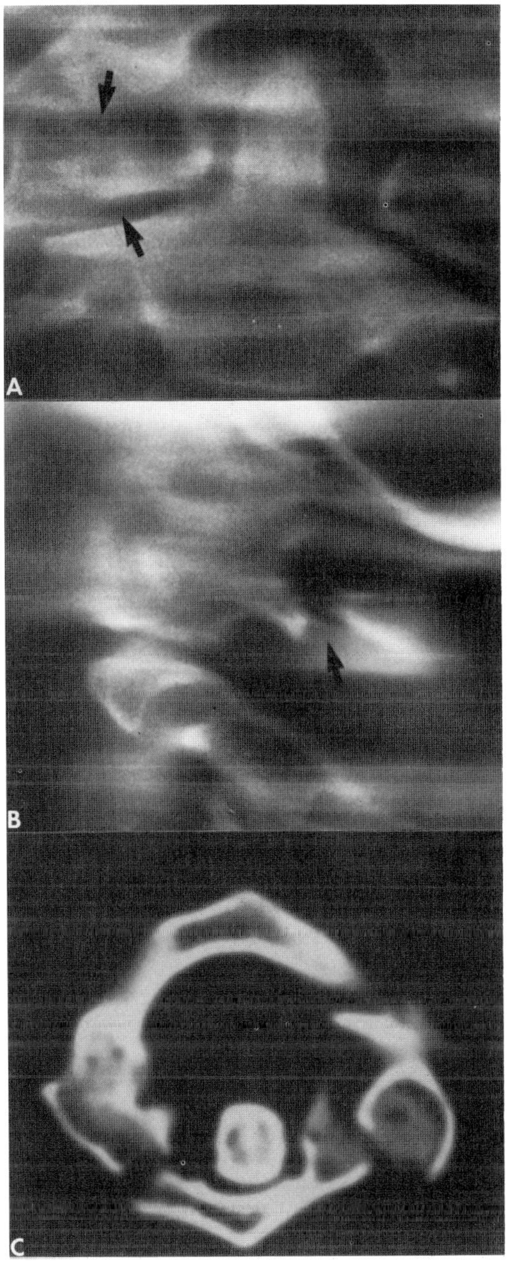

Figure 5

Patient with upper neck pain after a motor vehicle accident. AP (*A*) and lateral (*B*) tomograms demonstrate fracture of right lateral mass and posterior ring of C-1 (*arrows*). Note increased distance between odontoid and left lateral mass of C-1. *C*, CT scan demonstrates fractures and position of the fragments more clearly. Left anterior ring fracture was not evident on the tomogram.

post-injury period (48 hours), these studies are not useful because muscle spasm and guarding can result in false-negative examinations. Patients with suspected injury should be placed in a collar for several days prior to motion studies.

Magnetic Resonance Imaging MRI has superior soft tissue contrast and the ability to provide direct sagittal and coronal images, which offer certain advantages over CT and

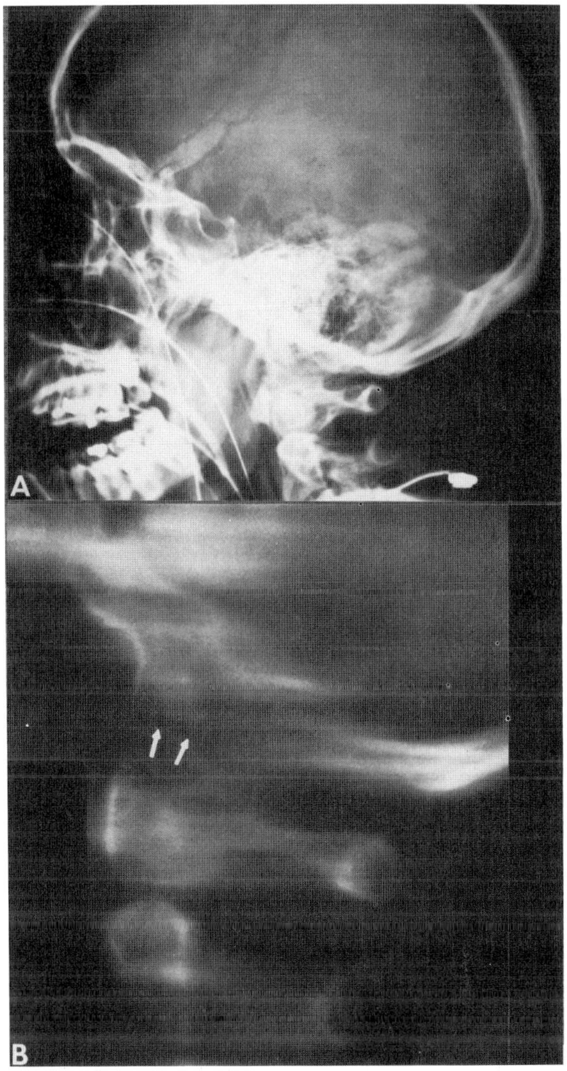

Figure 6

Lateral view of skull (*A*) and lateral tomogram (*B*) of craniovertebral junction. The transverse fracture (*arrows*) of the occipital condyle was not seen on CT because the fracture line was parallel to the plane of the image.

myelography. The vertebrae, disks, and spinal canal can be assessed without contrast material, and the entire anatomic region can be clearly displayed. Detection of more subtle causes of pain, such as paraspinal muscle tears, is also possible. MRI shows definite potential in studies of spinal and paraspinal injury. To date, because of scan time and stability questions, patients with complex or potentially unstable injuries have not been extensively studied in the acute setting. The role of MRI in spine trauma will be more clearly defined as clinical experience increases.

Pelvis and Hips

Identification of pelvis and hip injury requires a systematic imaging approach. Using an improper sequence of examinations may obscure significant information.

Anterior pelvic fractures usually are easily identified, es-

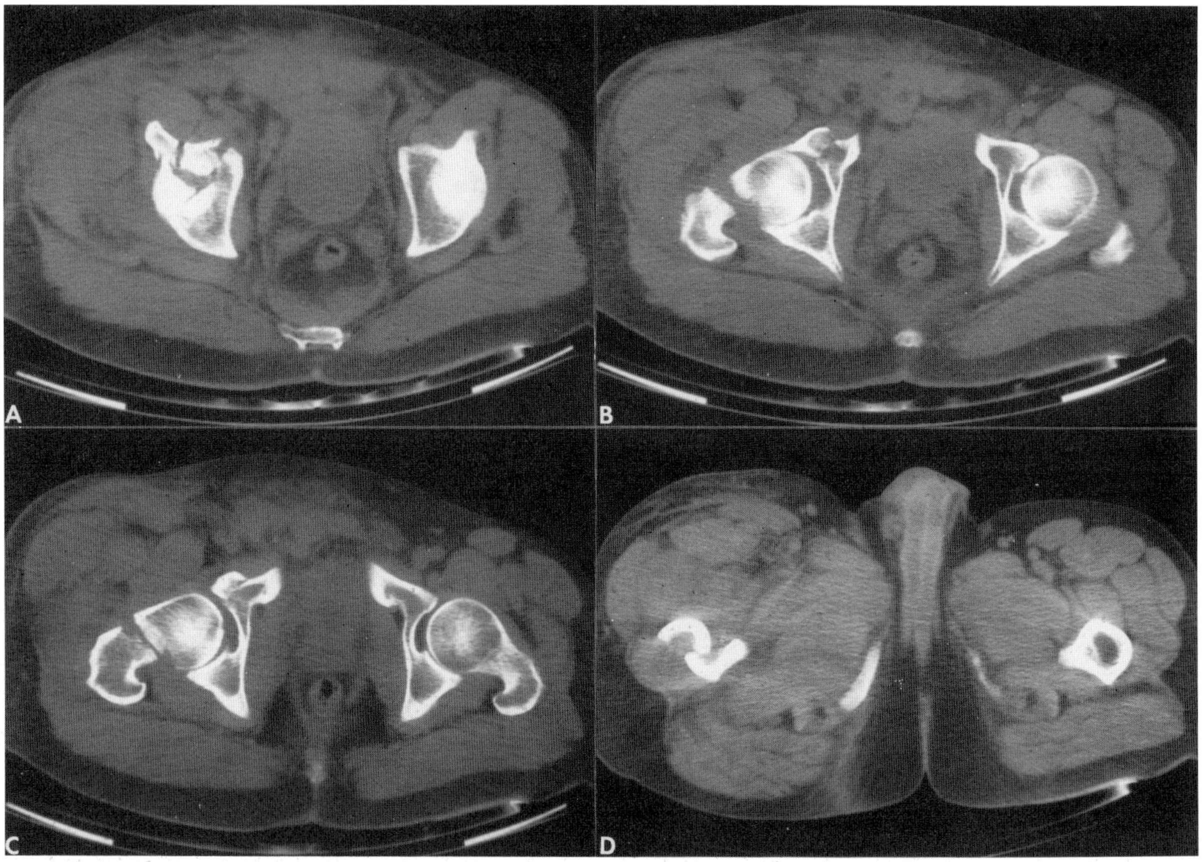

Figure 7
Complex fracture involving right acetabulum and femur. *A*, Position of the acetabular fragments is clearly defined. The dome and anterior column are involved and there is extensive hematoma. *B* and *C*, Femoral fracture extends into the subtrochanteric region (*D*).

pecially if displaced, on the AP view of the pelvis. Posterior fractures and sacral fractures are often more subtle and frequently overlooked. Therefore, in addition to a straight AP view, angled views (40° to head, 40° to feet) should be obtained. This will prevent overlooking subtle fractures, provide better evaluation of the sacrum and sacroiliac joints, and allow one to evaluate the degree of internal displacement of bone fractures. If hip trauma is suspected, Judet views are essential. Subtle central acetabular fractures can be easily overlooked (30% missed on the AP view). Judet views are also useful in patients with fracture-dislocation. In recent years, CT has provided valuable information in patients with posterior fractures. Questions regarding fragments or hip fracture-dislocation have also been answered with CT (Fig. 7). CT provides excellent bone detail as well as information regarding soft tissue injury. CT is particularly helpful after reduction of hip dislocation because the positions of fracture fragments and residual bone fragments in the joint are easily assessed. Recently, three-dimensional reconstruction has provided valuable information regarding the position of fragments. The information is not always superior but many find the images are particularly easy to assess (Fig. 2).

During radiographic assessment of complex pelvic fractures (double breaks in the ring) and displaced acetabular fractures, one must consider the potential complications and the imaging techniques that may be necessary for them. Complications of centrally displaced acetabular fractures and complex ring fractures are similar. The most significant complication is hemorrhage. More than 70% of patients require transfusions because of significant pelvic bleeding. Mortality rates greater than 20% are not uncommon. Detection of bleeding sites and control of hemorrhage can be accomplished with diagnostic angiography followed by embolization of bleeding sites. Bleeding sites are frequently multiple and usually difficult to detect and to repair surgically. Generally, the patients are significantly hypotensive so angiography should be considered early. In borderline cases, it is essential to decide if angiography will be needed prior to performing other contrast examinations (retrograde urethrography, cystography, excretory urography, etc.) that may obscure pelvic bleeding sites on the angiogram.

In evaluating lower genitourinary injury, a systematic approach is also required. Up to 20% to 40% of patients with displaced anterior pelvic fractures will have genitourinary injuries. Rupture of the urethra or bladder is most common. Examination should begin with a retrograde urethrogram, proceed to a cystogram if the urethra is intact, and then an excretory urogram to evaluate the upper genitourinary tract.

Distant injuries to the abdomen, chest, and head are not uncommon, and other fractures will be associated with pelvic fractures in 65% of the patients. Routine radiographs

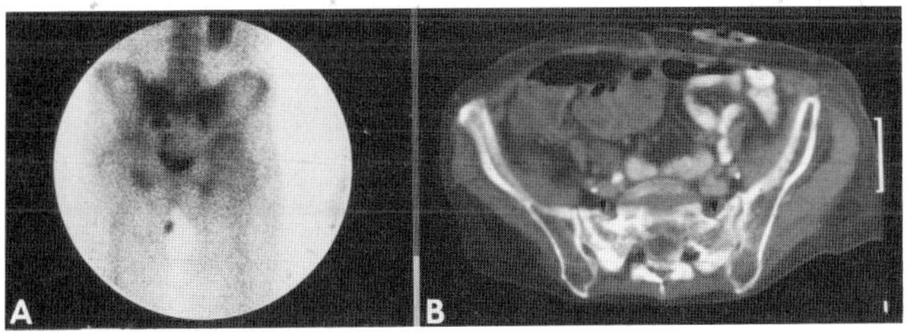

Figure 8

Pelvic and hip pain in 75-year-old woman. *A*, Posterior view of pelvis on a bone scan demonstrates classic H-type sacral insufficiency fracture. *B*, CT scan of pelvis demonstrates the fractures (*arrowheads*) through the sacral alae seen on the bone scan.

of these areas and occasionally abdominal CT may be needed. CT with oral and intravenous administration of contrast medium is particularly useful for evaluating the liver, spleen, pancreas, and kidneys as well as for detecting blood in the peritoneal and retroperitoneal spaces.

Radiographic evaluation of the upper femur is usually complete with AP and lateral or oblique views. Fractures of the femoral neck and intertrochanteric and subtrochanteric regions usually can be detected and assessed on these views.

Subtle stress or insufficiency fractures may be difficult to detect, and isotope bone scans may be helpful. In a retrospective study of fractures, 80% of bone scans were positive 1 day after fracture (95% of the bone scans in patients under 65 years of age were positive at 1 day) and almost 100% of fractures were positive within 3 days.

Insufficiency sacral fractures can occur in osteoporotic women. Very often the fractures are unsuspected because the clinical picture is confusing and radiographs are commonly negative. The bone scan shows a characteristic H-shaped pattern of uptake across the sacrum and sacroiliac joints (Fig. 8 *A*). Plain film tomography or CT may help to characterize these fractures (Fig. 8 *B*). In patients who

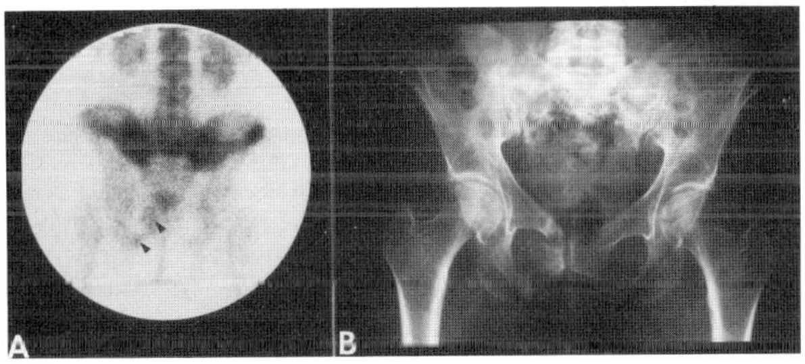

Figure 9

Sixty-five-year-old woman after radiation therapy for ovarian carcinoma. *A*, Posterior view of bone scan, demonstrating generalized decreased activity in lower pelvis. There is faint increased activity in the pubic ramus from a stress fracture (*arrowheads*) and increased uptake in the sacrum and extending through both sacroiliac joints to the anterior iliac crests bilaterally. This was secondary to an insufficiency fracture through the previously irradiated bone. *B*, Pelvic radiograph, demonstrating pathologic-appearing fracture in right pubic ramus and area of sclerosis extending from sacrum to both ilia which corresponds to area of increased uptake on bone scan.

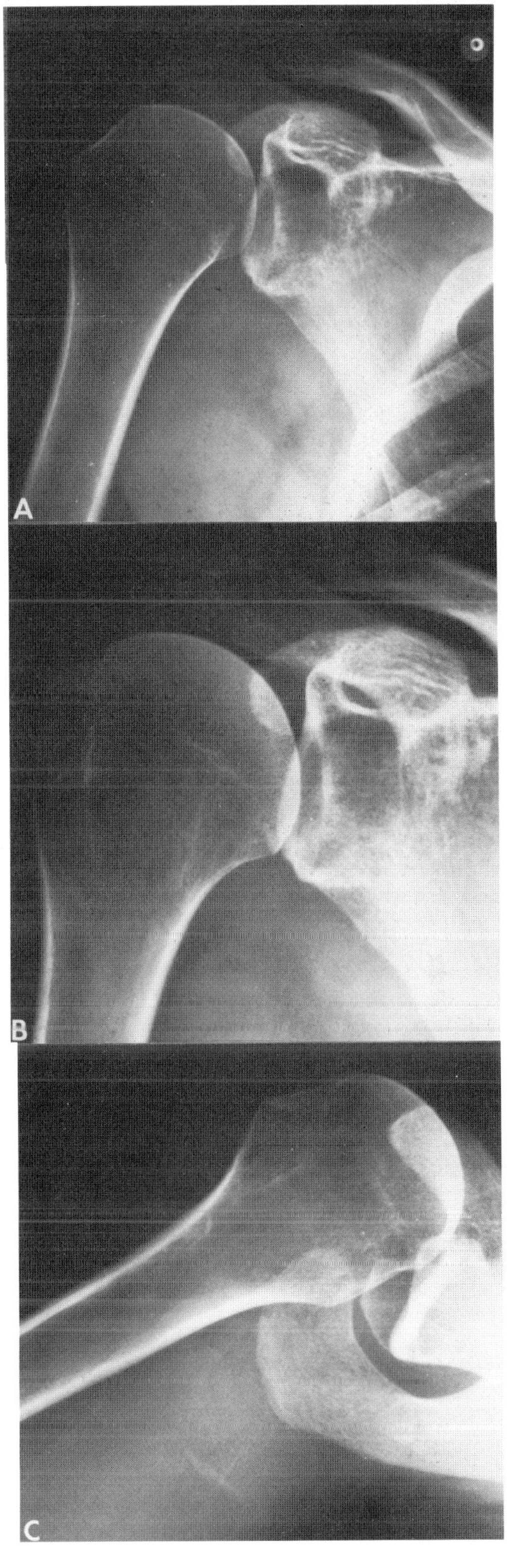

Figure 10

Anterior subluxation of right shoulder. The AP internal and external rotation views (*A* and *B*) do not demonstrate the abnormality clearly. On the axillary view (*C*), the anterior dislocation is obvious.

Table 5. Special Radiographic Views

Technique	Indication
Stryker notch view	Hill-Sachs deformity
West Point view	Hill-Sachs deformity Glenoid labrum fracture
Heinig view	Sternoclavicular joint
Bicipital groove view	Stenosis or subluxation of biceps tendon

have previous radiation exposure, the insufficiency fractures can be quite unusual and may extend beyond the sacrum (Fig. 9).

Long Bone Fractures

Occasionally, tomography is necessary to exclude subtle fracture or to obtain better definition of a stress fracture seen on the isotope scan. Stress fractures can be detected early with isotope studies, but this does not preclude the need for radiographs. In young (10 to 20 years old) runners, sarcomas and other pathologic problems can mimic stress fractures. In patients with atypical stress fractures, MRI may provide the most information regarding bone and soft tissue changes.

Articular Trauma

Radiographic evaluation of the joints is more difficult because of the complex bone and soft tissue injuries that can occur. Aside from routine and special views, further techniques such as arthrography, tomography, MRI, and CT may be required for complete evaluation.

Shoulder A three-film trauma series, including true AP (patient is oblique 40° posteriorly), axillary, and scapular lateral views, provides the basic anatomic information on patients with suspected shoulder trauma. Detection of fractures, especially subtle fractures such as of the coracoid process, can be accomplished easily. Also, dislocations (especially posterior dislocations) are easily identified with these views compared to more conventional AP internal and external rotation views (Fig. 10). Special views are summarized in Table 5. Complex shoulder injuries are best evaluated by CT.

Evaluation of the clavicle and its proximal and distal articulations may require additional techniques. Acromioclavicular joint separations are most easily demonstrated by weight-bearing stress views. Using a 14 × 17 inch film in the transverse position will include both acromioclavicular joints. This provides easy comparison and measurement of both joints and the coracoclavicular distance. Fractures and dislocations of the sternoclavicular joints are difficult to evaluate on routine films because of the overlapping bony structures. CT is ideal for evaluating the medial region of the clavicle, the sternoclavicular joint, and potential injury to the trachea and great vessels.

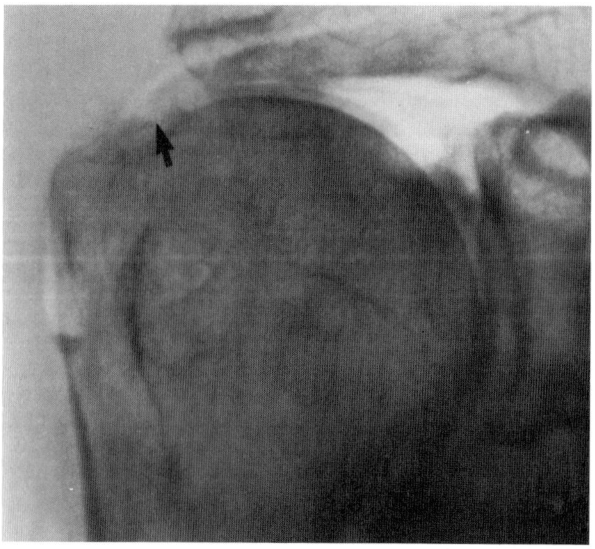

Figure 11

Air-contrast subtraction external-rotation arthrogram demonstrating a small linear tear (*arrow*) in the rotator cuff. The thickness of the cuff is easily assessed with air above and below it.

Soft Tissue Injuries Changes noted on routine views may provide clues to rotator cuff tears, impingement syndrome, and other articular abnormalities. The presence of bony eburnation inferior to the acromioclavicular joint should raise the question of impingement. Sclerosis or erosion of the greater tuberosity has been noted in 95% of patients with rotator cuff tears. A decrease in the humero-acromial distance (normally 0.8 to 1 cm on the external rotation AP view) is very common in patients with rotator cuff tears. Sclerosis and concavity of the inferior surface of the acromion can be seen in both impingement and rotator cuff tears. Arthrography and bursography may be required to evaluate chronic shoulder problems. The techniques should be tailored to the clinical problem. Single-contrast or air-contrast techniques alone or a combination with tomography or CT may be indicated. These decisions must be made prior to initiating the procedure. Air-contrast arthrotomography provides more accurate measurement of cuff tears and detection of glenoid labrum tears (Fig. 11). With glenoid labrum tears, CT may be even more useful. CT has also been useful in evaluating injury or displacement of the biceps tendon.

More recently, ultrasonography and MRI have been used to evaluate the rotator cuff and biceps tendon. One group reported a true-positive correlation in 31 patients, true-negative in 13, and false-negative in 3 of 47 patients who underwent ultrasonic evaluation of the rotator cuff prior to operation. Arthrography (41 patients) gave true-positive findings in 31, true-negative in 9, and false-positive in 1.

Elbow AP and lateral views of the elbow are usually sufficient in children. In adults, both oblique views are also obtained. The lateral view of the elbow is the most important. Soft tissue changes and the anterior humeral line can be evaluated and may provide the only clue to fracture. Displacement of the fat pads (especially posterior fat pads) and supinator fat stripe is 90% accurate in detection of subtle radial head fractures in adults. In children, the anterior humeral line is useful in detecting supracondylar or transcondylar fractures. A line drawn along the anterior margin of the humerus should pass through the middle third of the capitellum. Comparison views are also useful in children because of the often confusing appearance of the ossification centers. In certain situations, the radial head view is useful in patients with suspected fracture of the radial head. This view is obtained with the patient positioned exactly as for the lateral view; however, instead of angling the tube perpendicularly to the cassette, the tube is angled 45° off axis to produce a film that separates the radial head and ulna. This permits better evaluation of the radial head, radiocapitellar joint, and fat pads. In practice, this view is used infrequently.

With subtle fractures, especially osteochondral, a lipohemarthrosis may be the only indication of fracture. Lipohemarthrosis can be detected by using a cross-table technique with the elbow in the extended lateral position. Tomography and isotope studies occasionally may be helpful when other studies are negative but a fracture is still suspected. CT is less commonly used in the evaluation of elbow fractures.

Detection of soft tissue injury involving the capsule, muscles, tendons, and ligaments about the elbow can be difficult. Fluoroscopically monitored stress views can provide valuable information regarding ligament injuries. This examination requires careful comparison with the normal elbow. Injection of local anesthetic (4–5 ml of 1% lidocaine or bupivacaine) into the injured elbow may be required. An increase in the joint space of >1 mm compared to the normal side during varus or valgus stress is abnormal. Arthrography provides a more accurate assessment of capsule and ligament injuries. In most cases, double-contrast arthrotomography is used.

MRI may provide valuable information regarding periarticular hematomas and muscle and ligament tears.

Hand and Wrist The complex anatomy of the hand and wrist often leads to the need for special views. We routinely obtain PA, lateral, oblique, and scaphoid views. In addition to the bony anatomy, one should carefully evaluate the pronator and navicular fat stripes. Displacement or obliteration of these structures may be the only signs of distal radial or scaphoid fractures, respectively. Additional special views, fluoroscopic studies, and their applications are summarized in Table 6.

Evaluation of chronic post-traumatic wrist pain is an even more difficult problem. Subtle fractures and ligament injuries must be considered. Detection may require tomography, isotope studies (including high-resolution views as well as converging collimator or pinhole collimator magnification views), arthrography, MRI, or CT. Algorithm 2 suggests the imaging sequences needed for assessment of carpal injuries.

Recent advances in CT with three-dimensional reconstruction and MRI have provided valuable new information. MRI, with surface coil techniques, provides superb detail of the bone, articular cartilage, tendons, vessels, and nerves. Subtle fractures, soft tissue injury, and early osteonecrosis can be detected by using MRI (Fig. 12).

CT and MRI are also valuable in detection of subluxations of the distal radioulnar joint. The axial image plane is ideal for studying the relationship of the distal radius and ulna.

In suspected reflex sympathetic dystrophy, isotope bone scans may play an important role. Commonly, radiographs show only patchy osteopenia. Radionuclide bone scintigraphy may show increased flow during the radionuclide angiogram phase of the bone scan and may show early activity; however, the most sensitive indicator of reflex sympathetic dystrophy is increased tracer in the delayed image. Post-traumatic changes on bone scanning usually involve focal areas of increased uptake whereas changes related to reflex sympathetic dystrophy often involve diffuse increased uptake involving all of the bones of the hand and wrist. In one series, there was a 96% sensitivity and a 98% specificity for the diagnosis of reflex sympathetic dystrophy by the criteria of diffuse increased uptake in all portions of the hand and wrist on the delayed images.

Table 6. Special Radiographic Views of the Hand and Wrist

Technique	Indication
Brewerton view	Fractures of the metacarpal head
Burman view	Fractures of the 1st carpometacarpal joint
Carpal tunnel view	Fractures of hook of hamate bone, ventral trapezium, or pisiform
Dorsal tangential view	Dorsal chip fractures and soft tissue calcification
Dental film laterals of fingers	Subtle volar or dorsal plate injuries
Stress views	Ligament injury
Motion views	Subtle bony or ligament injury

Knee AP and lateral views meet the minimum requirement for post-traumatic radiography. In addition, we routinely obtain both oblique views. If the lateral view is obtained by using the cross-table technique, one may detect subtle intra-articular fractures. In these patients, a lipohemarthrosis will be evident.

There are numerous techniques for evaluating the patella and patellofemoral joint. In an acutely injured patient, it is best to use the simplest method possible. The Merchant and Settegast methods are commonly used and easily reproduced. The Merchant view is obtained with the knees flexed 45° over the end of the radiographic table. The patient can hold the cassette so that its bottom rests above the knee. The cassette is perpendicular to the tube which is angled 30° to horizontal. The Settegast technique is performed with the patient prone and the knee flexed 90°. The cassette is under the knee and the beam is angled 10° to 20° off vertical so it is perpendicular to the patellofemoral joint. Subtle abnormalities may require further views. Axial views taken at 30°, 60°, and 90° of flexion are useful in cases of suspected instability. Additional techniques may be indicated (Table 7).

Most fractures can be evaluated with routine views. Occasionally, tomography is needed to detect subtle osteochondral fractures or to evaluate the articular surface in tibial plateau fractures. Isotope scans are the most reliable technique for identification of stress fractures, subtle fractures, and osteonecrosis in the elderly.

Evaluation of the intracapsular and extracapsular soft tissue and cartilage of the knee is more complex. Arthrography is an accepted technique for evaluating the menisci. Popliteal cysts are easily demonstrated. However, accurate assessment of the cruciate and collateral ligaments is more difficult. Tomography and thermography have been somewhat more successful. CT has also been used, especially in conjunction with arthrography, to evaluate the cruciate ligaments, plicae, and patellofemoral malalignment. Accuracy of CT arthrography in these conditions is reported to approach 90% to 94%.

MRI without contrast medium can provide much of the same information as CT and arthrography (Fig. 13). Use of surface coils has increased spatial resolution so that even meniscal lesions are visible. In addition, MRI is effective in detecting muscle and ligament injury around the knee. Osteonecrosis can also be detected with greater accuracy than by conventional studies.

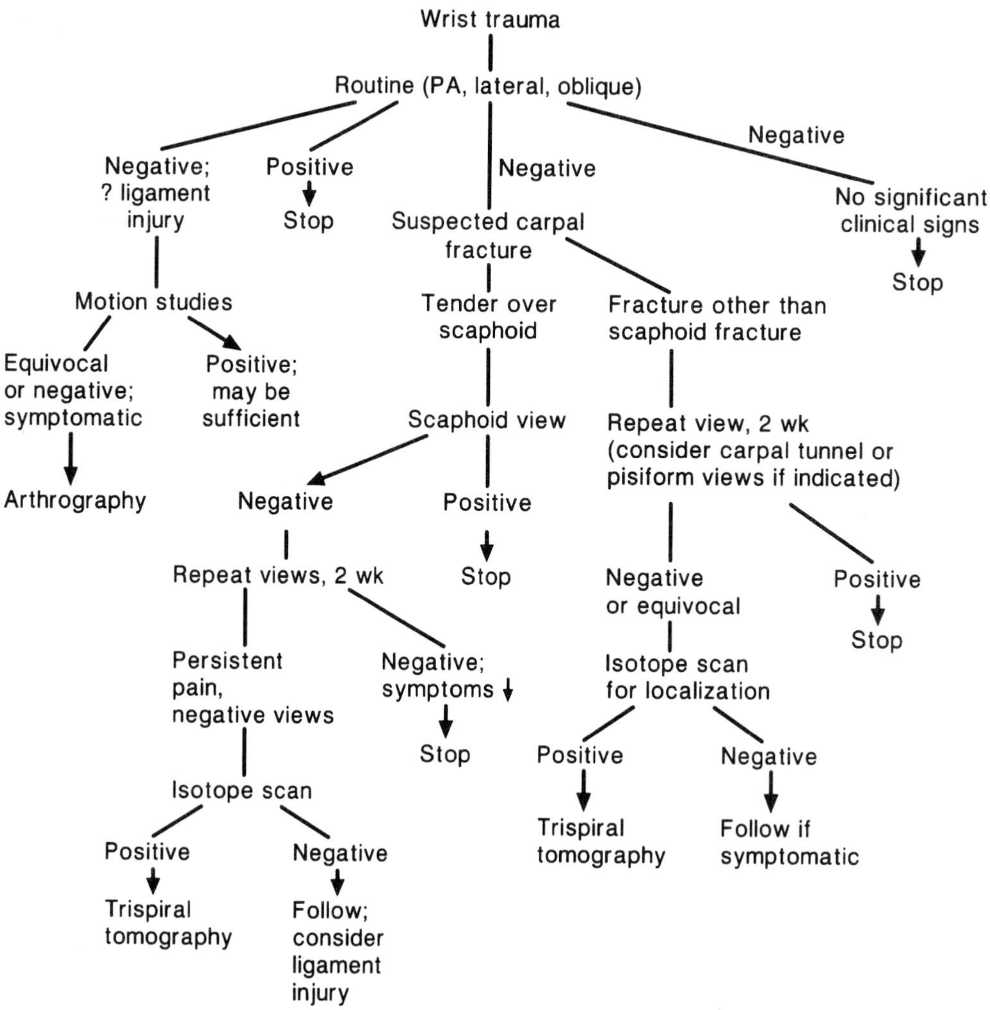

Algorithm 2

Selecting imaging sequences for carpal injuries. (From Berquist, T.H.: The hand and wrist. *In* Diagnostic Imaging of the Acutely Injured Patient, edited by T.H. Berquist, pp. 125–144. Baltimore, Urban & Schwarzenberg, 1985. By permission of Mayo Foundation.)

Foot and Ankle Like that of the hand and wrist, the anatomy of the foot and ankle can be difficult to demonstrate with routine views (AP, lateral, mortise of the ankle; AP, lateral, oblique of the foot). Certain views, such as the axial calcaneal view, are not difficult to reproduce. However, angled views of the midfoot and subtalar joint may be difficult to obtain. Therefore, we frequently use thin-section (3 mm) trispiral tomography to evaluate subtle or suspected lesions in the hindfoot and midfoot. Tomography is also essential for diagnosis and therapy planning in patients suspected to have talar dome fractures.

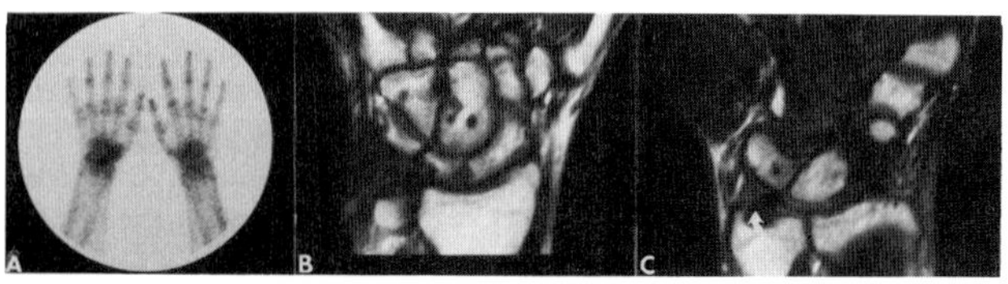

Figure 12

Patient with post-traumatic wrist pain. *A*, Isotope scan demonstrates increased uptake in the proximal carpal row. *B*, Coronal MRI of the wrist shows numerous degenerative cysts in the capitate and hamate. *C*, Coronal MRI in a different plane shows irregularity of the lunate and a triangular cartilage tear (arrow).

CT has been useful in evaluating post-traumatic and other deformities of the hindfoot and midfoot. The angles and articular relationships can be clearly demonstrated. Articular erosive changes, coalitions, and fractures may be more apparent than with other imaging techniques. Evaluation of soft tissue injury requires more specialized techniques. Stress views of the ankle can be valuable in demonstrating significant ligament injuries. However, the results are directly related to the experience of the examining physician and to the proper anesthesia of the joint. Arthrography and tenography are more reliable methods of evaluating ligament injury. Tenography also provides information concerning stenosis and subluxation of tendons.

Table 7. Special Radiographic Techniques for the Knee

Technique	Indication
Notch view	Osteochondral fractures of the femoral condyles
	Loose bodies
Patellar views	Fracture, subluxation
Stress views	Ligament injury
Varus-valgus	Medial and lateral ligaments
AP stress	Cruciate ligaments
Tomography	Subtle fractures
	Plateau fractures
Angiography	Vascular occlusion
Isotope scans	Stress fractures
	Osteonecrosis
MRI	Menisci
	Cruciate ligaments
	Medial and lateral collateral ligaments
	Periarticular muscle
	Patellar ligament
	Quadriceps tendon
Arthrography	Menisci
	Popliteal cysts
With CT	Cruciates and plicae
With xerotomography	Cruciate ligaments

MRI has added valuable information concerning soft tissue injury and osteonecrosis of the bones in the foot and ankle. The tendons and ligaments are easily demonstrated. Use of this noninvasive technique is especially easy for midline structures such as the Achilles tendon (Fig. 14). The perineal and flexor tendons also can be accurately demonstrated (Fig. 15).

Stress Fractures

It is well accepted that isotope scans are most useful in early diagnosis of stress fractures. Comparison radiographs, however, are necessary to exclude other causes of increased radioisotope uptake.

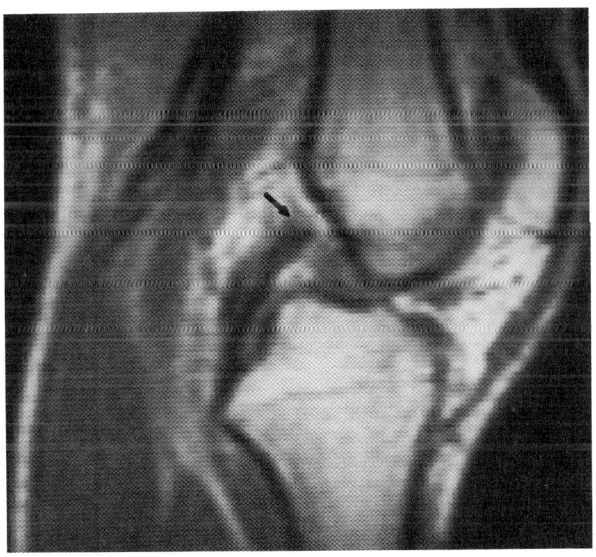

Figure 13

Sagittal MRI of the knee, demonstrating a tear (*arrow*) in the posterior cruciate ligament.

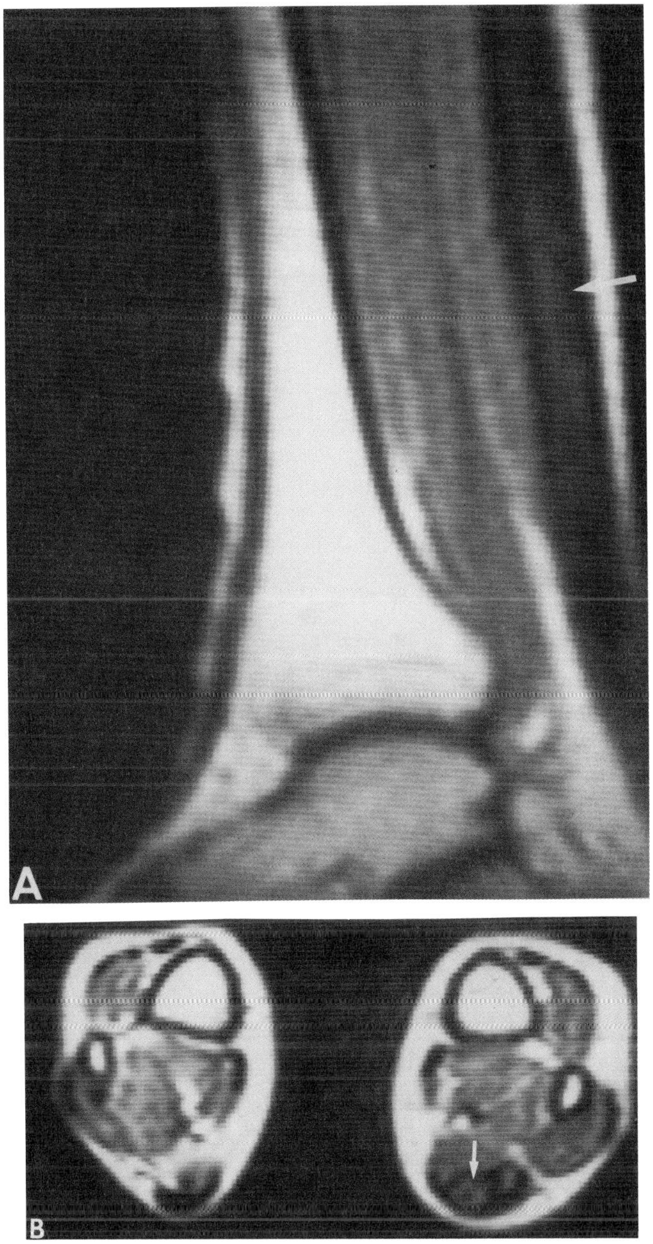

Figure 14

Sagittal (*A*) and axial (*B*) partial saturation sequences of the Achilles tendon show marked thickening and increased signal (*arrows*) due to a long incomplete tear.

Extra-articular Soft Tissue Injury

MRI has provided a valuable new tool for detection of soft tissue injury. Muscle tears and hematomas after trauma are easily identified. The appearance of blood is also quite specific, which allows differentiation from other pathologic conditions (Fig. 16).

Imaging of Joint Replacement and Reconstructive Procedures

Imaging of patients with arthroplasty and other metallic implants can be difficult, depending on the amount and

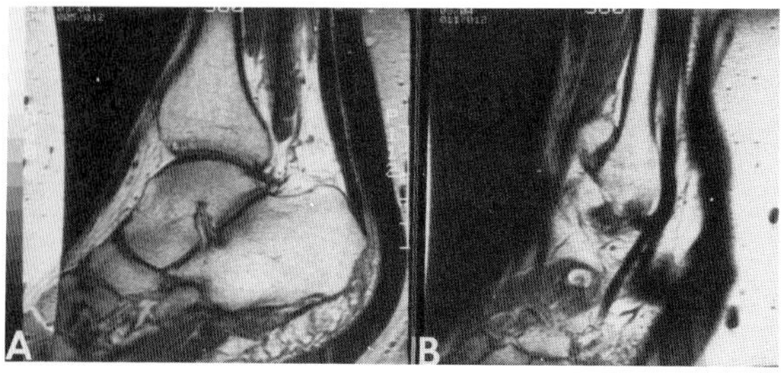

Figure 15

Sagittal surface coil images, demonstrating normal Achilles (*A*) and peroneal (*B*) tendons. Note the superior image quality with surface coils compared to Figure 14 which was done with conventional coils.

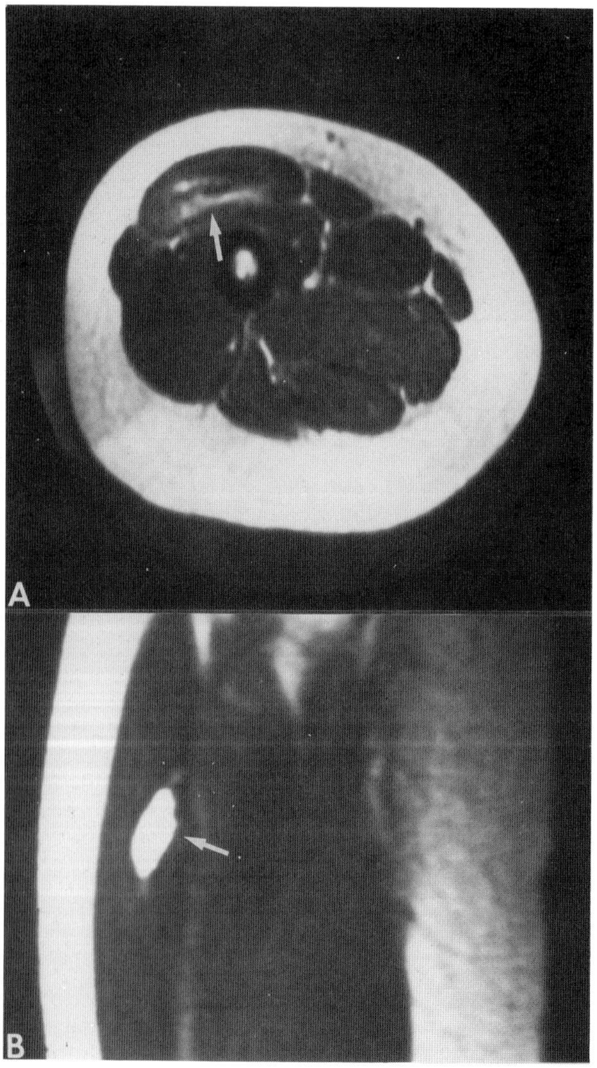

Figure 16

Axial (*A*) and sagittal (*B*) images show a tear (*arrow*) in the rectus femoris.

Table 8. Plain Radiographic Signs of Loosening and Infection in Total Joint Arthroplasty

Loosening	Infection
Position change	Endosteal scalloping
Increasing lucency at the bone-cement interface	Cortical osteoporosis
Lucency > 2 mm at bone-cement interface	Periosteal new bone
Cement fracture	Juxtacortical increase in soft tissue density
Component fracture	
Metal-cement lucency	
Cement voids	
Lytic areas around components or endosteal resorption	

configuration of the metal and whether opaque cement has been used. Patients are usually referred because of pain or loosening of components or because of a question of adequacy of reduction and stability in the case of internal fixation.

Patients with total joint arthroplasty most frequently are referred because of pain due to loosening or infection. Routine radiographic findings, especially serial examinations, provide valuable information (Table 8). Often, further studies are not necessary.

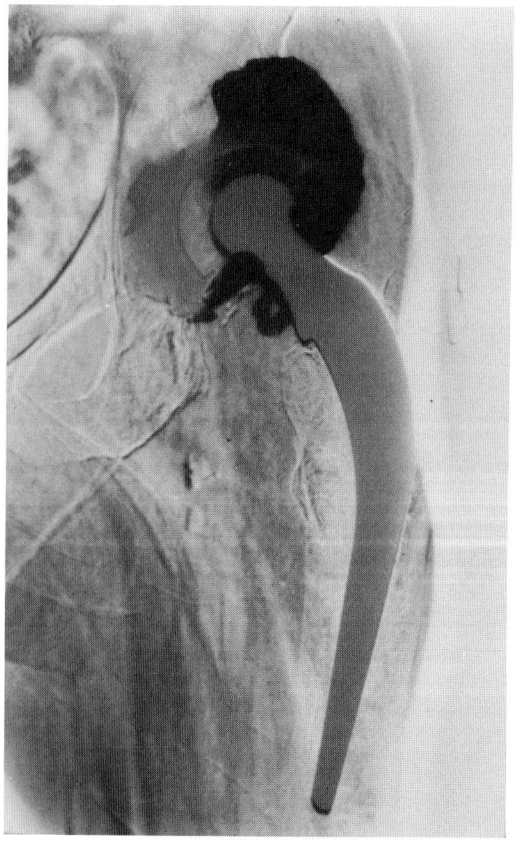

Figure 17

Subtraction arthrogram of left hip demonstrates a large bursa near the upper lateral margin. This is seen after recurrent dislocation and would not be evident on isotope scans or conventional radiographs.

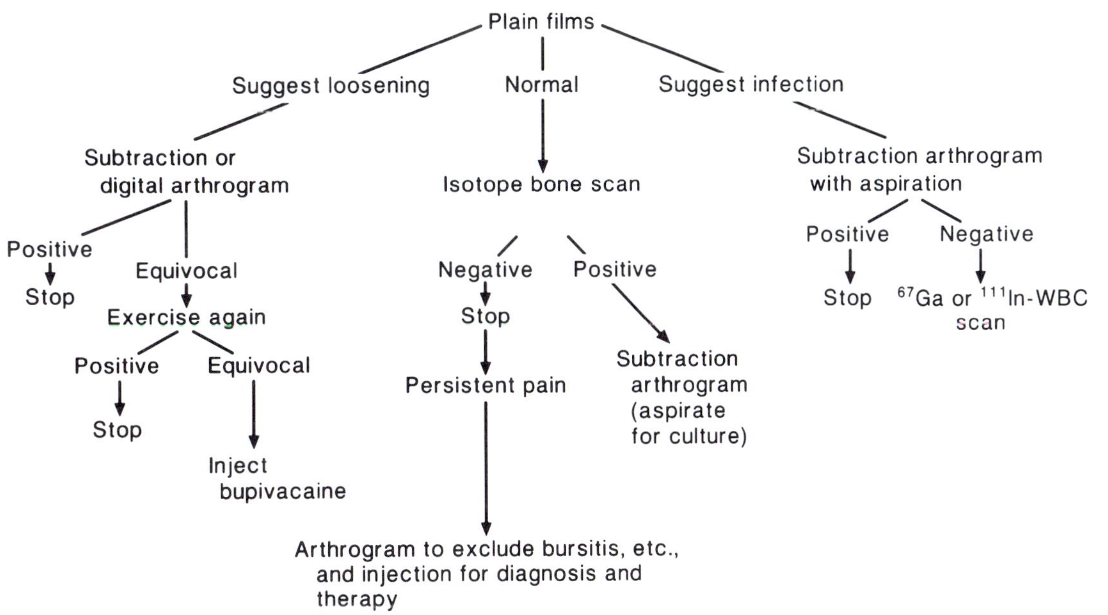

Algorithm 3
Diagnostic approach to painful joint prosthesis.

Subtraction arthrography is a versatile and valuable tool for evaluating a painful prosthesis. Evaluation of loosening or infection is especially accurate in the hip. Other causes of pain, such as bursitis or nonunion of the greater trochanter, also can be detected (Fig. 17). Diagnostic and therapeutic injection of anesthetic agent and aspiration for culture or other analysis also are possible. Accuracy of plain films, arthrography, and isotope studies in the detection of loosening and infection of total hip arthroplasties has been evaluated. In one study of 54 patients, subtraction arthrography was 96% accurate in identifying loosening of either the acetabular or femoral components and 94% accurate in evaluating infection when aspiration was included. Isotope bone scans were 77% accurate in diagnosis of acetabular loosening and 89% accurate in femoral component loosening. Gallium scans correctly identified infection in 77% of patients.

Radioisotope bone scanning with diphosphonates has been used for the evaluation of the painful hip for a number of years. One group showed that a minor increase in activity can be seen in asymptomatic patients more than 1 year after implantation of total hip prostheses. In their experience, marked changes (more than one grade) in activity compared to adjacent or contralateral sites were unusual and suggested loosening. Attempts have been made to categorize the type of uptake (whether diffuse or focal) and the site of uptake (whether involving the acetabular component as well as the femoral component or just localized to the tip of the femoral component) as a means of differentiating loosening from infection. In patients with painful hip prostheses, the pattern and the degree of uptake have not been helpful in differentiating loose aseptic prostheses from infected prostheses.

Small amounts of radioisotope (^{99m}Tc sulfur colloid) can be injected along with contrast agent at the time of arthrography. Because of the high target-to-background ratio, this technique may be more sensitive than routine arthrography for the detection of femoral component loosening. Further work in this area is needed for confirmation.

To determine whether painful prostheses are loose or infected, sequential ^{99m}Tc diphosphonate bone scanning and ^{67}Ga scanning have been performed. The criterion for infection is gallium activity more intense than technetium activity or gallium activity spatially noncongruent with technetium activity. In a series of 66 patients with surgical confirmation, this combination was helpful; however, the sensitivity was only 67% with a specificity of 79% and an accuracy of 73%. Other series have shown similar results.

In order to improve the specificity for diagnosing infection, ^{111}In-labeled autologous leukocytes have been injected to help evaluate potential sites of musculoskeletal sepsis. In a prospective study of 50 patients with suspected low-grade musculoskeletal sepsis, 15 had prosthetic components suspected of being infected. The technetium-gallium scan combination had a sensitivity of 57%, a specificity of 89%, and an accuracy of 75%. In the same 15 patients, the ^{111}In-labeled leukocyte scan had a sensitivity of 86%, a specificity of 100%, and an accuracy of 94%. Another group has reported no significant difference between the technetium-gallium and ^{111}In scans in chronic infections.

With a purified preparation of labeled polymorphonuclear leukocytes, with few if any platelets or lymphocytes, results may be excellent for acute osteomyelitis but relatively poor for low-grade chronic infections. ^{111}In-labeled leukocyte preparations that contain a mixed cell population may be more useful in the diagnosis of low-grade chronic infections because of the presence of leukocytes and other cellular elements (Fig. 18). ^{111}In-labeled leukocyte scanning may not be of great utility in the immediate post-traumatic or postoperative period because hematoma has been reported to show increased activity.

Algorithm 3 summarizes imaging approaches for patients with painful joint replacements.

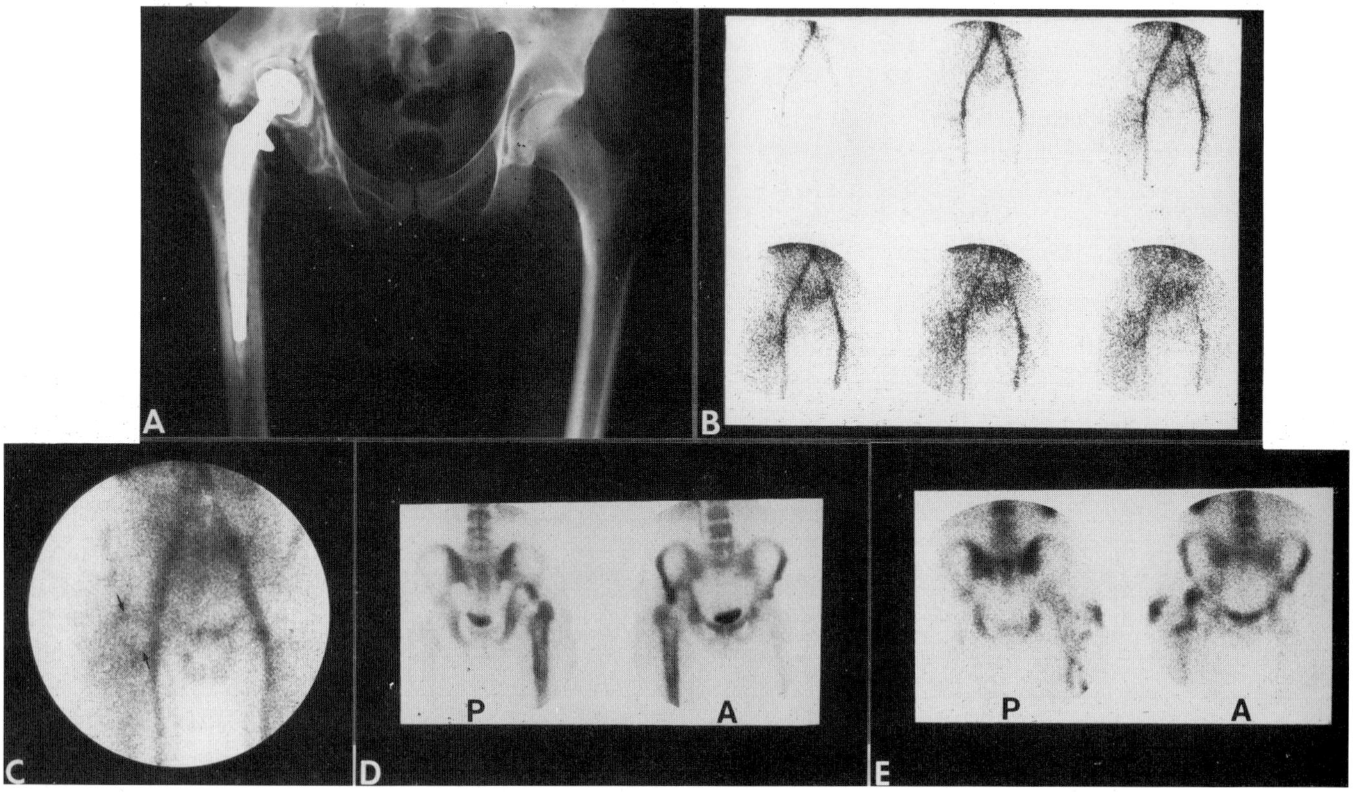

Figure 18

Fifty-five-year-old man with painful right total hip prosthesis. *A*, Radiograph demonstrates lucency about both the femoral and acetabular components. There is endosteal scalloping along the femoral component suggestive of infection. *B*, *C*, and *D*, Three-phase bone scan shows increased flow (*B*) to the region of the right upper femur with early activity (*C*) present in both the region of the pseudocapsule (*arrows*) and in the proximal thigh. The delayed bone scan (*D*) shows intense uptake in both the acetabular and femoral components. These findings would be consistent with an inflammatory response but would not differentiate loosening from infection. *E*, ^{111}In-labeled leukocyte scan shows an area of intense localization in the right acetabular component, along the right femoral component, and in the soft tissues lateral to the femur. At operation, this was an infected prosthesis. *A*, anterior; *P*, posterior.

Bone and Soft Tissue Tumors

Primary Bone and Soft Tissue Tumors

The emphasis in treating bone and soft tissue neoplasms has shifted to limb-salvage procedures. This requires ac-

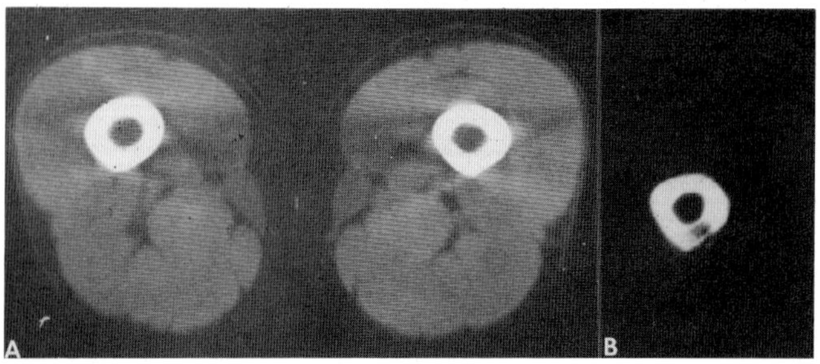

Figure 19

Lymphoma involving bone and soft tissues. CT scan with soft tissue setting (*A*) is normal. With setting for bone (*B*), cortical involvement is clear.

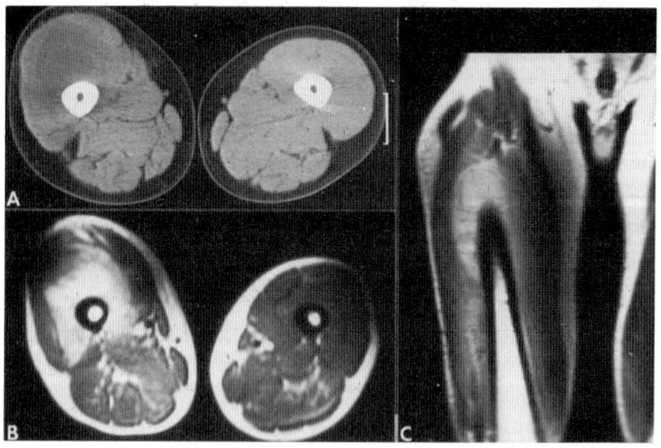

Figure 20

Soft tissue sarcoma. *A*, CT scan without intravenous contrast medium shows right thigh larger than left. The tumor intensity is slightly lower than muscle intensity. Axial (*B*) and coronal (*C*) MRI more clearly demonstrate lesion and its extent. Tumor intensity is higher than muscle intensity due to longer T_2 relaxation time.

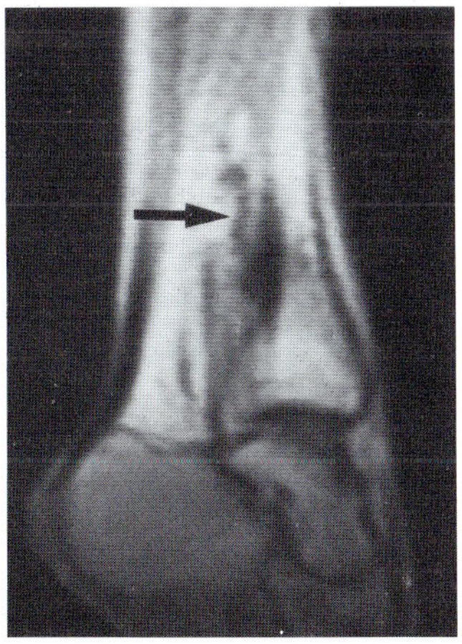

Figure 21

Arteriovenous malformation of the ankle. Sagittal MRI (T_E30, T_R500) shows the extent of the lesion and at least one serpiginous vessel (*arrow*) leading to the juxtacortical lesion. No contrast medium is needed to identify vessels by MRI.

curate identification of lesions and, even more importantly, determination of the extent of bone and soft tissue involvement. Imaging techniques play an important role in preoperative evaluation. Detection of local recurrence or distant metastasis after treatment is equally important.

Diagnosis and characterization of bone lesions often are possible with routine radiographs, occasionally with the aid of tomography. However, evaluation of soft issue involvement or detection of primary soft tissue lesions is difficult. Low kV and xerography techniques may be useful in detection of lipomas. Ultrasonography is useful in differentiating solid from cystic superficial lesions. However, until recently, CT has been the technique of choice for evaluation of bone and soft tissue tumors. It is important to study images with window settings for bone and for soft tissue. If this is not done routinely, lesions can be easily overlooked (Fig. 19). As experience increases, MRI is becoming the ideal technique for detection and determining the extent of involvement in these patients (Figs. 20, 21, and 22).

MRI has superior soft tissue contrast compared with CT. In addition, the ability to image in the coronal and sagittal planes provides valuable information regarding the extent of lesions. CT still provides valuable information in certain patients. For example, subtle calcifications may be helpful in characterizing the histology of lesions, and these findings are easily seen on CT but on MRI calcified material is seen as areas of no signal (black). Fine calcifications may not

Table 9. T_1 **Relaxation Times of Tissues**

Tissue	Time, msec
Normal marrow	278–404
Muscle	375–450
Osteosarcoma	400–500
Lymphoma	450–540
Hemangioma	455–533
Osteomyelitis	572–613
Hematoma	283–753

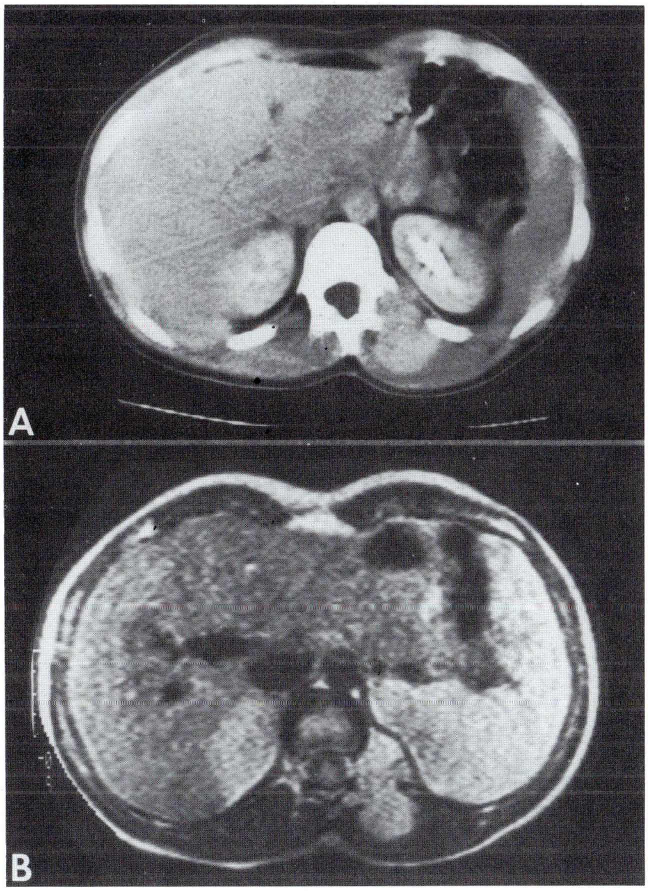

Figure 22

Paraspinal hemangioma. *A,* CT scan with contrast medium shows the lesion clearly. Cortical bone interferes with the epidural region at this window setting. *B,* MRI shows the lesion extending posteriorly to the lamina and into the epidural space.

be seen. It has been reported that MRI and CT are about equal in 50% to 60% of cases in regard to identification of lesions. In the remaining patients (approximately 40%), MRI is superior in detecting and determining the extent of lesions. When both of these techniques are used, additional studies such as angiography or digital angiography and arthrography (joint involvement) are rarely indicated.

The sensitivities of CT and MRI are well established. It was hoped that use of MRI would increase the specificity. However, to date, calculated T_1 and T_2 values have not been significant in differentiating benign from malignant lesions or in predicting their histologic features. The relaxation times of benign and malignant lesions overlap too greatly to be diagnostically useful (Table 9).

Despite the lack of specificity there are certain features that can be helpful in differentiating neoplasms. Lipomas are well-marginated, homogeneous, and of high signal intensity on both T_1 and T_2 weighted sequences. Benign lesions tend to be more homogeneous and well-marginated and may displace but do not encase vessels. Malignant lesions are inhomogeneous and irregular, encase vessels, and may involve the adjacent tissues (muscle from bone lesions, bone from soft tissue lesions). Exceptions to the rule are hemangiomas and desmoids. Hemangiomas fre-

Table 10. MRI Appearance of Bone and Soft Tissue Neoplasms

Lesion	Homogeneous	Well-marginated	Neurovascular encasement	Signal intensity
Bone tumors:				
Malignant	No (lymphoma may be exception)	No	Yes, if soft tissue involved	Mixed T_1 and T_2
Benign	Usually	Generally	No	High T_2; low T_1; occasionally mixed
Soft tissue tumors:				
Benign cysts	Yes	Yes, often capsule	No	High T_2; low T_1
Lipoma	Yes	Yes	No	High T_2; high T_1
Hemangiomas	No	No	Numerous vessels	High T_2; low T_1; may be mixed
Desmoids	No	<20%	Occasionally	Slight T_2 and T_1
Fibromas	Yes	Yes	No	Intermediate T_1 and T_2
Malignant	No	No, occasionally partially well marginated	Yes	Mixed T_2 and T_1

quently present with multiple vessels and may be irregular in appearance. Clinical history and the vascular appearance generally allow correct diagnosis (Fig. 22). Desmoids are aggressive fibrous lesions that generally are infiltrative or irregular and only slightly higher in intensity than muscle on T_2 weighted sequences or slightly lower in intensity than muscle on T_1 weighted sequences. Table 10 summarizes the MRI appearances of bone and soft tissue tumors.

Evaluation of patients after operation may be particularly difficult. Metal implants interfere with CT and conventional techniques after limb-salvage procedures. Fortunately, most orthopaedic appliances are nonferromagnetic and cause little if any artifact on MRI. Therefore, in these patients, MRI is the technique of choice in detecting recurrent tumor (Fig. 23). Differentiation of postoperative changes or scar tissue from tumors also can be difficult. In patients with organized scar tissue, MRI can easily differentiate scar from recurrence. On T_2 weighted scans, scar tissue will have a low signal intensity but recurrent tumor will have a high signal intensity.

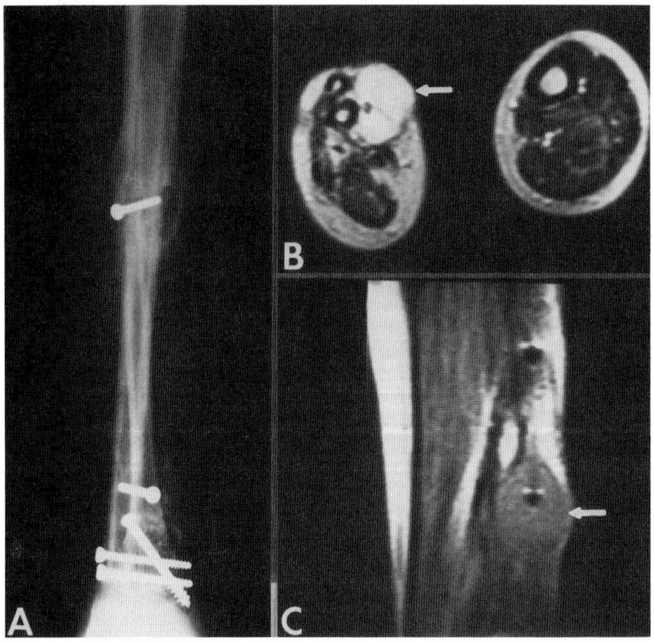

Figure 23

Recurrent sarcoma after partial resection of the tibia with fibular graft and screw fixation. *A*, AP radiograph of lower leg demonstrates the graft and metal screws; nothing suggests neoplasm. Axial T_2 weighted (T_E60, T_R2000) (*B*) and sagittal T_1 weighted (T_E30, T_R500) (*C*) MRI clearly show the recurrent tumor (arrows). There is minimal artifact from the metal.

Osteoid osteomas can often be identified on plain films. If the plain films are negative or equivocal, bone scanning should be performed. It is important to include areas significantly above and below the symptomatic area to avoid missing lesions that cause referred pain. After a lesion is located, further anatomic localization can be obtained with plain film tomography. At some institutions a dose of ^{99m}Tc MDP is given preoperatively and a small portable probe or gamma camera is used in the operating room for localization. After resection of the lesion the bone can be imaged to ensure that the affected area has been removed.

Algorithms 4 and 5 suggest imaging approaches to bone and soft tissue neoplasms.

Metastasis

Bone scans have been extremely useful in detecting metastases from soft tissue tumors and from primary bone tumors. Some patterns of uptake—such as multiple areas of increased uptake—are highly diagnostic of metastasis. However, solitary lesions must be correlated with radiographs to be certain that increased uptake is not due to benign disease. The combined data from seven series of patients with known primary malignancies show the following probabilities of a solitary lesion being due to metastasis: rib, 28%; extremity, 44%; skull, 54%; and spine or pelvis, 63%. Metastatic disease commonly involves the axial skeleton. In this region, MRI provides certain advantages. First, it is a very sensitive technique and can detect changes more easily than radiographs can. The anatomy is clearly displayed so that degenerative disease, osteoporotic compression fractures, and other pathologic conditions can be differentiated from metastasis. Second, sagittal images provide excellent detail of the cord and spinal canal. Therefore, obstruction can be detected without the need for CT with metrizamide or myelography in many cases. Localized areas in the extremities also can be studied more

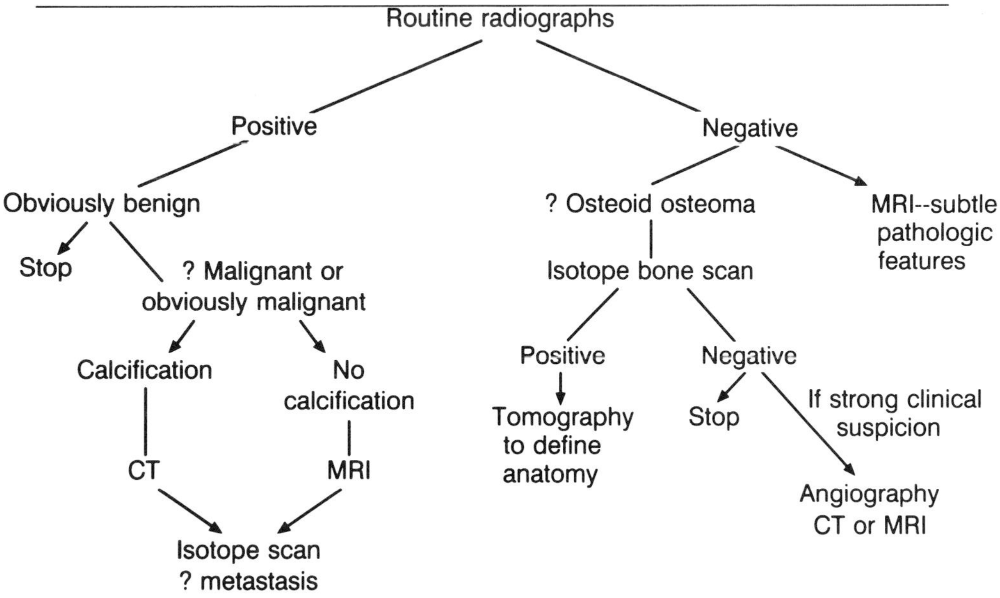

Algorithm 4
Imaging of bone tumors.

easily with MRI. However, a complete-body survey with MRI is impractical at this point due to the length of time this examination would take. CT remains the technique of choice for detection of pulmonary metastasis.

Infection

Musculoskeletal infections can occur with acute or insidious onset. Imaging of patients with suspected infection depends upon whether the infection involves nonviolated tissue or is present in an area of previous operation or fracture. Algorithms 6, 7 and 8 summarize imaging approaches to infection.

Nonviolated Tissue

The early changes of infection may be subtle on routine radiographs. Often, localized swelling of the superficial and deep soft tissues is the only finding. Bone or joint changes are often not evident for 10 to 14 days. Tomography may detect changes earlier.

The isotope bone scan has been shown to be very sen-

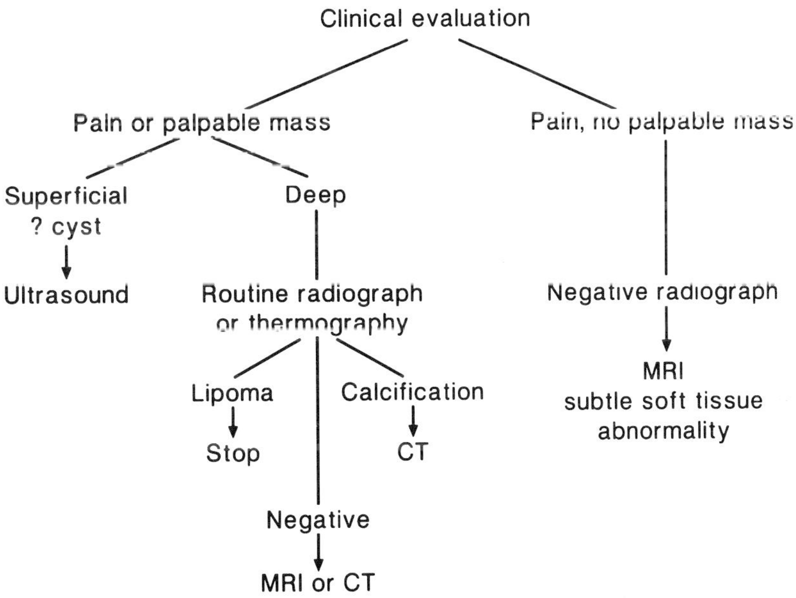

Algorithm 5
Imaging of soft tissue masses.

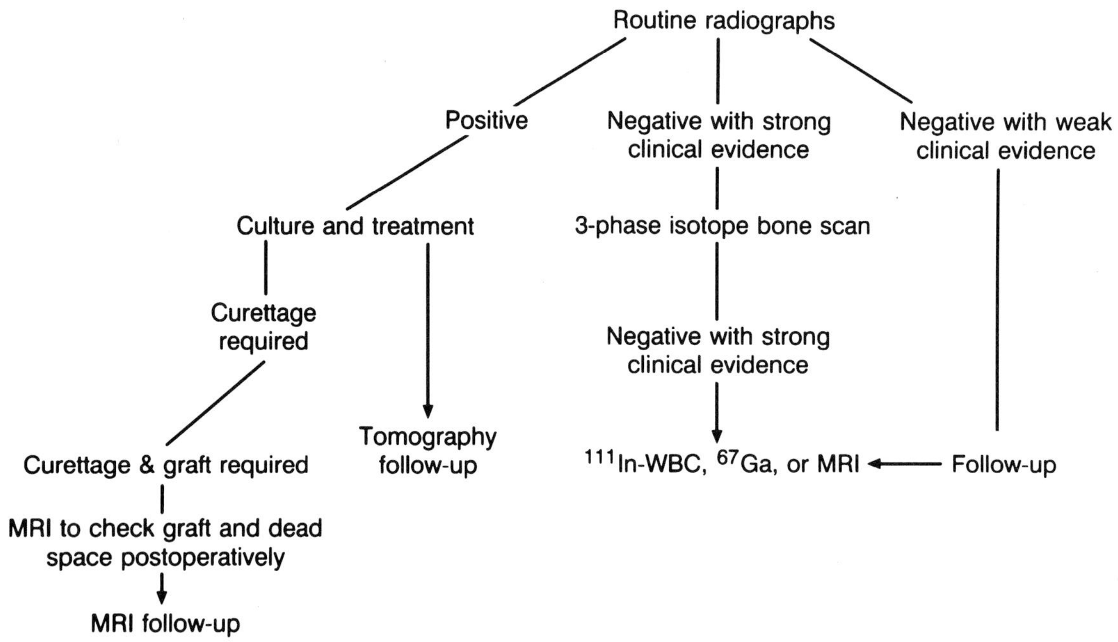

Algorithm 6

Imaging approaches to infection: osteomyelitis.

sitive for the detection of early osteomyelitis in adults as well as children. There has been some controversy about the ability of the bone scan to detect neonatal osteomyelitis. In a recent study, radioisotope bone scans were performed in 33 infants less than 6 weeks old and suspected to have osteomyelitis. Each of the 25 sites of proved osteomyelitis demonstrated abnormal tracer localization, including 10 sites positive by scintigraphy but negative radiographically. The authors stressed the need for high-quality scintigrams, especially around the growth plate complex. There have been reports of normal bone scans or photon-deficient bone scans in early osteomyelitis. If there is a strong suspicion that osteomyelitis is present, consideration should be given to following the bone scan

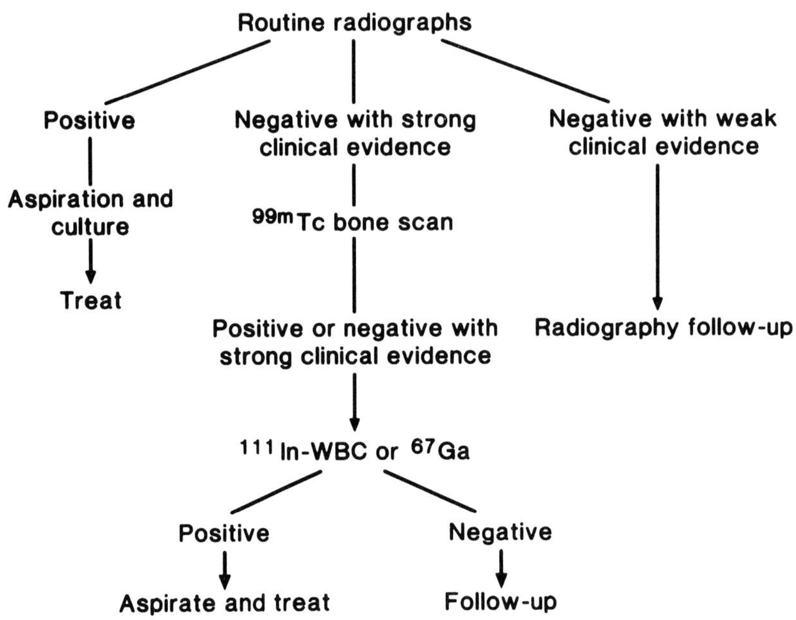

Algorithm 7

Imaging approaches to infection: joint space infection.

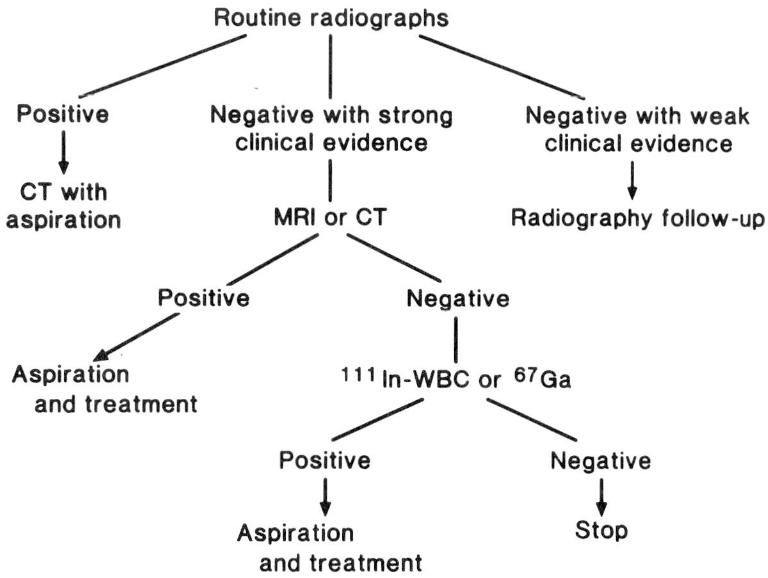

Algorithm 8

Imaging approaches to infection: disk space infection.

with a gallium scan or an ^{111}In-labeled leukocyte scan. MRI is also more sensitive than conventional radiographs but the comparison of isotope studies and MRI has not been completely evaluated in this regard.

Diagnosis of disk space infection can be particularly difficult. CT with or without metrizamide is very effective in demonstrating the degree of involvement of bone and soft tissue. When metrizamide is used, the spinal canal also can be accurately assessed. An additional benefit is CT-guided aspiration to identify the causative organism.

Recent work with MRI has demonstrated that disk space infection or vertebral osteomyelitis can be detected early and with a high degree of specificity. Sagittal images clearly define the level of involvement (Fig. 24). The degree of spinal canal involvement can also be accurately demonstrated. No contrast material is required.

Violated Tissue

Evaluation of patients who have had previous fracture (with or without metallic implants) or previous operation is difficult. Changes related to the trauma cause a confusing picture on MRI, and metal artifact reduces the value of tomography or CT significantly.

The use of combined isotopes has been especially valuable in patients who have had trauma or operation. Sequential technetium-gallium scintigraphy—with the criteria of moderate to high gallium uptake or incongruent technetium and gallium distributions—showed a sensitivity of 72%, a specificity or 86%, and an accuracy of 80% in one series of 159 patients. However, in another series of 30 patients with surgical confirmation, the sensitivity of the sequential technetium-gallium scan was only 48% with a specificity of 86% and an accuracy of 57%; the ^{111}In-labeled leukocyte technique had a sensitivity of 83%, a specificity of 86%, and an accuracy of 83%.

In pseudarthrosis, the gallium scan is often intensely positive, even when no infection is present. Early experience with ^{111}In-labeled leukocyte scanning shows that this study will be negative when there is no infection and will be positive when there is infection at a site of pseudarthrosis. Whether the ^{111}In-labeled leukocyte scan or the sequential technetium-gallium scan is used, the isotope technique provides additional valuable information in the work-up of patients suspected to have musculoskeletal sepsis in sites of violated bone.

Vascularized Grafts

Treatment of chronic osteomyelitis with vascularized fibular, omental, or muscle grafts is becoming more common. The goals of this procedure are to fill the dead space and to provide a vascular environment for healing. It is important to determine if the dead space is adequately filled and to determine if the grafts are viable. Isotope studies have been useful in evaluating the viability of free vascularized bone grafts when they are performed within the first 72 hours. Superior evaluation of the patency of the arterial supply of the graft is possible with digital subtraction angiography. To date, MRI has provided valuable information concerning residual dead space; the sagittal and coronal planes are particularly useful in this regard. Experience is too limited to be certain if MRI can accurately predict viability. However, as software improves and the role of spectroscopy evolves, this will become more clear. It appears that MRI will be most effective in evaluating muscle and omental flaps.

Miscellaneous Conditions

Imaging of many musculoskeletal problems is sufficient with routine radiographs. The newer modalities (CT, MRI, etc.) have added additional information in certain conditions other than those already discussed.

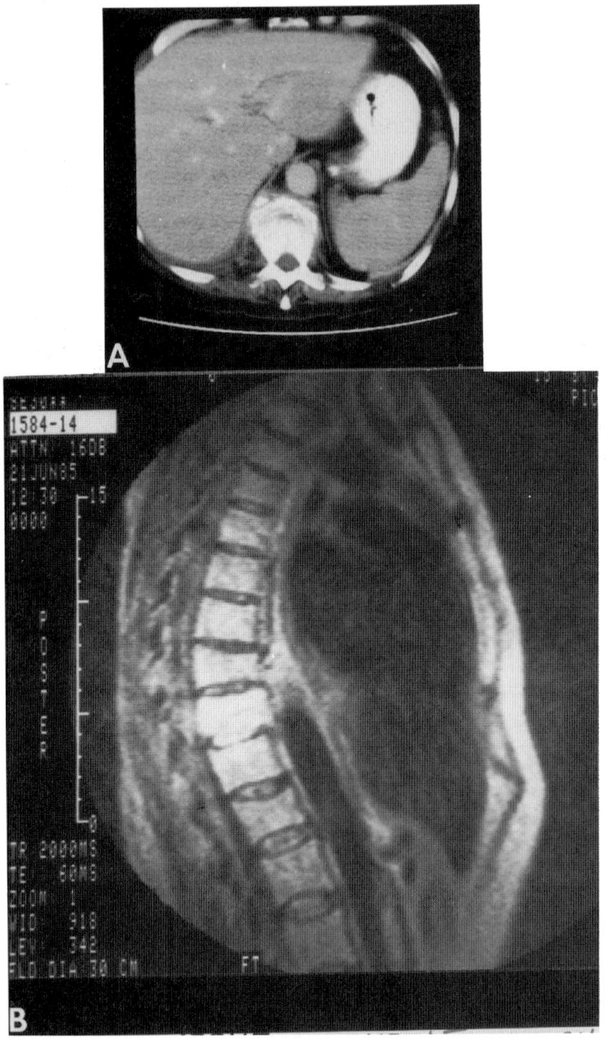

Figure 24

A, CT scan of the lower thoracic region demonstrating fragmentation of vertebral body due to brucellosis. There is little soft tissue reaction. *B,* Sagittal MRI (T_E60, T_R2000) shows compression of the vertebra with increased signal in the disk, due to infection.

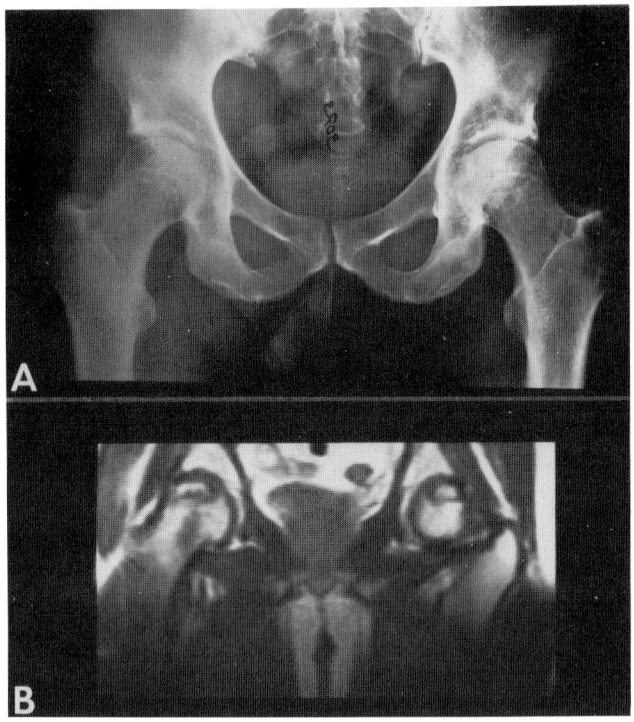

Figure 25

Osteonecrosis of the hips. *A,* AP view of pelvis shows normal right hip and some increased density of the left femoral head. An oblique frog-leg view would be helpful to be certain that the density was in the head and not due to bony overlap from the acetabulum. *B,* Coronal MRI shows bilateral osteonecrosis with sequestra (Ficat stage III).

Osteonecrosis

Osteonecrosis of bone has been detected with routine radiographs and isotope scans. CT has also been used in evaluation of osteonecrosis of the hips. MRI is a very sensitive technique for early diagnosis. The changes seen with MRI are similar to the findings noted on radiographs. However, MRI demonstrates osteonecrosis earlier and changes are more advanced than would be expected on radiographs. For example, if radiographs are normal or stage I (Ficat), the MRI image consistently will demonstrate a greater arch of involvement consistent with more advanced disease (Fig. 25). Although more work is needed, it appears that MRI is the technique of choice in evaluation of osteonecrosis, especially in the hip.

Myopathies

CT has been of some value in diagnosing neuromuscular disorders, especially if fatty replacement occurs. MRI shows infiltrative changes in local muscle groups or diffuse changes more clearly than CT. The appearance of inflammatory muscle disease is also fairly characteristic, which allows differentiation from neoplasm. Current software does not allow one to identify the type of myopathy specifically. In the future, ^{31}P spectroscopy may provide even more information, both in diagnosis and in evaluating the response to therapy.

Disk Disease and Related Disorders

Degenerative changes in the disk and disk herniation have been effectively studied with CT. In fact, CT with metrizamide and coronal and sagittal reconstruction is very effective in the study of other causes of low back pain, such as spinal stenosis. MRI is beginning to demonstrate its utility in this area as well. The normal disk has increased signal intensity on T_2 weighted images, due to its water content. As the disk degenerates, it loses both height and signal intensity. Sagittal images are particularly effective for evaluating disk changes and herniation. Oblique axial images will soon be available, which will increase the accuracy in diagnosing disk herniations.

MRI will have great impact in the future. High-resolution CT remains superior for evaluating subtle bone changes, osteophytes, and disk calcifications.

Spinal stenosis can be detected with CT and MRI (Fig. 26). The degree of spinal stenosis can be evaluated on sagittal MRI. Large osteophytes, hypertrophy of the ligamentum flavum, extrinsic defects in the dural sac, and the

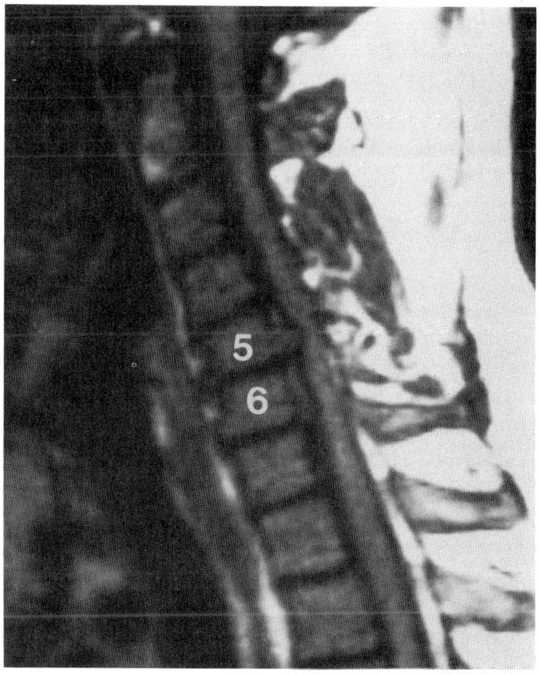

Figure 26

Cervical radiculopathy in middle-aged man. Sagittal MRI (T_E30, T_R500) shows spinal stenosis with cord compression at C-5 and C-6.

lateral recesses can be evaluated. More studies will be needed before the true role of MRI can be assessed accurately compared with CT and myelography.

Leg Length Discrepancy

A new technique was recently described for accurately assessing leg length discrepancy. CT digital radiography is accurate and can be performed quickly with conventional CT equipment. The radiation dose is a fraction of that from conventional techniques. Measurements are made using the CT cursor to select the measurement sites on a simple CT scout image of the extremities.

CT has also been useful in measuring other skeletal abnormalities such as the degree of femoral anteversion or retroversion and tibial torsion. Both CT and MRI provide valuable information about the configuration of the medullary canal in patients who require special surgical reconstruction procedures or custom-designed prosthetic devices.

Annotated Bibliography

Advances in Imaging Techniques

Collier, B.D.; Carrera, G.F.; Johnson, R.P.; Isitman, A.T.; Hellman, R.S.; Knobel, J.; Finger, W.A.; Gonyo, J.E.; and Malloy, P.J.: Detection of femoral head avascular necrosis in adults by SPECT. J. Nucl. Med. 26:979–987, 1985.

The article discusses the utility of single-photon emission computed tomography in the evaluation of patients suspected to have osteonecrosis. Emission computed tomography was more sensitive than planar imaging.

Jacobsson, H.; Larsson, S.A.; Vesterköld, L.; and Lindvall, N.: The application of single photon emission computed tomography to the diagnosis of ankylosing spondylitis of the spine. Br. J. Radiol. 57:133–140, 1984.

This article discusses single-photon emission computed tomography in the spine. The method allows specific anatomic localization of pathologic processes.

Larson, S.M.: Radiolabeled monoclonal anti-tumor antibodies in diagnosis and therapy. J. Nucl. Med. 26:538–545, 1985.

This review article discusses the use of monoclonal antibodies in diagnosis and its potential in therapy. Progress has been made in the use of monoclonal antibodies in patients with melanoma or lymphoma, and it is being tested in patients with breast carcinoma, prostate carcinoma, or colon carcinoma.

Pykett, I.L.; Newhouse, J.H.; Buonanno, F.S.; Brady, T.J.; Goldman, M.R.; Kistler, J.P.; and Pohost, G.M.: Principles of nuclear magnetic resonance imaging. Radiology 143:157–168, 1982.

The authors review the physics, scanning methods, and terms used in magnetic resonance imaging. Clinical pulse sequences are reviewed.

Richardson, M.L.; Genant, H.K.; Cann, C.E.; Ettinger, B.; Gordan, G.S.; Kolb, F.O.; and Reiser, U.J.: Assessment of metabolic bone diseases by quantitative computed tomography. Clin. Orthop. 195:224–238, 1985.

Various techniques for evaluating metabolic bone disease are reviewed with emphasis on quantitative computed tomography.

Totty, W.G., and Vannier, M.W.: Complex musculoskeletal anatomy: Analysis using three dimensional surface reconstruction. Radiology 150:173–177, 1984.

Reconstruction of computed tomographic images into a three-dimensional format resulted in improved understanding of spatial relationships, especially for nonradiologists.

Uri, G.; Wellman, H.; Capello, W.; Robb, J.; and Greenman, G.: Scintigraphic and x-ray arthrographic diagnosis

of femoral prosthesis loosening: Concise communication. J. Nucl. Med. 25:661–663, 1984.
The article describes the use of radionuclide arthrography in the evaluation of femoral prosthesis loosening. The results suggest that the radionuclide technique may be more sensitive than ones currently used.

Wahner, H.W.; Dunn, W.L.; and Riggs, B.L.: Assessment of bone mineral. Part 1 and Part 2. J. Nucl. Med. 25:1134–1141; 1241–1253, 1984.
The development and methods of bone mineral analysis are reviewed.

Wanebo, H.J.; Harpole, D.; and Teates, C.D.: Radionuclide lymphoscintigraphy with technetium 99m antimony sulfide colloid to identify lymphatic drainage of cutaneous melanoma at ambiguous sites in the head and neck and trunk. Cancer 55:1403–1413, 1985.
The article discusses the use of radionuclide lymphoscintigraphy to define the drainage patterns of cutaneous melanoma. It demonstrates the usefulness of defining unpredicted sites of tumor drainage.

Trauma

Berquist, T.H. (ed.): Imaging of Orthopedic Trauma and Surgery. Philadelphia, W.B. Saunders Company, 1986.
The anatomy, imaging techniques, and clinical details of adult trauma are reviewed. Evaluation of reduction and reconstructive techniques also is reviewed.

Keene, J.S.; Goletz, T.H.; Lilleas, F.; Alter, A.J.; and Sackett, J.F.: Diagnosis of vertebral fractures: A comparison of conventional radiography, conventional tomography, and computed axial tomography. J Bone Joint Surg. 64A:586–595, 1982.
Computed tomography is the examination of choice for vertebral trauma except that, in evaluation of the pars intra-articularis, conventional tomography was superior.

Mack, L.A.; Matsen, F.A., III; Kilcoyne, R.F.; Davies, P.K.; and Sickler, M.E.: US evaluation of the rotator cuff. Radiology 157:205–209, 1985.
Ultrasonography was compared with arthrography for evaluation of rotator cuff tears in 79 patients. Results of ultrasonography correlated with the findings at operation in 47 patients. The technique is nearly as accurate as arthrography and is noninvasive and less expensive.

Matin, P.; Lang, G.; Carretta, R.; and Simon, G.: Scintigraphic evaluation of muscle damage following extreme exercise: Concise communication. J. Nucl. Med. 24:308–311, 1983.
This article discusses the use of bone tracers in evaluating muscle damage after extreme exercise. It shows that it is possible to differentiate muscle injury from joint and osseous abnormalities in athletes.

Mino, D.E.; Palmer, A.K.; and Levinsohn, E.M.: Radiography and computerized tomography in the diagnosis of incongruity of the distal radio-ulnar joint. J. Bone Joint Surg. 67A:247–252, 1985.
True lateral views of the wrist are difficult to obtain, especially when the patient is in a cast. Computed tomography provides more accurate assessment of the distal radio-ulnar joint.

Schneider, R.; Yacovone, J.; and Ghelman, B.: Unsuspected sacral fractures: Detection by radionuclide bone scanning. A.J.R. 144:337–341, 1985.
The article describes sacral fractures in osteoporotic patients. The diagnosis is difficult, and the characteristic scintigraphic patterns aid in making this diagnosis.

Woodring, J.H., and Goldstein, S.J.: Fractures of the articular processes of the cervical spine. A.J.R. 139:341–344, 1982.
Tomography detected fractures of the articular processes in patients with neurologic symptoms. Routine films were negative.

Imaging of Reconstructive Procedures

Lyons, C.W.; Berquist, T.H.; Lyons, J.C.; Rand, J.A.; and Brown, M.L.: Evaluation of radiographic findings in painful hip arthroplasties. Clin. Orthop. 195:239–251, 1985.
Plain films, isotope studies, and subtraction arthrograms were reviewed. Subtraction arthrograms were most accurate in assessing loosening and provided a route for aspiration and anatomic assessment of other potential causes of pain.

Schneider, R.; Abenavoli, A.M.; Soudry, M.; and Insall, J.: Failure of total condylar knee replacement: Correlation of radiographic, clinical, and surgical findings. Radiology 152:309–315, 1984.
The radiographic features of failed total knee arthroplasty with a total condylar prosthesis are discussed. Causes of failure included infection, loosening, malalignment, and instability.

Steinbach, L.S.; Schneider, R.; Goldman, A.B.; Kazam, E.; Ranawat, C.S.; and Ghelman, B.: Bursae and abscess cavities communicating with the hip: Diagnosis using arthrography and CT. Radiology 156:303–307, 1985.
Abscess cavities and bursa communicating with the hip were identified with arthrography and computed tomography. Differentiation of bursae from other masses is important to avoid unnecessary operations.

Bone and Soft Tissue Tumors

Hudson, T.M.; Schiebler, M.; Springfield, D.S.; Hawkins, I.F., Jr.; Enneking, W.F.; and Spanier, S.S.: Radiologic imaging of osteosarcoma: Role in planning surgical treatment. Skeletal Radiol. 10:137–146, 1983.
Plain films provided the most diagnostic information. Computed tomography and angiography were most useful in preoperative assessment. Scintigraphy was rarely useful.

Weekes, R.G.; McLeod, R.A.; Reiman, H.M.; and Pritchard, D.J.: CT of soft-tissue neoplasms. A.J.R. 144:355–360, 1985.
The computed tomographic findings related to benign and malignant soft tissue tumors are reviewed. Computed tomography was excellent for identification and characterization (as benign or malignant) of lesions.

Zimmer, W.D.; Berquist, T.H.; McLeod, R.A.; Sim, F.H.; Pritchard, D.J.; Shives, T.C.; Wold, L.E.; and May, G.R.: Bone tumors: Magnetic resonance imaging versus computed tomography. Radiology 155:709–718, 1985.
The results of magnetic resonance imaging and computed tomography in detection and determining the extent of bone and soft tissue involvement are discussed. The former was superior to the latter except in identification of subtle calcification and pathologic fractures.

Infection

Berquist, T.H.; Brown, M.L.; Fitzgerald, R.H., Jr.; and May, G.R.: Magnetic resonance imaging: Application in musculoskeletal infection. Magn. Reson. Imaging 3:219–230, 1985.
Magnetic resonance imaging was sensitive in detecting infection but changes were often nonspecific. When combined with use of ^{111}In-labeled leukocytes, the anatomic detail and specificity were maximized.

Bressler, E.L.; Conway, J.J.; and Weiss, S.C.: Neonatal osteomyelitis examined by bone scintigraphy. Radiology 152:685–688, 1984.

In contrast to previous articles, this review shows that, with optimal scintigraphic technique, bone tracers can detect neonatal osteomyelitis as well as that in older children and adults.

McGahan, J.P., and Dublin, A.B.: Evaluation of spinal infections by plain radiographs, computed tomography, intrathecal metrizamide, and CT-guided biopsy. Diagn. Imag. Clin. Med. 54:11–20, 1985.

Computed tomography was most useful in diagnosis and aspiration of disk infection. With the addition of metrizamide as contrast agent, it was useful in evaluating the subdural and epidural spaces.

Merkel, K.D.; Brown, M.L.; Dewanjee, M.K.; and Fitzgerald, R.H., Jr.: Comparison of indium-labeled-leukocyte imaging with sequential technetium-gallium scanning in the diagnosis of low-grade musculoskeletal sepsis: A prospective study. J. Bone Joint Surg. 67A:465–476, 1985.

Sequential gallium-technetium scans were compared prospectively with scans made with ^{111}In-labeled leukocytes in 42 patients. The latter method was superior in detection of low-grade infection.

Modic, M.T.; Feiglin, D.H.; Piraino, D.W.; Boumphrey, F.; Weinstein, M.A.; Duchesneau, P.M.; and Rehm, S.: Vertebral osteomyelitis: Assessment using MR. Radiology 157:157–166, 1985.

Patients suspected to have vertebral osteomyelitis were studied with magnetic resonance imaging, radioisotopes, and radiographs. Magnetic resonance imaging was the most sensitive and specific technique.

Miscellaneous Conditions

Aitken, A.G.F.; Flodmark, O.; Newman, D.E.; Kilcoyne, R.F.; Shuman, W.P.; and Mack, L.A.: Leg length determination by CT digital radiography. A.J.R. 144:613–615, 1985.

Computed tomography digital radiography is accurate, is easily performed with commercial equipment, and can be accomplished with low radiation doses.

Modic, M.T.; Pavlicek, W.; Weinstein, M.A.; Boumphrey, F.; Ngo, F.; Hardy, R.; and Duchesneau, P.M.: Magnetic resonance imaging of intervertebral disk disease: Clinical and pulse sequence considerations. Radiology 152:103–111, 1984.

Anatomic pulse sequences used to study the spine and disk are reviewed. Magnetic resonance imaging shows significant potential in evaluation of disk disease.

Rosenthal, D.I.; Stauffer, A.E.; Davis, K.R.; Ganott, M.; and Taveras, J.M.: Evaluation of multiplanar reconstruction in CT recognition of lumbar disk disease. A.J.R. 143:169–176, 1984.

Axial, coronal, and sagittal computed tomographic scans were compared with myelograms in evaluating lumbar disk disease. The axial scans were the most sensitive. Reformatted images were only useful in complex cases when axial studies gave equivocal results.

16

Pediatric Reconstruction

The major advances in pediatric reconstruction of the upper extremity in the past 3 years have involved the use of microsurgical techniques for the reconstruction of congenital anomalies and for the repair of obstetric brachial plexus injuries.

Embryology

In the normal human embryo, the upper limb first becomes evident at 26 days of fetal life as a small bud of tissue on the upper lateral body wall, consisting of a mesodermal protuberance with an ectodermal covering. By the end of the fourth week (Fig. 1 *A*), the arm bud has grown longer and larger; the mesodermal tissue has condensed to form the humerus precursor; and the radius, ulna, and nerves are beginning to appear at the base of the bud. By the fifth week (Fig. 1 *B*), transverse surface lines divide the paddle-like hand from the forearm and the interdigital clefts appear; the humerus, radius, and ulna cartilage *Anlagen* appear and nerves reach the hand. By the sixth week (Fig. 1 *C*), metacarpals and phalanges are preformed in cartilage and nerve development is complete. By the seventh week (Fig. 1 *D*), muscles appear, the joints appear as clefts between the preformed bones, and the adult pattern is established, with all structures represented. These joints will not develop normally, however, without active fetal motion.

Further upper extremity development consists of increasing growth and maturity of the parts that are already present by the seventh week. At birth, the hand and upper extremity are similar to those of the adult except for the lack of ossification of the carpus and the hand epiphyses, a 30° flexion deformity of the elbow, and incomplete myelinization of the nervous system.

The vascular development of the upper limb arises in three separate but overlapping stages that occur between weeks 4 and 7 of fetal life. The first stage is characterized by a single main axial vessel, the subclavian-axillary-brachial-interosseous artery, that terminates in a hand plexus. In the second stage a median artery arises from the main stem and supplies the hand plexus. The third stage consists of the formation of the radial and ulnar arteries and involution of the median artery.

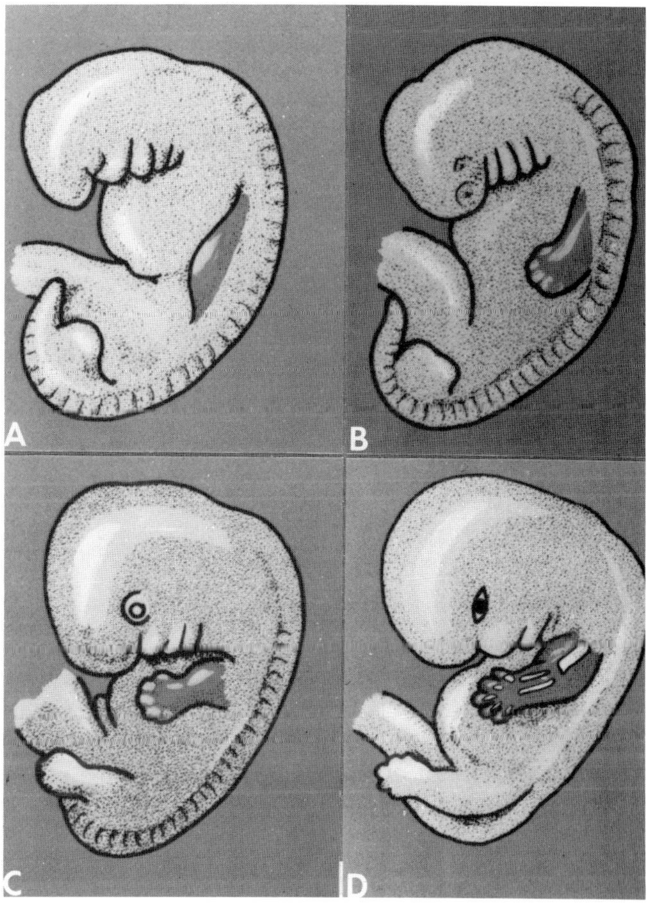

Figure 1

Embryologic development. *A*, Week 4. Limb bud appears; mesenchyme is covered with ectoderm; mesenchymal condensation into bone precursors has occurred. *B*, Week 5. Arm is developing; hand shows rays and fissures; future humerus, ulna, and radius are formed in cartilage. *C*, Week 6. Nerves are growing into buds; muscles are developed; digital clefts deepen and thumb diverges; skeleton is still differentiating as cartilage; metacarpals and proximal phalanges are present. *D*, Week 7. All soft tissue elements are differentiating; skeleton is completely "preformed" in cartilage.

Congenital Abnormalities

Localized Upper Extremity Disorders

Sprengel's Deformity Sprengel's deformity is the most common congenital anomaly of the shoulder. The scapular deformity causes abnormalities of the entire shoulder girdle including the glenohumeral joint and the clavicle. Normally, the scapula forms at the level of C-5 and descends to the level of T-5 between weeks 5 and 8 of fetal life. In Sprengel's deformity the scapula fails to descend normally (Fig. 2). Although the undescended scapula is the most obvious manifestation of the problem, there also is a high incidence of associated skeletal and soft tissue abnormalities not related to the shoulder, including scoliosis, cervical ribs, abnormal vertebral body segmentation, torticollis, renal abnormalities, and muscular hypoplasia, especially of the trapezius. In 30% of cases an omovertebral

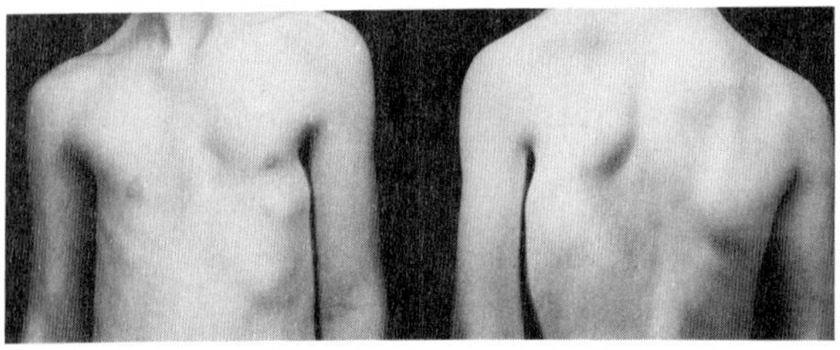

Figure 2
Sprengel's deformity.

body consisting of bone, cartilage, or fibrocartilage connects the superior angle of the scapula to the cervical spine. Because of the abnormal inferiorly oriented glenoid and aberrant attachments of the scapula, shoulder abduction is limited, adding functional impairment to the cosmetic deformity.

Because nonoperative methods have been unsuccessful, treatment is primarily surgical. Historically, there are two types of surgical treatment: procedures that attempt to improve cosmesis by resecting abnormal bony prominences; and those that attempt to lower the scapula by mobilizing it from its abnormal attachments and then reattaching the muscles with the scapula in a more normal position. Surgical treatment should be considered for children who have significant functional limitation and cosmetic deformity. The ideal age is between 3 and 8 years, although good results have been reported as late as age 15 years. The Schrock, Green, Jeannopoulos, and Klisic procedures divide and reattach the scapular muscles at their scapular insertion.

The Woodward procedure, first described in 1961, has achieved the greatest popularity, with good to excellent results reported in 80% of patients. The surgical technique consists of exposing and dividing the vertebral attachments of the trapezius, rhomboids, and levator scapula and resecting the omovertebral body, if any, and the deformed supraspinous portion of the scapula. The scapula is pulled inferiorly to the same level as the normal side and the detached muscles are resutured to their origins in the midline. The patient is then immobilized in a Velpeau type dressing for 2 to 3 weeks postoperatively. Complications include winging of the scapula and brachial plexus palsy; the latter may be due to compression of the plexus between the deformed first rib or a cervical rib and the abnormally straight clavicle. Osteotomy or morcellation of the clavicle or osteotomy of the coracoid may be necessary to prevent this complication.

Radial Clubhand Radial clubhand is characterized by varying degrees of deficiency of the radius, carpus, and thumb. It presents clinically as radial deviation of the hand and shortening of the forearm (Fig. 3). The ulna is shorter than normal and usually is deviated radially. The cause is unknown. The condition usually is not genetic, and most cases are sporadic. Half of the patients have bilateral defects.

There is a high incidence of associated extraskeletal abnormalities of which four are particularly significant: Holt-Oram syndrome; Fanconi's anemia; TAR syndrome; and the VATER association. In Holt-Oram syndrome there usually is an atrial septal defect or other cardiac abnormality that may require surgical correction before upper extremity surgery can be performed.

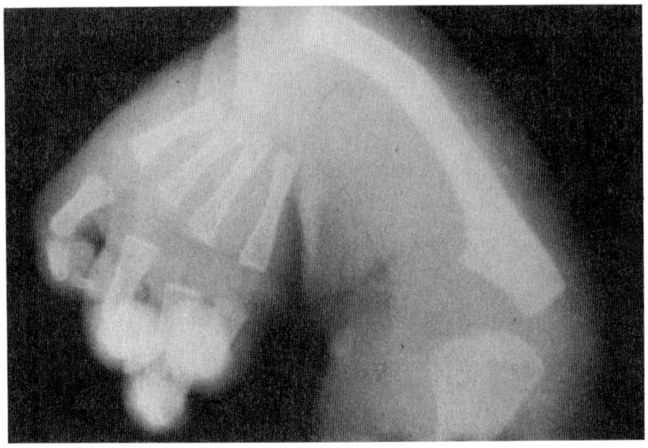

Figure 3
Radial clubhand.

In Fanconi's anemia, the patients are small at birth and have an uneven brownish pigmentation of the skin. All blood cells are decreased in number. This pancytopenia most often becomes apparent between 5 and 10 years of age and becomes progressively worse with increasing age. The prognosis is very poor, and death may occur at 2 to 3 years after the onset of the pancytopenia in some patients. Fanconi's anemia is an autosomal recessive disorder.

In TAR syndrome, the major findings are *t*hrombocytopenia and bilateral *a*bsence of *r*adii at birth. In contrast to Fanconi's anemia, the thrombocytopenia becomes less severe with age and the long-term prognosis is good. Most patients will have adequate platelet levels spontaneously by age 4 to 5. Therefore, surgery should be delayed in these patients.

The VATER association consists of an unexplained nonrandom occurrence of *v*ertebral segmentation and fusion abnormalities, *a*nal atresia, *t*racheoesophageal fistula, *e*sophageal atresia, *r*enal abnormalities, and *r*adial ray defects. Congenital heart disease is also present in half the reported cases. In spite of the problems, most of these patients can be treated successfully and surgical treatment for the upper extremity is justified in most of them.

Treatment All of the tissues of the forearm and radial side of the hand may be involved. The goals of treatment are to provide a well-aligned, stable hand on the forearm and thereby improve function as well as appearance. To be successful, treatment should begin at birth. This early treatment consists of manipulation of the hand to place it over the distal ulna and then holding it in the corrected position with carefully applied serial casts or splints. Treatment should be continued until the deformity is completely corrected or until correction has plateaued, in which case a light orthosis is used until the child is ready for operation.

Many surgical procedures have been described for radial clubhand. The goal of the current approach is centralization of the carpus over the distal end of the ulna by the first year of life. Recently, there has been a trend toward even earlier operation, which may improve correction but must be balanced against the possible increased risks of operation in young infants.

Some authors use radial and ulnar incisions to lengthen the skin on the radial side and shorten it on the ulnar side (Fig. 4 *A*). This has the advantage of providing good exposure of the tight structures on the radial side (which will be released) and the ulnar structures (which will be tightened). On the radial side, all soft tissue bands will have to be released except for the median nerve which will often be the tightest structure on this side and will be seen lying just deep to the deep fascia after skin incision. In some cases the median nerve will be combined with the sensory branch of the radial nerve to form a single median-radial nerve (Fig. 4 *B*). After soft tissue correction is obtained, the end of the ulna is squared off and fitted into a corresponding defect cut into the carpus, usually the capitate. A large Kirschner wire or Steinmann pin is then passed retrograde through the third metacarpal into the ulna (Fig. 5). If the ulna is very bowed, osteotomy is performed at the point at which the wire penetrates the ulnar cortex. The wire is left in place indefinitely and may have to be replaced if it loses purchase in less than a year postoperatively.

Recently, "radialization" has been proposed as a treatment for radial clubhand. There are two major differences from "centralization": the carpus is fixed ulnar to the long axis of the ulna and in ulnar deviation; and the extensor carpi radialis and flexor carpi radialis are transposed to the ulnar side of the wrist.

Postoperatively, splinting is continued until there is no further tendency for recurrence, usually several years.

Contraindications to surgical treatment include the severe associated cardiac and hematologic abnormalities mentioned above and a stiff, extended, ipsilateral elbow, which will prevent the "centralized" hand from reaching the mouth. Because many of these children are also missing a thumb or have defects of the thumb ray, index ray pollicization is often indicated. It is important to keep in mind that the radial digits—i.e., the index and middle fingers—are also abnormal and that pollicization of an abnormal index finger will not improve its motion.

Ulnar Deficiency This problem is much less common than radial deficiency. Ulnar deficiency occurs sporadically without a specific genetic pattern. It has been classified into four types: type I, hypoplasia or partial defect of the ulna; type II, total defect of the ulna; type III, total or partial defect of the ulna with humeroradial synostosis; and type IV, ulnar defect with congenital amputation at the wrist (Fig. 6). Although there are associated abnormalities, they are usually musculoskeletal, not systemic as in radial deficiency. Digital malformations occur in 89% of these cases. Radial head dislocation is common, and 68% of patients also have radial ray deficiencies. Ulnar deviation of the carpus usually is mild and does not require surgical treatment. The eventual function of the extremity depends more upon the condition of the hand and digits than on the condition of the forearm or elbow.

Treatment Primary treatment should be aimed at the digital deformities because these contribute the most to the lack of function. Syndactyly release and web deepening may be necessary. Resection of ulnar structures does not improve deformity or function in type II or type III deficiency. Treatment of the dislocated radial head should be individualized, and resection should be performed only after skeletal maturity. In general, treatment should be nonoperative for the elbow, forearm, and wrist.

Congenital Radio-Ulnar Synostosis This is a rare deformity resulting from failure of the separation of the proximal radius and ulna that normally occurs at approximately 5 weeks of fetal life (Fig. 7). The condition is thought to be hereditary. The involved forearms are almost always fixed in pronation. Derotation osteotomy can be considered for those patients fixed in pronation of 60° or more, if they are functionally handicapped. Some orthopaedists think that surgical correction is rarely indicated on functional grounds, regardless of forearm position. For those patients with bilateral deformity, treatment should be individualized. Complications of treatment include nerve palsy, vascular complications, and lack of full correction.

Madelung's Deformity This wrist disorder is characterized

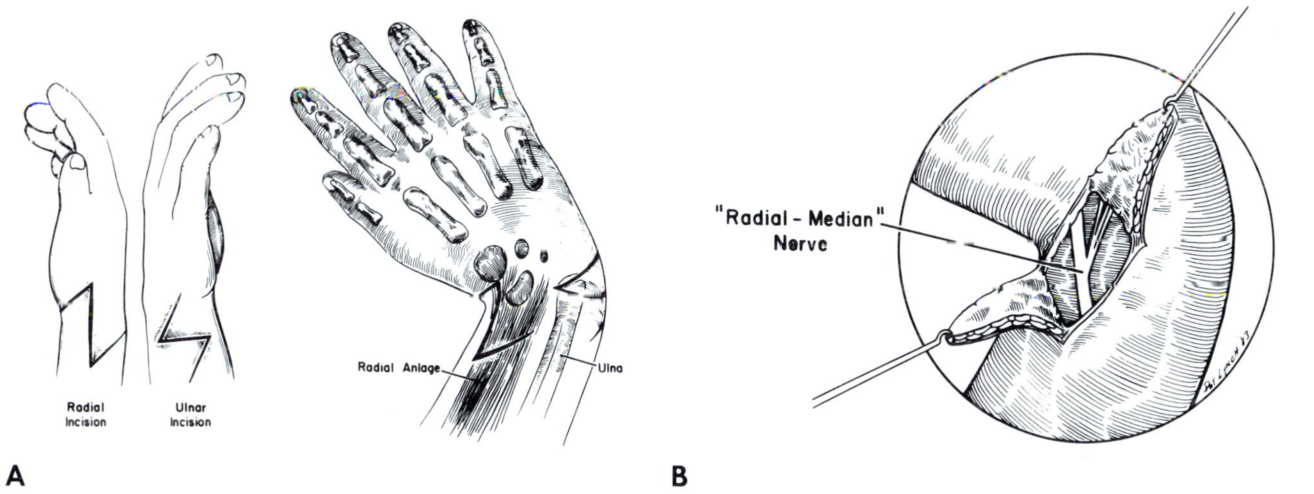

Figure 4

Radial clubhand. *A*, Surgical approach. *B*, Operative view, showing median nerve on radial side in subcutaneous tissue. (From Watson, H.K.; Beebe, R.D.; and Cruz, N.I. J. Hand Surg. [Am.] 9:541–547, 1984. By permission of the American Society for Surgery of the Hand.)

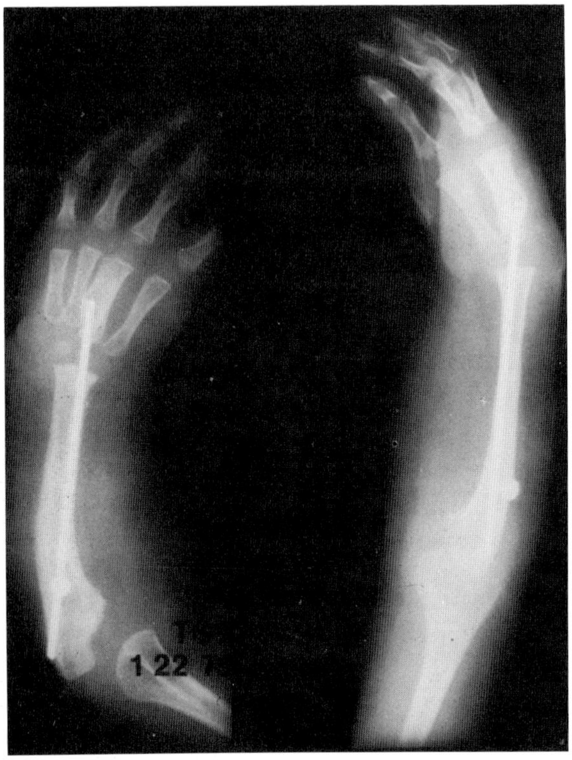

Figure 5

Correction of bowed ulna.

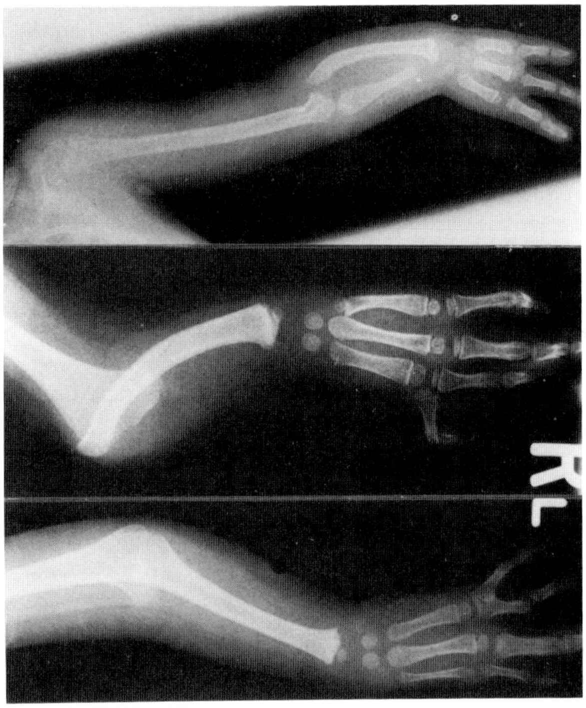

Figure 6

Types of ulnar deficiency. *Top,* Type I, hypoplasia or partial defect. *Middle,* Type II, total defect. *Bottom,* Total or partial defect of ulna with humeroradial synostosis. (From Swanson, A.B.; Tada, K.; and Yonenobu, K. J. Hand Surg. [Am.] 9:658–664, 1984. By permission of the American Society for Surgery of the Hand.)

by progressive ulnar and volar angulation of the distal radial articular surface due to failure of normal growth of the volar ulnar epiphysis of the distal radius. The carpus and ulna adapt to this deformity of the radius so that the carpus becomes V-shaped and the ulna becomes prominent. Madelung's deformity can be inherited as an autosomal dominant trait and is more common in females than males by a ratio of 4:1. It usually manifests itself in late childhood or adolescence. Clinical findings are deformity, decreased motion, and pain.

Treatment Many patients do not require treatment. For those whose symptoms are severe enough to require relief, a dorsal radial closing wedge osteotomy with distal ulna resection or ulnar shortening can be performed. No results of this procedure in large series have been published.

Congenital Pseudarthrosis of the Forearm This very rare condition is similar to congenital pseudarthrosis of the tibia. It usually presents as a nonhealing fracture of the radius and ulna in a child. Dislocation of the radial head can occur if the ulnar pseudarthrosis is not treated. Conventional treatment with bone grafting and internal fixation has not been successful. Success has been reported with free vascularized fibular bone grafts in two patients.

Syndactyly This is the most common congenital anomaly of the hand. It is due to failure of the side-to-side separation of the digits that usually occurs between weeks 5 and 7 of fetal life. Syndactyly is classified as "complete" if it involves the entire length of the digit and "incomplete" if involvement is only partial. If only the skin is involved, the syndactyly is classified as "simple"; if any other tissues are involved, it is "complex." The most common syndactyly involves the ring and middle fingers. If border digits

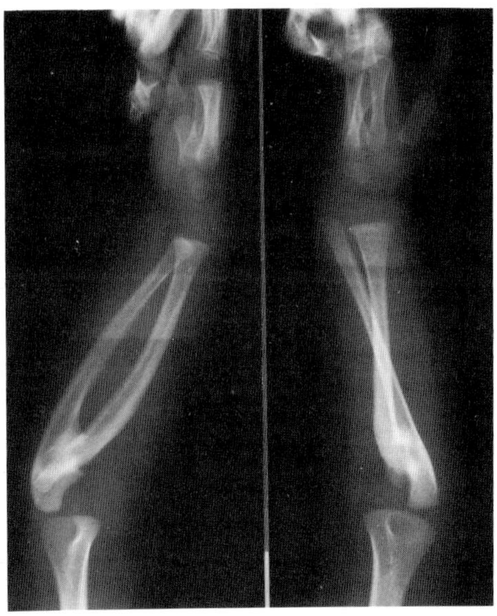

Figure 7

Congenital radio-ulnar synostosis.

are involved, they should be separated early to prevent flexion deformity of the longer digit.

Treatment Surgical treatment consists of release of the digits and resurfacing of the defects surgically created in the commissure and the adjacent sides of the digits. The commissure should always be resurfaced with local tissue, usually either opposing triangular flaps or a dorsally based quadrilateral flap. The bifurcation of the common digital artery usually is the most distal structure left intact in the web and almost never is it necessary to divide the digital artery itself. The sides of the digits are usually resurfaced with thinned local flaps on one side and full-thickness skin grafts harvested from the groin on the other side. Timing of the operation depends on the type of deformity and the digits involved. If the involved digits are of unequal length—such as ring-little or thumb-index syndactyly—they should be separated early to prevent flexion deformity of the longer digit with continued growth.

Complex syndactyly is more difficult and often requires staged operations including scar revision and osteotomy of the deformed digits. In Apert's syndrome (Fig. 8) (acrocephalosyndactyly) often only three fingers and a thumb can be constructed out of the complex syndactyly. In addition, there are severe deformities and stiffness of the digits with radial subluxation of the metacarpophalangeal joint of the thumb, and interphalangeal motion is limited if present at all.

Polydactyly The two most common types of polydactyly are preaxial (radial) and postaxial (ulnar).

Preaxial polydactyly, or duplication of the thumb, usually is sporadic in occurrence. The cause in unknown. There are significant functional as well as cosmetic considerations, not only because of the extra part but also because the adjacent digit is seldom normal. Therefore, the surgeon must examine the child carefully before any ablative surgery is planned. The parents must be told that a normal thumb will not necessarily result.

Treatment The most common defect is duplication of the distal and proximal phalanges of the thumb with a common metacarpal (Fig. 9) (type IV of Wassel) (Table 1). The radial side usually is less functional. At operation, it is important that neurovascular bundles be identified so that

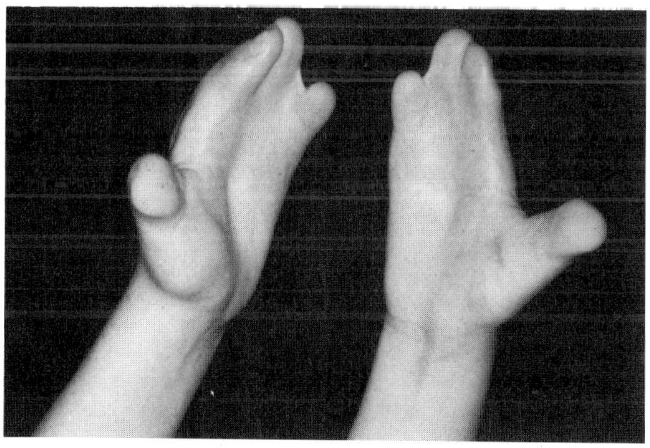

Figure 8

Apert's syndrome.

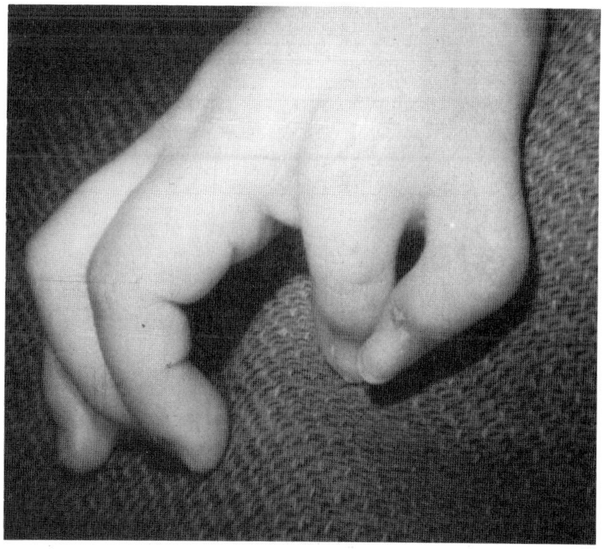

Figure 9

Preaxial polydactyly (type IV).

damage to them is avoided. Both collateral ligaments of the metacarpophalangeal joint may have to be reconstructed. It is also very important to reconstruct the extensor tendon because a zigzag deformity of the remaining digit will develop if the extensor mechanism is not rebalanced. The interphalangeal joint often is deformed. It can be treated by tailoring the articular cartilage with a knife, although this often will lead to interphalangeal joint stiffness. The skin is also involved in this deformity, and skin incisions should be planned accordingly.

Postaxial (ulnar side) polydactyly is less common than preaxial and sometimes is inherited as an autosomal dominant trait. Often it is a cosmetic problem rather than a functional one. When only skin is involved, surgical treatment is straightforward, consisting of removal of the extra digit. When bone is involved, it is necessary to be sure that enough skin from the ablated digit is allowed for closure and exposure of the neurovascular bundle as well as reconstruction of the metacarpophalangeal or interphalangeal joint of the remaining digit, if indicated.

Constriction Ring Syndrome This is a noninherited syndrome consisting of a partial or complete fibrous ring around the extremity at birth. The cause is unknown but is commonly thought to be related to fibrous amniotic bands as opposed to a germ plasm defect. Because amniocentesis may cause amniotic bands, it should be considered cautiously in subsequent pregnancies in a woman who has

Table 1. Types of Thumb Duplication (After Wassel)

Type	Description	Frequency, %*
I	Bifid distal phalanx	2
II	Duplicated distal phalanx	15
III	Bifid proximal phalanx	6
IV	Duplicated proximal phalanx	43
V	Bifid metacarpal	10
VI	Duplicated metacarpal	4
VII	Triphalangia	20

*Among 70 thumb duplications studied.

already had a child with constriction band syndrome. There is a high incidence of associated anomalies including clubfoot and cleft palate. The extent of the constriction varies, ranging from superficial and partial to deep and circumferential to complete intrauterine amputation of the part. The digits are involved much more commonly than the forearm and arm. If there is vascular, neural, or cosmetic compromise, surgical treatment should be considered.

Treatment There is almost complete unanimity of opinion that Z-plasty of the band in two or more stages is the technique of choice. One group recommends single-stage release for digital bands and has reported no increase in complications.

Congenital Amputation Although the term "congenital amputation" generally is used to describe a terminal limb deficiency present at birth (Fig. 10), the cause may be amputation of a formed distal part (as in constriction ring syndrome) or a failure of formation of the distal part. In the former, the proximal tissues are normal, but in the latter the tissues that remain may have various anomalies of bone, tendon, nerve, and vascular anatomy. This is particularly important in considering that, in addition to the increasingly sophisticated prosthetic solutions to amputation, there are several recently developed surgical techniques that can help a child with congenital limb deficiency. Digits that are present but too short can be augmented with lengthening by osteotomy and application of an external distraction device and subsequent immobilization until bone healing occurs. Lengthening of 2.5 to 3.8 cm usually is achieved. This technique is especially useful on the thumb and requires approximately 4 months of treatment. However, complication rates of over 50% have been reported.

Another technique helpful in selected cases is a free nonvascularized transfer of toe phalanges with intact periosteum and intact epiphyses. These phalanges have been reported to grow normally in 91% of cases when the operation is performed before the patient is 18 months old. The phalanx transfer-lengthening may be performed in a single stage or subsequent to a distraction lengthening as described above. In either case the length of the created digits will be limited by the soft tissues of the recipient bed. The procedure may be repeated to gain additional length as the patient grows. A third technique of digital reconstruction is microneurovascular transfer of the second or great toe. Several authors have reported good results with this procedure. In "on-top-plasty," an inadequate digit is transferred to a more functionally useful part, either on its neurovascular pedicle or as a free vascularized transfer.

For isolated compete congenital thumb loss, index finger pollicization is the treatment of choice. A high percentage of these patients will require a secondary procedure such as opponens-plasty; this was necessary in 45% of the patients in one recent series.

Relative lengthening and, to some degree, increased mobility of the deficient digits also can be obtained by web-space deepening with or without tendon transfers. Osteotomies and soft tissue realignment are sometimes indicated to improve the position and subsequent function of the digits. In the patient with total absence of a hand at the wrist, the Krukenberg procedure, which consists of separating the forearm bones and transferring tendons to allow independent motion of the radius and ulna, can be performed in certain cases. This is especially recommended for blind patients and patients who have no chance of having prosthetic devices.

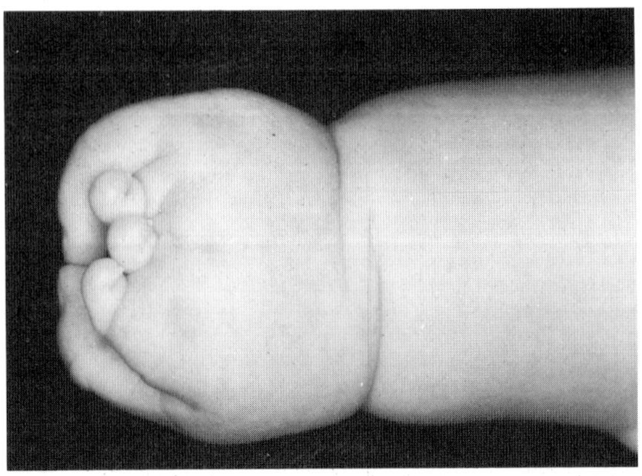

Figure 10

Congenital constriction band amputation with abnormal border digits.

Generalized Disorders With Upper Extremity Manifestations

Arthrogryposis This musculoskeletal disorder is characterized by congenital immobility of multiple joints secondary to congenital dysfunction of the muscles. It is not inherited. Histologically, there are two types, neuropathic and myopathic. In the neuropathic form, there is loss of the anterior horn cells in the spinal cord with consequent loss of muscular function. In the myopathic form, the muscles are the primary site of involvement and the neurologic structures are normal. Regardless of pathogenesis, the joint manifestations are similar: the shoulders are fixed in adduction and internal rotation; the elbows are fixed in extension or sometimes in flexion and pronation; the wrists are in flexion and ulnar deviation; the hands are either in metacarpophalangeal flexion/interphalangeal extension posture with the thumb in the palm or in flexion deformities of all the fingers at the interphalangeal joints; and the hands are more severely afflicted than the elbows and shoulders (a peripheral to central gradient).

Treatment The goals are first to decrease deformity of the part and second, if possible, to increase mobility. It is advantageous that most of these patients are intelligent and highly motivated and have normal sensibility. Although often involved, the shoulders seldom require treatment except when both are fixed in extreme internal rotation, in which case external rotation osteotomy of the humerus can be performed at the level of the deltoid insertion. The elbows should be considered together, so that if one is fixed in flexion and the other in extension, treatment may not be necessary. The usual problem is to gain elbow flexion on one side. Serial applications of casts for elbow contractures should begin at birth. After maximal benefit has been achieved, either closing wedge osteotomy of the distal humerus or joint capsulotomy, triceps release, and a tendon transfer to achieve flexion can be performed. The best muscle for transfer is usually the pectoralis major, although the latissimus dorsi also can be used.

For the wrist, closing dorsal radial wedge osteotomy proximal to the physis can be performed. Corrective osteotomy of the first metacarpal with first web reconstruction can be done for the thumb-in-palm deformity. Reconstruction to improve the position of the digits also can be done, but motion usually will not increase appreciably. Soft tissue procedures can be successful in selected cases.

Juvenile Rheumatoid Arthritis The manifestations of this systemic illness in the child are different from those in the adult. The shoulder and elbow are much less likely to be affected than the wrist and hand. The wrist usually assumes a flexed and ulnarly deviated posture and often will fuse in this position. Fingers tend to assume an extended and radially deviated posture at the metacarpophalangeal joints and extension deformity at the proximal interphalangeal joints. Although synovitis and tenosynovitis are common, they usually respond to nonoperative treatment including large doses of salicylates, splinting, and physiotherapy; surgical treatment, such as flexor tenosynovectomy, is occasionally indicated. It is important that the wrists be splinted at night so that, if they do fuse, they fuse in a functional position. Closing dorsal radial wedge osteotomy of the radius can be performed if the wrist does fuse in poor position. If the wrist is not yet fused, soft tissue reconstruction and synovectomy can correct malalignment. Synovectomy is rarely indicated in the small finger joints. After epiphyseal closure, arthrodeses and arthroplasties can be considered, just as in the adult. Intra-articular procedures often will increase stiffness, and surgical treatment is indicated much less commonly in the child than in the adult.

Cerebral Palsy This condition may be defined as a primarily musculoskeletal disturbance secondary to a fixed and nonprogressive brain lesion that occurred in the perinatal period. Within this diagnostic category are multiple varied manifestations. Most patients are not surgical candidates. The ones who can benefit from surgical treatment are spastic and have good voluntary control, good sensibility, and good intelligence and motivation. Because the basic problem is central, conventional tendon transfers are often not appropriate.

Treatment The shoulders are almost never operated on, although internal rotation deformity does occur and can be disabling. The elbow is usually flexed and the forearm is pronated. In severe contracture with the other criteria for operation met, the common flexor pronator origin can be released with or without Z-lengthening of the biceps and brachioradialis. If pronation is very severe and passive supination is possible, the pronator teres insertion also can be released. Rerouting of the pronator teres to make it a supinator has also been reported but the results are unpredictable and a fixed supination deformity is functionally much more disabling than a pronation contracture. The wrist and finger deformity usually is flexion at all levels, especially at the proximal interphalangeal joints.

There are three treatment groups defined according to severity:

Group I. Mild deformity. Digits can extend with the wrist in less than 20° of flexion.

Group II. Moderate deformity. Digits can extend with the wrist in less than 50° of flexion.

Group III. Severe deformity. The digits cannot be extended with the wrist in any position.

For group I, surgical treatment will not be indicated often. For patients in group II, musculo-aponeurotic release of the long flexors in the proximal third of the forearm combined with tenotomy of the flexor carpi ulnaris distally can be performed. If the patient has no active wrist extensors, instead of tenotomy the flexor carpi ulnaris can be transferred to the extensor carpi radialis brevis at the same time. It is important that the function of the flexor carpi radialis be preserved in these patients; otherwise, a permanent extension deformity of the wrist may result. It is also important that the digital flexors be sufficiently released so that the fingers can be actively extended out of the palm postoperatively with the wrist in neutral. An alternative to flexor carpi ulnaris-to-extensor carpi radialis transfer (Green-Banks) is extensor carpi ulnaris-to-extensor carpi radialis brevis transfer. The latter transfer may be less likely to overcorrect the wrist flexion deformity.

In the group III patients, whose digits cannot be passively or actively extended fully even with the wrist flexed, tenotomy of the long flexors in the distal forearm at different levels can be performed. With the digits extended, the proximal ends of the flexor digitorum sublimis are sutured to the distal ends of the flexor digitorum profundus. The wrist flexors are tenotomized. Proximal row carpectomy can help gain additional relative lengthening of the soft tissue. Arthrodesis of the wrist is seldom indicated in cerebral palsy because these patients depend on the enhanced tenodesis effect of wrist position to control the digits.

There are two types of thumb deformity: adduction of the first metacarpal, and adduction and flexion deformity at the metacarpophalangeal and interphalangeal joints—the so-called thumb-in-palm deformity. The former is due to spasticity of the adductor pollicis. This results in first metacarpal adduction with consequent hyperextension of the metacarpophalangeal joint. This can be corrected by release of the abductor pollicis brevis origin from the third metacarpal combined with augmentation of the abductor pollicis longus by tenodesis to the distal radius or brachioradialis transfer to the long abductor.

For the thumb-in-palm deformity, in which there is flexion contracture as well as adduction, several procedures are recommended. These include release of the adductor at its origin and lengthening of the flexor pollicis longus combined with rerouting of the extensor pollicis longus from the third to the first dorsal compartment. If necessary, augmentation of the abductor pollicis longus can be performed with the brachioradialis as above. Other procedures that can enhance function include capsulotomy or fusion of the metacarpophalangeal or the interphalangeal joints of the thumb.

Trauma

Fractures and Dislocations

Non-Growth-Plate Injuries Condylar fractures of the proximal or middle phalanx may displace proximally, leading to radial or ulnar deviation of the digit at the proximal or distal interphalangeal joint. If unrecognized, a fixed angular deformity of the joint may occur. This lesion is best treated by osteotomy through the old fracture site, with care to keep the collateral ligament attached to the condylar fragment and to preserve its blood supply.

Growth-Plate Injuries These are quite common. Fortunately, remodeling usually suffices and surgical treatment is not required. Fracture of the proximal humerus is most frequently Salter type II and represents the most common fracture of the shoulder in those 9 to 15 years old. Large degrees of angulation can be tolerated because of the large amount of glenohumeral motion and remodeling potential in this area. As a result, operation to correct late deformity is almost never indicated.

Supracondylar fracture of the humerus is the most common elbow fracture in children. The most frequent long-term complication is cubitus varus which rarely causes functional impairment. Lateral closing wedge osteotomy of the deformity may be considered if the cosmetic problem is very severe.

Occasionally, a lateral condylar fracture will not unite or will cause early closure of the lateral physis, and a valgus deformity will result. This can cause late ulnar palsy. Treatment for the ulnar nerve problem or osteotomy of the distal humerus may be indicated.

Wrist deformities—radial shortening and angulation—can result from distal radius Salter type II injuries complicated by physeal injury and premature physeal closure. To avoid additional physeal injury, repeated forceful manipulations of this fracture should be avoided. If significant, such wrist deformities can be corrected by radial osteotomy combined with ulnar shortening.

Birth Palsy

The incidence, approximately 2/1,000 live births, has not changed in the last 10 years, but the severity of the problem has decreased. The prognosis generally is excellent, with full recovery in 96% of such cases. Because 92% of the patients will recover in the first 3 months, it is recommended that no operation be performed sooner than that. Early treatment should be nonoperative positioning of the extremity in external rotation and abduction at the shoulder. Late deformities are typically internal rotation and adduction of the shoulder and flexion of the elbow. With time, these deformities become fixed with bony adaptation. The most common palsy is of the upper roots, but lower root and whole plexus palsy do occur and will affect the hand. Poor prognostic signs include recovery delayed beyond 6 months, Horner's syndrome, and lower or whole plexus palsy. After 1½ to 2 years, recovery has usually plateaued; reconstructive surgery can be considered after age 4 to 5 years.

Treatment There has been a report from France of good results after early nerve surgery for brachial plexus injury, but this has not yet been substantiated by other centers. Other treatment is directed at correction of residual deformity. At the shoulder, a combination of releases and tendon transfers after the method of Sever-L'Episcopo is recommended. This consists of pectoralis major and subscapularis lengthening and teres major and latissimus dorsi transfer to the posterior aspect of the humerus. Alternatively, external rotation osteotomy of the humerus can be considered in the older child. The flexion deformity of the elbow is only treated surgically if it is very severe—i.e., greater than 50°. In such patients, brachialis, biceps, and anterior capsule release can be helpful.

Upper Extremity Tumors

Juvenile Aponeurotic Fibroma

This is a benign soft tissue neoplasm found primarily in the hands and wrists of children or adolescents. There is a high incidence of local recurrence but the lesion never metastasizes. The tumor presents as a painless enlarging mass, usually in the palm of the hand or digits. Histologically, it consists of fibrous tissue with cartilage islands.

Treatment *En bloc* excision is used with frequent follow-up for possible recurrence. Recurrence is rare after puberty. Vital structures should be saved because this is not a malignant lesion.

Multiple Hereditary Osteochondroma

This benign lesion is a disorder of endochondral bone growth manifested by an abnormal metaphyseal bone prominence capped with cartilage and accompanied by defective metaphyseal remodelling and asymmetric retardation of longitudinal bone growth. Deformities of the forearm occur in 30% to 60% of these patients. The most common problem is ulnar shortening with consequent ulnar deviation of the wrist, ulnar bowing of one or both bones of the forearm, and dislocation of the radial head.

Treatment Removal of the lesion alone does not prevent the deformities, so distal hemiradial epiphyseodesis combined with ulnar lengthening and lesion removal should be performed early, before deformity occurs. Alternatively, radial osteotomy may be required if the patient presents after skeletal maturity.

Lymphangioma

This is a benign neoplastic proliferation of lymph vessels and lymphoid tissue which usually occurs in children. The tumor may develop anywhere in the body, including the extremities. When it involves the forearm and hand, deformity, compromised function, and pain may result from the soft tissue enlargement. Septic lymphangitis in the affected tissue is not uncommon.

Treatment Although the lesion can be excised, tumor recurrence, hypertrophic scars, and persistence of symptoms are common. Nonoperative measures such as elevation, elastic compression garments, analgesics, and antibiotics should be used first.

Annotated Bibliography

Congenital and Developmental Abnormalities

Buck-Gramcko, D.: Radialization as a new treatment for radial club hand. J. Hand Surg. [Am.] 10:964–967, 1985.

In this preliminary report, overcorrection of the hand into ulnar deviation is recommended to lessen the risk of recurrent deformity with growth.

Cleary, J.E., and Omer, G.E., Jr.: Congenital proximal radio-ulnar synostosis. J. Bone Joint Surg. 67A:539–545, 1985.

In a long-term review the authors found no correlation between degree of deformity and functional status and concluded that surgical treatment is seldom indicated.

Grogan, D.P.; Stanley, E.A.; and Bobechko, W.P.: The congenital undescended scapula. J. Bone Joint Surg. 65B:598–605, 1983.

Twenty-one patients underwent the Woodward procedure over the last 18 years at the Hospital for Sick Children in Toronto, Canada; mean follow-up was 8 years, 9 months. Eighty percent of the patients had excellent abduction and a mean lowering of the scapula of 2 cm. Complications were winging and temporary brachial plexus palsy, each in one patient.

Lamb, D.W.: Radial club hand: A continuing study of sixty-eight patients with one hundred and seventeen club hands. J. Bone Joint Surg. 59A:1–13, 1977.

A classic paper reports the author's extensive personal experience.

Lamb, D.W., and Scott, H.: Management of congenital and acquired amputation in children. Orthop. Clin. 12:977–994, 1981.

The incidence in Edinburgh is 1/3,000 live births. An attempt at prosthetic fitting was made for patients with amelia but this usually was unsuccessful. Best prosthesis users had below-elbow amputations. The amelia patients preferred to use their feet.

Manske, P.R.: Redirection of extensor pollicis longus in the treatment of spastic thumb-in-palm deformity. J. Hand Surg. [Am.] 10:553–560, 1985.

Twenty patients were treated with redirecting of the extensor pollicis longus to the first dorsal compartment combined with first web and thenar muscle release. All 20 patients improved.

Marcus, N.A., and Omer, G.E., Jr.: Carpal deviation in congenital ulnar deficiency. J. Bone Joint Surg. 66A: 1003–1007, 1984.

Seven of eight patients were treated nonoperatively. There was progression of the deformity only in the one patient who had surgical treatment.

Miura, T.: Congenital constriction band syndrome. J. Hand Surg. [Am.] 9:82–88, 1984.

Fifty-five patients were reviewed retrospectively; 35 patients had had bilateral constriction band syndrome. The author differentiates this anomaly from failure of formation of parts. The constriction band syndrome is usually bilateral and the part is normal proximal to the band. The failure-of-formation anomaly is unilateral, and the entire part may be poorly developed, especially with short metacarpals on the affected side.

Poznanski, A.K.: The Hand in Radiologic Diagnosis With Gamuts and Pattern Profiles. Vol. 1 and 2. Second edition. Philadelphia, W.B. Saunders Company, 1984.

This two-volume text surveys the entire range of hand problems as manifested in radiologic findings. Its approach is encyclopedic and includes radiologic findings for almost all diseases that affect the hand in adults and children. Additionally, there are pertinent comments about embryology and genetics.

Simmons, B.P.; Southmayd, W.W.; and Riseborough, E.J.: Congenital radioulnar synostosis. J. Hand Surg. 8:829–838, 1983.

Thirty-three patients were reviewed retrospectively. All had had rotational osteotomy to correct severe hyperpronation deformities. The authors recommended that, in bilateral cases, one side be left in neutral and the other side be placed in 10°–15° of pronation. There was a high incidence of complications related to the operation, including four neurovascular complications. The authors recommend that, if the deformity is greater than 60°, surgical treatment be considered. Eighty-two percent of the patients had good to excellent results.

Smith, R.J. (ed.): Symposium on congenital deformities of the hand. Hand Clin. 1:371–596, August 1985.

An up-to-date overview of selected congenital deformities of the hand. Especially good on embryology.

Swanson, A.B.; Swanson, G.D.; and Tada, K.: A classification for congenital limb malformation. J. Hand Surg. 8:693–702, 1983.

An international panel has constructed a classification scheme generally accepted by hand and upper extremity surgeons: I, failure of formation of parts; II, failure of differentiation of parts; III, duplication; IV, overgrowth; V, undergrowth; VI, congenital constriction band syndrome; and VII, generalized skeletal abnormalities. The purpose of this classification is to help with statistical evaluation and communication among upper extremity surgeons.

Swanson, A.B.; Tada, K.; and Yonenobu, K.: Ulnar ray deficiency: Its various manifestations. J. Hand Surg. [Am.] 9:658–664, 1984.

Fifty-six upper extremities in 65 patients were studied retrospectively both in Grand Rapids and in Japan. They were classified into four types: I, hypoplasia of the ulna or partial defect; II, total absence of the ulna; III, total or partial ulnar defect with humeroradial synostosis; and IV, ulnar defect with amputation at the wrist.

Tada, K.; Yonenobu, K.; Tsuyuguchi, Y.; Kawai, H.; and Egawa, T.: Duplication of the thumb: A retrospective review of two hundred and thirty-seven cases. J. Bone Joint Surg. 65A:584–598, 1983.

An extensive personal experience is reviewed with an excellent discussion of technical considerations.

Watson, H.K.; Beebe, R.D.; and Cruz, N.I.: A centralization procedure for radial clubhand. J. Hand Surg. [Am.] 9:541–547, 1984.

A technique for centralization for radial clubhand is presented that differs from the currently popular methods by avoiding carpal bone resection and performing Z-plasties on both sides of the wrist so that the ulnar Z-plasty removes skin and the radial Z-plasty provides skin. The centralization is held with a longitudinal 0.045-inch Kirschner wire for 6 weeks, after which it is removed. The procedures were done on patients less than 1 year old, usually at 6 months of age; mean follow-up was 10 years. Half of the patients had as much as 30° of recurrence.

Yonenobu, K.; Tada, K.; and Swanson, A.B.: Arthrogryposis of the hand. J. Pediatr. Orthop. 4:599–603, 1984.

In 45 patients, the worst deformity was usually distal. The hand deformities could be classified into two types: thumb-in-palm with intrinsic plus posture of the fingers (type I), and proximal interphalangeal flexion deformities of the fingers (type

II). Seventeen patients had surgical treatment, and all improved.

Zancolli, E.A.; Goldner, L.J.; and Swanson, A.B.: Surgery of the spastic hand in cerebral palsy: Report of the Committee on Spastic Hand Evaluation. J. Hand Surg. 8:766–772, 1983.

Patients with cerebral palsy affecting the upper extremity are not usually surgical candidates. However, with proper selection of patients, proper surgical procedure, and good technique, improvement in function can be obtained.

Trauma

Cunningham, M.W.; Yousif, N.J.; Matloub, H.S.; Sanger, J.R.; Gingrass, R.P.; and Valiulis, J.P.: Retardation in finger growth after injury to the flexor tendons. J. Hand Surg. [Am.] 10:115–117, 1985.

Four patients with unrepaired flexor tendon injuries in childhood showed significant growth retardation of the affected digit, compared with the normal side, long after the injury.

Lee, B.S.; Esterhai, J.L.; and Das, M.: Fracture of the distal radial epiphysis. Clin. Orthop. 185:90–96, 1984.

Ten children who had wrist deformity secondary to growth plate injury were studied. This problem was thought to be due to repeated forceful reductions.

Leonidas, J.C.: Skeletal trauma in the child abuse syndrome. Pediatr. Ann. 12:875–881, 1983.

One million children are reported to be victims of child abuse in the United States per year. When abuse is suspected, radiographs should include the skull, thoracolumbar spine, chest wall, and extremities. Fifty percent of these patients are under 2 years of age and most are under 5 years of age. The characteristic fractures that occur in this syndrome include multiple injuries at the metaphyseal/epiphyseal location.

Ogden, J.A.: Distal clavicular physeal injury. Clin. Orthop. 188:68–73, 1984.

Fourteen adolescent patients with this injury were studied. The injury is easily confused with acromioclavicular separation. Because of the remodeling potential in this age group, the radiographic appearance late is that of a duplicated clavicle.

Birth Palsy

Gilbert, A.; Khouri, N.; and Carlioz, H.: Exploration chirurgicale du plexus brachial dans la paralysie obstétricale: Constatations anatomiques chez 21 malades opérés. Rev. Chir. Orthop. 66:33–42, 1980.

Good results are found after early plexus exploration and repair with modern microsurgical techniques.

Greenwald, A.G.; Schute P.C.; and Shiveley, J.L.: Brachial plexus birth palsy: A 10-year report on the incidence and prognosis. J. Pediatr. Orthop. 4:689–692, 1984.

The incidence of birth palsy at the Kaiser Foundation Hospital in San Francisco between January 1972 and December 1982 was 2/1,000 live births, which is similar to previous reports in the literature. Thirty-eight patients were evaluated. The authors conclude that the incidence of birth palsy has not changed, but the severity has lessened considerably. Ninety-two percent of the infants recovered completely in the first 3 months, so it is recommended that the child be observed for this period before operation on the plexus is contemplated.

Iwasaki, A.; Kikuchi, M.; Eimoto, T.; Enjoji, M.; Yoh, S.; and Sakurai, H.: Juvenile aponeurotic fibroma: An ultrastructural study. Ultrastruct. Pathol. 4:75–83, 1983.

The pathology of this rare pediatric tumor is reviewed in detail.

Tumors and Infections

Blair, W.F.; Buckwalter, J.A.; Mickelson, M.R.; and Omer, G.E.: Lymphangioma of the forearm and hand. J. Hand Surg. 8:399–405, 1983.

All nine patients studied were symptomatic, with pain and deformity, at the completion of treatment at a mean follow-up of 11 years. Tumor recurrence, hypertrophic scars, and persistence of symptoms are frequent after surgical treatment for this lesion.

Feder, H.M., and Long, S.S.: Herpetic whitlow. Am. J. Dis. Child. 137:861–863, 1983.

By definition, this is herpes simplex infection of the fingertip. In children, it usually follows oral herpes by direct inoculation. Diagnosis is confirmed by hematoxylin-and-eosin staining of the vesicle fluid and finding viral giant cells. Viral culture may be helpful. Treatment is symptomatic, but acyclovir may be helpful.

Fogel, G.R.; McElfresh, E.C.; Peterson, H.A.; and Wicklund, P.T.: Management of deformities of the forearm in multiple hereditary osteochondromas. J. Bone Joint Surg. 66A:670–680, 1984.

The most common deformity in the upper extremity is ulnar deviation of the wrist with relative ulnar shortening secondary to radial overgrowth. These deformities usually progress. Eighteen patients underwent operation; at a 2-year follow-up, the only treatment that was effective was ulnar lengthening and radial epiphyseal arrest. Removal of the osteochondroma and ulnar lengthening alone was not effective in correcting the deformity.

17

Shoulder: Trauma

This chapter deals with fractures, instability, neurovascular injuries, and pediatric shoulder injuries. The fracture section includes fractures and fracture-dislocations of the proximal humerus and fractures of the humeral shaft, clavicle, and scapula. The instability section includes anterior, inferior, and posterior glenohumeral instabilities as well as failed repair of instability. Also, management of acromioclavicular and sternoclavicular dislocations is covered. The neurovascular section includes injuries to the axillary, suprascapular, and spinal accessory nerves and to the axillary artery.

Fractures

Fractures and Fracture-Dislocations of the Proximal Humerus

The classification of proximal humeral fractures and fracture-dislocations described by Neer is the most useful system for evaluation and treatment. It is critical to obtain anteroposterior and lateral radiographs in the scapular plane, and axillary radiographs if possible, to evaluate displacement of the fragments properly. Also, a thorough knowledge of the anatomy and tendon insertions of the rotator cuff on the proximal humerus is needed. The majority of proximal humeral fractures are minimally displaced and can be treated conservatively with immobilization. Care must be taken to administer physiotherapy properly; starting too late will result in a frozen shoulder and starting too early may result in nonunion, even of a nondisplaced fracture if it is not impacted and does not move as a unit.

Most displaced fractures require repair by closed reduction, open reduction and internal fixation, or a humeral head prosthesis. A two-part surgical neck fracture is probably the most amenable to closed reduction, but this may be prevented by interposed capsule, muscle, or the long head of the biceps. Also, the fracture may be too unstable to maintain reduction and may require percutaneous pinning or internal fixation. Three-part fractures are usually too unstable for closed reduction, and a forceful maneuver may result in further fragmentation. However, satisfactory results in 24 of 34 patients with three-part fractures treated by closed reduction have been reported. The better results were in older, more sedentary patients. Younger, active patients probably benefit more from operative repair.

Internal fixation of fractures of the proximal humerus can be difficult because of osteoporosis, comminution, complex anatomy, and unopposed muscle forces. In many instances, the poor quality of bone precludes rigid internal fixation. Heavy nonabsorbable sutures and 18- or 20-gauge wire are useful for internal fixation. A Rush rod may be needed for stability. The rotator cuff tissues are usually stronger than the tuberosity fragments, and wires or sutures should be passed through the cuff to assist immobilization and fixation. Because of poor bone quality, use of a plate and screws is not a good choice for fixation in most instances; the screws are not able to gain adequate fixation in the soft bone. This type of device is only indicated in younger patients with adequate bone. If a plate is used, proper positioning, size, and technique of application are essential (Fig. 1). Placing the plate too high on the greater tuberosity will result in impingement against the acromion.

In comminuted, osteoporotic, three-part proximal humeral fractures in older patients, internal fixation cannot achieve a stable reduction and early motion cannot be started, so a humeral head prosthesis is probably a better choice. Fixation of the tuberosities will be easier and early motion may be instituted. Closed reduction or open reduction with internal fixation of four-part fractures and head-splitting fractures of the proximal humerus usually results in malunion, nonunion, or osteonecrosis, leading

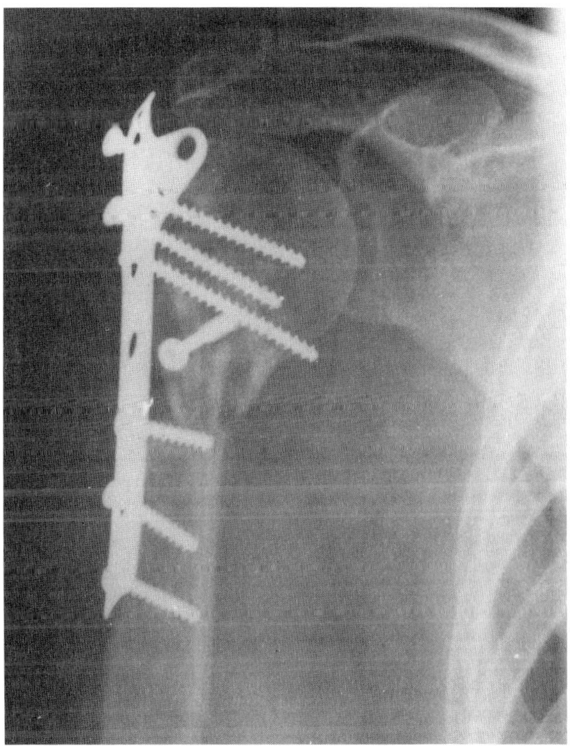

Figure 1

At 9 months after comminuted neck fracture, there is failure of the internal fixation device with loosening of the cortical screws in the soft cancellous bone of the head. The plate was placed too far above the greater tuberosity, causing impingement against the acromion and actually distracting the fracture.

to a painful and stiff joint. The use of a humeral head prosthesis is generally accepted as the treatment of choice (Fig. 2 *A*).

In recent years, several technical considerations for achieving a successful result from a humeral head replacement have been stressed. Because the deltoid is so important in shoulder function, it should not be removed from its origin because this weakens it. A long deltopectoral "deltoid on" approach avoids detachment of the deltoid origin but still allows adequate exposure. If more exposure is needed, the deltoid insertion should be removed because it can be reattached easily without weakening the muscle. It is important to restore proper length to the humerus with the prosthesis to preserve proper tension in the myofascial sleeve. The tendency to set the prosthesis against the remaining humeral shaft significantly shortens the humeral shaft and creates an unstable situation leading to inferior subluxation and inability to elevate the extremity because the deltoid is shortened and its function is compromised. Also, the prosthesis should be set at the proper angle of retroversion, generally between 30° and 40°. Cement is used when there is inadequate bony support.

The tuberosities are sutured or wired to both the fin of the prosthesis and the proximal humeral shaft. The split in the rotator cuff also should be closed with nonabsorbable sutures. Inadequate fixation of the cuff and tuberosities has been identified as a significant factor in early prosthesis failures. Also, the greater tuberosity should not be positioned above the head of the prosthesis or there will be impingement against the acromion. Furthermore, when there is a proximal shaft fracture, it is important to reconstruct this component prior to cementing in the prosthesis. Figure 2 *B* shows cerclage wire and no. 2 nonabsorbable nylon sutures used to secure the shaft fracture.

Fracture-dislocations of the proximal humerus remain difficult to diagnose and to treat. Recently, computed tomography has been found helpful in pinpointing the amount of glenoid and head involvement, in both acute and chronic situations. Anterior fracture-dislocations are easier to recognize and often require open reduction and internal fixation. Anterior two-part fracture-dislocations of the greater tuberosity usually can be reduced closed, but maintaining the greater tuberosity in a reduced position can be difficult and there should be frequent follow-up radiographs. Adequate healing or fixation of the greater tuberosity results in a stable situation without further instability. Three- and four-part anterior fracture-dislocations are quite unstable. Repeated attempts at closed reduction should be avoided. Generally, they require open reduction and operative repair by internal fixation. Injury to the axillary nerve and brachial plexus has been reported and must be evaluated carefully, both before and after operation. Myositis ossificans is rare but can occur, especially with a reduced dislocation.

Several recent reports have stressed the difficulty in diagnosis of a posterior fracture-dislocation. Often, only an anteroposterior radiograph is taken, and this can be quite deceiving. An axillary view is required to confirm the diagnosis (Fig. 3). Adequate physical examination, including testing of external rotation, is helpful but may be difficult because of pain. If there has been an electrical injury or a convulsive episode, a posterior dislocation should be sus-

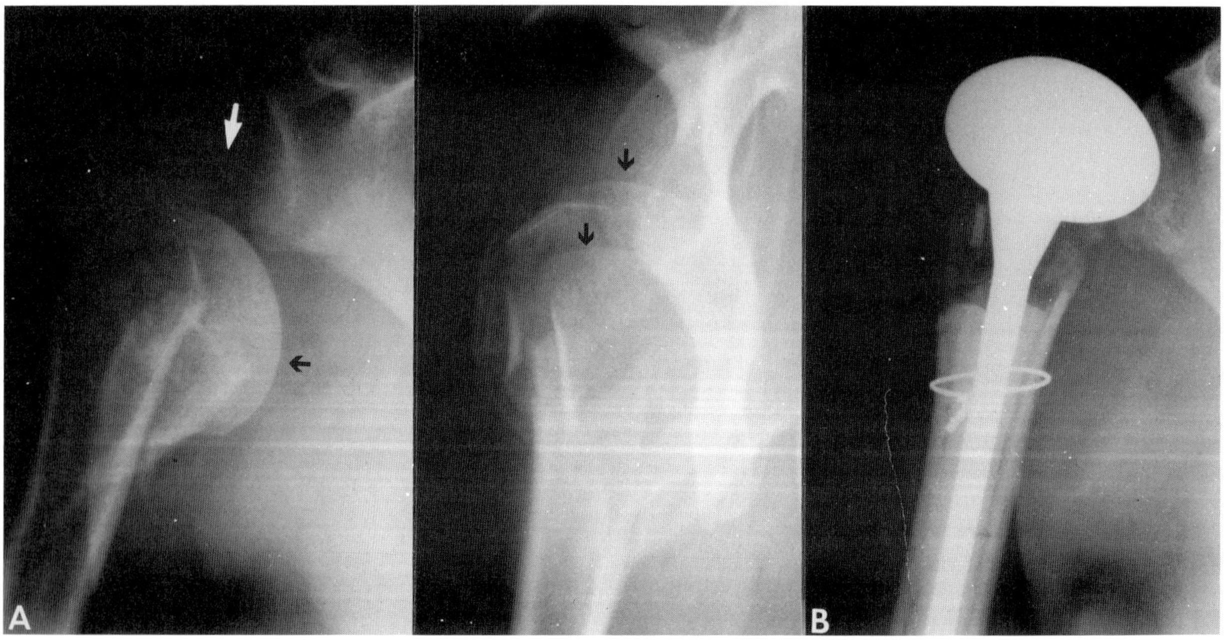

Figure 2

A, Anteroposterior (*Left*) and lateral (*Right*) radiographs in the scapular plane of head-splitting fracture with involvement of proximal humeral shaft. The greater tuberosity and 30% of the articular head are one fragment (*upper arrow*); the remaining articular head is another (*lower arrow*); and the lesser tuberosity is a third. The proximal shaft has an oblique fracture. *B*, Cemented Neer II prosthesis with cerclage wire fixation of the proximal humeral shaft fracture. The prosthesis has been set at the proper length to maintain the myofascial sleeve and avoid excessive deltoid shortening. The tuberosities have been securely attached to the prosthesis and the proximal shaft with no. 2 and no. 5 nonabsorbable nylon sutures. Cancellous bone graft from the head has been packed beneath the prosthesis. Because the repair was secure at operation, passive assistive motion was begun on postoperative day 3.

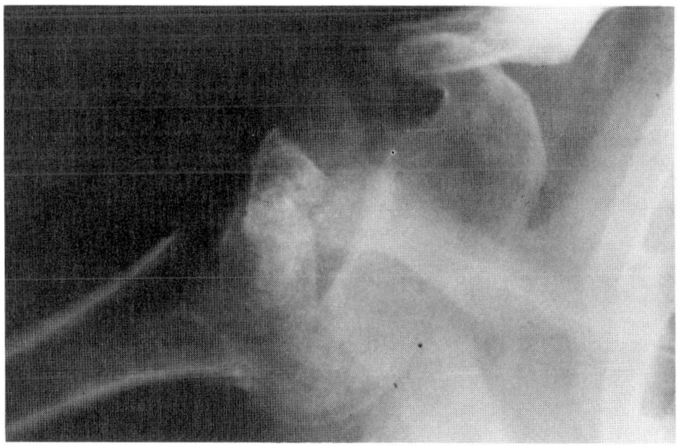

Figure 3

Axillary radiograph 6 months after injury in a missed posterior fracture-dislocation. The head is impaled on the posterior glenoid rim.

pected. Closed reduction usually is successful for two-part lesser tuberosity posterior fracture-dislocations because the lesser tuberosity fragment is small and does not lead to impingement or loss of strength. Three-part fracture-dislocations require open reduction and internal fixation. The greater tuberosity remains with the head and affords a significant blood supply. Four-part fractures require a prosthesis. The prosthesis may need to be in a little less retroversion, about 20°, if there is a tendency toward subluxation posteriorly.

Treatment of impression fractures of the articular surface differs with the size of the defect and the time of the diagnosis. If there is less than 20% head involvement and treatment is within 2 weeks after injury, a closed reduction may be adequate. The arm should be immobilized in external rotation after reduction of the posterior dislocation. For defects between 20% and 50%, the modification of the McLaughlin procedure using a screw for fixation is indicated, and the lesser tuberosity and subscapularis are transferred into the defect. Head defects greater than 50% require a prosthesis; if the glenoid is involved, it also may require a replacement.

Nonunion of proximal humerus fractures is not as rare as previously thought. There are several causes including inadequate or improper immobilization, traction, inadequate internal fixation (Fig. 1), interposition of soft tissues, and overly aggressive physiotherapy before the fracture moves as a unit.

Reconstruction poses a special problem because the bone is atrophic and soft and in some instances there has been previous internal fixation that must be removed. This further compromises the already soft bone. In these instances, infection must always be ruled out prior to further surgical treatment. Surgical repair should include internal fixation (usually wiring and an intramedullary rod) as well as iliac crest bone graft. A second procedure may be required to lyse adhesions and remove hardware so that motion may be improved.

Fractures of the Humeral Shaft

Most humeral shaft fractures are successfully treated by closed methods. The more frequently used techniques include the hanging cast, coaptation splints, sling and swathe, and functional bracing. The abduction splint, shoulder spica cast, and skeletal traction are rarely needed to maintain reduction. Although good results have been reported with the hanging cast, much patient cooperation and frequent supervision are necessary to avoid angulation and distraction which may lead to nonunion. Several recent reports show that functional bracing can give good results consistently. In one study there was rapid fracture union (mean, 7.5 weeks), early restoration of joint mobility, and only a 4% incidence of delayed union and nonunion. The orthotic device used had two polyethylene splints, a polyethylene hinge, three elastic webbing straps, and a shoulder strap for suspension. It can be applied early, usually 4 to 7 days after injury. Patient compliance and comfort were good.

Operative treatment is less frequent than closed reduction and in the past has been associated with a higher rate of complications including nonunion, infection, and radial nerve palsy. Recently, there have been some encouraging reports concerning open reduction and internal fixation; however, it remains a difficult procedure. The primary indications include humeral shaft fractures associated with multiple trauma, inadequate reduction by closed methods, nonunion, pathologic fracture, associated vascular injury, and progressive radial nerve palsy.

Good results after internal fixation with a compression plate and screws have been reported in several series including one series of 27 patients with a 100% union rate. Addition of iliac crest bone graft is indicated in nonunions and in fractures with significant comminution and bone loss. The results from intramedullary rod fixation are more variable. Fixation by a Rush rod inserted proximally is associated with a high rate of complications including delayed union, nonunion, reoperation, and painful adhesive capsulitis of the shoulder from proximal pin impingement. Open fractures treated with intramedullary fixation were associated with a higher rate of nonunion and infection. Better results have been found with use of Küntscher nails and multiple rods inserted distally in the condyles of the humerus.

Pathologic fractures can be especially difficult to treat because of significant bone loss and poor quality of the remaining bone. The best results have been reported with Rush rod fixation and cement at the pathologic fracture site to enhance stability. Important technical considerations are burying the proximal Rush rod tip below the rotator cuff in the posterior aspect of the greater tuberosity and protecting the radial nerve from the heat of the cement by placing Silastic sheeting around the shaft.

Radial nerve injury with fractures of the humeral shaft, especially of the distal shaft, is not infrequent and has been reported in as many as 18% of patients. Controversy still exists over early or late nerve exploration. Most nerve injuries are a neuropraxia or an axonotmesis and there will be recovery with time. Radial nerve laceration is more common in open fractures. The primary indication for early exploration is a progressive nerve palsy that may occur after closed reduction. Initial evaluation of the nerve is essential prior to any treatment.

Scapular Fractures

Fracture of the scapula is a less common injury of the shoulder girdle and usually is the result of a violent force. There can be a delay in diagnosis of this fracture because of the severity of associated bone and soft tissue injuries.

The mortality rate can be significant. The incidence of associated injuries can be quite high; it was 87% in one series of 62 scapular fractures. Furthermore, management of the associated injuries may be more difficult than management of the scapular fracture. The majority of these injuries involved the thorax and consisted of rib fractures (44%), clavicle fractures (39%), and pneumohemothorax (39%). A flail chest occurred in 18%. An especially severe injury is the combination of fractures of the scapula and the underlying first rib. Vascular and neurologic injuries are unusual with scapular fractures except that, with this combination, injuries to the brachial plexus and subclavian vessels must be considered because they can be compressed between the scapula and first rib.

Most fractures of the scapula can be treated conservatively—a sling for several weeks and exercises initiated as tolerated. Prolonged immobilization is not necessary. Certainly, the majority of body, spine, coracoid, acromion, and neck fractures can be managed in this manner. There are a few indications for open reduction and internal fixation, and they involve the glenoid surface. If unrepaired, glenoid rim fractures associated with a glenohumeral dislocation can result in a painful, stiff, and unstable shoulder. In young, active individuals, fractures of the body of the scapula that split the glenoid surface can be considered for open reduction, but there have been good results reported with closed treatment of significantly displaced fractures.

A new term, "scapulo-thoracic dissociation," has recently come into use for describing lateral displacement of the scapula and acromioclavicular separation with severe injury to the soft tissues. The cause is a severe blunt injury to the shoulder girdle, the force being applied to the anterolateral portion of the shoulder. The associated problems include injuries to the brachial plexus and subclavian vessels as well as multiple open and closed fractures of the ipsilateral upper extremity. It is important to make the diagnosis early by comparing the positions of the two scapulae on a chest radiograph: the involved scapula is significantly displaced laterally. Immediate evaluation of the vascular structures is needed to avoid fatal internal hemorrhage.

Fractures of the Clavicle

Fractures involving the clavicle are common injuries in the shoulder girdle region. In most instances, closed treatment is successful. Various closed methods have been described without consensus as to which is best. Comfort and pain relief should be the goals. Maintaining closed reduction of a displaced clavicle fracture is difficult. In most instances, a sling or sling and swathe is sufficient. A figure-of-8 dressing also may be helpful but alone does not support the arm. Less frequently, if these measures fail, a clavicular cast may be required for immobilization and reduction. However, in most instances, it is reasonable to accept the resultant bump and deformity because pain relief and function are quite good.

There are few indications for open reduction and internal fixation, and it is a procedure with a formidable rate of complication. Through the years, no particular method has emerged as superior. The indications for open reduction in displaced midclavicle fractures are open fracture, adjacent neurovascular injuries that require a stable clavicle, and improved cosmesis in younger women. However, operating to improve cosmesis must be approached cautiously because the deformity caused by a painless bump may be exchanged for a painful, unattractive scar or a painful nonunion after internal fixation. Fractures of the distal clavicle involving a tear of the coracoclavicular ligaments (Neer type II) often require open reduction and internal fixation.

Fortunately, nonunion of a clavicle fracture is uncommon. The most significant factors leading to a nonunion appear to be re-fracture, severe trauma, and interposition of soft tissue. Inadequate immobilization and previous surgical repair are other factors. Operative repair of nonunion is very difficult and has a high complication rate. In one series, the overall operative failure rate was 52%; it was more difficult to achieve union in an atrophic nonunion than in a hypertrophic nonunion. However, another recent report described union in all 10 patients, 8 with atrophic and 2 with hypertrophic nonunion; internal fixation (compression plate and screws) with iliac crest bone graft was used in all patients.

Instability

Glenohumeral Instability

Anterior Instability Acute primary anterior dislocation of the shoulder is a frequent injury. In two different series of primary anterior dislocations, the recurrence rates were almost identical.

In a multicenter Swedish study of 257 patients, an overall redislocation rate of 32% at 2-year follow-up was reported. In patients under 22 years of age the rate was nearly 50%, whereas in patients over 22 the rate was 25%. Immobilization had no effect on recurrence; however, the immobilization was for only 3 to 4 weeks. No specific rehabilitation/strengthening program was used. There were no recurrences of dislocations associated with a fracture of the greater tuberosity. Impression fractures in the posterior part of the humeral head (Hill-Sachs lesions), present in 55% of patients, were not associated with a significantly higher rate of dislocation.

In a study of 116 patients in Minnesota followed more than 4 years, a recurrence rate of 33% was found; most of the recurrences occurred within 2 years. The recurrence rate for patients under 20 years of age was 66%; none of the patients over 40 had a recurrence. Athletes had a much higher incidence of recurrence. Restricting athletic activity for more than 6 weeks seemed to have a beneficial effect on rate of recurrence.

Although the rate of recurrence was high in both of these series, it was less than reported previously. A significant number of patients, especially in the older group, did not have a recurrence. The data from these studies do not seem to justify operative repair after primary anterior dislocation. Furthermore, treating primary anterior dislocations with a restrengthening exercise program was successful in 15 of 20 midshipmen at the US Naval Academy. The treatment regimen included strengthening the muscles of internal rotation and adduction plus rigid restriction of activities until the goals of rehabilitation were met. This is quite significant because these patients were young and athletic, factors that increase the chance of recurrence. However, they were highly motivated with convenient access to rehabilitation and there was high compliance with the restrictions on their activity.

Obtaining adequate radiographic confirmation of recurrent anterior glenohumeral instability may be difficult. The two areas that must be evaluated are the posterolateral aspect of the humeral head and the anteroinferior aspect of the glenoid. The Hill-Sachs defect is best demonstrated by an anteroposterior view of the humerus in internal rotation or a Stryker notch view. An osseous Bankart lesion or a glenoid rim fracture is best documented by the West Point axillary and the Didiee view. However, difficulty in positioning the patient, superimposition of other bony or soft tissue structures, obesity, and large size of the patient, individually or in combination, can obscure the injury and make these views hard to interpret. Therefore, in addition to these routine radiographic views, axillary arthrotomography and double-contrast computed tomography of the glenohumeral joint have proved to be useful. The greatest utility seems to be in patients without clear-cut clinical signs of subluxation or dislocation but with pain, clicking, and vague shoulder discomfort suggestive of instability.

At present, double-contrast computed tomography is the preferred procedure. It is easy to perform and comfortable for the patient, whereas arthrotomography requires an oblique position which is quite uncomfortable (a shift of position can obscure the lesion). The dose of radiation in arthrotomography is 5 to 10 times higher than with computed tomography. Also, double-contrast computed tomography provides better image quality of both the glenoid rim and labrum. A tear of the glenoid labrum (Bankart lesion) not routinely seen in an axillary radiograph is readily seen; also, wearing and fraying of the labrum as well as cartilage erosion can be seen (Fig. 4 *A*). The extent of an osseous Bankart lesion or a glenoid rim fracture is more accurately quantified (Fig. 4 *B*). The same is true for Hill-Sachs lesions. Magnetic resonance imaging, a noninvasive method, may prove helpful in evaluating shoulder instability in the future when the technique is refined.

Many procedures have been described for correcting recurrent anterior dislocation and subluxation and recently good results have been reported in several large series with various repairs including the Bristow-Latarjet, Bankart, Putti-Platt, and Magnuson-Stack procedures, to name a few. It is difficult to recommend a single procedure as the best. Factors that have been stressed in achieving a successful procedure are adequate exposure and accurate surgical technique rather than the type of procedure. Some think that it is important to define the problem involved and to perform a procedure that corrects the deformity most anatomically.

One of the more popular procedures for repair of a recurrent anterior dislocating shoulder is the coracoid transfer, the Bristow-Latarjet procedure. It has been recommended for both adolescents (under 18 years old) and older patients. In one series of 34 patients under 18 years of age, only 2 had resubluxation; most of these patients were athletes with very active life-styles. The importance of precise operative technique for obtaining a successful result is stressed. The bone block must be placed inferior to the equator of the glenoid and less than 1 cm medial to its rim. Placement of the transplant more than 1 cm medial to the rim is associated with a higher incidence of redislocation or subluxation. Intra-articular placement of the bone block will lead to joint degeneration.

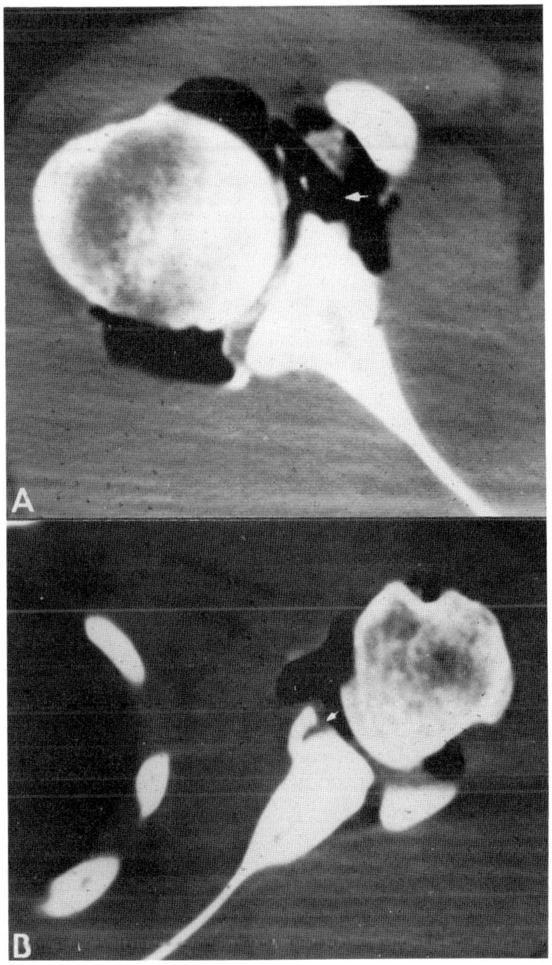

Figure 4

Double-contrast computed tomograms of the shoulder joint. *A*, Detachment of the anterior glenoid labrum (*arrow*) (Bankart lesion). *B*, Fracture of the inferior glenoid rim (*arrow*). This lesion may be difficult to visualize, even on a West Point axillary view, because of superimposition of adjacent structures and the size and positioning of the patient.

Another factor that must be considered is the use of metal implants about the shoulder joint; this can be a common source of complication. Broken, migrated, and misplaced screws and staples as well as intra-articular penetration are just a few of the reported problems leading to failure of the repair, reoperation, and joint degeneration (Fig. 5). Pain, decreased glenohumeral motion, crepitus, and radiating paresthesias can occur. Adequate exposure and careful placement of these implants are essential.

A persistent Bankart lesion is often the pathologic lesion contributing to recurrent anterior instability. Therefore, it seems logical to correct this as part of the surgical repair; 94% good and excellent results with a Bankart repair have been reported. When the labrum was not completely detached, a modified Bankart repair (capsulorrhaphy) was performed.

Rotational subcapital humeral osteotomy has been advised for recurrent anterior dislocation associated with a large Hill-Sachs lesion. Excellent results were obtained in more than 90% of patients in a large series. However, it is difficult to isolate the effect of the osteotomy because an integral part of the procedure is shortening of the subscap-

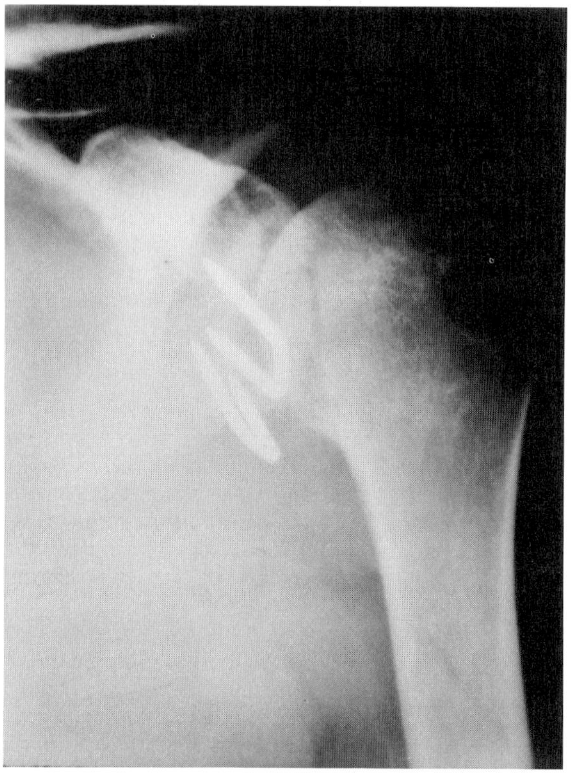

Figure 5

Anteroposterior radiograph of shoulder after Dutoit staple capsulorrhaphy with an intra-articular staple in a 28-year-old patient. There was significant articular damage to the head and glenoid, requiring total shoulder replacement.

ularis and capsule. Furthermore, a persistent Hill-Sachs lesion has not been identified by others as significant in contributing to a failure of a repair. Also, in many instances a second procedure is required to remove the hardware.

Inferior Instability Traumatic inferior dislocation of the shoulder (luxatio erecta) is rare but can be associated with significant complications. The mechanism of injury is usually a forceful hyperabduction of the arm, with the elbow flexed and the hand overhead. Reduction with adequate anesthesia may be accomplished by upward traction on the extended arm and countertraction on the top of the shoulder. The arm is carried through an arc to the side of the body. Repeated forceful attempts at reduction should not be tried. After reduction it is important to evaluate for fractures as well as injury to the brachial plexus and axillary artery. It is also important to realize that the rotator cuff may have been torn, but this is usually evaluated several weeks after initial injury if pain and weakness persist.

Posterior Instability Posterior instability of the humerus is not as common or as well understood as anterior instability but is being reported with more frequency. Unilateral traumatic posterior dislocation is still rare, but posterior subluxation, which may be associated with multidirectional instability, is becoming more common. The problem may be difficult to diagnose and treat. It is important to take a careful history so that a mechanism of injury can be established which may help clarify the diagnosis. Also, it is essential to identify "habitual posterior dislocators" because they may have underlying psychiatric problems and are less likely to respond to surgical repair.

The apprehension test for posterior instability is flexion of the shoulder beyond 90° with internal rotation and adduction. Forward elevation will also test for a posteroinferior component. Radiographic criteria are not as prevalent in recurrent posterior dislocation as in anterior. However, double-contrast computed tomography is helpful to evaluate the posterior labrum for tears or wearing. Evaluation under anesthesia is helpful to confirm the diagnosis and direction of instability and can be supplemented with a C-arm fluoroscopic examination in the axillary plane. Anterior and posterior displacement can be visualized with appropriate stress. Also, it is helpful to check the stability of the other shoulder for comparison.

The initial treatment of posterior instability should be conservative. The regimen includes avoidance of provocative activities such as sports and overhead lifting and educating the patient to avoid specific voluntary maneuvers that will cause posterior subluxation. Also, a strengthening program aimed at the external rotators and posterior deltoid should be started and closely monitored. Resistive exercises with rubber tubing, rotational exercises with 10-kg weights, and Cybex can be used.

Through the years, various types of procedures have been proposed to correct posterior instability, including soft tissue procedures such as the reverse Bankart and reverse Putti-Platt, extra-articular and intra-articular bone block procedures, glenoid osteotomy, and muscle transfers with capsulorrhaphy. Also, combinations of osseous procedures and capsulorrhaphy have been described. However, there have been few published reports on which to base an opinion as to the best procedure. In a retrospective study of 26 surgical procedures (17 posterior glenoid osteotomies, 6 reverse Putti-Platt applications, and 3 biceps tendon transfers) performed by several surgeons, a recurrence rate of 50% was found. There were five complications after the glenoid osteotomies; two were quite severe, resulting in degenerative arthritis of the glenohumeral joint. A recent report has suggested using a large intra-articular posterior bone block to correct instability. However, an intra-articular bone block can cause significant degeneration of the joint. It seems more advisable to consider an extra-articular bone block to act as a buttress for a soft tissue repair when there is bony insufficiency.

Great care should be taken in the selection of patients for surgical reconstruction of posterior instability because there is a high rate of recurrence and postoperative complications. The choice of conservative treatment—with the patient accepting the disability and adjusting his or her life-style—should be considered.

Posterior dislocation can be the major component in multidirectional instability, and operative repair for this problem generally has been successful. The procedure—inferior capsular shift from the posterior approach—advances the superior capsule inferiorly and overlaps this with the inferior capsule advanced superiorly. This not only obliterates the inferior pouch but also strengthens the posterior capsule because it is twice as thick. Furthermore, the infraspinatus is cut in such a way that it is overlapped and shortened. This also tends to buttress the posterior capsule. It is important to immobilize the arm in neutral or slight external rotation. Because this procedure has been reported to give long-term successful results, it seems reasonable to modify it for unidirectional posterior instability. The modification would be to perform less of an inferior capsular shift because there is no inferior pouch to obliterate and therefore there would be less overlap of the capsular flaps. Furthermore, if a bony deficiency were present, an extracapsular bone block from the scapular spine could be added.

Failed Repairs for Instability There have been several reports concerning recurrent instability after surgical repair, and this seems to be an increasingly prevalent problem. The two most commonly recognized pathologic lesions that cause failed repair are a persistent Bankart lesion and excessive capsular laxity. Both are present in more than 80% of failed repairs. Therefore, it seems important to recognize a Bankart lesion when the initial repair is performed and to correct it adequately.

In patients with excessive capsular laxity, an unrecognized multidirectional component may be present. Standard repairs will not correct this problem and are apt to fail. The primary lesion is a loose, redundant capsule with a large inferior pouch. This allows instability in three directions: inferior, anterior, and superior. Repairs such as the Magnuson-Stack, Putti-Platt, and Bristow-Latarjet only correct one component of the instability (Fig. 6). The same is true with posterior procedures such as bone blocks and glenoid osteotomies—they only correct the posterior component. The most appropriate procedure for multidirectional instability is the inferior capsular shift. Usually through one approach, either anterior or posterior depending on the greatest direction of instability, the redundant capsule on all three sides can be corrected. Occasionally, a second approach on the other side of the joint is required. For example, in a patient with posterior dislocation and antero-inferior subluxation, an inferior capsular shift from the posterior approach is performed but if a significant Bankart lesion along the anterior rim is discovered during the procedure, an anterior approach is required.

Other factors that are responsible for a failed repair include intra-articular or loose hardware, approach on the wrong side of the shoulder, scarred and weakened subscapularis, repair made too tight (results in arthritis or dislocation to the opposite side), missed loose bodies, infection, and neurovascular complications. The success of reoperation after previous failure is very encouraging. The procedure includes repairing a persistent Bankart lesion and performing a capsular shift to correct capsular laxity. If there is significant arthritis, humeral head or total shoulder replacement may be necessary.

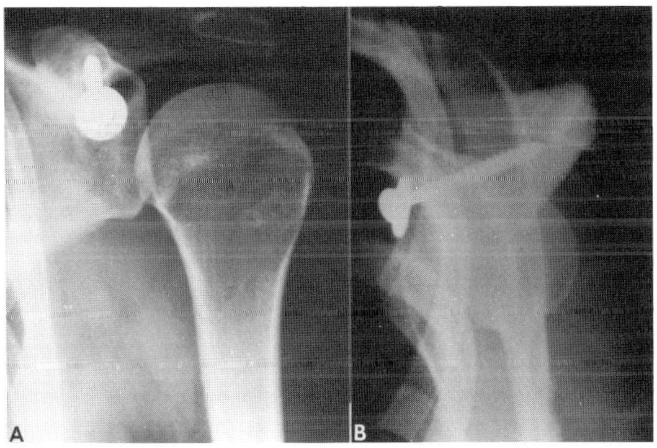

Figure 6

Recurrent multidirectional instability after a Magnuson-Stack procedure (the humeral staple has been removed) and a Bristow-Latarjet procedure. *A*, Anteroposterior radiograph shows screw and coracoid transfer malpositioned superiorly on the glenoid rim above the equator. The screw was loose and painful. *B*, Lateral radiograph in scapular plane, revealing posterior and superior protrusion of the screw. There was exquisite tenderness over the screw tip posteriorly.

Acromioclavicular Separation

Acromioclavicular separation has been associated with an active, athletic life-style. Acromioclavicular joint injuries are classified according to the amount of damage done to the ligament of the joint, the extra-articular ligaments (coracoclavicular ligaments), and the adjacent supporting muscles (deltoid and trapezius):

Type I, sprain of the acromioclavicular ligament with the joint intact.

Type II, tear of the acromioclavicular ligament with disruption of the joint; the coracoclavicular ligaments are sprained but intact.

Type III, tear of the acromioclavicular and coracoclavicular ligaments with joint dislocation and upward displacement of the clavicle; the coracoclavicular interspace is 25% to 100% greater than on the normal side; the deltoid and trapezius are detached from the distal end of the clavicle.

Type IV, essentially the same as in type III but the distal clavicle is anatomically displaced posteriorly into or through the trapezius muscle (Fig. 7); the skin may be tented posteriorly.

Type V, tear of the acromioclavicular and coracoclavicular ligaments with dislocation of the joint; the distal clavicle is grossly and severely displaced upward toward the base of the neck; the coracoclavicular interspace is 100% to 300% greater than on the normal side; the deltoid and

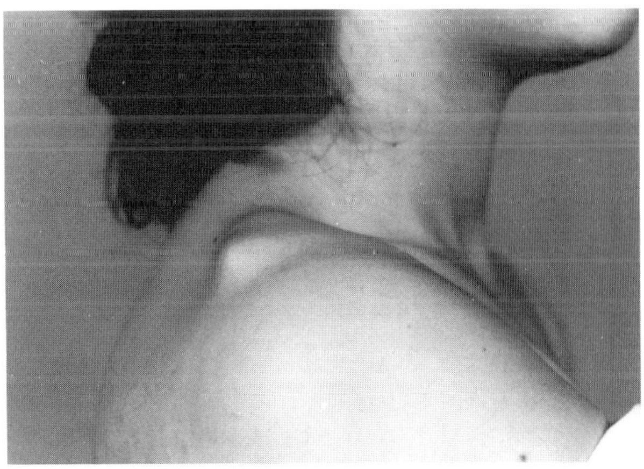

Figure 7

Type IV acromioclavicular separation with the unstable distal clavicle protruding posteriorly through the trapezius and tenting the skin.

trapezius are detached from the distal half of the clavicle; the skin may be tented.

Type VI, tear of the acromioclavicular ligament with dislocation of the joint; the distal clavicle is displaced downward and under either the acromion or the coracoid process; the coracoclavicular ligaments can be either intact or disrupted; the coracoclavicular interspace is reversed (this is a very rare injury).

The treatment of acute acromioclavicular separations continues to be extremely controversial. The trends fluctuate between nonoperative and operative approaches. Currently, most authors agree that all type I and II injuries initially should be treated nonoperatively. If pain and disability persist, surgical repair can be considered later. The current trend is toward treating acute type III injuries nonoperatively; this includes accepting the deformity, using a sling for support for a short time, and early institution of range-of-motion and strengthening exercises. Several large studies of young, active, athletic individuals have consistently revealed good results with conservative treatment. In a comparison of conservative treatment with operative repair (Bosworth screw technique), the interval to pain-free status (4.5 months versus 2.8 months) and the interval to return to sports (2.2 months versus 1.7 months) were shorter after conservative treatment. However, the choice between conservative and operative treatment still must be individualized to the patient. Type of work or sport, age, and dominant extremity of the patient must be taken into consideration.

When the dominant arm is injured in a patient involved in heavy manual labor or in a violent sport that requires strength overhead, operative repair may be more suitable. The more severe injuries (types IV, V, and VI) require operative repair. In type IV and V injuries there has been significant damage to the deltotrapezius aponeurosis with pronounced instability, and stabilization is required. Many types of operative repairs have been proposed, many with reported good results in reference to pain relief and function. There is no clear-cut evidence as to which type of repair is superior. It is important to reconstitute the coracoclavicular ligament to achieve vertical stability and also to avoid late arthritic changes in the acromioclavicular joint.

Sternoclavicular Joint

Injuries to the sternoclavicular joint are less frequent than acromioclavicular joint injuries and usually are the result of a motor vehicle accident or violent sport activity. Anterior sternoclavicular dislocations are more common than posterior, but posterior dislocations are harder to recognize and can have significant complications. In addition to pain, with a posterior dislocation there may be hoarseness, dyspnea, dysphagia, and numbness or weakness of the upper extremity. It is important to make an early diagnosis because closed reduction is more likely to succeed early after injury. Also, the potential for injury to the trachea, lungs, and great vessels must be considered. However, in contrast to the situation with an anterior dislocation, the clinical diagnosis may be difficult to make because it is hard to demonstrate on physical examination and the conventional radiographs of the sternoclavicular joint often are difficult to interpret. The 40° cephalic tilt view and tomography are helpful, but the best study is computed tomography which produces very clear osseous images that allow precise determination of the position of the medial clavicle and sternum. Furthermore, this technique reveals the relationship of the subclavian vessels, trachea, and esophagus to the sternoclavicular joint (Fig. 8).

For acute anterior sternoclavicular dislocations, it should be stressed that nonoperative treatment is indicated. Also, closed reduction is not indicated in this highly unstable injury because the reduction cannot be maintained. A sling may be worn for comfort. For posterior sternoclavicular dislocation, prompt closed or open reduction is required. If the diagnosis is made early, a closed reduction may be all that is needed. Adequate anesthesia is essential to relieve muscle spasm, and general anesthesia normally is used. The patient is placed on a table with a bolster or sandbag between the scapulae and traction is applied to the arm in abduction and slight extension. If this is unsuccessful, indirect traction with a sterile towel clip around the clavicle is attempted. If this is unsuccessful, open reduction is required. Whether by closed or open means, the reduction is usually stable. A figure-of-8 dressing or a sling is used for 4 to 6 weeks.

Neurovascular Injury

Vascular Injury

Injury to the axillary artery is infrequent, accounting for approximately 6% of arterial trauma, but it can occur after shoulder trauma. The injury is usually associated with penetrating or violent blunt trauma that causes multiple fractures. Also, risk is increased in older patients with arteriosclerosis because the vessel walls have lost elasticity and cannot stretch in response to trauma. Vascular injury also can occur after supposedly less serious injuries such as anterior dislocation and proximal humeral fractures, especially in the older age group. Pseudoaneurysm of the axillary artery has been reported after an acute dislocation and also after repair because of penetration of a screw used in a Bristow-Latarjet procedure. The most common location of the injury is the junction of the anterior circumflex and axillary arteries. Recent reports have stressed the

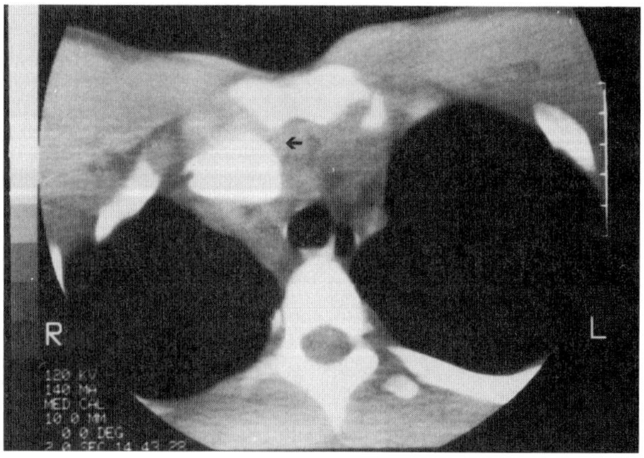

Figure 8

Computed tomogram of a posterior sternoclavicular dislocation, revealing clearly the sternum and clavicle as well as the trachea, esophagus, and lung fields. *Arrow,* medial clavicle posterior to sternum.

need to suspect vascular injury whenever there is a fracture near a major vessel, because the key to successful treatment is early diagnosis and repair and because physical examination of the axillary artery may be difficult when pain and muscle spasm prevent abduction.

It is important to check the radial pulse in the injured extremity. However, the presence of peripheral pulses may be due to collateral circulation and so is no guarantee that significant arterial injury has not occurred. Doppler ultrasonography can be helpful in detecting a pulse but also can be misleading because collateral circulation can create a pulse detectable by Doppler examination. Other signs include an expanding hematoma, pallor, and paresthesias. Paresthesias are probably the most reliable sign of inadequate distal circulation and should raise suspicion of a vascular injury. If an arterial injury is unrecognized, the complications can be catastrophic, including gangrene, amputation, and compressive neuropathies of the brachial plexus leading to permanent deficits unless there is early evacuation of the hematoma. Angiography should be performed to confirm the diagnosis and to establish the exact location and nature of the injury. Arterial repair should be done without delay and coordinated with the appropriate orthopaedic repair if necessary.

Neurologic Lesions

Axillary Nerve This is the most commonly injured nerve about the shoulder, yet it represents only about 1% of all peripheral nerve injuries. The axillary nerve courses on the inferior surface of the shoulder and is very susceptible to injury during anterior dislocation. This is especially true in a dislocation associated with a significant fall or traction injury. The other common causes are fracture and blunt trauma. It is important to get a complete electromyographic study when an axillary nerve injury is suspected because other nerves may be involved. In a recent study, electromyograms taken after an anterior dislocation revealed more extensive involvement of the brachial plexus than just the axillary nerve in several instances.

It is important to determine the cause of the axillary nerve palsy because there are significant differences in recovery. If the injury is secondary to a dislocation or traction injury, the chance for recovery is quite high. However, if the cause is blunt direct trauma the potential for recovery is diminished. Roughly half of the patients do not achieve satisfactory return of nerve function after trauma.

Suprascapular Nerve Isolated suprascapular nerve injury is uncommon and frequently is overlooked. The causes include penetrating injuries in the posterior cervical triangle, traction injuries, and fractures of the scapula that involve the base of the coracoid or suprascapular notch area. An association between traumatic rotator cuff tears and conduction latencies in the suprascapular nerve has been reported but this relationship remains unclear. Patients who have weakness of external rotation after trauma, especially older patients, should be evaluated for a complete-thickness rotator cuff tear with an arthrogram as well as an electromyogram to check the suprascapular nerve. In most instances, repair of the rotator cuff is followed by return of active external rotation and the suprascapular nerve lesion, if present, usually resolves.

The suprascapular nerve lesion resolves quickly in the first 5 months after injury and less rapidly between the 5th and 8th months. After this period of time, if a deficit persists and there is an obvious mechanical blockage, such as fracture callus or malunion in the area of the suprascapular notch, decompression of the nerve is warranted. Soft tissue constriction in the area of the suprascapular ligament also may occur, and release of this stricture may be necessary, but this is rare.

Spinal Accessory Nerve The spinal accessory nerve, cranial nerve XI, lies superficial in subcutaneous tissue on the floor of the posterior cervical triangle on its course to innervate the trapezius. It is susceptible to injury from penetrating trauma (such as a stab or gunshot wound) or blunt trauma (from a fall or motor vehicle accident) that puts traction on the nerve. However, the most common cause of injury is trauma from biopsy of a cervical soft tissue mass; during this procedure, the nerve may be scarred or cut. The resulting trapezius paralysis is a painful, deforming problem, causing drooping of the shoulder girdle, asymmetry of the neckline, winging of the scapula, and weakness of forward elevation. Accurate diagnosis can be difficult and requires thorough neurologic and electromyographic examinations. If the diagnosis is made early (within 1 year after injury), nerve exploration, with neurolysis, repair, or grafting if necessary, is indicated. The results are much better if the exploration is performed within 6 months after injury.

Orthopaedic reconstructive procedures should be considered after 1 year if pain persists and the deformity does not respond to conservative measures. The Eden-Lange procedure—transfer of the levator scapulae and rhomboid—is a dynamic transfer which substitutes for all three components of the trapezius: upper, middle, and lower. This procedure has been effective in relieving pain and improving function. Medial scapular retraction and upward rotation are enhanced, which corrects scapular drooping and winging.

Shoulder Trauma in Pediatric Patients

Little has been written recently concerning shoulder trauma in patients in the pediatric age group. Fractures of the humeral shaft in children are uncommon, compared to adults, and most are treated by closed reduction and immobilization. Fractures involving the proximal humeral physis are more frequent. Because approximately 80% of the growth of the humerus occurs at the proximal physis, the potential for remodeling is high, especially in the younger age groups. Therefore, immobilization is indicated in most instances. Closed reduction may be required in significantly displaced fractures in older adolescents near the end of their growth period. Open reduction and internal fixation is seldom indicated but may be required in the rare Salter IV fracture with articular involvement.

Clavicle fractures are quite common in children, and 80% of them occur in the shaft. The mechanism of injury is usually indirect, from a fall on an outstretched hand. Also, fracture of the clavicle during delivery is the most common birth injury. There is a high association with breech deliveries. The very few indications for open reduction include open fracture and neurovascular compromise. Internal fixation should be avoided. In general, conservative treatment with either a figure-of-8 bandage or a sling is sufficient for support and comfort.

Fractures of the scapula are also uncommon in children and generally are treated conservatively. Little has been written concerning acromioclavicular joint injuries in children, and their classification and treatment closely parallel those for injuries in adults.

Furthermore, sternoclavicular injuries are also considered with the adult injuries because the epiphysis of the sternal end of the clavicle does not ossify until age 18 years or older, and the physis does not close until age 23 to 25 years. Most injuries in children are either type I or type II epiphyseal separations that are best treated conservatively.

Annotated Bibliography

Fractures and Fracture-Dislocations

Proximal Humerus

Leyshon, R.L.: Closed treatment of fractures of the proximal humerus. Acta Orthop. Scand. 55:48–51, 1984.

The results in 42 patients with three- or four-part fractures of the proximal humerus treated only by closed methods were reviewed. All 8 with four-part fractures had poor results, and 10 of 34 with three-part fractures had poor results.

Stableforth, P.G.: Four-part fractures of the neck of the humerus. J. Bone Joint Surg. 66B:104–108, 1984.

A retrospective study of 32 patients with four-part shoulder fractures treated conservatively revealed persistent pain, stiffness, and dysfunction of the shoulder. A prospective study of 49 patients treated with a Neer prosthesis revealed that this reconstructive procedure usually restored comfort and function.

Tanner, M.W., and Cofield, R.H.: Prosthetic arthroplasty for fractures and fracture-dislocations of the proximal humerus. Clin. Orthop. 179:116–128, 1983.

Forty-nine shoulders in 48 patients had a Neer proximal humeral replacement for both acute and chronic displaced fracture-dislocations. Pain relief was satisfactory in all 16 with acute fractures and in 25 of 28 with chronic fractures. Function was better in patients treated earlier.

Humeral Shaft

Balfour, G.W.; Mooney V.; and Ashby, M.E.: Diaphyseal fractures of the humerus treated with ready-made fracture brace. J. Bone Joint Surg. 64A:11–13, 1982.

A method of treatment of diaphyseal fractures of the humerus with a polyethylene brace was developed. More rapid fracture union was obtained than with other methods of treatment, as was earlier restoration of joint mobility and increased comfort for the patient. Union was achieved in 41 of the 42 patients followed.

Foster, R.J.; Dixon, G.L.; Bach, A.W.; Appleyard, R.W.; and Green, T.M.: Internal fixation of fractures and nonunions of the humeral shaft. J. Bone Joint Surg. 67A:857–864, 1985.

A multicenter study reviewed the indications and results of internal fixation of the humeral shaft for fractures and nonunions. Compression plating resulted in a 100% union rate for fractures in multiply injured patients and an 80% union rate in nonunions. Intramedullary nailing also gave good results.

Stern, P.J.; Mattingly, D.A.; Pomeroy, D.L.; Zenni, E.J.; and Kreig, J.A.: Intramedullary fixation of humeral shaft fractures. J. Bone Joint Surg. 66A:639–646, 1984.

Seventy fractures of the humeral shaft treated by intramedullary fixation were reviewed. Complications developed in 67% and at least one additional procedure was required in 64%. Delayed union and nonunion were more common in open fractures and in those treated by a more extensive open reduction procedure. Adhesive capsulitis developed in 56% of patients treated with retrograde rods. Results can be improved by using proper timing and better techniques.

Scapula

Armstrong, C.P., and Van der Spuy, J.: The fractured scapula: Importance and management based on a series of 62 patients. Injury 15:324–329, 1984.

In 64 scapular fractures in 62 patients, a severe force usually was the cause and 87% had associated injuries. The mortality rate was 10%, with the combination of first rib fracture and scapular fracture being an especially severe injury. Conservative treatment is usually indicated except in active patients with scapular neck or glenoid fractures.

Oreck, S.L.; Burgess, A.; and Levine, A.M.: Traumatic lateral displacement of the scapula: A radiographic sign of neurovascular disruption. J. Bone Joint Surg. 66A:758–763, 1984.

A new term is introduced, "scapulo-thoracic dissociation," which is defined as lateral displacement of the scapula and acromioclavicular separation without an overlying partial or complete amputation through soft tissue. The cause is severe blunt trauma to the shoulder girdle which also causes injuries to the subclavian artery and vein and to the brachial plexus and multiple fractures of the ipsilateral upper extremity. If there is lateral scapula displacement on the chest radiograph, angiography is indicated.

Clavicle

Manske, D.J., and Szabo, R.M.: The operative treatment of mid-shaft clavicular non-unions. J. Bone Joint Surg. 67A:1367–1371, 1985.

Ten patients with nonunion of the clavicle (eight atrophic and two hypertrophic) were treated by open reduction, internal fixation with a compression plate and screws, and iliac crest bone graft. All patients achieved union at 10 weeks with minimal pain, full range of motion at the ipsilateral shoulder, and an acceptable cosmetic result.

Wilkins, R.M., and Johnston, R.M.: Ununited fractures of the clavicle. J. Bone Joint Surg. 65A:773–778, 1983.

Thirty-three cases of nonunion of the clavicle are reviewed; the two dominant predisposing factors were re-fracture and severe trauma. Surgical treatment to establish union was not reliably successful.

Instability

Glenohumeral

Aronen, J.G., and Regan, K.: Decreasing the incidence of recurrence of first time anterior shoulder dislocations with rehabilitation. Am. J. Sports Med. 12:283–291, 1984.

During a 3½-year period, 20 midshipmen at the US Naval

Academy sustained primary anterior shoulder dislocations and were treated by a restrengthening exercise program. The success rate was 75% with a 35.8-month follow-up.

Barry, T.P.; Lombardo, S.J.; Kerlan, R.K.; Jobe, F.W.; Carter, V.S.; Shields, C.L.; Yocum, L.A.; and Tibone, J.E.: The coracoid transfer for recurrent anterior instability of the shoulder in adolescents. J. Bone Joint Surg. 67A:383–387, 1985.

Thirty-six shoulders with recurrent anterior dislocation or subluxation in 34 patients <18 years old were treated with a modified Bristow-Latarjet procedure. Thirty had good or excellent results by objective criteria. There were no redislocations and two resubluxations. Two screws broke. The principal limitation was a mean loss of 10° of external rotation.

Hawkins, R.J.; Koppert, G.; and Johnston, G.: Recurrent posterior instability (subluxation) of the shoulder. J. Bone Joint Surg. 66A:169–174, 1984.

A retrospective survey of 50 shoulders with recurrent posterior instability revealed generally poor results of treatment, especially operative treatment (recurrence rate was 50% in 26 procedures). Seventeen posterior glenoid osteotomies were performed with a failure rate of 41%; degenerative arthritis developed in two patients. The authors advise careful selection of patients for operation.

Hovelius, L.; Eriksson, K.; Fredin, H.; Hagberg, G.; Hussenius, Å.; Lind, B.; Thorling, J.; and Weckstrom, J.: Recurrences after initial dislocation of the shoulder: Results of a prospective study of treatment. J. Bone Joint Surg. 65A:343–349, 1983.

Two hundred fifty-seven patients treated conservatively for a primary anterior dislocation of the shoulder were studied for recurrences during a 2-year period. All patients with a fracture of the greater tuberosity did not have redislocation but 32% of patients without a fracture did. Immobilization did not affect the rate of recurrence. Younger patients (under age 22 years) had a higher incidence of recurrence.

Hovelius, L.; Körner, L.; Lundberg, B.; Åkermark, C.; Herberts, P.; Wredmark, T.; and Berg, E.: The coracoid transfer for recurrent dislocation of the shoulder. Technical aspects of the Bristow Latarjet procedure. J. Bone Joint Surg. 65A:926–934, 1983.

One hundred twelve shoulders with recurrent anterior dislocations treated by the Bristow-Latarjet procedure had a redislocation rate of 6%; resubluxation occurred in 7%. No redislocation resubluxation occurred in the 40 patients with the following technical features: the transplant showed osseous or fibrous union at the scapula and was located inferior to the equator of the glenoid and less than 1 cm medial to its rim.

Kleinman, P.D.; Kanzaria, P.K.; Goss, T.P.; and Pappas, A.M.: Axillary arthrotomography of the glenoid labrum. A.J.R. 142:993–999, 1984.

Axillary arthrotomography performed in 67 shoulders was found to have a high degree of accuracy in identifying glenoid labrum defects. Its greatest utility is in patients without clinical signs of subluxation or dislocation but with pain, clicking, or vague shoulder discomfort secondary to a labral defect.

Norris, T.R., and Bigliani, L.U.: Analysis of failed repair for shoulder instability—A preliminary report. *In* Surgery of the Shoulder, edited by J.E. Bateman and R.P. Welsh, pp. 111–116. Philadelphia, Decker, 1984.

Forty-two patients with shoulder instability who had had 73 previous failed operations were evaluated. The most common causes for failure of a repair were a persistent Bankart lesion and unrecognized multidirectional instability. Reoperations were aimed at restoring anatomy, repairing Bankart lesions, and eliminating capsular redundancy.

Pavlov, H.; Warren, R.F.; Weiss, C.B., Jr.; and Dines, D.M.: The roentgenographic evaluation of anterior shoulder instability. Clin. Orthop. 194:153–158, 1985.

Radiographs of 83 patients with unilateral shoulder instability were evaluated. The Hill-Sachs and osseous Bankart lesions were considered pathognomonic radiographic signs of glenohumeral joint instability. An anteroposterior view in internal rotation and a Stryker notch view were best for demonstrating a Hill-Sachs defect. The osseous Bankart lesion was best documented on the Didiee and West Point axillary views.

Rowe, C.R.; Zarins, B.; and Cuillo, J.V.: Recurrent anterior dislocation of the shoulder after surgical repair. J. Bone Joint Surg. 66A:159–168, 1984.

Thirty-nine patients with unsuccessful surgical repairs for recurrent anterior dislocation of the shoulder were analyzed and treated. The most common pathologic lesions in this group were Bankart lesion, excessive laxity of the capsule, and Hill-Sachs lesion of the humeral head. Twenty-four patients had reoperations with successful results in 22.

Shuman, W.P.; Kilcoyne, R.F.; Matsen, F.A.; Rogers, J.V.; and Mack, L.A.: Double-contrast computed tomography of the glenoid labrum. A.J.R. 141:581–584, 1983.

Eleven patients with suspected anterior glenoid labrum damage underwent double-contrast shoulder computed tomography. The procedure was helpful in demonstrating attenuation, tears, and displacement of the labrum. This procedure is easy to perform, low in radiation dose, and accurate.

Simonet, W.T., and Cofield, R.H.: Prognosis in anterior shoulder dislocation. Am. J. Sports Med. 12:19–24, 1984.

One hundred sixteen patients treated for their first anterior glenohumeral dislocation were evaluated for recurrence. Thirty-three percent had recurrence of dislocation; the rate was higher among athletes and younger individuals.

Weber, B.G.; Simpson, L.A.; and Hardegger, F.: Rotational humeral osteotomy for recurrent anterior dislocation of the shoulder associated with a large Hill-Sachs lesion. J. Bone Joint Surg. 66A:1443–1450, 1984.

Rotational subcapital osteotomy of the humerus for recurrent anterior dislocation of the shoulder with a large Hill-Sachs lesion was performed on 207 shoulders. Shortening and overlap of the subscapularis and capsule was also performed to limit external rotation. Good to excellent results were noted in 90%. Poor results were secondary to redislocation, delayed union or nonunion, post-traumatic arthritis, and over-rotation at the osteotomy site. More than 10° of limitation of external rotation was present in 3.9%.

Zuckerman, J.D., and Matsen F.A., III: Complications about the glenohumeral joint related to the use of screws and staples. J. Bone Joint Surg. 66A:175–180, 1984.

Complications from the use of screws and staples in the surgical treatment of the glenohumeral joint in 37 patients were analyzed. Complaints were shoulder pain, decreased glenohumeral motion, crepitus, and radiating paresthesias. Forty-one percent of patients undergoing reoperation had significant articular injury. Adequate exposure and careful placement of these implants are essential.

Acromioclavicular

Bjerneld, H.; Hovelius, L.; and Thorling, J.: Acromioclavicular separations treated conservatively. Acta Orthop. Scand. 54:743–745, 1983.

Seventy patients with acute acromioclavicular separation treated conservatively were reviewed. All 37 patients with partial separations had good results, and only 3 of 33 with complete separations had unsatisfactory results. Conservative management is the initial treatment.

Galpin, R.D.; Hawkins, R.J.; and Grainger, R.W.: A

comparative analysis of operative *versus* nonoperative treatment of grade III acromioclavicular separations. Clin. Orthop. 193:150–155, 1985.

Two groups of patients with grade III acromioclavicular separations were compared. One group of 21 had conservative treatment with early activity and one group had operative treatment by a Bosworth screw technique. The group with conservative treatment compared favorably with respect to pain relief, strength, and throwing ability.

Sternoclavicular

Selesnick, F.H.; Jablon, M.; Frank, C.; and Post, M.: Retrosternal dislocation of the clavicle. J. Bone Joint Surg. 66A:287–291, 1984.

In four patients with retrosternal dislocations of the clavicle, computed tomography was useful in diagnosis as well as for delineation of surrounding soft tissues. Open reduction was necessary in three cases. Closed reduction is best under general anesthesia within 48 hours after injury.

Neurovascular Injury

Vascular

Gallen, J.; Wiss, D.A.; Cantelmo, N.; and Menzoin, J.O.: Traumatic pseudoaneurysm of the axillary artery: Report of three cases and literature review. J. Trauma 24:350–354, 1984.

Three cases of pseudoaneurysm of the axillary artery after trauma to the shoulder are reported. Delayed recognition may lead to compression neuropathies of the brachial plexus and permanent deficits. Early recognition of possible vascular injuries in shoulder trauma is essential to avoid this complication.

Gugenheim, S., and Sanders, R.J.: Axillary artery rupture caused by shoulder dislocation. Surgery 95:55–58, 1984.

A case of complete rupture of the axillary artery after anterior shoulder dislocation is reported. This is a rare injury and may be associated with a brachial plexus lesion. Radial pulse was present. A Dacron graft was used in the repair.

Neurologic

Bigliani, L.U.; Perez-Sanz, J.R.; and Wolfe, I.N.: Treatment of trapezius paralysis. J. Bone Joint Surg. 67A:871–877, 1985.

Trapezius paralysis is a painful, disabling problem for which conservative treatment is usually unsuccessful. Ten patients underwent operative reconstruction consisting of transfer of the levator scapulae and rhomboid. The results were excellent in seven, satisfactory in two, and unsatisfactory in one. All patients had improved function and correction of deformity, and nine patients had good pain relief.

Liveson, J.A.: Nerve lesions associated with shoulder dislocation: An electrodiagnostic study in 11 cases. J. Neurol. Neurosurg. Psychiatry 47:742–744, 1984.

Eleven patients had a nerve lesion proved by electromyography after shoulder dislocations. Axillary nerve injury was the most common, but the posterior cord and musculocutaneous nerve were also involved in several cases.

18

Shoulder: Reconstruction

Within the last 4 years, many new applications of radiography to diagnosis of shoulder diseases have been suggested and arthroscopy has emerged as a powerful diagnostic approach and a potential therapeutic tool. The spectrum of rotator cuff disease is a major topic. The frozen shoulder is still confusing, but it is becoming better defined. The pathology of shoulder arthritis is now known. Reconstruction for arthritis has become focused on the unconstrained resurfacing total shoulder replacement.

Related Research

Some aspects of anatomy have been restated as their applications to understanding disease processes and developing treatment plans have assumed more importance. For example, for better understanding of shoulder instability and of what is seen at arthroscopy, the anterior capsule-ligament complex has received close scrutiny. The anterior labrum is essentially the glenoid attachment of the inferior glenohumeral ligament (Fig. 1). The labrum varies greatly in size and shape and may tear in the portion within the joint with or without detachment from the glenoid neck, as occurs when the typical Bankart lesion is produced. The number and positioning of synovial recesses between the capsular ligaments vary. Most commonly there are recesses into the subscapularis bursa above and below the middle glenohumeral ligament; less commonly, there is only a recess above this ligament. Least common are the other variations in the capsular ligaments—one recess below the middle glenohumeral ligament, no recesses, or one large recess with no middle glenohumeral ligament present. A thick band representing the superior edge of the subscapularis often is seen above and anterior to the middle glenohumeral ligament at arthroscopy and can be confused with a glenohumeral ligament.

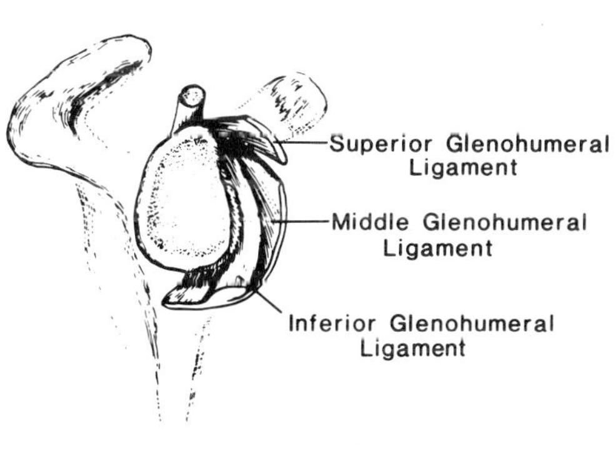

Figure 1

Glenoid attachments of the glenohumeral ligaments. Most of the attachment to the anterior and anterior-inferior regions of the glenoid rim comes from the inferior glenohumeral ligament. (From Matthews, L.S.; Terry, G.; and Vetter, W.L.: Shoulder anatomy for the arthroscopist. Arthroscopy 1:83–91, 1985. By permission of the Arthroscopy Association of North America.)

Shoulder motion and its patterns have been reassessed, as have certain elements of shoulder strength. Men and women have similar ranges of motion except that women have slightly greater arm rotation. Outward rotation is slightly greater on the dominant side. Surprisingly, there is little difference in motion with aging. Younger men have slightly greater flexion and outward rotation but less inward rotation compared with older men. Younger women have slightly greater abduction than older women. Codman's earlier observations of linkage in shoulder movement have been reinforced—medial rotation occurs with shoulder flexion, and lateral rotation occurs with shoulder abduction.

Muscle strength varies between men and women, between young and old, and between the direction of shoulder movements. Men are almost twice as strong as women (Fig. 2). Older people are weaker than younger ones by approximately 10% to 30%. Adductors are stronger than abductors, internal rotators are stronger than external rotators, and flexors may equal or be slightly stronger than extensors.

The 0 position of Saha continues to receive some attention. It is approximately 165° overhead and 45° in front of the coronal plane with the medial epicondyle of the humerus pointing forward and slightly medially. This is defined as the position at which the humeral and scapular axes coincide with the common axis of the surrounding cone of muscles. Over the years it has been used to reduce proximal humeral fractures, displaced epiphyseal injuries, or shoulder dislocations. Currently, some Japanese shoulder surgeons begin rehabilitation in this position with a bivalved cast or shoulder orthosis, and they report reasonable results.

For postoperative rehabilitation, several passive motion machines have been introduced. Early oral reports suggest that these may facilitate rehabilitation, but no published analyses are available. One study of early motion after axillary dissection suggests that more and longer wound drainage occurred and wound complications were more frequent. So the role of early (immediately to less than 2 days) motion for postoperative shoulder rehabilitation with or without the use of machines is not yet clear.

Throwing is a common sport activity. And epidemiologic reviews suggest that about 10% of sport injuries involve the shoulder. So it is natural that some research would be devoted to athletics. These studies detail the motion pattern or patterns of muscle activity. In flat-water kayaking, pushing with the upper extremity farther from the water occurs first by an integrated movement of the

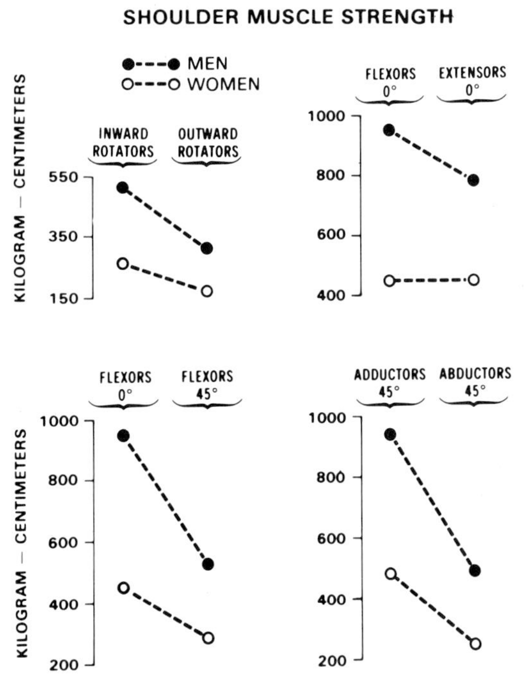

Figure 2

Mean values of maximum isometric torque for men and women generated by antagonistic shoulder muscle groups and by flexors at two joint positions. (From Murray, M.P.; Gore, D.R.; Gardner, G.M.; and Mollinger, L.A. Clin. Orthop. 192:268–273, 1985. By permission of J.B. Lippincott Company.)

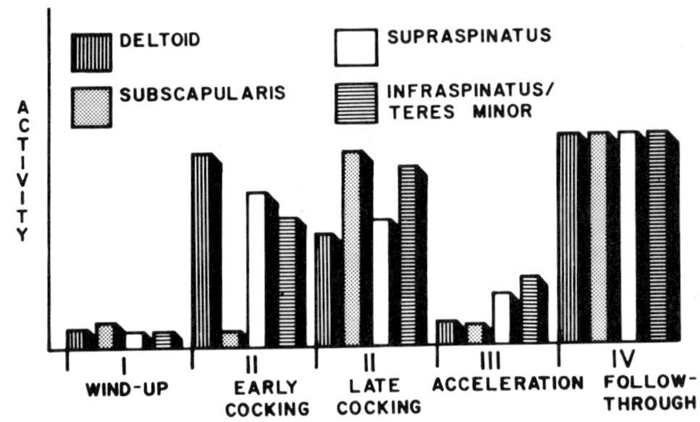

Figure 3

Muscle activity during the stages of a throw or pitch. (From Jobe, F.W.; Tibone, J.E.; Perry, J.; and Moynes, D. Am. J. Sports Med. 11:3–5, 1983. By permission of the American Orthopaedic Society for Sports Medicine.)

thrust wrist and elbow with minimal shoulder movement; this is followed by the pull coming from the extremity near the water and is accomplished by movement of this wrist, elbow, and shoulder and the opposite shoulder of the thrust side. Muscular activity in baseball pitching motions was analyzed by electromyography and high-speed photography. Wind-up had no consistent pattern of muscle use (Fig. 3). In cocking there was sequential activation of the deltoid and the rotator cuff muscles. It was surprising that there was almost no shoulder muscle activity during arm acceleration but most activity in follow-through when all muscles attempted to decelerate the arm.

Some workers, such as shipyard welders and steel plate workers, have a high frequency of shoulder symptoms. Myoelectric activity has been recorded for various work positions with varying hand weights. The degree of arm elevation is the most important variable influencing shoulder muscle load. The rotator cuff muscle activity is most sensitive to change in hand load. Thus, work situations ideally should be designed so that the arm can be kept close to the trunk and hand-held weight can be minimized. Static arm-use activities seem particularly likely to induce early shoulder symptoms.

Two articles have assessed shoulder function after ablative surgical procedures. After neck dissection, patients whose spinal accessory nerve was preserved had less pain and less functional disability and were stronger than those in whom the nerve was sacrificed. After resection of the clavicle for neoplasia, shoulder motion was full and strengths in internal rotation, external rotation, and extension were maintained; however, there was some weakness in shoulder abduction, adduction, and flexion.

Advances in Diagnosis

Plain Radiographs

Attempts continue to find the most efficient and effective ways to obtain radiographs of the injured shoulder. In one review of 172 patient evaluations, the anteroposterior view was almost twice as effective in detecting abnormalities as any other view. The axillary lateral and 60° anterior oblique views were of equal value in assessing dislocations or other injuries. In another series of 48 cases with abnormal findings, two greater tuberosity fractures were only seen on the anteroposterior view in external rotation and four other fractures were only visualized on the anterior oblique projection. It again was stated that the axillary view can be taken in emergency situations with the arm only abducted the width of the x-ray tube. Thus, as before, for shoulder trauma three views are recommended (the trauma series): anteroposterior view in external rotation or a posterior oblique view, anterior oblique view, and axillary view.

Stress radiographs have shown the normal shoulder to be remarkably stable, with mean subluxations of 0.8 mm anterior and 0.2 mm posterior in the awake, relaxed person. Thus, to evaluate shoulder instability fully, a general anesthetic may be necessary. An apical oblique projection (45° posterior oblique with a 45° downward inclination of the x-ray beam) has been suggested to confirm the presence or absence of a dislocation and reveal either intra-articular fractures or Hill-Sachs lesions.

The shoulder impingement syndrome may be suggested by flattening or sclerosis of the greater tuberosity or by bony excrescences arising from the anterior-inferior aspect of the acromion. In plain radiographic evaluation of rotator cuff disease, the subacromial space of 175 normal shoulders was between 9 and 10 mm, and a space of less than 6 mm was considered pathologic.

Arthrography

Arthrography is a mainstay in the diagnosis of shoulder disease including rotator cuff disease, some aspects of shoulder instability, and the frozen shoulder. Single-contrast studies continue to be quite useful. Double-contrast studies can be confusing to read but better outline the synovial lining characteristics, the articular cartilage, and, in certain instances, the size of rotator cuff tears. It has been suggested that the procedure of arthrography is more uncomfortable than previously believed, with up to three-quarters of the patients experiencing at least moderate discomfort within the first day or two afterward.

Pressure measurements made during shoulder arthrography have shown that normal joints initially have low pressures but the pressure increases as the injected volume increases—producing a biphasic pressure-volume curve. When rotator cuff tearing is present, the pressure remains low; but when a frozen shoulder is injected, the pressure increases quickly.

Pneumoarthrography is a consideration when the patient is sensitive to radiographic contrast agents. However, because of the low contrast between air and soft tissues, the exposure must be exact. An alternative for performing contrast arthrography in the patient sensitive to contrast medium is use of premedication, placement of an intravenous line, and having anesthesia personnel present with respiratory support equipment and appropriate medications.

The arthrogram is quite accurate in defining the presence or absence of a rotator cuff tear in a patient who has not undergone operation previously. Many authors have claimed that there is no correlation between the arthrographic findings and the size of the tear found at operation. Others think that, particularly with double-contrast studies with or without tomography, the arthrogram can in a general sense grade the amount of tendon tearing. Strapping weights to the patient's wrist and distracting the joint may enhance visualization of the rotator cuff. When the "geyser sign" is present (dye exiting from the joint through the subacromial bursa into the acromioclavicular joint), a full-thickness, chronic, and generally large rotator cuff tear is present.

In patients with shoulder pain and stiffness—often diagnosed as a frozen shoulder—the arthrogram can confirm this diagnosis and exclude associated rotator cuff tearing or a significant intra-articular synovitis (Fig. 4). A few reports state that joint distention during arthrography or arthrography combined with gentle manipulation has led to quick resolution of symptoms. No doubt this can occur but, during distention of the joint, the dye under pressure usually escapes medially from the subscapularis recess or out the biceps tendon sheath rather than forcefully stretching the main portion of the shoulder capsule and rotator cuff.

Subacromial bursography is of limited clinical usefulness. A normal bursogram may exclude scarring within the bursa, but it does not exclude acute or subacute tendon inflammation. Inability to obtain a bursogram may be due to technical inadequacy or previous bursal wall thickening with fibrosis. Little correlation has been found between bursographic findings and surgical histopathologic findings.

Computed Tomography

Computed tomographic scanning will define muscle atrophy, hypertrophy, or neoplasia. Combined with other imaging modalities, it will give detailed information for planning the surgical approach to a musculoskeletal tumor. Most recently, it has been used to study and to identify lesions in patients with subluxating or dislocating shoulders. As the scans progress from cranial to caudal, the glenoid articular surface twists to face more anteriorly. This is a normal occurrence but may prove to be more pronounced in some patients with shoulder instability. Computed tomography combined with double-contrast arthrography can identify not only glenoid labral tears and Hill-Sachs defects but also capsule enlargement and occult loose bodies.

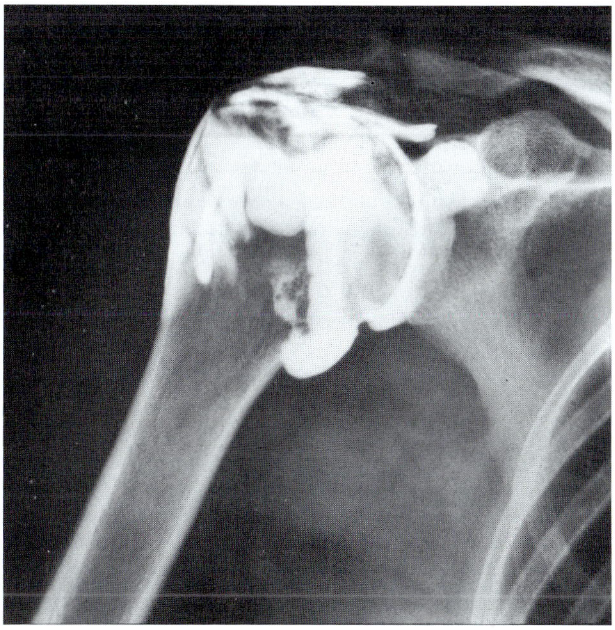

Figure 4

Arthrogram from 55-year-old woman presenting with 6-month history of shoulder pain and stiffness. The motion partially returned with physical therapy but pain persisted. Arthrography demonstrates contraction of joint volume with reduction in the size of synovial recesses and full-thickness tear of the supraspinatus tendon.

Ultrasonography

Ultrasonographic evaluation of the shoulder may be useful in the diagnosis of rotator cuff tearing and to some extent may diminish the need for arthrography. Bones are seen as bright, echogenic contours. Muscles are homogeneously hypoechogenic, and connective tissue septa and joint capsule are linear and highly echogenic. The ultrasound machinery is improving rapidly and the strong operator dependence that has existed is decreasing. Three centers have reported series in which ultrasonographic evaluations were compared with arthrography or surgical pathology. The accuracy of ultrasonography in identifying rotator cuff tearing is between 90% and 95%. The accuracy is less with smaller tears because tissue change within a nontorn tendon can mimic smaller tendon tears. This ability to define changes of tendon texture may prove valuable diagnostically. Ultrasonographic changes indicative of tendon tearing include a discontinuity in the normal homogeneous echogenicity of the cuff, nonvisualization of a segment of cuff, and alteration of the homogeneous cuff echogenicity by a central echogenic band.

Arthroscopy

Arthroscopy of the shoulder is an exciting and dynamic area. The shoulder undoubtedly will be second only to the knee in frequency of use of arthroscopy. The arthroscope can be placed from the front, the top, or the back of the shoulder, but the posterior portal is by far the most useful, allowing observation of almost all of the intra-articular structures with easy manipulation of the arthroscope and little chance of damage to critical neurovascular or other anatomic structures.

Arthroscopy has been used for many diagnostic and a few therapeutic reasons. One can evaluate the rotator cuff with arthroscopy, but a well-made arthrogram usually will suffice. Occasionally, it is helpful for determining the extent of arthritic involvement when a diagnosis is known or to obtain a synovial biopsy when the diagnosis of the type of arthritis is unknown. In acute septic arthritis, arthroscopy will allow thorough irrigation of the joint and accurate placement of drainage tubes. The frozen shoulder has been studied by arthroscopy. Some have recognized a contracted joint volume only, others have seen intra-articular adhesions, and still others have identified an active synovitis. Perhaps these are different stages of the process, but probably differences in problems can lead to the combination of shoulder pain and stiffness. It might be reasonable, if the diagnosis of frozen shoulder is in question, to obtain an arthrogram. If the arthrogram shows smooth synovium and a contracted joint volume, it is not necessary to investigate further. However, if the arthrogram reveals a significant synovitis, arthroscopy should be considered for synovial biopsy for diagnosis.

Arthroscopy seems to be most useful for the shoulder with instability. If the case is atypical and the history, physical examination, and radiographs are not clear in establishing the diagnosis, examination of both shoulders under anesthesia and arthroscopy of the involved shoulder will allow a complete assessment of joint laxity and visual identification of a Bankart or Hill-Sachs lesion. Some patients with recurrent subluxations or dislocations and a few without symptomatic instability complain primarily of locking and catching in the joint. In this case, a glenoid labrum tear with a flap into the joint can be identified with arthroscopy, and the flap can be removed.

Loose bodies can be removed through the arthroscope, and occasionally a synovectomy can be accomplished expeditiously through the arthroscope rather than by an open procedure. Developing techniques include stapling Bankart-type lesions with arthroscopic control, debriding inner surfaces of rotator cuff tears, and performing arthroscopic anterior acromioplasty; the value of these is uncertain.

Rotator Cuff Disease

Impingement Syndrome

Anterior acromioplasty (Fig. 5) was introduced as a method of treatment for the chronic impingement syndrome in the shoulder in 1972. It is clinically useful to consider lesions in three progressive stages (Table 1). In stage I, edema and hemorrhage, treatment is conservative and the prognosis for recovery is good. In stage II, repeated inflammation has led to bursal thickening with fibrosis in addition to recurrent tendinitis. If arthrography is negative and symptoms persist after ample conservative treatment for longer than 18 months, removal of the thickened bursa, division of the coracoacromial ligament, and possibly acromioplasty are considered. In stage III there is incomplete or complete tearing of the rotator cuff. Also, tearing of the biceps tendon may be present and bony changes will be seen on the anterior acromion and greater humeral tuberosity. Anterior acromioplasty is done for these patients when the rotator cuff is repaired. The distal clavicle is excised when there is arthritis and symptoms or when osteophytic enlargement of the joint with impingement on the supraspinatus tendon is present. These acromioclavicular changes are seen in approximately 50% of patients with rotator cuff tearing.

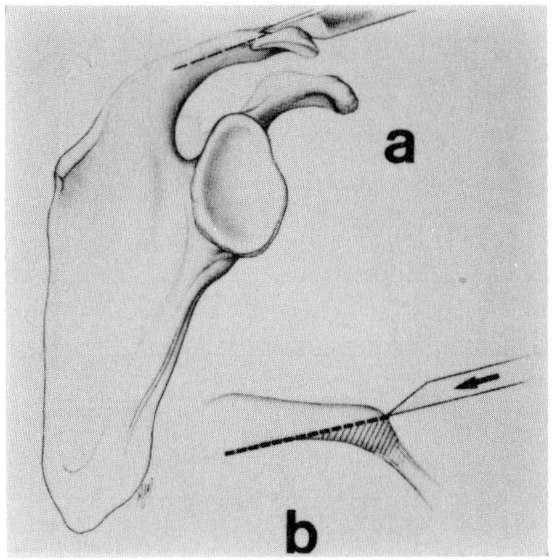

Figure 5
The technique of anterior acromioplasty. The objective is to produce a flat undersurface, *b*. (From Neer, C.S., II. Clin. Orthop. 173:70–77, 1983. By permission of J.B. Lippincott Company.)

In the absence of rotator cuff tearing, nonoperative treatment is undertaken for all patients with the impingement syndrome. The mainstays are rest or activity modifications, anti-inflammatory medications, gentle stretching and strengthening exercises, and occasional steroid injections. Some believe that it is necessary to isolate the individual rotator cuff muscles as much as possible to diagnose specific muscle weakness and to plan a specific rehabilitation program. Local steroid injections do diminish pain but also impair tissue metabolism. Injecting the subacromial-subdeltoid bursa in impingement lesions is more frequently successful than injection of trigger (or tender) points. Dimethyl sulfoxide, acupuncture, pulsed electromagnetic field therapy, and magnetic necklaces have been used for treatment of shoulder pain, but controlled studies suggest that little benefit was obtained.

Surgical treatment for the impingement syndrome (without rotator cuff tearing) has varied between coracoacromial ligament division and more complex procedures, often including many operative steps such as anterior acromioplasty, acromioclavicular arthroplasty, and biceps tendon tenodesis. It is disappointing that many of the reported series include patients with symptoms of only a few months'

Table 1. Neer's Classification of Impingement Syndrome

	Stage I: Edema and hemorrhage	Stage II: Fibrosis and tendinitis	Stage III: Bone spurs and tendon rupture
Typical age	<25 yr	25–40 yr	>40 yr
Differential diagnosis	Subluxation AC arthritis	Frozen shoulder Calcification	Cervical radiculitis Neoplasm
Clinical course	Reversible	Pain recurs with activity	Progressive disability
Treatment	Conservative	Consider bursectomy, division of C/A ligament	Anterior acromioplasty, rotator cuff repair

duration, and seldom are the operative pathologic or histopathologic findings reported in detail. Follow-up of these procedures is often short-term or intermediate in length. With these limitations, it is encouraging to note that pain relief is satisfactory in more than 90%. Limitation of motion or strength seldom is a problem before operation or afterward.

The results of surgical treatment for impingement in competitive athletes is unknown. Athletes usually will experience relief, or at least reduction, of their pain. However, athletes who are required to use their treated arm for skilled overhead throwing-like activities—such as pitching, serving in tennis, or swimming—often fail to regain previous levels of competitive ability. Over the next years, some of the uncertainties as to which athletes will benefit and how frequently performance will be improved by surgical treatment will be resolved.

For now it seems prudent to evaluate the patient to be sure that the signs and symptoms are consistent on repeated evaluations, to undertake a prolonged period of nonoperative treatment as suggested by the originator of the concept, and, only after this, to consider the operative alternatives. These alternatives will include removal of abnormal bursal tissue, coracoacromial ligament excision, and probably anterior acromioplasty. Excision of the distal clavicle should in all probability be done only when symptomatic synovitis or arthritis with osteophytic changes exists there. In the absence of a visible disease process, biceps tendon tenodesis may not be necessary at all. Reported results do not differ much from series to series, regardless of the extent of the procedure.

Rotator Cuff Tears

New material has been published on repair techniques for torn rotator cuffs. It is a practical possibility to approach the supraspinatus fossa from an anterior-superior exposure and to eliminate the need for the acromion osteotomy in the frontal plane suggested earlier by Debeyre. All rotator cuff tears are represented by five basic shapes, and the method of repair is based on the shape and size of the tear. Longitudinal tears are sewn tendon to tendon. Transverse tears are sewn tendon to bone. The most common tear includes both longitudinal and transverse components and requires sewing both tendon to tendon and tendon to bone. Large or massive tears with tissue deficiency have triangular or trapezoidal shapes and require a V-Y (MacLaughlin) repair or cranial transposition of adjacent subscapularis or infraspinatus tendons for repair. The use of staples for cuff repair has fallen from favor. Usually they must be removed, and results are less favorable than with suture repair. In one group of patients who had placement of human cadaver grafts as a supplement to their rotator cuff repair, pain relief was satisfactory and motion was maintained or slightly improved. This experience has not been confirmed in other clinical studies. Prosthetic grafting for tendon repair is presented in the literature only in an anecdotal way.

The results of surgical repair of the rotator cuff are better when the repair is accompanied by adequate decompression of the subacromial space. Pain relief is reasonably good (85% to 95%) despite the size of the repair. Return of strength relates to extent of tendon tearing, degeneration, and tissue scarring. The larger and more extensive the tear, the weaker the patients are postoperatively and the less motion they obtain. Preoperative deltoid weakness compromises the postoperative result. Chronic rotator cuff tears associated with an earlier shoulder dislocation have a poorer prognosis.

The timing and extent of postoperative physical therapy vary among reported series. The trend is for early passive movement within the limits of maintenance of the repair as determined at operation. Active movement is started when early tissue healing has occurred—usually at 4 to 6 weeks. The use of postoperative support continues to vary, and perhaps it should. Some repairs undoubtedly require more support than others.

Repeat repair of the rotator cuff is fraught with difficulty. Diagnosis may be difficult, and arthrography is confusing when surgical scarring is present. Certainly, massive tears are the ones most prone to failure, and repair of these tears is not easy at any time. If continuing pain seems to be due to continuing impingement, subacromial decompression may be helpful. If symptoms are related to recurrent tendon tearing, the potential for a satisfactory outcome is less favorable. Pain may be diminished in the majority who have a reoperation, but seldom is it eliminated. Gaining more strength and active motion is not likely. The importance of adequate initial repair is emphasized.

Cuff Tear Arthropathy

Occasionally, massive rotator cuff tears and non-rheumatoid shoulder arthritis coexist (Fig. 6 *Left*). When arthritis (loss of glenohumeral cartilage) occurs in association with massive rotator cuff tearing, there is usually a long history of preceding shoulder symptoms suggesting chronic tendon disease and also that the tendon involvement preceded the cartilage loss. In addition to the tendon and cartilage changes, bone loss in the humeral head, glenoid, and acromion is commonly a part of this cuff tear-associated shoulder arthritis. Both nutritional and mechanical factors

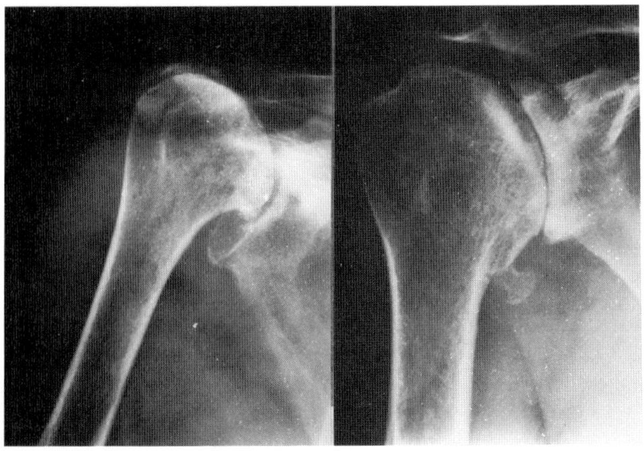

Figure 6

Left, Typical radiographic appearance of cuff tear arthropathy. Note upward subluxation of humeral head, loss of glenohumeral cartilage, and alterations of bony contour of glenoid, humeral head, and acromion. *Right,* Osteoarthritis of the shoulder has characteristic appearance, markedly different from that of cuff tear arthropathy. Central portion of humeral head is flattened with subchondral sclerosis, peripheral osteophyte formation, and joint space narrowing. On the anteroposterior view, humeral head is well centered in the glenoid.

have been identified as contributing to the development and progression of this problem. The term "cuff tear arthropathy" has been selected to best describe it.

In 1981 a syndrome with a similar clinical and radiographic presentation called the "Milwaukee shoulder" was reported. It included large rotator cuff defects, glenohumeral joint degeneration, and joint effusions containing few leukocytes, basic calcium phosphate crystals, particulate collagen of types I, II, and III, and collagenase and neutral protease activities. Recently, similar findings in knee joints have been reported, and a possible pathogenetic mechanism has been formulated. This theory espouses the importance of the crystals in leading to the destructive multitissue changes.

Cuff tear arthropathy and the "Milwaukee shoulder" may be the same or could represent two pathways to this end—a composite of severe tendon, cartilage, capsular, and bone disease. In any event, these extensive changes are difficult to treat. Currently, the preferred method is resurfacing total shoulder arthroplasty, rotator cuff reconstruction, and limited-goals rehabilitation. This syndrome, or these syndromes, is distinctly different from osteoarthritis of the shoulder. In osteoarthritis, the radiologic and pathologic changes are stereotypic and seldom include substantial rotator cuff disease (Fig. 6 *Right*).

Associated Suprascapular Neuropathy

In patients with shoulder pain and weakness with loss of active motion, there may be a suprascapular neuropathy or proximal brachial plexopathy coexistent with the rotator cuff disease. Together these lesions may make diagnosis difficult, especially after acute injury. In this setting, both arthrography and electromyography may be useful to define the problem. Nerve recovery is most rapid over the first 5 to 6 months but may or may not be complete. If a rotator cuff tear occurred or there was a substantial acute extension at the time of injury, waiting for neural recovery before repairing the tendons quite likely will have an adverse effect on the final outcome. Thus, early tendon repair is being considered more carefully when this combination of tendon and nerve injury coexists.

Calcific Tendinitis

Symptomatic calcific deposits in the rotator cuff formerly were common but they may be less frequent now. The classic hypothesis is that the tissues become avascular and necrotic, and secondarily there is a deposition of calcified material. A more recent idea suggests that the tendon may undergo cartilage metaplasia followed by an active cell-mediated calcification. On scanning electron microscopy, the deposits are extremely heterogeneous, and the crystals are larger than the typical apatite crystals—perhaps representing a calcium carbonate apatite.

Clinically, the patients are middle-aged—typically, younger than those with rotator cuff tears. In a recent series of patients, two-thirds were women. It is uncertain how often the symptoms will disappear spontaneously. It has been stated that, when a "fluffy" deposit is seen on the radiograph associated with an acute flare of pain, the frequency of remission is higher. This is proposed because active resorptive changes can be seen histologically in this type of deposit. Aspiration of the calcific material may be attempted, often with radiographic control of needle position. Irrigation of the deposit with saline containing a local anesthetic has been successful in relieving symptoms. However, the procedure itself may be quite painful. Before surgical removal is considered, other conditions that cause shoulder symptoms should be considered. However, after surgical removal, almost all patients will achieve relief of pain. Recovery from the operation may require 2 to 6 months.

Frozen Shoulder

Little attention has been focused on this problem in North America, despite its prevalence. The syndrome and its treatment are becoming better defined. Certain groups are more prone to develop this problem, including females, persons age 45 to 60 years, and patients with cardiac or cerebrovascular disease, thyroid dysfunction, or diabetes mellitus. It is a frequent problem after neurosurgical procedures; after mastectomy it is much less common than it once was. Personality may play a role. This entity has been attributed to an inflammation of the rotator cuff. More recently, it was proposed that this is an immune system-mediated response of the cuff tendon to an area of tendon necrosis. Decreased IgA and an increased incidence of HLA-B27 have been found in patients with a frozen shoulder. However, other investigators, and later the original investigators, have been unable to confirm the earlier findings. Other immunologic studies—immune complex levels, C-reactive protein, and altered lymphocyte transformations—may give temporarily abnormal results in some of these patients.

Arthrography characteristically will show the diminished capsular volume with diminution in size or elimination of the capsular recesses (Fig. 4). It will exclude an associated rotator cuff tear or an active proliferative synovitis. A technetium-99m bone scan will show increased uptake but is probably not useful or practical for following patients. The natural history is poorly documented. Earlier studies found either recovery within 2 years or continuing symptoms with some stiffness persisting after 3 or 6 years. In a recent study of 40 patients followed 40 to 48 months, mild and insignificant motion restriction remained in 11 but severe restriction (greater than 25% of movement) continued in 5. Between 10% and 20% develop this syndrome in the opposite shoulder.

Various anti-inflammatory medications have been compared for treatment of the frozen shoulder, and all had about the same efficacy in diminishing pain. Of course, they do little to change loss of movement. Transcutaneous electrical nerve stimulators and gentle prolonged traction may be useful adjuncts to the typical gentle physiotherapy mobilization program. Steroid injection may reduce pain early in the course but in general is less effective than in other aspects of rotator cuff disease.

A report in the *Journal of Traditional Chinese Medicine* described far superior results with a gradual stretching of the shoulder (84% complete recovery) compared with sudden tearing by force under brachial plexus block anesthesia (18% complete recovery). Investigators in West Germany used *brisement modéré*—a well-controlled application of force under general anesthesia—in 120 patients. Two patients had hemorrhagic effusion and two had large hematomas; there were no other complications. At a mean follow-up of 14 months for 81 shoulders, 75 had a good range of abduction, 61 a good range of internal rotation, and 54 a good range of external rotation. In Manchester, 78 frozen shoulders were treated with manipulation and local steroid injection; 83% had a full range of movement without pain within 8 weeks. Two acute dislocations occurred but neither became recurrent.

Operative treatment is almost never recommended. For the very unusual patient with prolonged shoulder stiffness, anterior and inferior capsular releases have been described. In 1981, surprisingly consistent success was reported in 20 shoulders with inferior shoulder capsule denervation. It is difficult to evaluate such a procedure when the natural course in the majority of patients is self-resolution.

In summary, the immune system may play a role in the development or perpetuation of the frozen shoulder. Rotator cuff tendon pathology is common, if not universally present. Arthrography can exclude rotator cuff tearing or an intra-articular hypertrophic synovitis. Conservative methods of treatment are the mainstay, and complete or nearly complete recovery is usually achieved. Manipulation is not necessary but may shorten the recovery period. Operative treatment is seldom necessary.

Arthritis

Acromioclavicular Joint

Degeneration of the acromioclavicular joint seems to be related to aging, with intra-articular disk degeneration preceding cartilaginous changes. The changes are more pronounced on the clavicular side of the joint. Distally pointing osteophytes that could be associated with rotator cuff impingement occur in approximately a quarter of those with more advanced joint degeneration. In a study of cadavers, the extent of degeneration was essentially equal bilaterally but in a radiographic study the arthrosis was more common on the right side. In a study of 620 joints, clinical symptoms became more frequent with increasing age, in general paralleling the radiographic progression of arthritis; however, many joints that displayed radiographic changes were not painful.

Osteolysis of the distal clavicle after trauma was described over 50 years ago and is now recognized to occur after certain stressful repetitive activities such as weight lifting. It may be associated with swelling about the joint; synovial hyperplasia appears to play an integral part in the resorptive process. Demineralization of the subchondral cortex of the distal clavicle may occur weeks to several years after a traumatic event.

Resection of the clavicle distal to the coracoclavicular ligaments is recognized to be successful in eliminating pain in patients with symptomatic degenerative joint disease of the acromioclavicular joint or continuing symptoms associated with clavicular osteolysis. In a review of 50 patients who had resection of the distal clavicle, poor results were found in 13 (25%) of the 51 shoulders. The initial results did not seem to change with time. There was no correlation between clinical results and radiographic appearance of new bone formation at the resection site. Nearly half of those with poor results had a history of psychiatric or alcoholic problems. Careful patient selection is essential.

Glenohumeral Joint

Radiographically, in rheumatoid arthritis of the shoulder, gross destruction is rare and progression of the disease is often sporadic and slow. Although the natural course is not predetermined in time, progression of the radiographic abnormalities is similar in many patients. These changes include osteoporosis, erosions at the superolateral part of the anatomic neck of the humerus, superior subluxation of the humeral head, cystic changes in the central and posterior aspect of the humeral head, and joint space narrowing. Cadaver and radiologic studies relate severity of change in osteoarthritis to increasing age, with equal frequencies of change in men and women and in right and left shoulders. Many patients with the radiographic changes of osteoarthritis are asymptomatic or have only mild symptoms. In osteoarthritis, osteophytes are located at the margin of the articular surface of the humeral head with greater involvement of the anterior and inferior aspects (Fig. 6 *Right*). Subchondral sclerosis is most evident in the middle and superior parts of the humeral head. Bony erosion predominates in the posterior-central part of the glenoid and superior anterior-central part of the humeral head.

Pigmented villonodular synovitis of the shoulder is rare. The radiographic appearance includes subchondral bone cysts and a relative lack of hypertrophic bone. On arthrography there is a hypertrophic synovitis with lobulated filling defects.

Polymyalgia rheumatica is a common disease of the elderly, and symmetric shoulder synovitis is common. The presenting complaints are aching and stiffness of the shoulder and pelvic girdles, malaise, and anorexia with some weight loss. Physical examination may reveal only minor limitation of motion with pain at the extremes. The radiographs usually are normal. Relevant laboratory findings include a markedly increased erythrocyte sedimentation rate, anemia, increased levels of immune complexes in the circulation, and, occasionally, abnormal results of liver function tests, especially increased alkaline phosphatase. This disease may be associated with temporal arteritis.

Shoulder joints are affected in 30% to 50% of patients with Lyme arthritis. In this disease, caused by a spirochete transmitted by a tick, there is a rash followed by an acute, migratory, arthritis of large joints. Joint involvement may become chronic and be similar in many ways to rheumatoid arthritis. Early administration of penicillin may prevent or minimize the arthritic involvement.

Pseudothrombosis—acute rupture of the capsule of the knee joint resembling deep calf vein thrombosis—has been well described. In a reported case, edema of the arm, resembling vascular obstruction, suddenly developed in a patient with rheumatoid arthritis. An arthrogram outlined the capsular distention and rupture. Swelling subsided with elevation of the limb. In another case, a massive synovial cyst of the shoulder with distal dissection and secondary ischemic necrosis of the biceps muscle developed in a 47-year-old man with paraplegia and loss of pain and temperature sensation in the arm.

Chronic repetitive trauma has been suggested as a cause of degenerative joint disease. Six cases of severe degenerative arthritis in tenacious, well-motivated amateur athletes were described; their histories suggested that repetitive trauma was the most important factor causing their arthropathy. Another article described 74 shoulders with a history of single or multiple dislocations and radiographic evidence of glenohumeral arthritis; neither the number of dislocations nor glenoid or humeral head defects were related to the severity of the arthritis. Shoulders with posterior dislocations and a delay in reduction or surgically treated shoulders in which metallic devices intrude into the joint frequently are involved by moderate or severe arthritis.

Reconstructive Surgery

Glenoidectomy had been advocated as a form of treatment for the significantly symptomatic rheumatoid shoulder. Reports on operation have been limited, and no new information has become available. The operation can no longer be advocated on the basis of its being a minor procedure because excision of the glenoid is not correctable if the result proves to be unfavorable.

Synovectomy and joint debridement is another option for the rheumatoid patient but is not commonly used. The only substantial report recently is from Norway: synovectomies were done in 29 shoulders, of which 24 had advanced intra-articular disease. Postoperatively, 19 patients had no pain and 7 had decreased pain. Range of motion did not change. In a patient with significant, continuing shoulder symptoms this option certainly should be considered; however, most of these patients also have joint surface destruction. This combination of active synovitis and cartilage loss suggests to most North American surgeons the need not only for synovectomy but also for prosthetic replacement of the destroyed surfaces, and the current literature reflects this feeling.

Ten years ago there were many designs of total shoulder replacement available. Now there are only a few, and almost all are relatively unconstrained, surface-replacement types of implants. In 1982, a decade of experience (in 273 shoulders) with an implant system of this type was reported: 194 shoulders could be fully evaluated at 24 to 99 months postoperatively; 150 of these patients were in a full exercise program and 129 (86%) obtained an excellent or satisfactory result. Those not in the full postoperative therapy program had a massive deficiency of bone or muscle and received rehabilitation with the idea of achieving somewhat limited goals: stability, 90° of elevation, 20° of external rotation. Of the 44 shoulders in this subclassification, 42 met these goals. There were 24 complications in the entire series, including 6 patients with instability and 5 with rotator cuff tears; 12 patients required a reoperation. No patient had symptomatic glenoid loosening. Radiolucent lines were present at the glenoid bone-cement interface in 30% of the shoulders. Overall, only four patients thought that they had not benefited from the procedure. In addition, this report emphasized the difficulty of the procedure, in part because of the variability in the involvement encountered. Much of the operative time is spent working with the soft tissues—protecting musculotendinous units, releasing contractures, and re-creating the delicate balance of mobility and stability of the shoulder. To achieve this stability, component version on bone (Fig. 7) and length in bone (Fig. 8) must mimic normal anatomy as closely as possible.

A series in which the unconstrained implant system was used in 73 patients for rheumatoid arthritis, osteoarthritis, or arthritis secondary to trauma has been reported. At 2 to 6½ years postoperatively, pain relief was satisfactory in 92%. Active abduction improved by a mean of 44°, to mean of 141° in osteoarthritis, 103° in rheumatoid arthritis, and 109° in traumatic arthritis. Complications developed in 13 shoulders, including rotator cuff tearing in 5 and symptomatic glenoid loosening in 3; reoperations were necessary in 5 patients. Five other glenoid components showed radiographic evidence of loosening, and 52 of the remaining 65 shoulders had some radiolucency at the glenoid bone-cement junction. Overall, 92% of the patients thought that they had benefited from the procedure.

Additional information was obtained from these two articles about the status of the rotator cuff in those who need total shoulder arthroplasty. Almost without exception the rotator cuff was intact in patients with osteoarthritis; it was thin in most patients with rheumatoid arthritis but actually torn in only about a third; in traumatic arthritis, bony deformities were present and tuberosity osteotomy and repositioning of the rotator cuff insertions were needed. This information coupled with the knowledge that approxi-

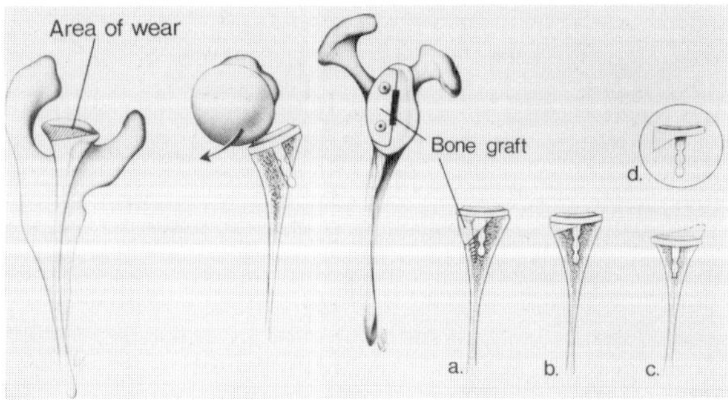

Figure 7

In patients who require total shoulder arthroplasty, the glenoid may be eroded unevenly. If the component is inserted without accounting for this, the shoulder may be unstable. Lesser amounts of erosion may be dealt with by filling the defect with bone cement (*b*) or grinding down the high side (*c*). A component with asymmetric thickness is available (*d*). For moderate to severe erosions, bone grafting of the glenoid before placing the component (*a*) is suggested as the best choice. (From Neer, C.S., II; Watson, K.C.; and Stanton, F.J. J. Bone Joint Surg. 64A:319–337, 1982. By permission of the journal.)

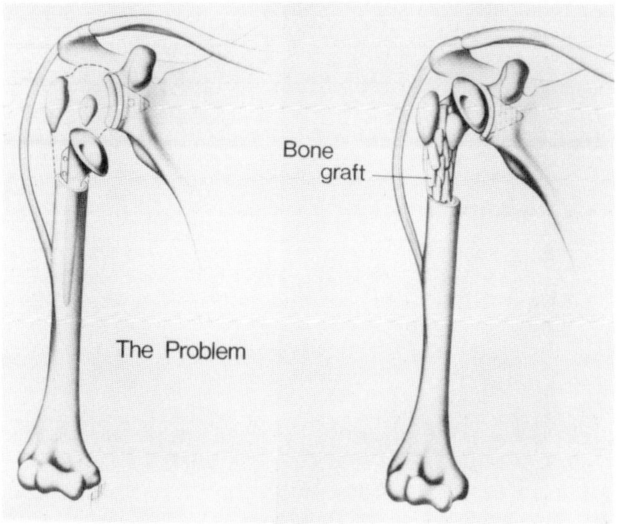

Figure 8

Excessive humeral shortening causes inferior subluxation with instability and relatively lengthens the deltoid, causing excessive weakness. To avoid these difficulties, the humeral component must be cemented to restore arm length. Bone graft fills the defect so that the tuberosities and rotator cuff can regain attachment to the humeral shaft. (From Neer, C.S., II; Watson, K.C.; and Stanton, F.J. J. Bone Joint Surg. 64A:319–337, 1982. By permission of the journal.)

mately half of the early constrained total shoulder designs failed by 2 years has turned interest toward the resurfacing total shoulder designs. However, a few patients with severe shoulder arthritis do have massive cuff deficiencies and may be considered potential candidates for a more constrained type of implant. A review, with longer follow-up, of experience with a modified, constrained, ball-in-socket type of implant system has recently been presented. In 78 patients followed for a mean of 46.5 months (range, 2 to 77 months), pain relief was noted in 67 (96%) of 70 shoulders analyzed. There were eight dislocations, two infections, one humeral loosening, three glenoid loosenings, and two broken glenoid screws; these necessitated 14 reoperations. For all patients, 50% had a radiolucency about the humeral stem, and 30% had a radiolucency about the glenoid screws and central post. The developer of this implant believed this type of prosthesis to be useful but seldom necessary and suggested that other, less extensive, shoulder reconstructions should be considered before this one is implanted.

A report from Belgium has appeared on an "isoelastic" (elasticity approximately equal to that of bone) plastic shoulder prosthesis. In 25 shoulders with a mean follow-up of 3 years, the result was excellent or good in 5 as scored by the physician. The patient thought the result was excellent or good in 18 of the shoulders. When the rotator cuff was repaired, active abduction averaged 106°; when no repair was done, it averaged 44°. There were three shoulders with subluxation, two with dislocation, two with infection, and three with loosening of the prosthesis.

Nothing has appeared recently in the literature about the use of a prosthesis for the proximal humerus without a glenoid component in patients with shoulder arthritis. In patients with chronic problems resulting from old fractures or fracture-dislocations of the proximal humerus and a reasonably well-preserved glenoid surface, approximately 90% can achieve satisfactory pain relief after placement of a proximal humeral prosthesis with tuberosity repositioning as necessary. Motion postoperatively is quite variable, depending on many factors including the degree of damage to the rotator cuff and capsule at the time of injury and the extent of scar formation. In one series of 28 shoulders, mean postoperative active abduction was 112° but ranged from less than 60° to 180°. Complications included rotator cuff mechanism stretching or tearing in nine shoulders. It was apparent that many problems would have been avoided if the operation had been done earlier—at the time of treatment of the fracture.

Reconstructive shoulder surgery after a failed shoulder arthroplasty is extremely difficult. In 40 humeral head and total shoulder arthroplasties requiring major revision, there was more than one factor contributing to the failure in almost every case. Prominent among the causes of failure were dense scar formation throughout the muscle planes, radical acromioplasty and other causes of deltoid weakness, a tight subscapularis, rotator cuff tearing and notably the loss of the external rotators in fixed-fulcrum implants, a prominent or retracted tuberosity, mechanical failure in fixed-fulcrum implants, loss of humeral length, uneven wear or central erosion of the glenoid, and infection. When infection occurs, the implant and cement are removed. If, after 1 year or more, the patient is dissatisfied, shoulder fusion is considered. In many of the other patients, an unconstrained total shoulder arthroplasty was done; the results of these revisions are not as favorable as those for other diagnostic categories.

Shoulder arthrodesis has a number of indications including paralysis of the rotator cuff and deltoid, shoulder sepsis with cartilage loss, unsuccessful operations for massive rotator cuff tears, and, occasionally, failed shoulder prosthesis. At arthrodesis the arm is positioned closer to the side than was formerly recommended. Abduction of 20° to 30°, forward flexion of 30°, and internal rotation of 45° to 50° are suggested. There are many alternatives in the surgical technique of arthrodesis, including internal fixation with a plate or plates and screws. A recent article reemphasized the value of external compression arthrodesis. In 16 shoulders treated by Charnley's original method, fusion was obtained in 15.

Infections

The diagnosis of infection about the shoulder may be difficult because it often occurs in association with other shoulder disease. Infection problems now usually are presented as case reports. Percutaneous catheter drainage of a septic shoulder joint has been successfully accomplished. Arthroscopy also may be useful in diagnosis and treatment of acute septic arthritis: excellent specimens for culture can be obtained, the joint can be thoroughly irrigated, and, if desired, drainage tubes can be placed. A case report described a young man who presented with septicemia and died; autopsy revealed a *Staphylococcus aureus* subscapular abscess and there was a history of a recent contusion to that area. In another reported case, an elderly man with tuberculosis was presented, emphasizing the difficulty in diagnosis and suggesting aspiration with arthrography as an important diagnostic step. A report from Hong Kong described five patients with tuberculosis who were treated with chemotherapy alone; all five became pain free and the sinuses healed.

Annotated Bibliography

Related Research

Herberts, P.; Kadefors, R.; Högfors, C.; and Sigholm, G.: Shoulder pain and heavy manual labor. Clin. Orthop. 191:166–178, 1984.

Elevation of the arm and use of hand tools of excessive mass causes intense electromyographic activity in shoulder muscles, especially the spinati. In certain work environments, symptoms from musculotendinous units are common, and static work seems to induce symptoms earlier.

Jobe, F.W.; Tibone, J.E.; Perry, J., and Moynes, D.: An EMG analysis of the shoulder in throwing and pitching: A preliminary report. Am. J. Sports Med. 11:3–5, 1983.

Wind-up has no consistent pattern of electromyographic activity. Cocking has a sequence of muscle activity—first the deltoid, then the supraspinatus, infraspinatus, and teres minor, and, finally, the subscapularis. In acceleration, there was little muscle activity; follow-through was the most active stage with all muscles active in attempting to decelerate the arm.

Murray, M.P.; Gore, D.R.; Gardner, G.M.; and Mollinger, L.A.: Shoulder motion and muscle strength of normal men and women in two age groups. Clin. Orthop. 192:268–273, 1985.

Shoulder motion was similar for men and women and for younger and older age groups. Women were weaker than men, and older subjects were weaker than younger subjects.

Advances in Diagnosis

Cofield, R.H.: Arthroscopy of the shoulder. Mayo Clin. Proc. 58:501–508, 1983.

In 74 arthroscopic examinations for various shoulder diseases, arthroscopy was an important diagnostic tool in the investigation of certain patients (32%), was optional for others (45%), and, in retrospect, was unnecessary in some patients (23%) in several diagnostic categories.

Mack, L.A.; Matsen, F.A., III; Kilcoyne, R.F.; Davies, P.K.; and Sickler, M.E.: US evaluation of the rotator cuff. Radiology 157:205–209, 1985.

In 79 patients, ultrasonography findings were correlated with arthrography or operative findings. Overall accuracy was 94%. There was less reliability with smaller tendon tears.

McGlynn, F.J., and Caspari, R.B.: Arthroscopic findings in the subluxating shoulder. Clin. Orthop. 183:173–178, 1984.

Arthroscopy is an accurate method for confirming this diagnosis. Glenoid labrum tears, Hill-Sachs defects, and increased humeral head translocations were identified.

Petersson, C.J., and Redlund-Johnell, I.: The subacromial space in normal shoulder radiographs. Acta Orthop. Scand. 55:57–58, 1984.

The normal mean subacromial space was 9.7 ± 1.5 mm in men and 9.2 ± 1.4 mm in women. An acromion-humeral head interval of less than 6 mm is pathologic.

Rotator Cuff Disease

Cofield, R.H., and Lanzer, W.L.: Rotator cuff repair, results related to surgical pathology (abstract). Orthop. Trans. 9:466, 1985.

Patients who require rotator cuff repair have a spectrum of tendon tear size, ranging from small to massive, and have five tendon tear shapes: longitudinal, transverse, longitudinal and transverse, triangular, and trapezoidal. The tear size and shape dictate the method of repair.

DeOrio, J.K., and Cofield, R.H.: Results of a second attempt at surgical repair of a failed initial rotator-cuff repair. J. Bone Joint Surg. 66A:563–567, 1984.

In 27 patients undergoing a second attempt at rotator cuff repair, 76% experienced a substantial diminution of their pain, but there was little change in the amount of active motion or strength.

Ha'eri, G.B., and Wiley, A.M.: Advancement of the supraspinatus muscle in the repair of ruptures of the rotator cuff. J. Bone Joint Surg. 63A:232–238, 1981.

The supraspinatus fossa may be exposed from an anterior-superior approach. When this surgical method was used, 77% of 18 patients had satisfactory results.

Haines, J.F., and Hargadon, E.J.: Manipulation as the primary treatment of the frozen shoulder. J. R. Coll. Surg. Edinb. 27:271–275, 1982.

Of 78 patients treated, 83% had a full range of pain-free motion within 2 months after manipulation.

Halverson, P.B.; McCarty, D.J.; Cheung, H.S.; and Ryan, L.M.: Milwaukee shoulder syndrome: Eleven additional cases with involvement of the knee in seven (basic calcium phosphate crystal deposition disease). Semin. Arthritis Rheum. 14:36–44, 1984.

Since the authors' initial reports in 1981, additional cases have been seen. The pathogenetic mechanism is postulated: basic calcium phosphate crystals are phagocytized by synovial cells, collagenase and neutral protease are released, and these enzymes "strip-mine" additional crystals and particulate collagen, which damages articular tissues and the rotator cuff.

Johansson, J.E., and Barrington, T.W.: Coracoacromial ligament division. Am. J. Sports Med. 12:138–141, 1984.

The coracoacromial ligament was divided in 41 shoulders of patients who experienced the painful arc syndrome. Preoperative duration of symptoms averaged 7 months (range, 2–24 months). At follow-up (8–76 months), 95% were judged to have had a satisfactory outcome.

Mudge, M.K.; Wood, V.E.; and Frykman, G.K.: Rotator cuff tears associated with os acromiale. J. Bone Joint Surg. 66A:427–429, 1984.

As pointed out by Neer, an ununited acromial ossification center may contribute to rotator cuff impingement and subsequent tendon tearing.

Neer, C.S., II: Impingement lesions. Clin. Orthop. 173:70–77, 1983.

Additional experience by the developer of the concept. There are three stages: 1) edema and hemorrhage, 2) fibrosis and tendinitis, and 3) tears, biceps ruptures, bone changes. The impingement "sign" and "test" are helpful in diagnosis. Acromioplasty is considered in the absence of rotator cuff tearing when disability persists for 1 year or longer.

Neer, C.S., II; Craig, E.V.; and Fukuda, H.: Cuff-tear arthropathy. J. Bone Joint Surg. 65A:1232–1244, 1983.

In association with a massive rotator cuff tear, 26 patients had loss of glenohumeral cartilage and destruction of subchondral bone. These changes seem to result from both nutritional and mechanical factors. Treatment is extremely difficult.

Neviaser, T.J.; Neviaser, R.J.; Neviaser, J.S.; and Neviaser, J.S.: The four-in-one arthroplasty for the painful arc syndrome. Clin. Orthop. 163:107–112, 1982.

Eighty-nine patients had coracoacromial ligament excision, acromioclavicular arthroplasty, anterior-inferior acromioplasty, and tenodesis of the biceps tendon. At 2 to 8 years, all patients had pain relief, and motion was improved in 81%.

Packer, N.P.; Calvert, P.T.; Bayley, J.I.L.; and Kessel, L.: Operative treatment of chronic ruptures of the rotator cuff of the shoulder. J. Bone Joint Surg. 65B:171–175, 1983.

Sixty-three repairs were done; 40 patients had good relief of pain. Results were better when subacromial decompression also was done.

Petersson, C.J., and Gentz, C.F.: Ruptures of the supraspinatus tendon: The significance of distally pointing acromioclavicular osteophytes. Clin. Orthop. 174:143–148, 1983.

Fifty-one percent of 47 shoulders in patients with supraspinatus ruptures and 54% of 54 cadavers with similar lesions had distally directed acromioclavicular osteophytes. This compares to 14% of patients and 10% of cadaver shoulders without rotator cuff lesions. Anterior acromion spurs were encountered but were much less common.

Post, M.; Silver, R.; and Singh, M.: Rotator cuff tear: Diagnosis and treatment. Clin. Orthop. 173:78–91, 1983.

In 59 shoulders repaired, there was no correlation between pain relief and extent of the cuff tear. Return of active abduction was inversely related to tear size.

Watson, M.: Major ruptures of the rotator cuff: The results of surgical repair in 89 patients. J. Bone Joint Surg. 67B:618–624, 1985.

In 89 surgical repairs, poorer results were associated with more preoperative steroid injections, deltoid weakness, and larger cuff defects. Results continued to improve for 2 years after operation.

Shoulder Arthritis

Cofield, R.H.: Total shoulder arthroplasty with the Neer prosthesis. J. Bone Joint Surg. 66A:899–906, 1984.

Of 73 shoulders, 92% achieved satisfactory pain relief. Postoperative active abduction averaged 120°. Complications developed in 13 patients, and 5 reoperations were necessary. Three glenoids were clinically loose, and five others showed radiographic changes of loosening.

Neer, C.S., II, and Kirby, R.M.: Revision of humeral head and total shoulder arthroplasties. Clin. Orthop. 170:189–195, 1982.

Forty humeral head and total shoulder arthroplasties were revised. More than one factor in failure was present in almost all cases. Reconstruction is difficult, and the results of revision are not as good as those of primary arthroplasty.

Neer, C.S., II; Watson, K.C.; and Stanton, F.J.: Recent experience in total shoulder replacement. J. Bone Joint Surg. 64A:319–337, 1982.

Of 150 patients in the full exercise program, 86% had an excellent or satisfactory rating. Only 4 of 194 shoulders were thought not to have benefited from the procedure. There were 24 complications; 12 required further surgery. Radiolucent lines were present at the glenoid bone-cement junction in 30%, but there was no clinical glenoid loosening.

Petersson, C.J.: Resection of the lateral end of the clavicle: A 3 to 30-year follow-up. Acta Orthop. Scand. 54:904–907, 1983.

Of 50 patients, 26% had a poor result. Nearly half of those with poor results had alcoholism or psychiatric disease. No correlation existed between the results and radiographic evidence of newly formed bone at the resection site.

Post, M., and Jablon, M.: Constrained total shoulder arthroplasty: Long-term follow-up observations. Clin. Orthop. 173:109–116, 1983.

A constrained total shoulder arthroplasty is rarely indicated. Design changes have minimized material failures. Of 78 shoulders, 15 have had major complications.

Samilson, R.L., and Prieto, V.: Dislocation arthropathy of the shoulder. J. Bone Joint Surg. 65A:456–460, 1983.

The development of arthritis after shoulder dislocation is rare and is often mild. Posterior dislocations with a delay in diagnosis, shoulders with limitation of external rotation, and shoulders in which surgically introduced metal penetrated the joint develop more severe arthritic changes. The number of dislocations was not related to the severity of the arthrosis.

Tanner, M.W., and Cofield, R.H.: Prosthetic arthroplasty for fractures and fracture-dislocations of the proximal humerus. Clin. Orthop. 179:116–128, 1983.

Pain relief was satisfactory in 25 of 28 shoulders with chronic fracture problems. Active abduction averaged 112°. Complications were more frequent in the chronic fractures than in acute fracture management and were related to tissue scarring and distortion of anatomy. If possible, prosthetic surgery should be performed early rather than late if such an indication exists.

Sports-Related Problems

Hill, J.A.: Epidemiologic perspective on shoulder injuries. Clin. Sports Med. 2:241–246, 1983.

Between 8% and 13% of athletic injuries involve the shoulder. Sports commonly associated with shoulder problems include baseball, swimming, football, wrestling, tennis, volleyball, and javelin throwing.

Advances in Anesthesia

Peterson, D.O.: Shoulder block anesthesia for shoulder reconstruction surgery. Anesth. Analg. 64:373–375, 1985.

Interscalene and upper thoracic paravertebral blocks were given to allow shoulder surgery. There were only two block failures (3.4%). There were no serious complications.

19

Elbow and Forearm: Trauma in Adult and Pediatric Patients

Introduction

The elbow and forearm provide a mechanism for positioning the hand in spacc. The treatment of trauma and its sequelae should be directed toward restoring painless and effective motion. This usually will involve accurate anatomic reduction and early mobilization. The role of radial head replacement and the necessity for removal of forearm plates remain areas of controversy. Recent studies suggest that −30° of elbow extension, 130° of elbow flexion, and 50° of forearm pronation and supination will permit most activities.

Anatomy and Biomechanics

Motion at the elbow and forearm occurs in two independent planes, both essentially uniaxial. Flexion and extension, through the ulnohumeral articulation, position the hand for reach to and from the body. Forearm rotation orients the hand for grip, opposition, and independent digital function.

Although the average normal range of motion is approximately 0° to 150° of flexion, the functional range of flexion is 30° to 130°. This allows not only the effective position for most activities of daily living but also the arc necessary for activities that require elbow motion (Fig. 1). Each patient will have individual requirements but, as shown in Figure 1, it is difficult to determine a single best position; therefore, fusion should be avoided. Loss of motion in the neck, wrist, and especially the shoulder further increases the need for elbow motion.

Forearm rotation occurs about an axis defined by a line from the center of the radiocapitellar joint to the distal articular surface of the ulna. The normal range of forearm rotation is approximately 85° of supination to 75° of pronation. Most activities of daily living require a range of 50° of supination to 50° of pronation (Fig. 2).

Malalignment of the radius and ulna has been shown to decrease the passive range of motion. Any angulation greater than 20° significantly decreases forearm rotation. Deformity at the midshaft causes greater relative limitation than deformity distally. The influence of the interosseous membrane on forearm rotation is not completely understood.

The stability of the elbow in the anteroposterior plane is conferred by the hemicircumferential articulation of the trochlea and olecranon coupled with the opposing pull of the flexors and the triceps. The anterior portion of the medial collateral ligament in concert with the radial head provides stability to valgus stress except that in full extension the anterior capsule contributes to support. Varus stress is resisted by the ulnohumeral articulation, lateral collateral ligaments, and anconeus.

Adult Fractures and Dislocations

Elbow Dislocations

Posterior elbow dislocation commonly occurs from a fall onto the outstretched hand. Associated injuries can include

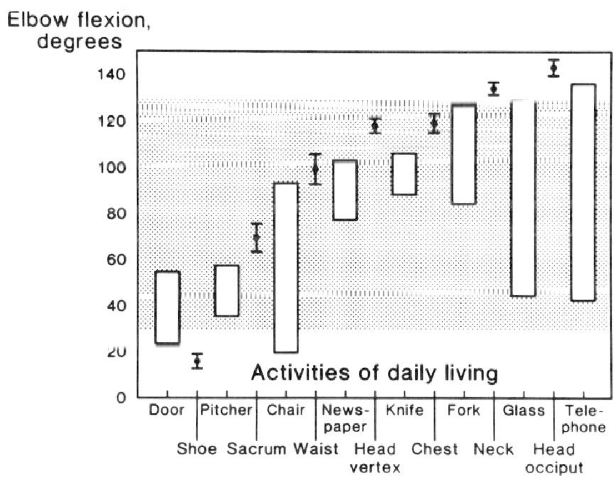

Figure 1

Normal elbow flexion positions for activities of daily living. Most functions can be performed between 30° and 130° of elbow flexion. (From Morrey, B.F.; Askew, L.J.; An, K.N.; and Chao, E.Y.: A biomechanical study of normal functional elbow motion. J. Bone Joint Surg. 63A:872–877, 1981. By permission of the journal.)

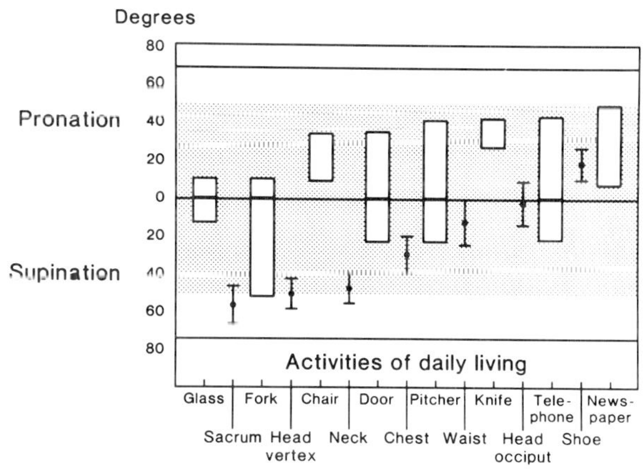

Figure 2

Routine daily activities requiring pronation and supination are performed between 50° of pronation and 50° of supination. (From Morrey, B.F.; Askew, L.J.; An, K.N.; and Chao, E.Y.: A biomechanical study of normal functional elbow motion. J. Bone Joint Surg. 63A:872–877, 1981. By permission of the journal.)

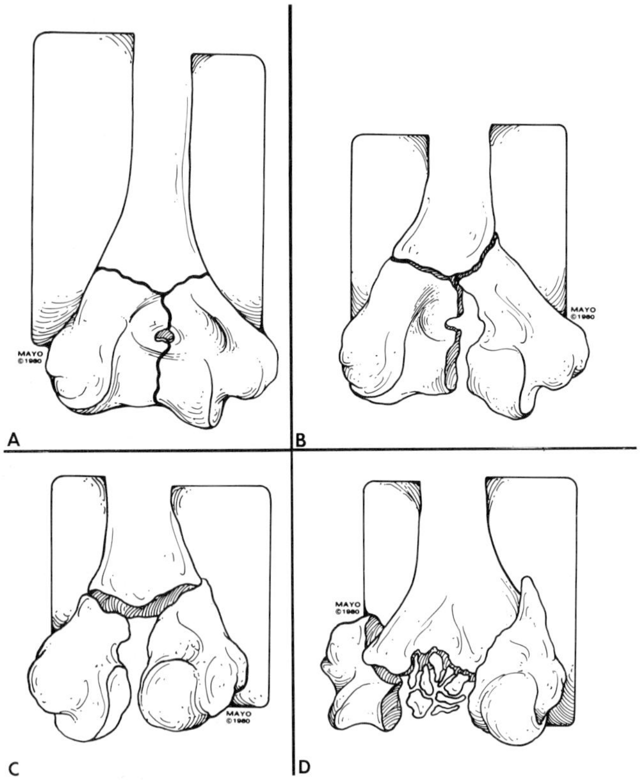

Figure 3

A, Type I—undisplaced T-condylar fracture of the elbow. *B,* Type II—displaced but not rotated T-condylar fracture. *C,* Type III—displaced and rotated T-condylar fracture. *D,* Type IV—displaced, rotated, and comminuted T-condylar fracture. (From Bryan, R.S.: Fractures about the elbow in adults. *In* AAOS Instructional Course Lectures. XXX:200–223. St. Louis, C.V. Mosby, 1981. By permission of Mayo Foundation.)

radial head fractures and distal radio-ulnar joint disruption. Gentle longitudinal traction followed by flexion after reduction is usually successful. If reduction is not possible or is unstable, careful examination of the radiographs may reveal a more significant bony lesion. Although most investigators think that there is complete disruption of the medial collateral ligaments and anterior capsule in most posterior and posterolateral dislocations, the incidence of late recurrent instability is rare. Therefore, open repair or reconstruction of the medial ligaments is rarely indicated. Motion generally can be initiated at 10 to 14 days after injury. Flexion contracture of 20° or less commonly occurs despite vigorous rehabilitation. This seldom imposes a functional disability. Longitudinal studies of simple elbow dislocations document little disability or dysfunction. Heterotopic bone formation or myositis ossificans is possible in a small percentage of patients.

The optimal treatment of dislocations associated with comminuted radial head fractures remains unknown. If radial head excision is dictated by severe comminution, the use of a silicone radial head prosthesis may add to stability and decrease stress on the damaged medial ligaments, but prosthetic material failure and associated synovitis may occur. No enhancement or benefit from ligament repair has been documented.

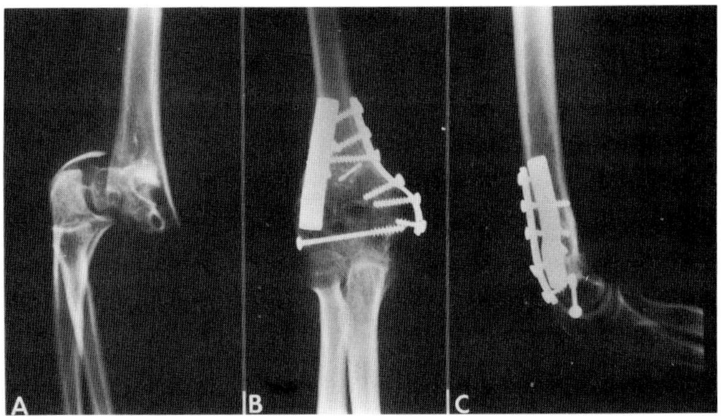

Figure 4

Maintenance of intra-articular reduction with screws and plates.

Supracondylar and T-Y Fractures

Supracondylar fractures in the adult without intra-articular involvement are uncommon and can be treated with external splinting if reduction can be maintained without compromise of the circulation. Alternatives include percutaneous fixation with smooth pins or open reduction and internal fixation.

A useful classification of intra-articular fractures of the distal humerus is shown in Figure 3. Type I fractures are rare and can be treated with 2 to 3 weeks of cast immobilization followed by gentle motion. Fractures with displacement and comminution, types II and III, are best treated with open reduction and internal fixation if technically possible. The goal of treatment is to establish skeletal stability and articular alignment to allow early motion and prevent contracture. Alternatives include olecranon pin traction followed by casting.

Type IV fractures are more difficult to treat because comminution makes stable reconstruction less likely. Elderly patients with severe comminution can be treated with olecranon pin traction. Motion can be started at the third week while the patient is in traction or has been fitted with a collar and cuff. In younger patients, stable reconstruction with internal fixation is desirable but is technically demanding.

Surgical exposures of the distal humerus include a form of triceps splitting or olecranon osteotomy. Some recommend olecranon osteotomy by tension band wiring with a single cancellous screw or K-wires. Use of a longitudinal screw alone has been associated with separation and nonunion. An alternative to olecranon osteotomy is the posterior approach (Bryan) in which the triceps tendon and olecranon fascia are incised medially and reflected laterally. The most stable configuration of internal fixation depends on the degree of comminution and individual screw purchase. Maintenance of intra-articular reduction with individual lag screws and augmentation with posterior or lateral plates (Fig. 4) seems to offer the most stable configuration.

Radial Head Fractures

Assessment of the patient with fracture of the radial head should include evaluation of the medial ligaments, capitellum, and distal radio-ulnar joint. The radiocapitellar view may be helpful for a more complete assessment of comminution and capitellar involvement. It is a modified lateral view of the elbow joint accomplished by angling the tube 45° toward the radial head, projecting it ventrally.

Radial head fractures have been classified according to the angulation and degree of comminution. Nondisplaced fractures (type I) have been shown by many to be best treated with a short period of immobilization, often in a sling, followed by motion as soon as tolerated. Comminuted fractures (type III) or those involving a significant portion of the articular surface should be treated by early excision.

The best management of displaced or slightly comminuted fractures (type II) remains in question. Each fracture requires individual assessment. Closed treatment with cast immobilization followed by motion at 1 to 3 weeks has been used by many with success. Emphasis should be placed on careful follow-up and reassessment for displacement. Open reduction with internal fixation is technically difficult and has not been uniformly successful. Excision should be considered only for patients with the majority of the articular surface involved or displacement greater than 3 mm.

Long-term studies of patients who have undergone radial head excision demonstrate proximal migration of the radius relative to the ulna. Controversy exists concerning the amount and significance of this migration. Pain at the distal radio-ulnar joint and loss of supination have been thought by some to be the result of this proximal shift; others have disagreed. The use of a prosthetic radial head replacement after isolated radial head fracture has been questioned because failure of the material and the related problems of silicone synovitis have been identified. Patients with associated elbow dislocation may require the prosthesis for stability.

Olecranon Fractures

Nondisplaced fractures of the olecranon can be treated with immobilization and motion at 3 weeks. Radiographs should be obtained after splinting and again a few days afterward to ensure that no displacement has occurred.

Displaced fractures of the olecranon that involve the joint or a significant fragment are best managed with open reduction and tension-band wiring with an intramedullary 6.5-mm cancellous screw or K-wires. Motion can be initiated as soon as tolerated. Intramedullary fixation with pins or lag screws without tension banding is not as stable.

Excision of the displaced fragments is an attractive alternative in the elderly patient. Up to 50% of the joint can be resected without decreasing stability. Care must be taken to ensure that the medial collateral ligament is not disturbed in the excision. Care also must be taken to retain the coronoid process and to suture the triceps tendon at the level of the remaining joint. Attachment of the triceps should be as close to the articular surface as is technically possible.

Radius and Ulna Fractures

Most closed displaced fractures of the radius and ulna are best treated with open reduction and internal fixation with compression plating according to the AO technique. Anatomic reduction, minimizing angulation and rotational deformity, influences the ultimate range of forearm rotation. Angulation of greater than 20° or rotation deformity has been shown *in vitro* to decrease supination and pronation significantly. Motion can be started a few days postoperatively, depending on the stability of fixation and degree of comminution.

Bone grafting may be necessary in cases of severe comminution. Use of plates five holes or longer significantly decreases the incidence of failure of fixation or nonunion. The incidence of synostosis is higher in a patient with head injury. Open fractures (grade I or II) of the radius and ulna can be plated as a delayed procedure several days after irrigation and debridement, as long as there is no evidence of infection or tissue necrosis.

Severe open injuries with extensive soft tissue and bone loss require initial stabilization with external fixation and early soft tissue coverage. Restoration of the bone deficit has been managed with tricortical iliac crest graft or free vascularized fibular transfer. The vascularized transfer has shown early incorporation and hypertrophy. A few patients may require conversion to a one-bone forearm.

Displaced isolated fractures of the radial shaft should also be treated with compression plating. Minimally displaced fractures of the middle or distal third of the ulna can be treated with casting or a fracture brace.

Monteggia fractures are best managed with compression plating of the ulna fracture and closed reduction of the radius. Maintaining reduction of the radial head dislocation is quite difficult without internal fixation of the ulna. The approach to Galeazzi fractures does not differ significantly. After anatomic reduction and compression plating of the fractured radius, attention can be directed to reduction of the distal radio-ulnar joint. Usually, this can be accomplished by casting in supination. Some prefer K-wire fixation in the distal joint.

Although elective removal of compression plates remains controversial, a specific concern in the forearm is re-fracture of the radius or ulna after plate removal. In a recent reported series, 7 re-fractures were noted in 23 patients, and caution was advised with regard to timing of plate removal and resumption of vigorous physical activity and torsional stress.

Pediatric Fractures and Dislocations

Elbow Dislocations

Posterior dislocation of the elbow in the child requires evaluation for signs of neurovascular compromise. Many authors have noted arterial lesions as well as entrapment of the median nerve. Careful assessment is necessary before and after attempts at reduction. Careful inspection of the radiographs with vigilance for associated medial epicondylar fractures is important. Knowledge of the timing and order of appearance of the centers of ossification is essential. The most common mistake is to confuse an entrapped medial condyle for a trochlear ossification center. Displaced epiphyseal fractures also can be confused with dislocations. Most dislocations are posterior and can be reduced with longitudinal traction followed by flexion. Any instability or failure of reduction must be investigated for possible avulsion of the medial epicondyle and entrapment in the joint (Fig. 5). As in the adult, the clinical outcome after an uncomplicated posterior elbow dislocation is excellent. Significant late sequelae of an uncomplicated dislocation are rare. Dislocations that come to medical atten-

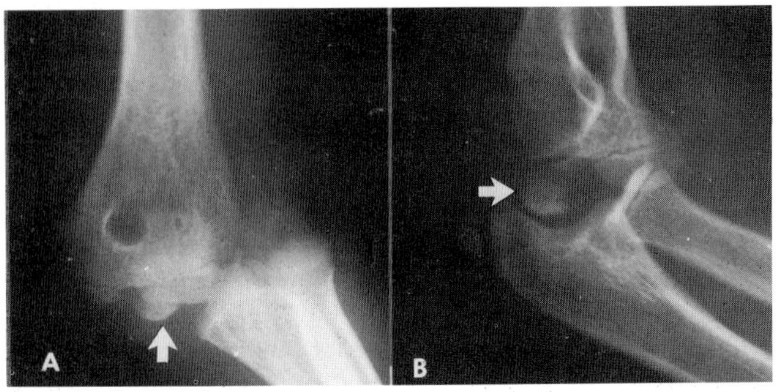

Figure 5

Posterolateral dislocation of the elbow with entrapment. *A*, Anteroposterior view, showing medial epicondyle within the elbow joint (*arrow*) which prevented a closed reduction. *B*, Lateral view, demonstrating fragment (*arrow*) between the humerus and olecranon. (From Wilkins, K.E.: Fractures and dislocations of the elbow region. *In* Fractures in Children, edited by Rockwood, C.A., Jr.; Wilkins, K.E.; and King, R.E., pp. 363–575. Vol. 3. Philadelphia, J.B. Lippincott Company, 1984. By permission of the publisher.)

tion late, 3 weeks or more after injury, should be reduced. Open reduction and temporary pinning may be necessary. This treatment produced a significant improvement in motion in children with dislocations that were discovered late (several weeks after injury).

Supracondylar Fractures

Proper management of the pediatric supracondylar fracture benefits from an algorithmic, systematic approach (Fig. 6). Injury to the brachial artery or median, radial, or ulnar nerve has been reported and must be suspected in each patient. Prompt assessment with angiography must be undertaken if vascular injury is suspected. If angiography delays exploration, it can be performed in the operating room. Digital subtraction angiography provides improved definition with less contrast agent. In the presence of vascular injury, immediate open reduction with pinning of the fracture and repair of the vessel is indicated. Most authors recommend observation in the hospital for any signs of increased compartment pressure.

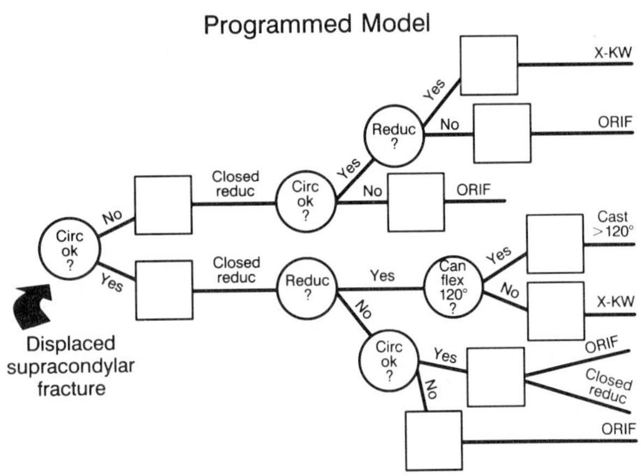

Figure 6

Example of algorithmic approach to displaced supracondylar fracture. Traction is an alternative to open reduction when vascular injury is not present. (From Millis, M.B.; Singer, I.J.; and Hall, J.E. Clin. Orthop. 188:90–97, 1984. By permission of J.B. Lippincott Company.)

Most injuries are displaced posteriorly and into extension. Flexion to 120° has been shown to be important for maintenance of reduction. If this amount of flexion is precluded by swelling or circulatory depression, traction or internal fixation of the fracture with K-wires should be considered. Careful assessment of the reduction, regardless of the method, is important. The varus-valgus alignment of the distal humerus must be restored to avoid cosmetic asymmetry from cubitus varus or valgus deformity.

Minimally displaced or angulated fractures usually can be managed with carefully molded splints or casts with the elbow in 120° of flexion. Care must be taken to ensure that loss of reduction does not occur as the swelling decreases and the cast immobilization becomes less effective.

Management of fractures that either are not amenable to closed manipulation or have not remained in acceptable alignment is still controversial. Those fractures with severe displacement should be treated with open reduction and pinning because traction usually will not improve alignment. If adequate reduction is achieved but cannot be maintained because of swelling, percutaneous pin fixation under fluoroscopic control can be performed. Alternatively, traction can be used until swelling diminishes enough to allow enough flexion in cast to maintain reduction. Recent studies indicate that most authors favor pin fixation over traction in these cases.

Cubitus varus is the most common complication after supracondylar fractures in children. This deformity is cosmetic and rarely functional. Corrective supracondylar osteotomy can improve appearance but is technically demanding, and careful preoperative planning is mandatory. Several techniques have been described; most utilize a closing wedge osteotomy with K-wire fixation.

Physeal Injuries

Medial Epicondyle and Condyle Isolated fractures of the medial epicondyle usually occur after age 9 years as a result of a valgus stress injury or posterior elbow dislocation. Entrapment in the joint can occur and should be treated with open reduction and pinning, even if discovered late. Before age 9, fractures that appear to involve the medial epicondyle can extend through the trochlear physis. For patients with unossified trochlear epiphyses, the presence of a metaphseal flake or "fat pad" may alert one to this possibility. Arthrography may be beneficial.

Medial condylar fractures can occur after age 8 years, usually before complete formation of the trochlear epiphysis. Although this injury is relatively rare, failure to diagnose it can result in severe growth deformity because of inadequacy of reduction. Tardy ulnar nerve palsy has also been associated with this injury. Open reduction with pinning is the treatment of choice.

Lateral Epicondyle and Condyle Lateral condylar fractures are common and occur in children after the appearance of the capitellar ossification center—usually after age 4 years. Fractures with displacement greater than 2 mm should be treated with open reduction and fixation with smooth pins. Fractures treated closed should be observed carefully for displacement. Although this fracture involves the physis, recent series have not documented frequent growth arrest or cubitus valgus deformity. Mild varus deformity is more common despite adequate reduction. Fractures of the lateral epicondyle are rare and usually occur in children more than 10 years old. Diagnosis can be difficult because of the irregular ossification pattern in this ossification center. Splint or cast immobilization for 3 to 4 weeks is usually sufficient.

Radial Head Fractures

Management of radial head fractures in children differs from that in adults in that a greater effort is made to preserve or reconstruct. Nondisplaced fractures of the radial head can be treated with a sling and early motion. Angulation greater than 30° often can be improved by closed manipulation. After closed manipulation, angulation of greater than 45° or severe displacement of the radial head may be better treated with open reduction. The use of internal fixation is controversial and should be avoided if possible. Severe comminution is quite rare, and excision should be reserved for treating failures of other methods.

Olecranon Fractures

Fractures of the olecranon in the child usually can be treated closed but, if significant displacement exists, open reduction with internal fixation may be necessary. Tension-band wiring can be used.

Radius and Ulna Fractures

Forearm fractures in children usually can be managed satisfactorily by closed manipulation and casting. In the very young, angulation of 15° can be accepted because remodeling will improve alignment with growth. However, in those over age 6, little change will occur in fractures of the diaphyseal region, and angulation of more than 10° should be remanipulated. For children over 12 years of age, open reduction with compression plating occasionally may be necessary to maintain adequate reduction. At any age, rotational malalignment will not improve with growth and will lead to malunion and limited motion if not recognized and corrected.

Malunions of the forearm in the older child can be cosmetically unpleasant as well as limiting to forearm rotation. Residual angulation greater than 20° significantly restricts pronation and supination. Correction of the deformity can be accomplished by osteotomy and compression plating or drill osteoclasis and casting. Significant improvement can be expected in forearm rotation with correction of the deformity.

Monteggia Fractures

Monteggia fractures usually can be managed by closed reduction. Occasionally, reduction of the radial head is not possible without intermedullary fixation of the ulnar fracture. Oblique fractures of the ulna are less stable than transverse fractures and may require intramedullary pinning to maintain reduction. Monteggia fractures treated late may require open reduction with reconstruction of the annular ligament (Fig. 7).

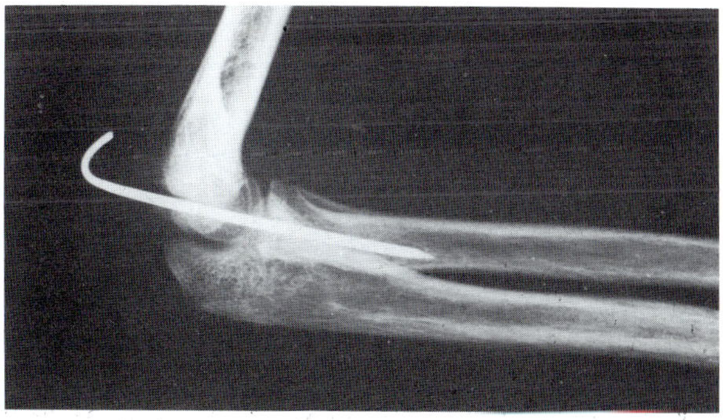

Figure 7

Reconstruction of the annular ligament by using fascia from the forearm. (From Fowles, J.V.; Sliman, N.; and Kassab, M.T. J. Bone Joint Surg. 65A:1276–1283, 1983. By permission of the journal.)

Soft Tissue Coverage

Open injuries of the elbow and forearm often require extensive soft tissue coverage. Skeletal stabilization should be achieved with external fixation and debridement of all necrotic and avascular tissue.

Extensive soft tissue defects in the upper extremity should be covered with composite grafts of muscle and skin. Local rotation flaps were used in the past with some success. However, with the advent of microsurgical technique and free tissue transfer, fewer rotation flaps are indicated (see Chapter 13).

Nonunions

Nonunions of fractures of the elbow are most common in the distal humerus and proximal ulna. In the young, active patient, rigid internal fixation with bone grafting and early motion often offers the best ultimate function. Elderly, less active patients with a distal humeral nonunion may be candidates for total elbow replacement. Nonunion of the olecranon can be treated with tension-band wiring and bone grafting in the young, active patient. Excision is an acceptable alternative when less than 50% of the articular surface is involved. Care must be taken to avoid excision of the medial collateral ligament.

Stiffness and Contracture

Maximizing the ultimate range of motion after trauma to the elbow requires a conscientious program of rehabilitation. Early postoperative motion—both active and gently passive, often with motorized devices—can limit the amount of permanent contracture. The stability of both the soft tissue envelope and the skeletal reconstruction usually determines the extent of motion permissible. Significant pain should be avoided because this points to a related incidence of ectopic bone formation. Traditional analgesics as well as local blocks may be useful.

Despite aggressive rehabilitation, permanent flexion contracture commonly occurs. Although 30° of contracture is probably well tolerated by most, further loss of extension begins to limit the length of reach and associated activities (Fig. 1).

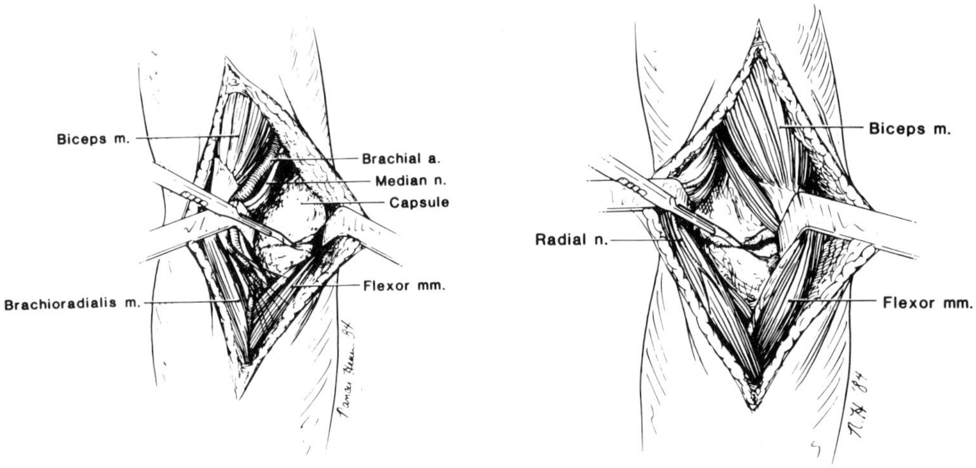

Figure 8

Medial portion of anterior part of the capsule is incised after retraction of brachial artery and median nerve laterally (shown here), or medially if that is easier. The anterior capsulotomy is completed by retracting biceps tendon medially and radial nerve laterally. Brachialis can be retracted to either side and is not cut. (From Urbaniak, J.R.; Hansen, P.E.; Beissinger, S.F.; and Aitken, M.S. J. Bone Joint Surg. 67A:1160–1164, 1985. By permission of the journal.)

After minor trauma and immobilization, contracture of the anterior capsule can cause loss of flexion despite normal bony and cartilaginous architecture. Malunion, intra-articular osteophytes, and spurring in any portion of the joint also can limit motion. Careful evaluation, with a detailed physical examination, often can reveal the pathologic anatomy. Computed tomography and standard radiographs with anteroposterior and lateral polytomography are helpful for complete evaluation.

Surgical intervention should be contemplated only after careful assessment of the patient's disability and goals. Equally important are the precise identification of the cause and the skill and experience of the surgeon. A long course of rehabilitation using continuous passive motion in the early stages and splinting, both static and dynamic, should be planned.

Results from anterior capsulotomy alone, followed by aggressive therapy, are encouraging. Even a small improvement in arc of motion can be beneficial (Fig. 8).

Replantation

Replantation after traumatic amputation at the elbow or forearm requires an experienced team of surgeons and therapists as well as a motivated patient. Revascularization is essential for any hope of limb survival and is often achievable. Nerve regeneration is the most important factor determining ultimate function. Primary nerve repair is preferred if possible.

Crush or avulsion injury may make replantation technically difficult and ultimate function unlikely. Long-term results of replantations at the elbow and forearm are dependent on ultimate function of the hand. Limb survival is reported to be between 50% and 70% in most series. The rate of good or excellent function is lower. An attentive plan of splinting and passive range-of-motion exercise is necessary to maximize the function of the hand.

Annotated Bibliography

General

Morrey, B.F.: The Elbow and Its Disorders. Philadelphia, W.B. Saunders, 1985.

This is an excellent general resource for the anatomy and biomechanics of the elbow. The management of trauma and reconstruction are well addressed.

Anatomy and Biomechanics

Morrey, B.F., and An, K.-N.: Articular and ligamentous contributions to the stability of the elbow joint. Am. J. Sports Med. 11:315–319, 1983.

A cadaveric biomechanical study of four elbows which quantifies some of the soft tissue and bony elements that provide stability of the elbow.

Adult Fractures and Dislocations

Elbow Dislocations

Josefsson, P.O.; Johnell, O.; and Gentz, C.F.: Long-term sequelae of simple dislocation of the elbow. J. Bone Joint Surg. 66A:927–930, 1984.

Review of 52 patients followed for a mean of 24 years. The major sequela of simple elbow dislocation was a minimal loss of extension. Valgus instability was present by examination in only seven patients and was asymptomatic.

Lansinger, O.; Karlsson, J.; Körner, L.; and Måre, K.: Dislocation of the elbow joint. Arch. Orthop. Trauma Surg. 102:183–186, 1984.

Seventy-two patients with elbow dislocations were reviewed at a mean of 5 years. Acute surgical repair of the medial collateral ligament did not afford better results in the clinically unstable elbow.

Intercondylar Fractures

Jupiter, J.B.; Neff, U.; Holzach, P.; and Allgöwer, M.: Intercondylar fractures of the humerus: An operative approach. J. Bone Joint Surg. 67A:226–239, 1985.

A review of 13 patients with fractures of the distal humerus treated with open reduction and internal fixation, including both the operative technique and the results.

Radial Head Fractures

Greenspan, A.; Norman, A.; and Rosen, H.: Radial head-capitellum view in elbow trauma: Clinical application and radiographic-anatomic correlation. A.J.R. 143:355–359, 1984.

The described "radiocapitellar view" provides better visualization of the capitellum and the radial head, especially the posterior portion.

Weseley, M.S.; Barenfeld, R.A.; and Eisenstein, A.L.: Closed treatment of isolated radial head fractures. J. Trauma 23:36–39, 1983.

Patients with Mason class I fractures did well with early motion. The majority of patients with Mason class II fractures did well without operative treatment.

Radius and Ulna Fractures

Hidaka, S., and Gustilo, R.B.: Refracture of bones of the forearm after plate removal. J. Bone Joint Surg. 66A:1241–1243, 1984.

Seven re-fractures occurred in 23 patients at times ranging from 2 to 40 weeks after plate removal. Three re-fractures were through the original fracture and four were through screw holes.

Stern, P.J., and Drury, W.J.: Complications of plate fixation of forearm fractures. Clin. Orthop. 175:25–29, 1983.

Major complications occurred in 28% of the patients. A higher rate of nonunion was associated with plates that utilized fewer than five screws.

Tarr, R.R.; Garfinkel, A.I.; and Sarmiento, A.: The effects of angular and rotational deformities of both bones of the forearm. J. Bone Joint Surg. 66A:65–70, 1984.

This *in vitro* study of cadaver forearms examined the effects of malalignment on forearm rotation. Combined angulation of 10° or less results in minimal limitation of pronation and supination due to bony impingement.

Pediatric Fractures and Dislocations

Elbow Dislocations

Carlioz, H., and Abols, Y.: Posterior dislocation of the elbow in children. J. Pediatr. Orthop. 4:8–12, 1984.

Review of 58 posterior dislocations of the elbow in children. Associated medial epicondylar fractures often required operation because of entrapment or severe displacement.

Fowles, J.V.; Kassab, M.T.; and Douik, M.: Untreated posterior dislocation of the elbow in children. J. Bone Joint Surg. 66A:921–926, 1984.

Open reduction of posterior elbow dislocations more than 3 weeks in duration resulted in increased motion and function.

Supracondylar Fractures

Jarvis, J.G., and D'Astous, J.L.: The pediatric T-supracondylar fracture. J. Pediatr. Orthop. 4:697–699, 1984.

Sixteen patients with T-supracondylar fractures of the elbow, the majority class II, were treated with open reduction and internal fixation. Satisfactory results were achieved in the majority of cases by using this approach.

Kekomäki, M.; Luoma, R.; Rikalainen, H.; and Vilkki, P.: Operative reduction and fixation of a difficult supracondylar extension fracture of the humerus. J. Pediatr. Orthop. 4:13–15, 1984.

Retrospective review of 45 supracondylar fractures in children. The majority were treated with open reduction and pinning; those treated with traction alone were more likely to have loss of the carrying angle.

Millis, M.B.; Singer, I.J.; and Hall, J.E.: Supracondylar fracture of the humerus in children: Further experience with a study in orthopaedic decision-making. Clin. Orthop. 188:90–97, 1984.

A useful algorithmic approach to the pediatric supracondylar fracture.

Morrissy, R.T., and Wilkins, K.E.: Deformity following distal humeral fracture in children. J. Bone Joint Surg. 66A:557–562, 1984.

Report of five cases of uncommon central proximal depression in the humerus after supracondylar fracture. Dissolution of the trochlea resulted in proximal migration of the ulna and a mild decrease in flexion.

Oppenheim, W.L.; Clader, T.J.; Smith, C.; and Bayer, M.: Supracondylar humeral osteotomy for traumatic childhood cubitus varus deformity. Clin. Orthop. 188:34–39, 1984.

Supracondylar osteotomy for cubitus varus deformity is undertaken for cosmetic reasons. The technical pitfalls and complications are described in 45 corrective osteotomies.

Physeal Injuries

Medial Humeral Condyle

Harrison, R.B.; Keats, T.E.; Frankel, C.J.; Anderson, R.L.; and Youngblood, P.: Radiographic clues to fractures of the unossified medial humeral condyle in young children. Skeletal Radiol. 11:209–212, 1984.

Fractures of the medial condyle in children may involve the joint. The presence of a fat pad sign or metaphyseal flake raises the probability of an intra-articular fracture.

Medial Epicondyle

Fowles, J.V.; Kassab, M.T.; and Moula, T.: Untreated intra-articular entrapment of the medial humeral epicondyle. J. Bone Joint Surg. 66B:562–565, 1984.

Elbow dislocation in children may be accompanied by unrecognized fracture and intra-articular entrapment of the medial epicondyle. Reduction or excision of the fragment leads to improved motion.

Lateral Condyle

Foster, D.E.; Sullivan, J.A.; and Gross, R.H.: Lateral humeral condylar fractures in children. J. Pediatr. Orthop. 5:16–22, 1985.

Fractures of the lateral humeral condyle with more than 2 mm of displacement are best treated with percutaneous pinning if adequate reduction is present or open reduction and pinning. Time to union is 6 to 8 weeks.

Fowles, J.V.; Sliman, N.; and Kassab, M.T.: The Monteggia lesion in children: Fracture of the ulna and dislocation of the radial head. J. Bone Joint Surg. 65A:1276–1283, 1983.

Fifteen cases were reviewed. Oblique fractures of the ulna required intermedullary pinning to maintain reduction.

Rutherford, A.: Fractures of the lateral humeral condyle in children. J. Bone Joint Surg. 67A:851–856, 1985.

Thirty-nine fractures of the lateral humeral condyle were reviewed. The best results occurred with accurate anatomic reduction. Careful observation of those fractures treated without pinning is necessary because of the tendency toward displacement.

So, Y.C.; Fang, D.; Leong, J.C.Y.; and Bong, S.C.: Varus deformity following lateral humeral condylar fractures in children. J. Pediatr. Orthop. 5:569–572, 1985.

Despite adequate reduction by either closed or open means, some loss of the carrying angle resulted. No significant functional or cosmetic deformity resulted.

Tibone, J.E., and Stoltz, M.: Fractures of the radial head and neck in children. J. Bone Joint Surg. 63A:100–106, 1981.

Results in 33 patients are reviewed. Poor results occurred in patients more than age 10 years. Angulation greater than 30° had a significant negative influence on the result.

Soft Tissue Coverage

Daniel, R.K., and Weiland, A.J.: Free tissue transfers for upper extremity reconstruction. J. Hand Surg. 7:66–76, 1982.

In 18 cases that utilized free tissue transfers, the latissimus dorsi muscle flap was most useful for soft tissue coverage.

Contracture

Urbaniak, J.R.; Hansen, P.E.; Beissinger, S.F.; and Aitken, M.S.: Correction of post-traumatic flexion contracture of the elbow by anterior capsulotomy. J. Bone Joint Surg. 67A:1160–1164, 1985.

After anterior capsulotomy alone, 11 patients with flexion contracture and no evidence of arthrosis had improvement of extension by a mean of 40°.

20
Elbow and Forearm: Reconstruction

Subjects covered in this section include basic science, diagnostic techniques, tendon problems, elbow synovectomy, radial head resection, muscle transfer procedures, nerve compression syndromes, and total elbow arthroplasty.

Basic Science: Articular and Ligamentous Stability of the Elbow Joint

Basic research regarding the mechanics of the elbow joint focused primarily on the value of the radial head in providing stability. To date, limited material has appeared in the literature but the results are consistent in demonstrating that the radial head provides about 30% of the first 3° to 5° of valgus stability of the elbow joint. The ultimate stability of the joint after radial head excision has not yet been defined.

Analysis of the degrees of stability offered by the articulating surfaces and the ligamentous structures of the elbow gave results that varied depending on the mode of load application. When valgus stresses were applied, the medial collateral ligament (MCL) played a dominant role, accounting for about 55% of the stability of the elbow. With varus stresses, the lateral collateral ligament (LCL) was much less important, contributing only 10% to 15% to the stability of the joint. A greater role in stabilizing the elbow to distractive forces was observed for the MCL (78%) compared with the LCL (10%). Anatomic investigations have identified an important element of the LCL complex, the "lateral ulnar collateral ligament." This structure originates from the lateral epicondyle and inserts on the tubercle of the crista supinatoris of the ulna. It provides varus stability to the ulna after the radial head has been excised. The radial collateral ligament complex originates at the lateral epicondyle at the axis of rotation and has been shown to be isometric during elbow flexion (Fig. 1). The MCL originates slightly posterior and distal to the axis of rotation and hence shows increased tension with increased elbow flexion (Fig. 2).

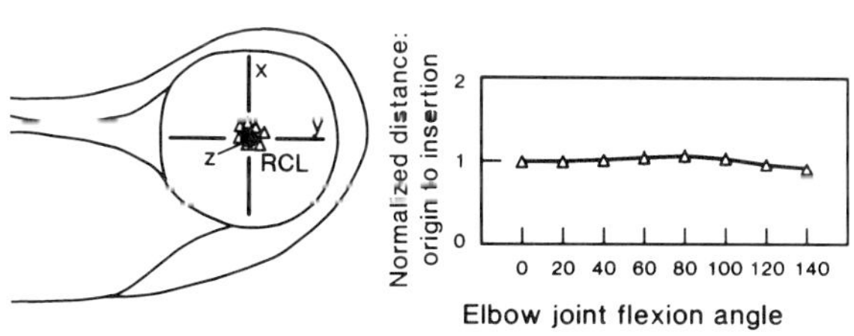

Figure 1

The radial collateral ligament (*RCL*) originates in the center of the lateral epicondyle. Therefore, it is isometric with respect to elbow position. Thus, reconstruction of this ligament should include an anatomic origin at the lateral epicondyle of the humerus.

Diagnostic Evaluation

The several complex-shaped articular surfaces found at the elbow create difficulties in the assessment of intra-articular lesions by standard radiographic methods. In a comparison of conventional radiography, arthrotomography, double-contrast arthrography, and conventional tomography, the greatest diagnostic information was gained from tomography. Arthrotomography rarely improved the diagnostic accuracy except when detection of purely cartilaginous bodies, the position of mineralized densities, or the status of articular cartilage was desired.

The use of arthroscopy as a diagnostic or therapeutic measure is slowly increasing. Patient selection is much more rigorous than for the knee, and reports to date emphasize the importance of understanding the anatomy of the elbow (Fig. 3), of experience with arthroscopy in general, and of recognition of the intended goals and limitations of the technique. Typically, the procedure is used diagnostically when a disparity exists between the objective findings and the subjective complaint. Removal of loose bodies is the best therapeutic use but limited debridement and partial

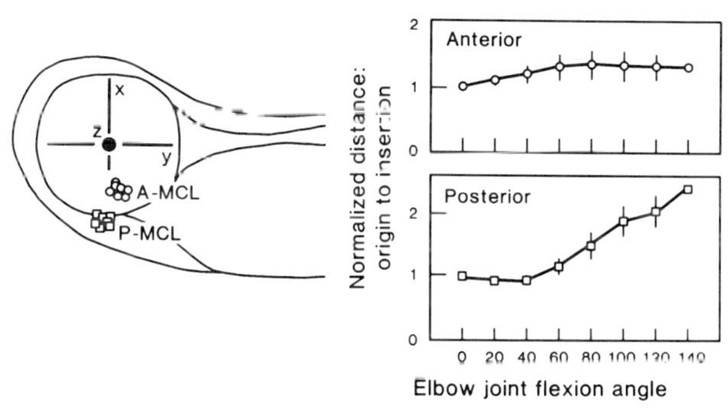

Figure 2

The anterior and posterior medial collateral ligaments (*A-MCL* and *P-MCL*) originate off the axis of rotation at the medial epicondyle; thus, with flexion there is a slight change in the length of the anterior cruciate ligament and a significant change in length of the posterior cruciate ligament. These data suggest that both elements of the collateral ligament complex should be reconstructed, even though the anterior portion is more essential, in order to restore stability in the most physiologic fashion.

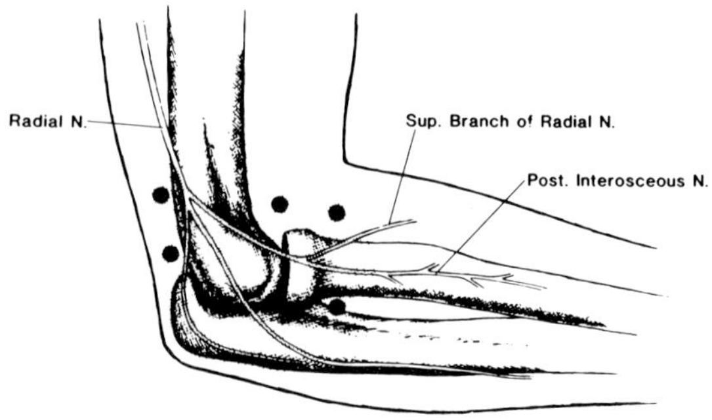

Figure 3

Several lateral portals are available for arthroscopy of the elbow. Note the relationship of these portals to the branches of the radial nerve. (From Guhl, J.F. Orthopedics 8:1290–1296, October 1985. By permission of Slack.)

synovectomy also may be effectively performed. In general, the procedure has been found to be effective in about 70% of the instances in which it was used.

Disorders of the Tendons

Several reports in the recent literature discussed the acute and subacute treatment of distal biceps tendon rupture. All indicated that a significant amount of impairment occurs if the tendon is not repaired; up to 40% of flexion and 40% of supination strength is lost. Loss of endurance is also a common problem in the patient not treated surgically. The use of two incisions to avoid injury to the radial nerve is the most popular surgical technique, although the anterior approach of Henry is still recommended by some. For orthopaedists relatively unfamiliar with an anterior exploration of the elbow, the two-incision technique is considered to be the safest approach. Early repair (within the first 7 to 10 days after injury) provides return of strength and function to nearly normal.

The problem in lateral epicondylitis most commonly is a degeneration or disruption of a component of the common extensor origin. The relationship of entrapment of the posterior interosseous nerve in the differential diagnosis of this condition continues to pose problems. The most definitive statement on this subject cites an incidence of concurrent radial nerve entrapment of about 5% in a population of patients with well-documented lateral epicondylitis. Pain elicited from resistance of extension of the middle finger has been described in the nerve entrapment syndrome. However, this test was not found to be as reliable a diagnostic test as pain elicited with resisted pronation and supination.

Several recent reports have described the surgical treatment of lateral epicondylitis in outpatients. Through a limited incision or simply with a pericutaneous release, approximately 90% satisfactory results have been achieved. Some have recommended that medial epicondylitis be treated in a similar fashion. Although these reports do seem promising, a desire to visualize the lesion persists. Furthermore, because of the possibility of nerve injury with percutaneous medial release, the formal surgical procedure remains the treatment of choice at this time.

Elbow Synovectomy

Elbow synovectomy still is done predominately for rheumatoid arthritis or, less frequently, in cases of fungal infection or arthroplasty in a hemophiliac when recurrent hemorrhage into the joint is a problem. As a general rule, range of motion is not improved after synovectomy although the use of continuous passive motion in the immediate postoperative period may increase the arcs of flexion and extension. Although often slow in developing, pain relief is the most predictable outcome. Relief from recurrent bleeding is observed postoperatively in the hemophiliac, and absence of recurrent effusions is an added benefit to the patient with rheumatoid arthritis. Regeneration of the joint synovium generally takes place within 90 to 100 days. Approximately a third of the patients with rheumatoid arthritis will have recurrence of the inflammatory synovitis 3 to 5 years postoperatively.

Synovectomy is generally reserved for stage I and II rheumatoid arthritis, although in a series of 35 patients with recurrent stage III and IV disease, 50% were rated as good to excellent postoperatively. Complications after synovectomy include problems of wound healing, superficial and deep infection, ulnar neuritis, and a loss of motion including the potential for ankylosis in relatively few situations. Synovectomy in the hemophiliac must be accompanied by administration of factor VIII for at least 8 to 10 days or until wound healing appears to be certain.

Radial Head Excision

Controversy remains as to whether radial head excision should be performed with synovectomy, especially in a rheumatoid patient. Some reports describe additional relief of pain when the radiocapitellar joint is decompressed by radial head excision. Other reports describe increased instability, especially to valgus stresses, after radial head excision (Fig. 4). Frequently, increased pain is noted over the medial aspect of the joint, presumably due to increased tensile stresses on the MCL complex but radiographs often show arthritic joint changes as well. Replacement of the radial head with a Silastic prosthesis may reestablish the buttressing effect across the radiocapitellar joint, thereby lessening the potential for valgus strain with lifting activities. Because of the potential for production of Silastic detritus, this replacement should not be considered when there is deformity or loss of cartilage over the capitellar articular surface. It is wise to advise the patient that it may be used as a temporary spacer and therefore a second operation often is required for its removal. Experimental studies have demonstrated that Silastic particles in the joint produce an inflammatory response similar to that seen in patients who have pain and synovitis after implantation of a Silastic prosthesis.

Interpositional Arthroplasty

The various nonmetallic materials used in interpositional arthroplasty include fascia lata, dermis, and thin sheets of silicone. Use of a 4-mm-thick silicone sheet to reconstitute destroyed articular surfaces in the elbow of hemophiliacs has given good short-term (30 months) results in a small series of patients (Fig. 5). Two-thirds of the patients noted complete relief of pain, and all exhibited a significant de-

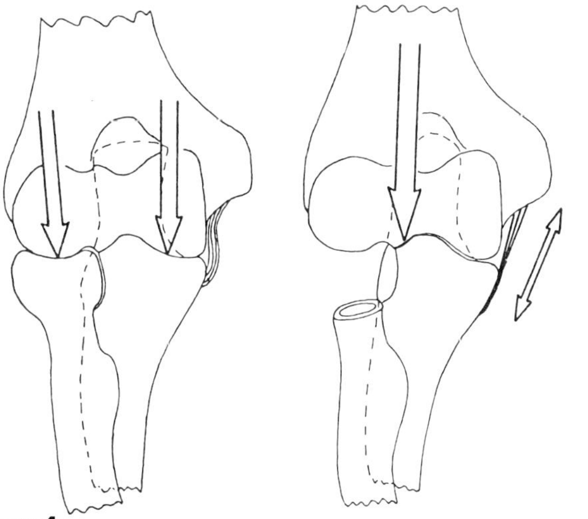

Figure 4

The radial head acts as an important buttress in preventing valgus stresses at the elbow when the hand lifts weight against gravity. Removal of the radial head increases the load on the humero-ulnar articulation and the tension observed in the medial collateral ligament. (From Rymaszewski, L.A.; Mackay, I.; Amis, A.A.; and Miller, J.H. J. Bone Joint Surg. 66B:109–113, 1984. By permission of the British Editorial Society of Bone and Joint Surgery.)

crease in recurrent hemorrhages. Radial head excision was performed in all cases. No instability was reported postoperatively. The technique of application of the silicone material includes contouring and suturing to the humeral surface.

Interposition of fascia lata should be done with caution in patients with rheumatoid arthritis. This can provide good pain relief but range of motion is often compromised and the postoperative balancing of deficient or stretched collateral ligaments and capsule remains an essential goal but one often difficult to achieve. Elbow ankylosis, with essentially no movement after trauma, septic arthritis, and traumatic myositis ossificans also are potential indications for fascial arthroplasty. In a series of 51 patients so treated, one-third regained a postoperative arc of motion of at least 90° and another 40% had an arc of 45° to 90°. Maximum recovery is often not achieved until 6 months postoperatively. Such treatment is particularly attractive over a prosthetic implant in a patient less than age 60 in whom heavy stresses will be placed on the elbow. However, some long-term failures have been observed with progressive resorption of the distal humerus, and interposition arthroplasty should be offered very cautiously to a young laborer.

One of the most promising variations of interposition arthroplasty is the placement of a pin across the axis of rotation and in the ulna to distract the joint (Fig. 6). Careful placement of the pin allows an arc of motion with a uniform distance (distraction) from the ulna, even during elbow motion. Thus, in difficult reconstructive procedures the patient may move the elbow through a reasonable arc of motion and avoid an early postoperative contracture. The pins are usually removed at 3 to 6 weeks. This technique has been used sparingly in the elbow and the knee for many years but has recently been reintroduced and popularized. The surgical technique is demanding and requires a second incision over the medial aspect of the joint to ensure that the ulnar nerve is adequately protected.

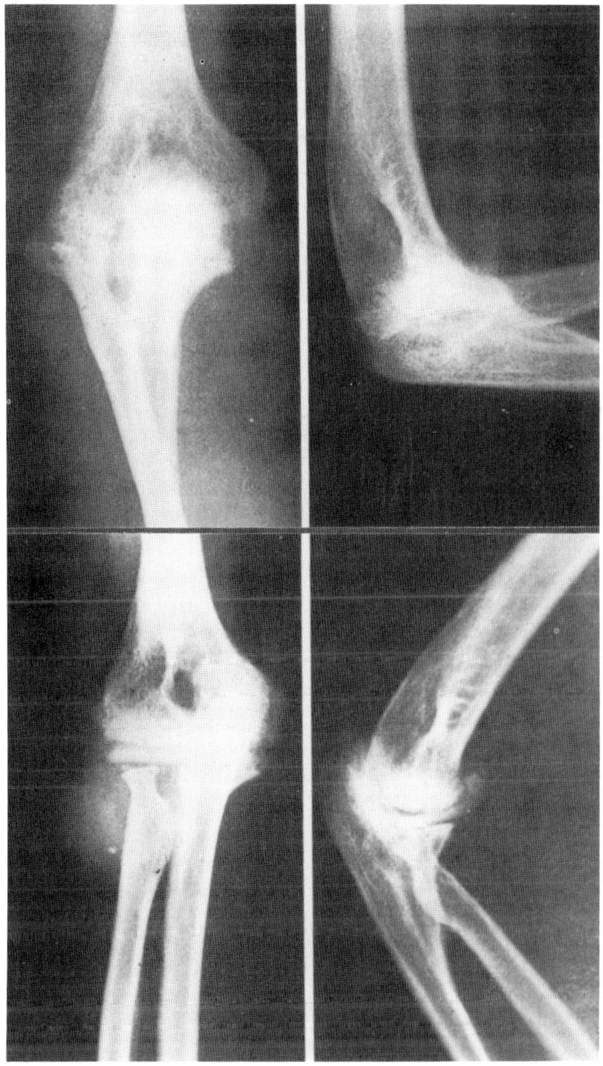

Figure 5

Preoperative (*Upper*) and postoperative (*Lower*) radiographs of an elbow badly destroyed by recurrent hemarthroses secondary to hemophilia. The joint space was reconstituted by insertion of a 3-mm-thick sheet of silicone. (From Smith, M.A.; Savidge, G.F.; and Fountain, E.J. J. Bone Joint Surg. 65B:436–440, 1983. By permission of the British Editorial Society of Bone and Joint Surgery.)

Wound problems and infection may occur with increased frequency with this procedure. It should be offered only with extreme caution and by those experienced in elbow reconstructive surgery.

Restoration of Motor Function at the Elbow

Elbow Flexion

Various methods have been described for the restoration of active elbow flexion: proximal and lateral advancement of the flexor pronator forearm mass; anterior transposition of the triceps tendon; transfer of the lower sternocostal margin of the pectoralis major into the tendon of the long head of the biceps; complete transposition of the pectoralis

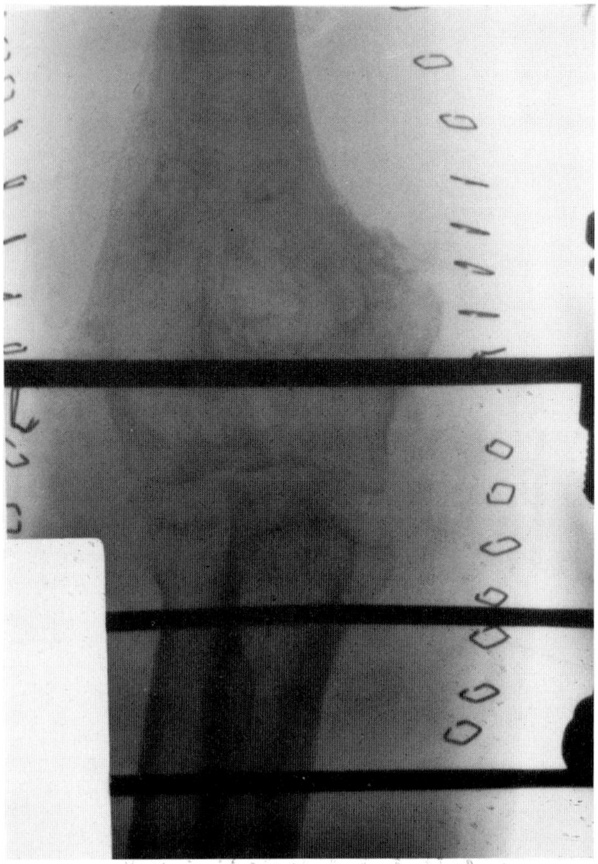

Figure 6

Distraction arthroplasty, showing pins in place. The joint has been distracted approximately 5 mm.

major on its neurovascular pedicle; transfer of the sternocleidomastoideus with a fascia lata extension; and free transfer of the latissimus dorsi with preservation of its neurovascular bundle.

Although each procedure offers the potential for improvement of forearm flexion against gravity, most carry some associated disadvantages. The flexor-plasty frequently provokes a flexion contracture, and forearm supination is not restored. Anterior transposition of the triceps eliminates active elbow extension, and transfer of the pectoralis major can give rise to internal rotation of the arm when flexion is initiated. Difficulty is also encountered in transferring the pectoralis major to the biceps without mobilization of the pectoralis minor because both muscles have a common neurovascular bundle from the medial pectoral nerve and the pectoral branch of the thoracoacromial artery.

Good results have been reported for restoration of elbow flexion by transfer of both pectoralis major and minor (Fig. 7). The transferred muscles retain their origin from the coracoid process and the lateral clavicle. The distal portion of the muscle unit is mainly composed of the sternocostal origin of the pectoralis major and a part of the anterior rectus abdominus fascia. Attachment to the distal third of the biceps muscle is then carried out.

Flexor-plasty using the latissimus dorsi is desirable because it is a powerful substitute for deficient forearm flexors and its neurovascular pedicle is sufficiently long to permit ease of transfer. The use of the latissimus dorsi transfer is indicated when an upper brachial plexus injury has occurred, because its innervation is from the sixth, seventh, and eighth cervical nerve roots.

Elbow Extension

Restoration of elbow extension can be achieved by transfer of the posterior third of the deltoid to the triceps. Although such a transfer converts a portion of the deltoid into a two-joint muscle, no functional loss at the shoulder has been perceived by the patients undergoing this procedure. Postoperatively, the patient is managed by plaster cast immobilization of the elbow at full extension for 6 weeks. A graduated program of increased flexion exercises is then instituted with an increase of no more than 15° of flexion per week over the second 6-week period. The restoration of elbow extension is beneficial in patients who have upper and lower extremity paralysis because such patients require extensor elbow function to propel a wheelchair and to raise themselves intermittently from a seated position to avoid sacral and ischial pressure sores.

Nerve Entrapment Syndrome

Entrapment neuropathies about the elbow include involvement of the median, ulnar, and radial nerves.

Median Nerve

Median nerve entrapment at or above the elbow can arise because of constrictive pressure from the ligament of Struther or from the lacertus fibrosus. Struther's ligament, a band coursing medially and inferiorly to the medial condyle, frequently is observed with a supracondyloid process. Because of the unyielding nature of these fibrous bands, hemorrhage, scarring, or muscle hypertrophy beneath these structures may give rise to median nerve entrapment. Incision of Struther's ligament or the lacertus fibrosus gives good results predictably.

Ulnar Nerve

Entrapment of the ulnar nerve at the cubital tunnel can arise from various causes including direct trauma, growth disturbance of the distal humerus (cubitus valgus), bony or synovial proliferation, ganglion, chronic external pressure, and compromised size of the tunnel because of encroachment by the two heads of the flexor carpi ulnaris and the ulnar collateral ligament. Surgical treatment is aimed at decompression by simple release of constricting tissues and subcutaneous or submuscular transfer. In a prospective study of 32 patients with the diagnosis of cubital tunnel syndrome, the factors that related most to an unsuccessful outcome were the presence of intrinsic muscle atrophy of the hand, decrease in motor conduction velocity, decrease in the evoked sensory perception, and presence of electromyographic fibrillation activity at rest. The most satisfactory postoperative results were achieved by subcutaneous or submuscular transfer of the ulnar nerve, although the final outcome was not as directly related to the type of procedure performed as to the presence or absence of the above factors.

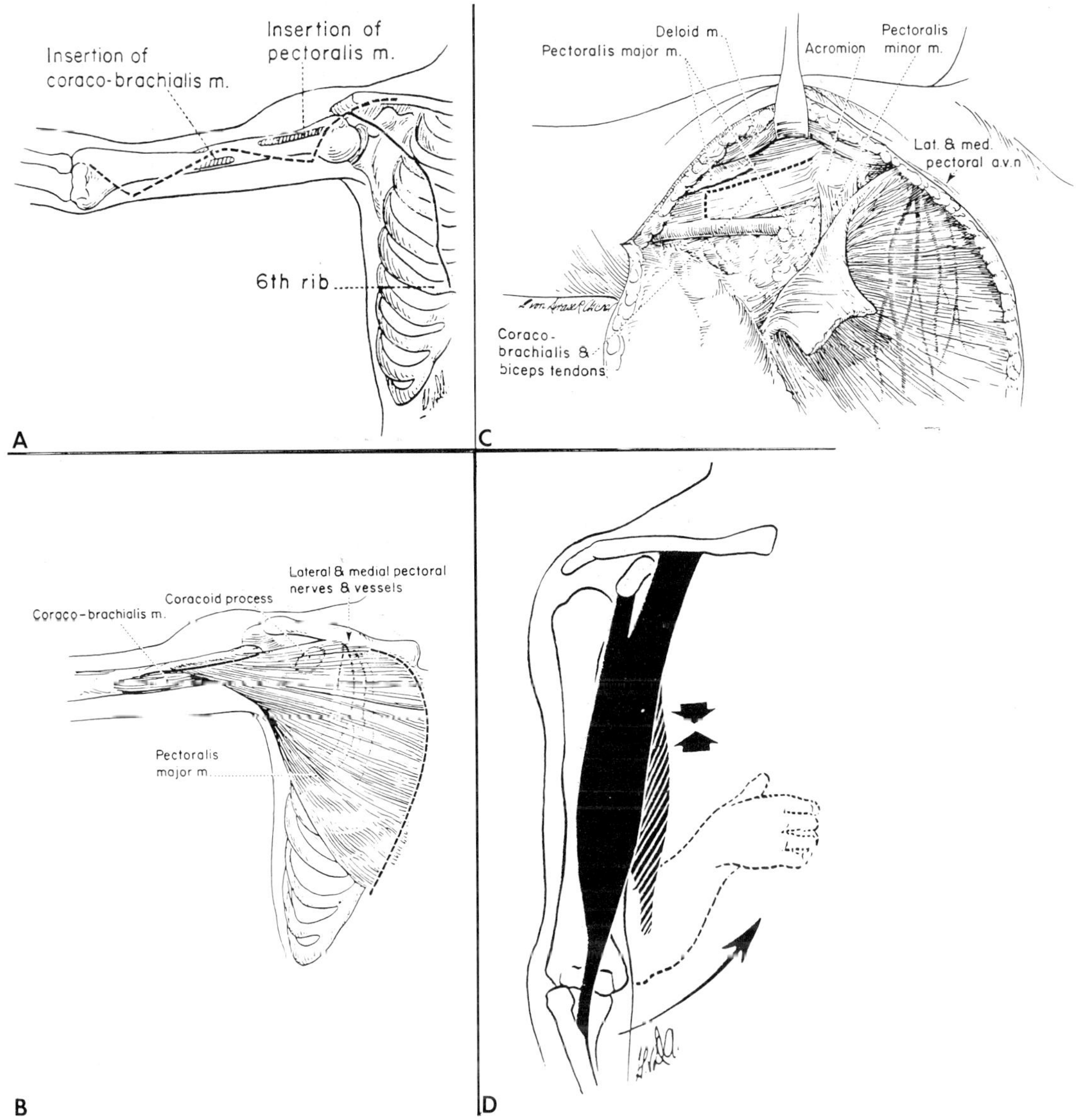

Figure 7

Restoration of elbow flexion by transfer of pectoralis major and minor. *A*, Skin incisions. *B*, Detachment of pectoralis major from its origin and insertion. *C*, Preparation of proximal coraco-brachialis and biceps tendons for attachment to pectoralis. *D*, Transferred pectoralis in extension and flexion (From Tsai, T.-M.; Kalisman, M.; Burns, J.; and Kleinert, H.E. J. Hand Surg 8:186–190, 1983. By permission of the American Society for Surgery of the Hand.)

Radial Nerve

Entrapment of the posterior interosseous nerve at the proximal fibrous margin of the supinator recently has been reported as occurring in conjunction with tennis elbow or as a cause of a failure to cure tennis elbow. The typical presentation is an aching pain in the forearm at approximately 3 cm distal and 1 cm anterior to the lateral epicondyle. Although the radial nerve does not have sensory fibers, the clinical presentation seems to document that aching pain referred to the region of the lateral epicondyle is possible with the radial nerve entrapment syndrome. The diagnosis is best made by localizing the symptoms and aggravating them with resisted pronation and supination. If the patient has localized tenderness over the lateral epicondyle, the diagnosis of lateral epicondylitis is appropriate. The two conditions coexist in about 5% of instances. Treatment for radial nerve entrapment syndrome consists of release of the proximal supinator which is the most common site of entrapment; this is successful in about 90% of instances.

Elbow Arthrodesis

Because the elbow acts as a linkage system, motion at the elbow is an absolute necessity for proper function of the entire upper extremity. There is no single optimal position for function. Thus, elbow arthrodesis is rarely indicated. Some form of arthroplasty designed to restore motion is far preferable to the arthrodesis in all but the most unusual circumstances such as in a laborer who requires significant flexion strength of the extremity or in instances of refractory sepsis.

Total Elbow Replacement

Severe arthritic involvement of the elbow can require a serious compromise in upper extremity function, particularly in activities of daily living. The elbow is the most critical joint in the upper extremity for providing the motion that permits the hand to be brought to the torso, head, or mouth. Extension at the elbow is also critical because this determines the lever arm length of the upper extremity. The arc of extension also determines whether personal hygiene will be possible in bathing of the lower trunk and lower extremities.

The essential arc of elbow motion for activities of daily living has been established as ranging from 130° to 30°. Pronation and supination, a function of elbow kinematics also shared by the wrist, is critical for activities of daily living. An arc of about 50° of each motion is considered necessary for daily activities. Dominant hand function requires pronation; the nondominant hand is generally aided by a certain arc of supination.

The history of total elbow replacement, commencing in 1970, has been fraught with design failures, high rates of aseptic and septic loosening, instability, recurrent dislocations, problems of wound healing, inadequacy of arc of motion, and transient or permanent ulnar neuropathies. Considerable bioengineering efforts have been undertaken to improve the design of total elbow prostheses. Concomitantly, research efforts have attempted to identify the magnitude of forces observed at the elbow with activities of daily living and the manner in which these joint reactive forces are dissipated across the elbow articulations.

Cadaver studies have demonstrated that hand-held weights will be magnified 4- to 8-fold at the elbow, the greatest forces occurring near full extension. The proportion of the joint reactive force shared by the radiocapitellar surface from a static axial load had been recognized as varying from 35% to 50%. However, in physiologic dynamic loading, the force transmission of the radio-humeral joint does not exceed body weight. Additionally, many activities of daily living—such as turning door handles, opening jar lids, etc.—produce significant rotational forces on the elbow. Therefore, a balance between the intrinsic stability of the prosthetic interface and the adjacent soft tissue envelope is critical if loosening and instability are to be kept to a minimum. Designs that have offered a greater degree of interface constraint have been associated with higher rates of mechanical loosening whereas designs giving lesser interface constraint have been characterized by higher rates of instability and dislocation. In recent years, the use of a semiconstrained or "sloppy hinge" type of articulation has allowed a more constrained elbow joint device to be used with a much lower incidence of bone-cement interface loosening.

Total elbow replacement continues to evolve as an increasingly dependable procedure. The learning curve for total elbow replacement, however, is complicated by the need for a very precise technique of insertion, a balancing of often deficient or absent soft tissue constraints, and the utilization of two prosthetic designs: 1) resurfacing that is both stable and capable of dissipating load stresses over the widest area of bony contact; and 2) semiconstrained which allows reconstruction for bone-deficient states and for revision procedures.

Techniques and Specific Case Reports

Prostheses

Experience with 19 surface replacement type total elbow replacements in 15 patients with rheumatoid arthritis revealed that, although two-thirds were pleased with the degree of pain relief postoperatively, half showed radiographic loosening of the ulnar component. Two patients required reoperation, one for prosthetic removal because of a deep infection and one to exchange a loosened humeral component. The prosthetic design—a concave metallic surface on the ulnar component with only a short intramedullary stem and a convex polyethylene nonmetallic reinforced humeral component without a stem—was thought to contribute, in part, to the development of radiolucencies (Fig. 8). Suggested revisions in prosthetic design include an exchange of the polyethylene and metallic surfaces between the ulnar and humeral components and the addition of an intramedullary stem for added fixation on the humeral side.

In contrast, with 44 long-stemmed total elbow prostheses inserted over a 12-year period commencing in 1970 in patients with the diagnosis of rheumatoid arthritis, "good" results were reported in 77%. The most predictable postoperative improvement was pain relief. There was no significant decrease in the arc of extension and only a slight increase in flexion postoperatively. The interface design of this prosthesis provided a single plane of motion, yet only one case of loosening was reported (Fig. 9). Other associated complications included five condylar fractures at the time of prosthetic insertion, four cases of persistent ulnar neuropathy, and four cases of wound breakdown. At present, this design is not thought to be appropriate because such constrained devices should have some "play" at the interface. The incidence of loosening of these devices appears to be dramatically decreased.

In a series of 153 patients undergoing total elbow replacement with an unconstrained surface replacement design, 90% reported "good" to "excellent" results. Both prosthetic components had intramedullary stems of adequate dimension. The prosthetic system also provided for proper tension of the soft tissue envelope about the elbow by providing ulnar components with 3-, 6-, and 9-mm plastic liners. Although the authors reported only one case of loosening over an 8-year period, numerous other problems arose, including a 7% dislocation rate, a 4% incidence of

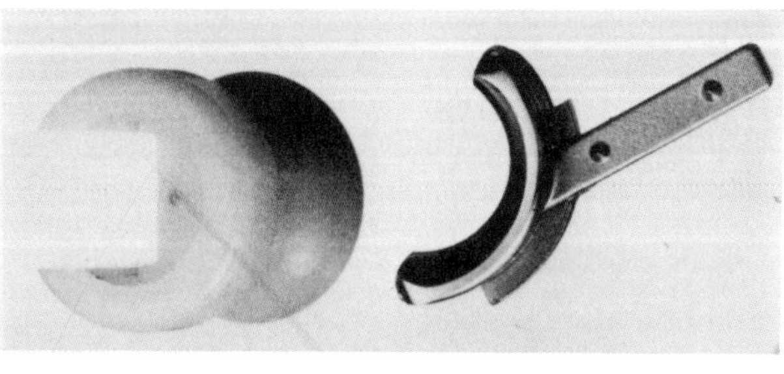

Figure 8

Elbow prosthesis that lacks long intramedullary stems for enhanced stability at bone/cement interface. (From Rydholm, U.; Tjörnstrand, B.; Pettersson, H.; and Lidgren, L. J. Bone Joint Surg. 66B:737–741, 1984. By permission of the British Editorial Society of Bone and Joint Surgery.)

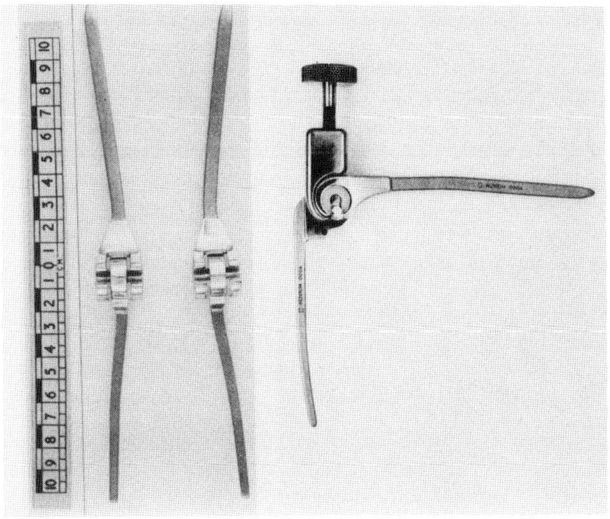

Figure 9

Highly constrained total elbow prosthesis (i.e., design permits only flexion and extension). The long anatomically shaped intramedullary stems enhance fixation. (From Johnson, J.R.; Getty, C.J.M.; Lettin, A.W.F.; and Glasgow, M.M.S. J. Bone Joint Surg. 66B:732–736, 1984. By permission of the British Editorial Society of Bone and Joint Surgery.)

permanent ulnar nerve sensory loss, and infection rates of 2% for superficial ones and 2% for deep ones. In a small subset of patients, a radial head replacement was used but 50% of these had a complete line of radiolucency about the radial component, and the incidence of radiolucency about the humeral components in such elbows was 4 times greater than in those in which a radial head had not been used. This increase in radiolucency suggested increased rotational moment forces generated about the humeral stem because of transmission of load between the radial head and the capitellar surface.

Salvage of Failed Total Elbow Prosthesis

Significant technical difficulties arise in providing any degree of stability and useful function to an elbow when removal of the prosthesis has become necessary. Two reports described use of an iliac wing graft to replace deficient bone in the region of the distal humerus. This technique is particularly useful when the medial and lateral condylar ridges have been preserved. The autogenous iliac graft is shaped so as to provide a convex surface for the olecranon and added length to the distal humerus, thereby reestablishing the proper tension to the triceps and the soft tissues about the elbow (Fig. 10). Fixation of the graft is with an AO plate or use of heavy (7/64 inch) threaded pins. Several patients were able to function postoperatively without an orthosis. However, in general, the results of nonseptic resection or graft reconstruction arthroplasty are not well defined. Significant instability remains a cause for concern.

Little is known about the results of reimplantation salvage of the failed total elbow arthroplasty. Experience at one institution has indicated a satisfactory result in 55% after the initial revision and an acceptable result in 80% after revision with a second implantation. The complication rate of revision surgery is about 60% and major complications occur in about 25%. These results have improved considerably in the last 5 years with the use of a specific semiconstrained device that allows some biologic incorporation and prevents axial rotation (Fig. 11).

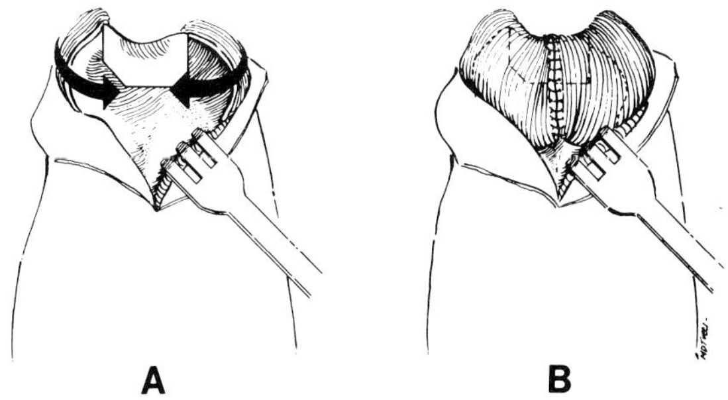

Figure 10

A, Large trochlear bony defect created by removal of a failed total elbow prosthesis is filled with an iliac wing bone graft precisely shaped so as to reconstitute the dimensions of the trochlea. The graft can be secured with a plate and screws or two 7/64 inch threaded Steinmann pins. *B*, Fascia lata or dermis is then placed over the bone graft surface. The medial and lateral collateral ligaments and capsular envelope often can be drawn posteriorly over the bony surface if laxity of these structures needs to be corrected.

Deep Sepsis After Total Elbow Arthroplasty

In a report on 156 total elbow replacements performed in 140 patients, a deep infection rate of 9% was noted. Significant risk factors associated with deep infection included presence of rheumatoid arthritis, history of a prior operative procedure, and the need for reoperation after prosthesis insertion. Among the 14 patients who had infection, 10 required a resection arthroplasty to arrest the infection and 8 of these had a satisfactory result; in the 2 other patients, delayed reimplantation of a total elbow was successful after control of the infection in 1 and 1 responded

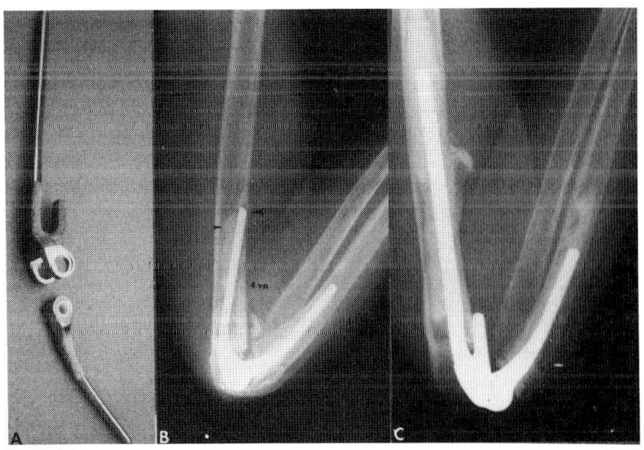

Figure 11

A, Newer semiconstrained elbow device with an anterior flange and a toggle hinge articulation. This anterior flange allows for primary replacement as well as for revision procedures. *B*, Constrained hinged prosthesis has loosened, with posterior displacement of the hinge and anterior tilt of the proximal stem (arrowheads). *C*, Flanged hinged revision prosthesis resists posterior forces at the articulation.

to debridement only. Although an infection rate of 9% after total elbow replacement appears to be higher than that reported elsewhere, prospective patients should be informed of this significant risk factor.

Annotated Bibliography

Basic Science

Morrey, B.F., and An, K.-N.: Articular and ligamentous contributions to the stability of the elbow joint. Am. J. Sports Med. 11:315–319, 1983.

A study of the stability offered by the various bony ligamentous and capsular structures composing the elbow disclosed the relatively greater role played by the medial collateral ligament in resisting valgus stresses, compared with the radial collateral ligament in varus stresses. In both varus and valgus loading patterns, significant stability is provided by the articulating surfaces.

Morrey, B.F., and An, K.-N.: Functional anatomy of the ligaments of the elbow. Clin. Orthop. 201:84–90, 1985.

An anatomic study demonstrated that the radial collateral ligament complex consists of an important ulnar humeral band which serves as an additional constraint to resist ulnar varus. This accounts for the typical varus stability observed, even after a lax radial collateral ligament due to radial head resection.

Diagnostic Modalities

Guhl, J.F.: Arthroscopy and arthroscopic surgery of the elbow. Orthopedics 8:1290–1296, October 1985.

Forty-five instances of elbow arthroscopy among 3,300 arthroscopic procedures over a 10-year period are reported. The technique is discussed in detail with emphasis on the value for removing loose bodies and limited debridement; the diagnosis of difficult cases is well presented.

Morrey, B.F.: Arthroscopy of the elbow. *In* AAOS Instructional Course Lectures. Edited by L.D. Anderson, pp. 102–107. St. Louis, C.V. Mosby, 1986.

The technique is mentioned briefly. A critical analysis of the indications and results demonstrates that the clinical diagnosis was confirmed in 31% and expanded in 38% of patients. Overall, the procedures were thought to have been helpful in 79% of patients.

Teng, M.M.; Murphy, W.A.; Gilula, L.A.; Destouet, J.M.; Edelstein, G.; Monsees, B.; and Totty, W.G.: Elbow arthrography: A reassessment of the technique. Radiology 153:611–613, 1984.

A review of 26 elbows evaluated by conventional radiography, arthrography, contrast arthrography, and conventional tomography disclosed that the last approach was the most beneficial single study in assessing the presence of intra-articular bodies, cartilage loss, or obscure fractures.

Tendon Disorders

Baker, B.E., and Bierwagen, D.: Rupture of the distal tendon of the biceps brachii: Operative versus non-operative treatment. J. Bone Joint Surg. 67A:414–417, 1985.

The use of a Cybex in studying 13 patients with rupture of the distal biceps demonstrates that the 3 patients not operated on had a significant loss of flexion and pronation strength. The two-incision technique is recommended and, when performed acutely, restores strength to almost normal.

Morrey, B.F.; Askew, L.J.; An, K.N.; and Dobyns, J.H.: Rupture of the distal tendon of the biceps brachii: A biomechanical study. J. Bone Joint Surg. 67A:418–421, 1985.

Ten patients studied in the biomechanics laboratory had a mean flexion loss of 30% and supination strength loss of 40% if the biceps was not repaired. With repair, normal arc of motion and essentially normal flexion and pronation strength were obtained. These authors recommend the two-incision technique.

Norman, W.H.: Repair of avulsion of insertion of biceps brachii tendon. Clin. Orthop. 193:189–194, 1985.

Sixteen cases with a mean follow-up of 8 years were reported. Some slight limitations in activities were reported but 14 of 16 patients returned to their previous occupations and activities. The recommendation to repair the injury surgically is strongly stated. These authors prefer the anterior radial approach with a pull-out suture.

Tennis Elbow

Baumgard, S.H., and Schwartz, D.R.: Percutaneous release of the epicondylar muscles for humeral epicondylitis. Am. J. Sports Med. 10:233–236, 1982.

Of 35 patients with lateral epicondylitis, 3 had an unsatisfactory result (10%). Interestingly, six patients with medial epicondylitis were so treated; five had an excellent result and one had an unsatisfactory result.

Neviaser, T.J.; Neviaser, R.J.; Neviaser, J.S.; and Ain, B.R.: Lateral epicondylitis: Results after patient surgery and immediate motion. Contemp. Orthop. 511:43–46, 1985.

A limited open procedure and direct visualization of the defect is recommended. The most notable contribution is that this rather typical surgical approach is conducted as an outpatient procedure under local anesthesia. All 33 patients had a good subjective result.

Yerger, B., and Turner, T.: Percutaneous extensor tenotomy for chronic tennis elbow: An office procedure. Orthopedics 8:1261–1263, October 1985.

The percutaneous outpatient technique for releasing the lateral common extensor tendon is discussed. In 144 patients, a satisfactory result was obtained in 90%.

Elbow Synovectomy

Brumfield, R.H., Jr., and Resnick, C.T.: Synovectomy of the elbow in rheumatoid arthritis. J. Bone Joint Surg. 67A:16–20, 1985.

In 35 patients with stage III or IV rheumatoid arthritis involvement who underwent elbow synovectomy and radial head excision, only 4 results were rated as "excellent" and approximately half were rated as "good" postoperatively. Although pain relief was observed, no improvement in range of motion was noted; one-third of the patients subsequently had active recurrent synovitis.

Linclau, L.A.; Winia, W.P.C.A.; and Korst, J.K.v.d.:

Synovectomy of the elbow in rheumatoid arthritis. Acta Orthop. Scand. 54:935–937, 1983.

Two-thirds of patients presenting with rheumatoid arthritis who underwent synovectomy of the elbow were judged to be satisfactory postoperatively. The outcome did not correlate with the disease stage or the length of follow-up.

Radial Head Excision

Rymaszewski, L.A.; Mackay, I.; Amis, A.A.; and Miller, J.H.: Long-term effects of excision of the radial head in rheumatoid arthritis. J. Bone Joint Surg. 66B:109–113, 1984.

A series of 40 patients with rheumatoid arthritis had a pattern of continued deterioration after synovectomy and radial head excision. Loss of the stabilizing effect of the radial head was thought to be the reason.

Worsing, R.A., Jr.; Engber, W.D.; and Lange, T.A.: Reactive synovitis from particulate silastic. J. Bone Joint Surg. 64A:581–585, 1982.

Silastic particles injected into the rabbit joint caused a proliferative synovitis that histologically resembled that observed in some patients with "reactive synovitis" after Silastic implant surgery.

Interpositional Arthroplasty

Deland, J.T.; Walker, P.S.; Sledge, C.B.; and Farberov, A.: Treatment of posttraumatic elbows with a new hinge-distractor. Orthopedics 6:732–737, June 1983.

This explains the concept of elbow distraction arthroplasty. The axis of rotation of the elbow closely resembles a hinge joint, and thus the location may be estimated as a line through the center of the projected joint seen on the lateral radiograph. By placing a pin through this landmark and pins in the ulna, elbow motion with uniform joint distraction may be accomplished.

Oyemade, G.A.A.: Fascial arthroplasty for elbow ankylosis. Int. Surg. 68:81–84, 1983.

In a review of 51 cases of elbow ankylosis treated with fascial arthroplasty, 75% of the patients had good results.

Smith, M.A.; Savidge, G.F.; and Fountain, E.J.: Interposition arthroplasty in the management of advanced haemophilic arthropathy of the elbow. J. Bone Joint Surg. 65B:436–440, 1983.

Six patients with hemophilic arthropathy at the elbow were treated by limited joint excision followed by insertion of an interpositional sheet of silicone. All patients noted good relief of pain, increased range of motion, and a reduction in recurrent hemarthroses.

Muscle Transfer Procedures

Lamb, D.W., and Chan, K.M.: Surgical reconstruction of the upper limb in traumatic tetraplegia: A review of 41 patients. J. Bone Joint Surg. 65B:291–298, 1983.

The authors review 41 patients with traumatic tetraplegia in whom various reconstructive tendon transfers were performed. The improvement in the functional status of the patients was uniform although, at times, minimal in nature.

Takami, H.; Takahashi, S.; and Ando, M.: Latissimus dorsi transplantation to restore elbow flexion to the paralysed limb. J. Hand Surg. [Br.] 9:61–63, 1984.

Transplantation of the latissimus dorsi was useful in restoring active elbow flexion in two patients who presented with brachial plexus lesions.

Tsai, T.-M.; Kalisman, M.; Burns, J.; and Kleinert, H.E.: Restoration of elbow flexion by pectoralis major and pectoralis minor transfer. J. Hand Surg. 8:186–190, 1983.

The authors report four patients who suffered brachial plexus injuries resulting in a loss of flexion of the elbow. Restoration of elbow flexion was achieved by transfer of the insertion of the pectoralis major and minor into the biceps. No neurovascular compromise of the pectoralis was noted.

Nerve Entrapment

Adelaar, R.S.; Foster, W.C.; and McDowell, C.: The treatment of the cubital tunnel syndrome. J. Hand Surg. [Am.] 9:90–95, 1984.

An assessment of treatment of the cubital tunnel syndrome by *in situ* release, submuscular transposition, and anterior subcutaneous transposition of the ulnar nerve revealed no variation in results. Two-thirds of the patients improved and one-third did not.

Gessini, L.; Jandolo, B.; and Pietrangeli, A.: Entrapment neuropathies of the median nerve at and above the elbow. Surg. Neurol. 19:112–116, 1983.

Three cases of median nerve entrapment above the elbow are described. One involved nerve entrapment because of Struther's ligament; the remaining two were caused by the lacertus fibrosus (one represented a hematoma secondary to trauma and the other, a hypertrophied brachial muscle). Soft tissue release provided satisfactory results in all three cases.

Werner, C.-O.: Lateral elbow pain and posterior interosseous nerve entrapment. Acta Orthop. Scand. [Suppl.] 174:1–62, 1979.

This extensive analysis of the clinical, laboratory, and long-term results of lateral epicondylitis emphasizes the differential diagnosis of radial entrapment syndrome, characterizes this pathologic process, and states that radial entrapment syndrome coexists with lateral epicondylitis in about 5% of instances.

Total Elbow Replacement

Ewald, F.C., and Jacobs, M.A.: Total elbow arthroplasty. Clin. Orthop. 182:137–142, 1984.

In the authors' 8-year experience with a nonconstrained resurfacing elbow prosthesis, only 1 case in 153 had loosening. Soft tissue complications, including dislocation, ulnar nerve neuropathy, and instability, remained to be resolved.

Greene, W.B.: Use of continuous passive slow motion in the postoperative rehabilitation of difficult pediatric knee and elbow problems. J. Pediatr. Orthop. 3:419–423, 1983.

The use of continuous passive motion at a very low rate of speed (one revolution per 12.5 minutes) proved effective in maintaining and enhancing elbow motion after surgical intervention in seven pediatric patients, of whom four presented with hemophilic changes. Hospital stays were decreased.

Gschwend, N.: Salvage procedure in failed elbow prosthesis. Arch. Orthop. Trauma Surg. 101:95–99, 1983.

A technique for reconstruction of the distal humeral condyles deficient after failure of total elbow replacement is described. Use of iliac wing grafts with AO plate fixation usually gave good results, with a mobile, useful elbow in four patients.

Johnson, J.R.; Getty, C.J.M.; Lettin, A.W.F.; and Glasgow, M.M.S.: The Stanmore total elbow replacement for rheumatoid arthritis. J. Bone Joint Surg. 66B:732–736, 1984.

The authors report on 50 total elbow replacements, performed in rheumatoid arthritis patients, in which a stemmed prosthesis was utilized. Forty-four patients were reviewed; 77% had good results. Complications included failure to develop an adequate arc of motion postoperatively, postoperative ulnar neuropathy, wound dehiscence, infection, and loosening. From an overall point of view, the procedure is recommended in patients with far-advanced destructive changes in the elbow.

Lowe, L.W.; Miller, A.J.; Allum, R.L.; and Higginson, D.W.: The development of an unconstrained elbow arthroplasty. A clinical review. J. Bone Joint Surg. 66B:243–247, 1984.

In a review of 47 elbow replacements performed in 44 patients, a high rate of loosening with a nonstemmed design is reported. Patients with post-traumatic arthritis also had poorer postoperative results. A subsequent design using an ulnar stem and humeral stem had a decreased rate of postoperative aseptic loosening.

Pritchard, R.W.: Anatomic surface elbow arthroplasty. A preliminary report. Clin. Orthop. 179:223–230, 1983.

The importance of utilizing a radial head replacement in nonconstrained total elbow arthroplasty is described. Load sharing and enhanced stability are thought to be the identifiable benefits.

Rosenberg, G.M., and Turner, R.H.: Nonconstrained total elbow arthroplasty. Clin. Orthop. 187:154–162, 1984.

Twenty-four of 28 surface replacements (condylar-capitellar design) with a mean of 35 months' follow-up were reported as satisfactory. Only one failure from loosening occurred, but four cases were complicated by postoperative dislocation.

Rydholm, U.; Tjörnstrand, B.; Pettersson, H.; and Lidgren, L.: Surface replacement of the elbow in rheumatoid arthritis: Early results with the Wadsworth prosthesis. J. Bone Joint Surg. 66B:737–741, 1984.

In 19 total elbow surface replacements in 15 patients with rheumatoid arthritis, two-thirds of the patients were pleased with the pain relief and range of motion when reviewed at an average follow-up of 30 months. More than half had radiographic loosening of the humeral component and two required reoperation, one because of loosening and one because of infection.

Soni, R.K., and Cavendish, M.E.: A review of the Liverpool elbow prosthesis from 1974 to 1982. J. Bone Joint Surg. 66B:248–253, 1984.

In 80 patients in whom the nonconstrained Liverpool elbow prosthesis was used, over half reported excellent results. Ten percent required a revision operation because of loosening and six patients, all with rheumatoid arthritis, required removal (in four, because of deep infection).

Surace, A., and Pietrogrande, V.: Total replacement of knee and elbow in hemophilia: Three cases. Int. Surg. 68:85–88, 1983.

Three cases of hemophilic arthropathy are discussed. In one case, total elbow arthroplasty was performed. Postoperatively, an improvement in the arc of motion in flexion and extension and in pronation and supination were noted.

Sepsis

Morrey, B.F., and Bryan, R.S.: Infection after total elbow arthroplasty. J. Bone Joint Surg. 65A:330–338, 1983.

The authors report 14 cases of deep sepsis after total elbow arthroplasty in 150 patients. The high rate of infection (9%) was attributed to the following factors: high-risk patients presenting with rheumatoid arthritis, history of prior operation, and need for additional operation after the arthroplasty, which appeared to predispose to deep infection. Resection arthroplasty was required to arrest the infection in 10 patients; 8 of these reported a satisfactory result.

21
Wrist and Hand: Trauma

Greater emphasis is currently being placed on accurate reduction and stabilization after Colles' fracture, particularly in younger patients. It is now clear that residual displacement and angulation of scaphoid fractures not only may predispose to nonunion but also may lead to radiographically evident post-traumatic arthritis. Accurate reduction and stabilization of scaphoid fractures and nonunions is currently recommended. Although replantation has been a major advance in the treatment of hand and finger amputations, replantation of a single amputated finger remains controversial. The most common cause for early failure after replantation is vascular thrombosis; salvage by reoperation occasionally is possible.

Carpal Vascular Anatomy

The carpal blood supply is an important factor in the incidence of osteonecrosis after carpal fractures and dislocations. By using latex injection techniques, the intraosseous arterial supply to the carpal bones has been defined and divided into three groups based on the number and location of entry vessels and the presence of intraosseous anastomoses.

The bones in the first group, including the scaphoid, the capitate, and 20% of the lunates, are supplied by single vessels and are at the greatest risk for osteonecrosis. Seventy percent of the scaphoid is supplied by a vessel entering through the dorsal ridge and extending proximally. Fractures often disrupt this vessel, explaining the significant incidence of proximal pole osteonecrosis after scaphoid fractures. Likewise, the capitate is supplied by a single vessel which enters distally and extends proximally into the neck and head and is subject to disruption after fractures through the neck of the capitate. The lunate is supplied by a single vessel 20% of the time, thus rendering it subject to osteonecrosis (Kienböck's disease).

The bones in the second group, trapezoid and hamate, have at least two areas of vessel entry but there may be a lack of intraosseous anastomoses. Osteonecrosis has not been reported in these bones.

In the third group the bones are the trapezium, triquetrum, pisiform, and 80% of the lunates. They receive nutrient arteries through two nonarticular surfaces which have intraosseous anastomoses and, thus, no large area of bone is dependent on a single vessel. These bones are protected from osteonecrosis.

Wrist Injuries

Colles' Fractures

Although most of these can be managed successfully by closed reduction and cast immobilization, external fixation of unstable fractures of the distal radius, particularly in young patients with associated soft tissue loss, has gained popularity. Satisfactory results may be obtained by using any type of quadrilateral frame. Two pins are placed at the bases of the index and middle finger metacarpals (60° to 90° to each other) and two pins are placed in the radius (8 cm proximal to the styloid to avoid damage to the sensory branches of the radial nerve) at a similar angle. Reduction is accomplished and a quadrilateral frame is applied (Fig. 1). The key to maintaining reduction and preventing radial shortening is anatomic alignment of the volar cortex of the radius. Despite satisfactory functional and anatomic results in the majority of patients, complications (particularly pin track infections) persist. Future improvements in pin design and insertion may minimize this complication. If satisfactory reduction cannot be achieved by closed means, open reduction may be necessary.

Persistent neuropathy of the median nerve is a common complication after fractures of the distal radius and probably occurs more frequently than is generally appreciated. Positioning the wrist in marked flexion and ulnar deviation (Cotton-Loder position) is generally condemned and contributes to median nerve dysfunction. Carpal canal pressure measurement with a wick catheter is a reliable technique for assessing median nerve dysfunction in patients with carpal tunnel syndrome. Of patients with Colles' fractures treated in 40° of wrist flexion, nearly 50% have carpal canal pressures that can lead to impairment of median nerve function. Thus, in patients with Colles' fractures who require wrist flexion to maintain reduction and who have evidence of median nerve dysfunction, the wrist should be positioned in a more neutral or slightly flexed position. If median dysfunction persists, one should consider a carpal tunnel decompression. If the fracture is unstable the fracture reduction should be maintained with pins and plaster cast or an external fixation device.

Scaphoid Fractures

It is generally accepted that early plaster cast immobilization of nondisplaced scaphoid fractures will lead to union; however, the treatment of acutely displaced fractures and nonunions and the role of internal fixation in the treatment of these fractures remains controversial.

Recent retrospective studies have shown that, in nearly all patients with untreated scaphoid nonunions, radiographically apparent osteoarthritis will develop and become progressively more extensive over time. During the first decade after fracture, resorption and sclerosis of the fracture margins and cyst formation are found. During the second decade, radio-scaphoid joint space narrowing and beaking of the radial styloid occur. Ultimately, most patients have generalized wrist arthritis and carpal collapse. This process is accelerated by the presence of a displaced

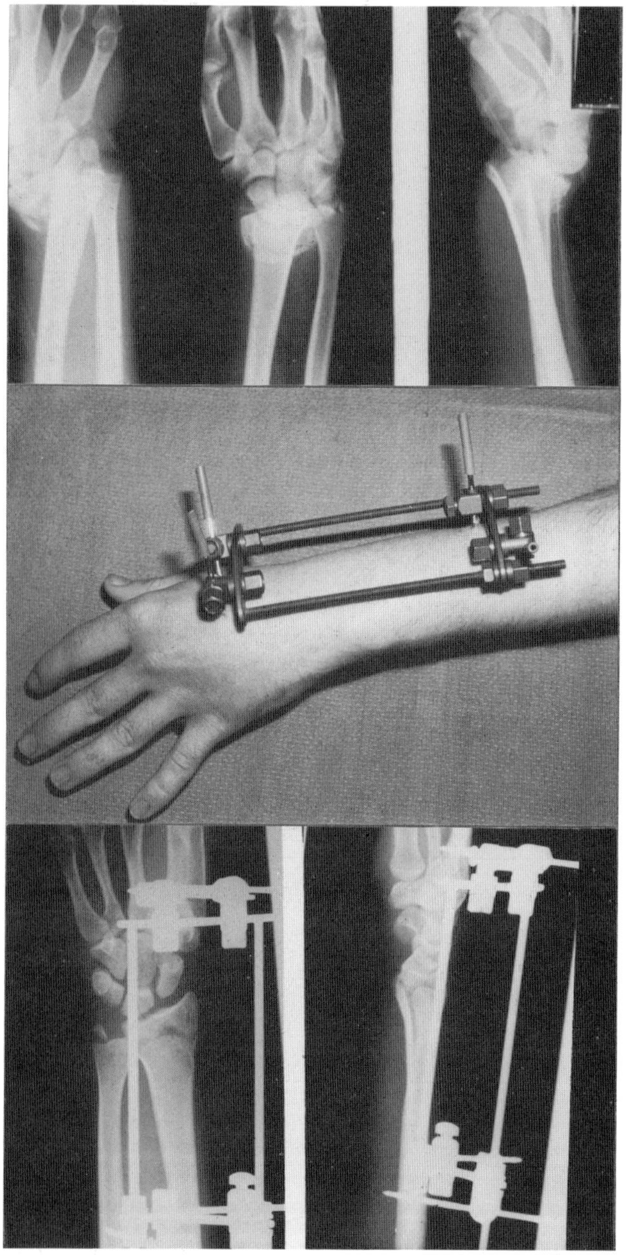

Figure 1

Top, Comminuted intra-articular fracture of distal radius and ulna. *Middle,* Quadrilateral frame for external fixation has been applied. *Bottom,* Radiographs show two threaded half-pins in radial shaft and single pins in the proximal index and middle metacarpals. Pins are in planes 60° to 90° to each other.

nonunion (cortical offset of more than 1 mm) or carpal instability as evidenced by more than 10° of lunate dorsiflexion (the angle formed by the longitudinal axis of the radius and the horizontal axis of the lunate).

Hence, even if asymptomatic, patients with scaphoid nonunions should be advised of the strong possibility of future osteoarthritis. For patients with symptomatic, unstable, or displaced nonunions, one should recommend treatment to secure union.

Many series have demonstrated that the Russe (palmar) approach to the scaphoid, in which the scaphoid is excavated and grafted with cortico-cancellous bone, is successful in 85% to 95% of nonunions. Occasionally, the scaphoid may shorten significantly, and this can lead to carpal instability. Reconstitution of the scaphoid length can be accomplished by measuring the length of the uninjured scaphoid, inserting a wedge-shaped cortico-cancellous graft (apex dorsal) of appropriate size, and stabilizing the graft with Kirschner pins (Fig. 2).

Screw fixation of scaphoid fractures has never gained popularity. It is technically difficult, and the failure rate in several series has been unacceptably high. To circumvent these problems, the Herbert bone screw was designed (Fig. 3). The screw is buried completely within the bone, rarely requires removal, and is designed with threads of different pitch at the trailing and leading ends so as to compress the fracture. Accurate insertion is facilitated through the use of a guiding jig. Results with this screw have been encouraging, particularly in acutely displaced fractures. One series found a union rate of 100%. It must be remembered, however, that success in the treatment of scaphoid non-

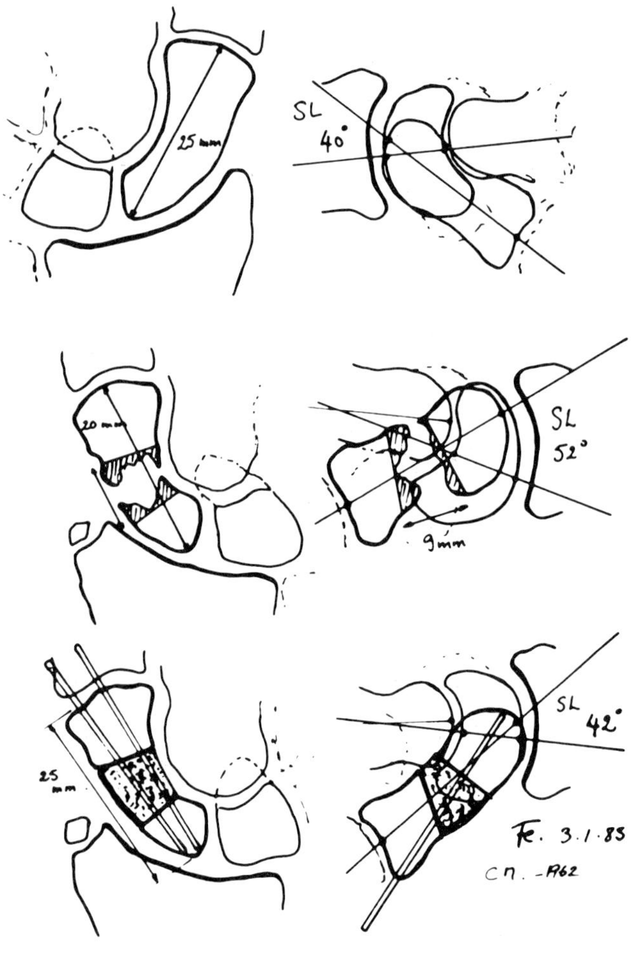

Figure 2

Preoperative planning. *Top,* Tracing of uninjured wrist and measurement of scaphoid length and SL angle. *Middle,* Calculation of size of resection area and form of graft. *Bottom,* Definitive diagram of operation. (From Fernandez, D.L. J. Hand Surg. 9:733–737, 1984. By permission of the American Society for Surgery of the Hand.)

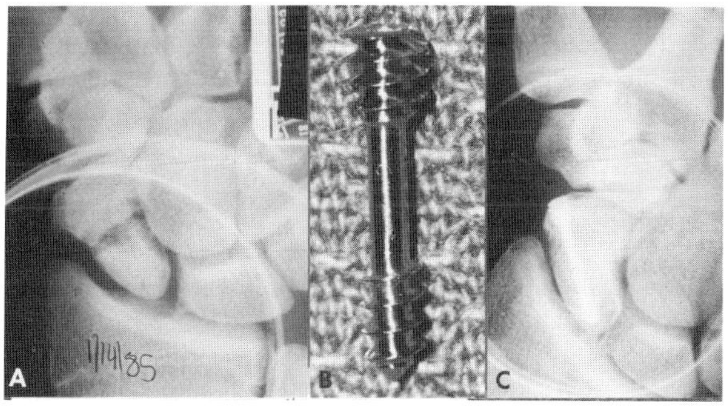

Figure 3

A, Nonunion of the scaphoid. *B*, The Herbert screw. *C*, Herbert screw with cortico-cancellous bone graft was inserted, and union occurred. External immobilization was discontinued 3 weeks postoperatively.

unions with the Herbert screw is comparable to but no better than results with the Russe technique.

Pulsed electromagnetic stimulation in combination with a long-arm-thumb spica cast is also being used to treat scaphoid nonunions. It has the advantage of being noninvasive. A union rate of 80% was reported for one series.

Small, sclerotic, fragmented, nonunited fractures of the proximal pole of the scaphoid usually are not amenable to screw fixation or bone grafting. When symptomatic, excision of the proximal pole is indicated; however, results of excision alone have not always been favorable. Replacement of the proximal pole with a hand-carved silicone spacer has been shown to be a satisfactory solution. Follow-up at a mean of 5 years has not shown carpal collapse or spacer fragmentation. Although this procedure appears preferable to excision alone or to salvage procedures such as complete scaphoid replacement with silicone, proximal row carpectomy, or wrist fusion, in the patient at risk for silicone synovitis (see Chapter 22) alternative forms of reconstruction including tendon or ligament interposition after proximal pole excision should be considered.

Lunotriquetral Instability

Intercarpal instability, particularly disruptions between the scaphoid and lunate, has received much attention recently. Injuries to the ulnar side of the carpus have not been well defined.

Lunotriquetral (LT) sprains vary from a partial tear of the ligaments between these bones to a complete disruption. With a partial tear, there is tenderness dorsally between the lunate and triquetrum. The LT ballottement test is positive (test is performed by fixing the lunate between the index finger and thumb of one hand and displacing the triquetrum and pisiform dorsally and palmarly with the other hand to produce pain or crepitus). With mild sprains, plain radiographs of the wrist are unremarkable. With complete LT disruption, a lateral radiograph of the carpus shows the lunate to be palmar flexed (distal lunate concavity facing palmarward) to give the volar intercalary segmental instability (VISI) pattern.

Treatment depends on the severity of the disruption. When it is recognized acutely, immobilization with plaster usually is successful. Chronic LT disruptions that are not responding to conservative management may require surgical intervention. In the absence of degenerative changes or carpal collapse, repair of the LT interosseous ligaments or LT fusion has given satisfactory results in most patients.

Fractures and Dislocations in the Hand

Intra-articular Fractures of the Metacarpal Head

Intra-articular metacarpal head fractures are usually produced by direct trauma. The index metacarpal head is the one most commonly injured because of its border position and lack of mobility. The size, direction, and degree of comminution of the fracture vary. Comminuted fractures occur most frequently. When the fracture is nondisplaced or highly comminuted, immobilization followed by protected motion is indicated. However, if there are large articular fragments, open reduction and internal fixation through a dorsal approach is indicated. If a stable reduction can be achieved, early active mobilization is recommended, and a satisfactory result usually will ensue.

Traumatic Bone Loss

Complex hand injuries with bone loss often result in marked stiffness. Failure to reconstitute the skeletal framework precludes reconstruction of joints and tendons which require bony stability to function properly.

Wounds with bone loss require skeletal stabilization as a part of the initial wound management. This can be achieved with spacer wires, transfixing wires, or an external fixator. Traditionally, bone grafting has been delayed by weeks or months because of fear of infection. However, it has become increasingly apparent that autogenous bone graft can be safely placed into wounds that are surgically clean at 3 to 10 days after injury if the wound can be immediately closed or covered with a local or distant flap. The advantages of delayed primary grafting include elimination of dead space caused by the bone loss, graft placement into a well-vascularized bed, greater ease in maintaining skeletal length, minimizing recovery time, and securing primary bone union which is conducive to preserving joint and tendon mobility.

Shaft Fractures of the Proximal Phalanx

Inadequate reduction of displaced shaft fractures of the proximal phalanx can lead to significant functional loss secondary to shortening, angulation, and malrotation. Fractures, particularly transverse ones, through the phalangeal base tend to angulate (apex palmar). Reduction usually is simple and is accomplished by axial traction through the middle phalanx while flexing the metacarpophalangeal joint to 60° to 80°. However, maintenance of reduction with plaster immobilization is difficult. Pseudoclawing (metacarpophalangeal hyperextension and proximal interphalangeal flexion) ensues if the reduction is lost. It has been shown recently that closed reduction and percutaneous Kirschner pin fixation can produce excellent results in most patients. The technique involves the administration of an appropriate anesthetic, closed reduction as described above, and percutaneous insertion of one or two longitudinal Kirschner pins through the metacarpal head and into the distal subchondral portion of the proximal phalanx. The fracture and adjacent digit are immobilized for 3 weeks; then the pin(s) is removed and active motion is initiated. By 6 weeks after fracture, satisfactory motion usually can be achieved.

Digital Performance After Phalangeal Fractures

Restoration of function after phalangeal fractures is influenced by three broad categories: patient factors, fracture factors, and management factors.

Patient factors such as motivation and general health may strongly influence the final result. In addition, recovery of total active motion is directly proportional to the patient's age. After age 50, patients with phalangeal fractures regain 50% of total active motion whereas before age 50, 70% is regained.

Extra-articular, noncomminuted fractures that are displaced minimally or not at all can be expected to gain more total active motion than intra-articular, comminuted, displaced phalangeal fractures. Likewise, concomitant injury to the soft tissue (skin, tendon, nerve, or artery) has a detrimental influence on fracture outcome.

The treating physician cannot modify these patient factors (age) or fracture characteristics, but the therapeutic regimen also influences the outcome. The major decision is whether or not to use internal fixation of the fracture. General indications for internal fixation include unstable fractures in which it is impossible to maintain satisfactory alignment with splinting, intra-articular or displaced periarticular fractures, and fractures associated with soft tissue damage. Early mobilization after a phalangeal fracture can be expected to produce a more favorable outcome than prolonged splinting; however, a satisfactory final total active motion can be expected if a fracture is immobilized for no more than 4 weeks. When mobilization is for more than 4 weeks, there is a precipitous decrease in total active motion.

Palmar Dislocation of the Proximal Interphalangeal Joint

Dorsal dislocations of the proximal interphalangeal joint occur frequently, are usually easy to reduce, and, more often than not, are stable after reduction. Palmar dislocations (base of middle phalanx dislocates palmar to head of proximal phalanx) are uncommon, are often irreducible, and are frequently unstable once reduction has been achieved. A recent study demonstrated that, in addition to disruption of the extensor mechanism where it inserts into the base of the middle phalanx, the palmar plate and one collateral ligament are disrupted. If the injury is recognized immediately, percutaneous pinning of the proximal interphalangeal joint in extension for 4 weeks followed by a program of range of motion exercises can give a satisfactory outcome. The majority of patients, however, present 2 to 3 months after injury with a loss of static and dynamic joint support which may result in symptomatic palmar subluxation, malrotation, a boutonniere deformity, or a fixed flexion contracture. Operative intervention is necessary to reduce the joint anatomically and to reattach the damaged soft tissue structures. Although improvement in proximal interphalangeal joint motion can be anticipated, full motion is rarely achieved regardless of treatment modality.

Mallet Fracture

A mallet fracture results when a variable-sized fragment of bone (with attached terminal extensor tendon) avulses from the dorsal base of the distal phalanx. Such fractures occur in approximately one-third of all mallet deformities and occur more frequently on the ulnar side of the hand. Therapeutic recommendations vary from no treatment to splinting to surgical intervention. Palmar subluxation of the terminal phalanx and a fracture involving more than one-third of the articular surface traditionally have been the most common indications for surgical treatment.

A nonrandomized, retrospective study to compare operative intervention with splinting (for a mean of 6 weeks, maintaining the distal interphalangeal joint in full extension) in mallet fractures with a mean follow-up of more than 3 years has been carried out. Age, digit involved, mechanism of injury, size of fragment, and palmar subluxation of the distal phalanx were not factors that influenced the outcome, regardless of treatment modality. Surgical treatment was difficult and did not have any distinct advantage over nonoperative treatment except for an irreducible epiphyseal-physeal injury. Anatomic reduction of the fracture was considered unnecessary for a satisfactory outcome (Fig. 4). Although half of the distal interphalangeal joints showed degenerative changes radiographically, none of the patients had pain and there was a mean range of motion of the joint of 65°. The major "complication" in both treatment groups was a bump over the joint but this had no functional significance. Thus, nonoperative treatment of mallet fractures, regardless of fragment size or subluxation, is considered safe and reliable; however, additional studies are necessary to determine the role of internal fixation in the management of fracture subluxations.

Acute Tendon Injuries

Despite recent advances in understanding of flexor tendon anatomy, healing, and nutrition, full functional restoration remains a challenge, particularly within "no-man's land" (metacarpophalangeal joint to superficialis insertion).

Primary tenorrhaphy of both tendons with postoperative controlled motion is the treatment of choice for clean flexor tendon lacerations in this area. Suture techniques for repairing the severed tendon ends vary but the majority call for a nonabsorbable core or grasping suture to approximate the tendon end-to-end atraumatically followed by a small

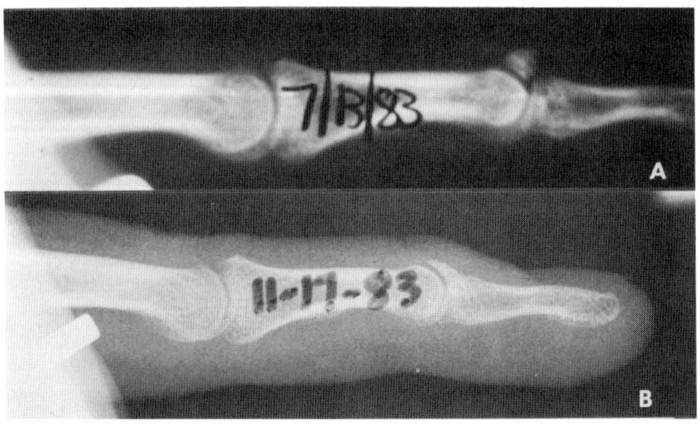

Figure 4

A, Lateral view of displaced mallet fracture involving 40% of the distal interphalangeal articular surface. *B*, Joint was splinted in extension for 6 weeks. Note healed fracture and full *active* extension.

circumferential suture to tidy the repair. Closure of the sheath is controversial. In the past, excision of a portion of the sheath was recommended to facilitate mechanical gliding of the tendons. More recently, sheath closure has been recommended because it prevents the ingrowth of restrictive adhesions and minimizes the chance for the repair to impinge (trigger) where the sheath has been cut.

Historically, flexor tendon repairs were immobilized for 3 to 4 weeks to avoid disruption of the repair. It was thought that extrinsic tendon adhesions were necessary for tendon healing. Experimentally, however, it has been demonstrated that extrinsic adhesions that are precipitated by sheath injury, tendon suture, or immobilization are not essential for tendon healing. Tendons that are mobilized after repair not only may heal without adhesion ingrowth but also may have a greater ultimate tensile load strength and greater mobility than immobilized tendons. Clinically, postoperative mobilization involves the application of a dorsal splint to block wrist and metacarpophalangeal joint extension but to allow full interphalangeal joint extension. Mobilization without producing tension on the repair is accomplished by allowing either active digital extension or passive digital flexion.

Nerve Grafting for Digital Nerve Defects

Laceration of a digital nerve is a frequent cause of loss of hand sensibility and is very disabling in patients whose occupation requires precise control of fingertips. The sensory deficit is even more disabling if both digital nerves are injured or if the radial digital nerve to the index finger is severed. Often, an injury will produce a segmental nerve defect. If a digital neurorrhaphy requires digital flexion to prevent postoperative disruption or repair is done under tension, it is nearly always doomed to failure. In such patients, a digital nerve graft may be necessary. The lateral antebrachial cutaneous nerve, located just deep to the cephalic vein in the antecubital crease, is an excellent donor nerve. It is locally convenient, produces minimal donor morbidity (loss of sensibility in the lateral forearm), and is a good size match because its fascicular area is similar to that of the digital nerve. In addition, because the nerve bifurcates 5 to 6 cm distal to the antecubital crease, it can be used as a Y graft to bridge a gap between a common digital nerve and two proper digital nerves. Other nerves such as the medial antebrachial cutaneous and the posterior interosseous (at the wrist) also can be used to bridge digital nerve defects.

Use of the lateral antebrachial cutaneous nerve to bridge a digital nerve defect produced nearly normal sensibility in two-thirds of patients followed for 14 months or more. The most important prognostic indicator for return of functional sensibility was age less than 20 years. The length of the graft and time interval from injury to grafting did not correlate well with the final results.

Replantation

Indications for replantation in the hand include amputation of the thumb, multiple digits, or part or all of the palm. With improved microsurgical techniques, most replantation centers achieve a survival rate of 80% or better. However, it is restoration of function rather than survival that is the major determinant of success.

Replantation of a single digit is controversial. Although usually aesthetically acceptable, it is argued that single digit replantation may impair overall hand function and cause unnecessary morbidity. Survival is more likely if one artery and at least two veins are anastomosed. Survival is highest in patients older than 10 years because young children have small-caliber vessels and are subject to anxiety which can produce peripheral vasospasm. If survival is achieved, nearly all proximal interphalangeal joint motion is preserved with replantation distal to the superficialis insertion whereas most proximal interphalangeal joint motion is lost in proximal digital replantation. Two-point discrimination is 10 mm (normal, less than 5 mm) and after the first 12 to 18 months patients rarely complain of cold intolerance. Additional surgical procedures are rarely necessary in distal digital replantation, and patients return to work in just over 2 months. Accordingly, single digit replantation distal to the superficialis insertion is justifiable whereas replantation proximal to the proximal interphalangeal joint generally is not.

A subcategory of the single digital amputation is the ring avulsion injury. This injury has been classified by severity: class I, circulation is intact; class IIA, arterial compromise but no tendon, bone, or nerve injury; class IIB, inadequate circulation with bone, tendon, or nerve injury; class III, complete degloving or amputation.

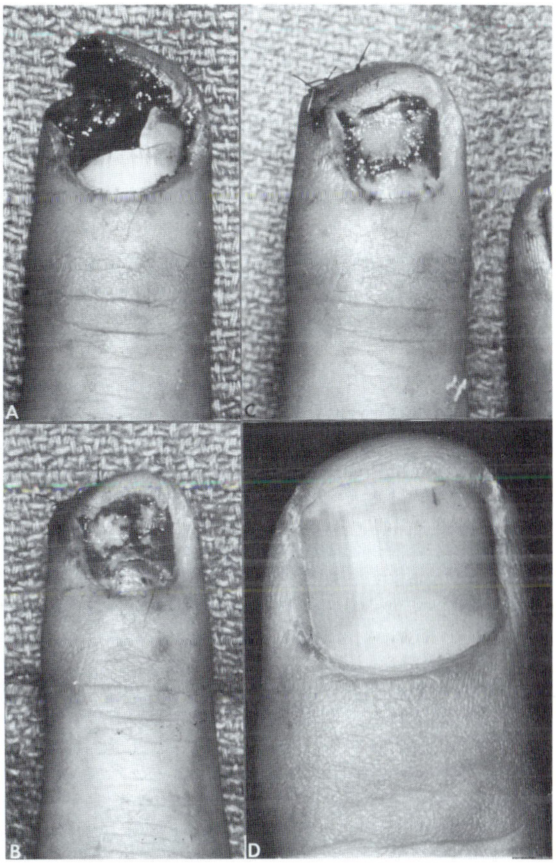

Figure 5

A, Crush injury to finger tip. *B*, Skin repaired, but cortical bone exposed. *C*, Splint nail bed graft from great toe in place. *D*, At 1 year after repair. (Courtesy of Elvin G. Zook, M.D., Springfield, IL.)

Although class IIB and III injuries often can be salvaged by microsurgical techniques, acceptable function is rarely restored and, except for unusual circumstances, primary amputation is recommended. On the other hand, successful revascularization after a class IIA injury (arterial damage alone) can provide a functionally normal digit. The injury is deceptively benign. The arterial injury may be overlooked because the digit has normal sensibility and range of motion as well as capillary refill, albeit delayed. The presence of a diminished digital temperature and the lack of a Doppler tone distal to the injury confirm the diagnosis and are strong indications for exploration and microsurgical arterial repair.

The most common cause for early failure after replantation is vascular thrombosis. Unless this complication is recognized and dealt with, survival is unlikely. It is recognized clinically if a digit becomes pale (arterial insufficiency) or mottled (venous occlusion) or has delayed capillary refill (more than 2 seconds). In addition, if the digital temperature falls to less than 30°C, vascular compromise should be suspected. Nonsurgical measures, including release of a tight dressing or sutures and pharmacologic manipulation (anticoagulation or stellate ganglion blockade), are usually unsuccessful. By far the most effective way to treat impending vascular failure is reexploration and vascular revision. Thrombosis can occur on either the arterial or venous side of the circulation. Salvage by thrombectomy usually is unsuccessful, but insertion of interposition vein grafts can be successful in 40% to 60% of the cases reexplored.

Infections

Optimal treatment of established hand infections is imperative to minimize functional morbidity. *Staphylococcus aureus* remains the major pathogen; however, 60% to 70% of infections are polymicrobial. Anaerobic organisms (particularly *Bacteroides* and *Peptostreptococcus* spp.) can be recovered from 30% to 40% of infections, especially after human bites. Appropriate cultures (aerobic and anaerobic) are mandatory for appropriate antimicrobial management of established wound infections, and specimens should be taken from deep tissues rather than from the wound surface.

In addition to anaerobes, *Eikenella corrodens,* a gram-negative organism, is also a common pathogen in human bite wounds; *Pasteurella multocida,* a gram-negative coccobacillus, is more common after animal bites. Herpetic whitlow is commonly confused with finger pulp space infection. Characteristic skin vesicles help in making the diagnosis. The infection occurs most frequently in health professionals, especially in the dental fields. Treatment is symptomatic. Antimicrobials and debridement are not necessary.

With the emergence of mixed infections, the initial selection of an antimicrobial agent is usually empiric and can be altered subsequently to conform with final culture results. Several recent studies have shown that a first- or second-generation cephalosporin with its broad-spectrum coverage of aerobes and anaerobes is a reasonable choice. Treatment solely with a broad-spectrum agent is not a substitute for surgical drainage and debridement which remain the key to successful treatment of pyogenic infections.

A number of factors contribute to the final outcome, including initial extent of the infection, associated illnesses (diabetes), and anatomic location of the infection. Treatment delay, particularly in infections arising in closed spaces (pulp space, palmar space, tendon sheath, joints), directly correlates with slow resolution and is associated with a high incidence of permanent impairment.

Nail Bed Injuries

Nail bed injuries, particularly those resulting from crush injuries, can produce significant functional and aesthetic

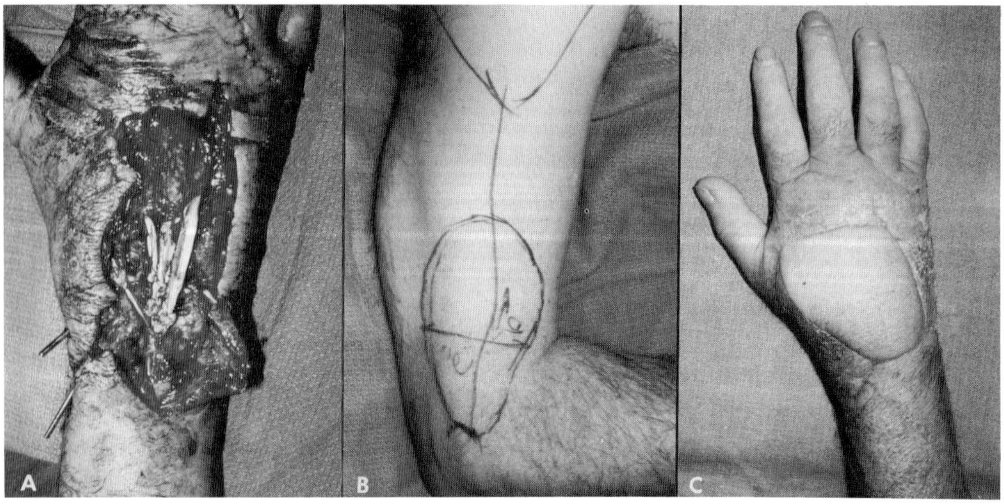

Figure 6

A, Cornpicker injury to hand with open wrist dislocation, multiple extensor tendon lacerations, and dorsal skin loss. *B,* After debridement, free vascularized lateral arm flap from distal lateral brachium provided immediate coverage of the exposed tendons. *C,* Stable coverage at 4 months postoperatively.

problems such as split nail, nail roughness, or lack of adherence of the nail to the underlying matrix. Such deformities can be minimized if the nail plate is removed and the damaged matrix is approximated, under magnification, with fine absorbable sutures. The nail plate should then be replaced not only to minimize postoperative discomfort but also to act as a splint for an underlying fractured distal phalanx and to serve as a template for nail bed approximation.

Sometimes a portion of the sterile matrix (the matrix distal to the lunula) is avulsed and, if it is not replaced, the nail will not adhere. Recent clinical and experimental studies have shown that thin split-thickness nail bed grafts harvested from an uninjured nail bed or from the great toe can be used to fill in the matrix defect and give excellent cosmetic results without producing donor morbidity (Fig. 5).

Soft Tissue Coverage

Large cutaneous defects in the hand require flaps for coverage if there is exposed bone, tendon, nerves, or vessels. Traditionally, pedicled flaps such as from the groin or abdomen have been used; however, these flaps require the hand to be buried in the groin or abdomen for 3 to 4 weeks, making mobilization of uninjured joints difficult and also slowing down the overall reconstructive process. In the past decade, free tissue transfer has become an alternative to conventional pedicle flaps (Fig. 6). Free tissue transfer is defined as the transfer of a composite of tissue with its vascular pedicle from one site in the body to a distant site with viability maintained by microvascular anastomoses between the vascular pedicle and recipient vessels. Free tissue transfer has several advantages. First, tissue can be moved from one place in the body to another during a single operative procedure, thus shortening the overall reconstructive process. Second, free tissue transfer brings a fresh blood supply to the injured bed, which may help minimize infection and promote healing of underlying fractures. Finally, depending on the choice of flap, additional tissue such as bone, tendon, or nerve can be included in the transfer. The major disadvantage of free tissue transfer is that the procedure is technically demanding and it requires a team thoroughly familiar with microvascular techniques and anatomy. Many donor flaps are available, each with advantages and disadvantages, but discussion of this topic is beyond the scope of this chapter.

Annotated Bibliography

Anatomy

Panagis, J.S.; Gelberman, R.H.; Taleisnik, J.; and Baumgaertner, M.: The arterial anatomy of the human carpus. Part II: The intraosseous vascularity. J. Hand Surg. 8:375–382, 1983.

Latex injection studies of the human carpus demonstrated three patterns of arterial vascularity. The scaphoid, capitate, and 20% of the lunates have a single artery, and this correlates clinically with a higher level of osteonecrosis in these bones.

Wrist

Fractures of the Distal Radius

Cooney, W.P.: External fixation of distal radial fractures. Clin. Orthop. 180:44–49, 1983.

A quadrilateral frame was used to stabilize unstable fractures of the Colles and Smith type, with 86% good or excellent results.

Gelberman, R.H.; Szabo, R.M.; and Mortensen, W.W.: Carpal tunnel pressures and wrist position in patients with Colles' fractures. J. Trauma 24:747–749, 1984.

Carpal tunnel pressures measured by the wick catheter method were increased in 23 patients with a Colles' fracture. Wrist flexion produced increased pressure, and it was suggested that median nerve dysfunction may result from plaster immobilization in excessive wrist flexion.

Scaphoid

Beckenbaugh, R.D.: Noninvasive pulsed electromagnetic stimulation in the treatment of scaphoid nonunion (abstract). Orthop. Trans. 9:176, 1985.

Fernandez, D.L.: A technique for anterior wedge-shaped grafts for scaphoid nonunions with carpal instability. J. Hand Surg. [Am.] 9:733–737, 1984.

Long-standing scaphoid nonunions often demonstrate scaphoid shortening and dorsal carpal instability patterns. Restoration of scaphoid length and carpal alignment can be achieved by insertion of a trapezoidal graft (apex dorsal) into the nonunion through an anterior approach, supplemented by internal fixation.

Herbert, T.J., and Fisher, W.E.: Management of the fractured scaphoid using a new bone screw. J. Bone Joint Surg. 66B:114–123, 1984.

A double-threaded compression screw was designed for fixing scaphoid fractures internally. The rate of union was 100% for acute fractures and 83% overall.

Mack, G.R.; Bosse, M.J.; Gelberman, R.H.; and Yu, E.: The natural history of scaphoid non-union. J. Bone Joint Surg. 66A:504–509, 1984.

Ununited scaphoid fractures, particularly when associated with carpal instability, will progress to carpal arthritis. It is recommended that such fractures be reduced and bone grafted, regardless of symptoms.

Ruby, L.K.; Stinson, J.; and Belsky, M.R.: The natural history of scaphoid non-union: A review of fifty-five cases. J. Bone Joint Surg. 67A:428–432, 1985.

Osteoarthritis developed in 97% of scaphoid nonunions present for more than 5 years. The patient should be warned of this.

Zemel, N.P.; Stark, H.H.; Ashworth, C.R.; Rickard, T.A.; and Anderson, D.R.: Treatment of selected patients with an ununited fracture of the proximal part of the scaphoid by excision of the fragment and insertion of a carved silicone-rubber spacer. J. Bone Joint Surg. 66A:510–517, 1984.

Excision of a small ununited proximal pole of the scaphoid and insertion of a silicone spacer allowed return to work and strenuous activities in 95% of patients. Pain relief was significant but grip and range of motion did not change appreciably.

Carpal Instability

Reagan, D.S.; Linscheid, R.L.; and Dobyns, J.H.: Lunotriquetral sprains. J. Hand Surg. [Am.] 9:502–514, 1984.

Lunotriquetral sprains must be considered when there is pain on the ulnar side of the carpus. The diagnosis often requires special studies (arthrogram or motion studies) and treatment depends on the severity of symptoms and the degree of lunotriquetral disassociation.

Metacarpal and Phalangeal Fractures and Dislocations

Metacarpal Head Fractures

McElfresh, E.C., and Dobyns, J.H.: Intra-articular metacarpal head fractures. J. Hand Surg. 8:383–393, 1983.

Intra-articular metacarpal head fractures occur most frequently in the vulnerable border metacarpals. Open anatomic reduction is stressed for large fracture fragments; however, with avulsions and comminuted fractures, treatment must be individualized.

Bone Loss

Freeland, A.E.; Jabaley, M.E.; Burkhalter, W.E.; and Chaves, A.M.V.: Delayed primary bone grafting in the hand and wrist after traumatic bone loss. J. Hand Surg. [Am.] 9:22–28, 1984.

Delayed primary bone grafting (within 10 days after injury) can be performed safely if the wound is surgically clean and there is stable skeletal fixation and secure soft tissue coverage.

Phalangeal Fractures

Belsky, M.R.; Eaton, R.G.; and Lane, L.B.: Closed reduction and internal fixation of proximal phalangeal fractures. J. Hand Surg. [Am.] 9:725–729, 1984.

Displaced extra-articular fractures of the proximal phalanx can be reduced closed by longitudinal traction and metacarpophalangeal flexion and immobilized with a Kirschner pin placed antegrade through the metacarpal head and across the fracture site. Good or excellent results were seen for 90% of fractures.

Strickland, J.W.; Steichen, J.B.; Kleinman, W.B.; and Flynn, N.: Factors influencing digital performance after phalangeal fracture. In Difficult Problems in Hand Surgery, edited by J.W. Strickland and J.B. Steichen, pp. 126–139. St. Louis, C.V. Mosby, 1982.

Four hundred fifteen phalangeal fractures were reviewed retrospectively to determine which factors affect digital motion adversely. The most important included immobilization for more than 4 weeks, concomitant tendon injury, increasing patient age, and comminuted fractures.

Anterior Proximal Interphalangeal Dislocation

Peimer, C.A.; Sullivan, D.J.; and Wild, D.R.: Palmar dislocation of the proximal interphalangeal joint. J. Hand Surg. [Am.] 9:39–48, 1984.

Palmar dislocations of the proximal interphalangeal joint cause disruption of the extensor mechanism, palmar plate, and collateral ligament. Surgical repair is usually indicated and gives satisfactory results; however, no patient regained full motion.

Mallet Fractures

Wehbé, M.A., and Schneider, L.H.: Mallet fractures. J. Bone Joint Surg. 66A:658–669, 1984.

Most mallet fractures can be treated nonoperatively. Lack of anatomic reduction, joint subluxation, fragment displacement, and size are not indications for operative treatment.

Flexor Tendon Injuries

Gelberman, R.H.; Vande Berg, J.S.; Lundborg, G.N.; and Akeson, W.H.: Flexor tendon healing and restoration of the gliding surface: An ultrastructural study in dogs. J. Bone Joint Surg. 65A:70–80, 1983.

Tendon healing is more rapid with early controlled passive motion than with immobilization after repair, supporting the concept that immediate mobilization improves the quality of the biologic repair within the tendon sheath.

Lister, G.D.: Incision and closure of the flexor sheath during primary tendon repair. Hand 15:123–135, 1983.

Sheath closure after tenorrhaphy within the digital flexor sheath is recommended to restrict the ingrowth of extrinsic adhesions which may interfere with tendon gliding.

Strickland, J.W.: Flexor tendon repair. Hand Clin. 1:55–68, February 1985.

Automatic techniques for primary repair of flexor tendons and postoperative controlled mobilization are outlined.

Acute Nerve Injuries

Tenny, J.R., and Lewis, R.C.: Digital nerve-grafting for traumatic defects. J. Bone Joint Surg. 66A:1375–1379, 1984.

The lateral antebrachial cutaneous nerve was used to bridge digital nerve defects. Age, rather than length of graft or time interval from injury to grafting, was the most important prognostic indicator of return of sensibility.

Replantation and Ring Avulsion Injuries

Moneim, M.S., and Chacon, N.E.: Salvage of replanted parts of the upper extremity. J. Bone Joint Surg. 67A:880–883, 1985.

Vascular occlusion after replantation often can be treated successfully by early exploration (within 11 hours after replantation), excision of the thrombosed vessel, and vein grafting. Thrombectomy was not recommended as a salvage procedure.

Nissenbaum, M.: Class IIA ring avulsion injuries: An absolute indication for microvascular repair. J. Hand Surg. [Am.] 9:810–815, 1984.

Class IIA ring avulsion injuries (digital artery compromise with intact bone, tendon, nerve, and veins) can be restored to near-normal function by arterial revascularization. Failure to recognize and treat this injury can result in loss of the digit.

Urbaniak, J.R.; Roth, J.H.; Nunley, J.A.; Goldner, R.D.; and Koman, L.A.: The results of replantation after amputation of a single finger. J. Bone Joint Surg. 67A:611–619, 1985.

Review of 59 single-digit amputations (excluding the thumb) demonstrated that replantation distal to the superficialis was justified but replantation proximal to the superficialis insertion was seldom justified.

Infections

Glass, K.D.: Factors related to the resolution of treated hand infections. J. Hand Surg. 7:388–394, 1982.

Delay in treatment (more than 2 days) was a major cause of delayed resolution of deep hand infections. Other factors associated with the rate of resolution were the adequacy of surgical drainage, efficacy of antimicrobial therapy, and absence of diabetes mellitus.

Stern, P.J.; Staneck, J.L.; McDonough, J.J.; Neale, H.W.; and Tyler, G.: Established hand infections: A controlled, prospective study. J. Hand Surg. 8:553–559, 1983.

Avoidance of complications in established hand infections requires more than treatment with a broad-spectrum antimicrobial. Other factors such as treatment delay, initial extent of infection, cause of infection, and extent of surgical debridement contribute to complications.

Nail Bed Injuries

Shepard, G.H.: Treatment of nail bed avulsions with split-thickness nail bed grafts. J. Hand Surg. 8:49–54, 1983.

After replacement of the nail matrix with a split-thickness nail bed graft taken freehand from either the great toe or injured nail bed, there was no nail deformity in 26 of 31 nail beds so treated. There was no donor site deformity.

Zook, E.G.; Guy, R.J.; and Russell, R.C.: A study of nail bed injuries: Causes, treatment, and prognosis. J. Hand Surg. [Am.] 9:247–252, 1984.

A detailed classification and treatment of 299 nail bed injuries is presented. Follow-up of 184 injuries revealed good or excellent results after surgical repair.

Acute Soft Tissue Loss

Hing, D.N.; Buncke, H.J.; Alpert, B.S.; and Gordon, L.: Free flap coverage of the hand. Hand Clin. 1:741–758, November 1985.

Large traumatic soft tissue defects in the hand can be covered by the transfer of arterialized skin flaps using microvascular techniques in a single operation, thus accelerating the overall rehabilitative process.

22

Wrist and Hand: Reconstruction

Reconstruction of the hand and wrist has benefitted from basic research including the introduction of three-dimensional reconstructions of computed tomograms and a more careful delineation of the biomechanics relevant to tendon transfer. Silicone synovitis and inflammatory reaction apparently secondary to microparticulate fragmentation of silicone implants have caused some tempering of enthusiasm for the use of such implants in the wrist. Because of the critical role of the distal ulna in wrist stability, in selected patients a limited resection of the articular surface of the distal ulna or a distal radio-ulnar joint arthrodesis may provide better wrist function than a Darrach resection.

Diagnostic Evaluation

Three-Phase Bone Scanning

Three-phase bone scans have proved helpful in defining reflex sympathetic dystrophy syndrome and separating it from focal skeletal disorders in the wrist and hand. The technique involves scanning during injection (radionuclide angiogram) and immediately afterward as well as the more conventional 3 to 4 hours after injection. The two early phases may be helpful in localizing a focal disorder in the wrist or hand. A diffusely positive late image, with *all* areas showing increased activity, is considered diagnostic of reflex sympathetic dystrophy, with both sensitivity and specificity greater than 95% (Fig. 1).

Three-Dimensional Computed Tomographic Image Reconstruction

Three-dimensional reconstruction of computed tomograms is an exciting application of modern technology. Similar devices are in use for planning reconstructive facial surgery and stereotactic neurosurgical dissections. Such techniques make possible accurate preoperative localization of a lesion and also provide the opportunity to plan reconstructive procedures such as osteotomy or prosthesis replacement more accurately. By using computer-assisted design techniques, an actual three-dimensional model of the area of interest can be constructed to aid in fabrication of custom prostheses. Mock surgical procedures can be carried out on the model so that the effect of specific reconstruction can be predicted more accurately.

Reconstruction of Bony Defects

Thumb

Reconstruction options for traumatic loss of the thumb include pollicization, metacarpal lengthening, osteoplastic reconstruction, and toe-to-hand transfer. Relative indications depend on the extent of thumb loss, the presence of associated injuries, and patient factors such as age and occupation. In general, however, for amputations proximal to the metacarpophalangeal joint, pollicization or toe transfer is preferred; for more distal levels, pollicization of a damaged digit, toe transfer, or osteoplastic reconstruction is preferred. Osteoplastic reconstruction can be in the form of conventional reconstruction (with iliac bone graft to restore length, groin flap for skin coverage, and neurovascular island pedicle flap to restore sensation) or a wraparound flap (bone graft is covered and sensation is provided by a free microvascular transfer of skin from the great and second toes) (Fig. 2). Recent reports have emphasized the use of the wraparound flap which does not sacrifice a finger or a complete toe and is aesthetically superior to conventional osteoplastic reconstruction. Metacarpal lengthening is an alternative for injuries at or just distal to the metacarpophalangeal joint in cases with good local soft tissue coverage, particularly in younger patients.

Joints

Free vascularized joint transfers are a treatment option to consider in the management of post-traumatic metacarpophalangeal or proximal interphalangeal joint loss. The tissue to be transferred can be harvested from the second toe or an injured, unsalvageable finger and is particularly useful in a pediatric patient when a functional epiphysis can be transferred as well as in a young, active patient when arthrodesis may be undesirable and arthroplasty may be unreliable. As much as 90° of motion in the transferred joint is possible, with an average of about 45° in the cases reported to date.

Bones

For the metacarpals, allograft replacement may be an alternative to conventional bone grafting in cases of segmental defect and provides an opportunity to replace the distal articular surface as well. In a series of 12 cases in which allograft was used as an intercalated graft for segmental metacarpal defects of 1.3 to 4.0 cm, only one nonunion was reported.

Reconstruction for Arthritis

Proximal Interphalangeal Joints

At present, arthrodesis, volar plate interposition, and silicone replacement arthroplasty remain the mainstays for reconstruction of the proximal interphalangeal joint. In selected cases, perichondrial resurfacing arthroplasty also may be indicated. In this technique, the damaged articular surface to be replaced is denuded of cartilage and resurfaced with rib perichondrium. If both sides of a joint are resurfaced, a silicone sheet is inserted to prevent ankylosis

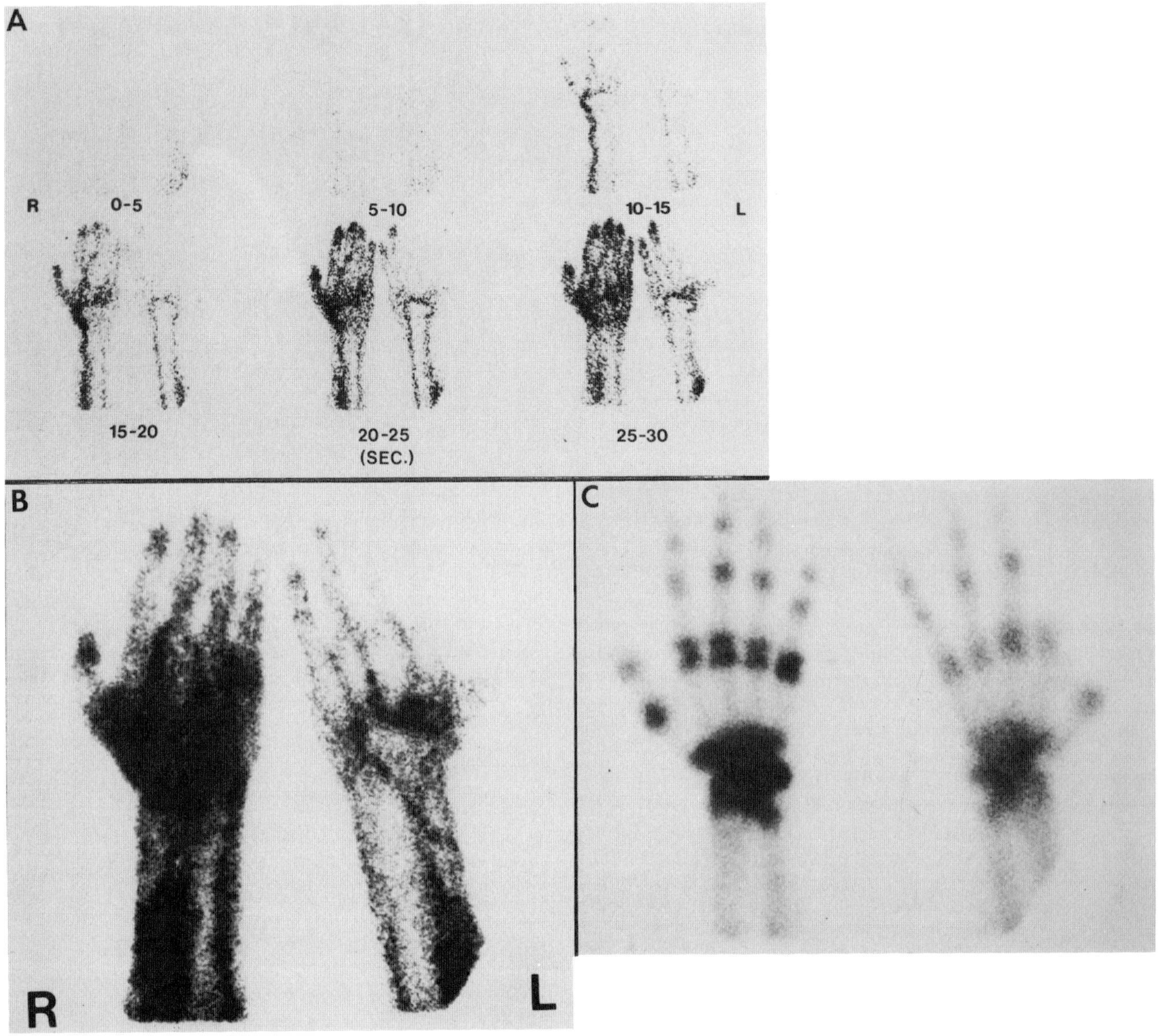

Figure 1

Diffusely abnormal three-phase bone scan. Clinical diagnosis: Reflex sympathetic dystrophy. *A,* Increased perfusion of wrist and digits in right hand compared with uninvolved left hand. *B,* Blood pool image. Diffusely increased relative vascularity in wrist and digits. *C,* Delayed image. Diffusely increased activity throughout radiocarpal, intercarpal, and carpometacarpal joints. (From Mackinnon, S.E., and Holder, L.E. J. Hand Surg. [Am.] 9:556–563, 1984. By permission of the American Society for Surgery of the Hand.)

in the early postoperative period. The sheet is removed at a second surgical procedure. The mean gain in motion in the series reported to date is 14° which is roughly the same as that provided by silicone replacement arthroplasty. The procedure is indicated particularly in patients under age 30 with degenerative or post-traumatic arthritis. Rheumatoid arthritis, old sepsis, and bony defects are considered to be contraindications to the technique, and arthrodesis or joint replacement is preferred.

Metacarpophalangeal Joints

Although silicone replacement arthroplasty remains the benchmark arthroplasty of the metacarpophalangeal joint, a new pyrolytic carbon resurfacing arthroplasty holds promise for the future. Unlike other finger joint replacements, this prosthesis is completely unconstrained and aims to resurface the joint anatomically. The pyrolytic carbon surface allows for biologic fixation. Because the implant is unconstrained, soft tissues must be adequate to provide joint stability or dislocation may occur. In stable joints, motion of up to 90° can be achieved.

Perichondrial resurfacing arthroplasty is also an alternative at the metacarpophalangeal joint level. As at the proximal interphalangeal joint, it is recommended that the procedure be limited to children or young adults with post-traumatic arthritis. A mean gain of 22° in metacarpophalangeal joint motion has been reported.

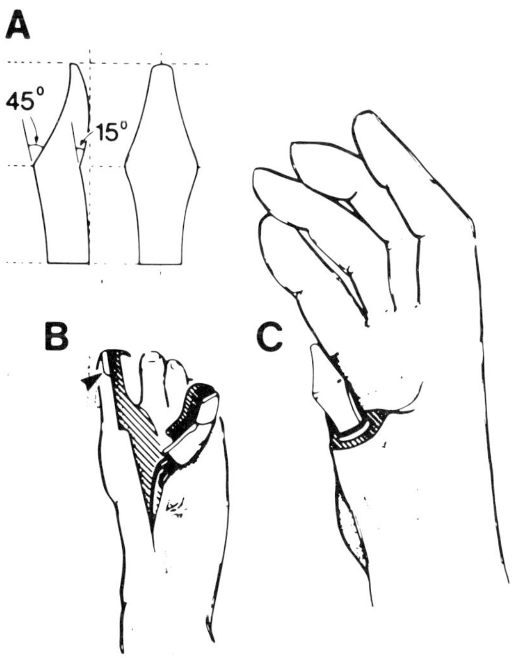

Figure 2

Neurovascular wraparound flap from big toe. *A,* Iliac crest bone graft is shaped to resemble combined distal and proximal phalanx. *B,* Toe flap is elevated with dorsal vessels and nerves; toe distal phalanx is shortened. Donor site coverage is from local flaps, skin grafts, and cross toe flaps. *C,* Graft is arthrodesed to remaining portion of thumb phalanx. Wraparound flap covers graft. (From Orthopaedic Knowledge Update I. Chicago, American Academy of Orthopaedic Surgeons, pp. 181–188, 1984.)

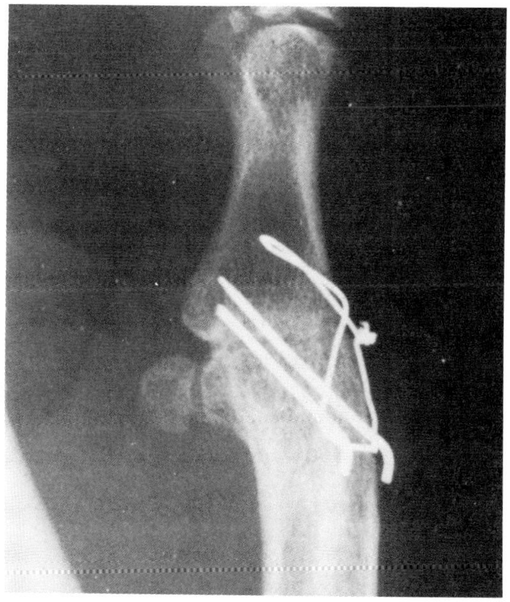

Figure 3

Patient had persistent thumb pain despite solid metacarpophalangeal fusion. Note radiographic appearance of osteophyte in the sesamoid-metacarpal joint surface. Good pain relief was achieved after excision of the sesamoid. (From Trumble, T.E., and Watson, H.K. J. Hand Surg. [Am.] 10:94–100, 1985. By permission of the American Society for Surgery of the Hand.)

Thumb

In the thumb, the sesamoids as well as the proximal phalanx articulate with the metacarpal head. A series of 36 patients with radial sesamoid-metacarpal degenerative arthritis successfully treated with simple sesamoidectomy has been reported. The condition may be confused with metacarpophalangeal joint disease. The differentiation is important in order to avoid unnecessary metacarpophalangeal joint surgery and to direct treatment to the appropriate area. A 45° supination radiograph of the thumb (Fig. 3) is helpful in visualizing the radial sesamoid-metacarpal joint surface. Results of excision generally are good.

Thumb Carpometacarpal Joint

Anatomic studies have shown the importance of the volar and dorsal intermetacarpal ligaments as the main stabilizers of the trapeziometacarpal joint. Long-term studies confirm that, in patients with mild to moderate trapeziometacarpal disease, reconstruction of the ligaments produces a high proportion of good and excellent results. Thumb metacarpal abduction osteotomy is another alternative in the patient with mild to moderate disease. Changing the axis of the thumb metacarpal seems to redirect the line of forces across the joint.

For patients with more advanced isolated trapeziometacarpal disease, trapeziometacarpal arthroplasty or arthrodesis may be considered. If arthroplasty is to be performed, care must be taken to ensure the stability of the restraining ligaments, particularly the intermetacarpal ligaments, to prevent postoperative subluxation. At this time, reported results are similar, comparative studies are few, and the indications for choosing among arthrodesis, cemented metal-plastic arthroplasty, silicone interposition arthroplasty, and tendon interposition arthroplasty of the trapeziometacarpal joint are unclear.

When both the trapeziometacarpal joint and the scaphotrapezial joint are involved, total trapeziectomy is indicated. Reported results of total trapeziectomy suggest little difference between silicone replacement and tendon interposition.

Wrist

A new acronym has appeared in the wrist surgeon's vocabulary—SLAC wrist or *scapholunate advanced collapse*—to describe a typical pattern of degenerative change associated with rotatory subluxation of the scaphoid or scaphoid nonunion in which degenerative changes begin at the radioscaphoid joint and progress to the capitolunate joint, sparing the radiolunate joint (Fig. 4). Proposed reconstruction includes capitolunate arthrodesis, usually combined with scaphoid excisional arthroplasty.

For the rheumatoid wrist, attention has turned to the problem of carpal subluxation, particularly that after distal ulnar resection. In this group of patients, the midcarpal joint may be relatively spared. If so, radioscapholunate or

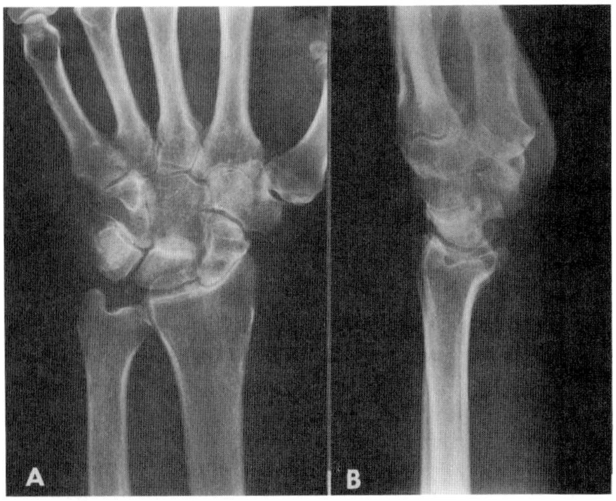

Figure 4

A, Typical appearance of scapholunate advance collapse (SLAC). Note degenerative changes in radioscaphoid and capitolunate with sparing of the radiolunate joint. *B,* Lateral view shows erosions in the radius and dorsiflexed posture of the lunate.

radiolunate arthrodesis may be considered as an alternative to total wrist replacement or total wrist fusion.

A number of reports have emphasized potential hazards of silicone replacement arthroplasty, particularly of the scaphoid or lunate. "Silicone synovitis" describes the generalized foreign body giant cell reaction and focal bony destruction secondary to fragmentation of silicone implants (Fig. 5). This reaction to the silicone apparently is not to it as a chemical compound but rather is a mechanical response to the small particles generated by implant wear. The incidence of the problem is unknown but the implant manufacturer has recommended that all patients who have or are considering silicone replacement arthroplasty be cautioned of the risk of silicone synovitis. The risk seems highest with scaphoid and lunate implants in young, physically active patients and when cysts or other degenerative changes are noted preoperatively. Use of K-wires or sutures passing through silicone implants for temporary postoperative stabilization is no longer advised because this may predispose to silicone synovitis. If diagnosis is delayed, destructive changes may spread to involve joints not immediately adjacent to the silicone implant. Once silicone synovitis is diagnosed, synovectomy and implant removal are indicated. Intercarpal arthrodesis, wrist arthrodesis, or proximal row carpectomy may also be necessary, depending on the circumstances. Large bone cysts may require grafting. In all cases reported thus far, the synovitis has not recurred after implant removal and synovectomy. Although silicone particles also have been found occasionally in lymph nodes in autopsy specimens, at present there is no evidence that the silicone particles have a systemic toxicity or are in any way oncogenic.

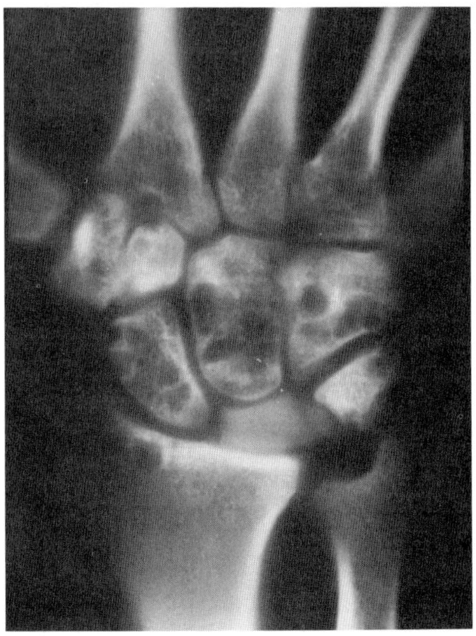

Figure 5

Radiographic appearance of silicone synovitis. Note fragmentation of lunate implant on this tomographic view with multiple cyst formation in the radius and remaining carpal bones.

The occurrence of other complications after silicone replacement arthroplasty is causing a general reevaluation of the indications for these procedures, particularly at the lunate and scaphoid. A recent study of scaphoid replacement found a high incidence of implant subluxation. Nearly a third of the patients required subsequent revision surgery. Average grip and motion were not significantly improved after operation, and carpal collapse and degeneration progressed after prosthetic implantation. A long-term study of lunate implants likewise found progression of degenerative changes postoperatively and emphasized the importance of carpal stability to the quality of results postoperatively. If such stability is not present preoperatively, intercarpal arthrodesis or other procedures may be helpful in restoring stability and "protecting" the implant from compressive stress.

Distal Radio-Ulnar Joint

The importance of the distal ulna to wrist stability is now clear. The ulna represents the proximal anchor for the triangular fibrocartilage complex (TFCC), acting as both volar and ulnar buttress against carpal migration. In young, active patients and patients with rheumatoid arthritis, distal ulnar resection may result in a form of radiocarpal instability with pain and weakness as the carpus slides ulnarly and volarly in response to removal of this buttress. For such patients at risk for this problem, treatment options for distal radio-ulnar joint disease should include hemi-resection arthroplasty (Fig. 6) and distal radio-ulnar joint arthrodesis with distal ulna shaft segmental resection to permit forearm rotation (the Lauenstein procedure) (Fig. 7). Both of these options preserve the triangular fibrocartilage complex and its stabilizing effect. A second problem with distal ulnar resection may be over-resection that causes distal ulnar instability or extensor tendon rupture. In some patients, a painful convergent snapping of the ulna on the radius may occur. No satisfactory treatment is available for this distal ulnar impingement syndrome at the present time, and the best recommendation is to minimize resection of the distal ulna.

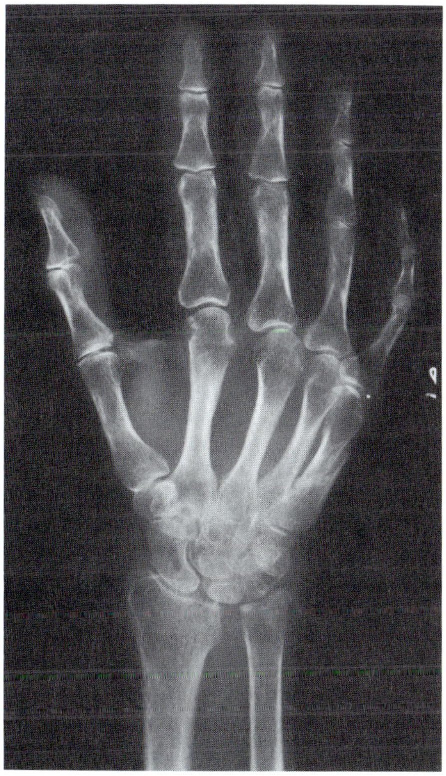

Figure 6

Hemi-resection arthroplasty of distal radio-ulnar joint in a 50-year-old woman with rheumatoid arthritis.

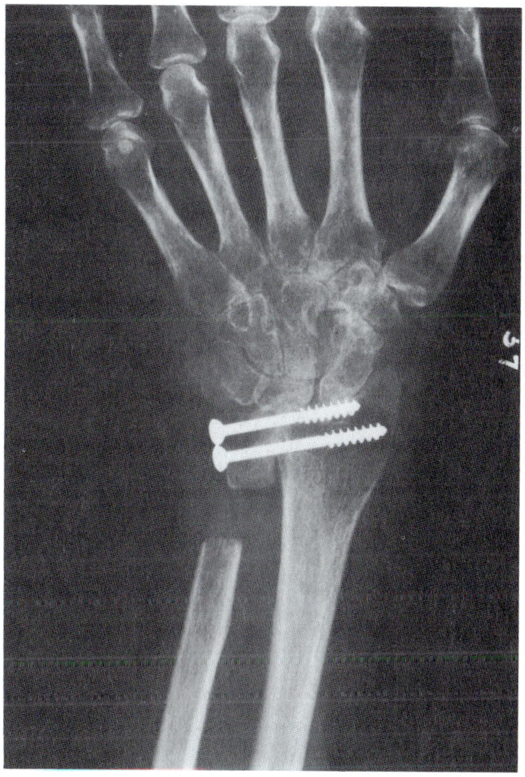

Figure 7

Arthrodesis of the distal radio-ulnar joint with proximal ulnar resection (Lauenstein procedure).

Reconstruction for Nerve Injury

Reconstruction after spinal cord injury remains a challenging problem. There is now general agreement on a classification of injuries that is based on sensibility (ocular or cutaneous) and number of functioning muscles distal to the elbow (Table 1). Treatment principles have become more uniform. It is essential to await neurologic stabilization, psychologic acceptance, and completion of basic rehabilitation before considering surgical reconstruction of the upper extremities. For this reason, it is inappropriate to consider upper extremity reconstruction in most patients until at least a year after injury. Some patients will never reach a stable point at which surgical upper extremity reconstruction can reasonably be considered. Adequate postoperative rehabilitation and social support must also be in place before reconstruction is performed.

It is now generally agreed that, for the quadriplegic patient, side rather than tip or chuck pinch is to be preferred and arthrodeses are generally avoided, especially in the insensate hand. In hands with cutaneous sensibility (functioning C-6 root or lower), thumb carpometacarpal joint arthrodesis may help to stabilize the thumb after transfers to restore active pinch.

In patients with group I function (Table 1), transfer of the brachioradialis to the wrist extensors combined with flexor pollicis longus tenodesis and thumb interphalangeal joint stabilization, as recommended by Moberg, has proved to be a reliable treatment option for many patients. Some patients in groups II and III may benefit from transfer of the brachioradialis to the flexor pollicis longus for active pinch. An alternative transfer for the thumb in this group would be to prolong the brachioradialis with a flexor digitorum superficialis graft through the carpal tunnel and then insert it as an opponens-plasty.

In groups IV and V, some patients may also benefit from tendon transfers to restore active finger flexion by using the brachioradialis, pronator teres, or extensor carpi radialis longus as the motor. Of course, if the extensor carpi radialis longus tendon is to be used as a transfer, it is extremely important to be absolutely certain that the extensor carpi radialis brevis is indeed functioning. Some

Table 1. International Classification (Modified) of Upper Extremity Involvement in Spinal Cord Injury

Group	Muscles functioning
0	Weak BR (≤grade 3*)
I	BR (≥grade 4*)
II	BR, ECRL
III	BR, ECRL, ECRB
IV	BR, ECRL, ECRB, PT
V	BR, ECRL, ECRB, PT, FCR
VI	BR, ECRL, ECRB, PT, FCR, finger extensors
VII	BR, ECRL, ECRB, PT, FCR, finger and thumb extensors
VIII	Lacks only intrinsics

BR, brachioradialis; ECRB, extensor carpi radialis brevis; ECRL, extensor carpi radialis longus; FCR, flexor carpi radialis; PT, pronator teres.
*Medical Research Council grade.

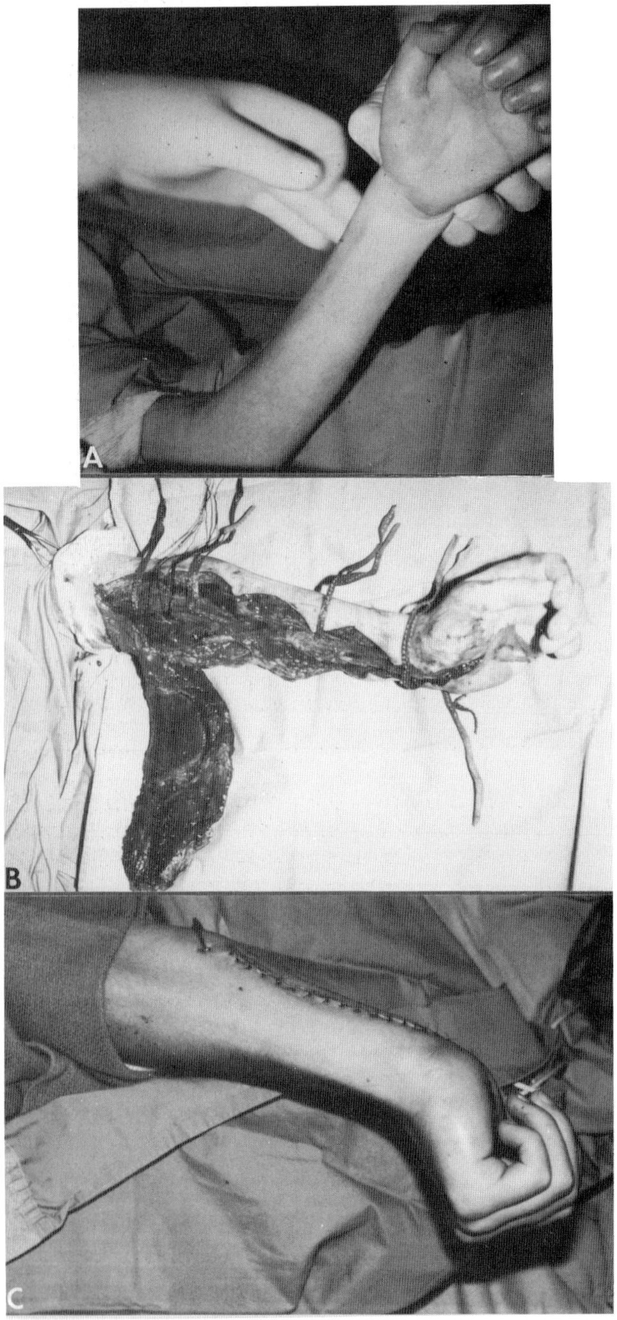

Figure 8

A, Patient had absence of hand flexor function and fixed flexion contracture after crush injury, with resultant Volkmann's ischemic contracture. *B,* Intraoperative view of free functioning latissimus dorsi transfer. *C,* Active finger flexion at tenolysis, 2 years postoperatively. (Courtesy of Michael B. Wood, M.D.)

patients with finger flexion transfers and absence of active finger extension will develop disabling flexion posture of the hand and therefore may also require extensor tenodeses. Patients in groups VI and VII have multiple options for reconstruction of active finger and thumb flexion and possibly some intrinsic function. Patients in group VIII lack only intrinsics and can be treated by standard

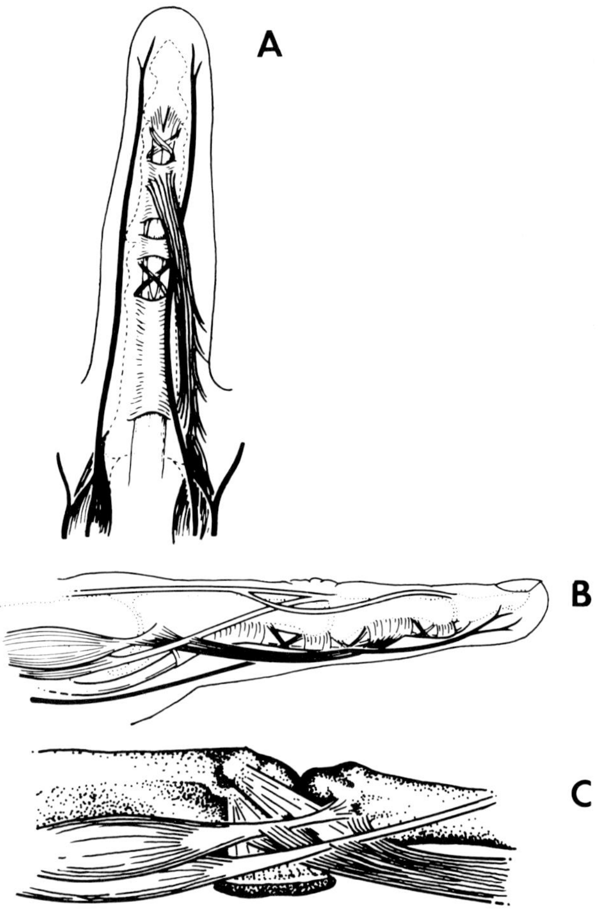

Figure 9

A, Lateral digital cord, palmar view. *B,* Lateral view, showing relationship to neurovascular bundle. *C,* Detailed view of origin of lateral digital cord from periosteum at base of proximal phalanx and collateral ligament of the metacarpophalangeal joint and intrinsic tendons. (From Strickland, J.W., and Bassett, R.L. J. Hand Surg. [Am.] 10:118–124, 1985. By permission of the American Society for Surgery of the Hand.)

techniques to restore intrinsic function as in cases of combined low median and ulnar palsies.

Reconstruction for Muscle and Tendon Deficit

Free functioning muscle transplantation has opened new vistas for the reconstructive surgeon faced with a difficult problem of lack of hand function due to devastating loss of flexor and extensor muscle mass as might occur after a severe crushing injury, burn, or blast injury. Innervated free muscle transfer has proved helpful in restoring muscle function in some cases (Fig. 8). Gracilis is most commonly used, but pectoralis major and latissimus dorsi also may be transferred in this way. Restoration of acceptable finger motion frequently can be achieved, usually with satisfactory strength. Setting of optimal muscle tension is in some respects the most challenging part of the procedure. Suture markers placed at 5-cm intervals along the donor muscle prior to harvest can be reset to that distance after trans-

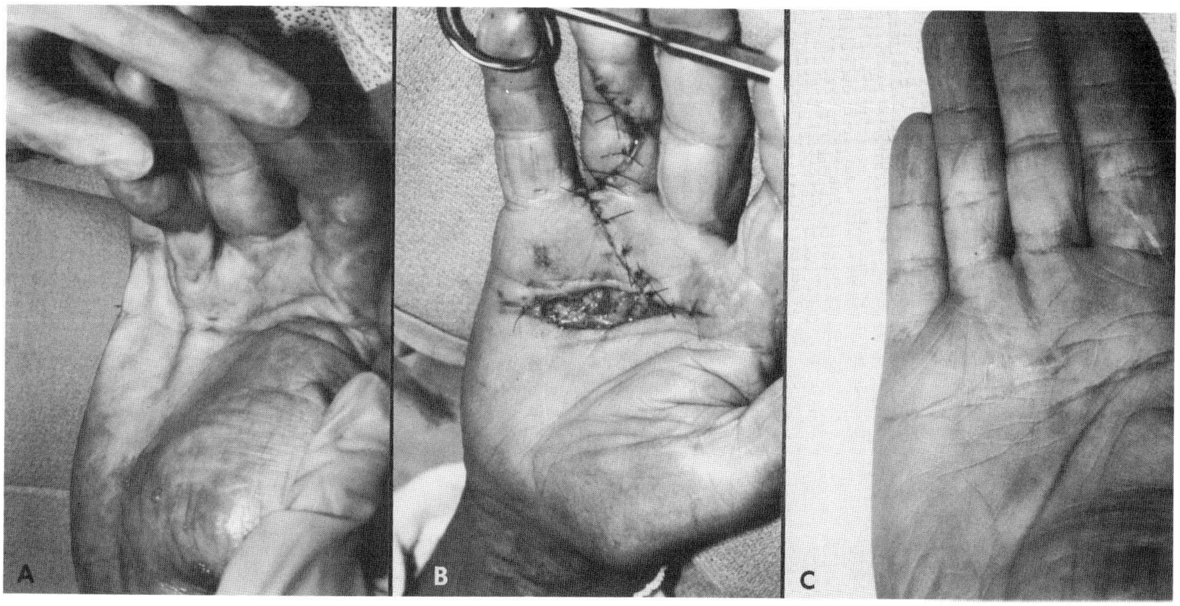

Figure 10

Open-palm method. Diseased tissue is excised through a combination of zigzag incisions in the fingers and a transverse incision in the palm. The palmar wound is not closed at operation but is permitted to heal by second intention. Active motion exercises, proper splinting, and a cooperative patient are necessary for this method to succeed. *A,* Appearance preoperatively. *B,* Immediately postoperatively. *C,* At 1 month postoperatively.

plantation, to at least approximate correct resting length. Of course, a suitable recipient motor nerve must be available. Ideally, the distance from nerve anastomosis to neuromuscular junction should be less than 2 cm to speed reinnervation before significant atrophy can occur. Functional reinnervation begins at about 2 to 4 months but usually requires 6 to 9 months to restore active motion. Strength gradually increases for up to 2 years postoperatively.

Dupuytren Contracture

Although the basic biology of the tissue in Dupuytren contracture has been fairly well described by light microscopy, electron microscopy, and biochemical analysis, the cause remains unclear and nonsurgical treatments of contracture remain unsuccessful. Late local recurrence and disease extension are common and represent significant problems for some patients. Refinements in the surgical management continue to develop, however. A better understanding of the anatomy of isolated digital cords and the mechanism of proximal interphalangeal contracture has been provided recently and should help lessen the risk of intraoperative mishap as well as increase the likelihood of more complete excision and contracture correction (Fig. 9). Controversy continues regarding the open-palm technique but comparative studies suggest a lower rate of complication and better ultimate motion when the transverse palmar incisions are left open (Fig. 10).

Lipofibromatous Hamartoma of Median Nerve

Lipofibromatous hamartoma of the median nerve remains a rare but challenging problem. There are two basic presentations. The more typical is a slowly enlarging soft tissue mass in the forearm or palm of a young adult, usually associated with median nerve sensory deficit. The lesion may also present as a progressive macrodactyly, usually in a child. There are two aspects to treatment: reducing the size of the enlarged tissues, and preserving or restoring sensibility. Because progressive nerve deficit may occur even after external decompression such as carpal tunnel release, some authors recommend microsurgical excision of this interfascicular tumor, but long-term results are not available and the procedure is a formidable one.

For isolated hamartoma of a digital nerve, neurectomy will decrease finger bulk and usually prevents recurrence or progression. Loss of sensibility usually is minimal because the involved digital nerve often is nonfunctional, and redundant innervated skin from the contralateral digital nerve can often be preserved selectively at the time of closure.

Reconstruction for Vascular Problems

Kienböck's Disease

Some disagreement persists regarding the relationship of negative ulnar variance to Kienböck's disease and the preferred treatment for Kienböck's disease, particularly in the early stages. Involvement is generally classified in four stages, according to severity: stage I, sclerosis; stage II, fragmentation; stage III, collapse; and stage IV, intercarpal and radiocarpal arthritis. For the first three stages, there are three basic approaches to treatment which can be used either alone or in combination: mechanical unloading of the lunate to prevent deformation or stimulation of the

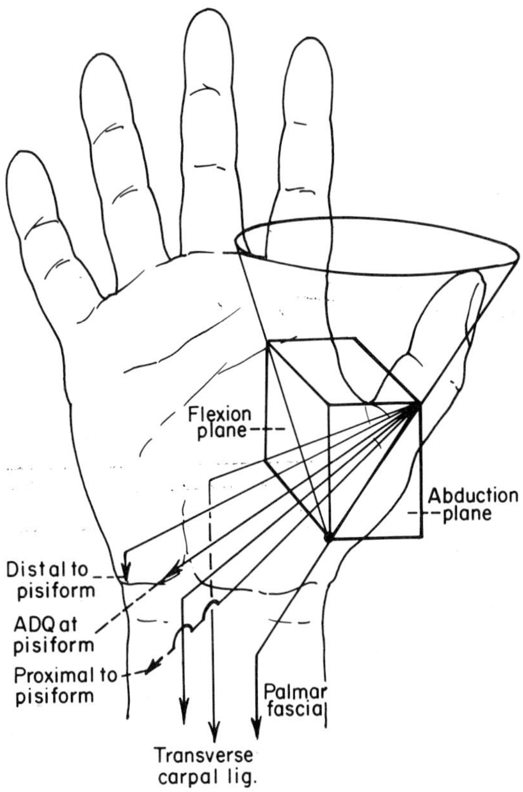

Figure 11

Potential pulley locations for opposition transfer move in a rough semicircle from the distal edge of the transverse carpal ligament to the pisiform to a relatively straight-line pull from the mid forearm. Pulley location and direction of action influence motion and strength. Abduction plane transfers provide greater motion; flexion plane transfers provide greater strength. (From Cooney, W.P.; Linscheid, R.L.; and An, K.-N. J. Hand Surg. [Am.] 9:777–786, 1984. By permission of the American Society for Surgery of the Hand.)

revascularization process for stages I and II; resection with tendon or silicone replacement of the lunate for stage III; and wrist arthrodesis and possibly arthroplasty for stage IV. Wrist denervation, a symptomatic measure, can be included with any of the above.

Mechanical unloading can be relative (i.e., adjusting the relative length of the radius and ulna by osteotomy) or absolute (i.e., decreasing the total load transmitted across the lunate by some form of fixed distraction). Scaphotrapezial trapezoid arthrodesis has the theoretical advantage of decreasing the compressive load transmitted to the lunate in this way because it creates a rigid lateral column through which force can be transmitted from the metacarpals around the lunate to the radius. It may also help to restore and to maintain carpal height. Reported results are promising.

Revascularization procedures for the lunate have been reported only sporadically. They include local muscle pedicle flaps, arterial implantation, and simple bone grafting. Noninvasive electrical stimulation also has been suggested. Currently, there is little documentation for the benefits of any of these approaches which purport to hasten revascularization in Kienböck's disease.

Although lunate replacement with a silicone implant is commonly performed for Kienböck's disease, concerns about silicone synovitis and progression of carpal collapse after implantation have tempered some of the enthusiasm for this technique. These considerations have increased the emphasis on the lunate-sparing surgery mentioned above. When the lunate is excised, soft tissue replacement may be a reasonable treatment alternative, particularly for patients at risk for silicone synovitis. Reported results of soft tissue replacement are similar to those for silicone replacement. Because of coincident carpal collapse, scaphotrapezial trapezoid arthrodesis or other intercarpal arthrodesis may be indicated at the time of lunate excision.

Biomechanics

Wrist

The range of wrist motion required for daily activities has been the subject of several recent investigations. It is clear from this work that the wrist is truly a triaxial joint, permitting not only flexion, extension, radial deviation, and ulnar deviation but also pronation and supination. The rotational component is difficult to quantitate but seems to range from about 2° to 12° for most activities. Other wrist motions can be measured externally more readily; one recent study suggests that 5° of palmar flexion, 30° of dorsiflexion, 10° of radial deviation, and 15° of ulnar deviation are sufficient for most activities of daily living. This information is useful in evaluating the potential effect of surgical procedures that may limit wrist motion. Radioscaphoid or radioscapholunate arthrodesis, for example, usually leaves ample palmar flexion but may not permit sufficient dorsiflexion postoperatively; some consideration might be given to positioning of the arthrodesis in slight dorsiflexion to compensate for this. Midcarpal arthrodesis and scaphotrapezial arthrodesis seem to provide sufficient motion to satisfy the functional range.

Tendon Transfers

Previous studies on forearm and hand muscle mass, fiber length, and cross-sectional area have now been combined with biomechanical measurements of tendon excursion and moment arms to permit biomechanically sound recommendations with regard to transfers to restore thumb opposition. Of the muscles commonly used for transfer, only the flexor digitorum superficialis and the extensor carpi radialis longus approximate the strength of the median thenar muscles. If restoration of strength is important, therefore, these motor tendons should be considered. The route of the transfer is also important. As Bunnell had noted, the transfer should pull from the general direction of the pisiform. Transfers with a more distal pull will add more strength but less motion. Those with a more proximal pull will add more motion but less strength (Fig. 11). The technique of insertion of opposition transfer has been the subject of controversy but at present it appears that a simple insertion into the abductor pollicis brevis tendon is the most effective. All the transfers studied have sufficient excursion to compensate for that of the lost median thenar muscles.

A clear understanding of the potential action of each of the host of opposition tendon transfers available, based on sound biomechanical evaluation, should permit a rational selection to suit the needs of the individual patient.

Annotated Bibliography

Diagnostic Evaluation

Mackinnon, S.E., and Holder, L.E.: The use of three-phase radionuclide bone scanning in the diagnosis of reflex sympathetic dystrophy. J. Hand Surg. [Am.] 9:556–563, 1984.

This technique is both highly sensitive and specific for reflex sympathetic dystrophy and is helpful in distinguishing that syndrome from other pain dysfunction syndromes.

Weeks, P.M.; Vannier, M.B.; Stevens, W.G.; Gayou, D.; and Gilula, L.A.: Three-dimensional imaging of the wrist. J. Hand Surg. [Am.] 10:32–39, 1985.

This exciting report gives a glimpse of the future when three-dimensional reconstruction techniques should make it possible to plan, accurately and preoperatively, the design and effect of osteotomies, arthrodeses, and other reconstructive procedures.

Reconstruction for Bone Problems

Lister, G.D.; Kalisman, M.; and Tsai, T.-M.: Reconstruction of the hand with free microneurovascular toe-to-hand transfer: Experience with 54 toe transfers. Plast. Reconstr. Surg. 71:372–384, 1983.

An excellent overview of this procedure which emphasizes not only technique but also clinical results and indications.

Nunley, J.A.; Goldner, R.D.; and Urbaniak, J.R.: Thumb reconstruction by the wrap-around method. Clin. Orthop. 195:97–103, 1985.

This single-stage procedure has some advantages over other forms of osteoplastic thumb reconstruction, both cosmetically and functionally. It shares with other types of osteoplastic reconstruction problems of graft resorption, however.

O'Brien, B.; Gould, J.S.; Morrison, W.A.; Russell, R.C.; MacLeod, A.M.; and Pribaz, J.J.: Free vascularized small joint transfer to the hand. J. Hand Surg. [Am.] 9:634–641, 1984.

Six of seven transplantations were successful, including all in children. The procedure is recommended as an alternative to arthrodesis or arthroplasty in young patients with significant post-traumatic joint destruction.

Treatment of Arthritis

Beckenbaugh, R.D.: Preliminary experience with a noncemented nonconstrained total joint arthroplasty for the metacarpophalangeal joints. Orthopedics 6:962–965, 1983.

A resurfacing joint arthroplasty for the metacarpophalangeal joints would be useful; this implant has many desirable features.

Bell, M.J.; Hill, R.J.; and McMurtry, R.Y.: Ulnar impingement syndrome. J. Bone Joint Surg. 67B:126–129, 1985.

Painful instability of the distal ulna stump after resection arthroplasty is difficult to manage. Caution is recommended when considering performing a Darrach resection in a young, active patient.

Bowers, W.H.: Distal radioulnar joint arthroplasty: The hemiresection-interposition technique. J. Hand Surg. [Am.] 10:169–178, 1985.

This arthroplasty has the advantage of addressing distal radio-ulnar impingement while preserving ulnar length and the mechanical function of the triangular fibrocartilage complex for wrist stability.

Darrow, J.C., Jr.; Linscheid, R.L.; Dobyns, J.H.; Mann, J.M., III; Wood, M.B.; and Beckenbaugh, R.D.: Distal ulnar recession for disorders of the distal radioulnar joint. J. Hand Surg. [Am.] 10:482–491, 1985.

In patients with symptoms consistent with ulnar carpal impingement, chondromalacia of the ulnar head, triangular fibrocartilage complex tears, and instability of the distal radio-ulnar joint, satisfactory results can be expected after ulnar shortening in approximately 75%.

Eaton, R.G.; Glickel, S.Z.; and Littler, J.W.: Tendon interposition arthroplasty for degenerative arthritis of the trapeziometacarpal joint of the thumb. J. Hand Surg. [Am.] 10:645–654, 1985.

Partial trapeziectomy with ligament reconstruction and tendon interposition provides good or excellent results in 92% of patients with isolated trapeziometacarpal arthritis.

Eaton, R.G.; Lane, L.B.; Littler, J.W.; and Keyser, J.J.: Ligament reconstruction for the painful thumb carpometacarpal joint: A long-term assessment. J. Hand Surg. [Am.] 9:692–699, 1984.

This study indicates that the early promising results of basal ligament reconstruction continue long-term. The procedure is indicated in patients who have isolated mild to moderate arthritic changes at the trapeziometacarpal joint with normal scaphotrapezial joints.

Kleinert, J.M.; Stern, P.J.; Lister, G.D.; and Kleinhans, R.J.: Complications of scaphoid silicone arthroplasty. J. Bone Joint Surg. 67A:422–427, 1985.

This multicenter study suggests a high complication rate for scaphoid silicone arthroplasty, with 13 of 33 patients having subluxation of the implant and 10 patients requiring revision surgery. Scaphoid silicone replacement arthroplasty does not seem to improve wrist motion or strength significantly and does not prevent progressive carpal collapse.

Nalbandian, R.M.; Swanson, A.B.; and Maupin, B.K.: Long-term silicone implant arthroplasty: Implications of animal and human autopsy findings. J.A.M.A. 250:1195–1198, 1983.

This article suggests that the foreign body giant cell reaction to silicone is a local one with no evidence of systemic dissemination of silicone particles in the human and animal tissue studied.

Seradge, H.; Kutz, J.A.; Kleinert, H.E.; Lister, G.D.; Wolff, T.W.; and Atasoy, E.: Perichondrial resurfacing arthroplasty in the hand. J. Hand Surg. [Am.] 9.880–886, 1984.

This procedure may be helpful in the treatment of post-traumatic arthritis in the younger patient, particularly at the interphalangeal joints.

Smith, R.J.; Atkinson, R.E.; and Jupiter, J.B.: Silicone synovitis of the wrist. J. Hand Surg. [Am.] 10:47–60, 1985.

The exact incidence of this problem is unknown but seems to be increasing with time. The Dow Corning Company now recommends caution in the use of these implants in young, physically active patients and patients with associated preoperative degenerative changes. They no longer recommend intraoperative temporary stabilization with K-wire or suture. The synovitis usually subsides after the implants are removed.

Trumble, T.E., and Watson, H.K.: Posttraumatic sesamoid arthritis of the metacarpophalangeal joint of the thumb. J. Hand Surg. [Am.] 10:94–100, 1985.

This previously unreported syndrome may be easily confused with thumb metacarpophalangeal joint arthritis. Clinical distinction is critical because metacarpophalangeal joint arthrodesis for patients with this syndrome would be both unnecessary and ineffective.

Watson, H.K., and Ballet, F.L.: The SLAC wrist: Scapholunate advanced collapse pattern of degenerative arthritis. J. Hand Surg. [Am.] 9:358–365, 1984.

A common pattern of sequential changes in degenerative arthritis of the wrist is identified and a rational treatment program is outlined.

Wilson, J.N., and Bossley, C.J.: Osteotomy in the treatment of osteoarthritis of the first carpometacarpal joint. J. Bone Joint Surg. 65B:179–181, 1983.

In early stages of trapeziometacarpal disease, extra-articular abduction osteotomy seems to be a reasonable treatment alternative to arthroplasty.

Reconstruction of Nerve Injury

Freehafer, A.A.; Kelly, C.M.; and Peckham, P.H.: Tendon transfer for the restoration of upper limb function after a cervical spinal cord injury. J. Hand Surg. [Am.] 9:887–893, 1984.

An excellent review of the current state of the art in this area.

House, J.H., and Shannon, M.A.: Restoration of strong grasp and lateral pinch in tetraplegia: A comparison of two methods of thumb control in each patient. J. Hand Surg. [Am.] 10:22–29, 1985.

Although arthrodeses generally are not recommended for restoration of function in tetraplegic hands, thumb carpometacarpal arthrodesis may be an exception, as pointed out in this article.

Reconstruction for Muscle Deficit and Tendon Injury

Manktelow, R.T.; Zuker, R.M.; and McKee, N.H.: Functioning free muscle transplantation. J. Hand Surg. [Am.] 9:32–39, 1984.

Innervated muscle transfer was used to restore hand motion in 12 patients with severely damaged forearm musculature. Eleven of 12 flaps survived and 9 of 12 were strong enough to provide full finger motion with grip strengths up to 27 kg (60 pounds).

Treatment for Tumors Specific to Wrist and Hand

Lubahn, J.D.; Lister, G.D.; and Wolfe, T.: Fasciectomy and Dupuytren's disease: A comparison between the open-palm technique and wound closure. J. Hand Surg. [Am.] 9:53–62, 1984.

Complications were fewer and motion better in the open-palm group.

Silverman, T.A., and Enzinger, F.M.: Fibrolipomatous hamartoma of nerve: A clinico-pathologic analysis of 26 cases. Am. J. Surg. Path. 9:7–14, 1985.

This benign lesion may or may not be associated with macrodactyly. It may occur in nerves other than the median nerve.

Strickland, J.W., and Bassett, R.L.: The isolated digital cord in Dupuytren's contracture: Anatomy and clinical significance. J. Hand Surg. [Am.] 10:118–124, 1985.

This article is useful in preoperative planning because it outlines the pathoanatomy of isolated digital involvement in Dupuytren's disease, based on clinical experience with 37 involved digits.

Treatment of Vascular and Metabolic Disorders Specific to Wrist and Hand

Ishiguro, T.: Experimental and clinical studies of Kienböck's disease. Excision of the lunate followed by packing of the free tendon. Nippon Seikeigeka Gakki Zasshi 58:509–522, 1984.

An anchovy type arthroplasty produced satisfactory results in 80% of patients at 3-year follow-up.

Swanson, A.B.; Maupin, B.K.; Swanson, G.D.G.; Ganzhorn, R.W.; and Moss, S.H.: Lunate implant resection arthroplasty: Long-term results. J. Hand Surg. [Am.] 10:1013–1024, 1985.

This detailed long-term follow-up of a group of 42 nonconsecutive patients followed a mean of 5 years found cyst formation in one-third of implants. It is suggested that silicone lunate replacement arthroplasty does not prevent progression of carpal collapse. Postoperative strength and motion were not reported.

Watson, H.K.; Ryu, J.; and DiBella, A.: An approach to Kienböck's disease: Triscaphe arthrodesis. J. Hand Surg. [Am.] 10:179–187, 1985.

This procedure, alone or in combination with lunate replacement arthroplasty, seems useful in the treatment of Kienböck's disease.

Biomechanics of Wrist and Hand

Cooney, W.P.; Linscheid, R.L.; and An, K.-N.: Opposition of the thumb: An anatomic and biomechanical study of tendon transfers. J. Hand Surg. [Am.] 9:777–786, 1984.

A study of the biomechanical consequences and clinical indications for the various thumb opposition transfers available.

Palmer, A.K.; Werner, F.W.; Murphy, D.; and Glisson, R.: Functional wrist motion: A biomechanical study. J. Hand Surg. [Am.] 10:39–46, 1985.

This is one of the first articles to address the topic of minimal functional requirements for wrist motion. It suggests that 5° of flexion, 30° of extension, 10° of radial deviation, and 15° of ulnar deviation are sufficient for most functional activities.

Rozing, P.M., and Kauer, J.M.G.: Partial arthrodesis of the wrist: An investigation in cadavers. Acta Orthop. Scand. 55:66–68, 1984.

This biomechanical study reviews the expected ranges of motion after various intercarpal and radiocarpal arthrodeses and is a useful reference for those who perform these procedures.

23

Cervical Spine: Pediatric and Reconstructive Aspects

This section reviews recent information on developmental anatomy, congenital and developmental problems, degenerative disorders of the cervical spine, inflammatory arthritis, infection, and surgical fabrications.

Developmental Anatomy

The development of the cervical spine is complex. Anomalies can result from failure of completion of development, as in failures of segmentation noted in Klippel-Feil syndrome, or from failure of the coalescence of secondary centers of ossification, as noted in os odontoideum. In C-1, there is ossification of both posterior neural arches with a posterior synchondrosis. The neurocentral synchondrosis forms on each side anteriorly and appears at 6 to 24 months of age. Sometimes the anterior center is multifocal. At 4 to 6 years of age, the posterior and anterior centers fuse and the space available for the spinal canal is determined at this time. In C-2, the dens forms from two primary centers of ossification which coalesce at 1 to 3 months of age. They are separated from the vertebral body by the dentocentral synchondrosis, and bipolar growth results. At 8 to 10 years of age, the ossiculum terminale forms at the apex of the dens. It fuses to the dens at 10 to 13 years of age. Failure of fusion of these centers is being reported in the clinical literature as a consequence of detection by computed tomography. These congenital defects can be mistaken for fractures. Posterior bifid C-1 arches are found in 5% of the population. Anterior bifid arches are much less common. In combination, these defects can represent a weak area, and atlantoaxial instability has been reported in this setting in a child in whom avulsion of the transverse ligament has been hypothesized.

Radiologic anatomy can be confusing in the cervical spine because of the superimposition of adjacent vertebral, craniofacial, and laryngeal structures. Normal variants include a bipartite superior articular surface of the atlas, pseudonotch of the atlas, absence or partial absence of the posterior arch of the atlas, backward "displaced" spinolaminal line of the axis (noted in 10% of children), posteriorly tilted dens, pseudosubluxation of the axis (normally found in children less than 10 years old), short C-5, notched articular process of C-7, and accessory ossicles. Posterior arch defects, including spondylolysis and absence of a pedicle, in the subaxial spine have been identified as congenital anomalies and may be confused with fractures. This type of anomaly is accompanied by a large foramen, absence of a pedicle, a displaced articular segment, and an abnormal transverse process.

The configuration of the cervical spinal canal can be indicative of intracanal expansile lesions. In children less than 10 years of age, gradual widening of the lower canal and ballooning of the mid canal are frequently observed. Occasionally this is seen at ages 10 to 18 years. This configurational variation is not noted in adults. Therefore, investigation for an intracanal lesion is not merited in children unless there are accompanying symptoms and signs. Adults with these findings should be investigated with computed tomography and myelography.

Awareness of these variations and anomalies is important in avoiding a misdiagnosis and pursuit of unindicated studies.

Congenital and Developmental Disorders

Anomalies in the cervical spine have been identified in association with other conditions. In patients with congenital scoliosis and kyphosis, 25% had segmentation defects in the cervical spine; 82 of 298 had a single level of failed segmentation, of which 52 were at C2-3. Anomalies can accompany facial malformations. In Apert's syndrome there is a high correlation of upper cervical spine anomalies with nondeforming failure of segmentation. Hemifacial microsomia, especially the Goldenhaar syndrome, has a high incidence of cervicothoracic scoliosis which can be progressive. Treacher-Collins syndrome has not been found to predispose to cervical anomalies.

Atlantoaxial instability may be found in various conditions. Instability may be caused by laxity of the transverse ligament in association with pharyngeal infection (Grisel's syndrome). Anatomic study of the pharyngeal veins has shown retrograde filling with lymphovenous anastomoses draining the posterosuperior pharynx. It is hypothesized that hyperemia accompanying infection causes laxity of the transverse ligament and subsequent anterior C1-2 subluxation or rotatory subluxation of C-1 on C-2. In addition to anterior C1-2 subluxation, rotatory subluxation of C1-2 is found in association with upper respiratory infection. Computed tomography has been useful in defining the existence of this subluxation because rotation may be difficult to determine on plain radiographs.

Patients with Down's syndrome have a tendency toward anterior C1-2 subluxation, and 25% have been estimated to have it. A recent study of 236 patients demonstrated that 40 had C1-2 instability and 7 of these 40 had neurologic findings. Another study demonstrated that instability is more likely to develop in boys over the age of 10 and that this group is more at risk for the development of myelopathy. Early identification and fusion will result in a good outcome. Long-standing myelopathy shows little improvement with fusion in patients with Down's syndrome.

Atlantoaxial instability can be found in atlanto-occipital fusion (associated with C2-3 fusion), basilar impression, and anomalies of the odontoid such as os odontoideum which may be developmental failure of fusion of the dens or a traumatic nonunion. Dysplastic development of the dens may be found in generalized bone dysplasias such as achondroplasia, spondyloepiphyseal dysplasia, Morquio's syndrome, and Larsen's syndrome. Instability is defined traditionally as an abnormal atlantodental distance; 5 mm is accepted by most surgeons as the upper limit of normal in children. Indications for fusion include painful or neurologically significant atlantoaxial instability. Clinically silent instability presents the greatest difficulty in decision making. Because persistent instability of 5 mm or more represents an absolute risk factor, it probably should be stabilized. Computed tomography can be useful in deciding whether instability is physiologically dangerous by demonstrating a flattened spinal cord behind the dens.

Subaxial instability is difficult to judge in a young child because of the laxity of the spine. Pseudosubluxation of C-2 on C-3 in flexion can be very pronounced. Determining the alignment of the posterior sublaminar line (Fig. 1) may be helpful in determining the presence of a physiologic subluxation. Radiologic criteria that have been used to determine traumatic ligamentous instability in children are an increase in the interspinous distance, a loss of parallelism between the articular processes, and widening of the posterior disk space. Surgical treatment is recommended in these cases only after prolonged immobilization.

Patterns of instability in children appear to be instability adjacent to fusions and instability at the level of defects. Klippel-Feil syndrome includes all congenital failures of segmentation, whether it be two segments, congenital block vertebrae, or the entire cervical spine. No symptoms are usually ascribed to these affected vertebrae, but a traumatic central cord syndrome in an adolescent with C2-3 Klippel-Feil syndrome has been reported.

Surgical fusion for instabilities in children can be very successful. Congenital defects may require modification of the usual techniques, such as lateral placement of wires in atlantoaxial fusions in the presence of posterior C-1 arch defects. Some authors have thought that passage of wire in children and adolescents may involve undue risk in the presence of congenital defects and recommend onlay fusions after decortication. Halo casts are necessary when this strategy is used. Cadaver allograft has been used for posterior fusion, but a report on seven fusions in children with allografts indicated that none fused successfully. Allograft is not recommended and autologous iliac crest is preferred.

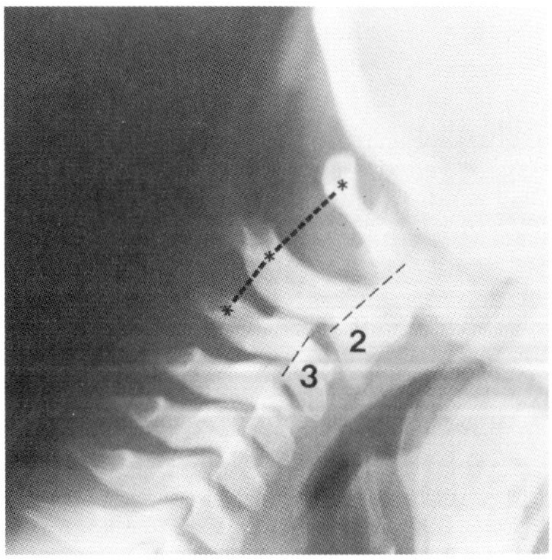

Figure 1

Pseudosubluxation of C-2 on C-3. Hypermobility is common in children under age 8 years. Specific measurements of the movement of the vertebral bodies (thin dotted line) are unreliable whereas the relationship of the posterior elements (thick dotted line) is more consistent. In flexion, the posterior arch of C-2 normally aligns itself in a straight-line fashion with C-1 and C-3. (From Orthopaedic Knowledge Update I, pp. 189–198. Chicago, American Academy of Orthopaedic Surgeons, 1984.)

Degenerative Disorders

Pain emanating from the cervical spine as a result of degenerative or spondylotic change is traditionally thought of as being produced by inflammatory change or by lesions of neural compression centered on the nerve root or the spinal cord with a spectrum of compression. Treatment is directed toward the relief of neural compression, stabilization of a degenerated motion segment, and reduction of inflammation either at the motion segment or at the nerve root. Acute cervical disk herniation invokes the classic concept of a neural compressive lesion at the root and spinal cord. An epidemiologic study has shown that cervical disk herniations are most common in the fourth decade of life, occur in a male-to-female ratio of 1.4:1, and have risk factors of frequent lifting, cigarette smoking, and diving from a board. Primary treatment is supportive and includes rest, immobilization, traction, and pain blockade; supportive medications include analgesics, muscle relaxants, and anti-inflammatory drugs.

The same therapies are used in the treatment of neck pain without radiculopathy. A double-blind prospective study of the influence of a single manipulation done under diazepam sedation for neck pain has shown no value to this intervention. Chronic cervical pain remains a difficult problem without definitive solutions. It is complicated by behavioral changes because of the psychosocial stresses of ongoing pain and disability. Because the biology is poorly understood and it is not a matter of a neural compressive lesion, imaging by myelography and computed tomography is of little value. Cervical discography is of little use because of age-related degeneration and nonspecificity of the test.

Cervical discometry is accomplished by placing needles into the disk space at the suspected symptomatic levels and adjacent levels, under local anesthesia and fluoroscopic control, through the anterolateral aspect of the neck anterior to the carotid sheath and lateral to the esophagus. Injury to these structures and infection are risks. Saline is injected at each space from a small syringe. Degenerative disks will accept greater than 0.5 ml under low pressure; normal disks will not, and injection will reproduce the symptomatic pain. Degenerative disks can be painful nonspecifically and so only reproduction of symptomatic pain is of significance. Some surgeons find abatement of pain with local injection of anesthetic agents.

Surgical intervention for neck pain and cervical radiculopathy is indicated when intractable pain lasts for an intolerable period and is unresponsive to nonoperative management. The majority of patients with cervical radiculopathy will not require surgical intervention. The natural history, however, is not known. More spondylotic disks may produce greater chronic pain. Some surgeons think that a radicular neurologic deficit should not be permitted to continue for long periods of time because root injury may become permanent and recovery will not occur. This becomes more urgent when intrinsic hand function or shoulder dysfunction occurs and the loss is functionally more disabling. There is no documentation to substantiate these suspicions, and these deficits surely do resolve on a case-by-case basis.

Controversy continues on two other points. The first is whether surgical intervention is indicated for chronic cervical pain in the absence of radiculopathy. Discometry appears to be the only method of value in localizing the pain. Patients with positive discometric results may be candidates for anterior cervical discectomy and fusion, but the success of this intervention staged in this manner is unproved. Anatomic compression of the root and cord can be visualized by myelography, computed tomographic scan, and contrast-enhanced computed tomographic scan (Fig. 2).

Once the lesion is localized and surgical intervention is planned, the second controversy is encountered and centers on the questions of anterior versus posterior decompression for cervical radiculopathy and of fusion or no fusion in anterior approaches. Both approaches can be effective, and the selection is based on the nature of the lesion, the surgical goals, and the experience and confidence of the surgeon in each area. The anterior approach has proved to be safe and effective for removing disks and disk fragments. Most orthopaedic surgeons will include fusion; many neurosurgeons think that fusion is not necessary. Reports of series of cases without fusion suffer from lack of long-term follow-up.

A prospective study of 63 patients with cervical disk herniations approached anteriorly, some with fusions and some without, showed that at 12-month follow-up the group without fusion did better. In another series of anterior discectomy with fusion for spondylosis and disk herniation, the fusion rate was 97%; pain relief was total in 78% and partial in 18%. Anterior interbody fusion appears to increase the risk of accelerated degenerative change at adjacent levels, but the literature does not provide any information as to the frequency or clinical significance of this problem.

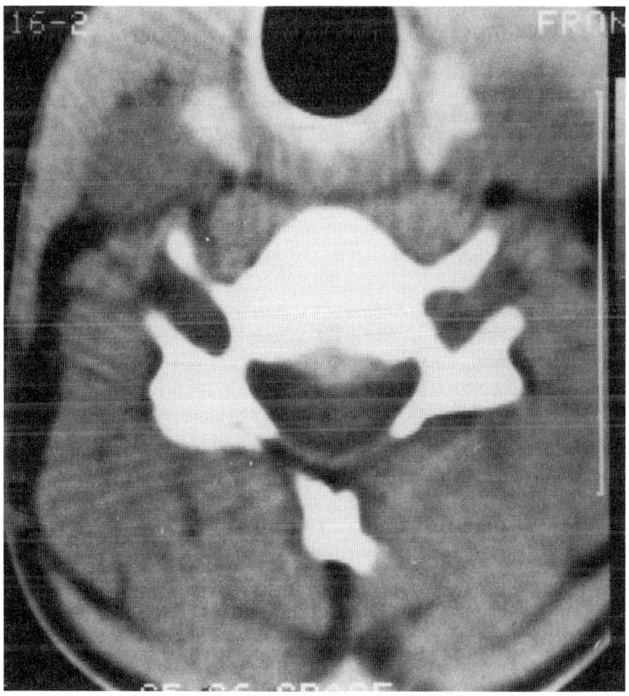

Figure 2

Transverse computed tomogram at C5–6, demonstrating a disk herniation with both cord and right root impingement in a patient with myeloradiculopathy.

Cervical spondylotic myelopathy (CSM) can be caused by developmental spinal stenosis, ossification of the posterior longitudinal ligament (commonly found in Japan), and spondylosis. Patients with myelopathy can present with various symptoms including neck pain, upper extremity pain, gait disturbance, weakness, sensory changes, motor ataxia, bowel and bladder disturbances, and outright quadriparesis and quadriplegia including cord syndromes. In 40 of 63 patients with refractory spondylosis, average canal sagittal diameter at the level of the pedicle was less than normal (17 mm). In nine patients with CSM, the anteroposterior compression ratio (defined as the ratio of the anteroposterior diameter to the transverse diameter) correlated with the degree of cord destruction. Developmental narrowing was more significant than spondylotic canal encroachment in the production of myelopathy. Canal narrowing caused demyelination and gray matter infarcts in the cord, whereas trauma from spondylosis provoked the clinical manifestations and final cord pathology.

The treatment of CSM is surgical. Controversy exists as to the choice of anterior versus posterior decompression and the type of anterior decompression involved. A report on microsurgical anterior osteophytectomy for CSM demonstrated that 91% of patients improved. In 6 of 10 patients who did not have fusion, arm and neck pain developed later. Fusion did not affect the recovery from the myelopathy. Posterior laminaplasty has been done for myelopathy of the three types. This operation expands the canal size and provides osseous protection of the cord, protects the dura from invasive scar formation by retaining the lamina, and retains stability by keeping the posterior elements (Fig. 3).

Canal expansion can be documented through postoperative computed tomography. In a series of 191 patients followed for up to 12 years, posterior operations gave better results than anterior procedures for more advanced myelopathies such as transverse lesions, Brown-Séquard syndrome, and motor syndromes. Patients with brachialgia or central cord syndromes did well with anterior procedures. The type of anterior or posterior procedure made no difference. Patients with a short duration of symptoms did better than those with more chronic symptoms. In another series of 95 patients with CSM, laminectomy was compared with anterior discectomy and fusion of the Cloward and Smith-Robinson type and subtotal spondylectomy and fusion. Subtotal spondylectomy, with resection of a large portion of the vertebral body, was a superior operation and up to three disk levels could be treated this way. If four or more levels were involved, laminectomy was recommended.

Inflammatory Arthritis

Anatomic abnormalities of the cervical spine involved in rheumatoid arthritis are a consequence of the destruction

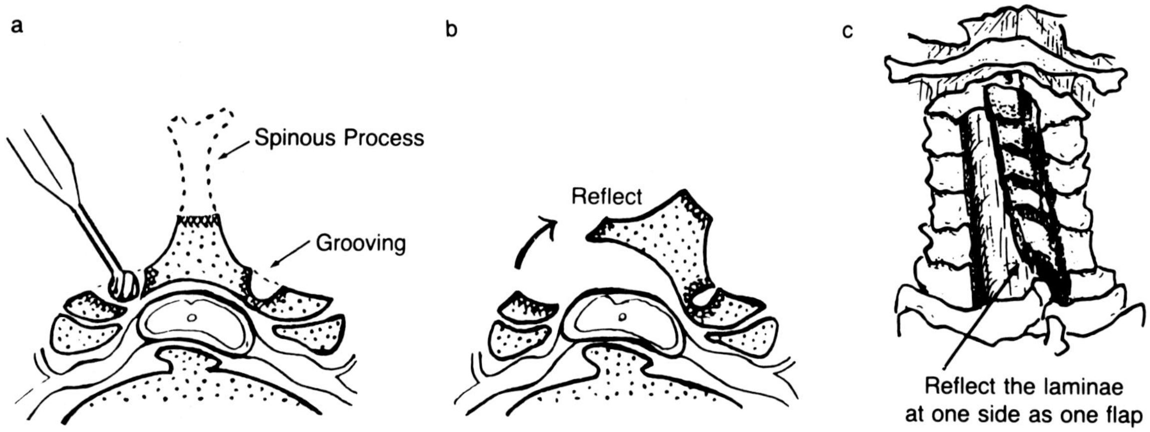

Figure 3

Method of canal-expanding laminaplasty. *a,* A groove is made on each side of the lamina with an air drill along an imaginary line separating the laminar arches from the articular processes. *b* and *c,* All of the laminae are then lifted as one flap. (From Kimura, I., et al. J. Bone Joint Surg. 66A:914–920, 1984. By permission of the journal.)

in joints, ligaments, and bone caused by synovitis. Such destruction causes subluxation, the nature of which is dependent on the structures involved. Clinical abnormalities include pain in the affected part and neurologic abnormality resulting from distortion of the spinal cord, roots, and vertebral artery that occurs with subluxation. Atlantoaxial subluxation (AAS) is ascribed to erosive synovitis in the atlantoaxial, atlanto-odontoid, and atlanto-occipital joints as well as the synovium-lined bursa between the odontoid and the transverse ligament. "Atlantoaxial impaction" (AAI)—also called pseudobasilar invagination, cranial settling, and vertical subluxation—describes the settling of the skull onto the atlas and of the atlas onto the axis. AAI results from erosion and bone loss in the atlanto-occipital and atlantoaxial joints. The subaxial cervical spine is affected via the facets, interspinous ligaments, and intervertebral disks (spondylodiscitis). Subluxations of all types have been noted in 43% to 86% of patients with rheumatoid arthritis.

AAS can be anterior, posterior, or lateral. Anterior AAS is the most commonly noted and has been found in 11% to 46% of postmortem studies of rheumatoid arthritis. Anterior AAS in adults is considered abnormal beyond an atlantodental distance of 3.5 mm, and subluxation beyond 10 mm implies loss of integrity of the transverse, alar, and apical ligaments. Computed tomography can be useful in assessing the presence of synovitis posterior to the dens and assessing the canal diameter, but a computed tomographic study of 33 patients showed no relationship among symptoms, signs, and radiologic abnormalities except when cord compression was clinically apparent. Anterior AAS is present in 19% to 71% of patients with rheumatoid arthritis.

Posterior AAS has been described, and it accounted for 6.7% of all AAS in one series. It was thought to be benign, but a report of four cases with myelopathy has shown that it can cause a posterior kinking of the spinal cord as it enters the foramen magnum. Contrast-enhanced sagittal imaging, computed tomographic sagittal reconstruction imaging, and magnetic resonance imaging can show this abnormality of cord configuration (Fig. 4).

Lateral AAS can be visualized on a frontal view in which the lateral masses of C-1 lie 2 mm or more laterally on those of C-2. Lateral AAS was found to account for 21% of all AAS, and 10% of a rheumatoid population was found to have nonreducible head tilts, all with lateral AAS and frequently with other accompanying deformities. Lateral AAS is found more commonly in patients with cord compression than in those without it.

AAI has been found in 5% to 32% of rheumatoid patients and accounted for 22% of all AAS. AAI can be measured by McGregor's line and the settling of C-1 on C-2 on lateral radiographs as in Ranawat's measurement in which the height of a line drawn from the center of the C-2 pedicle to a line drawn between the centers of the anterior and posterior arches of C-1 is determined (Fig. 5). Heights less than 13 mm are indicative of AAI. The measurement obviates the need to visualize the hard palate or the top of the odontoid on the radiograph. Tomography and computed tomography are most useful in defining this deformity.

Subaxial subluxations can be found at multiple levels, giving a "stepladder" appearance. These subluxations can be found in 10% to 20% of rheumatoid arthritis patients. Osteophyte formation is absent, and narrowing and subluxation at C2-3 and C3-4 are characteristic.

Cervical instability appears to occur early in the clinical course of rheumatoid arthritis. Risk factors include a history of corticosteroid use as part of medical therapy, seropositivity, the presence of rheumatoid nodules, erosive and mutilating disease, and being male. Patients with cervical rheumatoid arthritis are at risk for premature death, but not necessarily from cervical subluxation. Subluxations worsen with time, but neurologic progression is less marked. Risk factors for the development of cord compression have been identified as being male, having greater than 9 mm of anterior AAS, and the presence of AAI.

Nonsurgical management of patients with cervical rheumatoid arthritis is supportive. The definitive management is surgical and is indicated for patients with neurologic symptoms and sometimes for those with pain. Preopera-

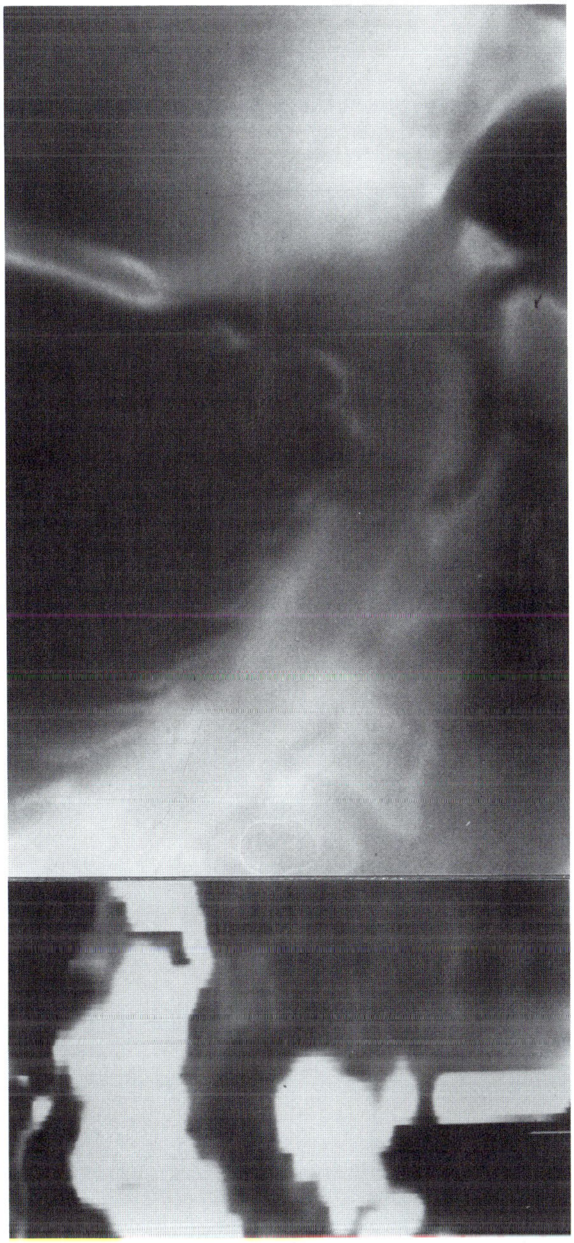

Figure 4

Posterior AAS. *Upper*, Contrast-enhanced sagittal tomography. *Lower*, Sagittal reconstruction computed tomography. The posterior kinking of the spinal cord is visualized.

tive halo traction is used to reduce subluxations and myelopathic changes. Posterior fusion at involved levels is the most common stabilization procedure. Some surgeons continue halo immobilization postoperatively; others use wire fixation and less cervical support. Nonunions are common (rates of 20% to 33% have been reported). In a recent series of 34 atlantoaxial fusions, the fusion rate was 58% with wire fixation and a collar used postoperatively. In another series, 9 of 10 patients had fusion with a halo cast used postoperatively. Prolonged halo immobilization in this group of patients is problematic because of their debilitated state, a condition in which halo immobilization and its

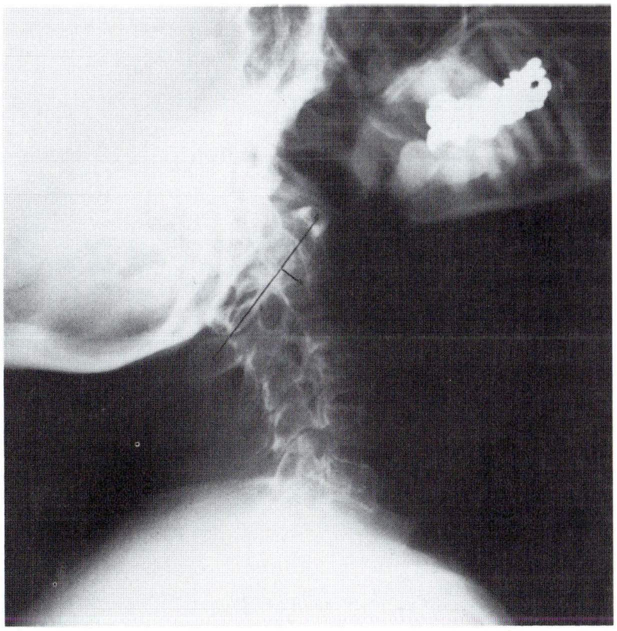

Figure 5

AAI in rheumatoid arthritis determined by Ranawat's line.

consequent decrease in mobility can lead to skin breakdown and respiratory infections. To avoid halo immobilization and overcome some of the difficulties presented by the poor quality of bone in the rheumatoid patient, some surgeons have used methyl methacrylate to enhance posterior cervical fusions in occipitocervical and long posterior fusions. Wound dehiscence and infection have been encountered, but satisfactory immediate stabilization is provided by the use of wire mesh and cement.

Juvenile rheumatoid arthritis does not commonly cause clinical problems in the cervical spine. An epidemiologic study identified 39 such patients in a population of 12,643–16,749 persons under 16 years of age. Eleven had cervical spine disease, clinically apparent in seven and radiologically apparent in four. In a study of 92 patients with juvenile rheumatoid arthritis, 29 (32%) had cervical involvement, 14 had pain and stiffness, 2 had torticollis, 5 had anterior AAS, and 4 had facet ankylosis. Two of the patients with AAS had myelopathy; it resolved in one. No AAI or subaxial subluxation was identified.

Patients with ankylosing spondylitis can develop rupture of the transverse ligament and subsequent AAS or spondylodiscitis with subluxation via a fracture commonly at the cervicothoracic junction. A chin-on-chest deformity can occur which can be corrected by cervicothoracic junction osteotomy. Spinal cord injury can occur in ankylosing spondylitis. A review of 105 patients revealed 13 with fractures and 8 of these had severe cord injury. Computed tomography is useful for evaluation, and operation is not often indicated. Immobilization in a halo vest to allow healing is adequate. A 29% mortality rate and 46% incidence of permanent neurologic deficit have been reported in ankylosing spondylitis with fracture and spinal cord injury.

Infection

Osteomyelitis of the cervical spine is not common. Fine-needle aspiration anteriorly can be used to establish the bacteriologic diagnosis. Use of an anterior approach is recommended to biopsy for diagnosis, to decompress the spinal canal, to drain abcesses, and to stabilize a segment if needed. Tuberculosis of the upper cervical spine has been noted to present with pain, stiffness, paralysis, and retropharyngeal swelling. Medical therapy and transoral decompression and fusion have been used. Tuberculosis in children has been noted to have more extensive involvement and abscess formation in the lower cervical spine; adults tend to have more localized disease and less pus formation: 43% of children had cord compression compared with 81% of adults. In a series of 107 adults with tuberculous spondylitis, 35% had negative bone scans, 70% had negative gallium scans, and 14% had negative tuberculin skin tests. Fifty-three required operation, and anterior drainage was the procedure of choice; 94% recovery from neurologic loss was achieved.

Surgical Fabrications

Surgical fabrications in the cervical spine have been designed to solve specific clinical problems. The anterior approach to the subaxial cervical spine is commonly used. The Smith-Robinson technique of fusion by using tricortical iliac crest graft is probably the most popular. Many neurosurgeons tend to use the Cloward technique. Cadaver allograft is being used but clearly suffers from a potential decreased rate of incorporation. In a review of 82,114 cases of cervical interbody fusion, 311 major complications were identified, including 70 myelopathies. Quadriparesis and quadriplegia accounted for 66% of the deficits, and Brown-Séquard syndromes were found in 30%. The cause of the deficit was usually not apparent to the surgeon, and reoperation was of little value in aiding recovery.

The transoral approach to the upper cervical spine is indicated in anterior element disease, anterior compression unrelieved by a posterior approach, and instability that cannot be treated by a posterior fabrication because of disease or the absence of posterior elements. The transoral approach has an infection rate as high as 50% associated with it. To avoid this problem and also to permit more extensive exposure, a lateral retropharyngeal approach to the upper cervical spine has been described; this is very demanding technically.

An anterior cervicothoracic approach, using a high axillary thoracotomy and an anterolateral cervical approach, has been described and used for cervicothoracic scoliosis. In this approach, the carotid sheath contents are brought anteriorly to avoid the thoracic outlet and the incisions are joined by breaking through the dome of the pleura.

In posterior approaches, modifications are made for defects such as atlantoaxial fusions in the presence of a bifid posterior arch of the atlas. Here, lateral wire placement held by the graft can be used to isolate the fusion satisfactorily to C1-2. C1-2 fusions are generally accomplished via Gallie or Brooks techniques. Gallie fusions use a wire passed around the posterior arch of the atlas and around the spinous process of C-2. Brooks fusions utilize wires passed under the arch of C-1 and laminae of C-2 on each side. This fabrication may give more control of C1-2 rotation, but this has not been proved in a cadaver study of this rotation. The Brooks technique involves an extra risk of neural injury from passage of the C-2 sublaminar wires.

Iatrogenic instability can be brought about by multilevel laminectomy. A study of deformity after multilevel laminectomy showed that adults over the age of 25 do not develop deformity unless there was also trauma to the vertebral body or facetectomy. Under age 25, and especially in children, deformity is a problem: 46% of children less than age 15 years had deformity after laminectomies at all levels of the spine; 100% of those undergoing cervical laminectomy had deformity which started between 2 and 74 months after operation. It is recommended that patients less than 25 years of age be followed yearly for 6 years postoperatively to detect instability that may require stabilization.

Methyl methacrylate has been used in situations of inadequate quality of bone, such as in tumor reconstructions and in rheumatoid arthritis. The goals are to give immediate stability and to avoid cervical orthoses. In nonmalignant situations, graft should be included for long-term stability. Mesh, spinous process, and sublaminar wires have been used for attachment of the methacrylate. In pathologic fractures from malignancy, graft should be included if survival is expected to be more than 6 months. Methacrylate alone may have immediate stability but weakens thereafter. A canine study of wire with graft or methacrylate demonstrated that the methacrylate had lost stability at 1 month postoperatively and was loosening by 2 months. Good-quality bone graft is just as stable initially as methacrylate. Definition of surgical goals and sound judgment are called for in the judicious use of these fabrications.

Annotated Bibliography

General

The Cervical Spine Research Society: The Cervical Spine. Philadelphia, J.B. Lippincott Company, 1983.
An excellent review of all aspects of the cervical spine.

Developmental Anatomy and Radiologic Anatomy

Kattan, K.R., and Pais, M.J.: Some borderlands of the cervical spine. I. The normal (and nearly normal) that may appear pathologic. Skeletal Radiol. 8:1–6, 1982.
A summary of radiologic findings that may be interpreted as abnormal because of superimposition of the adjacent vertebra, craniofacial and laryngeal structures, and nine pediatric anatomic variants.

Kattan, K.R., and Pais, M.J.: Some borderlands of the

cervical spine. II. The subtle and the hidden abnormal. Skeletal Radiol. 8:7–12, 1982.
A review of abnormalities of short sagittal diameter, vertebral body neoplasms, apophyseal osteophytes, trauma, and infection. At C3–7, canal diameter of less than 11 mm on lateral films is consistent with spinal cord compression.

Ogden, J.A.: Radiology of postnatal skeletal development. XI. The first cervical vertebra. Skeletal Radiol. 12:12–20, 1984.
At birth there is ossification of both posterior neural arches. The anterior neurocentral center ossifies at 6 to 24 months and may be multifocal. These fuse at 4 to 6 years and set the size of the spinal canal.

Ogden, J.A.: Radiology of postnatal skeletal development. XII. The second cervical vertebra. Skeletal Radiol. 12:169–177, 1984.
The dens has two primary ossification centers which coalesce at 1–3 months of age and are separated from the vertebra by the dentocentral synchondrosis. Bipolar growth results. At 8 to 10 years, the ossiculum terminale forms as a secondary center and fuses at 10 to 13 years.

Yousefzadeh, D.K.; El-Khoury, G.Y.; and Smith, W.L.: Normal sagittal diameter and variation in the pediatric cervical spine. Radiology 144:319–325, 1982.
Gradual widening of the lower cervical canal and ballooning of the mid canal is frequent in children less than 10 years of age and occasionally in the 10- to 18-year-old group. Myelography is not indicated in children unless symptoms are present. Widening of the lower canal in adults merits investigation to rule out tumor.

Congenital and Developmental Disorders

Burke, S.W.; French, H.G.; Roberts, J.M.; Johnston, C.E., II; Whitecloud, T.S., III; and Edmunds, J.O., Jr.: Chronic atlanto-axial instability in Down syndrome. J. Bone Joint Surg. 67A:1356–1360, 1985.
Atlantoaxial instability is more likely to develop in boys over age 10 and is secondary to ligamentous laxity. Accessory upper cervical ossicles can develop as avulsion fractures and are not associated with pathologic motion. Instability greater than 4 mm is more dangerous in the over-10 group.

Juhl, M., and Seerup, K.K.: Os odontoideum: A cause of atlanto-axial instability. Acta Orthop. Scand. 54:113–118, 1983.
Os odontoideum was found with post-traumatic neck pain, signs of medullary compression, and asymptomatically. Fusion is recommended if instability is present.

Koop, S.E.; Winter, R.B.; and Lonstein, J.E.: The surgical treatment of instability of the upper part of the cervical spine in children and adolescents. J. Bone Joint Surg. 66A:403–411, 1984.
Instability is noted adjacent to developmental fusions and at congenital vertebral defects. Autologous bone fusions on decorticated areas with halo-cast immobilization is recommended as the safest and most reliable procedure.

Parke, W.W.; Rothman, R.H.; and Brown, M.D.: The pharyngovertebral veins: An anatomical rationale for Grisel's syndrome. J. Bone Joint Surg. 66A:568–574, 1984.
Atlantoaxial instability after pharyngeal infection is accounted for by retrograde filling of veins in the posterosuperior pharynx with lymphovenous anastomoses.

Pennecot, G.F.; Leonard, P.; Peyrot Des Gachons, S.; Hardy, J.R.; and Pouliquen, J.C.: Traumatic ligamentous instability of the cervical spine in children. J. Pediatr. Orthop. 4:339–345, 1984.
Radiologic criteria of instability of increased interspinous distance, loss of parallelism between the articular processes, and posterior widening of the disk space were used. Fusion was recommended after long periods of immobilization.

Roach, J.W.; Duncan, D.; Wenger, D.R.; Maravilla, A.; and Maravilla, K.: Atlanto-axial instability and spinal cord compression in children: Diagnosis by computerized tomography. J. Bone Joint Surg. 66A:708–714, 1984.
A flat spinal cord on the computed tomographic scan was used as a criterion for surgical treatment.

Sherk, H.H.; Whitaker, L.A.; and Pasquariello, P.S.: Facial malformations and spinal anomalies: A predictable relationship. Spine 7:526–531, 1982.
Apert's syndrome showed a high correlation with upper cervical anomalies and nondeforming segmentation failures. Hemifacial microsomia, especially Goldenhaar syndrome, has a high risk of progressive cervicothoracic scoliosis.

Stabler, C.L.; Eismont, F.J.; Brown, M.D.; Green, B.A.; and Malinin, T.I.: Failure of posterior cervical fusions using cadaveric bone graft in children. J. Bone Joint Surg. 67A:370–375, 1985.
None of seven children who underwent fusion with cadaver bone had posterior cervical fusion. Autologous graft is recommended.

Winter, R.B.; Moe, J.H.; and Lonstein, J.E.: The incidence of Klippel-Feil syndrome in patients with congenital scoliosis and kyphosis. Spine 9:363–366, 1984.
Cervical segmentation defects were present in 25% of patients with congenital scoliosis or kyphosis. Of 298 patients, 82 had single-level defects and 52 were at C2–3.

Degenerative Disorders

Gore, D.R., and Sepic, S.B.: Anterior cervical fusion for degenerated or protruded discs: A review of one hundred forty-six patients. Spine 9:667–671, 1984.
Pain relief was total in 78% and partial in 18%. Fusion rate was 97%.

Kelsey, J.L.; Githens, P.B.; Walter, S.D.; Southwick, W.O.; Weil, U.; Holford, T.R.; Ostfeld, A.M.; Calogero, J.A.; O'Connor, T.; and White, A.A., III: An epidemiological study of acute prolapsed cervical intervertebral disc. J. Bone Joint Surg. 66A:907–914, 1984.
Acute prolapsed cervical disks occurred more in the fourth decade; male-to-female ratio was 1.4:1. Risk factors were frequent lifting, cigarette smoking, and diving from a board.

Rosenørn, J.; Hansen, E.B.; and Rosenørn, M. A.: Anterior cervical discectomy with and without fusion: A prospective study. J. Neurosurg. 59:252–255, 1983.
In a prospective study of 63 patients with cervical disk herniation, followed 3 to 12 months, patients without fusion did better than those with fusion.

Sloop, P.R.; Smith, D.S.; Goldenberg, E.; and Doré, C.: Manipulation for chronic neck pain: A double-blind controlled study. Spine 7:532–535, 1982.
A single manipulation done under diazepam sedation did no better than the control treatment in patients with spondylosis or nonspecific neck pain.

Cervical Spondylotic Myelopathy

Edwards, W.C., and LaRocca, H.: The developmental segmental sagittal diameter of the cervical spinal canal in patients with cervical spondylosis. Spine 8:20–27, 1983.
In patients with refractory cervical spondylosis, the sagittal

diameter was measured at the pedicle and the disk. The average midcervical diameter was 17 mm; 40 of 63 patients had less than the average diameter. Canal dimensions determine symptom production and neural compromise.

Hukuda, S.; Mochizuki, T.; Ogata, M.; Shichikawa, K.; and Shimomura, Y.: Operations for cervical spondylotic myelopathy: A comparison of the results of anterior and posterior procedures. J. Bone Joint Surg. 67B:609–615, 1985.

Posterior operation did better than anterior for patients with more advanced myelopathies such as transverse lesions, Brown-Séquard syndrome, and motor syndromes. Brachialgia, cord syndromes, and central cord syndromes had a satisfactory outcome with anterior operations. The type of anterior or posterior operation made no difference. Patients with a short duration of symptoms did better.

Kadoya, S.; Nakamura, T.; and Kwak, R.: A microsurgical anterior osteophytectomy for cervical spondylotic myelopathy. Spine 9:437–441, 1984.

Ninety-one percent of patients with CSM treated with this operation improved. Of 10 patients without fusion, 6 developed arm and neck pain. Fusion did not affect the resolution of the myelopathy.

Kimura, I.; Oh-Hama, M.; and Shingu, H.: Cervical myelopathy treated by canal-expansive laminaplasty: Computed tomographic and myelographic findings. J. Bone Joint Surg. 66A:914–920, 1984.

Laminaplasty allows osseous protection of the cord, can decrease scarring, and retains stability. In 24 patients with CSM, OPLL, and stenosis who were treated, results were excellent in 4 and good in 18. Computed tomography can show the expanded canal.

Ogino, H.; Tada, K.; Okada, K.; Yonenobu, K.; Yamamoto, T.; Ono, K.; and Namiki, H.: Canal diameter, anteroposterior compression ratio, and spondylotic myelopathy of the cervical spine. Spine 8:1–15, 1983.

The degree of cord destruction is correlated with the ratio of anteroposterior diameter to the transverse diameter (AP compression ratio). Developmental narrowing is the most important factor; spondylotic protrusion is less important. The former causes demyelination and gray matter infarcts, whereas trauma causes the symptomatic manifestations and further cord damage.

Yonenobu, K.; Fuji, T.; Ono, K.; Okada, K.; Yamamoto, T.; and Harada, N.: Choice of surgical treatment for multisegmental cervical spondylotic myelopathy. Spine 10:710–716, 1985.

Laminectomy, Cloward or Smith-Robinson fusion, and subtotal spondylectomy and fusion were compared in CSM. Subtotal spondylectomy did significantly better. Up to three levels can be approached this way. If four or more levels are involved, laminectomy is recommended.

Inflammatory Arthritis

Bryan, W.J.; Inglis, A.E.; Sculco, T.P.; and Ranawat, C.S.: Methylmethacrylate stabilization for enhancement of posterior cervical arthrodesis in rheumatoid arthritis. J. Bone Joint Surg. 64A:1045–1050, 1982.

Wire, mesh, and poly(methyl methacrylate) were used with iliac crest for occipitocervical and long cervical fusion in rheumatoid arthritis. Wound dehiscence and infection were problems, but an immediate internal splint and avoidance of external fixation were provided.

Castor, W.R.; Miller, J.D.R.; Russell, A.S.; Chiu, P.L.; Grace, M.; and Hanson, J.: Computed tomography of the craniocervical junction in rheumatoid arthritis. J. Comput. Assist. Tomogr. 7:31–36, 1983.

In 33 rheumatoid arthritis patients, low-attenuation lesions were found by computed tomography in 11 posterior to the dens, indicating transverse ligament synovitis and rupture. Cord compression was found in 3, dens erosion in 19, and subluxation in 20. No relationship among signs, symptoms, and radiologic abnormalities was noted except in cases of cord compression.

Fried, J.A.; Athreya, B.; Gregg, J.R.; Das, M.; and Doughty, R.: The cervical spine in juvenile rheumatoid arthritis. Clin. Orthop. 179:102–106, 1983.

Neurologic complications from the cervical spine are less common in juvenile rheumatoid arthritis than in adult rheumatoid arthritis. Of 92 patients, 31% had cervical involvement; 15% had limited motion, 14% had pain and stiffness, and 2% had torticollis. Five C1–2 instabilities were found, two with myelopathy. No AAI or subaxial subluxations were noted.

Kankaanpää, U.; Paukku, P.; Laasonen, E.; and Slätis, P.: Atlanto-axial subluxation (AAS) in rheumatoid arthritis. A comparison of clinical symptoms and radiographic changes. Acta Orthop. Scand. 54:529–530, 1983.

Of 42 patients with severe AAS, 25 had cord symptoms and 17 had pain in the neck and occiput. There was no relationship of the atlantodental distance, medullary canal width, Thiebaut-Wackenheim line, or McRae's line with neurologic symptoms.

Lipson, S.J.: Rheumatoid arthritis of the cervical spine. Clin. Orthop. 182:143–149, 1984.

Synovitis injures structures, producing AAS, AAI, and subaxial disease. Patients can die but usually do not from their cervical disease. Nonsurgical treatment is supportive. Posterior fusion is the most common surgical intervention.

Lipson, S.J.: Cervical myelopathy and posterior atlanto-axial subluxation in patients with rheumatoid arthritis. J. Bone Joint Surg. 67A:593–597, 1985.

Posterior AAS with myelopathy was noted in four patients with posterior kinking of the spinal cord as the cause. Contrast-enhanced sagittal imaging or computed tomographic sagittal reconstruction showed the configuration. Halo traction and occipitocervical fusion is the treatment of choice.

Weinstein, P.R.; Karpman, R.R.; Gall, E.P.; and Pitt, M.: Spinal cord injury, spinal fracture, and spinal stenosis in ankylosing spondylitis. J. Neurosurg. 57:609–616, 1982.

In 105 patients with ankylosing spondylitis, 13 had fractures, 8 had severe spinal cord injury, 2 had central cord syndrome without fracture, 3 had spinal stenosis, and 4 had pseudarthrosis. Computed tomography was used to define the canal, and a halo vest was used for treatment. Mortality rate was 29%, and 46% had permanent neurologic loss. No surgical treatment is recommended.

Infection

Hsu, L.C.S., and Leong, J.C.Y.: Tuberculosis of the lower cervical spine (C2 to C7). J. Bone Joint Surg. 66B:1–5, 1984.

In 40 patients, pain and stiffness were the most common symptoms. Children less than 10 years old had more extensive involvement with large abscesses. Above age 10, disease was more localized and there was less pus. Forty-three percent had cord compression. Drug therapy and anterior decompression with grafting gave good results for pain, cord compression, and upper airway obstruction.

Lifeso, R.M.; Weaver, P.; and Harder, E.H.: Tuberculous spondylitis in adults. J. Bone Joint Surg. 67A:1405–1413, 1985.

In 107 adults with tuberculous spondylitis, 35% had negative bone scans, 70% had negative Ga scans, and 14% had negative skin tests. Anterior decompression was the procedure of choice with grafting; all were done for neurologic deficits, instability, and failed medical therapy.

Surgical Fabrications

Bonney, G., and Williams, J.P.R.: Trans-oral approach to the upper cervical spine: A report of 16 cases. J. Bone Joint Surg. 67B:691–698, 1985.

This approach—indicated for anterior element disease, anterior compression unrelieved by a posterior approach, and instability not treated by a posterior operation—is described.

Clark, C.R.; Keggi, K.J.; and Panjabi, M.M.: Methylmethacrylate stabilization of the cervical spine. J. Bone Joint Surg. 66A:40–46, 1984.

Poly(methyl methacrylate) can be used in tumor, fracture, or rheumatoid arthritis, with graft and wire where appropriate. Debilitated patients with spinal cord injury are the best candidates, to avoid the use of orthoses.

Fidler, M.W.: Pathological fractures of the cervical spine: Palliative surgical treatment. J. Bone Joint Surg. 67B:352–357, 1985.

Posterior instrumentation with laminar wires was used with and without graft for metastatic tumor. Graft is used if survival is expected to be greater than 6 months.

Flynn, T.B.: Neurologic complications of anterior cervical interbody fusion. Spine 7:536–539, 1982.

In 82,114 cases, there were 311 major complications with 70 myelopathies of unknown source. Quadriparesis and quadriplegia accounted for 66% of the deficits, and reoperation was of little value in achieving recovery.

Whitehill, R., and Barry, J.C.: The evolution of stability in cervical spinal constructs using either autogenous bone graft or methylmethacrylate cement. A follow-up report on a canine in vivo model. Spine 10:32–41, 1985.

An experimental model using wire with graft or poly(methyl methacrylate) showed that cement loses stability after 1 month postoperatively and loosens by 2 months. Bone graft is superior to cement for long-term stability.

Yasuoka, S.; Peterson, H.A.; and MacCarty, C.S.: Incidence of spinal column deformity after multilevel laminectomy in children and adults. J. Neurosurg. 57:441–445, 1982.

In adults more than 25 years old, deformity did not occur after laminectomy unless there was trauma or facetectomy. In patients less than 15 years old, 46% of laminectomies at all levels resulted in deformity, and 100% of patients having cervical laminectomies developed deformity. Deformity started 2 to 74 months postoperatively. Yearly follow-up is recommended for 6 years after extensive laminectomy in all patients less than 25 years old.

24

Cervical Spine and Cord: Trauma

Cervical spine and cord injuries are still a major cause of disability, although their diagnosis and treatment have become more standardized over the past decade. The cause of cervical spine injuries is vehicular accidents in one-third of the cases and falls in one-third; the remaining third are related to some type of athletic injury or missile wound. The treating physician must understand the pathology of the cervical spine and cord to be able to institute a basic treatment plan and follow the patient through the rehabilitation process.

Pathology: Clinical and Experimental

By definition, a cervical fracture is interruption of the osseous architecture of the vertebra, either anteriorly or posteriorly, and a subluxation is abnormal motion of the contiguous joints without complete disruption of the joint. The term "facet dislocation" implies complete disruption of the ligament and capsular structures of the joint. The pathology of cervical spine and cord injuries may be divided into the categories of osseous, soft tissue, and central nervous system.

In a study of the pathology of 50 fatal craniospinal injuries, it was found that soft tissue injuries occurred by hemorrhage into the anterior musculature (as much as 700 ml) and that the vertebral artery was rarely damaged. The soft tissue hemorrhage was secondary to tearing of the radicular artery branches in the foramina. Cervical disk disruption was a common injury, occurring in 38% of this fatal injury series; complete herniation of the disk was uncommon. Ligament injuries occurred in combination—that is, with disk disruption and tearing of both anterior and posterior longitudinal ligaments—indicating that multiple forces were involved. Small spinal epidural hemorrhages were noted in only three cases and did not compress the spinal cord. Massive epidural hemorrhage only occurs in patients who have ankylosing spondylitis and sustain cervical spine injuries.

Injury to the cervical spinal cord occurs predominantly in the more vulnerable central gray matter, and its severity varies. The pathologic features of the spinal cord injury include the initial cord contusion (which may be incomplete), compression of the spinal cord by bone or disk fragments (resulting in microvascular ischemia), and distortion of the spinal cord by angular kyphosis. Incomplete spinal cord injuries, therefore, have the potential to recover to varying degrees, depending on the amount of initial damage and on the type of treatment of these lesions. Head and neck injuries may be commonly associated and so one should consider the head and neck as a unit when treating a patient who has sustained multiple trauma.

In a review of 300 cervical spine injuries, the autopsy findings in 48 cases indicated that only 3 of these involved total cord disruption; many other patients with clinical evidence of total cord lesions had incomplete contusions, indicating sparing of neural tissue. In addition, some patients had significant quadriparesis with anterior cord syndromes but had a normal spinal cord microscopically without evidence of gross cord disruption (Fig. 1). These findings indicate that ischemia and direct neural compression may play a role in the recovery from incomplete spinal cord injury. In addition, four patients who had unilateral facet dislocations had impairment of major radicular feeder vessels to the spinal cord associated with central cord necrosis, which would imply that early reduction of spinal fractures

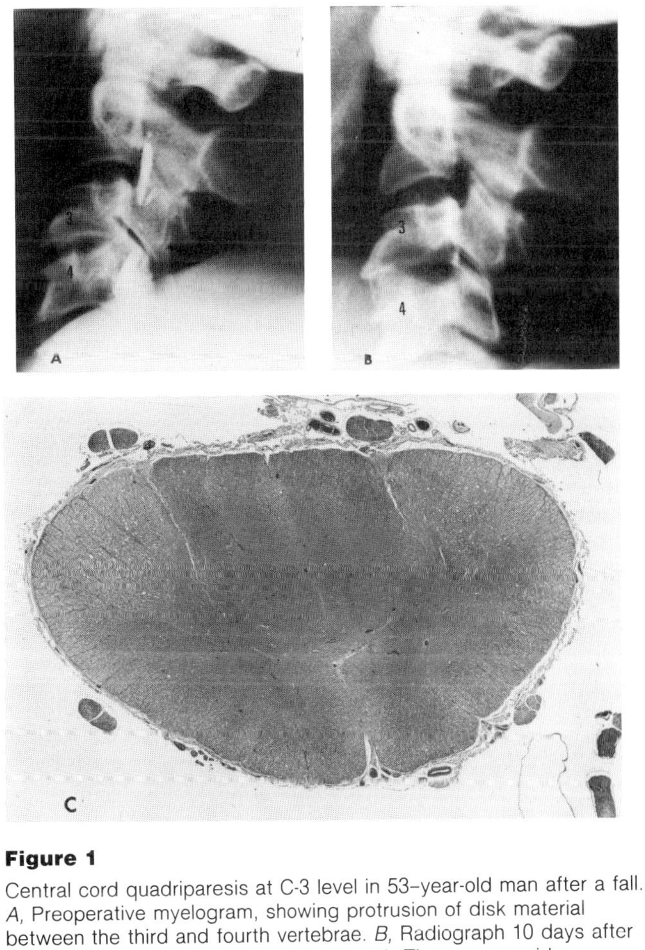

Figure 1

Central cord quadriparesis at C-3 level in 53-year-old man after a fall. *A*, Preoperative myelogram, showing protrusion of disk material between the third and fourth vertebrae. *B*, Radiograph 10 days after anterior discectomy and fusion (Robinson). There was rapid recovery of function but the patient died of a pulmonary embolus 10 months after injury. *C*, Histologic section of the spinal cord at the level of injury shows little more than peripheral vacuolization. (Hematoxylin and eosin, x5.) (From Bohlman, H.H. J. Bone Joint Surg. 61A:1119–1142, 1979. By permission of the journal.)

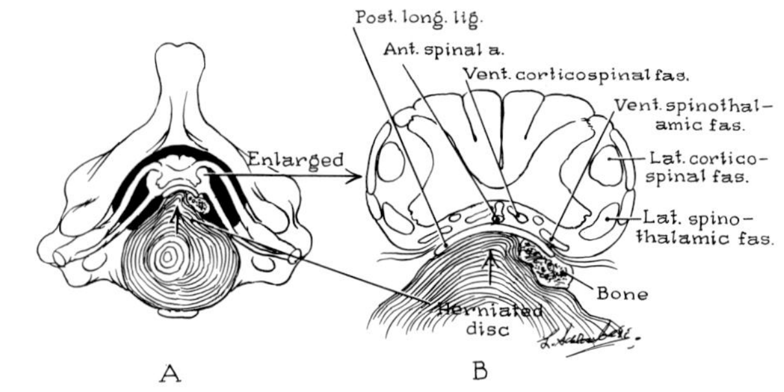

Figure 2

Anterior cord syndrome. A herniated disk or bone fragment compresses the anterior spinal artery and cord. This may produce ischemia of the anterior two-thirds of the cord and sparing of posterior column function (touch, position, and vibratory senses). (From Bohlman, H.H.: The neck. *In* Musculoskeletal Disorders: Regional Examination and Differential Diagnosis, edited by R.D. D'Ambrosia, pp. 178–244. Philadelphia, J.B. Lippincott Company, 1977. By permission of the publisher.)

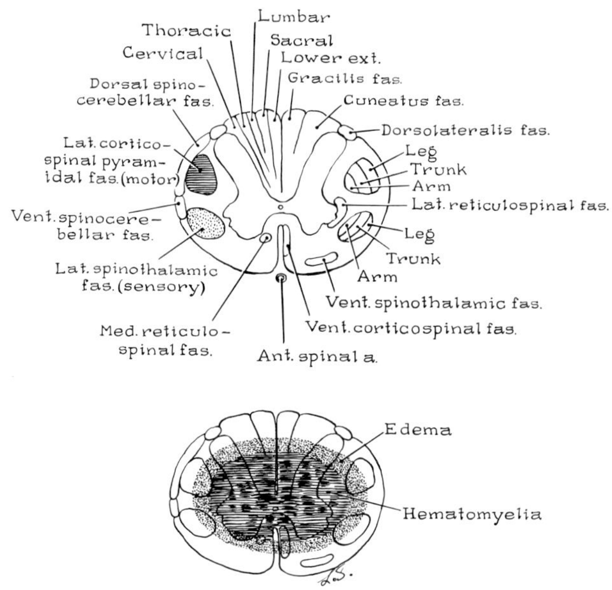

Figure 3

Central cord syndrome. Centrally placed tracks are affected by central edema or necrosis. Note that the most medial portion of the pyramidal track is for arm function. The upper extremity paralysis therefore is greater than the lower extremity paralysis. (From Bohlman, H.H. *In* Musculoskeletal Disorders: Regional Examination and Differential Diagnosis. [See Figure 2.] By permission of the publisher.)

would be beneficial from the standpoints of restoring vascular supply and of relieving pressure on the spinal cord.

In animal models of chronic anterior cord compression and in the weight-drop contusion model, central necrosis of the gray matter is the most common pathologic finding in association with varying degrees of demyelinization. Also, histologically normal spinal cord could be found after long-standing anterior compression. The anterior and central cord syndromes may represent varying degrees of the same pathologic process, including contusion of the central cord, microvascular ischemia, edema, and subsequent further necrosis of the spinal cord after long-standing compression.

There has been a misconception for many years that nonoperative treatment was best for spinal cord injuries and that, once the initial cord damage had occurred, function of the spinal cord could not be restored. In the past, laminectomy has been proposed for the treatment of spinal cord injuries. However, this operation produced a high rate of neurologic deficit and deaths. Therefore, it is contraindicated for the treatment of cervical spine injuries, with one exception—when there is massive epidural hemorrhage in a patient with ankylosing spondylitis and fracture of the cervical spine. Because compression of the spinal cord almost always occurs anteriorly, any decompressive operative procedure should be carried out from the anterior approach, with the rare exception of laminar fractures which may compress the spinal cord.

It has been demonstrated experimentally and clinically that, with incomplete spinal cord injuries, recovery to varying degrees is possible, depending on the amount of the initial cord contusion and on other factors such as bone and disk fragments compressing the neural tissue. If the spinal cord damage is incomplete and there is a bone or disk fragment compressing the spinal cord anteriorly, spinal cord function may be blocked for a long time without total destruction of the neural tissue. As in experimental animals, patients who sustain incomplete spinal cord injuries will recover neurologically to a certain point in time and then reach a plateau after which no further recovery of the spinal cord occurs unless the compressive elements are removed anteriorly, which may aid recovery of spinal cord function.

Clinical Experience

Long-term follow-up (2 to 12 years postoperatively) has been reported on 111 patients who underwent late anterior decompression for cervical spinal cord injury between 1973 and 1983. Approximately half of the patients had motor-complete quadriplegia and the other half had incomplete spinal cord injuries; all had plateaued in their neurologic recovery prior to late anterior decompression which was performed an average of 1 year after injury. Of the 54 patients who sustained motor-complete quadriplegia and had plateaued in their arm function recovery, 62% recovered one to three levels of further nerve root function after anterior decompression. Of the 57 with motor-incomplete spinal cord injury and who had decompression, 45 were unable to walk preoperatively; 36 of these were able to walk to some degree postoperatively. In addition, all of the patients with incomplete spinal cord injuries recovered one to three levels of nerve root function in the upper extremities. Therefore, further neurologic recovery can occur with anterior decompression in both motor-complete and incomplete spinal cord injuries.

Cervical spine injuries without neurologic deficit include osseous as well as ligament injury which must be assessed to determine if there is instability and, therefore, if surgical intervention is necessary. Upper cervical spine injuries are rarely associated with neurologic deficit, so the decision to operate usually is related to instability or the degree of osseous and ligament damage. The type of treatment carried out for lower cervical spine injuries (C-3 to C-7 levels) depends on the degree of vertebral body disruption and posterior osseous and ligament injury that has occurred.

Axial loading compression fractures of the lower cervical vertebrae may be treated with a rigid cervical orthosis and will heal uneventfully. However, more severe compression fractures may produce osseous fragment protrusion into the spinal canal, which necessitates skeletal traction for reduction and possibly anterior excision and arthrodesis to obtain stability.

A common severe cervical spine injury occurs when flexion results in tearing of the posterior ligament complex with subluxation or dislocation of the associated vertebra and anterior disk protrusion or disruption, in which case there is damage on both sides of the spinal cord. Late instability is much more common than frequently realized because ligament structures do not reconstitute normally, even after prolonged rigid external fixation. Therefore, unless spontaneous fusion occurs anteriorly after a reduced dislocation, chronic instability can occur and produce pain or paralysis. Some instances of anterior compression of the vertebral body and posterior ligament tearing will require both posterior and anterior stabilization.

General Patient Assessment

Treatment of the patient with a cervical spine and cord injury begins with initial evaluation and general assessment. However, the first priority is to save the patient's life. Therefore, if there have been multiple traumatic injuries, one must treat the hypovolemic shock, cardiovascular injuries, or obstructed airway and simultaneously stabilize the cervical spine in traction. Only after the patient is stabilized from a medical standpoint should any thought of surgical intervention be entertained. Suspicion and recognition of the cervical spine and cord injury should begin at the scene of the accident or no later than treatment in the emergency room. In the review of 300 cervical spine injuries, delay in diagnosis was very common; in 100 cases the diagnosis was missed in the initial emergency room setting. Generally, the failure to recognize cervical spine injuries was a consequence of associated head injury, multiple trauma, and alcohol intoxication.

After general physical examination to assess all organ systems, a careful neurologic evaluation must be performed to identify a specific nerve root or spinal cord injury. These examinations should be documented on neurologic data sheets. The most common neurologic syndromes that occur with lower cervical spine injuries are isolated nerve root paralysis, anterior cord syndrome, central cord syndrome, Brown-Séquard syndrome, and a complete cord syndrome or quadriplegia (Figs. 2 and 3). When a neurologic injury has been identified, skeletal traction should be immediately applied to support the head and neck in neutral alignment.

Meticulous neurologic examination must be carried out to look for any evidence of paralysis, either sensory or motor. If gross paralysis is present, one should observe for any sparing of sensory or motor function below the level of the cervical spine injury. The perianal region must be examined for sensation in the lower sacral dermatomes which may be the only neurologic sparing in an incomplete spinal cord injury. All voluntary motor contraction should be noted, as well as voluntary rectal sphincter tone. The latter is also evidence of sacral sparing. Frequently, the only evidence of motor function sparing is toe flexor contractions. Deep tendon reflexes are decreased or absent in the patient with acute spinal cord injury; however, if pathologic reflexes occur, such as clonus or positive Babinski reflex, this may indicate acute spinal cord compression in

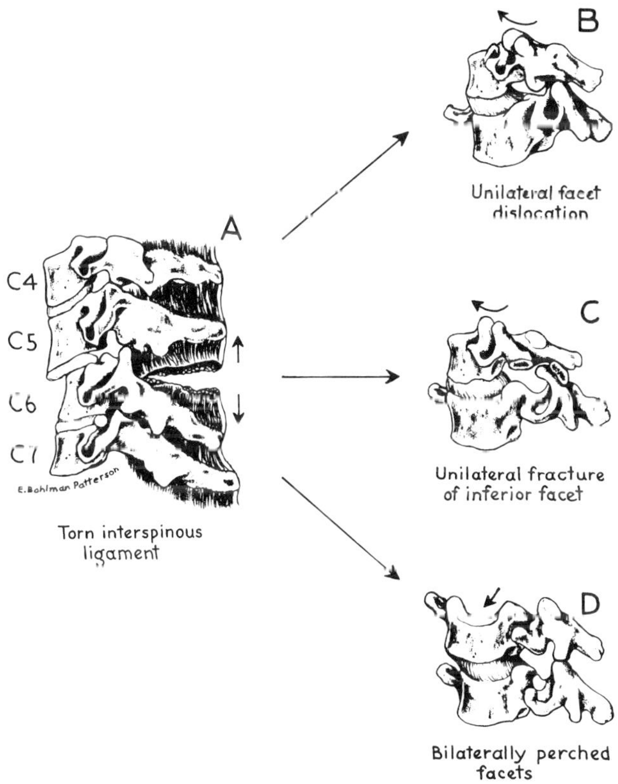

Figure 4

Types of fractures and dislocations of the articular processes that may cause moderate anterior subluxation. (From Bohlman, H.H. J. Bone Joint Surg. 61A:1119–1142, 1979. By permission of the journal.)

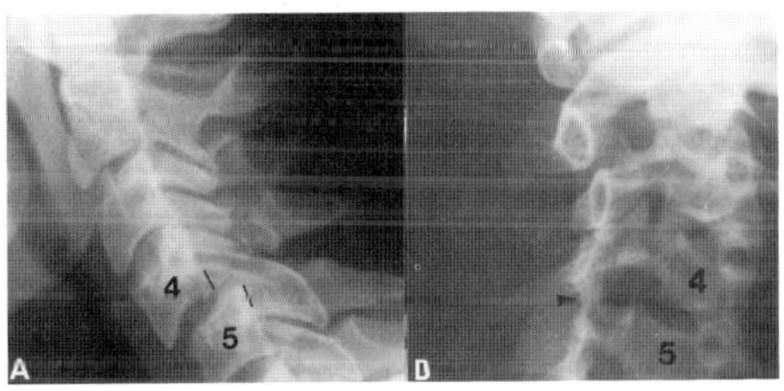

Figure 5

A, Lateral radiograph of patient who sustained moderate anterior subluxation of C-4 on C-5. Vertebral displacement is approximately one-third of the width of the vertebral body. In this situation, oblique views must be obtained to determine the specific pathology involving the posterior elements. *B*, Right oblique radiograph, demonstrating fractured C-5 facet, allowing the anterior subluxation. (From Bohlman, H.H.: Surgical management of cervical spine fractures and dislocations. *In* AAOS Instructional Course Lectures. XXXIV:163–187. St. Louis, C.V. Mosby Company, 1985. By permission of the publisher.)

a patient with incomplete cord injury and may be a good prognostic sign.

Initially, the spinal cord goes through a period of shock when there is very little or no physiologic function occurring; however, this state may resolve within 48 hours. If the bulbocavernosus reflex is present after 48 hours following injury, it is assumed that the patient is out of spinal cord shock. If at that time there is no documentation of any motor or sensory recovery below the level of the cervical spine fracture, then the patient can be diagnosed as having a complete spinal cord injury and no further distal recovery of motor function can be expected. If the patient has any spared motor or sensory function, then the diagnosis is incomplete spinal cord injury with varying potential for recovery.

Radiographic Assessment

Any patient with evidence of a head injury—either facial laceration or decreased level of consciousness—should have a lateral cervical spine radiograph made in the emergency room. Certainly, this also should be done for a patient suspected to have cervical spine injury. After that, routine anterior-posterior, oblique, and open-mouth odontoid views can be obtained. The lateral cervical spine radiograph can initiate the diagnosis of cervical spine injury because almost all of these patients will have some displacement of the osseous elements that is quite evident. Tomograms or computed tomography may be needed to define specifics of the fracture.

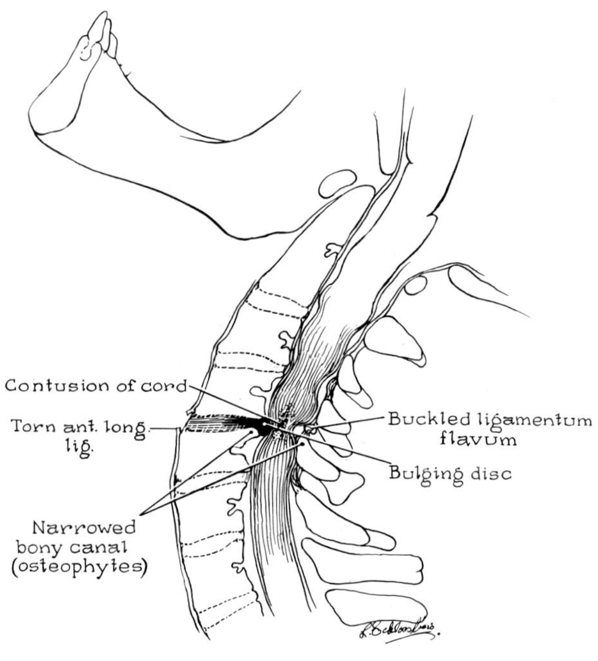

Figure 6

Hyperextension with cervical spondylosis produced by frontal head injury. Note that ligamentum flavum buckles inward against the posterior spinal cord; bulging disk compresses the cord anteriorly. The combined forces contuse the cord. The disk is also disrupted. (From Bohlman, H.H. *In* Musculoskeletal Disorders: Regional Examination and Differential Diagnosis. [See Figure 2.] By permission of the publisher.)

Atlanto-occipital dislocations are rare, but these patients can survive with improved emergency care and transport. These are diagnosed by separation of the atlas from the occipital condyles with either anterior or posterior displacement of the skull. In addition, there will be a large amount of soft tissue swelling anterior to C-2 evident on the lateral radiograph.

Fractures of the axis and atlas can be detected by open-mouth odontoid and lateral views. Tomograms may be helpful to define the type of fracture of the axis and to classify this injury. Fractures and dislocations of the lower cervical spine are classified according to whether they involve posterior elements, anterior elements, lateral elements, or a combination of these. On the lateral radiograph, one of three major types of vertebral body displacement is usually evident: 1) slight (1 to 3 mm) posterior subluxation of the upper vertebra on the lower; 2) moderate (3 to 5 mm) anterior subluxation of the upper vertebra on the lower; or 3) maximal anterior dislocation (5 mm or greater) (Figs. 4 to 8). A slight posterior subluxation usually occurs with extension injuries or frontal facial lacerations and is commonly associated with cervical spondylosis. In this instance, a fracture occurs through the ossified disk space, tearing the longitudinal ligaments and producing the retrolisthesis on the lateral radiogram. Moderate anterior subluxation usually indicates some disruption of the posterior ligament complex, which may be unilateral facet dislocation, unilateral facet fracture, or bilateral perched facets. These entities may be associated with incomplete quadriparesis or nerve root compression. Maximal anterior dislocation indicates complete bilateral dislocated osteoarticular facets and is usually associated with complete quadriplegia which is evident on clinical examination. Choice of the appropriate treatment method for these injuries depends totally on identifying the type of injury that has occurred. For example, bilateral perched facets may be easy to reduce with skeletal traction; however, a unilateral dislocated facet may be extremely difficult to reduce without surgical intervention.

Operative Treatment

The major considerations in treatment of cervical fractures and dislocations are 1) immobilization, 2) medical stabilization, 3) spinal alignment, 4) operative decompression if there is proved cord compression, and 5) spinal stabilization. The treatment plan must be based on the pathology involved for each specific injury and may have great bearing on the ultimate stability and neurologic recovery as well as on enhancement of the rehabilitation process in these patients.

Many fractures of the upper cervical spine can be treated without surgical intervention, but there are specific indications for stabilization. Injuries of the occipital-cervical joint are rare with survival but should be stabilized with a cervical occipital arthrodesis if they occur (Fig. 9). All ligament structures are torn between the occiput and the atlas with cervical occipital dislocations and, therefore, stabilization is necessary as soon as feasible, regardless of whether the patient has an incomplete or a complete spinal cord injury.

Fractures of the atlas rarely require internal fixation, with

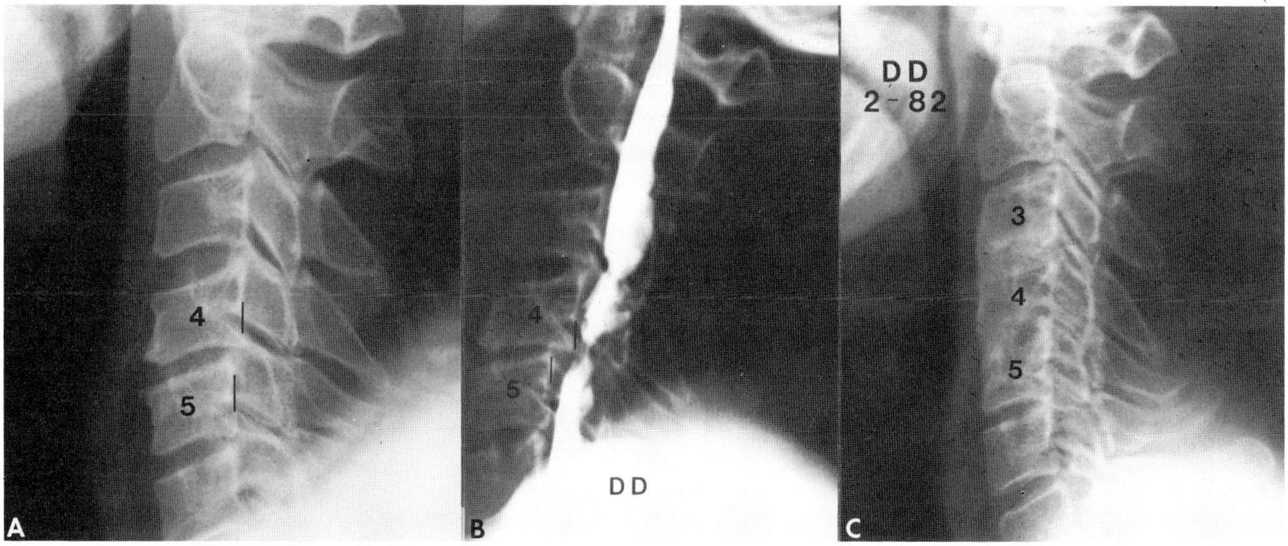

Figure 7

Patient who sustained a central cord quadriparesis after a surfing accident. *A,* Lateral radiograph of cervical spine. Note slight reverse subluxation of C-4 on C-5 and relatively narrow cervical spinal canal at that level. *B,* Lateral myelogram, demonstrating anterior cord compression at C3-4 and C4-5. *C,* Lateral radiograph 2 years after anterior cervical discectomy and fusion at C3-4 and C4-5 levels. The patient recovered total motor function and was ambulatory without aid. (*A* from Bohlman, H.H., Ducker, T.B.; and Lucas, J.T. *In* The Spine, edited by R.H. Rothman and F.A. Simeone, pp. 661–756. Vol. 2. Second edition. Philadelphia, W.B. Saunders Company, 1982. By permission of the publisher. *B* and *C* from Bohlman, H.H. *In* AAOS Instructional Course Lectures. [See Figure 5.] By permission of the publisher.)

the exception of those that produce tearing of the transverse ligament and atlantoaxial subluxation (Fig. 10). In this instance, it is better to apply a halo cast or vest, allow the atlas fractures to heal, test for stability at 2 or 3 months, and then, if atlantoaxial subluxation greater than 5 mm at the atlantodental interval persists, perform a posterior atlantoaxial arthrodesis. Although traumatic tearing of the transverse ligament is rare, it does produce instability, and a posterior arthrodesis should be performed primarily. Fractures that involve the lateral mass of the atlas and the articular surface of the atlantoaxial joint may require late arthrodesis because of pain or spastic torticollis, but most of these can be treated with a rigid orthosis. Posterior atlantoaxial dislocation is rare, but it can occur with survival and requires skeletal traction for reduction and posterior arthrodesis because of severe ligament disruption. Anterior atlantoaxial dislocation may occur as the result of a transverse ligament tear or secondary to dysplasia of the odontoid process which becomes manifest after a traumatic episode.

Posterior atlantoaxial arthrodesis is indicated to prevent future cord injury. Fractures of the odontoid process can be treated with rigid external fixation—a two-poster rigid brace or a halo vest. However, type II fractures of the odontoid through the waist of the dens heal poorly, and generally a primary posterior atlantoaxial arthrodesis is used in most of these patients (Fig. 11). It is important not to overdistract odontoid fractures with halo fixation because this may lead to nonunion. If the odontoid fractures are displaced initially, skeletal traction is instituted to reduce the fracture, followed by arthrodesis or halo fixation. Almost all pedicle fractures of the axis will heal with conservative management. If they are nondisplaced, a two-poster rigid orthosis is utilized. However, with displacement, skeletal traction is instituted for 2 to 3 weeks to obtain reduction and early callus formation; then, a halo vest is utilized for 2 months. A very unstable pedicle fracture of the axis may occur when the longitudinal ligaments and disk are completely disrupted between the second and third vertebrae. This injury is probably secondary to a combined flexion-extension force, and the fracture is extremely unstable and cannot be held in the reduced position even with halo fixation. In this situation, skeletal traction can be used for 2 to 3 weeks and then an anterior C-2 to C-3 arthrodesis is performed; otherwise, late instability may occur (Fig. 12).

Surgical intervention for patients with lower cervical spine injuries depends on the presence of instability and neural compression. In patients sustaining fractures and dislocations without neurologic deficit, the concern is whether there is anterior or posterior instability. Flexion injuries produce major tearing of the posterior ligament complex and should be treated in general with a posterior arthrodesis, including cortico-cancellous iliac graft wired into place (Fig. 13). Late instability secondary to flexion injuries was common in the review of 300 cervical spine injuries with long-term follow-up: 21 patients had chronic instability secondary to posterior ligament tearing. Twelve other patients with osteoarthritis had hyperextension injuries with disruption of the anterior longitudinal ligament and a disk with chronic instability. White's criteria for instability are used to determine when fusion is necessary. Axial loading injuries or compression fractures of the vertebral body may produce marked kyphotic deformity and require anterior resection of the vertebral body and iliac grafting to maintain alignment and stability.

Patients who sustain lower cervical spine injuries between C-3 and T-1 with neurologic deficit require imme-

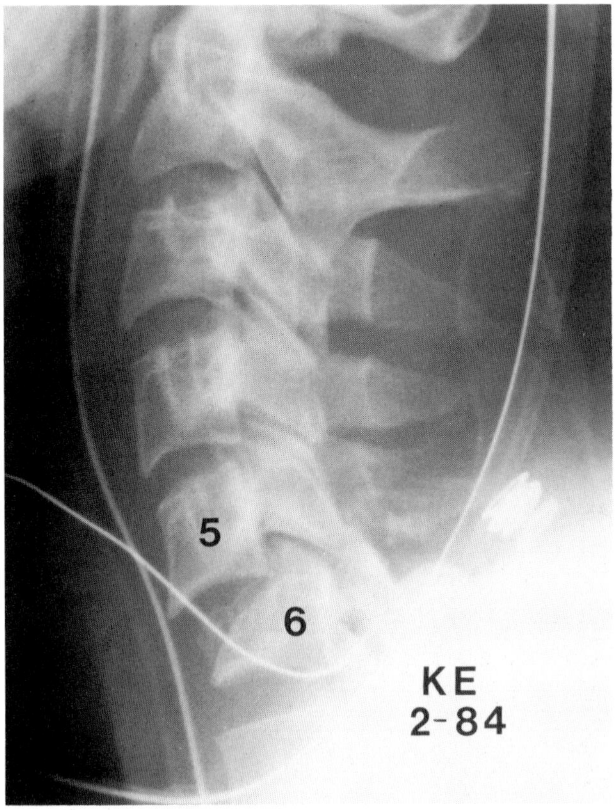

Figure 8

Lateral radiograph of 21-year-old man who sustained a complete bilateral facet dislocation of C5-6 in car accident, resulting in complete quadriplegia. Note 50% displacement of the vertebrae. (From Bohlman, H.H. *In* AAOS Instructional Course Lectures. [See Figure 5.] By permission of the publisher.)

diate skeletal traction to realign the spine and to restore the spinal canal diameter. This is the first stage in decompression of the spinal cord. It is no longer believed that patients should have skeletal traction instituted over a period of days or weeks to attempt reduction of fractures and dislocations in association with neurologic deficit. The more severe the fracture or dislocation, or the greater the axial loading injury, the more severe the neurologic deficit noted in the review of cervical spine injuries. Because one cannot tell if the spinal cord injury is complete within the first 48 hours, complete dislocation of the cervical vertebra should be reduced as soon as possible to relieve pressure on the spinal cord. Reduction of flexion injuries and total dislocations with early institution of skeletal traction at no more than 50 pounds is attempted. If this fails within the first few hours after injury, posterior open reduction and iliac grafting are performed. Thus, the patient can be ambulated in a two-poster orthosis in a sitting position on the following day and begin the rehabilitation process.

After posterior open reduction and fusion, a cervical myelogram is obtained to assess the spinal canal for intrusion of bone or disk fragments anteriorly. For patients with incomplete spinal cord injuries with lesser degrees of flexion injuries—that is, unilateral facet dislocation or fractured or perched facets—reduction in skeletal traction and arthrodesis posteriorly are used as soon as possible. Patients with cervical spine fractures and isolated nerve root lesions initially are placed in skeletal traction and then assessed as to whether there is compressive pathology anteriorly or posteriorly. If there is a fractured facet posteriorly impinging on the nerve root, a posterior foraminotomy and fusion is carried out (Fig. 14); if there is an anterior disk fragment compressing the nerve root, anterior discectomy and fusion is performed. The nerve root will recover as long as it is decompressed and stabilized. Unilateral facet dislocations may be difficult to reduce in skeletal traction and usually require open reduction and posterior fixation.

Cervical myelography with computed tomography is carried out on all patients who have incomplete neurologic deficits preoperatively. In patients who sustained an axial loading injury with compression fracture anteriorly and have an incomplete neurologic deficit, early anterior decompression by corpectomy and iliac grafts is performed as soon as the patient is stable and able to undergo operation, if anterior cord compression is proved (Fig. 15). Only if the patient is recovering neurologic function rapidly and there is no evidence of cord compression is a conservative program used without surgical intervention.

Uncommonly, a patient may sustain a lower cervical spine injury with both severe flexion and axial loading, in which case the posterior ligaments are completely torn and there is anterior osseous compression of the spinal cord by bone fragments. In this situation, posterior cervical arthrodesis, anterior corpectomy, and iliac grafting for decompression are used. Although extremely rare, a posterior reduction accomplished under general anesthesia occasionally can pull a large disk fragment back into the spinal canal and compress the spinal cord in the patient with incomplete spinal cord injury, increasing the neurologic deficit. To avoid this situation, spinal cord monitoring during the procedure is important in these high-risk patients.

Patients over age 50 years with preexisting cervical spondylosis most commonly have a central cord syndrome, or even complete quadriplegia, after hyperextension cervical spine injury. Almost all of these patients have a retrolisthesis of the upper vertebral body on the lower, secondary to the hyperextension force that tears the longitudinal ligaments and disrupts the intervertebral disk. This may be a very unstable fracture that is subtle on roentgenographic examination. These patients should be placed in skeletal traction initially. If a patient with incomplete neurologic deficit does not improve rapidly, cervical myelography and computed tomography are performed to determine if there is spinal cord impingement. Very often this is the case, and the patient will have a soft disk fragment or spondylitic bar compressing the spinal cord which necessitates anterior discectomy and fusion at the appropriate levels. Even with late decompression, years after injury, in this situation major neurologic recovery can occur.

The timing of operative treatment for anterior decompression of the spinal cord injury will vary to some degree, but in general it is the obligation of the treating physician to free the patient of any pathologic process that may continue to compress the spinal cord and produce further malfunction of it. Therefore, a decision regarding decompression should be attempted within the first few hours or days after spinal cord injury, if the patient's other medical and neurologic conditions permit this. Steroids are not used in the treatment of spinal cord injuries because there is no clinical proof that they improve neurologic re-

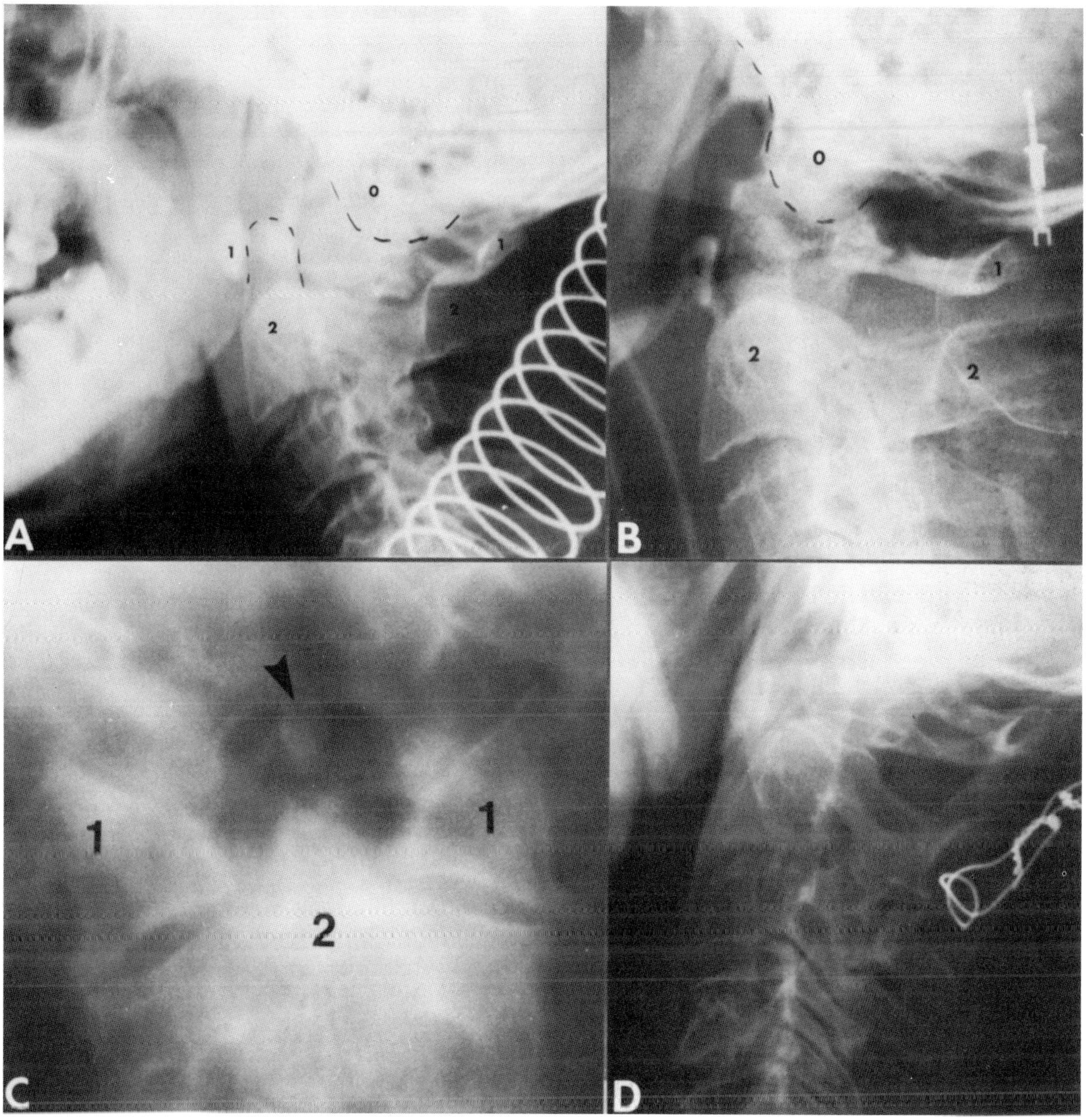

Figure 9

A, Lateral cervical radiograph, demonstrating posterior atlanto-occipital dislocation and fracture of the posterior arch of the atlas. Basion is grossly posterior to the odontoid process. The lateral mass of the atlas also appears to be dislocated slightly posterior in relationship to the odontoid process but this is due to the rotation of the head as shown by the asymmetric position of the mandibular rami. *B,* True lateral radiograph of cervical spine centered at level of the atlas, showing reduction of the atlanto-occipital dislocation. *C,* Anteroposterior laminagram at 10 weeks after fusion, demonstrating avulsion of apex of odontoid process which probably includes the bone attachment of the alar ligaments. *D,* Lateral radiograph of the cervical spine at 11 months after fusion, showing a solid fusion from the occiput to C-3 with the occiput and cervical spine in their normal relationship. (From Elsmont, F.J., and Bohlman, H.H.: Posterior atlanto-occipital dislocation with fractures of the atlas and odontoid process: Report of a case with survival. J. Bone Joint Surg. 60A:397–399, 1978. By permission of the journal.)

covery and there is a high incidence of complications such as gastrointestinal hemorrhage and death.

Fractures of the cervical spine in patients with ankylosing spondylitis present unusual problems, unlike fractures in other patients. These fractures will heal uneventfully with rigid immobilization after initial skeletal traction for reduction for approximately 3 weeks. One problem that may arise in the patient with ankylosing spondylitis is a preexisting kyphotic deformity of the cervical spine. In this case, after the fracture, the kyphosis straightens out during the tong traction in the horizontal position, which produces a retrolisthesis of the upper portion of the spine on the lower and can add to cord or root compression. Therefore, the patient may have to be placed in skeletal traction in the sitting position in bed. Another problem that occurs with these patients is massive epidural hemorrhage; this

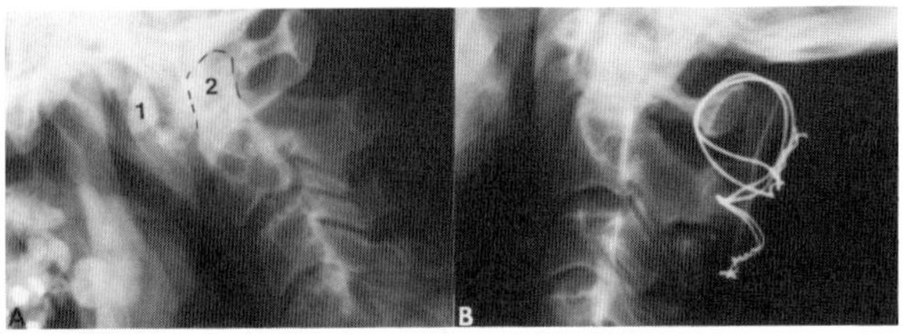

Figure 10

Driver of a truck that was struck by a train. *A*, Anterior dislocation of the axis on the atlas without fracture. This is evidence of a ruptured transverse ligament. *B*, Lateral radiograph after atlantoaxial arthrodesis. (*A* from Bohlman, H.H. *In* Musculoskeletal Disorders: Regional Examination and Differential Diagnosis. [See Figure 2.] By permission of the publisher.)

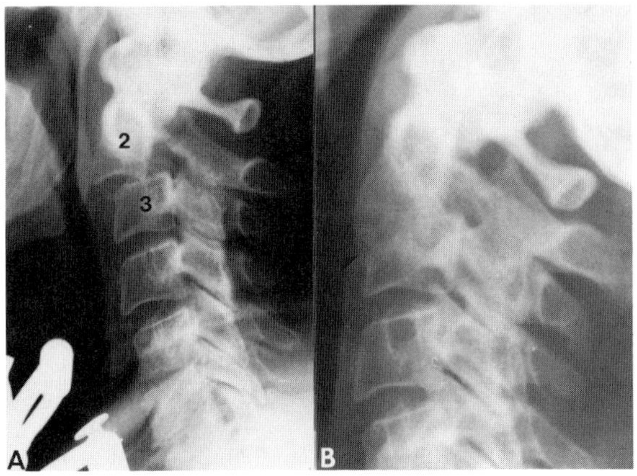

Figure 12

Lateral radiographs of the cervical spine. *A*, Gross instability of C-2 on C-3 at 6 weeks following a fall. There is disruption of disk and longitudinal ligaments and pedicle fractures of the axis, resulting in subluxation even though the patient was in a halo vest. *B*, At 11 months after anterior cervical arthrodesis, the axis pedicles and vertebral bodies of C-2 and C-3 have united. (From Bohlman, H.H. *In* AAOS Instructional Course Lectures. [See Figure 5.] By permission of the publisher.)

does not occur in any other cervical spine fracture. In the review of 300 cervical spine injuries, 8 patients had ankylosing spondylitis and 4 developed massive epidural hemorrhage; some of these had ascending paralysis which occurred if the patient was not properly immobilized. Also found in the patient with ankylosed spine is restrictive lung disease which may produce significant pulmonary problems such as difficulty in clearing of secretions and decreased oxygenation. Treatment is vigorous pulmonary toilet and, occasionally, tracheostomy; ordinarily, operation on the spine is not required except that massive epidural hemorrhage and ascending paralysis may be an indication for laminectomy.

Gunshot wounds of the cervical spine and cord are treated without operative intervention unless there is compression of the spinal cord. If a missile traverses the spinal canal, the spinal cord damage that occurs is evident by clinical examination and no further operative intervention is necessary. However, gunshot wounds that transect the esophagus may be considered to be open contaminated fractures and should be debrided. In addition, if the patient presents with incomplete quadriparesis and the bullet or a major bone fragment is present in the spinal canal and is still compressing the spinal cord, myelography and computed tomography are indicated. If the bullet is predominantly in the posterior aspect of the spinal canal, a laminectomy is performed to remove the missile, followed by a posterior fusion. If the bullet remains anterior to the spinal cord, it is removed from the anterior approach, followed by arthrodesis. If bullets are left within the confines of the spinal canal, lead can be absorbed into the system but, more important, a foreign body reaction occurs over

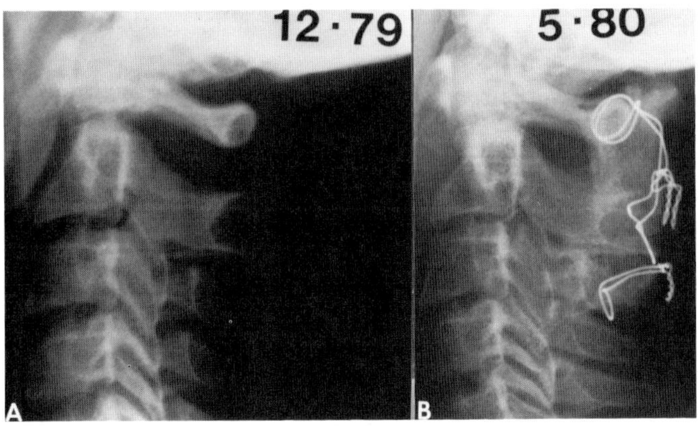

Figure 11

A, Lateral radiograph shows fracture through the waist of the odontoid process. *B*, Lateral radiograph at 6 months after atlantoaxial arthrodesis. (*A* from Bohlman, H.H., et al. *In* The Spine. [See Figure 7.] By permission of the publisher. *B* from Bohlman, H.H. *In* AAOS Instructional Course Lectures. [See Figure 5.] By permission of the publisher.)

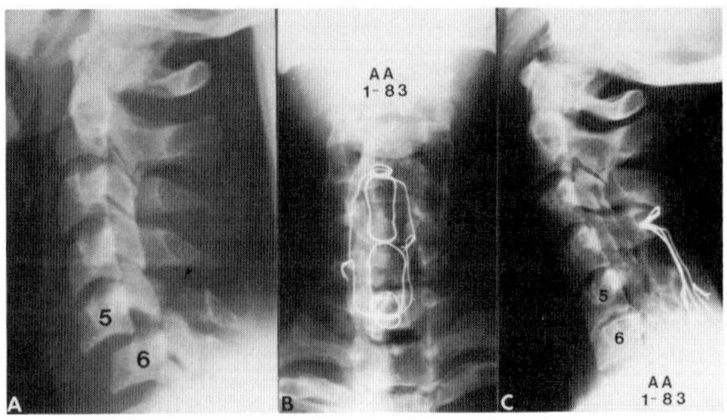

Figure 13

A, Lateral radiograph of cervical spine, demonstrating a complete dislocation of C-5 on C-6 caused when patient was sucked into a jet engine. This resulted in complete C-6 quadriplegia. *B*, Anteroposterior radiograph of cervical spine 6 years after posterior cervical arthrodesis utilizing the triple-wire technique and iliac graft. Immediate stability was obtained so the patient could be upright in a rigid two-poster orthosis. *C*, Postoperative lateral radiograph of cervical spine, demonstrating maintenance of the reduction and stability. (From Bohlman, H.H. *In* AAOS Instructional Course Lectures. [See Figure 5.] By permission of the publisher.)

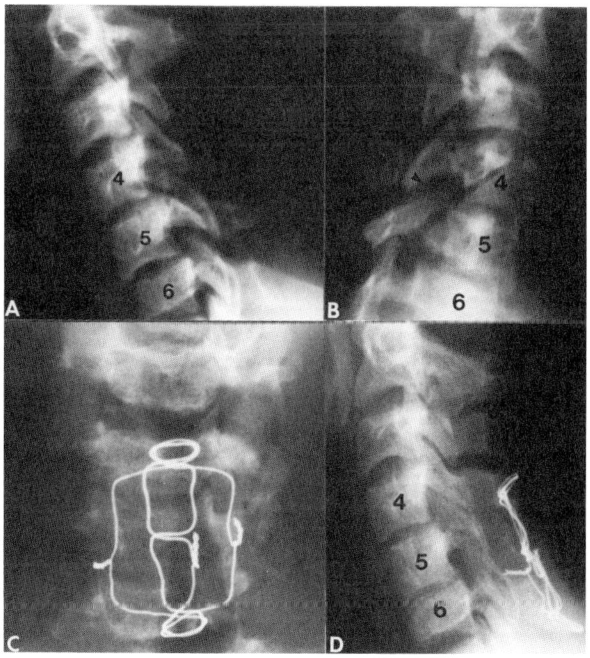

Figure 14

Neck injury in 16-year-old boy who dived into an ocean wave. *A*, Lateral cervical radiograph shows right C-5 root injury and moderate anterior subluxation of C-4 on C-5 and C-5 on C-6. *B*, Right oblique cervical radiograph, demonstrating fracture of the pedicle of C-5 with the facet occluding the foramen, compressing the C-5 nerve root. *C*, Anteroposterior radiograph at 19 months after posterior foraminotomy to decompress the nerve root and posterior fusion to stabilize the spine from C-4 through C-6. *D*, Lateral radiograph of cervical spine after posterior arthrodesis. (From Bohlman, H.H. *In* AAOS Instructional Course Lectures. [See Figure 5.] By permission of the publisher.

a period of months and years and further compression of the spinal cord, with deterioration of neurologic function, may occur from a mass of scar tissue.

Operative Techniques

There are many different operative techniques for accomplishing cervical occipital, atlantoaxial, and lower cervical arthrodesis in the patient with cervical spine trauma. The technique of anterior discectomy and arthrodesis by the Smith-Robinson method is well established and published. The technique of anterior cervical corpectomy with iliac fusion has been described. There are some important points with regard to various arthrodesis techniques that can be applied to the patient who has sustained a cervical spine fracture.

Cervical occipital fusion is best accomplished by utilizing a well-molded, thick cortico-cancellous iliac graft that is wired to the occiput through a small hole through the outer cortex of the skull approximately 2 cm superior to the foramen magnum. If possible, the atlas ring is incorporated into the graft with a second wire, and a third wire is passed through and around the spinous process of the axis; all wires are tied down over the iliac graft on either side of the cervical spine. This procedure can be performed with local or general anesthesia.

Atlantoaxial arthrodesis may be carried out with a 20-gauge wire loop passing under the arch of the atlas, incorporating it as a Gallie fusion, and an additional separate wire passed through and around the spinous process of the axis; again, two thick cortico-cancellous iliac grafts are tied down to the laminae. The need for external fixation by halo vest or cervical orthosis depends on the specific situation. The use of methyl methacrylate in trauma patients has disadvantages: it merely takes up room in the soft tissues, does not lock to cortical bone, and frequently is associated with postoperative infections and failure.

Posterior cervical arthrodesis of the lower cervical spine from C-3 to T-1 may be carried out with either local or general anesthesia. For this procedure the patient is placed in the prone position after intubation, either on a turning frame and skeletal traction or in a Mayfield headrest firmly locking the head. After preparation of the skin, the subcutaneous tissue and musculature is injected in the midline with a solution of epinephrine in saline (1:500,000) to control bleeding. If the cervical dissection is kept exactly in the midline, bleeding is easily controlled and sharp dis-

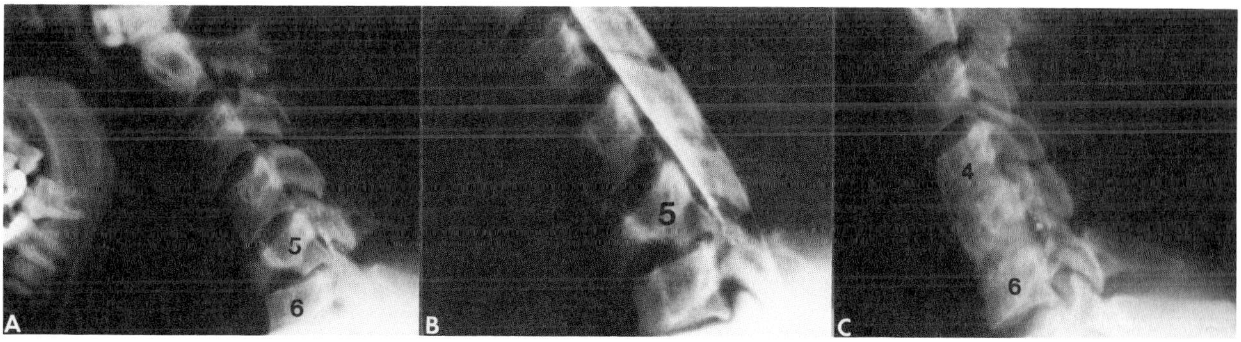

Figure 15

Axial loading injury of C-5 (vehicular accident) resulting in anterior cord quadriparesis in 21-year-old man. *A*, Lateral radiograph of cervical spine. Note compression fracture of C-5 with bone protrusion into the spinal canal. *B*, Lateral myelogram of the cervical spine demonstrating increase in kyphosis secondary to torn posterior ligaments and anterior unstable compression fracture, with cord compression. *C*, Lateral radiograph of cervical spine after anterior corpectomy of C-5 and iliac graft extending from C-4 to C-6. This resulted in recovery of neurologic function, stabilized the spine, and corrected the kyphosis. (*B* and *C* from Bohlman, H.H. *In* AAOS Instructional Course Lectures. [See Figure 5.] By permission of the publisher.)

section can be carried down to the spinous processes and laminae without manipulating the spine. Once the cervical spine is exposed, a power burr is used to drill holes through the bases of the spinous processes, external to the spinal canal. Open reduction of dislocations is accomplished by burring away some facet joint. Then, a 20-gauge wire is passed through and around the spinous process above and below and twisted down on itself, holding the reduced vertebrae together. A 22-gauge wire is passed through and around the spinous process below, and a 22-gauge wire is passed through and around the spinous process above. Two cortico-cancellous grafts are obtained, drill holes are placed in both ends of these grafts, and the individual grafts are tied down onto the lamina on either side of the cervical spine by using the free ends of the wires. Once this triple-wire fusion fabrication has been accomplished, immediate stability of the spine is achieved and the patient may be ambulatory in a two-poster rigid orthosis without need for a halo vest. Decortication of the lower cervical spine is not necessary. Passing sublaminar wires to fix bone grafts in the cervical region may cause radiculopathy and further cord compression, necessitating removal of the wires.

Anterior corpectomy, or vertebrectomy of the lower cervical spine fracture, is carried out by the Smith-Robinson approach to the cervical spine (Fig. 16). Once the fracture level has been identified, the anterior longitudinal ligament is incised on either side of the fractured vertebra, and the disks are removed with curets and pituitary rongeurs (Fig. 17 *A*). High-intensity headlight and magnifying loupes are

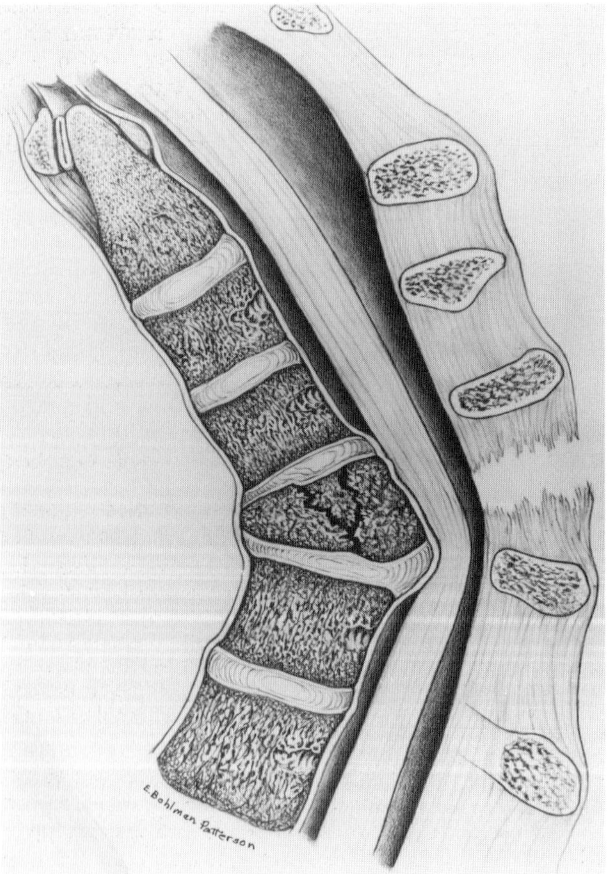

Figure 16

Anterior corpectomy. Typical compression fracture with protrusion of disk material, presence of bone fragments, and kyphotic deformity causing compression of the anterior aspect of the cord. (From Bohlman, H.H. J. Bone Joint Surg. 61A:1119–1142, 1979. By permission of the journal.)

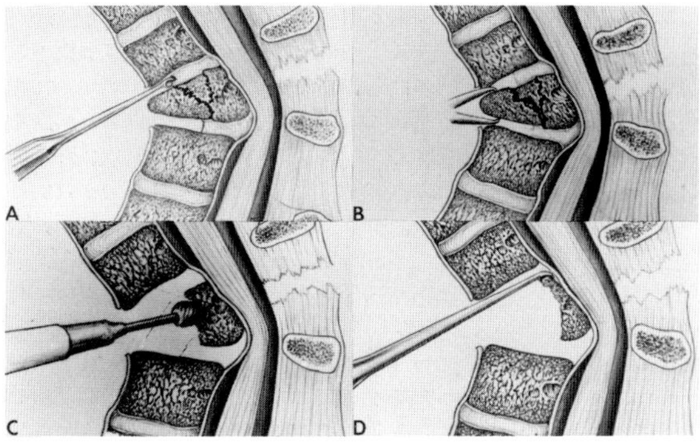

Figure 17

A, Lateral view of cervical spine, showing initial removal of disk material on either side of the crushed vertebral body which serves as a guide to identify the extent of the crushed bone superiorly and inferiorly, as well as posteriorly. *B*, Hand rongeurs are used to remove first portion of the crushed vertebral body. *C*, Part of remaining crushed vertebral body is removed with power burr, back to the posterior longitudinal ligament, to identify the extent of bony protrusion. *D*, Remaining posterior vertebral cortex is removed by using a curet to peel the bone from the longitudinal ligament. (*A* and *B* from Bohlman, H.H. *In* AAOS Instructional Course Lectures. [See Figure 5.] By permission of the publisher. *C* and *D* from Bohlman, H.H., and Eismont, F.J. Clin. Orthop. 154:57–67, 1981. By permission of J.B. Lippincott Company.)

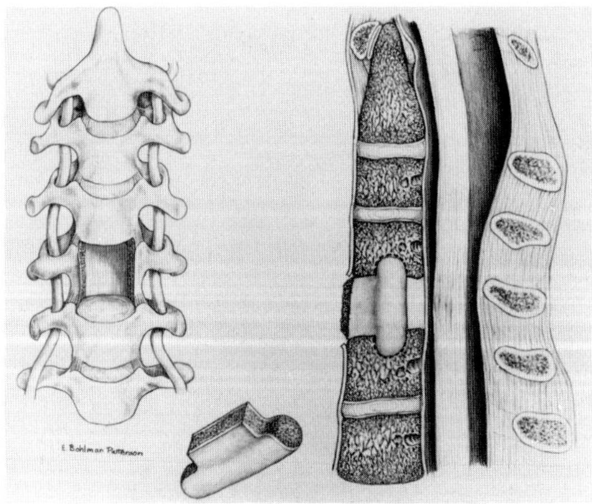

Figure 18

Anterior view of cervical spine, showing the extent of vertebral body resection to the posterior longitudinal ligament, sparing the lateral cortices to protect the vertebral arteries. The posterior longitudinal ligament is not violated, and no instruments enter the spinal canal. A full-thickness iliac crest graft is inserted to replace the resected vertebra. The cortical surface of the crest is placed posteriorly. This procedure corrects the kyphotic deformity and relieves the spinal cord compression. (From Bohlman, H.H. J. Bone Joint Surg. 61A:1119–1142, 1979. By permission of the journal.)

utilized in carrying out the decompression. The crushed vertebral body is partially removed with a Leksell rongeur and curets to approximately half the depth of the vertebral body (Fig. 17 *B*). Further disk material is removed from either side of the crushed vertebra back to the posterior longitudinal ligament that identifies the posterior aspect of the vertebral body above and below. In almost all instances of cervical axial loading injuries, bone fragments lie anterior to the posterior longitudinal ligament, and therefore the posterior ligament usually is not disrupted. There is no reason to inspect the spinal canal *per se;* only the crushed vertebral body is removed. Removal of the remaining body is carried out with a power diamond burr and small curets until the entire posterior longitudinal ligament has been freed and begins to bulge anteriorly in the decompression site (Fig. 17 *C* and *D*).

When the decompression is complete, a small concavity is placed in the vertebral body end plate above and below, and a full-thickness, three-sided cortico-cancellous iliac graft is inserted with the three-sided cortex placed posteriorly. The graft is tamped into place and countersunk, leaving the cancellous portion of the graft exposed anteriorly where it is smoothed off flush with the anterior vertebral body surface so that it will not impinge on the esophagus (Fig. 18). Wires, screws, or plates are not used for anterior corpectomy because bone remodeling will expose metallic fixation devices and they may loosen and erode through the esophagus.

Controversies in Surgical Treatment

Use of methyl methacrylate is not recommended for fixation in cervical trauma. It has created a high incidence of wound infection, loosening of the device, and loss of fixation. The methyl methacrylate does not adhere to cortical bone, and the wire fixation utilized with this method ordinarily loosens with time unless the fracture spontaneously heals anteriorly. It is not necessary to use cement because cortico-cancellous iliac bone offers the best chance of immediate fixation and long-term stability.

Anterior plates or screws are not recommended for fixation of the cervical spine because the screws penetrate the inner cortex of the vertebral body, and therefore the spinal canal, endangering the neural structures. Screws and plates also may loosen and migrate anteriorly to produce an esophageal fistula. The use of pedicle screws to fix the posterior cervical spine carries a risk of damaging the nerve roots and vertebral artery and this method of fixation is not necessary.

Summary

The physician who treats cervical spine and cord injuries should have a thorough understanding of the pathology and mechanisms of injury. Based on these principles, one can make a rational decision as to when surgical intervention is necessary and what operative procedure or procedures are necessary for decompression and stabilization of the cervical spine. One principle is establishing immediate stability and decompression in order to ambulate the patient with cervical spine and cord injury, which avoids many of the problems that may occur with prolonged bed rest. The ultimate goal of surgical intervention is to produce rapid rehabilitation without many of the complications seen in the past.

Annotated Bibliography

Anderson, L.D., and D'Alonzo, R.T.: Fractures of the odontoid process of the axis. J. Bone Joint Surg. 56A:1663–1674, 1974.

Forty-nine odontoid fractures were classified into three types: including 2 avulsion fractures at the odontoid tip (type 1), 15 basilar fractures through the waist of the odontoid (type 2), and 32 axis body fractures (type 3). Type 2 fractures most commonly (36%) resulted in nonunion when treated conservatively.

Assenmacher, D.R., and Ducker, T.B.: Experimental traumatic paraplegia: The vascular and pathological changes seen in reversible and irreversible spinal-cord lesions. J. Bone Joint Surg. 53A:671–680, 1971.

The authors report the vascular and pathologic changes seen in reversible and irreversible experimental spinal cord injuries in 31 monkeys. The reversible lesion showed an initial vascular disturbance that resolved with time and the cord was normal histologically in 5 days. The irreversible lesion included pathologic circulatory disruption with increased time and included venous dilatation, vascular stasis, marked intramedullary hematoma formation, and edema of the cord at 5 days and went on to liquefactive necrosis.

Bohlman, H.H.: Acute fractures and dislocations of the cervical spine: An analysis of three hundred hospitalized patients and review of the literature. J. Bone Joint Surg. 61A:1119–1142, 1979.

Two hundred sixteen patients lived and 51 died within 4 months after injury; 33 were lost to follow-up. Important findings were that laminectomy resulted in a high mortality rate and loss of motor function and that steroid therapy did not improve neural recovery in quadriplegics and was associated with gastrointestinal hemorrhage. Closed or open reduction followed by posterior fusion for subluxations or dislocations and anterior decompression or fusion for vertebral compression fractures offered the best chance of recovery of neural function and restoration of stability.

Bohlman, H.H.: Complications of treatment of fractures and dislocations of the cervical spine. *In* Complications in Orthopaedic Surgery, edited by C.H. Epps, Jr., pp. 681–712. Vol. 1. Second edition. Philadelphia, J.B. Lippincott Company, 1986.

The author details the various complications that occur during the treatment of cervical spine injuries, including misdiagnoses, regional complications such as gastrointestinal hemorrhage, pulmonary problems, and central nervous system complications. Other complications that occur are secondary to nonoperative as well as operative treatment, including sepsis, respiratory distress, central nervous system complications, the use of methyl methacrylate, and complications of arthrodesis techniques.

Bohlman, H.H.: The neck. *In* Musculoskeletal Disorders: Regional Examination and Differential Diagnosis, edited by R. D'Ambrosia, pp. 219–286. Second edition. Philadelphia, J.B. Lippincott Company, 1986.

The author reviews the various types of cervical spine injuries with illustrative cases, as well as the differentiation of various cervical spinal cord syndromes occurring with trauma.

Bohlman, H.H.; Ducker, T.B.; and Lucas, J.T.: Spine and spinal cord injuries. *In* The Spine, edited by R.H. Rothman and F.A. Simeone, pp. 661–756. Vol. 2. Second edition. Philadelphia, W.B. Saunders Company, 1982.

The authors review the pathologic basis of spinal and spinal cord injuries, both experimental and clinical. Early emergency treatment including initial medical care and diagnosis is reviewed as well as a classification of the types of spine and cord injuries. Specific treatment of the patient with spinal cord injury includes immobilization, medical stabilization, spinal alignment, and anterior decompression of the spinal canal. Surgical techniques are described.

Bohlman, H.H., and Eismont, F.J.: Surgical techniques of anterior decompression and fusion for spinal cord injuries. Clin. Orthop. 154:57–67, 1981.

The authors describe the indications for spinal cord decompression and fusion as well as the surgical technique of cervical vertebral body resection (corpectomy). Patients with cervical spinal cord injuries may be at a higher risk for surgery if they: 1) have high cervical cord injuries (C-5 or above); 2) have chronic obstructive pulmonary disease; 3) are over 60 years of age; and 4) are severely depressed.

Burke, D.C.: Hyperextension injuries of the spine. J. Bone Joint Surg. 53B:3–12, 1971.

The author describes a pathologic analysis of 51 extension injuries of the cervical spine as well as other injuries. He points out that certain groups of extension injuries may appear as flexion injuries. The first group are extension-disruption injuries without dislocation and are manifest by slight posterior subluxation of the upper vertebrae on the lower with tearing of the longitudinal ligaments. Extension and disruption may occur in ankylosing spondylitis with separation of the vertebral column. Hyperextension injuries may masquerade as flexion injuries in the upper as well as lower cervical spine, and the final radiograph may show forward luxation of the upper vertebra on the lower one; all ligament structures are torn.

Davis, D.; Bohlman, H.; Walker, A.E.; Fisher, R.; and Robinson, R.: The pathological findings in fatal craniospinal injuries. J. Neurosurg. 34:603–613, 1971.

The authors describe 50 fatal cervicospinal injuries, detailing the soft tissue, osseous, and neural pathology of the cervical region. Disruption was found in 38% of the cases. Vertebral body compression fractures were rare; two-thirds of the cases involved upper cervical spine and cord injuries between the occiput and C-3. Vascular structures were rarely damaged, especially the vertebral artery, and ligaments were torn in combinations attesting to the multiple forces involved in the injuries.

Doppman, J.L., and Girton, M.: Angiographic study of the effect of laminectomy in the presence of acute anterior epidural masses. J. Neurosurg. 45:195–202, 1976.

Anterior cord compression was produced with a balloon, and laminectomy was performed in 16 monkeys to decompress the simulated acute epidural mass in front of the spinal cord. Acute anterior epidural masses larger than 4 mm in diameter could not be decompressed adequately via the posterior approach.

Ducker, T.B.; Bellegarrigue, R.; Salcman, M.; and Walleck, C.: Timing of operative care in cervical spinal cord injury. Spine 9:525–531, 1984.

The emphasis of this review is on bone pathology, not on neurologic syndromes. When neurologic deficits do increase, this is more often an indication for further diagnostic studies to see if the alignment is proper, to rule out further compression, or to increase medical support if the cardiovascular status has deteriorated. When there has been a dramatic and sudden worsening of the neurologic deficit, as occurs in 3% of patients after the initial injury, the most common etiologic factor has been vascular insufficiency and further infarction of an already damaged cord. This has been substantiated by repeated diagnostic studies without compressive pathology and two pathologic specimens. Strict attention must be paid to the guidelines of care for spinal cord injury: 1) immobilization; 2) general medical support; 3) alignment; 4) diagnostic procedures; 5) decompression only when necessary; 6) stabilization only when required.

Eismont, F.J., and Bohlman, H.H.: Posterior methylmethacrylate fixation for cervical trauma. Spine 6:347–353, 1981.

Five cases of cervical instability after trauma were reviewed after being treated with posterior methyl methacrylate fixation at other hospitals. Three patients had infections, and reduction was lost postoperatively in two others. A total of four reoperations was required. The disadvantages of this technique of treatment of post-traumatic cervical instability are emphasized.

Eismont, F.J.; Clifford, S.; Goldberg, M.; and Green, B.: Cervical sagittal spinal canal size in spine injury. Spine 9:663–666, 1984.

This study investigated the relationship between cervical spine sagittal canal diameter and neurologic injury in cases of spinal fracture-dislocation. A group of 98 patients with such injuries was reviewed: 45 had no neurologic deficits, 39 had incomplete quadriplegia, and 14 had complete quadriplegia. Spinal canal sagittal diameter was measured in all, and large diameter and small canals were defined. Small canals were correlated significantly with neurologic injury; large canals provided protection from neurologic injury in cervical fracture dislocation.

Evans, D.K.: Dislocations at the cervicothoracic junction. J. Bone Joint Surg. 65B:124–127, 1983.

Dislocations of the cervicothoracic junction are frequently missed. Experience with this rare injury over 27 years at the spinal injuries unit in Sheffield confirms that nearly two-thirds were not properly diagnosed on admission. Only 2 of the 14 dislocations studied were reduced by conservative methods, and both were associated with fractures of the posterior bony elements. Open reduction is necessary to replace pure dislocations at the C-7 to T-1 level. It seems likely that the spinal cord lesion is not influenced by reduction of the displacement. The three patients who had an incomplete lesion of the spinal cord made excellent neurologic recoveries, although none of the dislocations was reduced. It is concluded that on theoretical grounds it is justified to embark on operative reduction of displacements at this spinal level only if the cord lesion is incomplete and nerve root recovery therefore is possible or if the operation can be performed soon after the injury.

Fielding, J.W.; Cochran, G.V.B.; Lawsing, J.F., III; and Hohl, M.: Tears of the transverse ligament of the atlas: A clinical and biomechanical study. J. Bone Joint Surg. 56A:1683–1691, 1974.

This is a mechanical and clinical study of the strength of the atlantoaxial ligaments in laboratory testing of 20 autopsy specimens in correlation with a clinical series of 11 patients with traumatic transverse ligament rupture and anterior subluxation of the atlas on the axis. Transverse ligament failure occurred in the body of the ligament with a mean force of 84 kiloponds and in no instance did the odontoid process fracture prior to failure of the ligament. Typically, the alar ligaments stretched but did not break during the 12-mm displacement.

Herkowitz, H.N., and Rothman, R.H.: Subacute instability of the cervical spine. Spine 9:348–357, 1984.

This article describes a new entity, subacute instability of the cervical spine. It is defined as the development of radiographic evidence of cervical instability within 3 weeks after a cervical spine injury when initial adequate radiographs show no bony or soft tissue abnormality. Six patients who conformed to this definition are reported. Each was found to have neurologic deficit and radiographic evidence of instability of the cervical spine on repeat examination when none was present initially. There were four unilateral facet dislocations (two C5–C6, one C6–C7, one C4–C5), one perched facet (C5–C6), and one extension subluxation (C4–C5). The subacute instability is thought to be due to elastic and plastic deformation of the ligamentous structures and disks of the cervical spine. It is hoped that injuries of this nature will be discovered so that appropriate treatment can be rendered before a fixed deformity develops.

Kobrine, A.I.; Doyle, T.F.; and Rizzoli, H.V.: Spinal cord blood flow as affected by changes in systemic arterial blood pressure. J. Neurosurg. 44:12–15, 1976.

The hydrogen clearance method was used to measure focal spinal cord blood flow in the rhesus monkey over a wide range of mean arterial blood pressures to test the hypothesis of autoregulation. The spinal cord blood flow remained constant and in the normal range with a mean arterial pressure varying from 50 to 135 mm Hg, indicating the presence of autoregulation. Below 50 mm Hg, the spinal cord blood flow decreased with further decreases in mean arterial pressure.

Kobrine, A.I.; Evans, D.E.; and Rizzoli, H.V.: Experimental acute balloon compression of the spinal cord: Factors affecting disappearance and return of the spinal evoked response. J. Neurosurg. 51:841–845, 1979.

The findings suggest that the major pathologic substrate for neural dysfunction after anterior compression of the spinal cord, acute or slow, is physical injury to the neural membrane, irrespective of blood flow changes. Also, the neural membrane will or will not recover, depending on the rapidity and length of time of compression.

Marar, B.C.: Hyperextension injuries of the cervical spine: The pathogenesis of damage to the spinal cord. J. Bone Joint Surg. 56A:1655–1662, 1974.

Forty-five patients who had sustained hyperextension injuries of the cervical spine were analyzed by clinical and roentgenographic features. Autopsy was performed in four patients who died; the injury was induced in seven cadavers. The cord appeared to be damaged by an anterior-posterior squeezing effect produced between a backward-subluxing vertebral body at the disk space level or through complete fracture of the vertebral body just below the pedicle. The mechanism of injury is a combination of hyperextension and backward shearing forces.

Marar, B.C.: The pattern of neurological damage as an aid to the diagnosis of the mechanism in cervical-spine injuries. J. Bone Joint Surg. 56A:1648–1654, 1974.

One hundred twenty-six cases of injuries of the cervical spine were analyzed with regard to the clinical patterns and neurologic damage and the roentgenographic patterns of skeletal injury. These patients were divided into five groups: 1) total motor and sensory loss; 2) motor loss of variable degree in the upper extremities or in all four extremities with patchy sensory loss; 3) complete motor loss in extremities with hypoesthesia below but no loss of position or vibratory sense; 4) motor power weakness in all four extremities or in the upper extremities alone with no sensory loss; and 5) a Brown-Séquard syndrome. Flexion injuries occurred in group 1. In group 2 a central cord syndrome occurred with hyperextension injury. In group 3 the anterior cord syndrome occurred with burst fractures and flexion injuries with retropulsed bone. In group 4 a type of anterior cord syndrome occurred with flexion injuries and fractures of the arch of the axis.

Mazur, J.M., and Stauffer, E.S.: Unrecognized spinal instability associated with seemingly "simple" cervical compression fractures. Spine 8:687–692, 1983.

This paper describes 27 patients who had apparently stable compression cervical vertebral fractures. All were treated with cervicothoracic orthoses. None was initially treated in a halo device or surgically. Twenty patients were stable and healed. One patient spontaneously stabilized within 6 months with anterior bony ankylosis in a kyphotic position. Six patients had persistent progressive post-injury instability related to posterior ligament rupture. As muscle spasm diminished, the patients could be given a more reliable flexion-extension radiographic examination, unmasking the hidden posterior instability. Five of the six who demonstrated this instability were disabled because of pain.

Reale, F.; Delfini, R.; Mazzarella, F.; and Gambacorta, D.: Traumatic dislocation of the cervical spine without neurological deficit: Eleven cases. J. Neurosurg. Sci. 27:191–195, 1983.

The authors present 11 cases of traumatized patients without neurologic deficit in spite of a gross dislocation of the cervical spine. To explain this discrepancy, various parameters were taken into account. The vertebral canal has been noted to be abnormally wide in these cases (average, 19.8 mm). The authors suggest that the great width of the vertebral canal has in some way prevented the spinal cord of these patients being damaged by the dislocation.

Schatzker, J.; Rorabeck, C.H.; and Waddell, J.P.: Fractures of the dens (odontoid process): An analysis of thirty-seven cases. J. Bone Joint Surg. 53B:392–405, 1971.

The anatomy and blood supply to the odontoid are described as pathologic bases for nonunion in 63% of 37 patients with odontoid fractures treated by closed methods. Posterior displacement of the odontoid had a significantly high nonunion rate. The blood supply reaches the dens through the accessory ligaments and in some cases through the apical ligament.

Stauffer, E.S., and Kelly, E.G.: Fracture-dislocations of the cervical spine: Instability and recurrent deformity following treatment by anterior interbody fusion. J. Bone Joint Surg. 59A:45–48, 1977.

This report is of six patients with fracture dislocations of the cervical spine treated with an anterior dowel or Cloward interbody fusion. All had postoperative instability with recurrence of angular deformity, and all were shown to have disruption of the posterior ligaments. Therefore, an anterior fusion should not be performed as a primary surgical treatment for fractures of the cervical spine when there is evidence of disruption of the posterior ligaments.

Torg, J.S., and Das, M.: Trampoline and minitrampoline injuries to the cervical spine. Clin. Sports Med. 4:45–60, 1985.

This paper: 1) examines the world's literature documenting cervical spine injuries; 2) attempts to identify common factors regarding patient characteristics, environment, injury mechanisms, and pathology; 3) reviews policy statements and safety guidelines of various medical and athletic administrative bodies; and 4) evaluates what effect, if any, these policies and guidelines have had on documented injuries. On the basis of this review, it seems that the American Academy of Pediatrics was ill-advised in altering its position on the use of trampolines. Both the trampoline and the minitrampoline are dangerous devices when used in the best of circumstances, and their use has no place in recreational, educational, or competitive gymnastics.

White, A.A.; Southwick, W.O.; and Panjabi, M.M.: Clinical instability in the lower cervical spine: A review of past and current concepts. Spine 1:15–27, 1976.

Clinical instability of the cervical spine was defined by biomechanical analysis (sectioning of various ligament complexes in the cervical spine and measuring vertebral displacement). Instability was defined as more than 3.5 mm of horizontal displacement of one vertebra in relation to an adjacent vertebra measured on the lateral radiograph or more than 11° of rotation difference from that of either adjacent vertebra measured on a resting lateral or flexion-extension radiograph.

25
Thoracolumbar Spine: Pediatric Aspects

This chapter deals with congenital and developmental diseases and deformities of the spine in children and adolescents. The techniques of evaluation and diagnosis are discussed and the current methods of treatment are outlined.

Congenital Deformity of the Spine

Natural History

The prognosis for congenital scoliosis depends on the type of congenital deformity present, its location in the spine, and the age of the patient at presentation. A progressive spinal deformity is rarely produced by either block vertebrae, which are secondary to bilateral failure of segmentation, or wedged vertebrae. Single hemivertebrae may produce a progressive spinal deformity; however, their behavior is unpredictable, making radiographic follow-up necessary. Double hemivertebrae that are ipsilateral and adjacent to one another are more likely to produce a progressive scoliosis that requires treatment (Fig. 1 *A*). Unilateral unsegmented bars are the most frequent congenital cause of progressive spinal deformity. The deformity produced by a unilateral unsegmented bar is relentlessly progressive; once a unilateral unsegmented bar is identified, fusion is required to prevent a severe deformity. If a unilateral unsegmented bar is associated with a contralateral hemivertebra, the progression of the deformity is even more rapid and, if untreated, the ultimate deformity is even more severe.

Both the location of the congenital abnormality and the patient's age at onset affect the prognosis. An upper thoracic location has the best prognosis, followed by the lumbar spine. Congenital deformities in the lower thoracic or thoracolumbar spine are the most likely to progress. Hemivertebrae at the lumbosacral junction produce an oblique takeoff of the lumbar spine which induces the development of a secondary lumbar or thoracolumbar curve that becomes progressive and severe with an associated severe clinical deformity (Fig. 2). The earlier the onset of the clinical deformity, the worse the prognosis of the curvature. In general, if the clinical deformity appears in the first year of life, the curvature will be progressive and will require surgical fusion.

Treatment

The treatment of a given congenital spinal deformity depends to a great extent on the prognosis for the anomaly. As soon as a unilateral unsegmented bar is diagnosed, a fusion should be performed to prevent progression of the deformity. Double hemivertebrae usually progress and therefore most likely will require surgical treatment; unilateral hemivertebrae are less predictable in their behavior and require observation to determine if fusion is needed.

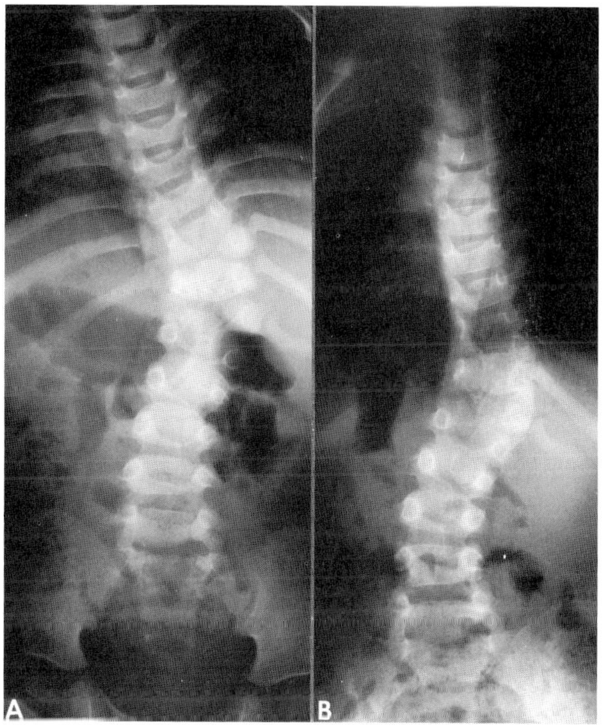

Figure 1

Congenital scoliosis in 12-month-old boy. *A*, Anteroposterior radiograph of the spine, showing two ipsilateral and adjacent hemivertebrae that have produced a progressive scoliosis. *B*, Anteroposterior radiograph of same child 3 years later. Treatment was simultaneous anterior interbody fusion and posterior fusion on the convex side only. The fusion extended from the normal vertebral body above the upper hemivertebra to the normal vertebral body below the lower hemivertebra. There is a solid anterior and posterior fusion on the convexity only and, as a result of the localized arrest of growth on the convexity, there has been improvement in the scoliosis.

When other factors influencing prognosis such as age and location are taken into consideration, the prognosis for an individual hemivertebra is easier to determine.

Surgical treatment of a congenital spinal deformity depends on both the patient's age and the severity of the deformity. It is generally recommended that posterior fusion be performed early in the case of a progressive congenital scoliosis. The fusion should be performed either when a definitely progressive type of deformity—e.g., an unsegmented bar—is identified or once a deformity has proved to be progressive. The posterior fusion should be

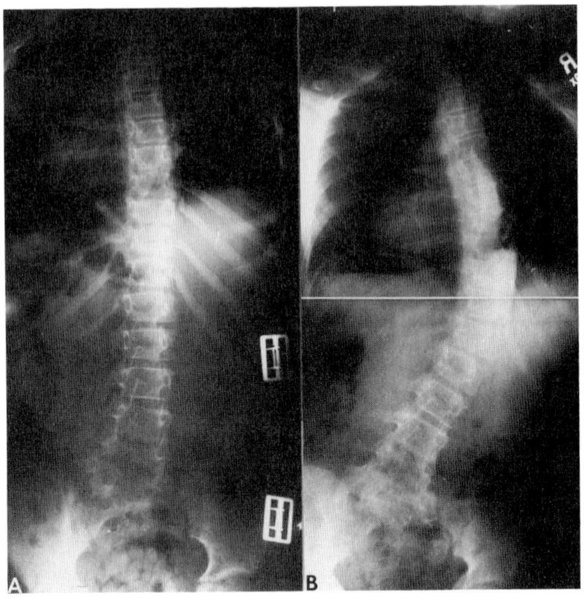

Figure 2

Radiographs from a girl with a hemivertebra at the lumbosacral junction that produced severe curvature of the thoracolumbar spine. *A*, Anteroposterior radiograph of the spine at age 6 years, showing a hemivertebra on the left side at the lumbosacral junction. There is a small curvature above this congenital deformity. *B*, At age 10 years, thoracolumbar scoliosis has progressed to above the level of the hemivertebra.

performed on both the convex and the concave side of the spinal deformity because fusions performed only on the convex side tend to bend with time. When the posterior fusion is on the convex side only, there is continued growth of the vertebral bodies, especially on the concave side. This can be overcome by performing an anterior interbody convex fusion at the same time that the posterior convex fusion is performed. Use of this simultaneous fusion has been recommended by several authors and is generally accepted as the preferred method of treating a progressive congenital curve in a small child. The anterior interbody fusion prevents progression of the curve by arresting the growth of the vertebral bodies on the convex side of the curve. This procedure also allows for progressive correction of the curvature if growth continues in the concavity of the deformity (Fig. 1 *B*). In older children with congenital scoliosis, instrumentation and correction of the deformity may be performed if tethering of the spinal cord has been ruled out by myelography or magnetic resonance imaging.

Congenital kyphosis is potentially more ominous than congenital scoliosis because of the danger of paraplegia developing if the kyphosis is neglected. Treatment depends on the type and severity of the deformity and on the age of the patient. If the lesion is progressive, the treatment is spinal fusion. Posterior fusion alone may be effective if the kyphosis is less than 55° in a growing child. If the deformity is greater than 55°, both anterior and posterior fusion will be required. The anterior fusion should be a combination of a strut graft and an interbody fusion. An anterior unsegmented bar will be produced in the growing child if an interbody fusion is not added to strut grafting, because the growth of the unfused vertebral bodies has not been arrested. The further growth of the vertebral bodies posterior to the strut graft will allow progression of the kyphosis. Vertebral growth is arrested by performing an interbody fusion extending to the limits of the strut graft. A strut graft should be placed as close to the vertebral bodies as possible because pseudarthrosis is more likely to develop if the graft is more than 4 cm from the apical vertebra. Correction of a congenital kyphosis carries with it the risk of paraplegia. A congenital kyphosis may be corrected intraoperatively if great caution is used, but correction should never be attempted preoperatively with traction because the spinal cord will be stretched over the kyphosis, which is fixed, thereby producing paraplegia.

Adolescent Idiopathic Scoliosis

Etiology

Many authors report disturbances in function of the posterior columns of the spinal cord in patients with adolescent idiopathic scoliosis. Some authors have reported a decrease in perception of vibratory stimuli, as well as a decrease in proprioception, in both the upper and lower extremities in these patients. These symptoms indicate that, if a lesion does exist, it will be located above the cervical cord. Other authors have noted a disturbance of vestibular function in these patients. The sagittal plane deformity has received much more attention in recent years. When one looks at the apex of a thoracic scoliosis, one finds that the spine is truly lordotic. The posterior deformity that one sees is actually the rotational deformity of the ribs on the convex side of the scoliosis. The lordosis of the apex of a scoliosis has been shown to be the first change that one sees in a child who has a straight spine that goes on to scoliosis. This small area of lordosis of the spine produces a rotational instability of the spine which then evolves into a scoliotic curve.

Screening

Screening for scoliosis at school has been advocated and even mandated in some states. Recently, the cost-effectiveness of this program has been questioned, although it is still thought by most that this screening is worthwhile. Many children have been referred for treatment with minor curves that require no treatment, but the use of the scoliometer may allow screening personnel to determine more accurately which children should be referred. The scoliometer is an inclinometer that measures the rotational deformity of the scoliosis at the apex of the curvature. If the scoliometer indicates that there is an angle of elevation of 5°, the patient is referred to a physician. In addition, this screening method has a false-negative rate of only 0.1%. Those patients with scoliosis severe enough to require treatment will exhibit a visible trunk asymmetry by age 10; consequently, screening should concentrate on children at this age.

Natural History

The natural history of adolescent idiopathic scoliosis has been the subject of many papers in the past few years. For many years, it was assumed that all curves progressed. Recently, however, it has been discovered that only some curves progress, and criteria have been established for determining the probability of progression. It is known, for example, that scoliosis has a greater tendency to progress if the spine still has potential for growth. The importance of this factor has been recognized, and the appearance and growth of the iliac apophyses have been used as predictors of remaining skeletal growth (Risser sign).

In a review of 727 patients with curves of 5° to 29°, 23.2% of these patients had curves that progressed. Also, progression was related to the type and magnitude of the curve. In addition, age, the Risser sign, and the presence or absence of menarche at presentation were important factors to consider when predicting curve progression. The younger the patient—as determined by the Risser sign, bone age, and absence of menarche—and the greater the curve severity, the greater the chance of progression. Based on this information, a nomogram that uses age, menarche status, and curve magnitude to predict the chance of progression of an individual curve was developed. In addition, it was found that a child with scoliosis is more likely to require treatment if a parent has scoliosis.

Others also have shown that progression is related to the patient's age at the time of presentation. Previously, it was believed that scoliosis did not progress in adults; recently, however, this has been shown to be incorrect. In more than 100 patients followed for a mean of 40 years, curves of 30° or less at the time of skeletal maturity had little chance of progression and curves greater than 50° at maturity had a significant chance of progression. Although this information provides a good general guideline for counseling patients, each curve should be assessed individually. Contradictory findings have been reported on the effect of pregnancy on progression of scoliosis in adults. Some authors have indicated that early and multiple pregnancies increase the chance of progression, whereas others have found no increase in progression of scoliosis after pregnancy and no greater chance of progression even with early and multiple pregnancies.

Treatment

Bracing The Milwaukee brace was originally used for scoliosis of minor degrees of curvature in adolescents. In recent years, the criteria for bracing have become more rigidly defined. At the present time, most physicians think that bracing should be reserved for immature patients with curves of 25° or more that have shown at least 5° of progression. In skeletally immature patients, curves of at least 30° are braced even if there has been no evidence of progression. Lesser curves in immature patients are not treated but are observed for progression. If the scoliosis progresses beyond 25°, a brace is prescribed. By using these criteria, physicians can eliminate much unnecessary bracing. Exercise treatment may be prescribed as an adjunct to bracing; however, by itself, exercise is not effective in preventing progression of scoliosis.

The upper limit of degree of curvature for bracing is less well-defined than the lower limit. However, it is known that curves of 50° or more are likely to progress after maturity, and most physicians use 40° to 45° of curvature as the upper limit for bracing.

Because bracing for scoliosis has been shown to decrease thoracic kyphosis, it is important to determine whether or not a relative thoracic lordosis exists. The patient with a thoracic hypokyphosis may require spinal fusion sooner than the patient with an equal but relatively kyphotic curve.

The Milwaukee brace has largely been replaced by underarm braces which seem to be as effective in treating curves with apices at T-8 or lower, and they have certain advantages over the Milwaukee brace. Both the Milwaukee brace and the newer braces depend upon pressure from thoracic and lumbar pads to lessen the curve. In addition to exerting lateral pressure on the curve, however, newer orthoses such as the Boston orthosis decrease lumbar lordosis, which also produces some reduction of the scoliotic curvature.

Patient compliance with these braces has been assumed to be very high until recently, when poor compliance was reported in several studies. These reports of poor compliance prompted a study of part-time bracing which revealed that patients who used their braces part-time had results almost equal to those in a similar group of patients who used their braces full-time. Part-time (16 hours a day) use of braces allowed the patients to continue with normal daily activities. It is widely recognized that bracing does not correct scoliosis; rather, bracing is used to prevent progression of the curve until skeletal maturity.

Electrical Stimulation The use of electrical stimulation for the control of adolescent idiopathic scoliosis has been well-publicized, especially by the lay media, because of the attractiveness of this method. Electrical stimulation has been reported to be as effective as bracing. However, other investigators have not achieved these results; they have found that electrical stimulation may not change the natural history of adolescent idiopathic scoliosis. Unpublished reports presented at the 1985 meeting of the Scoliosis Research Society have also questioned the efficacy of electrical stimulation in preventing curve progression.

Radiation Hazard Patients with scoliosis are often subjected to significant amounts of radiation during their lifetime due to the need for radiographs of their spines to determine progression of spinal curvature. The amount of radiation exposure may be reduced in several ways. First, only those radiographs that are absolutely necessary should be taken. Second, bending films should be obtained only preoperatively. In addition, proper shielding and collimation can reduce the radiation exposure of the breasts, gonads, and thyroid gland. High-speed rare earth screens can be used to reduce the total radiation dosage. Finally, use of posterior-anterior projection delivers a lower dose to the patient than does use of the anterior-posterior view.

Surgical For years, use of the Harrington distraction rod combined with a thorough posterior extra- and intra-articular fusion has been the standard surgical treatment for adolescent idiopathic scoliosis. This treatment is followed by immobilization of the patient in a cast or brace for 4 to 9 months. This technique has had excellent success for 25 years. The incidence of neurologic injury is less than 1%, the pseudarthrosis rate is less than 5%, and the average curve correction is greater than 40%. For a new procedure to become standard, it must provide a significant improvement on these results.

The level of the spine to which fusion extends has been discussed in several recent papers. It has been reported that fusion of only the thoracic curve is necessary in double curves in which the lumbar curve is only slightly smaller and is more flexible on bending. The bottom of the fusion should extend to the stable vertebra (the vertebra that is bisected by a line drawn through the middle of the spines of the sacrum); this may not be the same as the neutral vertebra. The lower level of fusion in lumbar curves should not extend to the lower lumbar region unless absolutely necessary. In adults who have undergone spinal fusion for scoliosis, the lower the level of fusion, the higher the incidence of back pain. Fusion should rarely, if ever, extend to L-5, and L-4 should be spared if at all possible.

The use of anterior instrumentation for lumbar and thoracolumbar curves has been shown to increase the amount of curve correction and to eliminate the necessity of fusing the lower lumbar levels. Both the Dwyer and the Zielke system have been used for this procedure. Theoretically, the Zielke system provides more derotation of the spine than the Dwyer system. The Zielke system has also been reported to decrease lumbar lordosis less than the Dwyer system, but a statistically significant difference has not been demonstrated. If the two systems do reduce lumbar lordosis to different degrees, the difference may be less significant if the spine is only instrumented to the L-3 level. Short fusions of three segments, from T-12 to L-3, have successfully corrected the scoliosis and significantly corrected the rotational deformity of the spine without fusing to the level of L-4 (Fig. 3). One as yet unanswered question is whether the pseudarthrosis rate is acceptably low with anterior instrumentation and fusion.

Other recently developed systems of surgical instrumentation seem to afford good correction and are rigid enough to obviate the need for postoperative immobilization. The addition of the device for transverse traction (DTT) developed by Cotrel to the combination of the distraction rod and the compression rod has been shown to increase the strength of the instrumentation. However, the compression device also increases the thoracic lordosis, which is undesirable because of the presence of the already problematic thoracic hypokyphosis. Segmental spinal instrumentation using contoured Luque rods secured to the spine with sublaminar wires affords stable fixation and excellent curve correction. An increased incidence of neurologic injury due to the passage of sublaminar wires has been reported with this device, however. The Harrington rod has been used with sublaminar segmental wiring, but this appears to carry an even greater risk of neurologic injury than does segmental instrumentation with Luque rods.

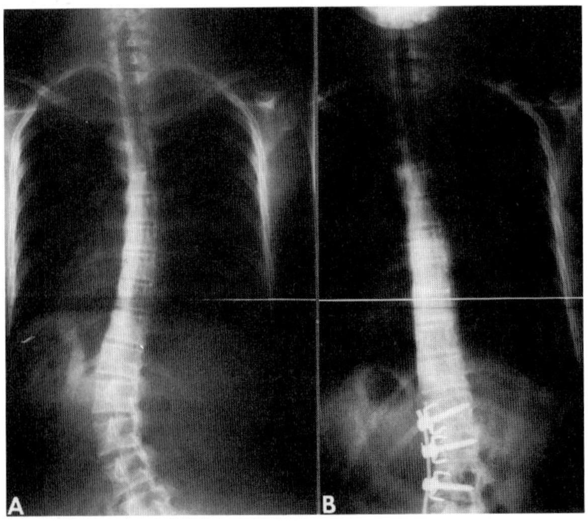

Figure 3

Left lumbar scoliosis in a 16-year-old girl. *A*, Anteroposterior radiograph of the spine, demonstrating left lumbar scoliosis that has produced decompensation to the left. *B*, Postoperative anteroposterior radiograph, showing correction of the scoliosis by Dwyer instrumentation. The lumbosacral spine is straight without fusion below L-3.

The interspinous process segmental spinal instrumentation devised by Drummond appears to provide the desired segmental fixation without the passage of sublaminar wires. Drummond's technique features the use of a button-wire implant which is passed through the base of the spinous process after holes are made with specially designed awls. Two wires are passed through each spinous process except for those at the top and bottom of the curve. The Harrington distraction rod is inserted through the wires on the concave side of the curve and then secured in the routine fashion except that a bifid hook is used at the top to prevent hook migration. The lower hook should have a longer shoe to prevent dislodgement. A Luque rod is then shaped to fit on the convex side of the curve. Next, both rods are secured by twisting the wires, which increases the curve correction and also increases the stability of the fixation. This is a simple technique which increases operative time very little while increasing the strength of fixation and thus eliminating the need for postoperative immobilization (Fig. 4). To date, no neurologic complications have been reported.

The complication of neurologic injury is a feared one. One new technique, the measurement of somatosensory-evoked potentials (SSEP) during operation, has been used to help prevent neurologic injury. The accuracy of this modality has not yet been firmly established. Because inhalation agents block neural transmission in the posterior columns of the spinal cord, accurate measurement of the SSEP requires the use of balanced anesthesia. Temperature and blood pressure have also been shown to affect evoked potentials. The wake-up test, as described by Stagnara, is frequently used to determine the presence of neurologic injury. More recently, the clonus test has been used for the same purpose. Clonus is normally seen in all patients undergoing general anesthesia, during both induction and wake-up. The clonus test is analogous to the wake-up test except that it requires no patient cooperation. Both feet are tested for clonus; the presence of clonus indicates an intact neural pathway, and its absence is indicative of neurologic injury.

The rib hump produced by the rotational deformity of the spine in scoliosis usually is not completely corrected by the standard spinal fusion. Rib resection has been recommended as a means of correcting the rib hump. The ribs in the deformity are resected from the transverse process to the axillary line. Care must be taken to avoid entering the pulmonary cavity. The ribs regenerate quickly but are flatter than before operation, thereby correcting the hump. This procedure can be performed through either a midline incision, especially if the incision is shaded slightly toward the convexity, or a separate incision parallel to the midline incision.

Several problems are associated with the surgical correction of adolescent idiopathic scoliosis. Intraoperative blood loss may be excessive. To combat this, specialized spinal frames which allow complete suspension of the abdomen during operation can be used. These frames appear

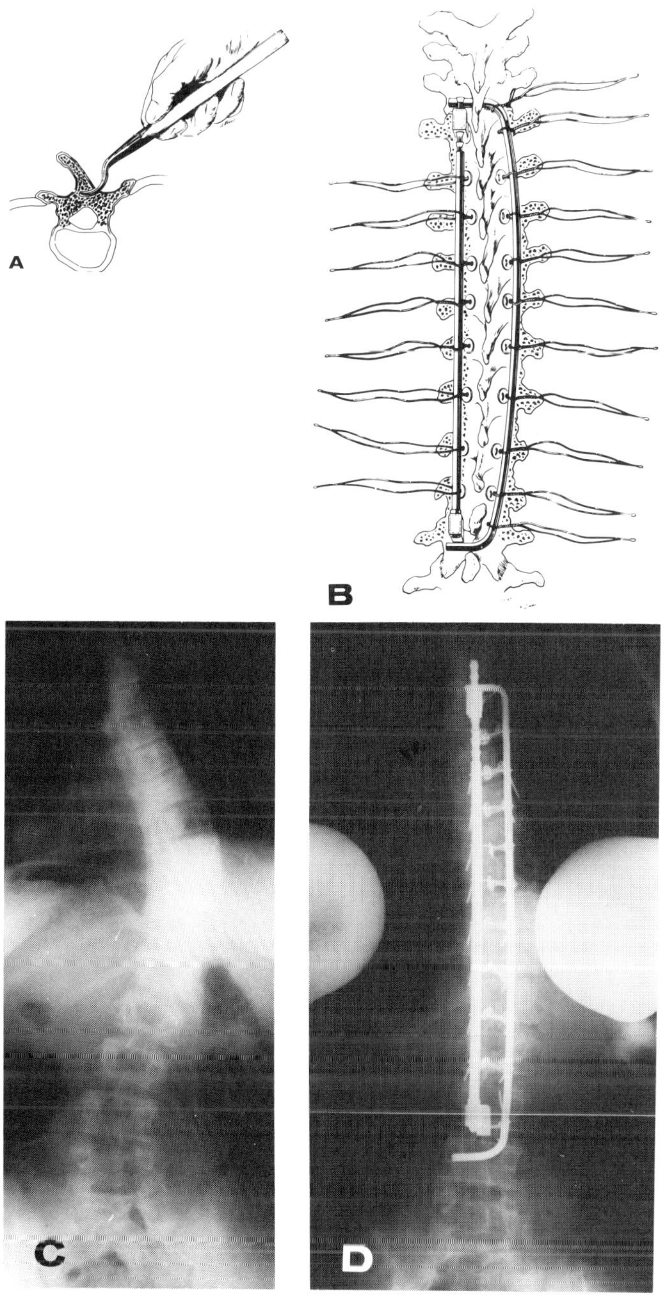

Figure 4

Surgical technique for interspinous process segmental spinal instrumentation. *A*, Holes are made through the base of the spinous processes with awls. The awls pass through the thickest portion of the spinous process but remain out of the spinal canal. *B*, Double button-wire implants are passed through the spinous processes. The Harrington rod passes through the wires on the convex side and is fixed to the spine with a bifid upper hook and a lower hook that has a longer shoe to prevent dislodgement. The Luque rod is passed through the wires on the convexity. The wires are twisted to secure both rods to the spine. *C*, Preoperative anteroposterior radiograph, demonstrating a 45° right thoracic scoliosis. *D*, Postoperative anteroposterior radiograph, demonstrating significant correction of the curvature, to 22°. Both rods are securely wired to the spine by using double button-wire implants. (*A* modified from Drummond, D., et al. J. Pediatr. Orthop. 4:397–404, 1984. By permission of Raven Press.)

to prevent compression of the intra-abdominal venous system, thereby decreasing venous blood loss. Hypotensive anesthesia has also been shown to decrease blood loss significantly. Because the spinal cord has an autoregulatory mechanism that increases cord blood flow when systemic blood pressure is decreased, it appears to be protected from vascular injury when hypotension is induced in this way. In addition, the use of autologous blood can significantly decrease or entirely eliminate the need for bank blood.

Physicians occasionally may encounter the superior mesenteric artery syndrome postoperatively. This syndrome is associated with weight loss which decreases the fat content in the retroperitoneal area. This complication is treated with nasogastric suction and hyperalimentation until sufficient weight has been gained to prevent recurrence of the obstruction. Occasionally, surgical release of the second portion of the duodenum is necessary.

It has been shown that there is an increased incidence of back pain in the adult when fusion is extended to the lower lumbar spine. It is therefore recommended that spinal fusions for scoliosis do not cross the L4-5 disk and, if possible, go no lower than L-3. Contouring of the Harrington rod seems to be important in the maintenance of the normal lumbar lordosis. The use of square-ended rods contoured to conform to the normal sagittal shape of the spine is recommended. Even with the use of these contoured rods, the lumbar spine is flattened when distraction is applied. Other, newly developed devices may help eliminate this problem. Among these devices is a compression system for the lumbar spine that tends to maintain the lordosis when used with a Harrington distraction rod. The Cotrel-Dubousset system, recently developed in France, at this point seems to have the best chance of supplanting the standard Harrington system. The Cotrel-Dubousset system consists of two very well contoured rods that maintain the sagittal architecture of the spine while providing excellent correction of the scoliosis. Segmental fixation is accomplished with multiple hooks on both the convex and concave sides of the spine. The security and strength of fixation are sufficient to obviate the need for postoperative immobilization.

Infantile Idiopathic Scoliosis

The incidence of infantile idiopathic scoliosis is consistently higher in Great Britain than in the United States. It has been postulated recently that this scoliosis is related to positioning of the infant. European children are routinely placed in the supine position whereas American infants are usually placed in the prone position. When infants are in the supine position or, more correctly, turned slightly from supine, excessive force appears to be placed on the immature spine, producing scoliosis. English children are increasingly being placed prone, and the incidence of infantile idiopathic scoliosis is decreasing in England.

Infantile and juvenile scoliotic curves that are relentlessly progressive are very difficult to treat. Some authors have suggested that the use of instrumentation of the spine without fusion will provide stabilization and allow for growth. Unfortunately, this approach has met with little success. The use of segmental instrumentation with Luque rods also has been unsuccessful because of rod breakage and spontaneous fusion in the area of the spinal exposure. The use of a subcutaneous Harrington rod, which involves exposure of the spine only at the ends of the rod for hook insertion, has met with limited success as well, both because the rod has to be distracted periodically and because the spine must be braced until growth has ceased.

Neuromuscular Scoliosis

Cerebral Palsy

Scoliosis is common in children who have cerebral palsy. The risk and severity of progression of the curvature are related to the severity of the neurologic deficit; children who are severely involved neurologically are more likely to have a severe, progressive scoliosis. Treatment of neuromuscular scoliosis depends on the functional status of the patient. Custom-molded seating inserts that conform exactly to the patient's body and allow upright positioning can be fabricated, but they will probably not prevent progression of the curvature. If the curvature is progressive and is severe enough to threaten the patient's ability to sit, surgical stabilization should be considered. The decision to stabilize the spine surgically should be made jointly by the patient's physician, family or caretakers, and therapists.

The decision to treat neuromuscular scoliosis surgically can be a difficult one because the standard posterior spinal fusion has a high pseudarthrosis rate. Combined anterior and posterior fusion will produce better correction and will decrease the rate of pseudarthrosis. More recently, the use of Luque rods with segmental instrumentation has been shown to afford even better correction than the combined anterior and posterior fusion, without the need for postoperative immobilization. In addition, the pseudarthrosis rate seems to be lower with the use of segmental instrumentation. If a fixed pelvic obliquity is associated with the scoliosis, the spinal fusion should extend to the sacrum. With segmental instrumentation, the spine is instrumented to the sacrum and the rods are secured to the pelvis by using the Galveston technique (Fig. 5). The Luque rods are contoured to the pelvis and to the spine and are inserted into the pelvis through holes predrilled between the inner and outer tables of the pelvis approximately 1 to 2 cm above the sciatic notch to a depth of approximately 6 to 8 cm. These contoured rods are then segmentally wired to the posterior elements of the vertebrae included in the fusion. This technique provides excellent correction of the curvature and eliminates the need for postoperative immobilization.

Myelodysplasia

In patients with spina bifida, scoliosis may be either congenital or paralytic. Congenital curves are the direct result of congenital abnormalities of the spine. The treatment for congenital curves in the patient with spina bifida is similar to the treatment for congenital scoliosis without a paralytic component: that is, if the curvature becomes progressive, a localized fusion should be performed early to prevent further progression. The paralytic scoliosis is the result of paralysis rather than of bony abnormalities of the spine. The treatment for paralytic scoliosis is also dependent on progression of the curvature. In evaluating the patient with spina bifida, the physician must carefully determine the cause of the progression. Tethering of the cord, very common in children with spina bifida, may cause a progressive scoliosis; it also may produce either a deterioration of neurologic function or an increase in the spasticity of the lower extremities. Any change in the neurologic picture in the extremities of a patient with spina bifida should alert the physician to the possibility of an underlying tethering of the spinal cord. The presence of tethering can be determined by myelography and magnetic resonance imaging. Hydromyelia and brainstem compression from the Arnold-Chiari malformation, both of which can be detected by magnetic resonance imaging, can produce deterioration of neurologic function. Hydrocephalus also must be considered when there is neurologic deterioration because it is the most common cause of a changing neurologic picture in patients with spina bifida.

In children with spina bifida, progressive curvatures of the spine do not respond well to bracing; if the curvature is severe, it will require spinal stabilization and fusion. To increase the chance of achieving a solid arthrodesis, many authors recommend the use of both anterior and posterior fusion. The combination of anterior instrumentation and posterior Harrington instrumentation appears to decrease the ever-present lumbar lordosis and to increase the fusion rate. More recently, combining Luque segmental instrumentation with the Galveston technique of fixing the rods to the pelvis has been shown to increase the chance of fusion and to yield fewer complications than other techniques, without the need for postoperative immobilization (Fig. 5). Good results with anterior release and fusion with-

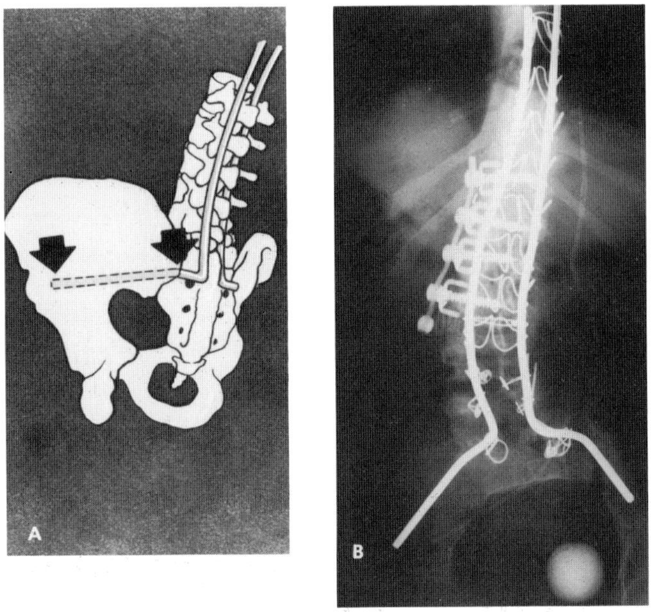

Figure 5

Galveston technique of segmental fixation of Luque rods to the pelvis. *A,* Site of insertion of the rods into the pelvis just anterior to the posterior superior iliac spine. They pass about 1–2 cm above the sciatic notch, to a depth of 6–8 cm. It is important to keep the rods between the two cortices of the ilium throughout their entire depth of insertion. *B,* Anteroposterior radiograph of the spine of a 14-year-old boy with spina bifida after instrumentation to the sacrum by the Galveston technique. Button-wire implants have secured the rods in the low lumbar spine. The patient had undergone a first-stage anterior release and fusion. Dwyer apparatus had been used to enhance the security of the fixation and to decrease the severe lumbar lordosis. (*A* from Allen, B.L., Jr., and Ferguson, R.L. Spine 9:388–394, 1984. By permission of Harper & Row Publishers.)

out instrumentation in combination with posterior fusion using Luque rods and segmental instrumentation have been reported.

Spinal Muscular Atrophy

There are three forms of spinal muscular atrophy. Type I, or Werdnig-Hoffmann, has onset from birth to 6 months, and the prognosis for survival is guarded. Type II, or chronic Werdnig-Hoffmann, has onset from 6 months to 5 years. The mildest form, type III or Kugelberg-Welander, has onset from 2 to 17 years. Spinal muscular atrophy is an autosomal recessive disease typified by loss of anterior horn cells of the spinal cord. In children with this disease, a progressive scoliosis frequently develops which may compromise their ability to sit. The treatment of the curvature is surgical; bracing has not been shown to be effective. Although a brace may slow the progression of a given curve, it will not prevent the progression altogether, and pulmonary function may deteriorate to the point such that operation is impossible. It is therefore recommended that spinal stabilization and fusion be performed as soon as the curvature reaches 50°.

Duchenne Muscular Dystrophy

Duchenne muscular dystrophy is a relentlessly progressive sex-linked recessive disease. Children with this disease usually lose their ability to ambulate by age 12 to 14 years. Once confined to a wheelchair, approximately 50% to 80% of these children develop a collapsing scoliosis that eventually becomes extremely severe. This scoliosis limits the children's ability to sit, which further compromises an already deteriorating pulmonary status. Bracing is poorly tolerated in this population and, although braces may slow the rate of curve progression, they will not prevent it. The use of a brace actually may slow curve progression while pulmonary function deteriorates to a degree such that operation is impossible. Bracing therefore is not recommended in these patients unless there is some contraindication to surgical stabilization of the spine. Even though most children with Duchenne muscular dystrophy develop a progressive scoliosis that will require fusion, prophylactic fusion of all spines is not recommended. Once a curve reaches 25°, however, spinal fusion should be performed as long as the pulmonary function is adequate. Fusion will enable the patient to sit; the pulmonary function of the patient will continue to deteriorate but not as rapidly as it would if the scoliosis were to progress.

Spinal stabilization is best accomplished with the use of Luque rods and sublaminar segmental instrumentation. The spine should be instrumented from T-2 or T-3 to the sacrum. One must instrument and fuse to the upper thoracic spine because a curve will develop above the upper level of the fusion if it extends only to the midthoracic region. Fixation to the pelvis is accomplished with the Luque rods inserted into the ilium by the Galveston technique. Recently, a single-unit rod has been developed for correction of the spine in patients with muscular dystrophy. This single rod is actually fashioned from two Luque rods that are joined at the top. It is designed to prevent recurrence of the pelvic obliquity that may develop with settling when two independent Luque rods are used.

Friedreich's Ataxia

The incidence of scoliosis in patients with Friedreich's ataxia is very high. The severity of the spinal deformity parallels the severity of the disease itself. Bracing has proved to be ineffective in preventing progression of the spinal curvature; however, as in other progressive neuromuscular diseases, the use of bracing may delay the progression of the curvature until pulmonary function is too poor to allow for surgical correction of the spine. A patient with Friedreich's ataxia should be observed for progression of the scoliosis, and the spine should be fused if the curve progresses to 50° to 60°.

Miscellaneous Spinal Problems

Quadriplegia

Quadriplegic children have a very high incidence of scoliosis. The incidence and the severity of the deformity are inversely proportional to the age of the patient at the time of onset of the quadriplegia. Bracing will help the child to sit upright, and it may help slow the progression of the scoliosis; however, the curve will progress despite bracing, although at a slower rate than if bracing were not used. For progressive curves, surgical stabilization eventually will be necessary.

Osteogenesis Imperfecta

The incidence of scoliosis in patients with osteogenesis imperfecta is very high, perhaps 50% or more. Bracing has proved to be ineffective in preventing progression, and the braces themselves produce deformities of the soft ribs. Spinal fusion has been advocated for curves that progress beyond 50°. The use of instrumentation allows some correction of the curve and enhances the fusion rate. The improved spinal alignment improves sitting balance.

Neurofibromatosis

In patients with neurofibromatosis, scoliosis may be either dystrophic or nondystrophic. The dystrophic form can be recognized by the bony anomalies seen on radiographs. These anomalies include pencilling of the ribs, scalloping of the vertebral bodies, and adjacent soft tissue masses. Nondystrophic curves should be treated in the same manner as idiopathic scoliosis. Dystrophic curves are more difficult to treat because they usually do not respond to bracing. If progressive scoliosis is not associated with a kyphosis, the spinal deformity may be corrected with posterior instrumentation and arthrodesis which usually yield good results. On the other hand, if an associated kyphosis exists, posterior fusion alone carries a high risk of pseudarthrosis. If the angle of the kyphosis is not sharp, an anterior fusion followed by a posterior fusion with instrumentation usually will produce a solid arthrodesis. However, if there is a sharp, angular kyphosis, the spinal deformity may progress in spite of a solid anterior and posterior fusion.

Laminectomy

Laminectomy of the growing spine has been found to be associated with a very high incidence of spinal deformity; both kyphosis and scoliosis are associated with this treatment. A child who has undergone this operation will require prolonged follow-up and may require a spinal fusion. If there is an associated kyphosis, both anterior and posterior fusion will have to be performed. Posterior instrumentation is made more difficult in these children by the lack of posterior elements.

Bone Tumors

Osteoid osteomas may occur in the posterior elements or the pedicles of the spine. These tumors typically produce pain as a result of the high concentration of prostaglandins that they produce. Scoliosis frequently develops with the lesion located at the apex of the concavity of the curvature. If the diagnosis is made early enough and treatment (surgical resection) is carried out promptly, the scoliosis will regress spontaneously. Delay in treatment, on the other hand, may result in a progressive structural curve. Because osteoid osteomas may be difficult to localize, interoperative technetium-99m scanning with a sterilized probe may be necessary. If the lesion is localized in a pedicle, complete removal by a direct surgical approach should cure the lesion without destabilization of the spine. Osteoblastomas, which are histologically related to osteoid osteomas but are much larger, occur in the posterior elements. They may produce a scoliosis, but their removal usually will result in regression of the curve.

Giant cell tumor, an uncommon tumor of the spine, usually involves the vertebral body. Complete surgical excision and grafting is the recommended treatment. Irradiation is not recommended because of the possibility of producing a sarcoma. Aneurysmal bone cysts may occur in either anterior or posterior elements of the spine. The treatment for this lesion is complete excision of the cyst and grafting.

Eosinophilic granuloma of the spine usually produces a very characteristic picture on a lateral radiograph (Fig. 6). This so-called vertebra plana, rarely reported in conditions such as leukemia and blastomycosis, is almost definitively diagnostic of eosinophilic granuloma. The earliest stages of this lesion, however, may have the appearance of a lytic lesion on the radiograph. Treatment requires establishment of the diagnosis by biopsy of the spinal lesion or other lesions if present. Occasionally, biopsy may be avoided if the lesion is thought to be radiographically characteristic and there are no systemic or laboratory signs of other diseases. Because the lesion is self-limiting, the treatment is observation unless the lesion is producing a neurologic deficit, in which case low-dose irradiation of the lesion (500 to 900 rads) is justified to prevent paraplegia.

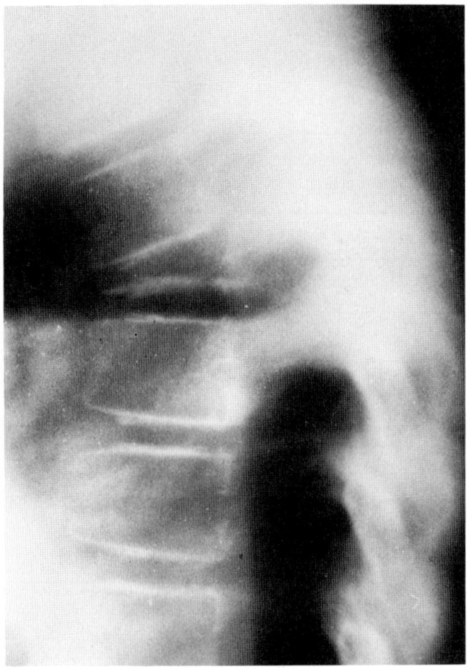

Figure 6

Lateral radiograph of thoracic spine of a child with an eosinophilic granuloma of T-4. There is a typical vertebra plana deformity. Note preservation of the disks above and below the lesion.

Back Pain

Infection

Disk space infection, or discitis, is an inflammatory lesion of the intervertebral disk that occurs in children. Its cause has been the subject of debate, although most authors believe it to be infectious. The infection probably begins in one of the contiguous vertebral end plates, and the disk is infected secondarily. Severe back pain that begins insidiously is characteristic of the disease. Although most children will continue to walk in spite of the pain, very young children may refuse to ambulate. The characteristic finding is extension of the spine and the child's complete refusal to flex the spine. Children with discitis usually are not systemically ill. They rarely have an elevated temperature, and their peripheral leukocyte count is frequently normal; however, the sedimentation rate is usually increased. Lateral radiographs of the spine usually will reveal disk space narrowing with erosion of the vertebral end plates of the contiguous vertebrae (Fig. 7). On occasion, lateral tomography is necessary for better definition of the lesion. Technetium bone scanning has been recommended as being helpful in localizing a lesion that is difficult to diagnose clinically. However, because false-negative bone scans do occur, the diagnosis of disk space infection should not be excluded simply because a bone scan is negative. Magnetic resonance imaging seems to be helpful in identifying a disk space infection. The appropriate treatment of these lesions has been the subject of controversy. All authors recommend plaster-cast immobilization, a treatment that seems to be effective by itself in many cases. Some authors think that antibiotics also should be given because this condition most likely is an infection of the disk (the organism involved is probably *Staphylococcus aureus*). In treating this lesion, aspiration biopsy usually is not necessary. A biopsy may be indicated in adolescents, especially if drug abuse is suspected, because of the possibility of organisms other than *S. aureus* being present.

Vertebral osteomyelitis has a very different presentation than does disk space infection, and it is much less common. Children with vertebral osteomyelitis are systemically ill, exhibiting increased temperature and leukocyte count. The causative organism usually is *S. aureus*. Long-term antibiotic therapy is required in the treatment of this infection and, if significant bone destruction is present, anterior de-

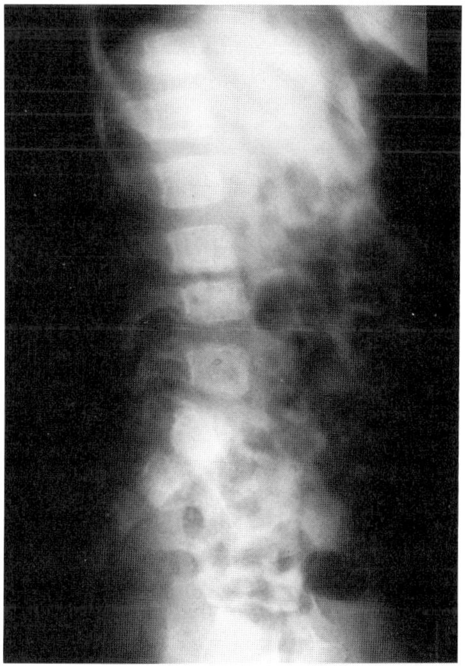

Figure 7

Disk space infection at L3-4 in 2-year-old child. Lateral radiograph of the spine, demonstrating marked narrowing of the disk space and erosion of the adjacent vertebral end plates.

bridement and fusion probably will be required to prevent kyphosis.

Although still rare, tuberculosis of the spine is becoming more common in the United States. Pott's disease may produce paraplegia in adults, but neurologic deficit is uncommon in children. Treatment depends on the extent of bony involvement; if there is minimal bone destruction, antituberculosis therapy and plaster-cast immobilization may be all that are necessary. On the other hand, if significant bone destruction exists, anterior debridement and fusion are required.

Disk Herniation

Disk rupture is uncommon in children and adolescents: only 2% of all herniated disks occur in this age group. The onset of symptoms is frequently more insidious than in adults; however, a history of trauma is often present. Most authors have found fewer objective neurologic deficits in children than in adults. Children often experience little or no back pain, but they usually have sciatica. Unless there is an extruded disk fragment, conservative treatment is frequently effective. Early surgical results are good, but these results seem to deteriorate with time.

Spondylolisthesis and Spondylolysis

Spondylolisthesis is an acquired disease in most patients, although there does seem to be a genetic predisposition in the development of a pars interarticularis defect. Spondylolisthesis does not occur at birth, but it has been found in children as young as 1 year old (Fig. 8). Although heredity plays a role in the development of a pars interarticularis defect, it is not the only causative factor. Children

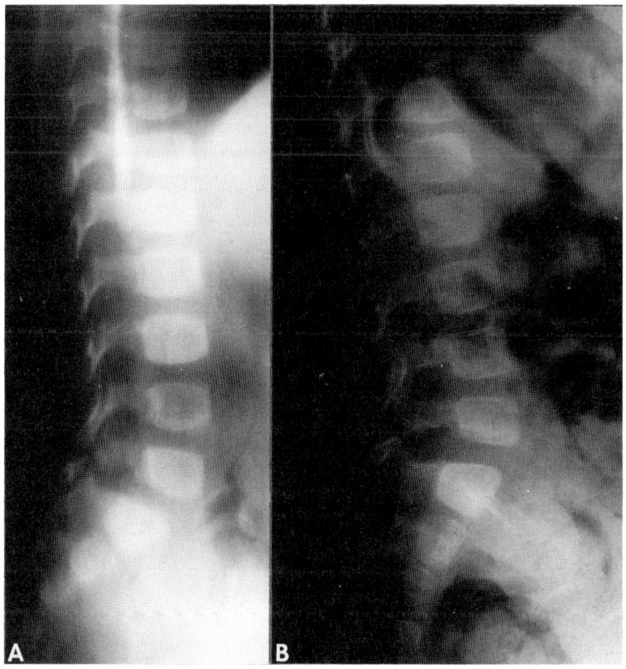

Figure 8

Spondylolisthesis in a 17-month-old girl who presented with acute back pain and refusal to walk after a fall. *A*, Lateral tomogram of the lumbosacral spine, demonstrating grade I spondylolisthesis with an obvious defect in the pars interarticularis bilaterally. *B*, Lateral radiograph 9 months later, showing healing of the spondylolysis. The patient had been immobilized in a cast for 3 months.

and adolescents involved in sports such as gymnastics and football are much more likely to develop a spondylolisthesis than is the public at large. This is most likely due to the hyperextension forces exerted on the lumbosacral spine in these activities. Some individuals have a pars interarticularis that is hereditarily weaker than the average and thus is more likely to develop a stress fracture if exposed to repetitive hyperextension stress.

The treatment of a symptomatic spondylolysis is controversial because there is little likelihood of progression to a frank slip. Most authors recommend treatment if the lesion has been recently acquired. The probability of healing can be determined with bone scintigraphy. If increased uptake can be seen on bone scan, healing of the stress fracture is possible. Immobilization or simple avoidance of the inducing stress may be all the treatment needed to allow healing.

Although a spondylolisthesis may progress during childhood, progression is unlikely. Children with this condition should be followed periodically with standing lateral radiographs of the lumbosacral spine to monitor for progression of the slip. The treatment of the spondylolisthesis depends on symptoms and the degree of the slip. In most instances, conservative treatment usually is effective. Once the patient is asymptomatic, normal activities, including contact sports, may be allowed.

Most patients will respond well to conservative treatment and will be able to return to normal activities without symptoms. Some patients, however, will require surgical treatment. One indication for operation is intractable pain in spite of an adequate trial of conservative treatment. The

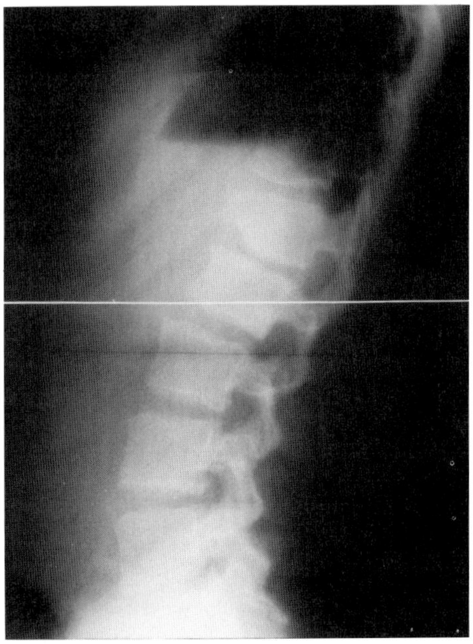

Figure 9

Lateral radiograph of the thoracolumbar spine of an adolescent boy with back pain, demonstrating Scheuermann's disease of the upper lumbar spine. Note the anterior inferior defect of L-1 that is characteristic.

recommended surgical procedure is posterolateral fusion from L-4 or L-5 to the sacrum. Postoperative immobilization is not required. Another indication for fusion is progression of the slip beyond 50%. Again, the fusion should be posterolateral between L-4 and the sacrum, and those patients fused because of progression should wear a pantaloon spica postoperatively. A combined anterior and posterolateral fusion may be necessary for a slip; a very high slip angle indicates a severe kyphosis at the lumbosacral junction. Reduction of the slip has been tried, but this procedure is probably indicated only for the very severe slip that produces significant physical deformity.

Scheuermann's Disease

Scheuermann's disease of the thoracic spine is defined as an excessive thoracic kyphosis with wedging of 5° or more of at least three adjacent apical vertebrae. Kyphosis in this area is rarely painful, and treatment is indicated if the deformity is cosmetically unacceptable. Thoracic kyphosis within a range of 20° to 50° is considered normal. If treatment is indicated in an immature patient, a Milwaukee brace is used; the brace should be worn until skeletal maturity. An underarm orthosis also may be used. Surgical treatment is rarely necessary because the kyphosis does not progress after skeletal maturity.

Scheuermann's disease of the thoracolumbar spine is frequently associated with pain. The radiographic picture is that of anterior deficits in the affected vertebral bodies (Fig. 9). The lesion may be mistaken for a more serious condition such as a tumor or infection. The radiographic picture is characteristic, however. The anterior portion of the affected vertebral body or bodies has a defect under the ring apophysis. Treatment for this disease is conservative, and most patients are asymptomatic within several months. Occasionally, a short period of cast or brace immobilization is necessary for complete resolution of the pain.

Miscellaneous Causes of Back Pain

Scoliosis does not cause back pain in children. If a scoliosis is associated with pain, the physician should look carefully for an entity causing both the scoliosis and the pain. A bony lesion such as an osteoid osteoma or an osteoblastoma may produce a scoliosis. A herniated disk is another painful condition that is capable of producing a secondary scoliosis. Intraspinal lesions such as spinal cord tumors and syringomyelia frequently present with painful scoliosis. Widening of the interpedicular distance on the anteroposterior radiograph will suggest the presence of an underlying lesion. Myelography, computed tomography, and magnetic resonance imaging usually are required to demonstrate the underlying problem.

Acute disk space calcification is a self-limiting disease of unknown cause. The patient usually presents with pain and decreased spinal motion in the area of the lesion, most commonly the cervical spine. Evidence of inflammation such as an increased sedimentation rate is usually present. The disease will run its own course, and many patients are asymptomatic within a month.

The patient with juvenile rheumatoid arthritis may present with back pain. This pain is usually localized in the upper cervical region. Ankylosing spondylitis, on the other hand, may present as back pain of insidious onset. Reiter's disease may also affect the lumbosacral spine and present as back pain.

Annotated Bibliography

Congenital Deformity of the Spine

Andrew, T., and Piggott, H.: Growth arrest for progressive scoliosis: Combined anterior and posterior fusion of the convexity. J. Bone Joint Surg. 67B:193–197, 1985.

This study confirms an earlier report by Winter that anterior epiphyseodesis and fusion combined with posterior convex fusion is effective in arresting the progression of severe congenital scoliosis in young children.

Bradford, D.S.; Ganjavian, S.; Antonious, D.; Winter, R.B.; Lonstein, J.E.; and Moe, J.H.: Anterior strut-grafting for the treatment of kyphosis: Review of experience with forty-eight patients. J. Bone Joint Surg. 64A:680–690, 1982.

Anterior strut grafting with rib is effective in producing a solid arthrodesis in patients with congenital kyphosis if the strut is not more than 4 cm from the apical vertebra. It should be combined with anterior interbody fusion and posterior fusion in the growing child.

McMaster, M.J., and Ohtsuka, K.: The natural history of congenital scoliosis: A study of two hundred and fifty-one patients. J. Bone Joint Surg. 64A:1128–1147, 1982.

An excellent classification of congenital scoliosis, this article shows the chance of progression of the deformity for the different types of abnormalities. The prognosis is worse with unilateral unsegmented bars, especially those associated with a contralateral hemivertebra. The prognosis is also age- and location-dependent.

Winter, R.B.; Moe, J.H.; and Lonstein, J.E.: Posterior spinal arthrodesis for congenital scoliosis: An analysis of the cases of two hundred and ninety patients, five to nineteen years old. J. Bone Joint Surg. 66A:1188–1197, 1984.

The authors report that *in situ* arthrodesis of congenital scoliosis is effective in preventing progression of the scoliosis in the majority of the patients. This should be performed early, before severe deformity develops. Instrumentation of congenital scoliosis can be performed safely if the existence of tethering of the spinal cord has been ruled out.

Winter, R.B.; Moe, J.H.; and Lonstein, J.E.: The surgical treatment of congenital kyphosis. A review of 94 patients age 5 years or older, with 2 years or more follow-up in 77 patients. Spine 10:224–231, 1985.

Posterior fusion alone may be effective for kyphosis less than 55°; but, for curves greater than 55°, anterior and posterior fusion is necessary.

Adolescent Idiopathic Scoliosis

Etiology

Barrack, R.L.; Whitecloud, T.S., III; Burke, S.W.; Cook, S.D.; and Harding, A.F.: Proprioception in idiopathic scoliosis. Spine 9:681–685, 1984.

This is one of many reports demonstrating abnormal proprioception in patients with adolescent idiopathic scoliosis. Scoliotic subjects showed asymmetry in their ability to reproduce angles between their two knees and an absolute deficit in their ability to reproduce angles, compared with controls.

Screening

Bunnell, W.P.: An objective criterion for scoliosis screening. J. Bone Joint Surg. 66A:1381–1387, 1984.

This report describes the use of the scoliometer, a device for measuring the angle of trunk rotation in a patient with scoliosis. This measurement is reproducible and is accurate for identifying curves of 20° or more.

Drummund, D.; Ranallo, F.; Lonstein, J.; Brooks, H.L.; and Cameron, J.: Radiation hazards in scoliosis management. Spine 8:741–748, 1983.

Radiation exposure of patients with scoliosis can be reduced by utilizing posterior-anterior views and with techniques such as proper collimation, gonadal shielding, beam filtration, and kVp technique. In addition, the use of rare earth intensifying screens and fast film can significantly reduce patient exposure.

Natural History

Lonstein, J.E., and Carlson, J.M.: The prediction of curve progression in untreated idiopathic scoliosis during growth. J. Bone Joint Surg. 66A:1061–1071, 1984.

In this report, the incidence of curve progression is related to the pattern and magnitude of the curve, the patient's age, the Risser sign, and the menarchal status. The authors developed a nomogram into which an individual patient's curve can be plotted to serve as a guide for prognosis.

Weinstein, S.L., and Ponseti, I.V.: Curve progression in idiopathic scoliosis. J. Bone Joint Surg. 65A:447–455, 1983.

The authors relate progression of scoliosis after maturity to the magnitude of the curve at maturity. In general, curves less than 30° did not progress after skeletal maturity, whereas curves greater than 50° did progress.

Treatment

Allen, B.L., Jr., and Ferguson, R.L.: The Galveston technique of pelvic fixation with Luque-rod instrumentation of the spine. Spine 9:388–394, 1984.

The authors describe their technique of Luque rod instrumentation to the pelvis for fixation and fusion to the sacrum in patients with neuromuscular scoliosis. This technique has proved to be the most effective means of stabilizing the lumbosacral joint and seems to provide the highest rate of fusion.

Bradford, D.S.; Tanguy, A.; and Vanselow, J.: Surface electrical stimulation in the treatment of idiopathic scoliosis: Preliminary results in 30 patients. Spine 8:757–764, 1983.

Results reported here are not as good as those reported by others. The authors conclude that significant improvement in the curves under treatment was unlikely, that progression may have been stopped in some curves, that curves less than 30° had the best results, and that curves that do not respond to electrical stimulation are not likely to respond to a brace.

Brown, J.C.; Axelgaard, J.; and Howson, D.C.: Multicenter trial of a noninvasive stimulation method for idiopathic scoliosis: A summary of early treatment results. Spine 9:382–387, 1984.

The early results of a large study, involving 54 investigators, of the LESS method of surface electrical stimulation for the treatment of adolescent idiopathic scoliosis are reported. In 72% of the patients, scoliosis was either reduced or stabilized.

Cochran, T.; Irstam, L.; and Nachemson, A.: Long-term anatomic and functional changes in patients with adolescent idiopathic scoliosis treated by Harrington rod fusion. Spine 8:576–584, 1983.

Back pain was found statistically significantly more often in patients in whom fusion was carried down to L-4 or L-5. The authors also found retrolisthesis in 24 patients when the distal hook site was at L-4 or L-5. All of these patients had back pain.

Drummond, D.; Guadagni, J.; Keene, J.S.; Breed, A.; and Narechania, R.: Interspinous process segmental spinal instrumentation. J. Pediatr. Orthop. 4:397–404, 1984.

The method described utilizes a button-wire implant that passes through the base of the spinous process. The wires are then secured to a Harrington distraction rod on the concavity and to a Luque rod on the convexity. Passing the wire through the spinous process avoids need for sublaminar passage and its possible risks. The compression and tension tests showed excellent strength.

Hefti, F.L., and McMaster, M.J.: The effect of the adolescent growth spurt on early posterior spinal fusion in infantile and juvenile idiopathic scoliosis. J. Bone Joint Surg. 65B:247–254, 1983.

The authors found that, in patients who underwent spinal fusion prior to the adolescent growth spurt, the vertebral bodies continued to grow. This anterior growth gave rise to loss of correction, increased vertebral rotation, and recurrence of the rib hump.

King, H.A.; Moe, J.H.; Bradford, D.S.; and Winter, R.B.:

The selection of fusion levels in thoracic idiopathic scoliosis. J. Bone Joint Surg. 65A:1302–1313, 1983.

The authors describe the criteria for a selective thoracic fusion for combined thoracic and lumbar curves when the thoracic curve equals or is greater than the lumbar curve and when the thoracic curve is at least as flexible as the lumbar curve. The lower level of the fusion should be to the stable vertebra—the vertebra that is bisected by a line drawn through the center of the sacrum and perpendicular to the iliac crests.

Malcolm-Smith, N.A., and McMaster, M.J.: The use of induced hypotension to control bleeding during posterior fusion for scoliosis. J. Bone Joint Surg. 65B:255–258, 1983.

This is the report of a controlled double series of patients who underwent spine fusion with either normotensive or hypotensive anesthesia. The intraoperative blood loss was 3 times greater in the normotensive group. There was a subsequent 55% reduction in blood replacement in the hypotensive group.

Miller, J.A.A.; Nachemson, A.L.; and Schultz, A.B.: Effectiveness of braces in mild idiopathic scoliosis. Spine 9:632–635, 1984.

The authors retrospectively compared two groups of patients who had mild scoliosis. One group was treated with bracing, and the other was not treated. Seventy-five percent of the control group did not have progression of their scoliosis. This is one of many recent reports that question the necessity of using bracing for minor curves. The authors did brace patients with curves of 15° or greater, a much more liberal bracing criterion than most use at the present time.

Moe, J.H.; Purcell, G.A.; and Bradford, D.S.: Zielke instrumentation (VDS) for the correction of spinal curvature: Analysis of results in 66 patients. Clin. Orthop. 180:133–153, 1983.

The authors describe the technique of insertion of the Zielke anterior device for scoliosis correction and report the results they obtained with the device. They think that the Zielke device allows better curve correction over a shorter fusion area than posterior instrumentation systems allow in lumbar and thoracolumbar curves. The device also allows for excellent correction of derotation of the spine.

Wilber, R.G.; Thompson, G.H.; Shaffer, J.W.; Brown, R.H.; and Nash, C.L., Jr.: Postoperative neurological deficits in segmental spinal instrumentation: A study using spinal cord monitoring. J. Bone Joint Surg. 66A:1178–1187, 1984.

This study showed a higher incidence of neurologic injury than found in studies of patients treated without sublaminar wire passage. The risk of neurologic injury was also increased when intraoperative correction exceeded preoperative bending correction and when the surgeon lacked experience in the passage of sublaminar wires.

Infantile Idiopathic Scoliosis

McMaster, M.J.: Infantile idiopathic scoliosis: Can it be prevented? J. Bone Joint Surg. 65B:612–617, 1983.

This article reports a marked decline of this condition in Great Britain where it once was very prevalent. The author suggests that it may have been caused by placing infants in the lateral position, and that it can be prevented by having infants lie in the prone position as is done in the United States.

Neuromuscular Scoliosis

Aprin, H.; Bowen, J.R.; MacEwen, G.D.; and Hall, J.E.: Spine fusion in patients with spinal muscular atrophy. J. Bone Joint Surg. 64A:1179–1187, 1982.

In this study, bracing was found to be ineffective in preventing progression of the scoliosis. To prevent curve progression, a long posterior fusion was deemed necessary. Spine fusion may slow the rate of deterioration of pulmonary function.

Cady, R.B., and Bobechko, W.P.: Incidence, natural history, and treatment of scoliosis in Friedreich's ataxia. J. Pediatr. Orthop. 4:673–676, 1984.

The incidence of scoliosis in Friedreich's ataxia is very high and the curve tends to progress even after maturity. Bracing is ineffective, and spine fusion should be performed early for progressive curves. Delaying the operation may allow deterioration of pulmonary function to a point such that the patient is unable to tolerate spinal fusion.

Ferguson, R.L., and Allen, B.L., Jr.: Staged correction of neuromuscular scoliosis. J. Pediatr. Orthop. 3:555–562, 1983.

The authors advocate combined anterior and posterior fusion in patients with neuromuscular scoliosis; however, they do not use anterior instrumentation. They state that anterior release and fusion followed by gravity tong traction prior to the second-stage posterior fusion is effective in curve correction and in obtaining a solid arthrodesis.

Lonstein, J.E., and Akbarnia, B.A.: Operative treatment of spinal deformities in patients with cerebral palsy or mental retardation: An analysis of one hundred and seven cases. J. Bone Joint Surg. 65A:43–55, 1983.

In this study, posterior fusion alone was found to be effective for thoracic curves. However, the authors recommend combined anterior and posterior fusion because this produced the best correction and yielded the best rate of solid arthrodesis. They utilized anterior instrumentation in addition to the posterior instrumentation.

Osebold, W.R.; Mayfield, J.K.; Winter, R.B.; and Moe, J.H.: Surgical treatment of paralytic scoliosis associated with myelomeningocele. J. Bone Joint Surg. 64A:841–856, 1982.

The authors recommend combining anterior instrumentation and fusion with posterior instrumentation and fusion for patients with paralytic curves associated with spina bifida. The fusion rate with this method was better than that obtained with posterior fusion alone.

Sussman, M.D.: Advantage of early spinal stabilization and fusion in patients with Duchenne muscular dystrophy. J. Pediatr. Orthop. 4:532–537, 1984.

Most patients with Duchenne dystrophy will develop a severe spinal curve. The author recommends early correction and stabilization with segmental instrumentation and fusion. He cautions against the use of bracing as a temporizing measure, because it may slow the curve progression just until the pulmonary function is too severe to allow spinal fusion.

Neurofibromatosis

Hsu, L.C.S.; Lee, P.C.; and Leong, J.C.Y.: Dystrophic spinal deformities in neurofibromatosis: Treatment by anterior and posterior fusion. J. Bone Joint Surg. 66B:495–499, 1984.

The authors state that there are two types of spinal deformities seen in patients with neurofibromatosis—dystrophic deformities and nondystrophic deformities. The nondystrophic may be treated as one would treat idiopathic scoliosis, but the dystrophic scoliosis, especially kyphoscoliosis, requires aggressive treatment. The kyphoscoliosis requires both anterior and posterior fusion; however, the curve may progress in spite of a solid fusion.

Bone Tumors

Ransford, A.O.; Pozo, J.L.; Hutton, P.A.N.; and Kirwan,

E.O'G.: The behaviour pattern of the scoliosis associated with osteoid osteoma or osteoblastoma of the spine. J. Bone Joint Surg. 66B:16–20, 1984.

Painful scoliosis may be caused by an osteoid osteoma. Although removal of the lesion usually results in regression of the scoliosis, prolonged delay in treatment may allow development of a progressive structural scoliosis.

Savini, R.; Gherlinzoni, F.; Morandi, M.; Neff, J.R.; and Picci, P.: Surgical treatment of giant-cell tumor of the spine: The experience at the Istituto Ortopedico Rizzoli. J. Bone Joint Surg. 65A:1283–1289, 1983.

Complete surgical excision of the tumor is recommended. Arthrodesis may be required; however, the authors caution against the use of radiation.

Back Pain

DeOrio, J.K., and Bianco, A.J., Jr.: Lumbar disc excision in children and adolescents. J. Bone Joint Surg. 64A:991–996, 1982.

Pain, especially sciatic, was the most common complaint of the patients studied. However, there was less loss of neural function than has been reported in adult patients. The rate of recurrence at the same level was equal to that seen in adults; however, the rate of protrusion at another level was higher.

Fredrickson, B.E.; Baker, D.; McHolick, W.J.; Yuan, H.A.; and Lubicky, J.P.: The natural history of spondylolysis and spondylolisthesis. J. Bone Joint Surg. 66A:699–707, 1984.

The authors report on a prospective study of 500 children. The incidence of spondylolisthesis was 4.4% at age 6 and 6% in adulthood. They found that slipping may increase during the time of growth but that it rarely increases after age 16. They recommend no treatment for the asymptomatic slip, and they allow full participation in sports for the asymptomatic child.

Infection

Eighth Report of the Medical Research Council Working Party on Tuberculosis of the Spine: A 10-year assessment of a controlled trial comparing debridement and anterior spinal fusion in the management of tuberculosis of the spine in patients on standard chemotherapy in Hong Kong. J. Bone Joint Surg. 64B:393–398, 1982.

This study showed that patients treated with radical debridement and anterior grafting had earlier bony fusion and no increase in kyphosis compared to patients treated with debridement without grafting. The recommendation is to combine radical debridement of a focus of spinal tuberculosis with anterior grafting if the necessary facilities are available.

Scoles, P.V., and Quinn, T.P.: Intervertebral discitis in children and adolescents. Clin. Orthop. 162:31–36, 1982.

In many cases, the cause of discitis is undoubtedly an infection; however, the authors state that antibiotic therapy is not always necessary. They recommend cast immobilization and state that needle aspiration is not necessary as routine treatment.

26

Thoracolumbar Spine: Trauma

The two main determinants of treatment in spinal injuries are the patient's neurologic status and the mechanical stability of the spinal column. Of the two, neurologic status is of primary importance. In those patients who have intact neurologic function, its preservation is vital; in those patients with compromised neurologic function, anything reasonable that can be done to enhance recovery is warranted.

Accurate assessment of mechanical stability is important because motion in the unstable spine can worsen a neurologic deficit. With spinal injury, the terms "stable" and "unstable" have no precise definitions. In common clinical usage, a spinal injury is considered stable if the injury will heal in a few months without significant alteration in position after nonoperative ambulatory management in a body brace or cast. Unstable injuries are those that will probably fail to heal or will angulate, translate, or settle with nonoperative treatment. Accurate assessment of the injured structures and of the probable mechanism of injury assists in predicting the behavior of thoracolumbar injuries.

Rationales for treatment of spinal injuries in adults and children based on these two determinants, in both the acute and chronic stages, are considered in this section.

Injuries in Adults

Acute Injuries

Spine Stability There are numerous classification systems for thoracolumbar injuries. The most useful is that advocated by Denis in which the spinal elements are subdivided into three columns: 1) the anterior column, consisting of the anterior longitudinal ligament, anterior anulus fibrosus, and anterior half of the vertebral body; 2) the posterior column, consisting of the pedicles, facet joints, lamina, spinous processes, and intraspinous and supraspinal ligaments; and 3) the middle column, consisting of the posterior longitudinal ligament, posterior anulus fibrosus, and posterior half of the vertebral body. In general, fractures behave in a stable manner if the middle column is intact and in an unstable manner if it is disrupted. There are exceptions to this rule, as follows.

In the upper thoracic spine—that is, above T-8—an injury may disrupt the middle column but the fracture still may be stable if the sternum and ribs in the area of the injury are intact. The chest wall tends to splint or support the injury site. The middle column can be disrupted at the lumbosacral junction—L-4 and L-5—but if the posterior elements are relatively intact the fracture may be stable because a significant amount of weight-bearing occurs through the posterior laminar elements. Physiologic lordosis prevents excessive weight-bearing in the middle column elements. Another exception to the middle column rule of stability is in distraction injuries; the Chance fracture is the classic example. In these injuries, the middle column is disrupted but, if the injury site goes through the vertebral body rather than the intervertebral disk space, interdigitation of the cancellous bone gives some degree of immediate stability. Rapid healing in the cancellous bone ensures early healing, and these fractures tend to behave in a stable manner. These injuries are seen most often in association with seat belt use.

In significant wedge-compression fractures at the thoracolumbar junction, the middle column can appear to be intact but, if there is gross disruption of the interspinous ligaments, the fracture may be unstable, settling into painful kyphosis. Noting these exceptions to the middle column theory of spinal stability gives the clinician a useful tool for classifying the behavior of injuries as stable or unstable.

Good-quality plain radiographs continue to be the best diagnostic modality for analyzing the extent of injury to the spinal column. An extremely useful radiographic sign of middle column disruption is widening of the interpedicular distance in the anteroposterior radiograph; this distance cannot widen without disruption of the middle column. Computed tomography is helpful in further defining the injury site, especially in burst fractures when elements of the posterior vertebral body compromise the spinal canal. It is least useful in injuries in a transverse plane through the vertebral body, as with distraction injuries. Very often, the tomographic cuts are above or below the injury site, giving the false impression of intact anatomic elements. Care must be taken in interpreting scans in distraction and shear-type injuries.

Several types of injury patterns deserve special mention because of their common occurrence and clinical implications.

Axial Compression Fractures (Burst) These are the result of compression forces on the vertebral body with compression failure in both the anterior and middle columns. Burst fractures are frequently associated with neurologic deficit that is reversible if the spinal canal is adequately decompressed. These injuries appear to be occurring more frequently in recent reports.

Flexion-Distraction (Seat Belt-Type) Injuries These injuries are the result of a distraction force exerted near the thoracolumbar junction as a result of acute flexion of the torso across a seat belt. Compression of the abdominal contents by the seat belt results in a fulcrum of rotation anterior to the vertebral elements. Tension failure occurs in the posterior column, the middle column, and, depending upon the exact site of the fulcrum, either in the anterior column or anterior to it. In a Chance fracture, the fulcrum is anterior to the vertebral column with distraction injury to all three columns. This fracture will be stable if managed conservatively. If the fulcrum of rotation falls in the vertebral body with comminution and compression of the anterior column, the fracture is unstable.

Fracture Dislocations This injury was widely discussed by Holdsworth. In these injuries, all three columns are compromised as a result of a combination of forces which may involve compression, tension, rotation, and shear. Although the spine is often angulated and deformed when initially evaluated radiographically, even this degree of deformity does not reflect the amount of displacement that probably occurred at the time of injury. The shear component in these injuries frequently results in irreversible damage to the neural elements. Although these injuries involve severe damage to the spinal column, the injury site often will heal in a stable manner with prolonged bed rest or immobilization. It is these injuries that generate the greatest divergence of opinion between the American and the British concept of treatment of spinal injury. In the United States, these injuries usually are surgically stabilized early whereas in Great Britain they are treated nonoperatively. There is ample evidence that nonoperative treatment can result in a stable spine. However, with operative intervention there is a much higher incidence of bony union in these injuries with earlier attainment of rehabilitation goals and less overall cost.

Neurologic Injury The most devastating aspect of spine injury is damage to the neural elements. In the fortunate patient with no neurologic deficit after injury, it is mandatory to protect the neural elements. Accurate assessment of spinal column stability and appropriate treatment, especially of unstable injuries, are extremely important. At the other end of the spectrum are those patients who have sustained irreversible neural damage. For these patients, rapid restoration of spinal column stability and early implementation of a rehabilitation program are the primary treatment goals. There are a few patients who will present with neurologic deficit that has the potential for some recovery. These patients require careful assessment and planning to obtain the best result.

It is difficult to evaluate the effectiveness of treatment of neural injuries because the potential for recovery varies between cord and nerve roots and between anatomic locations of the injury. Like the brain, an injured cord has poor potential for recovery. The cauda equina behaves more like peripheral nerves and has good potential. At the thoracolumbar junction, mixed injuries occur. The following description of the clinical state after spinal cord injury is helpful in understanding this problem.

Spinal Shock Immediately after injury to the neural elements, there is a transient period of total loss of motor, sensory, and reflex functions from the area of injury distally. This is analogous to the unconscious state that occurs after blunt trauma to the brain. Spinal shock is a transient phenomenon that may persist for up to 72 hours, and during this period the severity of cord injury cannot be assessed accurately. The end of spinal shock is determined clinically by return of the bulbocavernosus or anal reflex. Until this reflex has returned, it is not possible to separate complete from incomplete paraplegia.

Complete Paraplegia Total loss of motor and sensory functions distal to the site of injury after the end of spinal shock indicates that the cord has been transected anatomically or physiologically. The prognosis for return of neurologic function distal to the site of injury is extremely poor. The term "complete paraplegia" is reserved for injuries in the area of the spinal cord and is not used for injuries in the area of the cauda equina.

Incomplete Paraplegia Patients who have any neurologic function distal to the site of injury after the period of spinal shock have incomplete paraplegia. These patients have the potential for variable degrees of neurologic recovery. After spinal shock, the patient may present with any one of numerous signs of incomplete anatomic or physiologic transection of the cord. There may be scattered dermatomes with preservation of sensation or of weak motor function. Most frequently in severe injuries, incomplete paraplegia is noted by sacral sparing. There will be preservation of perianal skin sensation or voluntary rectal sphincter control. Anatomically, incomplete paraplegia indicates that certain neural elements have not been anatomically and physiologically transected; neural function may have stopped temporarily because of the response to swelling and edema and may return as the injury process reverses.

Prognosis Establishing an accurate prognosis for neural injury is extremely important for the individual patient and for evaluating the efficacy of treatment programs. The most important step in establishing prognosis in individual cases is serial physical examinations. However, the variability in the natural history of recovery after neural injury is so great that adequate assessment of various treatment programs will only be accomplished with pooled data from large numbers of spinal cord injury cases evaluated and treated in a controlled manner at multiple spinal cord injury centers. Computed tomography, which is extremely useful in evaluating damage to the spinal column, is of little value in evaluating the extent of neural tissue damage. Electromyography and spinal cord evoked potentials similarly are of little value in prognosticating for neural injuries. Magnetic resonance imaging currently is being evaluated as a tool in establishing the degree of neural damage, but its place is not as yet established.

Treatment There is no question that there is no effective treatment for patients with anatomically or physiologically severed neural elements. However, there is considerable controversy as to the effectiveness of various treatment modalities for anatomically intact but injured neural elements. One school of thought is extremely nihilistic, holding that damage to the neural elements occurs at the time of injury and nothing can be done to enhance recovery over and above immobilization of the torso by conservative means until stability of the spinal column is restored by the natural healing process.

Since early times, operative treatment to enhance neurologic recovery has been tried. Laminectomy not only has proved to be ineffective after closed injuries of the spine but also often has caused additional injury. Laminectomy makes the spinal column more unstable, resulting in further neurologic damage. Spinal cord cooling and various drug treatment regimens including steroids have been advocated to decrease swelling in the area of injury and perhaps to enhance neural recovery. To date, none of these modalities has enough proved clinical efficacy to merit widespread use.

Experimentally and clinically, evidence is accumulating that, for neural elements damaged primarily by compression, as occurs in burst fractures, neural recovery can be improved by adequate decompression of the spinal cord. It formerly was thought that postural reduction of the injured spinal column or reduction with dual Harrington rods would accomplish spinal cord decompression by anatomically restoring the spinal canal. There is now ample evidence that neither of these techniques reduces compression on the cord.

In burst fractures, a posterolateral or an anterolateral approach to the anterior vertebral elements may be necessary to ensure spinal cord decompression. It is unknown which approach is most efficacious. In the area of the spinal cord and conus medullaris, it is extremely important not to attempt spinal cord decompression via the posterior approach and laminectomy. Manipulation and retraction of the damaged neural elements will cause further neural injury. The advantage of the posterolateral technique is that it can be combined with posterior instrumentation for immediate stabilization. The advantage of the anterolateral approach is that it permits more complete visualization of the anterior neural elements and the extent of the burst fracture, but it renders the spine extremely unstable and requires some type of anterior instrumentation or supplementation with a secondary posterior procedure.

The treatment goal in patients whose injury pattern and clinical course suggest the possibility of neurologic recovery should be to ensure that, at the site of injury, there are no osseous or soft tissue elements impinging on the spinal cord and mechanical integrity is immediately restored to the spine. Restoration of mechanical integrity of the spinal column ensures that there is no abnormal motion at the site of injury as the patient is mobilized and decreases the swelling that results from the body's reaction to fractures.

Treatment Rationale The initial treatment of patients with spinal injury is no different from that for any major injury. The airway must be adequate, the circulatory status must be supported, and the patient must be evaluated for treatment of life threatening bleeding or organ damage. Often, the site of spinal column injury is obvious but it should be remembered that about 20% of patients with major fracture dislocations of the spinal column at one area have other areas of the spinal column also significantly damaged. An adequate history is necessary to help establish the mechanism of injury. The initial neurologic examination should be complete and well-documented. Serial examinations will be of most help in establishing the patient's prognosis.

Urinary retention is always present, and an indwelling catheter should be inserted to prevent overdistention of the bladder after the patient is first seen. An intermittent catheterization program is extremely helpful in the long-term management of the patient but does not need to be instituted in the acute phase—the first 7 days.

Even though sophisticated diagnostic studies and other pressing medical matters dominate the patient's treatment in the initial phase, it must be remembered from the very outset that prophylactic skin care in these patients is extremely important. Position changes and use of padding to prevent decubitus ulcers must be started immediately.

The two primary determinants of the patient's treatment will be the spinal column stability and the neurologic status. The following is a rationale for treatment based on these two determinants.

Neurologically Intact; Spinal Column Stable This most typically is seen in the patient who has had a compression fracture. In these patients the spinal column is stable and treatment of symptoms is all that is needed. If the patient is young and in good general physical condition, restriction of activity may be sufficient as treatment, after a short period of observation to ensure that ileus and urinary retention are not present. In a few patients it may be necessary to immobilize the torso with an orthosis for 2 to 3 months.

In distraction-type injuries such as seat belt injuries and Chance fractures, there is the possibility that these fractures can displace during the first few weeks if some immobilization of the torso is not instituted. For that reason, these patients should be immobilized in an orthosis or a body cast and observed closely, especially for neurologic status. These injuries consolidate rapidly. After an initial 2 to 3 weeks of continuous orthosis wear, the patient usually can be allowed out of the device daily for bathing. A restricted activity regimen should be followed for 2 to 3 months.

Neurologically Intact; Spinal Column Unstable In these patients, early operative intervention usually is indicated to ensure healing of the spinal column in an acceptable position in a short period of time and to allow early rehabilitation. For some patients in this category, nonoperative treatment may be elected. However, great care should be taken with patients whose burst fractures compromise more than 50% of the spinal canal. Conservative treatment of these patients can result in progressive neurologic loss in a significant number.

The standard technique of restoring spinal column stability is with posterior dual Harrington distraction rods. The rods are loaded by four-point bending and prevent the spine from flexing into more kyphosis. The most frequent clinical mode of failure with dual Harrington distraction rods has been cut-out or dislodgment of a hook. The implants can be supplemented by segmental wiring, and there is biomechanical evidence that these constructs are stronger than dual Harrington distraction rods alone. The techniques have the added risk of passage of the sublaminar wires in an area where spinal cord damage and swelling already may be present. Attempts at Luque instrumentation in spinal cord injury have been fraught with many problems, principally relating to the fact that Luque instrumentation will not hold a distraction force on the spine and thus permits settling. Alternatives to the Harrington system by modification with a locking hook mechanism are being offered.

The disadvantage to any posterior instrumentation is that, to gain enough length for four-point bending of the posterior rods, the spine must be immobilized at least two levels above and below the injury site. This is a distinct problem with injuries in the lower lumbar spine because the vital motion segments from L-4 to the sacrum are immobilized. All authors emphasize the importance of contouring the posterior instrumentation systems to maintain sagittal body contours in the lumbar spine. There has been considerable discussion regarding the concept of instrumentation over four or five motion segments while fusing only the short segment of the spine that is injured. The efficacy of "rodding-long and fusing-short" is questioned because of the known effects of stripping the posterior elements on the neurovascular supply to the erector spinae. Additionally, the immobilized facet joints undergo degenerative changes, whether fusion takes place or not.

For injuries of the lumbar spine below L-2, anterior instrumentation has been offered as a means of fixing only one level above and below the injury site. This instrumentation is relatively new, has not been widely used, and is controversial because of potential vascular complications that can occur when it is used on the left side of the vertebral column.

Another recently offered but unproved alternative to the long posterior instrumentation is single-level instrumentation above and below the injury site posteriorly with either internal or external skeletal fixation devices. Fixation to the vertebra is by Schanz-type pins passing from the lamina through the pedicle and into the vertebral bodies. These transpedicular fixation systems have been characterized biomechanically as showing adequate stabilization. Clinical experience with them, however, is extremely short, and the obvious potentials for damage to nerve roots, visceral organs, and vascular structures prohibit early endorsement of the concept.

Neurologically Compromised; Spinal Column Stable This is a rare combination in adults but is seen in children. The initial evaluation should include a complete characterization of the neural elements and spinal canal at the level of neural injury. If there is no impingement on the neural elements by extruded disk material or bony fragments, management should be like that described above for patients who are neurologically intact with stable spinal columns—symptomatic conservative treatment. If there is encroachment on the neural elements by disk or bony fragments, surgical intervention is indicated. The surgical approach probably will render the spinal column unstable, necessitating internal fixation.

Neurologically Compromised; Spinal Column Unstable Many interrelated factors must be taken into account to achieve optimal treatment. If analysis of the patient's history, neurologic findings, and radiographs shows that the neural injury is irreversible, then the sole determinant of treatment is restoring spinal column stability. This is frequently seen in thoracic fracture-dislocations in which there is a shear component to the injury and it is obvious from the initial radiographs and from the immediate and complete neurologic deficit that the patient has anatomically or physiologically transected spinal canal contents. If the fracture-dislocation is at T-7 or above and there has been no fracture of the ribs bilaterally or of the sternum, the spinal column is stable and only conservative treatment is needed. If there is a similar injury below T-7, the fracture will be unstable. Posterior instrumentation and fusion with dual Harrington rods or the equivalent is indicated.

If the patient presents with a neurologic deficit that is partially reversible—that is, the typical burst fracture patient with an unstable spinal column—several approaches are reasonable. Posterolateral decompression of the neural elements with immediate posterior instrumentation with dual Harrington rods is one alternative. Another is anterolateral decompression with anterior spinal instrumentation. A third is anterolateral decompression in an extracavitary manner utilizing tricortical iliac grafts anteriorly to prevent kyphosis. Often, these patients will require a secondary posterior instrumentation with dual Harrington rods.

The timing of operative intervention in patients with neural deficits remains controversial. Intuitively, and in animal experiments, it appears that early operative intervention offers the best chance of neural recovery. Attempts to prove this in clinical studies have not been fruitful. There is no clear-cut evidence that early operative intervention enhances neural recovery to a greater degree than later intervention does.

Chronic or Old Injuries

Deformity Patients with old unrecognized or inadequately treated unstable thoracolumbar injuries often present for treatment because of progressive deformity and pain. The most frequently noted deformity is kyphosis, often associated with some degree of scoliosis. Kyphosis at the thoracolumbar junction necessitates compensatory lumbar lordosis, and these patients frequently have as much pain in the compensatory curve as they have at the site of injury. These are fixed deformities, and surgical treatment requires initial mobilization of the spine to allow correction of the deformity followed by stabilization and adequate bone grafting. It is important to correct the deformity in order to reestablish torso balance and sagittal plane spinal contours. In addition, the weight-bearing function of the anterior vertebral elements is best served when excessive kyphosis and scoliosis is corrected. Attempts to fuse deformities *in situ* often leave the fusion mass poorly positioned and subject to tensile forces that cause failure.

Correction of the deformity restores the vertebral bodies to near the weight-bearing line of the torso and this, coupled with adequate anterior fusion, leaves a fusion mass that can resist late deforming forces that are still present. With fixed deformities of the spine, it usually is necessary to mobilize the vertebral elements on both anterior and posterior sides of the spinal column. It always is advisable to accomplish anterior and posterior fusion in these situations to ensure long-term stability.

Late-developing deformity in patients with complete neurologic deficit at the level of the injury site usually can be corrected by a single-stage posterior and posterolateral approach to the spinal column. A closing wedge osteotomy around the neural elements or even after transection of the nonfunctioning spinal cord with a direct posterior approach to the vertebral bodies allows complete correction of the deformity and placement of graft material for anterior and posterior fusion. Instrumentation can be accomplished posteriorly with heavy Harrington compression rods or segmental spinal instrumentation. Heavy Luque squares and sublaminar wires are extremely stable in these situations.

The patient with intact neurologic function and significant spinal deformity presents a greater challenge. The anterior and posterior vertebral elements still have to be mobilized to allow correction of the deformity but care must be exercised to protect the contents of the spinal canal. Staged surgery has been the traditional approach: anteriorly to mobilize the vertebral bodies and a second procedure posteriorly for spinal instrumentation. Recently, single-stage operative procedures with simultaneous anterior and posterior approaches have been advocated for these patients. The advantage of the single-stage procedure is that the deformity can be corrected under direct visualization of the spinal canal contents. This, coupled with spinal cord monitoring, appears to provide sufficient safety to the contents of the spinal canal. When the spine is approached both anteriorly and posteriorly at the same time, it is possible to instrument the spine in the corrected position both anteriorly and posteriorly. This makes an extremely rigid construct and aids anterior and posterior fusion.

Significant pain usually accompanies progressive deformity. Occasionally, one sees patients who have mechanical-type pain at the site of injury with little deformity present (less than 40° of kyphosis and less than 20° of scoliosis). In these patients, especially if the deformity is above L-2, posterior *in situ* fusion with or without instrumentation is adequate treatment.

It is extremely important to differentiate between chronic mechanical pain that results from spinal column instability and the chronic pain syndrome seen in patients with significant neural deficits. The latter patients usually present with nonmechanical deep burning pain at the site of injury and may have radiation of the pain into the lower extremities and around the torso. They are seldom helped by surgical intervention. Numerous techniques have been proposed for these patients, including spinal canal decompression, deformity correction, and surgical and chemical rhizotomy. To date, nothing has proved to be effective.

Neurologic Deficit There have been several reports of both pain relief and improved neurologic function after late anterior decompression and stabilization. These patients, who initially had incomplete paraplegia, either had not been treated initially or had been treated inadequately. Often, they had had laminectomy without instrumentation or laminectomy with posterior instrumentation and failure to decompress the spinal canal. In patients presenting up to 18 months after injury, both relief of pain and improved motor function were achieved when adequate spinal canal decompression, deformity correction, and spinal stabilization were performed.

Injuries in Children

Acute Injuries

Fortunately, these injuries do not occur with the same frequency in children as they do in young adults. This may relate to the anatomy and physiology of the child but probably is more related to the fact that children do not engage in the type of activities so frequently associated with spinal cord injuries. A unique feature of acute spinal cord injuries in children is the incidence of neurologic compromise without radiographic demonstration of spinal column injury. Up to 20% of children presenting with paraplegia or quadriplegia may be in this category. When in the thoracolumbar spine, the neurologic deficit usually is in the upper thoracic area. About half of the children who present with spinal cord injury without a demonstrable spinal column injury have a history of late onset of paralysis (up to 4 days after the initial episode of injury). It is probable that the spinal column separated through the soft tissue elements with deformity and damage to the cord at the time of injury and then subsequent swelling and perhaps vascular compromise resulted in the permanent neurologic deficit.

Acute injuries in children are managed in the same way as those in adults. The same rationale for treatment based on spinal column stability and neurologic deficit applies.

Chronic or Old Injuries Therapy for chronic deformity and pain in the postpubertal patient is little different from that in the adult. In prepubertal patients with spinal cord injury, however, late deformity below the level of injury occurs in most patients. The degree and severity of deformity are almost directly related to the immaturity of the patient at the time of injury. In patients with paraplegia who are skeletally immature, the effect of gravity on the growth plates of the spine and the failure of the torso musculature to support the spine in a normal manner result in progressive kyphoscoliosis. Initially, the deformities are not fixed and do not require treatment. With time, both the severity and the increasing rigidity of the curve will necessitate surgical intervention. Although postural bracing while the patient is in a wheelchair intuitively is appealing, there is little evidence that it delays or prevents the deformity. Most of these patients will require spinal instrumentation and fusion as their curves approach 60° and become more fixed. Posterior segmental spinal instrumentation and fusion has been a great asset in these patients. It is extremely important to restore the spinal column to its normal sagittal plane contours and to correct any scoliosis that is present. Often, the fusion must be carried into the pelvis, and here Luque rods used with a Galveston technique of sacral fixation are helpful. When iliac wings are inadequate for fixation into the sacrum, the Luque rods may be contoured to fit over the ala of the sacrum and then up the spinal column.

Annotated Bibliography

Injuries in the Adult

Acute Injuries

Ahn, J.H.; Ragnarsson, K.T.; Gordon, W.A.; Goldfinger, G.; and Lewin, H.M.: Current trends in stabilizing high thoracic and thoracolumbar spinal fractures. Arch. Phys. Med. Rehabil. 65:366–369, 1984.

Data from the National Spinal Cord Injury Research Center on 1,385 patients show that the number of patients being treated surgically was relatively unchanged between 1973 and 1979 but use of spinal stabilization with dual Harrington rodding increased markedly. The surgically treated patients continue to have the shortest hospital stays, in both acute and rehabilitation settings.

Angtuaco, E.J., and Binet, E.F.: Radiology of thoracic and lumbar fractures. Clin. Orthop. 189:43–57, 1984.

Computed tomography is the superior technique for evaluating the neural canal in spinal fractures. Intrathecal administration of contrast medium at the time of the initial scanning often is necessary for evaluating a confusing neurologic picture.

Bohlman, H.H.; Freehafer, A.; and Dejak, J.: The results of treatment of acute injuries of the upper thoracic spine with paralysis. J. Bone Joint Surg. 67A:360–369, 1985.

Laminectomy is contraindicated for incomplete lesions of the upper region of the thoracic spinal cord, and anterior decompression with fusion offers the best chance of recovery of neurologic function. No patient with complete lesions in the upper thoracic spine had neurologic recovery.

Denis, F.: The three column spine and its significance in the classification of acute thoracolumbar spinal injuries. Spine 8:817–831, 1983.

Currently, this is the most widely used and clinically relevant classification system for thoracolumbar fractures. The middle column consists of the posterior wall of the vertebral body, posterior longitudinal ligament, and posterior fibrous ring. When the middle column is intact, the fracture is likely to be stable; when broken, the fracture is unstable.

Denis, F.; Armstrong, G.W.; Searls, K.; and Matta, L.: Acute thoracolumbar burst fractures in the absence of neurologic deficit. A comparison between operative and nonoperative treatment. Clin. Orthop. 189:142–149, 1984.

The surgically treated patients did better in terms of neurologic function, pain, and return to work than those not treated surgically. Seventeen percent of the nonsurgically treated patients had neurologic problems.

Denis, F.; Ruiz, H.; and Searls, K.: Comparison between square-ended distraction rods and standard round-ended distraction rods in the treatment of thoracolumbar spinal injuries. A statistical analysis. Clin. Orthop. 189:162–167, 1984.

Dual square-ended distraction rods offer better contouring for maintenance of lumbar lordosis than do traditional Harrington rods.

Dunn, H.K.: Anterior stabilization of thoracolumbar injuries. Clin. Orthop. 189:116–124, 1984.

The author describes an implant system for anterior stabilization of the spine at a single level above and below the injury site. In the treatment of 48 consecutive patients, no major complications occurred and the overall results were satisfactory. Short-level instrumentation and immediate stability after anterior decompression are the major advantages in comparison with posterior instrumentation.

Dunn, H.K.: Anterior spine stabilization and decompression for thoracolumbar injuries. Orthop. Clin. North Am. 17:113–119, 1986.

Anterior decompression for spinal cord injury offers a significantly better chance of neurologic recovery than does conservative treatment or posterior instrumentation with dual Harrington rods.

Eismont, F.J.; Green, B.A.; Berkowitz, B.N.; Montalvo, B.M.; Quencer, R.M.; and Brown, M.J.: The role of intraoperative ultrasonography in the treatment of thoracic and lumbar spine fractures. Spine 9:782–787, 1984.

The adequacy of spinal cord decompression was evaluated by ultrasonography at the time of posterior instrumentation. If adequate decompression has not been accomplished by the posterior procedure, then posterolateral or anterior intervention can be immediately carried out.

Frankel, H.L.; Hancock, D.O.; Hyslop, G.; Melzak, J.; Michaelis, L.S.; Ungar, G.H.; Vernon, J.D.S.; and Walsh, J.J.: The value of postural reduction in the initial management of closed injuries of the spine with paraplegia and tetraplegia. Paraplegia 7:179–192, 1969.

In this series of 612 patients with spinal injuries, nonoperative therapy was evaluated in terms of neurofunctional results. A good baseline comparison of operative methods to the nonoperative Guttmann method is provided.

Gaines, R.W.; Breedlove, R.F.; and Munson, G.: Stabilization of thoracic and thoracolumbar fracture-dislocations with Harrington rods and sublaminar wires. Clin. Orthop. 189:195–203, 1984.

Seventeen patients with unstable fractures were treated with dual Harrington rods segmentally wired to the spine. No external bracing was used postoperatively. All patients healed without failure of instrumentation.

Golimbu, C.; Firooznia, H.; Rafii, M.; Engler, G.; and Delman, A.: Computed tomography of thoracic and lumbar spine fractures that have been treated with Harrington instrumentation. Radiology 151:731–733, 1984.

In patients who had dual Harrington rod instrumentation for burst fractures and who failed to recover neurologic deficit, computed tomography revealed a significant incidence of failure of spinal canal decompression by dual Harrington rodding alone.

Jacobs, R.R., and Casey, M.P.: Surgical management of thoracolumbar spinal injuries. General principles and controversial considerations. Clin. Orthop. 189:22–35, 1984.

The "rodding-long, fusing-short" technique of posterior instrumentation for unstable injuries is advocated. Internal fixation protects neural elements. Properly contoured posterior instrumentation can provide spinal canal decompression. The authors think that motion occurs in the nonfused but instrumented segments with a low incidence of postoperative pain.

Jacobs, R.R.; Schlaepfer, F.; Mathys, R., Jr.; Nachemson, A.; and Perren, S.M.: A locking hook spinal rod system for stabilization of fracture-dislocations and correction of deformities of the dorsolumbar spine. A biomechanic evaluation. Clin. Orthop. 189:168–177, 1984.

The authors offer an improved design over dual Harrington rods. The implants are stronger, offer better control with contouring, and have a locking hook to prevent disengagement from the lamina with flexion.

Kahanovitz, N.; Bullough, P.; and Jacobs, R.R.: The effect of internal fixation without arthrodesis on human facet joint cartilage. Clin. Orthop. 189:204–208, 1984.

In eight patients treated with the "rodding-long, fusing-short" technique for thoracolumbar injuries, biopsy of the unfused facets showed gross and histologic evidence of osteoarthritis. Internal fixation of the spine without arthrodesis is not an innocuous procedure and may be a predisposing factor in the development of symptomatic spinal arthritis.

Kaneda, K.; Abumi, K.; and Fujiya, M.: Burst fractures with neurologic deficits of the thoracolumbar-lumbar spine: Results of anterior decompression and stabilization with anterior instrumentation. Spine 9:788–795, 1984.

Anterior instrumentation is described for fixation of burst fractures at a single level above and below the injury site. Twenty-six of 27 patients improved by 1 Frankel grade after anterior instrumentation and fusion. A new instrumentation system is described.

Keene, J.S.: Radiographic evaluation of thoracolumbar fractures. Clin. Orthop. 189:58–64, 1984.

Computed tomography should be the first choice among the methods used to augment standard radiography in the assessment of thoracolumbar fractures. It is more accurate in assessing the integrity of the spinal canal and the radiation exposure is only 1/10th that of conventional tomography.

Kostuik, J.P.: Anterior fixation for fractures of the thoracic and lumbar spine with or without neurologic involvement. Clin. Orthop. 189:103–115, 1984.

The author describes anterior instrumentation with a modified Hall-Dwyer screw and Harrington distraction rod used anteriorly. The implant has been used in 31 cases without major complications.

Magerl, F.P.: Stabilization of the lower thoracic and lumbar spine with external skeletal fixation. Clin. Orthop. 189:125–141, 1984.

An external skeletal fixation system for spine fractures is described in which Schanz screws are placed in the vertebral bodies transpedically. Sixty-five patients have been treated since 1977 and results have been satisfactory.

Munson, G.; Satterlee, C.; Hammond, S.; Betten, R.; and Gaines, R.W.: Experimental evaluation of Harrington rod fixation supplemented with sublaminar wires in stabilizing thoracolumbar fracture-dislocations. Clin. Orthop. 189:97–102, 1984.

Dual Harrington distraction rods were tested in the calf spine model for fracture stability with and without sublaminar wires. Sublaminar wires improved stability in all planes and especially in rotation.

Sturm, J.T., and Perry, J.F., Jr.: Injuries associated with fractures of the transverse processes of the thoracic and lumbar vertebrae. J. Trauma 24:597–599, 1984.

Benign-appearing transverse process fractures are associated with a high incidence of significant trauma to the abdominal viscera, suggesting that great energy was expended in generating these fractures. This should alert physicians to look for more severe injuries.

Trafton, P.G., and Boyd, C.A., Jr.: Computed tomography of thoracic and lumbar spine injuries. J. Trauma 24:506–514, 1984.

Burst fractures at T-12 or L-1 with 50% or more decrease of the midsagittal neural canal had significant risk of progressive neurologic loss in the post-injury period. Seven of 48 patients had progressive loss. Computed tomography was extremely helpful in characterizing the injuries.

Wenger, D.R., and Carollo, J.J.: The mechanics of thoracolumbar fractures stabilized by segmental fixation. Clin. Orthop. 189:89–96, 1984.

The mechanics of fixation with Harrington rods, Luque rods, and wired-in Harrington rods, based on previous calf spine models, are summarized. The Luque system is weak because it cannot hold a distraction force; the Harrington instrumentation is weak because it attaches to only the end vertebrae. The combined system of wiring in the Harrington distraction rod is a significant improvement over the Luque or Harrington system alone.

Willén, J.; Dahllöf, A.-G.; and Nordwall, A.: Paraplegia in unstable thoracolumbar injuries: A study of conservative and operative treatment regarding neurological improvement and rehabilitation. Scand. J. Rehabil. Med. [Suppl.] 9:195–205, 1983.

A rehabilitation score to allow comparison of patients was developed in a small series. Conservatively treated patients were compared to patients treated with laminectomy and instrumentation. At 1 month after injury, the Harrington group was considerably better than the other two groups. However, at 3 months, the conservatively treated group was similar to the Harrington group. The laminectomy and fusion group remained behind the other two groups, even at 2-year follow-up, confirming the disadvantages of a laminectomy.

Willén, J.; Lindahl, S.; Irstam, L.; and Nordwall, A.: Unstable thoracolumbar fractures: A study by CT and conventional roentgenology of the reduction effect of Harrington instrumentation. Spine 9:214–219, 1984.

Harrington instrumentation restored general spinal alignment. However, a cross-sectional area of the spinal canal remained diminished by 26% postoperatively on evaluation by computed tomography. Early operation was more effective than later operation, and surgical intervention within 3 days after injury is recommended.

Chronic Injuries

McAfee, P.C.; Bohlman, H.H.; and Yuan, H.A.: Anterior decompression of traumatic thoracolumbar fractures with incomplete neurological deficit using a retroperitoneal approach. J. Bone Joint Surg. 67A:89–104, 1985.

Thirty-seven of 42 patients with motor deficit improved by at least one class of motor strength, and 14 of 30 nonambulatory patients became ambulatory. Twelve of 32 patients with conus injuries regained bowel and bladder functions. The degree of neurologic recovery after anterior decompression appeared to be better than that previously reported after techniques that do not decompress the spinal canal. Stabilization of the spine with anterior tricortical iliac grafts alone generally was not satisfactory and needed supplementation with dual Harrington rods posteriorly.

Mudge, K.; Van Dolson, L.; and Lake, A.S.: Progressive cystic degeneration of the spinal cord following spinal cord injury. Spine 9:253–255, 1984.

Cysts can form in the spinal cord several years after traumatic paralysis and present as progressive neurologic loss. Early deep treatment with decompression and shunting can result in restoration of newly lost function.

Whitesides, T.E., Jr.: Traumatic kyphosis of the thoracolumbar spine. Clin. Orthop. 128:78–92, 1977.

Persistent and progressive kyphosis can impede rehabilitation by causing progressive neural loss, inhibiting potential neural recovery, and causing a painful deformity that precludes a supine, sitting, or standing posture.

Injuries in the Child

Acute Injuries

Asher, M.A., and Jacobs, R.R.: Pediatric thoracolumbar spine trauma. *In* The Pediatric Spine, edited by D.S. Bradford and R.M. Hensinger, pp. 105–117. New York, Thieme-Stratton, 1985.

This is a good review of the subject.

Kleinman, P.K., and Zito, J.L.: Avulsion of the spinous processes caused by infant abuse. Radiology 151:389–391, 1984.

Avulsion fractures of the spinous process are often present in abused children. They are probably the result of violent shaking.

Pang, D., and Wilberger, J.E., Jr.: Spinal cord injury without radiographic abnormalities in children. J. Neurosurg. 57:114–129, 1982.

Among children with spinal cord injury without radiographic abnormality, 52% have delayed onset of paralysis up to 4 days after injury. Most recall transient paresthesia, numbness, or subjective paralysis. There is a review of the possible mechanisms of neural damage.

Chronic Injuries

Mayfield, J.K.; Erkkila, J.C.; and Winter, R.B.: Spine deformity subsequent to acquired childhood spinal cord injury. J. Bone Joint Surg. 63A:1401–1411, 1981.

In this study, spine deformities developed in all juvenile patients with spinal cord injuries. Eighty-six percent had progression of deformity. Collapsing kyphosis and hyperlordosis were noted in 57% and 18% of the patients, respectively.

27

Thoracolumbar Spine: Reconstruction

The primary goals in reconstructive surgery of the thoracolumbar spine are 1) preservation or improvement of neurologic function, 2) maintenance or restoration of spinal stability, and 3) preservation of the maximum number of vertebral levels of motion (particularly the lower lumbar and lumbosacral joints).

Magnetic Resonance Imaging

Because of its ability to visualize soft tissue structures in greater detail than any previous radiographic modality, magnetic resonance imaging has been heralded as one of the greatest advances in recent years in the diagnosis of thoracolumbar pathology (Table 1). It is particularly useful in the diagnosis of spinal disorders because it can visualize the spinal cord and cerebrospinal fluid without intrathecal administration of a contrast agent. Other advantages are no radiation exposure and provision of direct sagittal, coronal, and oblique views. Disadvantages of magnetic resonance imaging compared with computed tomography include poorer image resolution and slightly increased imaging time; it cannot be used for patients with intracranial aneurysm clips or cardiac pacemakers.

Table 1. Comparison of Contrast (Metrizamide) Computed Tomography (CT) and Magnetic Resonance Imaging (MRI)

Metrizamide CT	MRI
Utilizes ionizing radiation (approximately 3 to 5 rads per examination)	No radiation exposure; no known biologic hazards
Requires subarachnoid puncture (cisternal or lumbar) and introduction of contrast material to delineate CSF from neural tissue	Noninvasive; no contrast agent required
Computer reformatting of data collected by axial images required to visualize in sagittal or coronal planes	Direct sagittal, coronal, and oblique imaging
For each change in cervical spine position, a complete sequence of axial images is required for reconstructed images	Readily allows for functional flexion-extension cuts
Resolution 1 mm or better with current technology	Resolution 2 by 3 mm with current technology (head coil)
Usually requires overnight hospitalization because of frequency of side effects	Can be done on an outpatient basis
Few contraindicating factors (allergy to contrast agent)	No patients with cardiac pacemakers or ferromagnetic implants (in particular, intracranial aneurysm vascular clips)
Imaging time on the order of seconds	Each image requires 2 to 7 minutes

Adult Scoliosis

In contrast to idiopathic scoliosis in the adolescent, which is usually corrected to prevent progression of deformity, the most common presenting symptom of scoliosis in the adult is pain.

The role of scoliosis in the production of mechanical back pain is controversial. Incidence of back pain is not increased compared with a group of age-matched controls. However, the clinical course of back pain in adults without spinal deformity is different from that in adults with scoliosis—improvement in 64% of adults without scoliosis versus persistence or increased severity of pain in 83% of adults with scoliosis. The back pain increases with increasing age and degree of scoliotic curvature. In patients with scoliosis, surgical treatment significantly decreases pain ($P < 0.0001$) whereas conservative treatment does not. At 5-year follow-up, 83% of surgical patients had sufficient pain relief to make the surgical treatment worthwhile.

The clearest indication for operation in adult scoliosis is neurologic compression—*radicular* pain arising either from the concavity of the major curve or the concavity of the fractional lumbosacral curve (Fig. 1). Scoliotic deformity has been demonstrated to progress after skeletal maturity. For thoracic curves greater than 60° or lumbar curves greater than 40°, the general rule of thumb is a constant rate of progression of 1° per year (Fig. 2). More disabling than curve progression is lateral translation or rotational olisthy which occurs at the inferior end of the lumbar curve. Superimposition of degenerative changes and facet hypertrophy predisposes the adult scoliosis patient to spinal stenosis. A specific history should be obtained concerning neurogenic intermittent claudication and pain exacerbation on thoracolumbar extension with pain relief on thoracolumbar flexion.

Neurosurgical decompression of compressed lumbosacral nerve roots will lead to rapid sagittal (iatrogenic spondylolisthesis) and coronal (lateral olisthy) spinal subluxation (Fig. 3). The recommended treatment of spinal stenosis and scoliosis with radiculopathy is a combination of 1) correction of the curvature, 2) decompression of the compressed nerve roots, and 3) fusion to prevent iatrogenic loss of spinal alignment. Localization of the nerve root compression is based on the history of radicular pain distribution (L-5 dermatomal paresthesia associated with a lumbosacral fractional curvature, for example) and high-resolution computed tomography and myelography.

There are several important mechanisms of neurologic compression in deformities: 1) lateral recess stenosis, 2)

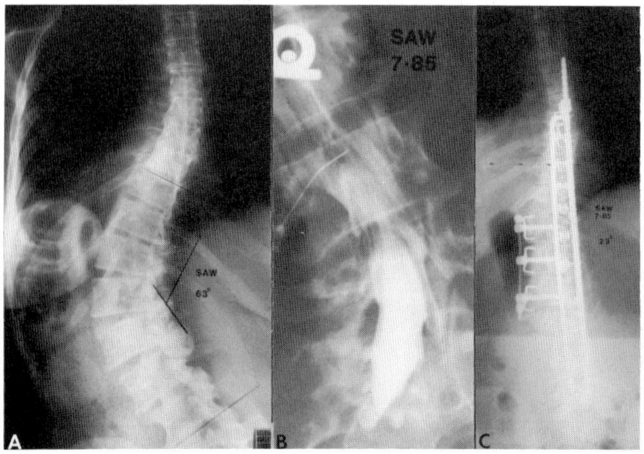

Figure 1

Adult scoliosis with radiculopathy in a 47-year-old woman. She had classic symptoms of neurogenic claudication in the left leg in L-5 nerve root distribution, paresthesias and radicular pain with standing, and inability to walk 7.5 m comfortably. *A,* Left thoracolumbar idiopathic scoliosis at presentation. *B,* Myelogram shows left L4-5 nerve root compression by fractional lumbosacral curve. *C,* Two-stage reconstruction (anterior discectomies and Dwyer instrumentation via a transthoracic retroperitoneal approach; then, posterior segmentally wired Harrington and Luque rods by the Wisconsin instrumentation technique) provided complete relief of radicular pain.

pedicular kinking and nerve root traction, 3) herniated intervertebral disk at the inferior end of the deformity, 4) progressive myelopathy due to spinal cord compression if the predominant deformity is kyphosis, and 5) malrotated pedicles at the apical vertebrae.

The recent advances in surgical correction of scoliosis have been directed toward segmental instrumentation to provide 1) more rigid internal stabilization, 2) better rotational correction of the deformity, and 3) limitation of the levels of fusion and instrumentation to as few lumbar vertebrae as possible (Fig. 4). Long-term studies of patients who had undergone posterior instrumentation and fusion for scoliosis showed no increase in disability, provided the fusion extended to the upper lumbar spine. However, if the fusions extended below L-3 there was a definite tendency toward chronic low back disability and pain—62% for fusions extending down to L-4 and 82% for fusions extending down to L-5. Anterior Dwyer or Zielke instrumentation with anterior discectomies and fusion can provide correction of a rigid adult scoliosis and preserve the inferior lumbar vertebral motion segments, preventing low back disability.

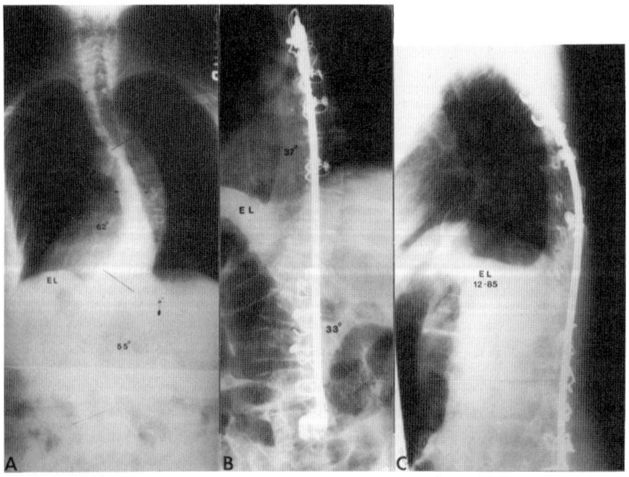

Figure 2

Progression of idiopathic scoliosis in an adult. *A,* A 55-year-old woman presented with a history of a 6.4-cm loss of height over 5 years, accompanied by osteoporosis. She had a painful 62° right thoracic and a 55° left lumbar curve. *B* and *C,* After a 6-month treatment for osteoporosis, posterior stabilization with double upper hooks and segmentally wired Harrington instrumentation was performed.

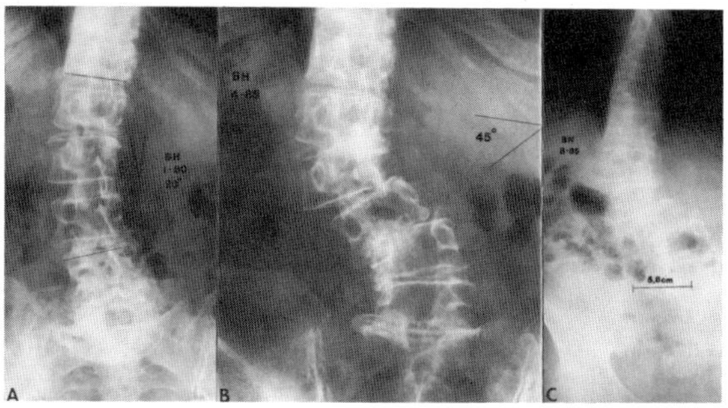

Figure 3

Iatrogenic postlaminectomy scoliosis and spondylolisthesis. *A,* A 70-year-old woman presented with spinal stenosis and underwent wide decompression laminectomies (performed elsewhere). *B,* Within several years later, leg weakness due to grade 1 iatrogenic spondylolisthesis of L3-4 and grade 2 spondylolisthesis of L4-5 with 45° of scoliosis from L-1 to L-3. *C,* Spine is laterally translated 5.8 cm out of balance, malaligning her thoracic cage with her pelvis.

In a report on 30 adult patients 20 to 72 years old (mean, 42 years) with idiopathic scoliosis and radicular symptoms, 17 needed operative procedures; 10 had Dwyer procedures. In an analysis of 100 patients treated by Dwyer instrumentation, patients older than 40 years did as well as those younger than 40, with no increase in incidence of complications.

The problems that can develop in patients previously treated for scoliosis include 1) pseudarthrosis, 2) loss of lumbar lordosis due to failure of rod contouring to the normal lumbar lordotic curvature, and 3) failure of fusion and technical complications in patients with prior lumbosacral fusion. A fused segment can become progressively out of balance due to a pseudarthrosis or progression of a curvature below the major deformity. Posterior multiple osteotomies usually are necessary to obtain correction. Correction of the thoracolumbar kyphosis is usually achieved at the L3-4 level below the level of the spinal cord, similar to "spontaneously fused" thoracolumbar kyphosis in ankylosing spondylitis. Correction and stabilization can be performed in two-stage operative procedures with intervening halo-gravity traction. However, combining the anterior or posterior osteotomy with posterior stabilization in one procedure is preferred. In a prospective study of 37 patients undergoing staged anterior and posterior spinal reconstructive procedures, with stringent cri-

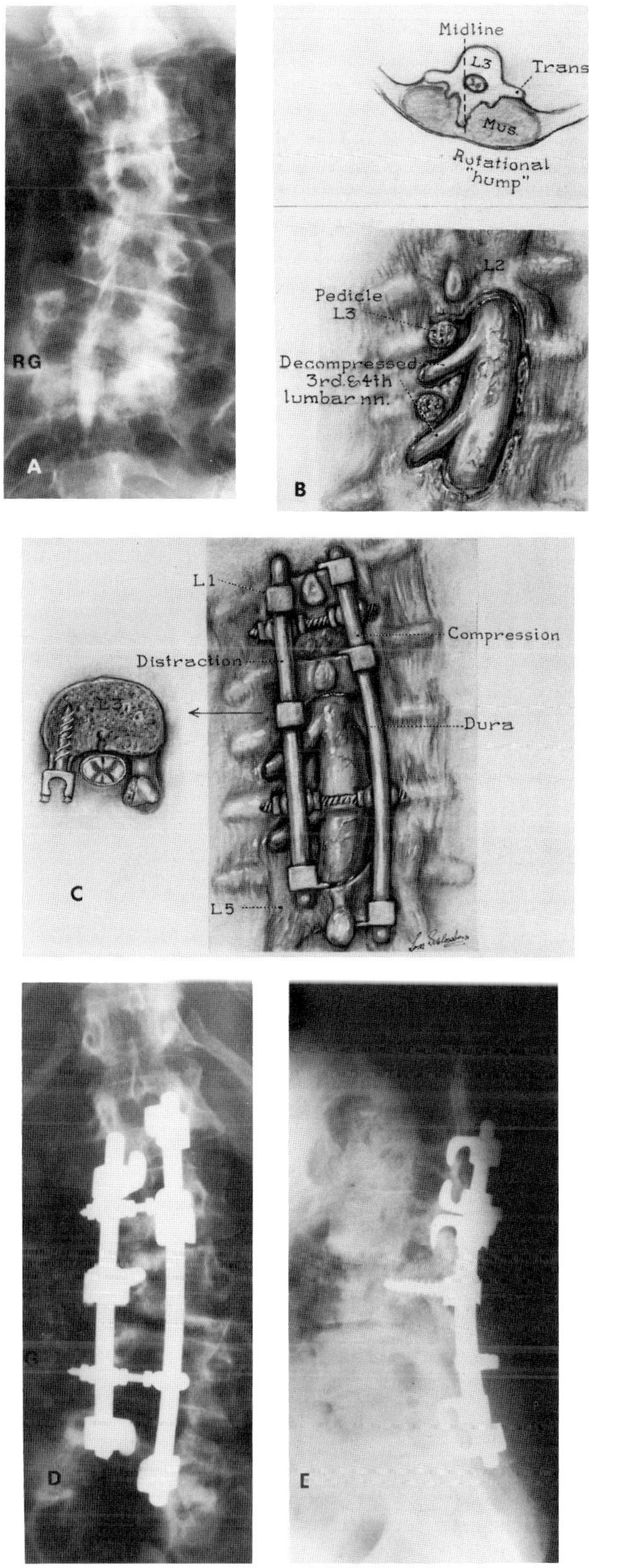

Figure 4

Decompression and segmental stabilization of adult scoliosis. *A,* A 42-year-old woman presented with left leg pain in femoral distribution (L-3 and L-4) and right leg pain in sciatic distribution (L-5 and S-1). *B,* Complete decompression of the left L-3 and L-4 nerve roots was performed. trans, transverse process. *C,* The scoliosis was stabilized and partially corrected with Cotrel-Dubousset instrumentation providing segmental purchase of L-3 via transpedicular fixation. *D* and *E,* Postoperative radiographs. The patient's radicular symptoms resolved immediately after operation.

teria for nutritional and immunologic incompetency (serum albumin < 3.5 g/dl and total lymphocyte count < 2,000/μl), 87% of the patients became malnourished at some time during hospitalization. For this reason, it is better to combine the reconstructive procedures in one operation and to obtain enough stability to allow rapid postoperative ambulation in the adult.

The Morbidity Committee of the Scoliosis Research Society reported, in 1978, a 15% instrumentation failure rate in all patients fused down to the sacrum; the failure rate in adults was 30%. Among 45 skeletally mature patients having spinal fusion extending to the sacrum, 35 (78%) had at least one significant postoperative complication. Thirteen of 22 patients with loss of lordosis required corrective osteotomies. Two patients had pseudarthrosis and five patients had neurologic complications. Due to high complication rates and long-term disability, fusion and instrumentation across the lumbosacral joint should be avoided in the treatment of scoliosis in adult patients except in unusual circumstances.

Post-Traumatic Kyphosis and Incomplete Paraplegia

The indications for operation for late post-traumatic thoracolumbar kyphosis include increasing kyphotic deformity, pain, and increasing neurologic deficit. Usually these are fixed deformities and will not be corrected, and therefore neurologic improvement can not be expected with posterior procedures alone. Even iatrogenic kyphosis from inappropriate post-traumatic laminectomies usually requires initial anterior surgery for correction. The delayed development of kyphosis after fractures of the thoracolumbar spine usually represents failure of the initial treatment to take posterior ligamentous injury into account. Despite casting or bracing, ligamentous injuries of the middle and posterior columns in translational or flexion-distraction injuries result in progressive kyphosis. A two-stage treatment is recommended—initial anterior decompression followed by posterior stabilization procedures (Harrington, Luque, or Cotrel-Dubousset instrumentation).

Anterior spinal exposure (transthoracic, T1-8; transthoracic-retroperitoneal, T11-L1; or retroperitoneal, L2-5) is the key to thoracolumbar reconstructive surgery for kyphosis. The operation for anterior transthoracic decompression and fusion is performed through a right thoracotomy to avoid the great vessels. It is best to approach the fracture level through a superior rib level rather than inferiorly. After self-retaining chest retractors are placed, the parietal pleura is split longitudinally along the vertebral bodies and the exposed segmental vessels are ligated with silk sutures. Once the periosteum is reflected, the fractured vertebrae are visualized. Hemorrhage is minimized by performing complete discectomies and anterior releases before performing corpectomies. All displaced bone and soft tissue anterior to the posterior longitudinal ligament at the kyphosis is completely debrided. Anteriorly directed pressure is exerted by the operative assistant at the posterior apex of the gibbus to correct the deformity as much as possible before an anterior fibular rib or iliac strut graft is inserted.

In the lower thoracic and upper lumbar segments, the only variation is the necessity of transecting the diaphragm to provide exposure. The general rule is to leave approximately 2 cm of peripheral diaphragm at its insertion into the chest wall to facilitate reattachment at closure; additionally, the portion of the diaphragm peripheral to the transection is denervated, so this margin is kept to as small a rim as possible.

Anterior retroperitoneal exposure is performed for kyphosis with an apex below L-1 and the approach is made through the periosteal envelope of the 12th rib. The transversalis fascia and perirenal fascia as well as the peritoneal and renal viscera are mobilized anteriorly. The anterior margin of the psoas muscle is mobilized posteriorly after the appropriate segmental vessels are ligated. Improved visualization of the dura and nerve roots can be achieved by resecting the pedicles of the involved vertebrae. However, due to the neuroforaminal and anastomotic plexus at each level, this does cause epidural venous bleeding. The decompression and iliac strut fusion technique is identical to the transthoracic technique. The wound is closed over suction drains. Before the posterior stabilization procedure the patient can be mobilized out of bed with a halo-gravity traction wheelchair.

Transpedicular Approaches and Fixation

The greatest single advance in spinal reconstruction in the past several years in the United States has been the adoption of transpedicular techniques from Europe (Fig. 5). Michele and Krueger should be credited with the first description of the transpedicular approach to the vertebral body. Recent enthusiasm for transpedicular techniques gives one the impression that it is a revolutionary idea, but Michele and Krueger's work was published in 1949. Judet described the technique of biopsy of the vertebral body from a posterior spinal incision via an interosseous route through the pedicle in 1960.

In general, posterior approaches are more familiar to orthopaedic surgeons and they provide more alternatives for spinal stabilization.

In the United States, a 3-year experience with transpedicular screw/posterior plate fixation in 152 cases has been reported. The deep wound infection rate was 6.2%, and reoperations were necessary in 34 cases (52 procedures)—a 22% reoperation rate—for pseudarthrosis, infection, nerve root compression, screw fatigue fracture, or cerebrospinal fluid drainage. In general, this is a very exacting technique but it offers great potential stability of lumbosacral fixation in the adult. However, North American investigators are currently at the initial portion of the "learning curve" for transpedicular techniques and long-term follow-ups are not available.

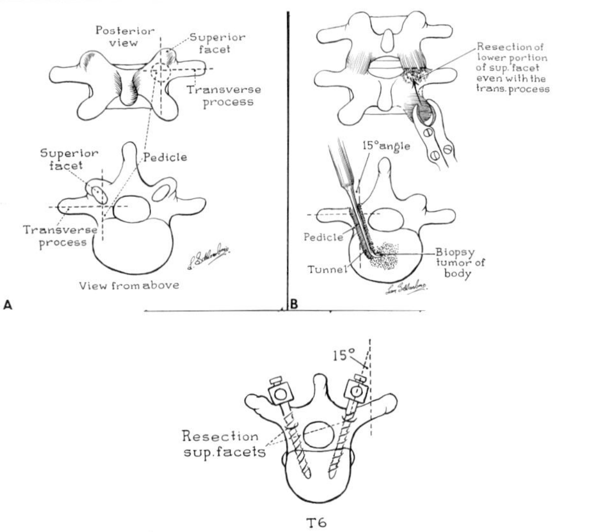

Figure 5

Transpedicular fixation. *A*, At every level of the thoracolumbar spine, the transverse processes are in the same transverse plane as the pedicles. *B*, Most investigators recommend probing rather than drilling through the pedicle to ensure intraosseous placement. Fluoroscopic visualization is helpful for orientation in obtaining biopsies of the vertebral body. *C*, Use of an angle of 15° with the sagittal plane, starting from the superior articular processes, can aid in the placement of fixation devices.

Metastatic Tumors

With improved chemotherapeutic and radiation therapy techniques, the incidence of and morbidity from tumors metastatic to the spine have been increasing. In a detailed study of 322 patients with metastatic bone disease, the seven most common sites of tumor origin with spinal metastasis were breast (31.2%), lung (21.8%), prostate (20.1%), kidney (6.7%), bladder (3.4%), colon (5.6%), and head and neck (2.2%). More than half of the patients with metastatic bone disease have involvement of the spine, and neurologic deficit occurs in 20% of these patients. Hypernephroma has the strongest propensity to occur with spinal cord impingement secondary to an occult primary malignancy.

Reconstructive spinal surgery is important as palliation for metastatic malignancies of the spine. Transthoracic-retroperitoneal or retroperitoneal approaches provide access for anterior decompression for incomplete neurologic deficit. The indications for vertebral body resection for epidural compression are 1) neural relapse after previous radiotherapy, 2) the need for tissue diagnosis, 3) treatment of a radioresistant tumor, 4) pathologic fracture-dislocation, and 5) neurologic deterioration while the patient is receiving radiation therapy.

In a series of 40 patients presenting with neurologic deficit, after anterior decompressions 80% had enough motor recovery to regain the ability to walk and 93% regained bowel and bladder sphincter control. In the past it had been customary not to consider operation if paraplegia had been present for 48 to 72 hours. Two patients who had been paraplegic for extended periods (up to 14 days) regained the ability to walk and regained sphincter control after anterior decompressions. Therefore, recovery from incomplete neurologic deficit after great lengths of time is possible if anterior decompression is performed.

The stabilization of anterior corpectomy defects for tumors is usually achieved with combinations of bone graft, methyl methacrylate, and metal fabrications (longitudinal Steinmann pins, Dwyer-Hall rods, Zielke devices). In the largest series of patients reported, there were only 5 instances of dislodgement of anterior fabrications in 95 patients who underwent anterior reconstruction. For more than two levels of involvement, a second-stage posterior Harrington or segmentally wired Harrington rod instrumentation is recommended after anterior decompression and stabilization (Fig. 6).

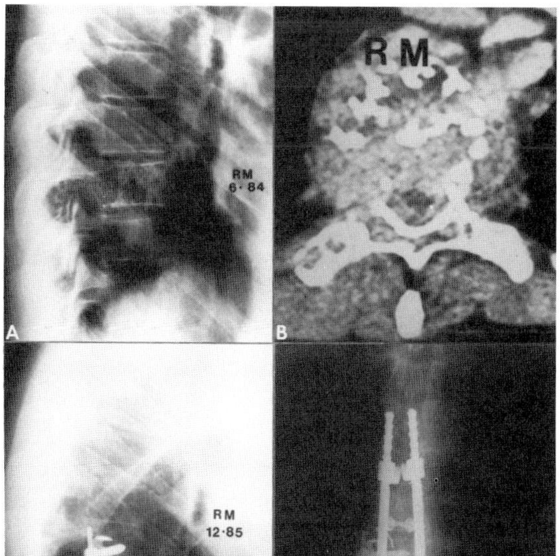

Figure 6

Reconstruction for neoplasms. *A,* A 45-year-old man had been treated unsuccessfully by radiation therapy for a tumor of T-9. *B,* At presentation, he had a spastic paraparesis from a plasmacytoma involving the anterior and posterior elements of T-9. *C* and *D,* Anterior transthoracic decompression and Dwyer-Hall rod stabilization was performed with posterior decompression (Harrington stabilization). This was as complete a vertebrectomy as is surgically possible. The patient regained independent ambulatory abilities over the next 2 months; at 12 months postoperatively he was neurologically normal with no evidence of recurrence.

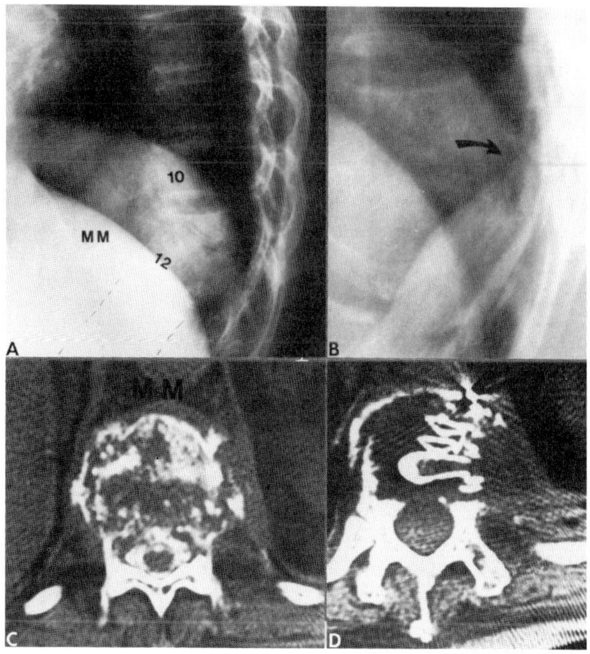

Figure 7

Pyogenic vertebral osteomyelitis with spinal cord compression. *A,* A 68-year-old woman had a history of loss of bowel and bladder function and paraparesis (grade 3/5 muscle strength in lower extremities) of 3 weeks' duration. *B,* Myelogram, showing erosion of T-11 vertebral body with complete obstruction of contrast medium at the *anterior* portion of the spinal canal at T11-12. *C,* Corresponding computed tomogram, showing extent of bony destruction (often the computed tomogram shows a paravertebral abscess, but not in this case). *D,* Transthoracic anterior decompression disclosed *Proteus* vertebral osteomyelitis. Note that the anterior decompression extends across the anterior aspect of the spinal canal from right to left to the base of the opposite pedicle. Stabilization was achieved with iliac and rib strut grafts. The patient underwent 6 weeks of intravenous antibiotic therapy. Ambulation was recovered gradually over this 6-week period and eventually neurologic recovery (including bowel and bladder function documented by pre- and postoperative cystometrograms) was complete.

Infections

Pyogenic Vertebral Osteomyelitis and Discitis

The largest reported series of nontuberculous spinal infections included 61 patients with pyogenic and fungal vertebral osteomyelitis with paralysis. Factors that predisposed to paralysis were 1) diabetes, 2) rheumatoid arthritis, 3) increased age, and 4) cephalad level of infection. Deterioration was noted after posterior laminectomy and destabilizing procedures that had been performed elsewhere prior to referral. The cause of paralysis was almost always anterior to the neural elements. The decompressive procedure of choice for incomplete paralysis was either transthoracic or retroperitoneal biopsy, discectomy, debridement, and anterior decompression (Fig. 7). The anterior approach provided exposure also for draining associated psoas and paraspinal abscesses. Provided the spine was adequately debrided and the patients were given appropriate intravenous antibiotic therapy, spine fusion could be performed safely with autogenous iliac bone graft placed in the site of infection. Costotransversectomy was recommended only as a life-saving procedure for biopsy and drainage of abscesses in patients too sick to undergo thoracotomy.

Tuberculosis of the Spine

In this era, this diagnosis is not often considered. Tuberculosis of the spine can mimic other infections or tumorous conditions. The tuberculous pus causes erosion of the vertebral bodies and can strip the anterior longitudinal ligament and periosteum of the adjacent vertebrae. There is usually a perispinal mass that gravitates inferiorly, may form skip lesions or psoas abscesses, or can extend posteriorly through the posterior lumbar triangle. Excellent results have been reported updating earlier descriptions of Hodgson and Stack's "Hong Kong operation." With or without Pott's paraplegia, an extensive anterior debridement of abscesses, sequestrated bone, and intervertebral disks is recommended. Under the cover of antituberculous chemotherapy, extensive anterior (usually transthoracic) debridement is performed and anterior strut grafts are inserted in order 1) to obtain tissue for diagnosis, 2) to decompress the spinal cord anteriorly, 3) to drain abscesses, and 4) to prevent post-infection kyphosis.

Thoracic Disk Herniation

Thoracic disk herniations are usually diagnosed late because of their infrequent occurrence and the difficulty of radiographic visualization. Early complaints are chest pain, back pain, or vague sensory dysfunction. By the time of diagnosis, most patients have gait disturbances, leg weakness, bowel and bladder abnormalities, and myelopathy. Predisposing factors are Scheuermann's disease and disk calcification. The radiologic method of choice is either magnetic resonance imaging or high-resolution computed tomographic myelography. Because the myelographic dye does not pool where there is thoracic kyphosis, the myelographer can miss a thoracic disk herniation.

The best surgical treatment for herniated thoracic disks is a formal anterior discectomy with generous removal of bone (hemicorpectomies) superiorly and inferiorly to provide adequate visualization. Laminectomy is associated with iatrogenic neurologic injury, and even wide posterolateral approaches can be hazardous because they provide only limited exposure. In a report on 16 patients treated by anterior decompression between 1972 and 1984, 14 had significant paralysis preoperatively; 10 recovered with mild residual spasticity, and 2 required walking aids.

Annotated Bibliography

Adult Scoliosis

Brown, R.H.; Nash, C.L., Jr.; Berilla, J.A.; and Amaddio, M.D.: Cortical evoked potential monitoring: A system for intraoperative monitoring of spinal cord function. Spine 9:256–261, 1984.

The report describes the intraoperative use of a somotasensory evoked potential system to monitor spinal cord function during 300 orthopaedic thoracolumbar reconstructive procedures. There were no false-negative results. In this series, three neurologic deficits were documented intraoperatively and confirmed postoperatively. In four cases, changes in evoked potentials led to changes in operative procedure, and there was no subsequent neurologic deficit. Intraoperative spinal cord monitoring has become the "state of the art" in thoracolumbar reconstruction surgery. Further refinements in the United States will probably involve the use of electrodes that stimulate the dura directly, with monitoring of efferent motor pathways.

Cummine, J.L.; Lonstein, J.E.; Moe, J.H.; Winter, R.B.; and Bradford, D.S.: Reconstructive surgery in the adult for failed scoliosis fusion. J. Bone Joint Surg. 61A:1151–1161, 1979.

Fifty-nine patients required salvage operations after surgical procedures for adult scoliosis. The indications for operation were pain (78%), loss of correction (68%), and dyspnea (36%). The complication rate after revision surgery using Harrington instrumentation was high (71%). The procedure was one-stage in 16 cases and combined with halo-traction and multiple osteotomies in 43 cases. Complications included pseudarthrosis, wound infection, urinary tract infection, loss of lumbar lordosis, and pressure sores.

Jackson, R.P.; Simmons, E.H.; and Stripinis, D.: Incidence and severity of back pain in adult idiopathic scoliosis. Spine 8:749–756, 1983.

The incidences of back pain in a referred group of 197 adults with idiopathic scoliosis and in a comparable control group of 180 adults without known spinal deformity were the same. However, the severity, persistence, and progression of pain were greater for the scoliotic patients. Pain increased with age and degree of scoliosis curvature ($P < 0.0005$). Pain came mainly from the concavity of either the major or compensatory curve and included discogenic, facet joint, and radicular origins. Surgical treatment significantly decreased pain ($P < 0.0001$); conservative therapy did not. At a mean follow-up of 5 years, 83% of surgical patients had sufficient pain relief to make surgery worthwhile.

Kaneda, K.; Satoh, S.; Nohara, Y.; and Oguma, T.: Distraction rod instrumentation with posterolateral fusion in isthmic spondylolisthesis: 53 cases followed for 18–89 months. Spine 10:383–389, 1985.

Fifty-three cases of isthmic spondylolisthesis were treated with distraction rod instrumentation and posterolateral fusion with or without nerve root decompression; mean follow-up was 39 months. Thirty-one cases without neurologic deficit were treated with instrumentation and fusion only; 22 cases with neurologic compression underwent foraminotomy and decompression of the fibrocartilaginous mass and the ragged bony edge of the pars interarticularis defect. The solid fusion rate (judged by stringent radiographic criteria) was 91%, and clinical results were superior to those of conventional methods without instrumentation.

McAfee, P.C.; Werner, F.W.; and Glisson, R.R.: A biomechanical analysis of spinal instrumentation systems in thoracolumbar fractures: Comparison of traditional Harrington distraction instrumentation with segmental spinal instrumentation. Spine 10:204–217, 1985.

Sixty-one biomechanical tests performed on 25 cadaveric spine segments showed that Luque segmental spinal instrumentation provides the greatest rotational stability whereas segmentally wired Harrington distraction instrumentation provides the greatest axial stability. Segmental instrumentation dramatically increases thoracolumbar reconstructive stability by distributing stress along a greater number of vertebral segments, prevents hook dislodgement, and prevents deformation within the instrumented segment of the thoracolumbar spine. In clinical practice, postoperative bracing is minimized.

Simmons, E.H.: Surgery of the spine in rheumatoid arthritis and ankylosing spondylitis. *In* Surgery of the Musculoskeletal System, edited by C.M. Evarts, pp. 85–151. Vol. 2, Section 4. New York, Churchill Livingstone, 1983.

This is the best available summary of the indications and techniques for cervical, thoracic, and lumbar osteotomy for reconstruction of kyphosis secondary to ankylosing spondylitis. Acceptable complication rates have been achieved through meticulous operative planning. Local anesthesia is used to permit continuous monitoring of neurologic function. The author relates a wealth of information derived from a personal series of 67 osteotomies of the cervical spine and 57 osteotomies of the lumbar spine.

Simmons, E.H., and Jackson, R.P.: The management of

nerve root entrapment syndromes associated with the collapsing scoliosis of idiopathic lumbar and thoracolumbar curves. Spine 4:533–541, 1979.

The treatment of neural compression associated with adult scoliosis in 30 patients is described. Root entrapment in the sciatic distribution was most common and arose on the side opposite the major curve, coming from the concavity of compensatory lumbosacral curves. Root entrapment in a femoral nerve distribution came from the concavity of the major curve. The mechanisms of compression were neuroforaminal stenosis and pedicular kinking. Anterior Dwyer instrumentation was the most effective method of surgical correction and required involvement of fewer vertebral levels in the fusion compared to posterior instrumentation techniques.

Tamaki, T.; Noguchi, T.; Takano, H.; Tsuji, H.; Nakagawa, T.; Imai, K.; and Inoue, S.: Spinal cord monitoring as a clinical utilization of the spinal evoked potential. Clin. Orthop. 184:58–64, 1984.

"Invasive" intraoperative spinal cord monitoring was performed on 229 patients in Japan. Recording electrodes were placed in the subarachnoid space at the level of the conus medullaris, and stimuli were delivered to the rostral spinal cord at the thoracic epidural space. Simultaneous monitoring of evoked potentials revealed that this method was more sensitive than the wake-up test.

Weinstein, S.L., and Ponseti, I.V.: Curve progression in idiopathic scoliosis. J. Bone Joint Surg. 65A:447–455, 1983.

A classic study of the natural history of idiopathic scoliosis with long-term follow-up of patients into adulthood.

Post-Traumatic Kyphosis and Incomplete Paraplegia

Bohlman, H.H.; Freehafer, A.; and Dejak, J.: The results of treatment of acute injuries of the upper thoracic spine with paralysis. J. Bone Joint Surg. 67A:360–369, 1985.

The surgical technique of thoracotomy and transthoracic anterior spinal cord decompression for incomplete neurologic deficits is described. The same operative technique with exposure of the spinal cord is useful for treating infections, tumors, and post-traumatic incomplete paraplegia.

McAfee, P.C.; Bohlman, H.H.; and Yuan, H.A.: Anterior decompression of traumatic thoracolumbar fractures with incomplete neurological deficit using a retroperitoneal approach. J. Bone Joint Surg. 67A:89–104, 1985.

The operative technique for anterior decompression of the thecal sac from T-12 to L-4 via a retroperitoneal-extrathoracic approach is described. The exposure is used for anterior decompression for neoplasms, infections, and fractures with incomplete paralysis.

Micheli, L.J., and Hood, R.W.: Anterior exposure of the cervicothoracic spine using a combined cervical and thoracic approach. J. Bone Joint Surg. 65A:992–997, 1983.

Four cases are described in which a combined anterior cervical and transthoracic approach for good exposure was of benefit in the treatment of cervicothoracic and upper thoracic kyphotic disorders.

Pang, D., and Wilberger, J.E., Jr.: Tethered cord syndrome in adults. J. Neurosurg. 57:32–47, 1982.

Although usually symptomatic during the growth spurt, tethered cord syndrome was found in 23 adult patients due to trauma to the lumbar area, narrowing of the spinal cord, or additional tugging of an already tight conus. Progressive sensorimotor deficits in the lower extremities as well as bladder and bowel dysfunction were common findings. Surgical treatment provided gratifying relief of pain and motor weakness but was disappointing in regard to resolution of bowel and bladder dysfunction.

Roberson, J.R., and Whitesides, T.E., Jr.: Surgical reconstruction of late post-traumatic thoracolumbar kyphosis. Spine 10:307–312, 1985.

Of 34 patients undergoing operation for late post-traumatic thoracolumbar kyphosis, 18 underwent anterior decompression. The postoperative neurologic status was unchanged in 13 and improved in 5 of these 18. The entire procedure, including opening and closing the chest, was done by the orthopaedist.

Transpedicular Approaches and Fixation

Michele, A.A., and Krueger, F.J.: Surgical approach to the vertebral body. J. Bone Joint Surg. 31A:873–878, 1949.

Recent enthusiasm for the transpedicular approach leaves the impression that it is a revolutionary "new" idea. This 40-year-old in-depth anatomic study describes the transpedicular approach to the thoracolumbar vertebral bodies.

Metastatic Tumors

Siegal, T.; Tiqva, P.; and Siegal, T.: Vertebral body resection for epidural compression by malignant tumors: Results of forty-seven consecutive operative procedures. J. Bone Joint Surg. 67A:375–382, 1985.

All patients in the series presented with neurologic deficit, and the indications for anterior decompression were neural relapse after radiation therapy, need for tissue diagnosis, presence of a radioresistant tumor, neurologic deterioration while receiving radiation therapy, and pathologic fractures. After anterior decompression and stabilization with methyl methacrylate, bone graft, anterior Harrington instrumentation, or combinations of these, 80% were able to walk, 18% were paraparetic, and 1 patient was still paraplegic. Normal urinary and bowel control were regained after 93% of the procedures.

Infections

Eismont, F.J.; Bohlman, H.H.; Soni, P.L.; Goldberg, V.M.; and Freehafer, A.A.: Pyogenic and fungal vertebral osteomyelitis with paralysis. J. Bone Joint Surg. 65A:19–29, 1983.

A retrospective review of 61 patients with vertebral osteomyelitis revealed that the associated diseases of diabetes mellitus and rheumatoid arthritis as well as increased age and a more cephalad level of infection predisposed to paralysis. For patients who had spinal cord compression, the results were best after treatment by anterior spinal decompression (thoracotomy or retroperitoneal approach) and stabilization. Costotransversectomy was useful for culture, biopsy, or drainage of a perispinal abscess in a severely debilitated patient who could not tolerate thoracotomy. Laminectomy was condemned because in nearly all cases the site of neural compression was anterior to the neural elements.

Thoracic Disk Herniation

Tsuyama, N.: Ossification of the posterior longitudinal ligament of the spine. Clin. Orthop. 184:71–84, 1984.

Although statistically more prevalent among Orientals and in the cervical spine, ossification of the posterior longitudinal ligament can cause myelopathy in the thoracolumbar spine and can affect non-Orientals. In a series of 207 patients with this condition, 42% were unable to walk without support. The ossification develops in four modes: 1) a *continuous* mass extending over several vertebrae, 2) *segmental* behind each vertebral body, 3) a *mixture* of types 1 and 2, and 4) *localized* or circumscribed.

28
Lumbar Spine

Back Pain

Epidemiology

People in the industrialized nations seek help for back pain in epidemic proportions. Up to 90% of the adult population eventually suffers from back problems, and as many as 25% of those 30 to 50 years of age report having back trouble. Back problems are the most common cause of disability during the most productive working years, severely affecting the lives of those disabled and of their families. Practitioners worldwide are attempting to prevent back injuries or to provide many varied and sometimes expensive treatment programs. Most attempts lack either a scientific basis or any evidence that they actually prevent back pain or disability.

In North America, back pain has become one of the most common and expensive health-care problems and is easily the most costly of orthopaedic ailments. In 1976 it was estimated that back problems cost more than $14 billion per year. More recently, costs were estimated to exceed $30 billion per year.

Disability

Most information about industrial job-related back problems is based on absenteeism data or insurance company reports. This information is retrospective and has been termed "potentially misleading." Back injury data concerning work factors, individual factors, and environmental factors have been found to be controversial at best. Industrial disability data do indicate that 2% of the industrial workers in the United States report back injury every year. However, 90% of back injuries account for only 20% of the back injury-related compensation costs. The 10% who recover slowest account for 80% of the costs and provide an obvious target for prevention efforts. Even if effective prevention methods were available, they would need to be administered to 1,000 workers with the hope of affecting the 2 workers who account for 80% of the back injury costs for that population.

Recent data indicate that our greatest opportunity to change the job-related back problem is to approach the prevention of chronic back disability by monitoring care to eliminate inappropriate treatment.

Prevention of Back Pain

Most attempts to curb back problems have aimed at prevention of injuries. These preventive approaches have included preemployment screenings (such as radiography of the lumbar spine or specialized testing) and educational programs to eliminate hazards to the back at the work site. To date, there is no scientific substantiation that back injury prevention is cost-effective because the cost of back problems continues to rise unimpaired.

Back pain prevention seems to be a formidable task for a number of reasons. First, few people escape back pain during adult life, raising the question as to whether back pain can be considered to be a "disease" rather than a naturally occurring process. Second, although there are many causes of back symptoms, 85% of the time we cannot verify the pathoanatomic cause and must term most problems "idiopathic." Third, back problems are common to all occupations, whether sedentary or requiring heavy use of the back; some data actually show that lumbar disk hernias are more common in sedentary workers than in those with more demanding jobs. Fourth, the onset of back problems is not commonly associated with an accident or unusual activity.

Fortunately, most patients recover rapidly, irrespective of treatment. Fifty percent to 60% of patients with back pain recover within 1 week. Even for the 2% to 3% of the population with sciatica, half recover within 1 month. For all types of back conditions, 90% of patients recover from their symptoms within a 3-month period. The major problem seems to lie in those 1 out of 10 who are disabled for 3 months or longer.

Pretreatment Considerations

Many problems of the lumbar spine and its surrounding structures, as well as general health problems, have been reported to cause back symptoms. Despite technical advances in medicine, the patient's history most often provides the best clues to ruling out or detecting a potential source of symptoms.

The patient's perception about the onset and location of symptoms, about how they interfere with activities and life-style, and about previous treatment commonly guide the work-up for disk hernia, stenosis, or instability as a potential cause of neural compromise or pain. When combined with the medical history, family history, and review of systems, the history is still the most sensitive means of detecting referred nonregional and systemic causes of back symptoms. In only 12% to 15% of the cases can a pathoanatomic diagnosis be verified as the cause of delayed recovery. From a physical standpoint, 85% of the time the diagnosis must be considered idiopathic, and a rapid recovery is expected.

Psychosocial factors can delay recovery from a back problem. Thus, questioning the patient about who is responsible for the present problem and what the patient wants and expects from treatment can help to detect the potential for using back pain as a solution to psychosocial problems. Such suspicions can be verified by the pain drawing, use of the Waddell tests for nonorganic causes of low back pain, and a search for inconsistencies on the physical examination. These tools can predict the response to treatment and alert one to the potential need for psychologic testing or consultation as a part of further work-up.

Treatment

The first step in preventing disability through use of acute treatment is to avoid unnecessary debilitation of the patient. Bed rest, commonly used in the treatment of back problems, is not without significant risks. Bed rest has been found to decrease bone density in the spine and may slow recovery because of the effect rest has on skeletal muscle. No data are available to indicate that more than a few days of bed rest is helpful in treating back problems.

Methods Proved Scientifically To Decrease Disability Until 1977, no treatment methods could scientifically claim to speed recovery or provide future protection from back problems. Then, Bergquist-Ullman and Larsson reported their experience with a prospective trial of three different treatment methods. At the Volvo plant in Gothenburg, Sweden, 210 consecutive employees claiming to have back problems that interfered with their ability to work were randomly selected for one of three treatment programs. The results indicated that teaching patients about their backs, including what to expect and how to stay active yet control mechanical stress on the back, returned people to work sooner than standard physical therapy or placebo treatment; standard physical therapy including manipulation was found to be no more effective than placebo treatment. Those who received the education program also received an evaluation of the work site by specially trained physical therapists prior to returning to work.

Many authors have produced variations of the Swedish Back School program. Some are complex and costly, involving as much as 15 hours of classroom time. The simpler programs seem better accepted by patients. There is no hard evidence that these programs can prevent or decrease the incidence of back pain. They aim to give the patient a basic understanding of back problems so that the patient will not be afraid of back pain in dealing with everyday situations. The Swedish Back School is the only program proved to be effective, and then only when combined with a return-to-work visit that customizes the information to the patient's livelihood. It has not been found effective alone or for patients with chronic problems.

In 1979, Cady et al. reported a prospective study indicating that fitness can provide future protection from back problems. The initial data found physical fitness, with heavy emphasis on cardiovascular endurance, to reduce the risk of back injury in firefighters. In a subsequent follow-up study, a cardiovascular fitness program was found to improve not only stamina and endurance but also test results for strength and flexibility. More important, workers compensation costs were 25% lower for firefighters who significantly increased their cardiovascular fitness without significantly increasing their strength and flexibility.

The combined therapeutic potential of these methods was reported in a recent study in a sector of Gothenburg, Sweden. A treatment program consisting of previously proved methods was provided for all individuals off work for 4 to 6 weeks because of back problems. This included the Swedish Back School program, fitness training emphasizing improvements of endurance through speed-walking, jogging, or cycling, a return-to-work evaluation by a physical therapist specially trained in ergonomics, and a judicious surgical work-up. As part of this program, local physicians were educated in the techniques being applied to their patients. This team approach utilizing an orthopaedic surgeon, an orthopaedic nurse, and a physical therapist reduced the long-term disability by 50%. It was estimated that in a countrywide program in Sweden, which has a population of about 8 million, this approach could save $15 million per year.

Thus, the application of three principles is now proved to prevent chronic back pain disability: 1) an education program tied to a return-to-work evaluation, 2) the judicious use of surgery, and 3) the use of cardiovascular endurance training as a means of restoration of physical condition. The cornerstone of the nonoperative treatment is an education program. Detailed information can be easily provided about what to expect from the back in the future and about the relationship between back symptoms and mechanical stress on the back as measured by intradisk pressure. Information about stress placed on the back by side lying (the intradisk pressure being 80% of the stress of standing) and sitting unassisted (140–180% of the interdisk pressure of standing) usually can provide patients with sufficient assurance to avoid the debilitating effects of bed rest and to remain active during convalescence. Furthermore, the education program can cover how to perform the activities of daily living while limiting the mechanical stress on the back. The major emphasis is usually on the mechanics of lifting and should simply stress the need to keep objects as close to the abdomen as possible and to avoid twisting or excessive bending to help control symptoms.

Unproved Treatments Drug therapy is a common adjunct to help control symptoms. There are three major categories of drugs in common use: anti-inflammatory medication, analgesics, and muscle relaxants. Anti-inflammatory agents are used because of the belief that inflammation contributes to pain production. Various anti-inflammatory agents are available. None is more effective than aspirin or plain acetaminophen, which are effective and inexpensive. If the response is not satisfactory, a nonsteroidal anti-inflammatory medication can be tried. All of these medications are utilized in conjunction with, but do not replace, control of the mechanical stress on the spine during early convalescence. In some cases, after an initial recovery a patient will experience intermittent recurrent attacks or complain of aching; in these cases, relief may be provided by maintenance doses of anti-inflammatory medication.

Analgesic medication may be very important in the acute phase. The goal is to help the patient get symptoms under control. Early control of symptoms with 30 to 60 mg of codeine is commonly recommended, although not scientifically verified. If strong medication is necessary, it should be used for only short periods. As the pain decreases, nonnarcotic analgesics should be substituted as soon as possible.

Muscle relaxants are not recommended. Generally, muscle spasm is secondary to primary back problems, and if the mechanical stress on the back can be controlled the muscle spasm will subside.

Traction The application of pelvic traction to the lumbar spine has been a popular treatment. The theory is that stretching the lumbar spine distracts the vertebrae so that the protruded disk is allowed to return to a more nearly normal position. It has been determined that a distraction force of 60% of the body weight is needed just to reduce the interdisk pressure at L-3 by 25%. Such forces cannot be applied practically. Clinically, double-blind studies on the effect of traction on patients with and without sciatica have not demonstrated any significant benefit. In a study of patients with herniated disks, for one group weights were used in the traction bags and for the other no weights were used. No statistically significant difference was found between the two groups in terms of relief of symptoms. Traction has been justified only to keep the patient in bed and to create a positive psychologic effect for expectation of recovery. Hospitalization is not necessary for administering traction; if chosen, it can be administered at home.

Manipulation Spinal manipulation is another modality used to treat low back problems. The principle involved is that malalignment of the spinal structures can be corrected by manipulation; the assumption is that malalignment is the cause of the patient's pain. Several clinical randomized trials to determine the efficacy of manipulation have shown that patients felt some immediate relief but did not have long-term benefit.

Spinal manipulation probably is not indicated for patients with acute radiculopathy. In such cases, there have been reports of manipulation leading to increased neurologic findings and paralysis.

Braces and Corsets External support of the lumbar spine with a corset or brace is indicated only for a short period at most, early during the patient's recovery. A properly fitted garment sometimes aids the patient in regaining mobility. As recovery progresses, the brace should be abandoned in favor of increasing the patient's activity and conditioning. There are two regimens that are commonly advocated: 1) isometric flexion exercises, and 2) hyperextension exercises. They are purported to reduce the frequency and intensity of low back pain episodes, although there has been no scientific evidence to support these contentions. The isometric flexion exercises are based on Williams' theory that, by reducing lumbar lordosis, back pain is decreased. Results of three controlled studies make this concept questionable.

Other Physical Therapy Modalities There are many other treatment modalities used for low back pain. These all are variations of heat, cold, or massage. They are well tolerated and pleasant. Most patients experience some immediate relief of symptoms but, unfortunately, no long-standing effect has ever been verified. There is no evidence that any of these regimens offers long-term benefits or adds to the efficacy of other treatment modalities. For most patients, a self-administered home program usually can be designed that is more convenient and expresses to the patient the relative importance of such a program in comparison to more-established methods.

Early Treatment Summary While injections, traction, bracing, forms of heat and cold, and various medications are advocated by some to help for a short time, their effectiveness in shortening the period of disability has not been proved. Such is also the case with joint manipulation, abdominal strengthening exercises, back stretching exercises, and the McKenzie extension exercise techniques. An epidemiologic study indicates that building back muscle endurance may be helpful in those asymptomatic enough to tolerate the activity.

The best information available indicates that cardiovascular fitness training seems to be the most important element in providing future protection and improving functional capacity. Walking, cycling, swimming, and even jogging have been demonstrated to be less stressful on the back than sitting, according to intradisk pressure measurements. The advantage that this approach has over the many unproved treatment methods is that it can be tolerated well by patients with back pain alone or with a significant component of sciatica. Endurance training to improve functional capacity and provide future protection from back problems is most strongly justified by prospective studies.

Timing of Surgical or Special Study Work-Up Fifty percent of patients recover from back pain in 7 days and from sciatica by 4 weeks. Thus, special studies and surgical work-up performed before 4 weeks are commonly obviated by the natural history for half of the patients, especially between the ages of 20 and 50 years. Patients under age 20 tend not to have idiopathic back pain and a firm diagnosis is possible in about 60% of these. Thus, earlier diagnostic work-up is easier to justify in younger patients (less than age 20) or older ones (more than age 50) when the incidence of tumor and infection begins to increase.

In the middle group, even radiologic examination can easily be delayed for 1 month because only once in every 2,500 sets of lumbosacral spine radiographs is something found that was not suspected from the history and physical findings.

Patients who have had 4 weeks of controlled activity and medication but continue to have difficulty functioning are those who defy the natural history of the disease as experienced by more than 50% of patients. If pain persists, one must consider a work-up to seek anatomic, physiologic, and psychosocial reasons for the delay of recovery. Conservative management for sciatica and radiculopathy is similar to that for general back problems but natural history data indicate that progress is slower when these are limb problems.

Acute Lumbar Radicular Syndromes

Over the course of the past 4 years, a tremendous amount of work has been focused on the lumbar spine. Many physicians are interested in acute lumbar radicular syndromes because they offer a high potential for use of invasive therapeutic procedures.

This section deals with the diagnosis and treatment of acute lumbar radiculopathies. Definition of these conditions and the history, physical examination, and diagnostic tests necessary to identify them will be discussed first. Then, an approach to the evaluation and treatment of radiculopathies will be presented in a standardized protocol format. Controversial or new material will be interjected where appropriate.

Definition of Lumbar Radicular Syndrome

Radicular pain can be defined as that caused by compression of an inflamed nerve root along its anatomic course. In the lumbar spine this most frequently occurs at the L-5 and S-1 nerve roots, resulting in pain, numbness, and tingling distal to the knee. The most common cause of compression of a nerve root in the under-40 age group is a herniated nucleus pulposus.

A herniated disk can be defined as herniation of the nucleus pulposus through the fibers of the anulus fibrosus. The perforations usually arise through a defect just lateral to the posterior midline, where the posterior longitudinal ligament is weakest.

Disk herniations at L5-S1 will usually compromise the S-1 nerve root; herniation at the L4-5 level most often affects the L-5 nerve root. Variations in nerve root configuration (double roots) as well as in the position of the herniation itself can modify these relationships. An L4-5 disk rupture at times can affect the S-1 as well as the L-5 nerve root, and in extreme lateral herniations the nerve exiting at the same level as the disk will be involved.

Not every patient with a disk herniation has significant discomfort. Although a large herniation in a capacious spinal canal may not be apparent clinically (because there is no compression of the neural elements), a minor protrusion in a small canal may be crippling (because there is not enough room to accommodate both the disk and the nerve root).

Infrequently, a disk herniation can occur high in the lumbar canal at L2-3 and L3-4 but this is uncommon. With a "high" disk the pain will not radiate below the knee and must be differentiated from referred pain. Referred pain can be defined as pain in mesodermal tissues of the same embryologic origin. The muscles, tendons, and ligaments of the buttocks and posterior thighs have the same embryologic origin as those of the low back. Therefore, a local injury (strain) to the low back with referral to the thigh can be confused with symptoms from a high disk.

In patients over 40 years of age, the spinal canal normally becomes smaller. Degeneration of both the facet joints and the intervertebral disks leads to narrowing. The canal is rimmed by large osteophytes that develop as a result of the excessive load on the intervertebral disks. The facets are hypertrophic, and the ligamentum flavum becomes redundant. These combined changes in the spinal canal and neural foramina result in decreased volume which, if severe enough, causes direct mechanical pressure on the neural elements, resulting in a radiculopathy. This process is referred to as spinal stenosis and is covered in another section.

History, Physical Examination, and Diagnostic Tests

History Pain, numbness, and tingling in the involved leg are the most common symptoms of an acute lumbar radiculopathy. The pain will radiate in the distribution of the affected nerve root, usually will be described by the patient as sharp or lancinating, and will progress from proximal to distal in the involved leg. The onset may be insidious or sudden and may be associated with a tearing or snapping sensation in the low back. In some instances when sciatica develops, the back pain may markedly decrease because once the annulus has ruptured it is no longer under tension. The intensity of the leg pain can vary: it may be so severe that the patient will be unable to ambulate and will feel his back "locked," or the discomfort may be limited to a dull ache that increases in intensity with ambulation.

Physical Examination On physical examination, the back generally will show a decreased range of motion, with the patient leaning to one side. On ambulation, the patient will walk with the involved leg flexed so as to put the least possible pressure on the extremity.

The neurologic examination may yield objective evidence of nerve root compression. When the S-1 nerve root is compressed, the patient can have gastrocnemius/soleus weakness. The Achilles reflex often is diminished or absent, and atrophy of the calf may be apparent. Sensory loss is confined to the posterior aspect of the calf or lateral side of the foot.

Compression of the L-5 nerve root may lead to weakness in extension of the great toe and, less often, to weakness of the everters and dorsiflexors of the foot. The sensory deficit may occur over the anterior tibia and the dorsomedial aspect of the foot down to the great toe. Primary reflex changes are uncommon, but sometimes a change in the posterior tibial reflex can be elicited. The absence of this reflex, however, must be asymmetric for it to have any clinical significance.

Involvement of the L-4 nerve root may lead to quadriceps weakness. This can present as weakness of knee extension or the complaint of an unstable knee. Atrophy of the thigh musculature can be marked, and the sensory loss will be over the anteromedial aspect of the thigh. The patellar tendon reflex is affected.

One must remember that there may be no objective neurologic findings because the involved nerve often remains functional. In addition, a neurologic deficit may have little temporal relevance because it may relate to a prior attack at a different level. To be significant, reflex changes, weakness, atrophy, or sensory loss must conform to the rest of the clinical picture.

Nerve root sensitivity can be elicited by any method that creates tension on the nerve (tension sign). The straight leg raising test in either the sitting or lying position is the one most commonly used (Fig. 1 *A* and *B*). This test is considered positive when the patient's radicular symptoms are reproduced; the production of back pain does not indicate a positive test. For example, when the S-1 or L-5 nerve root is involved, a straight leg raising test should reproduce pain below the knee and possibly down into the foot to be positive. The contralateral straight leg raising test is the most specific of the tension signs. It is performed by extending the uninvolved leg and is positive when leg pain is produced in the symptomatic leg. For "high" disks (L2-

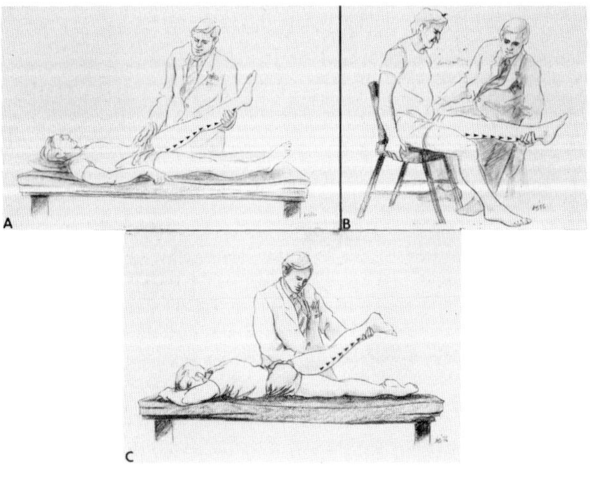

Figure 1

Leg raising tests. *A* and *B*, Straight leg raising test in supine or sitting position. *C*, Reverse straight leg raising test; patient is in prone position.

3 and L3-4), the reverse straight leg raising test may be positive. This is performed with the patient prone and, again, is positive when leg pain is reproduced (Fig. 1 *C*).

Diagnostic Tests In general, diagnostic tests should be used to confirm the information gathered from a thorough history and physical examination. To appreciate the true value of any diagnostic test, one must know its specificity (false-positives) and sensitivity (false-negatives). Each test has a particular role in the temporal sequence of making a diagnosis. None of the tests discussed below should be used for general screening because most of them are overly sensitive and relatively unselective. A great many of the iatrogenic disasters in the management of acute lumbar radiculopathies can be attributed directly to overreliance on diagnostic findings with no positive clinical correlation.

Plain Radiographs In most cases the diagnosis of a herniated disk can be made on the basis of the history and physical examination. Plain radiographs of the lumbosacral spine usually will not add any information but must be obtained to rule out other pathologic conditions such as infection or tumor.

Computed Tomography Computed tomography (CT) has become quite useful for evaluating abnormalities of the lumbosacral spine. It creates cross-sectional images of the spine at various levels and, with reformatting, one also can obtain coronal and sagittal sections. The CT scan assesses not only the bony configuration but also the soft tissue in graded shadings, so that ligaments, nerve roots, free fat, and intervertebral disk protrusions can be evaluated as they relate to their bony environment.

The CT scan can be an extremely valuable diagnostic tool if used appropriately to confirm clinical findings derived from the history and physical examination. It is important to understand that the scan should be used for confirmation, not for primary diagnosis. Recent studies reveal the potential pitfalls of making clinical decisions on CT scan findings isolated from the patient's complete clinical picture.

CT scans of the lumbar area of 53 normal subjects with no history of back trouble were submitted to three expert interpreters. Of the scans reviewed, 34% were read as abnormal, but there was agreement among the interpreters in only 11% of the cases. The implication is that a patient with a history and physical findings not indicative of a spinal lesion has a 1-in-3 chance of having an abnormal CT scan. If a major therapeutic decision (i.e., to operate) is made based only on the scan results, there is a 30% chance that the patient will undergo an unnecessary operation. However, if the patient's history and clinical findings are indicative of spine pathology, the CT scan frequently can be a helpful confirming diagnostic tool.

Myelography Myelography is the established method for evaluating neural compression when an invasive spinal procedure is contemplated. At this time, metrizamide, a water-soluble dye, is the contrast agent of choice but better contrast materials such as iohexol soon will be available. The newer agents are reported to have fewer side effects such as seizures and nausea and vomiting.

The myelogram, like the CT scan, should be used as a confirmatory study. An abnormal myelogram without substantiating history and physical findings is not meaningful. It is known that 24% of asymptomatic people will have an abnormal myelogram (iophendylate [Pantopaque] contrast). The trained spine surgeon usually reserves the myelogram for preoperative assurance—to confirm the location of the damaged disk or to check for a congenitally anomalous nerve root, tumor, or double disk. If the myelogram is used as a "screening test" in the absence of objective clinical findings, exploratory surgery and disaster are the frequent results. Patients who undergo myelography without positive physical findings (tension sign or neurologic finding) are reported to have a significantly higher chance of side effects from the procedure itself (nausea, vomiting, or increased back pain).

A particular advantage of the myelogram is that it can evaluate the lower thoracic spine. Intradural extramedullary tumors in the lower thoracic area can present as acute radiculopathies. When an appropriate lesion is not found in the lumbosacral area, the lower thoracic spine should be scrutinized for the presence of an occult spinal tumor.

Finally, the metrizamide myelogram compares favorably with the CT scan in blind diagnosis of herniated lumbar disks. A group of patients with surgically confirmed herniated lumbar disks underwent both preoperative metrizamide myelography and CT. Each test was then evaluated blindly by a neuroradiologist. Myelography was more accurate than CT—83% versus 72%.

Electromyography The electromyogram (EMG) determines if the nerve supply to the involved muscles is intact. An abnormal EMG can demonstrate impaired nerve transmission to a specific muscle and isolate the nerve root involved. After 21 days of significant pressure on a nerve root, signs of denervation with fibrillation can be observed in the EMG.

The EMG is not a screening tool. In the evaluation of the average low back problem, it rarely provides any information that cannot be derived from careful physical examination (with much less trouble and cost). It may even confuse the picture because an EMG may be abnormal from other causes such as diabetes, previous peripheral nerve involvement, or trauma.

Thermography Thermography records changes in skin temperature; areas that are "hotter" than normal are believed to represent locations of increased pain. The exact role of the thermogram in the diagnosis of low back problems is not yet clear. The prospective studies performed to date have demonstrated no diagnostic value for thermography in cases of back and leg pain (these studies included patients with acute lumbar radicular syndromes as well as those with back pain alone).

Interpretation of thermograms should be standardized. Prospective studies must be conducted to correlate the findings of thermography with those of myelography and CT scans. The specificity and sensitivity of the thermogram need further definition. A number of such investigations are now under way; when the results are available, the value and role of thermography will be clarified, but at present its usefulness is in question.

Magnetic Resonance Imaging Magnetic resonance imaging (MRI) is now coming into general use as a diagnostic tool. The image is obtained by evaluation of the differences in proton density of the tissues studied. This approach is noninvasive—in contrast to CT scans and myelography—because it uses no ionizing radiation or contrast agents and can provide direct multiplanar images.

MRI technology for the lumbar spine is still being developed. Large clinical studies are under way to evaluate the specificity and sensitivity of this test. It holds great promise as an imaging method because of its high theoretical limits in image detail and its very low attendant risks. As the technology advances and more clinical experience is accumulated, the true place of MRI in the diagnostic arsenal will be established.

Treatment Protocol

This treatment protocol is organized into the format of an algorithm (Fig. 2). Webster's dictionary defines an algorithm as "a set of rules for solving a particular problem in a finite number of steps." The algorithm is an organized pattern of decision-making and thought processes that have proved useful in caring for patients with acute lumbar radicular syndromes. It has been expanded for the entire spectrum of problems in the lumbar spine.

The primary objective for the physician is to return the patient to his regular activity as quickly as possible. In achieving this goal he must be concerned with making efficient and precise use of diagnostic studies, avoiding ineffectual surgical procedures, and making therapy available at a reasonable cost to the patient and to society. The algorithm follows well-delineated rules established as the consensus of a broad segment of qualified spine surgeons. It allows the patient to receive the most helpful diagnostic and therapeutic measures at optimal times. For example, not every patient who presents with clinical findings of a herniated disk requires a CT scan; only after initial treatment fails is this study appropriate. The algorithm outlines the *appropriate* diagnostic studies and treatment at the *appropriate* time.

Cauda Equina Compression The protocol begins with the universe of patients who present with signs and symptoms of an acute lumbar radiculopathy. They will have undergone an initial evaluation—medical history and physical examination—with resultant demonstration of appropriate findings. The first major decision is to rule in or out the presence of cauda equina compression syndrome. Significant compression of the cauda equina or truly progressive motor weakness is the only major surgical emergency to be found in patients with an acute radiculopathy.

The compression usually is due to extrinsic pressure on the caudal sac by a massive, centrally herniated disk. The symptom complex includes low back pain, bilateral motor weakness of the lower extremities, bilateral sciatica, saddle anesthesia, and even frank paraplegia with bowel and bladder incontinence.

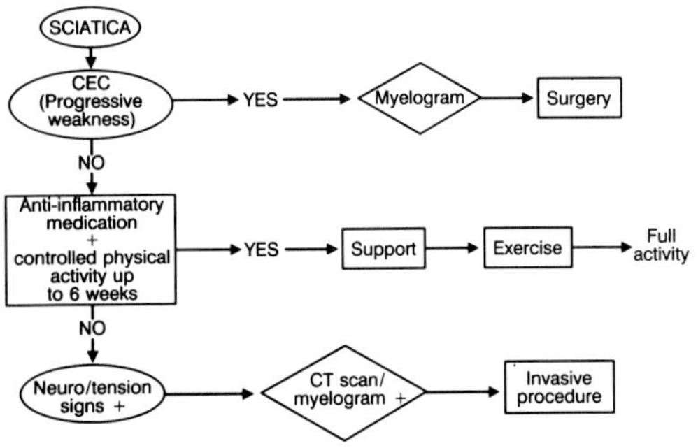

Figure 2
Algorithm for treatment of lumbar radicular syndromes.

Once this diagnosis is suspected, the patient should undergo myelography immediately and, if it is positive, emergency surgical decompression. The major need for prompt surgical intervention is to arrest the progression of neurologic loss; the chance of actual return of neurologic function after operation is slight. Although the incidence of cauda equina compression syndrome in the total population of patients with acute radiculopathies is very low, it is the only entity that requires immediate operative intervention.

Conservative Care The remaining patients should be started on a course of conservative therapy. Some of them will need an invasive procedure, but at this stage there is no way to predict which individuals will respond to conservative therapy and which will not.

The early treatment of an acute radiculopathy is a waiting game. The passage of time, the use of anti-inflammatory medication, and bed rest are the modalities that have proved safest and most effective. The vast majority of these patients will respond to this approach. With today's emphasis on quick solutions, many patients are pushed too rapidly toward more complex (i.e., invasive) treatment. This "quick fix" has no place in the treatment of patients with acute radiculopathy. In most cases, surgical treatment does not return people to heavy work and, in the long run, the best chance of getting a patient back to full activity is the nonoperative approach. Traction, braces and corsets, exercises, and physical therapy have limited roles in the management of acute radiculopathy.

Rest (Controlled Physical Activity) Over the years, rest has evolved as one of the most important elements in the treatment of lumbar radiculopathies. The purpose of rest is to allow any inflammatory reaction that is present to subside. The relief achieved may or may not be permanent. The amount of rest prescribed varies for each patient.

When patients first present with acute symptoms they may require a short period of bed rest—2 to 7 days. As their symptoms are relieved, the patients are strongly encouraged to take short walks but to do as little sitting as possible. As time passes, each patient's physical activity is tailored to increase movement without incurring return of symptoms. Complete bed rest for long periods (more than 2 weeks) has a deleterious effect on the body in general and should be monitored closely. Thus, the physician must strictly control the patient's physical activity during the course of treatment. Methods of conservative management for sciatica are similar to those for back pain but response is slower.

Drug Therapy Drug therapy is an adjunct to controlled physical activity. There are three major categories of drugs in common use: anti-inflammatory agents, analgesics, and muscle relaxants. If the inflammation can be relieved, the patient's pain usually will subside.

Various anti-inflammatory agents are available. None appears to be superior on the basis of scientific studies. The patient should be started on adequate doses of aspirin which is effective and inexpensive. If the response is not satisfactory, other anti-inflammatory agents such as naproxen (Naprosyn), ibuprofen (Motrin), or indomethacin

(Indocin) can be tried. All of these medications are utilized in conjunction with rest for acute pain; they do not *replace* adequate rest. In some cases, after an initial recovery a patient will experience intermittent recurrent attacks or complain of chronic low backache; in these cases, many will be relieved by a maintenance dose of an anti-inflammatory drug.

Invasive Procedures At this juncture, the patients have had up to 6 weeks of rest and medication. If pain persists, one must consider some type of invasive procedure.

Epidural Injections If leg pain persists, one may consider epidural injections of steroids, which can be done on an outpatient basis. Theory holds that anti-inflammatory medication (steroids) placed directly into the epidural space will be more effective than oral medication in reducing inflammation. However, a recent double-blind study has shown that use of steroids plus procaine (Novocain) worked no better than procaine alone in relieving symptoms: in both study groups, 40% of the population had a significant decrease in symptoms. Nevertheless, an epidural injection is worth trying; the chance of success is 40% and the morbidity is relatively low, particularly compared with either of the next steps—chemonucleolytic injection or operation.

If the injection is effective in alleviating the patient's leg pain, a program of exercises is begun and the patient is encouraged to return to as normal a life-style as possible. In most cases, heavy work (lifting more than 25 kg repetitively) is not recommended because these patients will be prone to recurrences. This treatment regimen usually will be complete in less than 3 months. The majority of patients with an acute radiculopathy will respond and not have to undergo any major invasive treatment.

Should epidural injections prove ineffectual, some more potent type of invasive treatment should be considered. The patient group then is divided into those with probable herniated disks and those with symptoms secondary to pressure on the neural elements by bone.

The physician must carefully reevaluate the patient for a neurologic deficit and a positive tension sign. For those patients with either, a metrizamide myelogram should be considered. If the myelogram is positive and is consistent with the physical findings, an invasive procedure is a viable option. The CT scan also is helpful and in some instances, if clearly positive, can replace the myelogram. If all criteria are present, and an invasive procedure is indicated, the choice must be made between the use of chemonucleolysis and surgical removal of the herniated disk.

Chemonucleolysis This is the injection of an enzyme (chymopapain) into the nucleus pulposus to dissolve it and thus relieve the pressure on the neural elements. It has been in use for several years. The actual technique has been refined, and the current recommendation is to perform it under local anesthesia without diskography. Skin testing for allergy should be done. The indications for chemonucleolysis are the same as those for operation; this procedure should not be done by anyone who does not perform routine spine surgery such as laminectomy for a herniated disk. Chemonucleolysis is not indicated when a bony lesion is present or in the patient who has undergone multiple operations.

Results of chemonucleolysis have been controversial. Surgical treatment for an acute soft herniated disk will give good to excellent results in 90% to 95% of cases. In a recent prospective double-blind study, 77% of patients treated with chymopapain were assessed as moderately improved compared with 47% of saline-treated patients. Thus, chymopapain appears to give better results than a placebo, but compared with surgical treatment its effectiveness and safety are still unresolved and its results do not seem as good. The exact indications for chemonucleolysis are not clear, and questions remain about its safety. Its role will not be determined until more surgeons gain experience using it and adequate research is done.

There is no question that the use of chemonucleolysis should be approached with the same seriousness as operation. The complications can be grave (paralysis and death), and the technique is challenging. One of the more serious errors is failure to meet the strict criteria for its use: leg pain, a positive tension sign or neurologic deficit, and a positive contrast study. In other words, the indications for its use should be the same as those for a major surgical procedure.

Surgical Treatment Operation has proved to be safe and efficient in treating patients who have herniated disks. There is consistent documentation that, for surgical treatment to be effective, the surgeon must find unequivocal operative evidence of nerve root compression. This mechanical nerve root compression must be firmly substantiated, not only by neurologic examination but also by radiographic data before the laminectomy. There is no place for "exploratory" back surgery. If the patient has neither a neurologic deficit nor a positive straight leg raising test, then regardless of radiographic findings there is not enough evidence of nerve root compression to proceed with surgery. Twenty-five percent of asymptomatic patients have positive myelograms, and 35% have positive CT scans. Patients without objective findings have poor results from surgery. Those who meet these criteria for lumbar laminectomy will have a satisfactory outcome: 95% of them can expect good to excellent results.

The technique for performing a laminectomy for an acute herniated disk has been well described. The essential steps are gaining access to the epidural space without injuring the neural elements and then extending the exposure laterally so that the edge of the nerve root is visualized before it is retracted (Fig. 3). There should be no blind probing to find the nerve root; this can lead to injury and subsequent symptoms. In performing a laminectomy the surgeon should use a headlight and as much magnification as is necessary for him to see clearly. High-powered loupes (greater than 3.5 magnification) or a microscope generally is not required.

At the conclusion of a laminectomy, the surgeon should have excised bone or soft tissue as necessary to remove all extrinsic pressure on the neural elements. The surgical details must be tailored to the individual patient, depending on the local anatomy and pathology.

For routine removal of a disk, no form of fusion is indicated (including posterior lumbar interbody fusion). Fusion is only necessary if there are objective signs of instability as described for lumbar spinal segment instability.

Chronic Lumbar Radicular Syndromes

Management of the patient who has had multiple unsuccessful lumbar spine operations continues to challenge the

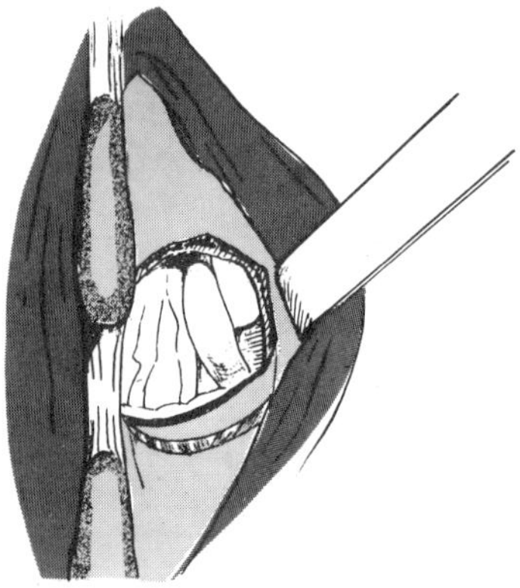

Figure 3

Approach for laminectomy. Exposure should extend to permit visualization of lateral edge of nerve root.

orthopaedist. Several investigators have shown that the primary cause for such "low back loser" patients revolves around the selection criteria for the initial surgical procedure (Fig. 4). Although prevention is the ideal long-term solution to this complex problem, treatment for the established condition is still required because of the current magnitude of the problem. Indeed, authors of recent publications have provided a ray of optimism by suggesting that intensive, disciplined, conditioning programs may entice nearly 80% of these patients to resume productivity. Nearly all orthopaedists, regardless of subspecialty, continue to see patients who suffer from chronic musculoskeletal pain. Thus, the pitfalls inherent in the assessment and management of these patients must be recognized to lessen the likelihood for inappropriate treatment.

Most authors accept the definition of chronic pain as the concept of a "disabling pain syndrome, present for at least 6 months, that has not responded to traditional treatment approaches. . . ." The important feature of this definition is the disabling nature of the pain complaint, thereby excluding those patients who have long-term "chronic" complaints but have noted no significant alteration in the quality of their life or in their vocational productivity. The discussion in this section will focus on chronic benign pain complaints, intentionally excluding the management of chronic pain resulting from malignancies or demyelination of the central nervous system.

Chronic pain must be clearly differentiated from acute pain because nearly all treatments that are effective in patients who suffer from acute pain are contraindicated in patients who experience chronic pain. Chronic benign pain may be viewed more appropriately as "pain behavior" because the usual biomedical model of pain does not accurately describe the clinical observations of patients who suffer from chronic benign pain. Pain behavior represents a compilation of nociception (tissue damage), depression, anxiety, and other factors that interact to produce the manner in which the patient behaves in the clinical environment (e.g., office or hospital). Thus, in chronic pain patients, the severity of pain behavior (e.g., grimacing, crying, demanding narcotics) does not correlate with the degree of tissue damage (Fig. 5). Because many factors determine pain behavior, a thorough assessment of these patients must be implemented, including a thorough psychosocial evaluation.

Diagnosis

Previous medical records, including the description of any surgical procedures, should be reviewed prior to formulating any additional assessment or treatment strategies. Interview features that may assist in identifying chronicity include: pain over a wide area of the body; deeper, more central pain; high level of anxiety; and a low activity level.

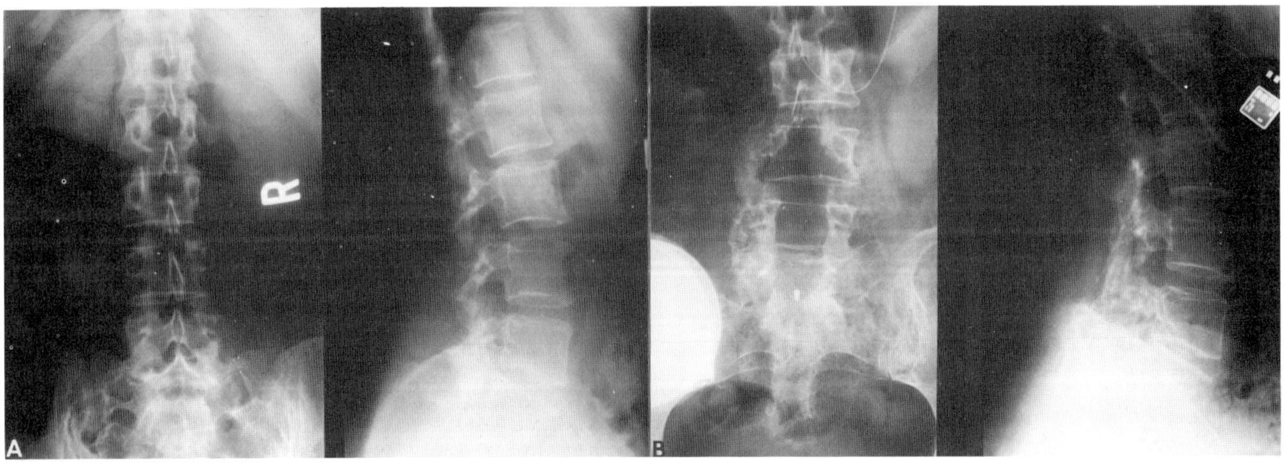

Figure 4

A, Anteroposterior and lateral radiographs of the lumbosacral spine of a 45-year-old woman prior to operative intervention. The indications for the subsequent surgical procedures were elusive. *B*, Anteroposterior and lateral radiographs of same patient as in *A*, 5 years later, after numerous surgical procedures. Use of an electrical stimulating device is also apparent. Osteopenia of the spine, secondary to disuse and multiple interventions, is now evident. In spite of all these aggressive attempts to minimize pain, the patient is even worse off compared with her preoperative status. Selection criteria remain of paramount importance in the proper selection of patients for lumbar spine surgery.

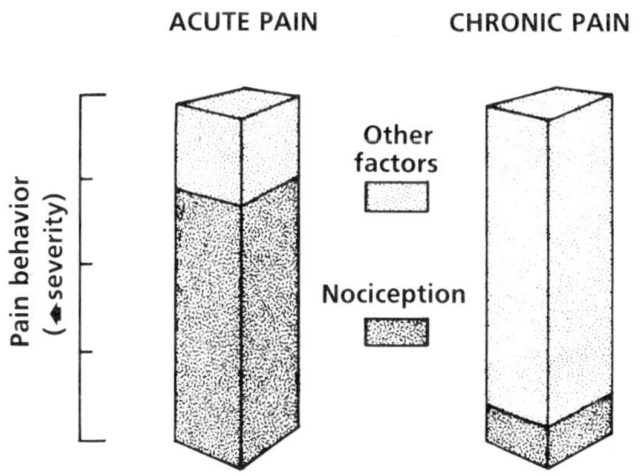

Figure 5

Diagram depicting the relative contributions of nociception to acute pain and to chronic pain.

In addition, a careful and complete assessment of medications used is important because the majority of chronic pain patients develop a dependency on narcotics or tranquilizers. The pain-free interval after each surgical procedure should be recorded. Pain-free intervals of less than 1 year suggest that the procedure was not appropriate (e.g., wrong level, wrong diagnosis) or that the patient did not meet the appropriate criteria for the procedure chosen (e.g., symptom amplification, disincentives).

The usual thorough physical examination must be performed. Recent modifications in the examination should be incorporated in the evaluation of patients suffering from acute or chronic low back pain. When inappropriate physical findings are identified, traditional management strategies are unlikely to succeed (Table 1). Gait assessment will also provide insight in cases of low back pain. Patients who have received disability payments or ingested narcotics develop nonorganic gait patterns that are significantly different from those of patients with organic disorders.

Psychologic assessment is useful in the evaluation of any patient who is not improving rapidly on an accepted nonoperative treatment protocol. The assessment of psychologic factors is imperative in a patient who suffers from chronic low back pain or has undergone one lumbar spine procedure. Nonresponders to lumbar spine surgery have been found to be much more psychiatrically disturbed and socially disabled than are responders. Other authors have reported that disabled patients with low back pain formed a distinctive subgroup characterized by significant elevations of hypochondriasis and hysteria scores on the MMPI. An appropriate psychologic assessment of such patients would include a pain drawing (Fig. 6), MMPI objective method for the assessment of depression (e.g., Beck inventory, Zung scale), and consultation with a clinical psychologist or psychiatrist interested and knowledgeable in the management of chronic pain.

Electrodiagnostic studies provide useful information in the assessment of patients who report recalcitrant low back pain. The standard EMG identifies approximately 70% of patients who have a herniated lumbar disk and approximately 80% of patients who have proved lumbar spinal stenosis. The EMG also aids in preoperative planning for surgical intervention.

No consistent evidence exists to suggest that low back pain patients have increased paraspinal EMG activity. Therefore, any treatment based on such a hypothesis remains experimental. Likewise, no diagnostic subgroup of low back pain patients produces a single unique pattern of EMG signal. Thus, the hypothesis of a relationship between the strength of paraspinous muscle contractions and the reported intensity of chronic low back pain remains unverified.

Dermatomal somatosensory evoked potentials (DSSEP) have remained controversial as a means of selecting patients for lumbar spine surgery. Authors have both recommended and challenged the validity of these evoked potential techniques.

Additional assessment of patients may include the bone scan, CT scan, myelogram, and MRI. These studies have been discussed in the section on acute lumbar radicular syndromes. Only the features that differ from the prior discussion will be presented. The bone scan is useful in the overall evaluation of patients who report chronic back

Table 1. Nonorganic Physical Signs in Low Back Pain

Category	Test	Comment
Tenderness	Superficial palpation	Inordinate, widespread sensitivity to light touch of the superficial soft tissues over the lumbar spine is nonanatomic and suggests amplified symptoms
	Nonanatomic testing	Tenderness is poorly localized
Simulation (to assess patient cooperation and reliability)	Axial loading	Light pressure to the skull of standing patient should not significantly increase symptoms
	Rotation	Physician should rotate the standing patient's pelvis and shoulders in the same plane—this does not move the lumbar spine and should not increase pain
Distraction	Straight leg raising	Physician asks the seated patient to straighten the knee—patients with true sciatic tension will arch backward and complain; these results should closely match those of the traditional, recumbent straight leg raising test
Regional		Diffuse motor weakness or bizarre sensory deficits suggest functional regional disturbances if they involve multiple muscle groups and cannot be explained by neuroanatomy principles
Overreaction		Excessive and inappropriate grimacing, groaning, or collapse during a simple request is disproportionate

Adapted from Waddell, G.; McCulloch, J.A.; Kummel, E.; and Venner, R.M.; Nonorganic physical signs in low-back pain. Spine 5:117–125, 1980.

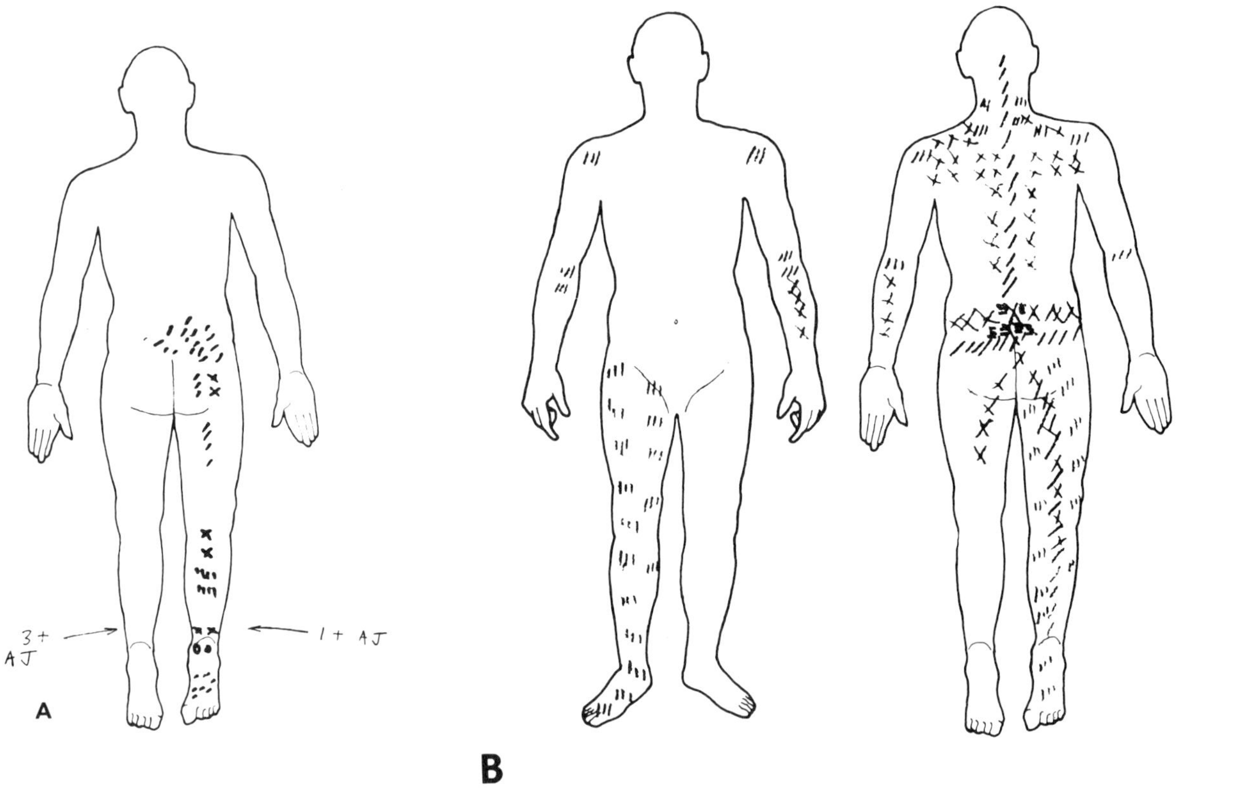

Figure 6

Pain drawings. *A*, By patient who had a clear-cut herniated disk at L5–SI on the right. Note the precise anatomic distribution of the symbols. *B*, By a 52-year-old man who had undergone one lumbar disk procedure without relief. Note the nonanatomic distribution of the pain and the endorsement of multiple symbols. This drawing correlated very well with results of more formal psychologic evaluations of the patient. Additional surgical intervention was not indicated because no objective findings were discovered. Although the pain drawing does not rule out organic processes, important psychologic factors can be identified more easily with this technique.

complaints because unsuspected pathologic processes will be discovered in approximately 2% of patients (Fig. 7). CT after lumbar myelography changed the diagnosis in 7% of 214 patients who complained of back and lower extremity symptoms. Important additional information was also provided in an additional 12% of these patients. Lumbar myelography with metrizamide remains the established standard for the complete assessment of the neural elements and vertebral canal. Iohexol, a new contrast agent for myelography, causes fewer adverse reactions than metrizamide. Extended clinical trials of iohexol are in progress. Flexion-extension views during myelography have been recommended to identify associated lateral recess stenosis in patients with lumbar disk herniations. MRI is a newer, noninvasive imaging technique that can identify lumbar disk herniations and spinal stenosis. This technique also is extremely useful in evaluating intramedullary spinal cord lesions such as syringohydromyelia and cystic tumors. Further controlled studies of this extremely sensitive technique are needed to define the true clinical value of MRI.

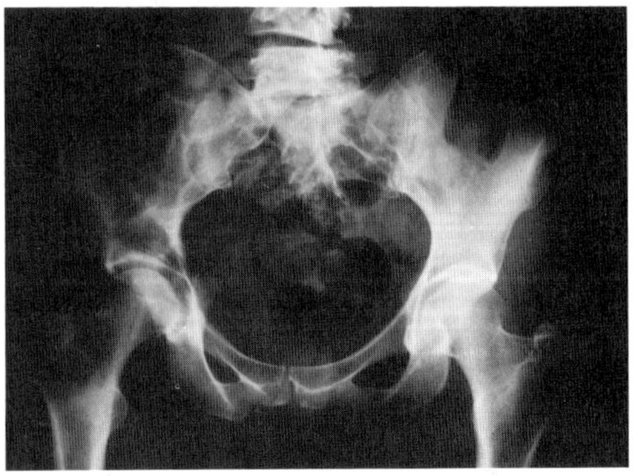

Figure 7

Anteroposterior view of the pelvis in a 50-year-old man who underwent lumbar discectomy and decompression for "pain" in the buttocks and greater trochanteric region. Note the large lytic area in the proximal femur on the left side. Careful assessment of individuals with chronic complaints is essential to identify occult metastasis properly. Many patients will exhibit degenerative changes of the spine. Therefore, the astute observer must continue to search for causes of discomfort other than the usual degenerative changes.

Treatment

The vast majority (>95%) of patients who suffer from chronic benign pain syndromes are not candidates for surgical intervention. Before recommending operation, the surgeon must identify a specific pathologic process that appears to be contributing significantly to the patient's pain behavior. The most common indications for "salvage" spine surgery include: recurrent disk herniation, segmental instability, progressive deformity, central and lateral spinal stenosis, and a combination of these processes. The complaint of pain alone without one of these specific causes should be treated with strategies other than surgical.

Most patients with chronic benign pain syndromes are best managed through a program that emphasizes behavior modification and conditioning. In two separate studies, 58% and 80% of the patients were returned to productivity. The factors believed to account for the chronicity of the low back pain included deconditioning, fear, and poor biomechanics.

Although the concept of Back School has been shown to be effective in acute and subacute low back pain episodes, no benefits accrued to patients with chronic low back pain who were evaluated in a prospective, controlled study. The patients were all followed for 1 year after being involved in the Swedish Back School program.

Many other treatment regimens have been purported to be successful in managing patients who suffer from chronic low back pain but these studies are not reviewed here because no controls were provided and thus no conclusions could be drawn or supported (Fig. 8). The need for controls in the evaluation of treatments of low back pain is apparent from a study in which equal results were obtained from detuned diathermy and from two other common treatments. Even more surprising, the benefits of the placebo treatment were still present after 12 weeks. This study supports the plea for improved methodologic rigor in studies of the treatment of low back pain.

Lumbar Spinal Stenosis

The clinical syndrome of lumbar stenosis likely represents a wide spectrum of clinical presentations—from the middle-aged patient with a single nerve root involved by lateral recess stenosis to the elderly patient with marked multilevel central and lateral stenosis. The histories obtained from patients with lumbar stenosis are consistently inconsistent. Patients report localized gluteal claudication-type symptoms as well as symptoms that are relieved by walking. Only approximately 50% of patients report the classic unilateral or bilateral sciatica that worsens after they walk a few yards. The most appropriate interpretation of these various complaints is that a key feature of spinal stenosis is that the clinical symptoms change with position.

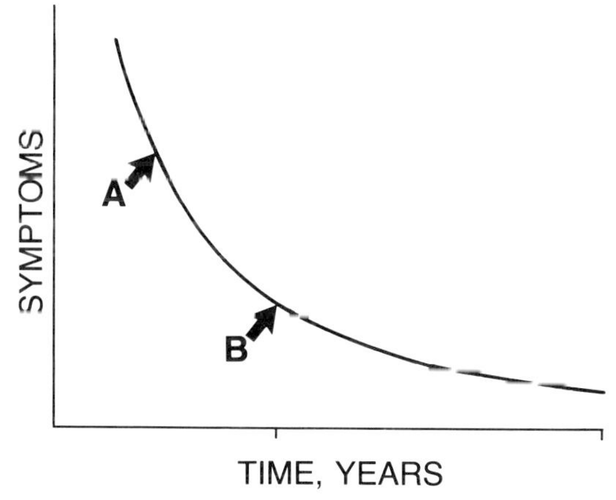

Figure 8

Diagram of the natural history of low back pain. A percentage of patients who are managed at point A will appear to have improved when evaluated at point B. Importantly, however, the improvement has nothing to do with the type of intervention. This emphasizes the necessity to assess control populations when evaluating treatment strategies for patients who suffer from low back complaints.

Physical findings are generally minimal, resulting in a discrepancy between symptoms and findings. Patients often may be mislabeled as "hysterics." The most common physical findings include pain with extension of the lumbar spine and weakness of the extensor hallucis longus. Sciatic tension signs are lacking except in selected patients with a unilateral lateral recess entrapment syndrome. Elderly patients often will walk with a forward-flexed "stooped" posture, possibly due to a relative increase in the vertebral canal volume in this position. Because aortic-iliac vascular outflow obstruction with vascular claudication is the chief differential diagnosis, the vascular tree should be assessed carefully.

Radiographs generally reveal degenerative changes consistent with age, although metastatic lesions, degenerative spondylolisthesis, and significant lumbar scoliosis may be observed. Further assessment is required only if the patient perceives a significant impairment of quality of life. Impaired quality of life represents the chief indication for elective surgery in this condition, and then only after appropriate nonoperative management has been tried.

The most important psychologic issue to address in the elderly is depression. Depression often can be manifested by multiple somatic complaints, including back and leg pain. Formal consultation should be considered for any patient who appears depressed or who does not have the characteristic physical findings on thorough evaluation.

The EMG is positive in approximately 80% of patients with lumbar spinal stenosis. The true value of the EMG, however, is in preoperative planning. Involved nerve roots should be inspected carefully at operation. Bone scanning should be considered to diminish the chance of encountering an unusual presentation of a metastatic neoplasm. The lumbar myelogram and the CT scan confirm the diagnosis. Dimensions of the bony vertebral canal do not reliably identify patients with acquired spinal stenosis. The anteroposterior diameter and the cross-sectional area of the dural sac as determined by myelography or high-resolution CT reliably identify patients with lumbar stenosis. The most accurate objective anatomic measurement for acquired degenerative lumbar spinal stenosis is cross-sectional area of the dural sac less than 100 mm^2 (this correlates well with an anteroposterior diameter of 10 mm). The anteroposterior diameter is more easily determined from careful inspection of the myelogram or high-resolution CT scan.

Good results consistently average 85% after surgical decompression for lumbar spinal stenosis, with follow-up of 4 years. Approximately 8% of patients have increasing symptoms after operation, and 5% require additional intervention. The precise surgical procedure for patients with spinal stenosis remains undecided although most authors favor extensive multilevel decompressions without fusion. Laminaplasty procedures and routine stabilization procedures will require additional validation. Stabilization in addition to decompression is probably the treatment of choice for patients with symptomatic degenerative spondylolisthesis.

Redundant nerve roots, as observed on myelograms, have been reported in patients with significant central lumbar spinal stenosis. The myelographic appearance of redundant roots is a characteristic tortuosity of all of the rootlets within the cauda equina. The collapse of multiple disk spaces from advancing degenerative changes with subsequent relative lengthening of the nerve roots has been implicated as a factor in the pathogenesis of this process. Patients with redundant nerve roots have neuronal losses that support a friction neuritis. Longitudinal incisions of the dura have been recommended, in addition to bony decompression, for patients with extensive redundant nerve roots. More data are required to validate this treatment approach.

Lumbar Spinal Segmental Instability

Lumbar segmental instability is present when physiologic loads produce abnormal spinal motion, either rotational or translational. Radiographic studies with dynamic views in the frontal (lateral bending) and lateral (flexion-extension) planes will identify these abnormal motions. When they are clearly identified, surgical stabilization of the lumbar spine may be considered if nonoperative management fails to afford pain relief. Translation motion at one spinal motion segment that exceeds 3 mm at L3-4 or L4-5 or 5 mm at L5-S1 or angulation of one motion segment of more than 10° defines the truly unstable motion segment. The stabilization approach recommended will depend upon numerous factors including previous surgical experience and the background and preferences of the surgeon. The dictum of *primum non nocere* must be weighed in the decision-making process. Reports extolling the virtues of any given method must be examined critically for data from a suitable control group for comparison with the method in question.

Lumbar Spondylolysis and Spondylolisthesis

A recent landmark study on the natural history of spondylolysis and spondylolisthesis suggested that a child with these conditions can be permitted to enjoy a normal childhood and adolescence without restriction of activities and without fear of progressive olisthy or disabling pain. The incidence of spondylolysis with or without spondylolisthesis was 4.4% at age 6 compared with about 6% in adulthood. The male/female ratio was 2:1 at age 6 and in adulthood. Slipping may increase up to age 16, but rarely. Even the listhesis was not symptomatic in the population group studied.

Lumbar spondylolisthesis was thoroughly reviewed in Orthopaedic Knowledge Update I. Newer information has evolved primarily in the area of treatment. With the development of newer and more stable spinal implant systems, surgical reduction of most deformities has become technically feasible. However, incidence of complications, long-term follow-up, and surgical indications remain as key issues not fully defined at this time.

Miscellaneous

Pregnancy Among a series of 48,760 consecutive deliveries, only 5 pregnant patients with symptoms and signs of lumbar disk herniation were identified, an incidence of 1:10,000. The five patients all were managed nonoperatively during their pregnancy. After uneventful deliveries, all five underwent successful surgical treatment.

Referred Pain Three patients were reported who presented with back and leg pain secondary to involvement of the femoral nerve by abdominal aortic aneurysms. Such reports reemphasize the need for thorough assessments of patients who have lumbar radicular complaints.

Annotated Bibliography

Back Pain

Andersson, G.B., Jr.: Epidemiologic aspects on low-back pain in industry. Spine 6:53–60, 1981.

Most data on industrial back pain may be misleading. They are obtained retrospectively from absentee records or insurance reports. Therefore, controversies continue about the relationship of back pain, disk hernia, and long-term disability as they relate to heavy physical work, static work postures, frequency of bending and twisting, lifting and forceful movements, repetitive work, and vibration. The same controversies exist as they relate to age, sex, anthropometry, posture, muscle strength, fitness, spine mobility, psychosocial factors, psychiatric problems, social factors, and radiographic findings.

Biering-Sorensen, F.: One-year prospective study of low back trouble in a general population. Prognostic value of low back history and physical measurements. Dan. Med. Bull. 1985.

Recurrence of back pain is associated with weak trunk muscles, decreased flexibility of back and hamstrings, early onset of back pain in life, the presence of sciatica, and previous medical treatment. The first episode of back pain during the 1-year follow-up was associated with poor back muscle endurance and a high degree of back flexibility.

Cady, L.D., Jr.; Thomas, P.C.; and Karwasky, R.J.: Program for increasing health and physical fitness of fire fighters. J. Occup. Med. 27:110–114, 1985.

A physical fitness program emphasizing endurance and stamina (aerobic exercise) increased strength, flexibility, and aerobic capacity in firefighters. More importantly, the 14-year program found a 25% decrease in workers compensation costs in those who significantly increased their physical work capacity (aerobic fitness) without significantly increasing their muscular strength or spinal flexibility.

Dzioba, R.B., and Doxey, N.C.: A prospective investigation into the orthopaedic and psychologic predictors of outcome of first lumbar surgery following industrial injury. Spine 9:614–623, 1984.

The success of treating industrial back problems is decreased in patients who have poor proficiency in English, increased number of nonphysical signs (Waddell), a high hypochondriasis scale on the MMPI, and an abnormal pain drawing.

Frymoyer, J.W.; Newberg, A.; Pope, M.H.; Wilder, D.G.; Clements, J.; and MacPherson, B.: Spine radiographs in patients with low-back pain: An epidemiological study in men. J. Bone Joint Surg. 66A:1048–1055, 1984.

Degenerative changes in the lumbar spine increase with age. Spurs and joint space narrowing were not found to correlate with occupation, lifting, or exposure to vibration. Congenital and developmental changes and aging changes of the spine occur in frequencies that do not support the use of radiographs as a back pain predictive tool for individual cases.

Frymoyer, J.W.; Pope, M.H.; Clements, J.H.; Wilder, D.G.; MacPherson, B.; and Ashikaga, T.: Risk factors in low-back pain: An epidemiological survey. J. Bone Joint Surg. 65A:213–218, 1983.

Only 30% of more than 1,200 individuals ages 18–56 claimed they had never experienced back pain, and almost 25% claimed they have had or were having severe back pain. Those with severe pain were more likely to report limb symptoms and heavy lifting and vibration on the job and were more likely to be cigarette smokers than those with moderate or no back pain.

Kelsey, J.L., and White, A.A., III: Epidemiology and impact of low-back pain. Spine 5:133–142, 1980.

Back pain affects 80% or more of the adult population and is the most common cause of disability for people under age 45. Those not working because of back pain for 6, 12, and 24 months have a 50%, 25%, and 0% chance, respectively, of returning to a productive life-style. Herniated disk is the most common problem in the group 30–39 years old and is more associated with sedentary than with active occupations. Degenerative joint disease is most closely linked to a natural aging process, and its relationship with symptoms has not been established. Traumatic spondylolisthesis is rare and slip of 25–30% is not documented as being more closely associated with back pain than in cases without spondylolisthesis.

Krølner, B., and Toft, B.: Vertebral bone loss: An unheeded side effect of therapeutic bed rest. Clin. Sci. 64:537–540, 1983.

Recumbency decreases the mineral content of bone. When the recumbency period is short, re ambulation can increase bone mineral content in the spine. Recurrent bed rest periods may predispose patients to spinal osteoporosis.

Nachemson, A., and Bigos, S.J.: The low back. *In* Adult Orthopaedics, edited by R.L. Cruess and W.R.J. Rennie, pp. 843–937. Vol. 2. New York, Churchill Livingstone, 1984.

Five hundred ninety-seven up-to-date references on all aspects of low back pain and sciatica.

Nachemson, A.L.: The natural course of low back pain. *In* Symposium on Idiopathic Low Back Pain, edited by A.A. White, III, and S.L. Gordon, pp. 46–51. St. Louis, C.V. Mosby Company, 1982.

Only 2–3% of adults with back pain have sciatica. With back pain and sciatica, both resolve rapidly, although the recurrence rate is as high as 60%, especially with leg symptoms. A pathoanatomic diagnosis can be made in no more than 15% of cases.

Robertson, L.S., and Keeve, J.P.: Worker injuries: The effects of workers' compensation and OSHA inspections. J. Health Polit. Policy Law 8:581–597, 1983.

OSHA inspections for work hazards were found to decrease the number of objective injuries but increase the number of subjective injuries, the most common of which is back pain. It may be better to promote back health in industry with wellness programs rather than through prevention of health hazards.

Snook, S.H.: Low back pain in industry. *In* Symposium on Idiopathic Low Back Pain, edited by A.A. White, III, and S.L. Gordon, pp. 23–38. St. Louis, C.V. Mosby Company, 1982.

Annually, 2% of industrial workers report back pain, and 10% of the cases are responsible for approximately 80% of back compensation costs. Eighty-four percent of the workers who reported disabling back injuries had no definite diagnosis and the majority were not able to associate the onset of their symptoms with an unusual circumstance or accident. High-risk jobs include trucking, material handling, and nursing. Factors such as type of treatment, compensation, and recurrence of symptoms can increase absenteeism.

Valkenburg, H.A., and Haanen, H.C.M.: The epidemiology of low back pain. *In* Symposium on Idiopathic Low Back Pain, edited by A.A. White, III, and S.L. Gordon, pp. 9–22. St. Louis, C.V. Mosby Company, 1982.

Twenty-five percent of this large study population had been unfit for work at least once and 2–4% had changed jobs because of back problems. Forty percent of the population age 35 and older had radiographic evidence of lumbar aging changes, termed "degenerative arthritis," that did not relate well to symptoms or history of symptoms.

Weber, H.: Lumbar disc herniation: A controlled, prospective study with ten years of observation. Spine 8:131–140, 1983.

Between 85% and 90% of surgically treated and nonsurgically treated patients with disk hernias were asymptomatic after 4 years. Less than 2% of the subjects in both groups were symptomatic at the end of 10 years. Those who were unable to work and received disability benefits had obvious psychosocial problems. Even with improved physical condition, none was motivated to give up the insurance benefits. There was no evidence that muscle weakness of unknown duration was an indication for operation for disk hernia.

Wiesel, S.W.; Feffer, H.L.; and Rothman, R.H.: Industrial low-back pain: A prospective evaluation of a standardized diagnostic and treatment protocol. Spine 9:199–203, 1984.

Unbiased medical surveillance using a standard protocol led to changes in physician and patient behavior, resulting in decreased disability and cost savings with the promotion of good medical practice.

Wiesel, S.W.; Tsourmas, N.; Feffer, H.L.; Citrin, C.M.; and Patronas, N.: A study of computer-assisted tomography. I. The incidence of positive CAT scans in an asymptomatic group of patients. Spine 9:549–551, 1984.

CT scans showed that almost 20% of asymptomatic subjects under 40 years of age had a herniated nucleus pulposus. Fifty percent of the subjects over 40 years of age had abnormal findings, most commonly herniated disk, facet degeneration, and spinal stenosis.

Acute Lumbar Radicular Syndromes

Natural History

Weber, H.: Lumbar disc herniation: A controlled, prospective study with ten years of observation. Spine 8:131–140, 1983.

One hundred twenty-six patients with herniated lumbar disks were randomized between surgical and conservative treatments. At 1 year, those in the surgical group had less pain, but after 4 years there was no statistically significant difference in relief of symptoms between the two groups.

Epidemiology

Frymoyer, J.W.; Pope, M.H.; Clements, J.H.; Wilder, D.G.; MacPherson, B.; and Ashikaga, T.: Risk factors in low-back pain: An epidemiological survey. J. Bone Joint Surg. 65A:213–218, 1983.

Evaluation of 1,121 men in a family practice revealed that 30.1% had never had low back pain, 46.3% had moderate low back pain, and 23.6% had severe low back pain. Risk factors associated with severe low back pain included jobs requiring repetitive heavy lifting, use of jackhammers or machine tools, and operation of motor vehicles.

Pathophysiology

Kirkaldy-Willis, W.H.: The relationship of structural pathology to the nerve root. Spine 9:49–52, 1984.

Lumbar spine nerves may be entrapped in a number of different anatomic areas which are described. Symptoms vary with the area of entrapment, each requiring specific treatment.

Nachemson, A.: Lumbar spine instability: A critical update and symposium survey. Spine 10:290–291, 1985.

An overview of instability is presented, with the hard information currently available and focus on areas that need further investigation. The bibliography is up-to-date.

Neidre, A., and MacNab, I.: Anomalies of the lumbosacral nerve roots: Review of 16 cases and classification. Spine 8:294–299, 1983.

Sixteen cases of lumbar nerve root anomalies are reviewed and a classification system is presented. Lumbar radiculopathy is the most common symptom. Diagnosis and treatment are reviewed.

Patient Evaluation

Bell, G.R.; Rothman, R.H.; Booth, R.E.; Cuckler, J.M.; Garfin, S.; Herkowitz, H.; Simeone, F.A.; Dolinskas, C.; and Han, S.S.: A study of computer-assisted tomography. II. Comparison of metrizamide myelography and computed tomography in the diagnosis of herniated lumbar disc and spinal stenosis. Spine 9:552–556, 1984.

A prospective blind study comparing the efficacies of myelography and CT in diagnosing spine problems is presented. The authors conclude that the former is more accurate than the latter in diagnosis of both herniated lumbar disk and spinal stenosis.

Eisen, A., and Hoirch, M.: The electrodiagnostic evaluation of spinal root lesions. Spine 8:98–106, 1983.

The available electrophysiologic techniques found helpful in identifying nerve root lesions are surveyed. There is a 70–80% correlation among clinical, myelographic, and electrophysiologic findings. Electrophysiology is found to have limited value in postlaminectomy assessment.

Frymoyer, J.W.; Newberg, A.; Pope, M.H.; Wilder, D.G.; Clements, J.; and MacPherson, B.: Spine radiographs in patients with low-back pain: An epidemiological study in men. J. Bone Joint Surg. 66A:1048–1055, 1984.

Three groups of patients—no back pain, moderate pain, and severe pain—underwent radiography and the positive findings were evaluated for significant association with low back pain. The conclusion was that plain radiography of the spine is of little use in determining causes of low back pain.

Mayer, T.G.; Tencer, A.F.; Kristoferson, S.; and Mooney, V.: Use of noninvasive techniques for quantification of spinal range-of-motion in normal subjects and chronic low-back dysfunction patients. Spine 9:588–595, 1984.

An inclinometer is demonstrated that can separate the components of the compound motion of the hip and spine. This provides the physician with a simple method of obtaining an accurate, quantitative measure of the range of motion of the lumbar spine.

Southwick, S.M., and White, A.A.: Current concepts review: The use of psychological tests in the evaluation of low-back pain. J. Bone Joint Surg. 65A:560–565, 1983.

The most commonly used psychologic tests are reviewed and their roles in evaluation of low back pain are presented.

Wiesel, S.W.; Tsourmas, N.; Feffer, H.L.; Citrin, C.M.; and Patronas, N.: A study of computer-assisted tomography: I. The incidence of positive CAT scans in an asymptomatic group of patients. Spine 9:549–551, 1984.

The incidence of positive CT scans in a group of asymptomatic patients was found to be 35.4%. In patients under 40 years of age, 19.5% had normal scans, with a herniated nucleus pulposus in every case. In patients over 40, 50% had abnormal findings; the most frequent diagnoses were herniated nucleus pulposus, facet degeneration, and stenosis.

Witt, I.; Vestergaard, A.; and Rosenklint, A.: A comparative analysis of x-ray findings of the lumbar spine in patients with and without lumbar pain. Spine 9:298–300, 1984.

Lumbar spine radiographs of 238 patients with low back pain and sciatica were compared with those of 66 patients without low back pain. No difference between the two groups could be demonstrated in incidences of spondylosis and disk degeneration.

Treatment

Bell, G.R., and Rothman, R.H.: The conservative treatment of sciatica. Spine 9:54–56, 1984.

A standardized approach to the conservative treatment of sciatica is presented. The cornerstones are bed rest and anti-inflammatory drugs; as patients respond, they are encouraged in good low back hygiene with exercises.

Bradford, D.S.; Oegema, T.R., Jr.; Cooper, K.M.; Wakano, K.; and Chao, E.Y.: Chymopapain, chemonucleolysis, and nucleus pulposus regeneration: A biochemical and biomechanical study. Spine 9:135–147, 1984.

Intervertebral disks of dogs were injected with chymopapain. Initially, there was disk narrowing with loss of normal biochemical and biomechanical properties; however, at 3 months after injection these properties began to reverse and approach those of the uninjected controls. The observations suggest that chymopapain has a profound but reversible effect on normal canine intervertebral disks.

Cuckler, J.M.; Bernini, P.A.; Wiesel, S.W.; Booth, R.E., Jr.; Rothman, R.H.; and Pickens, G.T.: The use of epidural steroids in the treatment of lumbar radicular pain: A prospective, randomized, double-blind study. J. Bone Joint Surg. 67A:63–66, 1985.

A double-blind study comparing the results of epidural injection of methylprednisolone and procaine and of physiologic saline and procaine failed to show any significant difference in outcome between the two groups. Patients had a clinical diagnosis of either acute herniated nucleus pulposus or spinal stenosis.

Dan, N.G., and Saccasan, P.A.: Serious complications of lumbar spinal manipulation. Med. J. Aust. 2:672–673, 1983.

Seven cases of serious complications after lumbar spinal manipulation are described, including massive cauda equina compression and vertebral pedicle fracture. The article emphasizes that lumbar spine manipulations are not without potentially serious risks.

Deburge, A.; Benoist, M.; and Boyer, D.: The diagnosis of disc sequestration. Spine 9:496–499, 1984.

Sequestration of a disk herniation is a potential cause of failure of chemonucleolysis and thus its recognition is important. After review of 98 patients, the authors found no characteristic clinical signs or pathognomonic features to identify disk sequestration.

Deyo, R.A.: Conservative therapy for low back pain: Distinguishing useful from useless therapy. J.A.M.A. 250:1057–1062, 1983.

Fifty-nine therapeutic trials were examined for adherence to good methodologic criteria. Flexion exercises, administration of each of three drugs, one traction method, and certain manipulations all were supported by single studies of reasonable validity, but the importance of the results and their applicability to particular types of low back pain were unclear. No valid trials supporting use of corsets, bed rest, transcutaneous nerve stimulation, and conventional traction were found.

Fraser, R.D.: Chymopapain for the treatment of intervertebral disc herniation: The final report of a double-blind study. Spine 9:815–818, 1984.

Sixty patients with unilateral sciatica resulting from lumbar herniated nucleus pulposus were entered in a double-blind study. Two years after injection, 77% of patients treated with chymopapain were found to be moderately improved compared with 45% of saline-injected patients. In the chymopapain group, 57% were pain-free compared with 23% in the saline group.

Gallinaro, P., and Cartesegna, M.: Three cases of lumbar disc rupture and one of cauda equina associated with spinal manipulation (chiropraxis) (letter to the editor). Lancet 1:411, 1983.

Four complications of lumbar spinal manipulation are presented.

Godfrey, C.M.; Morgan, P.P.; and Schatzker, J.: A randomized trial of manipulation for low-back pain in a medical setting. Spine 9:301–304, 1984.

A single-blind study was performed to test the efficacy of spinal manipulation. Both treated and control patients improved rapidly during the observation period. On re-test, there was no statistically significant difference between the two groups in any of the measured variables.

Hall, B.B., and McCulloch, J.A.: Anaphylactic reactions following the intradiscal injection of chymopapain under local anesthesia. J. Bone Joint Surg. 65A:1215–1219, 1983.

Among 4,282 patients treated with chymopapain under local anesthesia, 15 (0.35%) suffered an anaphylactic reaction and were treated appropriately, with no deaths or known sequelae. The advantage of local anesthesia is that the patient remains responsive and can give an early warning of the subjective symptoms of anaphylaxis.

Inoue, S.-I.; Watanabe, T.; Hirose, A.; Tanaka, T.; Matsui, N.; Saegusa, O.; and Sho, E.: Anterior discectomy and interbody fusion for lumbar disc herniation: A review of 350 cases. Clin. Orthop. 183:22–31, 1984.

Of the patients studied, 94.3% had bony union. The authors thought that the good clinical results could be attributed to restoration of disk height and correlation of spinal alignment. They suggested that this procedure is indicated in young adults and physical laborers who have low back pain and sciatica and in patients who have spinal instability.

Konings, J.G.; Williams, F.J.B.; and Deutman, R.: The effects of chemonucleolysis as demonstrated by computerized tomography. J. Bone Joint Surg. 66B:417–421, 1984.

In patients with herniated nucleus pulposus, CT scans were performed before chemonucleolysis and 3 months afterward. In 20 of the 28 patients with positive scans, the compression produced by the herniated nucleus pulposus was eliminated or reduced. After injection, diffuse bulging of the annulus developed in 23 of the 28. The authors conclude that chemonucleolysis is an effective treatment for herniated nucleus pulposus but is not indicated when neural compression is due to a bulging annulus.

Lin, P.M.; Cautilli, R.A.; and Joyce, M.F.: Posterior lumbar interbody fusion. Clin. Orthop. 180:154–168, 1983.

The authors think that posterior interbody fusion (PLIF) dynamically decompresses neural structures by holding the vertebral bodies apart and fusing them into a single-motion segment. Follow-up of 465 PLIF cases demonstrated a fusion rate of 88% and satisfactory clinical results in 82%.

Tile, M.: The role of surgery in nerve root compression. Spine 9:57–64, 1984.

Before operating, the surgeon must have a precise neurologic diagnosis, clinically based and with corroborating radiographic, electrodiagnostic, and nerve block evidence. The important concept is "Think nerve root." Surgical management must be tailored to the individual patient on the basis of local anatomy and pathology and on whether there is disk herniation or lateral bony entrapment.

Chronic Lumbar Radicular Syndromes

Anatomy and Physiology

Hansson, T.; Bigos, S.; Beecher, P.; and Wortley, M.: The lumbar lordosis in acute and chronic low-back pain. Spine 10:154–155, 1985.

No increased prevalence of lumbar lordosis was observed in patients with acute or chronic low back pain.

Hansson, T.; Sandström, J.; Roos, B.; Jonson, R.; and Andersson, G.B.J.: The bone mineral content of the lumbar spine in patients with chronic low-back pain. Spine 10:158–160, 1985.

The bone mineral content of the lumbar spine varied inversely with the duration of the low back pain. The longer low back pain persisted, the lower the bone mineral content of the lumbar vertebrae.

Neidre, A., and MacNab, I.: Anomalies of the lumbosacral nerve roots: Review of 16 cases and classification. Spine 8:294–299, 1983.

The authors highlight the anatomic variation of the lumbosacral nerve roots. Because 50% of these anomalies were discovered at repeat exploration, nerve root anomalies should be suspected in cases of failed disk surgery.

Parke, W.W., and Watanabe, R.: The intrinsic vasculature of the lumbosacral spinal nerve roots. Spine 10:508–515, 1985.

This study supports the concept that spinal nerve roots are structurally, vascularly, and metabolically unique regions of the nervous system. Peculiarities of their intrinsic vasculature may account for suspected "neuroischemic" responses to pathologic mechanical stresses and inflammatory conditions associated with degenerative disease of the lower spine.

Rydevik, B.; Brown, M.D.; and Lundborg, G.: Pathoanatomy and pathophysiology of nerve root compression. Spine 9:7–15, 1984.

The functional changes induced by compression can be caused by mechanical nerve fiber deformation but also may be a consequence of changes in nerve root microcirculation, leading to ischemia and formation of intraneural edema. Intraneural edema and demyelination seem to be critical factors for the production of pain in association with nerve root compression.

Spencer, D.L.; Irwin, G.S.; and Miller, J.A.: Anatomy and significance of fixation of the lumbosacral nerve roots in sciatica. Spine 8:672–679, 1983.

The authors show how pressure can be applied to the extrathecal nerve root by a disk herniation without compression of the nerve root against the posterior elements. Dural ligaments, described in the article, were implicated in the pathogenesis of the sciatica syndrome.

Imaging Techniques

Bell, G.R.; Rothman, R.H.; Booth, R.E.; Cuckler, J.M.; Garfin, S.; Herkowitz, H.; Simeone, F.A.; Dolinskas, C.; and Han, S.S.: A study of computer-assisted tomography. II. Comparison of metrizamide myelography and computed tomography in the diagnosis of herniated lumbar disc and spinal stenosis. Spine 9:552–556, 1984.

Metrizamide myelography is more accurate than CT in the diagnosis of both herniated lumbar disks and spinal stenosis, remaining the diagnostic study of choice.

Gehweiler, J.A., Jr., and Daffner, R.H.: Low back pain: The controversy of radiologic evaluation. AJR 140:109–112, 1983.

The efficacy of oblique radiographs was evaluated in a prospective study. The authors show that 12% of patients had an abnormality detected on oblique views that were not observed on the standard anteroposterior and lateral views.

Han, J.S.; Kaufman, B.; El Yousef, S.J.; Benson, J.E.; Bonstelle, C.T.; Alfidi, R.J.; Haaga, J.R.; Yeung, H.; and Huss, R.G.: NMR imaging of the spine. AJR 141:1137–1145, 1983.

MRI was shown to be extremely useful in evaluating intramedullary spinal cord lesions such as syringohydromyelia and cystic tumors.

Hindmarsh, T.; Ekholm, S.E.; Kido, D.K.; Sahler, L.; and Sands, M.: Lumbar myelography with iohexol and metrizamide: A double-blind clinical trial. Acta Radiol. [Diagn.] (Stockh.) 25:365–368, 1984.

The frequency of adverse reactions was lower with iohexol. Extended clinical trials are now in progress.

Modic, M.T.; Pavlicek, W.; Weinstein, M.A.; Boumphrey, F.; Ngo, F.; Hardy, R.; and Duchesneau, P.M.: Magnetic resonance imaging of intervertebral disk disease: Clinical and pulse sequence considerations. Radiology 152:103–111, 1984.

MRI is a promising, newer imaging technique that can identify disk herniations and bony stenosis.

Pyhtinen, J.; Lähde, S.; Tanska, E.-L.; and Laitinen, J.: Computed tomography after lumbar myelography in lower back and extremity pain syndromes. Diagn. Imag. 52:19–22, 1983.

CT scans of the lumbar spine after myelography changed the diagnosis in 7% of 214 patients. Important additional information was provided in an additional 12%.

Wiesel, S.W.; Tsourmas, N.; Feffer, H.L.; Citrin, C.M.; and Patronas, N.: A study of computer-assisted tomography. I. The incidence of positive CAT scans in an asymptomatic group of patients. Spine 9:549–551, 1984.

Over 35% of asymptomatic people were found to have abnormal CT scans, and over 19% of those study subjects under age 40 were diagnosed as having herniated nucleus pulposus. In patients over age 40, 50% had an abnormal finding, with the most common diagnoses being canal stenosis and facet degeneration. Correlation of CT findings with the clinical findings was urged.

Wilmink, J.T.; Penning, L.; and van den Burg, W.: Role of stenosis of spinal canal in L4–L5 nerve root compression assessed by flexion-extension myelography. Neuroradiology 26:173–181, 1984.

The authors emphasized the association of lateral recess stenosis in patients with soft disk herniations.

Outcome Predictors

Neoplasms

Barcena, A.; Lobato, R.D.; Rivas, J.J.; Cordobes, F.; de Castro, S.; Cabrena, A.; and Lamas, E.: Spinal metastatic disease: Analysis of factors determining functional prognosis and the choice of treatment. Neurosurgery 15:820–827, 1984.

Life expectancy and functional results are dependent on tumor biology. Radiotherapy alone is often the treatment of choice. Only 42% of the patients required surgery.

Ker, N.B., and Jones, C.B.: Tumours of the cauda equina: The problem of differential diagnosis. J. Bone Joint Surg. 67B:358–362, 1985.

Most of the 32 patients reviewed in this article were initially misdiagnosed as having an intervertebral disk herniation. The authors believe that all surgical explorations of the spine, even in the presence of a typical clinical picture of a lumbar disk herniation, should be preceded by adequate myelography.

Chronicity

Murphy, K.A., and Cornish, R.D.: Prediction of chronicity in acute low back pain. Arch. Phys. Med. Rehabil. 65:334–337, 1984.

Patients whose acute pain became chronic complained of pain over a wider area of the body, had deeper, more central pain, were highly anxious, and had a lower activity level.

Turner, J.A.; Robinson, J.; and McCreary, C.P.: Chronic low back pain: Predicting response to nonsurgical treatment. Arch. Phys. Med. Rehabil. 64:560–563, 1983.

Physicians' predictions of pain relief and return to normal activities, the Activities Discomfort Scale (ADS), and the hypochondriasis scale of the MMPI each was associated significantly with patient's rating of return to normal activities after treatment. The authors concluded that the ADS may be useful in identifying poor-risk patients.

Electrodiagnostic Studies

Aminoff, M.J.; Goodin, D.S.; Barbaro, N.M.; Weinstein, P.R.; and Rosenblum, M.L.: Dermatomal somatosensory evoked potentials in unilateral lumbosacral radiculopathy. Ann. Neurol. 17:171–176, 1985.

The authors raise doubt about the ultimate utility of these evoked potential techniques in the evaluation of patients with suspected radiculopathies.

Dvonch, V.; Scarff, T.; Bunch, W.H.; Smith, D.; Boscardin, J.; Lebarge, H.; and Ibrahim, K.: Dermatomal somatosensory evoked potentials: Their use in lumbar radiculopathy. Spine 9:291–293, 1984.

The authors recommend this measurement as a useful adjunct in the selection of patients for lumbar spine surgery.

Nouwen, A., and Bush, C.: The relationship between paraspinal EMG and chronic low back pain. Pain 20:109–123, 1984.

The authors conclude that no consistent evidence exists to suggest that low back pain patients have elevated paraspinal EMG activity. Therefore, any treatment based on this hypothesis is experimental.

Sherman, R.A.: Relationships between strength of low back muscle contraction and reported intensity of chronic low back pain. Am. J. Phys. Med. 64:190–200, 1985.

No diagnostic subgroup of low back pain patients produced a single unique pattern. No single aspect of the EMG signal (surface electrodes) had predictive value for any individual subject.

Physical Examination

Keefe, F.J., and Hill, R.W.: An objective approach to quantifying pain behavior and gait patterns in low back pain patients. Pain 21:153–161, 1985.

The gait of patients receiving disability payments or taking narcotics differed significantly from that of those who were not.

Psychologic Factors

Bouras, N.; Bartlett, J.R.; Neil-Dwyer, G.; and Bridges, P.K.: Psychological aspects of patients having multiple operations for low back pain. Br. J. Med. Psychol. 57:147–151, 1984.

Nonresponders after one lumbar spine procedure were more psychiatrically disturbed and socially disabled than responders. The authors recommend psychiatric examination for patients being considered for a second lumbar spine procedure.

Frymoyer, J.W.; Rosen, J.C.; Clements, J.; and Pope, M.H.: Psychologic factors in low-back-pain disability. Clin. Orthop. 195:178–184, 1985.

Disabled patients had significant elevations of hypochondriasis and hysteria scores on the MMPI. These patients formed a distinctive subgroup.

Biomechanical Factors

Facet Joints

Lorenz, M.; Patwardhan, A.; and Vanderby, R., Jr.: Load-bearing characteristics of lumbar facets in normal and surgically altered spinal segments. Spine 8:122–130, 1983.

This study shows that the absolute facet loads remain relatively constant with increasing segmental compressive loads such that the facet load expressed as percentage of load applied to the segment decreases with increasing axial loads. Significant variation in the load-bearing characteristics of the L2–3 and L4–5 segment levels may be attributed to differences in the facet anatomy relative to the anatomic planes of the body.

Yang, K.H., and King, A.I.: Mechanism of facet load transmission as a hypothesis for low-back pain. Spine 9:557–565, 1984.

Normal facet joints carried 3–25% of the applied load. In degenerative conditions, the load transmitted through the facet joints could approach 47%. The data also show that an overloaded facet joint will cause rearward rotation of the inferior facet, resulting in the stretching of the joint capsule. Although this hypothesis could represent a source of low back pain, further investigations are necessary to prove it.

Intervertebral Disks

Bradford, D.S.; Oegema, T.R., Jr.; Cooper, K.M.; Wakano, K.; and Chao, E.Y.: Chymopapain, chemonucleolysis, and nucleus pulposus regeneration: A biochemical and biomechanical study. Spine 9:135–147, 1984.

The authors used a canine model to show that *in vivo* injection of chymopapain into the intervertebral disk resulted in disk space narrowing at 2 weeks. Nevertheless, the nucleus retained the ability to synthesize proteoglycans. At 3 months after chymopapain injection, the disk showed an increase in disk height and return of nuclear material and proteoglycan aggregate. Six months after injection, these features approached normal. Biomechanical changes included a reduction in compression stiffness and an increase in creep rate. These alterations returned to normal at approximately 3 months. The authors conclude that chemonucleolysis with chymopapain would be less likely to alter proteoglycan biochemistry and the biomechanical properties of the disk permanently than would surgical excision in experimental animals.

Panjabi, M.M.; Krag, M.H.; and Chung, T.Q.: Effects of disc injury on mechanical behavior of the human spine. Spine 9:707–713, 1984.

The effects of injury to the intervertebral disk were investigated by using three-dimensional flexibility and creep measurements of functional spinal units. Sagittal plane symmetry was disturbed, resulting in asymmetric facet joint movements. The authors dispute the previously espoused "self-scaling" mechanism of the disk.

Seligman, J.V.; Gertzbein, S.D.; Tile, M.; and Kapasouri, A.: Computer analysis of spinal segment motion in degenerative disc disease with and without axial loading. Spine 9:566–573, 1984.

The center of rotation of the spinal motion segment is an indicator of spinal instability. The motion segment does not move about a single fixed axis of rotation but rather about a locus of instantaneous axes of rotation, the centrode. Computer analysis of spinal motion provided a highly reliable and quantifiable method of detecting early changes in spinal motion in degenerative disk disease prior to well-recognized radiographic changes.

Wakano, K.; Kasman, R.; Chao, E.Y.; Bradford, D.S.; and Oegema, T.R.: Biomechanical analysis of canine intervertebral discs after chymopapain injection: A preliminary report. Spine 8:59–68, 1983.

Three weeks after chymopapain injection into canine intervertebral disks, significant reductions were seen in disk height and compressive stiffness, but the creep rate was increased substantially. These changes began to reverse 3 months after injection. The authors suggest that chymopapain causes a disk to change its material properties, but such effects appear to be time related.

Specific Disorders

Coccygodynia

Postacchini, F., and Massobrio, M.: Idiopathic coccygodynia: Analysis of fifty-one operative cases and a radiographic study of the normal coccyx. J. Bone Joint Surg. 65A:1116–1124, 1983.

The authors reviewed 51 patients with this elusive diagnosis. The radiographic features of the sacrum are also discussed.

Aging

Lavsky-Shulan, M.; Wallace, R.B.; Kohout, F.J.; Lemke, J.H.; Morris, M.C.; and Smith, I.M.: Prevalence and functional correlates of low back pain in the elderly: The Iowa 65+ Rural Health Study. J. Am. Geriatr. Soc. 33:23–28, 1985.

Over 75% of subjects had sought treatment for lower back pain; more than 5% had had lumbar spine surgery. Substantial functional and clinical burdens were borne by the rural elderly as a result of low back pain.

Pregnancy

LaBan, M.M.; Perrin, J.C.S.; and Latimer, F.R.: Pregnancy and the herniated lumbar disc. Arch. Phys. Med. Rehabil. 64:319–321, 1983.

Five pregnant patients with symptoms and signs of lumbar disk herniation were identified among a series of 48,760 consecutive deliveries, an incidence of 1:10,000. The five patients were managed nonoperatively during pregnancy. After their uneventful deliveries, all five patients underwent successful surgery.

Lumbar Disk Herniation

Herron, L.D., and Turner, J.: Patient selection for lumbar laminectomy and discectomy with a revised objective rating system. Clin. Orthop. 199:145–152, 1985.

The authors present a revised rating scale for selecting patients for lumbar discectomy. The rating scale was highly predictive of the result in 106 consecutive patients.

Hudgins, W.R.: Computer-aided diagnosis of lumbar disc herniation. Spine 8:604–615, 1983.

In a blind evaluation, an expert could not detect a significant difference between the output of the computer and the diagnoses and treatment plans of 10 clinicians.

Spengler, D.M., and Freeman, C.W.: Cited in Spengler, D.M.: Lumbar discectomy: Results with limited disc excision and selective foraminotomy. Spine 7:604–607, 1982.

The authors improved their ability to identify patients with objective surgical findings by using a standardized preoperative assessment scale based on objective data from four categories: neurologic signs, sciatic tension signs, psychologic factors (MMPI), and myelographic findings.

Lumbar Spinal Stenosis

Bolender, N.-F.; Schönström, N.S.R.; and Spengler, D.M.: Role of computed tomography and myelography in the diagnosis of central spinal stenosis. J. Bone Joint Surg. 67A:240–246, 1985.

Dimensions of the bony vertebral canal do not reliably identify patients with acquired spinal stenosis. The anteroposterior diameter of the dural sac as determined by myelography or from high-resolution CT scans was the most reliable method of recognizing lumbar stenosis, with a diameter of 10 mm being the critical anteroposterior dimension of the dural sac.

Hall, S.; Bartleson, J.D.; Onofrio, B.M.; Baker, H.L., Jr.; Okazaki, H.; and O'Duffy, J.D.: Lumbar spinal stenosis: Clinical features, diagnostic procedures, and results of surgical treatment in 68 patients. Ann. Intern. Med. 103:271–275, 1985.

Surgery was extensive, with 72% of patients having three or more laminae removed. At follow-up (mean, 4 years), 84% of the patients had good to excellent results.

Lassale, B.; Deburge, A.; and Benoist, M.: Résultats à long terme du traitement chirurgical des sténoses lombaires opérées. Rev. Rhum. Mal. Osteoartic. 52:27–33, 1985.

Satisfactory results were obtained in 83%; 87% reported substantial functional improvement. Worsening was observed in 8%, and 5% required a second surgical procedure.

Tsuji, H.; Tamaki, T.; Itoh, T.; Yamada, H.; Motoe, T.; Tatezaki, S.; Noguchi, T.; and Takano, H.: Redundant nerve roots in patients with degenerative lumbar spinal stenosis. Spine 10:72–82, 1985.

The redundant nerve roots have neuronal losses resulting from a longer duration of stenosis that suggests a sort of friction neuritis. The authors believe that satisfactory operative results can be achieved only after thorough decompression including a dural incision.

Lumbar Spinal Instability

Dupuis, P.R.; Yong-Hing, K.; Cassidy, J.D.; and Kirkaldy-Willis, W.H.: Radiologic diagnosis of degenerative lumbar spinal instability. Spine 10:262–276, 1985.

Radiographic study of symptomatic patients with dynamic views obtained in the frontal and lateral planes will identify unstable states in the office.

Lumbar Spondylolysis and Spondylolisthesis

Fredrickson, B.E.; Baker, D.; McHolick, W.J.; Yuan, H.A.; and Lubicky, J.P.: The natural history of spondylolysis and spondylolisthesis. J. Bone Joint Surg. 66A:699–707, 1984.

The authors performed a prospective radiographic study to determine the incidence of spondylolysis, spondylolisthesis, or both. The incidence of spondylolysis at age 6 was 4.4% and increased to 6% in adulthood. The male/female ratio of affected subjects remained 2:1. Children with spondylolysis or spondylolisthesis can be permitted to enjoy a normal childhood and adolescence without restriction of activities and without fear of progressive olisthy or disabling pain.

Referred Pain

Wilberger, J.E., Jr.: Lumbosacral radiculopathy secondary to abdominal aortic aneurysms: Report of three cases. J. Neurosurg. 58:965–967, 1983.

These three patients presented with back and leg pain secondary to involvement of the femoral nerve. This report emphasizes the need for considering aortic aneurysm in older patients with back and lower limb symptoms.

Infection

Romanick, P.C.; Smith, T.K.; Kopaniky, D.R.; and Oldfield, D.: Infection about the spine associated with low-velocity-missile injury to the abdomen. J. Bone Joint Surg. 67A:1195–1201, 1985.

The authors reviewed 20 patients with low-velocity missile injuries to the abdomen and the spine. Perforation of the colon by a low-velocity missile before the missile fractured the spine was associated with a high incidence of infection. Although no precise treatment plan could be formulated on such retrospective data, the authors suggest that early operative intervention may be indicated for gunshot wounds that penetrate the colon prior to striking the spine.

Education

Low Back School

Lankhorst, G.J.; Van de Stadt, R.J.; Vogelaar, T.W.; Van der Korst, J.K.; and Prevo, A.J.H.: The effect of the Swedish Back School in chronic idiopathic low back pain: A prospective controlled study. Scand. J. Rehabil. Med. 15:141–145, 1983.

No benefits accrued to patients with chronic low back pain after 1-year follow-up. The authors recommend using this concept for patients in the acute and subacute pain categories.

Lindequist, S.; Lundberg, B.; Wikmark, R.; Bergstad, B.; Lööf, G.; and Ottermark, A.-C.: Information and regime on low back pain. Scand. J. Rehabil. Med. 16:113–116, 1984.

Although no demonstrable financial impact of Low Back School was observed, the authors conclude that the initial treatment of low back pain should be limited to advice about back care, a few days of rest, and prescriptions for analgesics when needed.

Treatment

Crawshaw, C.; Frazer, A.M.; Merriam, W.F.; Mulholland, R.C.; and Webb, J.K.: A comparison of surgery and chemonucleolysis in the treatment of sciatica: A prospective randomized trial. Spine 9:195–198, 1984.

Failure rates in the two chymopapain groups were 52% and 47%; failure in the surgical group was 11%. Surgical salvage for chymopapain failures was usually delayed and unrewarding. Seven of 11 patients were classed as having a poor result. The authors believe that failure of chymopapain treatment is predictable at 1 month. Early operation was recommended to prevent chronic scarring after chymopapain failure.

Deyo, R.A.: Conservative therapy for low back pain: Distinguishing useful from useless therapy. J.A.M.A. 250:1057–1062, 1983.

Classic article documenting need for improved methodologic rigor in studies on the treatment of low back pain.

Ejeskär, A.; Nachemson, A.; Herberts, P.; Lysell, E.; Andersson, G.; Irstam, L.; and Peterson, L.-E.: Surgery versus chemonucleolysis for herniated lumbar discs: A prospective study with random assignment. Clin. Orthop. 174:236–242, 1983.

The authors discontinued the study because of the high failure rate in the patients treated with chymopapain.

Gibson, T.; Grahame, R.; Harkness, J.; Woo, P.; Blagrave, P.; and Hills, R.: Controlled comparison of shortwave diathermy treatment with osteopathic treatment in non-specific low back pain. Lancet 1:1258–1260, 1985.

The need for controls in studies of treatment of subjects who suffer from low back pain is emphasized. Detuned (turned off) diathermy was as effective as the other two modalities examined. Moreover, the benefits were still apparent 12 weeks after treatment.

Godfrey, C.M.; Morgan, P.P.; and Schatzker, J.: A randomized trial of manipulation for low-back pain in a medical setting. Spine 9:301–304, 1984.

In this well-controlled study, again no significant improvement was observed in patients who underwent manipulation.

Guck, T.P.; Skultety, F.M.; Meilman, P.W.; and Dowd, E.T.: Multidisciplinary pain center follow-up study: Evaluation with a no-treatment control group. Pain 21:295–306, 1985.

The long-term efficacy of a multidiscipline pain management center was evaluated by comparing 20 treated patients with 20 control patients not treated. At 1–5 years of follow-up, 60% of the treated patients met all of the criteria for success but none of the untreated patients did so. The results of this study clearly support the efficacy of inpatient multidiscipline treatment for chronic pain.

Lichter, R.L.; Hewson, J.K.; Radke, S.J.; and Blum, M.: Treatment of chronic low-back pain. A community-based comprehensive return-to-work physical rehabilitation program. Clin. Orthop. 190:115–123, 1984.

Using the described approach, the authors succeeded in returning 58% of patients to productivity. Deconditioning, fear, and poor biomechanics appeared to account for the chronicity of low back pain.

Nachemson, A.; Schultz, A.; and Andersson, G.: Mechanical effectiveness studies of lumbar spine orthoses. Scand. J. Rehabil. Med. [Suppl.] 9:139–149, 1983.

Good reference article to understand efficacy of various commonly used orthoses.

Wiesel, S.W.; Feffer, H.L.; and Rothman, R.H.: Industrial low-back pain: A prospective evaluation of a standardized diagnostic and treatment protocol. Spine 9:199–203, 1984.

The authors document that good medical care leads to cost savings in treating job-related low back pain. Unbiased medical surveillance leads to changes in behavior of both treating physicians and patients. The authors conclude that the outcome for most low back pain patients in industry is not as grim as previously perceived.

Philosophy

Nachemson, A.: Work for all: For those with low back pain as well. Clin. Orthop. 179:77–85, 1983.

The deleterious effects of long-term absence from activity and work are emphasized. Early, gradual, biomechanically controlled return to activity and work for the 80% of patients without objective findings is recommended.

Nachemson, A.: Recent advances in the treatment of low back pain. Int. Orthop. 9:1–10, 1985.

A stimulating state-of-the-art review article that focuses on the epidemic of low back pain.

29

Pelvis, Hip, and Femur: Pediatric Aspects

Congenital Problems

Dislocation of the Hip

This term actually applies only to a small number of abnormal hips. Most otherwise normal infants do not have a truly dislocated hip at birth. Only the occasional one with an antenatal dislocation or with a teratologic dislocation actually has true dislocation at birth. In the large majority of infants with abnormal hips, the hip can be subluxated or dislocated by appropriate manual examination. In some unusual circumstances, the hip can be very unstable and it will be difficult to determine whether the problem is a reducible dislocation or an unstable dislocatable hip. The basic underlying cause in these instances of instability most likely is a lax capsule, and the distinction between a subluxatable hip and a dislocatable hip is largely a matter of the degree of capsular laxity.

The so-called instability test of Barlow can identify those hips that can be displaced either partially (subluxatable) or completely (dislocatable) from the acetabulum. In the rather uncommon reducible hip dislocations that are present at birth in otherwise normal children, the femoral head is reduced in the acetabulum by the Ortolani maneuver, often referred to as the "jerk of entry." Adducting the thigh redislocates the femoral head, and this has been called the "jerk of exit."

Another term frequently used is "dysplasia." This usually refers to acetabular dysplasia but it also can be applied to abnormalities of the proximal femur. With a long-standing dislocation or subluxation of the hip, seldom is the growth of the proximal femoral component entirely normal, and there often is some degree of angular or rotational deformity. Acetabular dysplasia can be primary or secondary—the former being an inherited defect of the acetabulum, and the latter occurring through continuous abnormal pressure upon the developing acetabulum because of a persistent abnormal relationship between it and the femoral head.

A subluxatable or a dislocatable hip at birth frequently resolves in the first few days of life so that the Barlow test is no longer positive. The natural history of the dislocatable hip is shown in Figure 1. A crucial factor is the position in which the hip was held by its external environment. For example, it has been shown that in normal fetuses the hip can be dislocated over a period of hours by pressure applied with the hip either adducted or extended. Thus, treatment should be directed at reversing these forces.

Other abnormalities are known to occur in association with congenital dislocation of the hip. Patients having any of these abnormalities are termed high-risk infants. Among the most common is idiopathic muscular torticollis. The association of dislocation and acetabular dysplasia with torticollis may reach 15%, and many now recommend routine radiography of the pelvis in such children in addition to a carefully performed clinical examination. If the hip is normal on physical examination, the radiograph is best obtained at 3 to 4 months of age, after ossification of the ossific nucleus and when the radiograph has greater validity. Radiographs of newborns may be misleading.

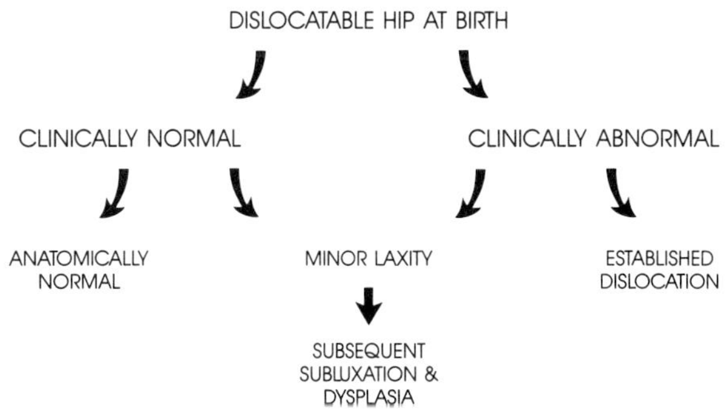

Figure 1

Natural history of dislocated hip at birth. At birth, hip may be assumed to be normal anatomically except for loose capsule which allows femoral head to be completely displaced from acetabulum. If femoral head is kept in acetabulum, it will become normal. If the femoral head is kept out of the acetabulum it will become an established dislocation with subsequent acetabular and femoral dysplasia. Capsule may tighten partially, keeping femoral head from dislocating completely but allowing it to slide partially out of the joint. This may occur to different degrees and will result in acetabular and femoral dysplasias of variable severity.

Organized screening programs for congenital dislocation of the hip have not been widespread in the United States, although all children born in a hospital are assumed to have been examined during the period they were in the newborn nursery. It was believed that all dislocated hips could be identified in the nursery; however, results to date indicate that this is not true. The reasons for these missed cases are not well established and must reflect the difficulty in establishing the presence of an unstable hip in the neonatal period. The most important factor to emerge from these studies is the need for continued examination of the infant throughout the first several months of life in order to discover the dislocated hip before walking age.

Ultrasonography is being evaluated to detect dislocation or subluxation of the hips. Some have shown that this technique is effective in detecting dislocations. Whether or not all radiologists will have the skill to do this and whether or not the time spent is worthwhile compared with a radiograph remains to be determined. Ultrasonography may have some value by reducing the need for repeated radiography (and increased exposure to radiation) during treatment. It has also been shown to be helpful in diagnosis when the child is in a cast or a Pavlik harness.

The goal of treatment for congenital dislocation of the

hip is well established but may be forgotten in the details of treatment. To obtain a stable and concentric reduction of the hip is the foremost goal (Fig. 2). Initially, in children under age 6 months, this may be done best by holding the hip in a physiologic position that encourages reduction. Currently, the Pavlik harness is perhaps the most popular form of treatment for these infants. It is physiologic, allowing motion of the joint and producing the desired position of flexion while at the same time limiting adduction. It is important that the Pavlik harness be properly applied so that forced abduction is avoided. Excessive abduction can cause an increased incidence of osteonecrosis. In addition, medial instability of the knee has been reported to result from improper positioning of the splint. It also must be remembered that these young children grow very rapidly; thus, all straps must be loosened as growth occurs, in order to avoid these complications as well as possible inferior dislocation of the hip.

When the Pavlik harness is used, stable reduction of the hip must be demonstrated early in the treatment (the first 2 to 4 weeks). If it does not occur, other methods such as closed reduction and cast application, with or without preliminary traction, are appropriate.

Use of triple diapers is totally inadequate to achieve reduction. The Frejka pillow does not produce the desired amount of flexion. Rigid devices such as malleable splints likewise often do not produce as much flexion as desired and have the danger of producing rigid abduction. Severe abduction with these (exceeding 45° to 60°) during treatment must be avoided. It has been shown that flexion of the hip does not interfere with the blood flow to the femoral head, whereas greater degrees of abduction decrease the blood flow and could produce osteonecrosis.

Occasionally it is difficult to determine accurately whether the reduction is concentric and stable. When doubt exists, an arthrogram may be indicated. Whether or not interposed soft tissue will resorb with time after a stable reduction remains an area of controversy. A recent large series has shown that, whenever the hip stands out as a result of soft tissue interposition, the hip joint probably will not develop normally. How much laterality can be accepted, however, has not been precisely determined. Nevertheless, it is essential to achieve a concentric stable reduction if the best results are to be obtained.

Occasionally, closed reduction either fails completely or is not concentric. Such patients are candidates for open reduction. For the child 12 to 18 months old, there is controversy over the best approach to reduction—open or closed? It is well established, however, that open reduction is always preferable when extreme unphysiologic positioning of the hip is required in order to maintain a reduction or when there is nonconcentricity of reduction.

The medial approach for open reduction of the hip has been reported to have a risk of osteonecrosis due to interruption of the medial circumflex artery. This can be largely avoided by carefully preserving the vessels, but the surgeon must be skilled in order to do so. In addition, it should be realized that the purpose of the medial approach is to remove or release those structures that prevent reduction. This includes the hourglass constriction of the capsule, a contracted iliopsoas tendon, the transverse acetabular ligament, occasionally an infolded limbus, and even an enlarged ligamentum teres. The anterior approach has the advantage of permitting removal of these same obstructions and at the same time permitting the capsulorrhaphy that will help to stabilize the reduction of the hip.

The value of preliminary traction before open reduction of the hip in the older child is being reevaluated. There is evidence that in older children open reduction may be a more conservative approach, especially when femoral shortening is implemented at the same time. This approach avoids prolonged hospitalization, and it can correct any proximal femoral deformities that are present. One study has shown that the incidence of osteonecrosis and the rate of redislocation may be substantially decreased by such an approach.

After treatment for the dislocated hip, regardless of age and treatment, follow-up care is extremely important in order to ensure normal development. The acetabulum may fail to develop normally. This may be the result of primary acetabular dysplasia or persistent subluxation of the hip. Many studies have shown that the acetabulum has remodeling capacity beyond 4 years of age and perhaps even until 8 years of age, provided that the femoral head remains concentrically located in the acetabulum and is stable. Two series have demonstrated that rotational osteotomy of the femur may stimulate such development. These studies suggest that persistent excessive femoral anteversion decreases the stimulus to develop the acetabulum after reduction of the hip.

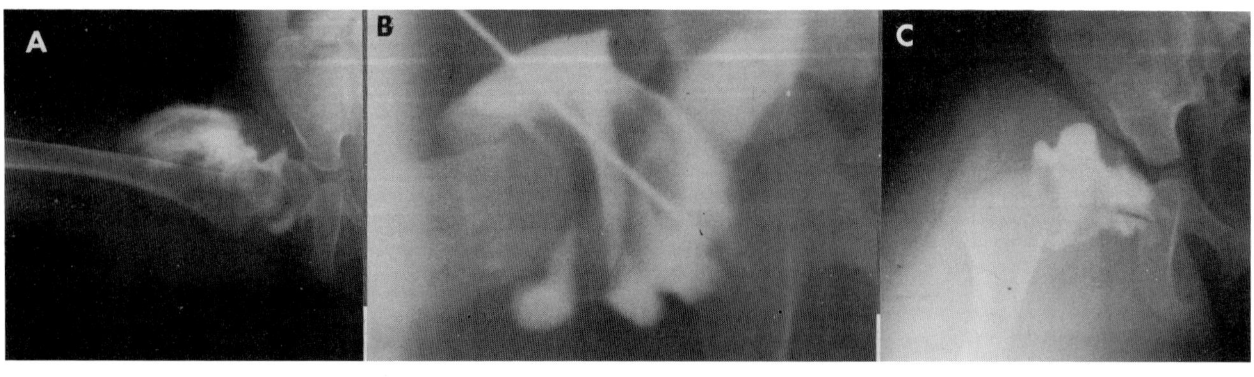

Figure 2

Arthrograms after closed reduction of congenital dislocation of hip. *A*, Good reduction. *B*, Adequate reduction with 4-mm-wide medial dye pool. *C*, Poor reduction with 9-mm dye pool. (From Race, C., and Herring, J.A. J. Pediatr. Orthop. 3:166–172, 1983. By permission of Raven Press.)

The need for routine pelvic osteotomy at the time of open reduction has also been seriously challenged by these studies. Pelvic osteotomy may be needed, and several types of osteotomy can be used, depending on the anatomic abnormality. However, published studies continue to emphasize how difficult the correct execution of these osteotomies can be.

Computed tomographic scanning can be very valuable in the evaluation of congenital dislocation of the hip. It can demonstrate adequacy of reduction well because the cast will not interfere. Its ability to show whether specific abnormalities exist, however, remains controversial as investigators report conflicting evidence regarding the configurations of the acetabulum and the proximal femur.

Proximal Femoral Focal Deficiency, Coxa Vara, and Congenital Short Femur

Perhaps no bone in the body manifests as much variation as the femur does, especially in its proximal portion. Proximal femoral focal deficiency (PFFD), coxa vara (both congenital and developmental), and congenital short femur represent a spectrum of the abnormalities that occur in this bone. In children born with PFFD, it is recognizable at birth. Congenital coxa vara may be recognized at birth or later, depending on the associated abnormalities. Developmental coxa vara is manifested at a later stage in life, usually around school age when children exhibit a waddling (Trendelenburg) gait. Congenital short femur also is variable in severity and may not be accurately identified until growth makes the limb length discrepancy noticeable.

One of the major problems in many of these anomalies is the coxa vara that often is associated with them. It is important to recognize which of these varus deformities will be progressive and which possibly will be self-correcting. In congenital coxa vara the angle formed by Hilgenreiner's line and a line through the epiphysis is a valuable guide (Fig. 3). An angle greater than 60° usually requires surgical correction; an angle less than 45° usually corrects spontaneously. Between these is a "gray zone." When associated with PFFD, progression of the coxa vara usually is not common whereas in developmental coxa vara, progressive varus is more likely.

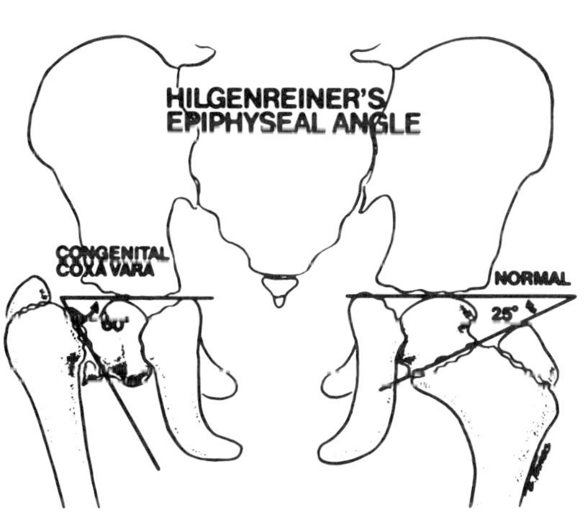

Figure 3

Determination of the Hilgenreiner epiphyseal angle, by using Hilgenreiner's line as the horizontal axis and a line through the defect adjacent to the metaphysis axis. (From Weinstein, J.N.; Kuo, K.N.; and Millar, E.A. J. Pediatr. Orthop. 4:70–77, 1984. By permission of Raven Press.)

Numerous classifications of PFFD, such as those of Aitken and Amstutz, have been devised for the deformity seen in the various disorders. A recent classification divides patients with PFFD and similar disorders into two groups—those who will require some form of amputation and those whose lower limbs may be preserved. Most of the patients in this latter group have a congenital short or hypoplastic femur. The knee is unstable in the anterior and posterior directions due to incompetence of the cruciate ligaments, and the head and neck of the femur may not be seen initially on radiographs but they are present as cartilaginous *Anlagen*. The varus deformity is nonprogressive. These patients have problems with limb length discrepancy. If the leg below the knee is normal, the overall discrepancy may be approximately 20%, or 15 to 20 cm, at skeletal maturity. In many of these patients, the limb can be lengthened successfully. In the group with true PFFD, various segments of the upper femur may be missing or hypoplastic. The aim of treatment in this group is to convert the limb to a prosthetic type. This usually requires knee arthrodesis and ankle disarticulation with possible reconstruction of the hip.

Developmental Problems

Legg-Calvé-Perthes Disease

This disease is most appropriately considered to be osteonecrosis of the femoral head. Although the necrosis implies that the cause is an interruption of vascularity, this has not yet been demonstrated conclusively.

The histopathologic characteristics in Legg-Calvé-Perthes disease are those of new bone laid down on dead bone. There is evidence suggesting that several episodes of necrosis have occurred, followed by new bone formation. Despite all of the circumstantial evidence pointing to systemic factors, such as low birth weight, small stature, and decreased bone age, nothing specific is known about the cause of this disorder.

One of the most interesting theories, however, is that there is a lack of the growth hormone metabolite somatomedin. It has been noted that this metabolite is decreased in children with Legg-Calvé-Perthes disease. This coincides well with some anthropomorphic measurements, including small stature, in certain parts of the body. The findings, in fact, are exactly opposite to those of acromegaly.

One popular theory is that Legg-Calvé-Perthes disease is due to an episode of synovitis that produces increased intracapsular pressure, thus partially or completely occluding the vascular supply to the femoral head. Experimental evidence in animals, however, does not support this thesis because it appears that the force necessary to do this and the duration for which the force must act are not attainable under physiologic circumstances (Fig. 4). In addition, a previous episode of synovitis has been recorded in only a small minority of patients.

Although the diagnosis of Legg-Calvé-Perthes disease appears to be obvious in the presence of the classic radiographic appearance, the differential diagnosis is very important. Many conditions, such as multiple epiphyseal

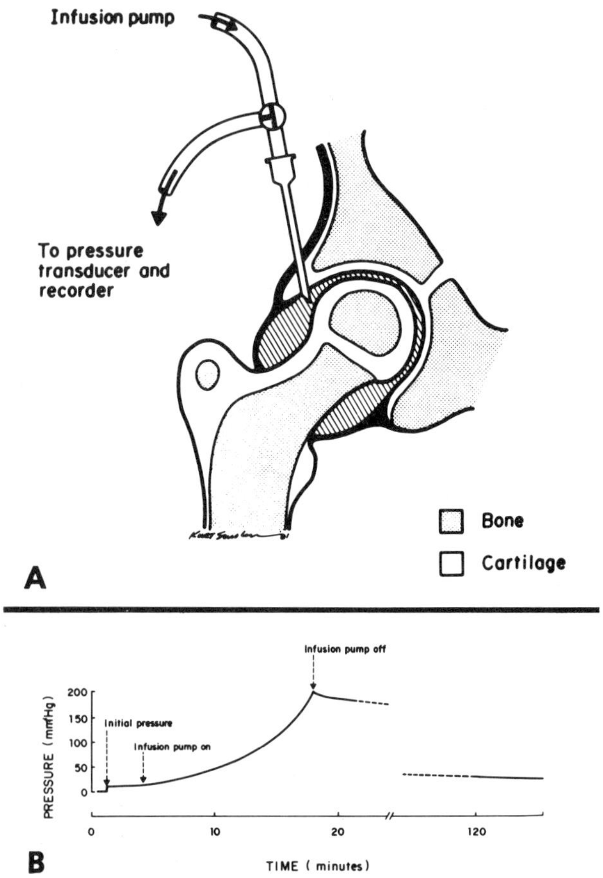

Figure 4

A, Diagram of method of tamponade production and monitoring of intra-articular pressure in pig's hip. *B,* Pressure in hip. (From Gershuni, D.H.; Hargens, A.R.; Lee, Y.-F.; Greenberg, E.N.; Zapf, R.; and Akeson, W.H. J. Pediatr. Orthop. 3:280–286, 1983. By permission of Raven Press.)

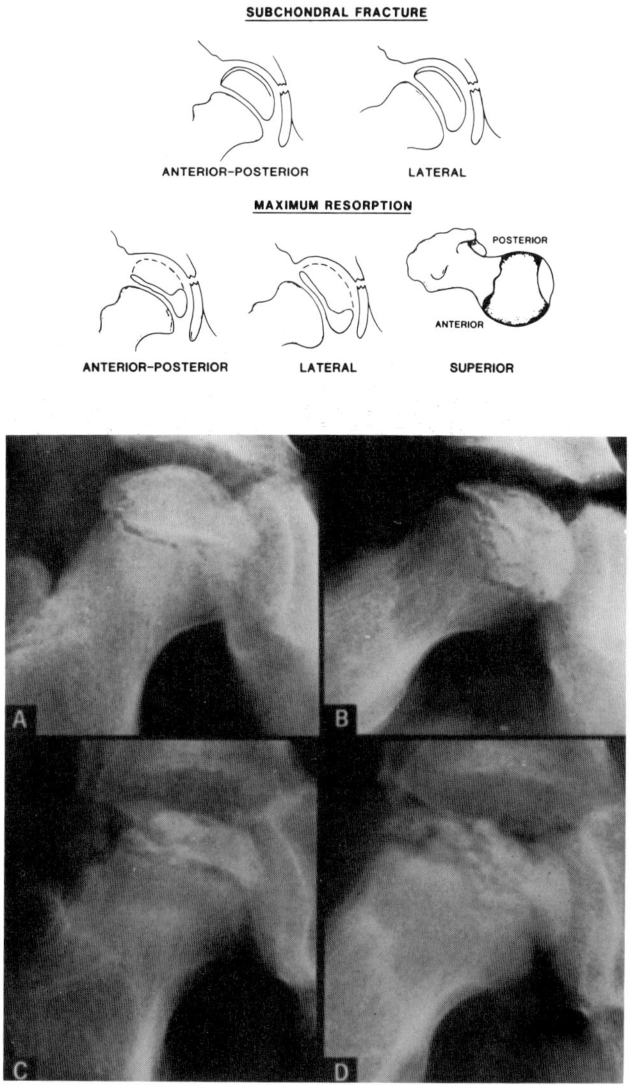

Figure 5

Upper, Schematic representation. *Lower, A* and *B,* Anteroposterior and lateral radiographs of right femoral head of 9-year-old boy with early Legg-Calvé-Perthes disease. On the anteroposterior radiograph the subchondral fracture extends to the lateral margin of the femoral head. *C* and *D,* Radiographic appearance 10 months later, at the stage of maximal resorption. (From Salter, R.B., and Thompson, G.H.: Legg-Calvé-Perthes disease: The prognostic significance of the subchondral fracture and a two-group classification of the femoral head involvement. J. Bone Joint Surg. 66A:479–489, 1984. By permission of the journal.)

dysplasia, spondyloepiphyseal dysplasia, and pseudoachondroplasia congenita and tarda, as well as other forms of osteonecrosis, may mimic this disorder. Two major features help to differentiate Legg-Calvé-Perthes disease from other conditions: even when both hips are involved, they are usually asymmetric, and the maturation of the pelvis is normal.

The value of bone scanning in Legg-Calvé-Perthes disease is controversial. Whether or not bone scanning can identify Legg-Calvé-Perthes disease accurately prior to any radiographic changes and whether or not it can accurately demonstrate the amount of femoral head involvement are not yet established. The subchondral fracture, when present, is a reasonably accurate reflection of the extent of the disease (Fig. 5). To demonstrate this best, the radiograph is taken with the patient in the frog position with 45° of flexion rather than 90° of flexion. If the subchondral fracture extends halfway across the head of the femur, it can be assumed that the involvement of the head will be the same. Thus, a good prognostic index can be obtained rather early, and it may influence treatment. Magnetic resonance imaging is being explored for the diagnosis of Legg-Calvé-Perthes disease. It has two advantages in that it gives an arthrogram-like image of the hip and, at the same time, has the ability to differentiate necrotic from live marrow. Its clinical usefulness is yet to be established, however.

Although Legg-Calvé-Perthes disease has often been thought to have a minimal effect on the longevity of the hip, a recent study indicates that there is a high incidence of degenerative hip disease developing in later years. At the average age of 56 years, only 40% had good hip function (Iowa hip rating of 80 or better); a large percentage of these patients had undergone total hip arthroplasty or had serious hip problems. On the other hand, only a small percentage of patients who had Legg-Calvé-Perthes disease appear to have pain as a predominant symptom within the first 3 decades of life.

The natural history of Legg-Calvé-Perthes disease clearly implicates one factor that portends a poor result in later life—age at onset of the disease. Those with onset at age 8 or less generally have done well; those whose age at onset is more than 8 generally do poorly. In addition, the length of follow-up is important because, the longer the patients are followed, the greater is the likelihood that they will have hip disease. It would appear that a follow-up of at least 40 years, and preferably more, is necessary in order to determine the ultimate outcome of Legg-Calvé-Perthes disease.

The treatment of Legg-Calvé-Perthes disease is still based on the principle of femoral head containment with motion. The concept of containment is that, if the cartilage model of the femoral head is kept spherical by containment within the acetabulum and is subject to physiologic motion, ossification will then occur in this cartilage model, thus producing congruency of the femoral head within the acetabulum.

The majority of patients who have group I or group II Legg-Calvé-Perthes disease and maintain good motion can be just observed without any special treatment. However, those children who present with group III or IV Legg-Calvé-Perthes disease most likely will need treatment. For these children, use of a brace is a well-accepted method of treatment, with the Atlanta Scottish Rite orthosis currently being the one most commonly used. This brace produces abduction and some flexion of the hip while at the same time permitting good mobility of the child and interfering little with function. However, it produces no inward rotation. The use of the brace requires that full motion, especially full abduction, be obtained prior to and during wearing of the brace. The brace may be unsuitable for children 10 years old or older.

Petrie's cast treatment is another form of treatment that is very successful in maintaining abduction and hip function, although it is difficult to obtain patient compliance and acceptability. It provides a reasonable alternative for the patient who does not accept the brace treatment but who is not a candidate for or refuses surgical treatment.

Surgical treatment for Legg-Calvé-Perthes disease has been used selectively for the past 15 years. Initially it was thought to have a salubrious biologic effect on healing of the necrotic head; however, this has now been challenged by a recent study that showed healing to be no quicker in those who underwent operation than in controls treated nonoperatively. One of the potential problems implicit in proximal femoral varus rotation osteotomy is increased shortening of the limb. Frequently, patients with group III or IV disease, who have the most serious hip involvement, are those who are most likely to have early closure of the epiphyseal plate. Thus, the production of varus for treatment purposes may produce a permanent neck shaft varus deformity. This results in coxa vara, trochanteric "overgrowth," and shortening of the limb. The role of pelvic osteotomy for Legg-Calvé-Perthes disease is not clearly defined. One of the drawbacks is the difficulty of performing this procedure.

One of the most common operations done for the residual effects of Legg-Calvé-Perthes disease is distal transfer of the greater trochanter. This operation is usually necessary in children age 8 years or more who have had arrest of the physeal growth of the femoral head. At this stage, early surgical arrest of the trochanter does not produce the desired biomechanical neck/trochanter relationship, and therefore lateral and distal transfer of the trochanter often becomes necessary. This should be done only in patients who are symptomatic with evidence of abductor pain on fatigue or who have a positive Trendelenburg test.

Slipped Capital Femoral Epiphysis

Slipped capital femoral epiphysis is a disorder of the proximal epiphysis of the femur that occurs during puberty. In this disorder, the growth plate becomes weakened and the epiphysis displaces from the neck of the femur. The femoral head remains in the acetabulum, thus migrating posteriorly on the neck of the femur. In the late stages of this process, the femoral shaft begins to migrate superiorly and the femoral head rotates more inferiorly.

Although the cause of slipped capital femoral epiphysis is unknown, much attention has been given to the hormonal aspects of this disease because it occurs during puberty, a time of sexual maturation and hormone change. The most common associated endocrinopathy is hypothyroidism. There is a strong familial pattern in slipped capital femoral epiphysis. Recent reports clearly demonstrate that the incidence among family members is much higher than that in the general population.

A causal role of the immune system in this disorder has recently been proposed. Although the mechanism by which this acts remains unclear, it appears that the synovitis associated with this disease involves an immune complex, an observation that differs from the synovitis in most other orthopaedic diseases. The role played by this mechanism in the pathology of the disease is not yet understood.

Osteonecrosis and chondrolysis are the principal causes of a bad result from slipped capital femoral epiphysis. Osteonecrosis is a rare complication in an untreated chronic case, although it occurs frequently in the acute case. Chondrolysis occurring prior to treatment likewise is unusual and it most commonly follows treatment for slipped capital femoral epiphysis.

The treatment of slipped capital femoral epiphysis has changed substantially in the past 30 years. Prophylactic pinning of the opposite asymptomatic hip has been abandoned. The opposite hip manifests an epiphyseal slip 25% of the time, and in approximately 10% to 15% of these the problem will be apparent at the time of the initial diagnosis.

In situ pinning of the slipped capital femoral epiphysis is currently the most accepted form of treatment. Proper attention to the anatomy of slipped capital femoral epiphysis will allow accurate *in situ* pinning. Many of the complications and mistakes of this form of treatment have been well analyzed. The problem of unrecognized pin penetration and the possible consequence of chondrolysis are now well known. To what extent pin penetration can contribute to chondolysis is not clearly established, but the fact that pin penetration can occur and be unrecognized on routine radiography is important.

Because of recent reports outlining the problems of pin penetration, capital femoral epiphysiodesis is gaining some support. It has the disadvantage of being a much larger operation than *in situ* pinning; it requires cast immobilization and is fraught with the same dangers as *in situ* pinning in that the bone graft, like a pin, can miss the epiphyseal plate or can penetrate the joint.

Acute slips have a higher incidence of osteonecrosis, most likely due to the sudden displacement of the femoral head and disruption of the vessels. Whether or not the necrosis can be prevented by prompt reduction of the head or other methods of treatment is controversial.

In severe displacement of the femoral head, proximal femoral osteotomy has been commonly recommended. However, recent evidence has demonstrated that substantial remodeling of the femoral head and neck can occur after *in situ* pinning, and it has been concluded therefore that osteotomy need not be done as frequently as in the past. In addition, there is evidence that those patients who have had osteotomy may have more complications than those who have had a severe slip pinned *in situ*. Osteotomy must be considered, however, for the patient who has a severe slip with deformity and reduced hip motion. The osteotomy may be performed in the region of the femoral neck, but a high incidence of osteonecrosis may be associated with it. Intertrochanteric osteotomy is by far the most common method used to correct displacement of the femoral head and has the advantage of safety. However, an increased incidence of chondrolysis, which frequently appears to be mild and transient, has been associated with this osteotomy.

In the treatment of chondrolysis, the clinician should maintain a degree of optimism. The literature indicates that at least one-third of these patients will do very well with the standard methods of treatment consisting of traction, motion, and oral administration of salicylates. An additional large percentage will obtain a reasonably symptomatic result despite some reduction of hip motion.

In salvaging the severe problems relating to chondrolysis or osteonecrosis, arthrodesis is the treatment of choice. It is the one solution that produces a stable, nonpainful hip that later can be converted to an arthroplasty. Recent follow-up studies have shown that hip fusion holds up well for many years when done in young patients. Arthroplasty, or total hip replacement, should be used only for those who have severe bilateral involvement.

Infection

Hip

Infection of the hip in an infant or child is a major problem. In part this is due to difficulty in diagnosis, especially in the neonate in whom early diagnosis is of extreme importance. The reason for this is the unique anatomy of the femoral head.

In infancy, before the epiphyseal plate is formed, the vessels from the metaphysis penetrate directly into the cartilage precursor of the femoral head. Infection in this area in the neonate or infant quickly destroys the epiphyseal growth centers and ruptures into the joint, destroying or deforming the joint. After epiphyseal plate formation, the time frame is slightly different but the consequence is the same if diagnosis is not made promptly because the metaphysis of the femoral neck, where osteomyelitis frequently begins, is intra-articular.

The early diagnosis of osteomyelitis of the femoral neck and septic arthritis of the hip relies on the clinician's acuity, especially in the neonate because the signs of infection often will be absent. Neonates with sepsis frequently are examined without complete orthopaedic evaluation of the hip joints which frequently are involved in these infants. Because of the neonate's inability to produce the inflammatory response to infection, the complete blood cell count and temperature may be normal and the signs of irritation in the hip joint may be minimal. Likewise, bone scanning frequently will fail to detect areas of infection in the neonate because of the lack of the inflammatory response.

The treatment of this condition is not controversial. Prompt surgical drainage along with administration of an appropriate antimicrobial agent is the preferred treatment. Whether or not the joint is drained through the anterior or posterior approach remains a matter of preference. Advantages of the anterior approach are that the hole in the capsule will be anteriorly where the hip is unlikely to dislocate, the incision is away from the blood supply which runs in the posterior retinaculum of the hip, and the patient is in the supine position during operation. Needle aspiration of the hip cannot replace surgery for drainage, not only because debridement of the hip is inadequate but also because repeated aspiration of the infant's hip can be difficult.

Selection of antimicrobials before culture results are available is difficult (Table 1). In the neonate, several organisms are possible. In the infant, *Haemophilus influenzae* and *Staphylococcus aureus* must be considered. In both, coexisting meningitis may be present, and therefore the antimicrobial should be one that can cross the blood-brain barrier.

Sacroiliac Joint

Osteomyelitis or septic arthritis in the sacroiliac region is difficult to diagnose. One common source of confusion is septic arthritis of the hip. However, this can be differentiated by the fact that, with sacroiliac involvement, the rotation of the hip in flexion remains free in internal rotation and often is somewhat painful on forced external rotation (when the sacroiliac joint is strained). This is in contrast to the septic hip, in which internal rotation produces pain and is limited. Technetium bone scanning is extremely valuable in localizing the area of involvement

Table 1. Most Likely Organisms Causing Bone and Joint Infections in Different Age Groups

Organism	Antimicrobial agent*
Neonate	
β-Streptococci	Ampicillin and gentamicin
Gram-negative bacteria	
Candida	
Staphylococcus aureus	
Any other	
Infant	
S. aureus	Cefuroxime
Haemophilus influenzae	
Child	
S. aureus†	Oxacillin
(*Neisseria gonorrhoeae*)	Nafcillin
	Cefazolin
	Cephaprin

*Infants frequently will not show signs of meningitis which may be present at the same time as joint sepsis. Therefore, meningitis must either be ruled out by spinal tap or an antimicrobial that crosses the blood-brain barrier must be used.
†*S. aureus* is the only organism consistently causing acute hematogenous osteomyelitis in children.

in infections about the pelvis where examination is difficult and plain radiographs frequently fail to demonstrate soft tissue swelling.

Treatment of sacroiliac osteomyelitis or septic arthritis usually does not require surgical drainage. Aspiration of the joint to obtain an organism, although frequently difficult and requiring general anesthesia, is very helpful (will most frequently yield *S. aureus*) in those cases in which the course is not typical, the resolution of the disease is not prompt, or unusual findings are noted on radiographs or physical examination. Most often, sacroiliac sepsis can be treated by the use of an antistaphylococcal antimicrobial agents. The morbidity from this particular disorder is low.

Trauma

Traumatic dislocation of the hip in children differs substantially in some respects from dislocation in the adult. Dislocation of the hip occurs with a less violent force in young children than in older children. A fall from a bicycle is a rather common cause of dislocation in children. In the older child and adolescent, however, the dislocation may be associated with the same concomitant clinical problems that are seen in adults—namely, head, chest, and abdominal trauma.

Children with trisomy 21 often suffer from dysplasia and dislocation of the hip. It has been estimated that approximately 1 child in 20 with trisomy 21 will have a dislocated hip by age 10 years. The dislocation frequently requires little force. Most often it is associated with an anatomic abnormality such as acetabular dysplasia along with excessive capsular laxity. Recommended treatment is open reduction, capsular plication, and pelvic or femoral osteotomy.

In reducing the traumatically dislocated hip in children, gentleness is essential in order to avoid the reported complication of displacement of the femoral capital epiphysis.

In a review of 33 children with traumatic dislocation of the hip, the most frequent complication encountered was soft tissue interposition, often requiring arthrotomy. Osteonecrosis occurs much less commonly than in the adult, and redislocation of the hip likewise is less common because the posterior acetabular rim rarely is fractured and the reduced hip therefore is basically stable.

Hip Fracture

Fracture of the hip in childhood is similar in many features to dislocation of the hip in that it often occurs with less violent force in the younger child. Most often, fracture occurs with pathologic conditions of the proximal femur such as severe osteopenia or benign neoplasm but it can occur from apparently minor injuries as well. When it occurs as a result of a motor vehicle accident or other severe trauma, the usual concern for concomitant head, chest, and abdominal trauma must be exercised.

Transepiphyseal fractures of the femoral neck in childhood carry a guarded prognosis because of the substantially increased incidence of osteonecrosis. Therefore, prompt reduction with internal fixation is advised. Transcervical fractures will be displaced in 80% of cases and they require accurate closed reduction and internal fixation. If accurate reduction cannot be obtained closed, open reduction is preferred. Cervicotrochanteric fractures or basal neck fractures are treated according to the same guidelines.

Intertrochanteric fractures, the least common of all, account for only 10% of all hip fractures in childhood and have the fewest complications. Traditionally, traction is the recommended treatment for these; however, many children, especially when older, do better with internal fixation and earlier mobilization.

Osteonecrosis is a serious complication of fracture of the proximal femur in childhood and occurs frequently. It appears to be related to displacement of the fracture more than to any other single factor. Nonunion and malunion with coxa vara often result from basal neck fractures and transcervical fractures. When present, they are best treated by a valgus-producing osteotomy to decrease the shear stresses and achieve compression of the proximal fragment on the distal fragment.

Femoral Shaft Fracture

Fracture of the femoral shaft is one of the most common serious fractures that children incur. The classic treatment of this fracture—traction until early callus forms, and then spica cast immobilization—has been challenged, partly because of economic circumstances and partly because of continued reports on the efficacy of early cast immobilization for these fractures. In infants and young children, a long spiral fracture is often easily reduced and immobilized in the spica cast within a day or two after injury. In the older child, between ages 2 and 10, most femoral shaft fractures can be reduced and effectively held in a cast within a few days after injury. Healing is prompt, angulation can be minimized by good cast application (under general anesthesia if necessary), and growth stimulation of the involved limb usually compensates for overriding that may be present (Fig. 6).

The use of internal fixation for fractures of the diaphysis of the femur in childhood is being explored. This is especially important in patients with head injury. The tendency to underestimate the recovery in such children often results in neglect of their associated femoral fractures. After recovery from their brain injury, some children are left with an overly shortened or deformed femur because of inadequate treatment. The use of an external fixator or an intramedullary rod in these children obviates many of the problems and does not interfere with subsequent growth of the limb.

Despite the common occurrence of these fractures, complications are rare. However, the clinician must be aware of them. Intimal tear of the femoral artery due to the fracture will result in vascular embarrassment in the foot and leg. This may not be apparent for several hours to days. Angular deformity and shortening must be watched for. Contrary to common belief, rotational deformity has been shown to correct itself substantially when the fracture occurs in young children.

Paralytic Problems

Cerebral Palsy

Children affected with cerebral palsy—especially spastic quadriplegia and, less frequently, spastic diplegia or hemiplegia—frequently will experience subluxation or dislocation of the hip. This is due to a combination of factors. Foremost among these is abnormal muscle balance with spastic adduction and flexion of the hip in the absence of

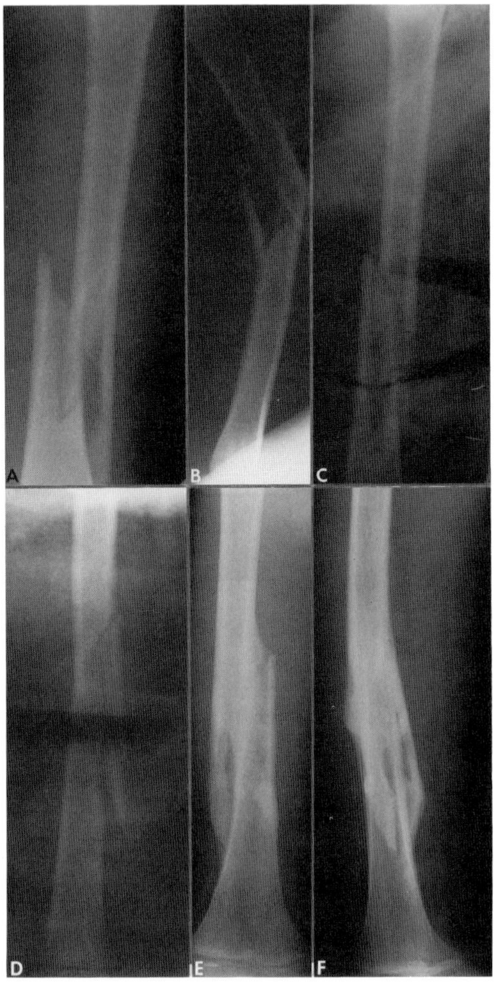

Figure 6

Anteroposterior and lateral radiographs of 9-year-old boy. *A* and *B*, Comminuted spiral oblique fracture of midfemur. *C* and *D*, Reduction achieved on day after fracture. Wedging of the cast was done to correct posterior and lateral angulation. *E* and *F*, At 3 months after fracture there has been no increase in the 1 cm of shortening accepted at the time of casting. (From Henderson, O.L.; Morrissy, R.T.; Gerdes, M.H.; and McCarthy, R.E. J. Pediatr. Orthop. 4:16–21, 1984. By permission of Raven Press.)

voluntary functional abductors and extensors. The result is a hip that gradually extrudes, causing acetabular dysplasia and subsequent subluxation and dislocation.

In treating this disorder, physical therapy appears to be of little value, and in older patients with established subluxation it may be harmful. Prophylactic bracing usually is futile because of the extremely strong muscular forces involved and the inability to brace the patient constantly without interfering with subsequent development. Muscle-release operations have proved effective early, prior to or just at the beginning of lateral migration of the femoral head as demonstrated radiographically. Whether or not it is best to perform adductor myotomy and tenomyotomy or to transfer the adductor muscles posteriorly has been a matter of controversy. Several recent studies suggest that there is no difference in the long-term outcome.

In the later established subluxation, with severe femoral anteversion, coxa valga, or acetabular dysplasia present, surgical correction of deformities is advisable. It is possible, and probably preferable, to correct all of the difficulties at the same time in those patients who have severe subluxation. If the hip is dislocated, femoral shortening may be necessary to bring the head back into the acetabulum. Muscle release should be carried out to ensure that good abduction of the hip is possible. Capsulorrhaphy should be done and the bony anatomy on both sides of the joint should be corrected. Salters' innominate osteotomy should be used cautiously because it often will decrease coverage posteriorly and increase it anteriorly where it is not needed. In many children who are sitters or who have flexion contractures, dislocation will occur posteriorly and thus this operation has substantial drawbacks compared with the Pemberton osteotomy, the shelf procedure, or the Chiari osteotomy in the older child.

In performing surgical muscle release in the adductor region of the child with cerebral palsy, complications are infrequent. A recent report of bilateral femoral head osteonecrosis after adductor and iliopsoas release warns of the position of the medial circumflex artery which supplies the femoral head. Just as in the medial approach to open reduction of the congenitally dislocated hip, this vessel may be injured in this approach, causing osteonecrosis.

Myelomeningocele

In myelomeningocele the hip is a frequent source of difficulty and controversy. Subluxation and dislocation are most common when it is at low lumbar level, and in these patients the incidence of subluxation or dislocation exceeds 50%. In those with higher levels of paralysis, the incidence of dislocation is often less and not of the same significance. In children with lower levels of paralysis, and in whom active abduction or extension is present, the incidence of dislocation decreases dramatically. It is the marginal walker who is most likely to experience subluxation or dislocation.

Whether or not the dislocation influences the patient's ability to walk is a matter of controversy. Recent studies indicate that hip dislocation *per se* does not appear to be a factor in determining the long-term likelihood of ambulation. Nevertheless, there are no studies that address the energy consumption of walking with and without a dislocated hip. The factors that appear to be most important in ambulation are motivation, presence or absence of obesity, and subsequent musculoskeletal deformity.

If the decision is made to treat a subluxating or dislocating hip, all anatomic abnormalities must be corrected, preferably at the same time. Foremost among these is the abnormal pull of the muscles on the hip. Recent reports indicate that posterior iliopsoas muscle transfer may be helpful in myelodysplasia in order to stabilize the hip. It should be performed only if all of the bony abnormalities of the acetabulum and proximal femur have been corrected. Correction of all abnormal anatomic factors may require acetabular osteotomy, femoral osteotomy, muscle transfer, and capsulorrhaphy.

Annotated Bibliography

Congenital Problems

Congenital Dislocation of the Hip

Berkeley, M.E.; Dickson, J.H.; Cain, T.E.; and Donovan, M.M.: Surgical therapy for congenital dislocation of the hip in patients who are twelve to thirty-six months old. J. Bone Joint Surg. 66A:412–420, 1984.

Fifty-one consecutive congenitally dislocated hips, all in children between 12 and 36 months of age, were studied prospectively. Acetabular osteotomy was done only as needed based on intraoperative assessment. Only two femoral shortenings were performed, and only three patients needed subsequent surgical treatment at follow-up.

Blockey, N.J.: Derotation osteotomy in the management of congenital dislocation of the hip. J. Bone Joint Surg. 66B:485–490, 1984.

One hundred seventeen congenitally dislocated hips treated by closed reduction and femoral rotational osteotomy, but not acetabular osteotomy, were analyzed 18 to 27 years after operation. The author suggests that rotational osteotomy may be sufficient to stimulate proper acetabular development.

Clarke, N.M.P.; Harcke, H.T.; McHugh, P.; Lee, M.S.; Borns, P.F.; and MacEwen, G.D.: Real-time ultrasound in the diagnosis of congenital dislocation and dysplasia of the hip. J. Bone Joint Surg. 67B:406–412, 1985.

In 259 hips examined by real-time ultrasonography, no dislocations were missed; there were three false-negatives and four false-positives. Results were not quite as good when patients were examined in a cast or Pavlik harness.

Gillespie, R., and Torode, I.P.: Classification and management of congenital abnormalities of the femur. J. Bone Joint Surg. 65B:557–568, 1983.

A classification is proposed for all of the femoral congenital abnormalities. One group of patients are those who have functional joints and are candidates for salvage of the limb. The second group are those with true proximal focal femoral deficiency whose legs cannot be equalized and in whom the treatment goal is to prepare the limb for better fitting of a prosthesis.

Iwasaki, K.: Treatment of congenital dislocation of the hip by the Pavlik harness: Mechanism of reduction and usage. J. Bone Joint Surg. 65A:760–767, 1983.

Two groups of children were treated with a Pavlik harness, one as inpatients and one as outpatients. The osteonecrosis rate was 28% for inpatients and 7.2% for outpatients.

Race, C., and Herring, J.A.: Congenital dislocation of the hip: An evaluation of closed reduction. J. Pediatr. Orthop. 3:166–172, 1983.

A series of congenital dislocated hips treated by closed reduction was assessed on the basis of criteria judging the adequacy of reduction. The less adequate the reduction, the more time was necessary to hold the reduction, the worse was acetabular remodeling, and the worse was the result at follow-up.

Schoenecker, P.L., and Strecker, W.B.: Congenital dislocation of the hip in children: Comparison of the effects of femoral shortening and of skeletal traction in treatment. J. Bone Joint Surg. 66A:21–27, 1984.

Two groups of open reduction of the hip are compared: one using femoral shortening and the other using preoperative traction. Osteonecrosis and redislocation rates were higher in the traction group.

Weinstein, J.N.; Kuo, K.N.; and Millar, E.A.: Congenital coxa vara. A retrospective review. J. Pediatr. Orthop. 4:70–77, 1984.

A concept of measuring the degree of coxa vara by an angle formed by Hilgenreiner's line and the epiphyseal plate is described. The authors correlate this with the need for corrective surgery.

Developmental Problems

Legg-Calvé-Perthes Disease

Clancy, M., and Steel, H.H.: The effect of an incomplete intertrochanteric osteotomy on Legg-Calvé-Perthes disease. J. Bone Joint Surg. 67A:213–216, 1985.

Fifty-three patients, over a 10-year period, had incomplete femoral osteotomy for Legg-Calvé-Perthes disease. The time for healing in these patients was no different than that in a control group treated nonoperatively.

Gershuni, D.H.; Hargens, A.R.; Lee, Y.-F.; Greenberg, E.N.; Zapf, R.; and Akeson, W.H.: The questionable significance of hip joint tamponade in producing osteonecrosis in Legg-Calvé-Perthes syndrome. J. Pediatr. Orthop. 3:280–286, 1983.

Utilizing a pig model, the authors were unable to produce osteonecrosis or to obtain pressures sufficiently high to produce osteonecrosis by induction of synovitis or infusion of plasma into the hip joint.

McAndrew, M.P., and Weinstein, S.L.: A long-term follow-up of Legg-Calvé-Perthes disease. J. Bone Joint Surg. 66A:860–869, 1984.

A long-term review of 37 hips affected by Legg-Calvé-Perthes disease showed that greater time of follow-up led to an increasing incidence of arthroplasty and osteoarthritis. The major determinant as to who did well in the long term was age at onset of disease, with age 8 years being the dividing point.

Slipped Capital Femoral Epiphysis

Bennet, G.C.; Koreska, J.; and Rang, M.: Pin placement in slipped capital femoral epiphysis. J. Pediatr. Orthop. 4:574–578, 1984.

The authors were unable to demonstrate any effect of pin penetration on chondrolysis in 148 slipped epiphyses examined. They did note, however, that pin penetration was more common than was initially thought from routine radiographs.

Ingram, A.J.; Clarke, M.S.; Clark, C.S., Jr.; and Marshall, W.R.: Chondrolysis complicating slipped capital femoral epiphysis. Clin. Orthop. 165:99–109, 1982.

Chondrolysis complicated 24% of 329 slipped epiphyses reviewed. Factors that increased the risk were: being female, being black, acute-on-chronic slip, open reduction, femoral neck osteotomy, trochanteric osteotomy, and pin penetration.

Morrissy, R.T.; Steele, R.W.; and Gerdes, M.H.: Localised immune complexes and slipped upper femoral epiphysis. J. Bone Joint Surg. 65B:574–579, 1983.

Synovial fluid from 10 of 11 patients with slipped capital femoral epiphysis revealed immune complex by the Raji cell assay in the C1q-binding assay. This was not found in other diseases with synovitis that were studied, suggesting that the synovitis in slipped capital femoral epiphysis is different.

Rennie, A.M.: The inheritance of slipped upper femoral epiphysis. J. Bone Joint Surg. 64B:180–184, 1982.

A review of 214 cases of slipped capital femoral epiphysis establishes that the incidence is higher in families of patients with this disorder than would be expected in the general population.

Weiner, D.S.; Weiner, S.; Melby, A.; and Hoyt, W.A., Jr.: A 30-year experience with bone graft epiphysiodesis in the treatment of slipped capital femoral epiphysis. J. Pediatr. Orthop. 4:145–152, 1984.

A large series of bone graft epiphysiodesis is reviewed. In four patients, slip recurred; there were two cases of osteonecrosis and one case of cartilage necrosis.

Hip Infection

Fabry, G., and Meire, E.: Septic arthritis of the hip in children: Poor results after late and inadequate treatment. J. Pediatr. Orthop. 3:461–466, 1983.

Long-term follow-up of children with septic arthritis of the hip shows that older children tend to do better; neonates do very poorly. The major factor in outcome is the time elapsed between the onset of symptoms and the beginning of adequate treatment.

Trauma

Hip Dislocation

Bennet, G.C.; Rang, M.; Roye, D.P.; and Aprin, H.: Dislocation of the hip in trisomy 21. J. Bone Joint Surg. 64B:289–294, 1982.

Children with Down syndrome are at risk for dislocation of the hip with almost 1 in 20 children having a dislocation by age 10. Correction of the anatomic abnormalities is recommended.

Offierski, C.M.: Traumatic dislocation of the hip in children. J. Bone Joint Surg. 63B:194–197, 1981.

The most common complication in this series of traumatic hip dislocations in children was interposition of soft tissue, requiring open reduction. Other complications resulted from missed injuries in the child with multiple injuries.

Hip Fracture

Malkawi, H.; Shannak, A.; and Amr, S.: Surgical treatment of pathological subtrochanteric fractures due to benign lesions in children and adolescents. J. Pediatr. Orthop. 4:63–69, 1984.

From a review of 12 children with pathologic subtrochanteric fractures, the authors conclude that these fractures are best treated by internal fixation which allows more thorough resection of the tumor.

Morrissy, R.T.: Fractured hip in childhood. *In* AAOS Instructional Course Lectures. XXXIII:229–241, 1984. St. Louis, C.V. Mosby, 1984.

This review article summarizes the major series on fractured hip in childhood and analyzes the results. Recommendations are given for treatment of various types of fracture in childhood.

Femoral Shaft Fracture

Hägglund, G.; Hansson, L.I.; and Norman, O.: Correction by growth of rotational deformity after femoral fracture in children. Acta Orthop. Scand. 54:858–861, 1983.

Repeated anteversion measurements in a series of femoral shaft fractures studied over a 10-year period shows that rotational deformity can correct itself.

Henderson, O.L.; Morrissy, R.T.; Gerdes, M.H.; and McCarthy, R.E.: Early casting of femoral shaft fractures in children. J. Pediatr. Orthop. 4:16–21, 1984.

In a prospective series, it is shown that, with early selective cast treatment, femoral shaft fractures in childhood can be treated adequately, at lower cost, and with no increase in complications.

Ziv, I., and Rang, M.: Treatment of femoral fracture in the child with head injury. J. Bone Joint Surg. 65B:276–278, 1983.

In a series of children with head injury and fractured femur, 84% of the children who had been in deep coma eventually were able to walk. Malunion was present in 6 of 34 fractures treated by traction and in none of the 16 that had intramedullary fixation.

Paralytic Problems

Cerebral Palsy

Schultz, R.S.; Chamberlain, S.E.; and Stevens, P.M.: Radiographic comparison of adductor procedures in cerebral palsied hips. J. Pediatr. Orthop. 4:741–744, 1984.

A series of adductor tenotomy and myomotomies and adductor transfers was compared. In follow-up, there appeared to be no difference between the two procedures in their effectiveness in reducing the lateral migration of the hip.

Zuckerman, J.D.; Staheli, L.T.; and McLaughlin, J.F.: Acetabular augmentation for progressive hip subluxation in cerebral palsy. J. Pediatr. Orthop. 4:436–442, 1984.

A technique of acetabular augmentation that significantly decreases the CE angle is reported in cerebral palsy patients. The results of this technique over a 13-year period have been good.

Myelomeningocele

Asher, M., and Olson, J.: Factors affecting the ambulatory status of patients with spina bifida cystica. J. Bone Joint Surg. 65A:350–356, 1983.

Neurologic level remains the most significant factor in ambulation. Other factors that made a difference in the low lumbar levels were motivation, obesity, and musculoskeletal deformity.

Lee, E.H., and Carroll, N.C.: Hip stability and ambulatory status in myelomeningocele. J. Pediatr. Orthop. 5:522–527, 1985.

Based on a review of 66 unstable hips, the authors recommend that an unstable hip be reduced in a child who potentially could walk. The recommended technique is to correct all anatomic problems at the same operation.

30 Trauma: Pelvis and Acetabulum

The topics included in this chapter are anatomy of the pelvis, overall management of patients who have pelvic injury, and orthopaedic management of patients with pelvic and acetabular fractures.

Anatomy

Skeletal

The pelvis is divided into the false and the true pelvis. The false pelvis is that portion above the arcuate and iliopectineal lines and promontory of the sacrum; it houses the caudal extent of the abdominal viscera. The true pelvis is below the iliopectineal and arcuate lines and promontory of the sacrum and contains the reproductive organs as well as the distal segments of the urinary and digestive systems.

Biomechanically, the pelvis can be considered to be a system of tie arches that support the spine in the upright position; forces are transmitted from the femoral heads along the arcuate line to the sacroiliac joints and then to the spinal column. This tie arch is supported by a tension-band type of arch through the iliopectineal line and symphysis pubis. In the sitting position, forces are transmitted from the ischial tuberosities through the ischium and arcuate lines to the sacrum and spine. This main arch is connected by an accessory tie arch made up of the pubis and the inferior pubic rami.

The innominate bone is described as formed by the ilium and the anterior and posterior columns. The acetabulum can be described as being situated in the "open arms of an inverted Y" formed by the anterior and posterior columns which are joined together inferiorly by an ischiopubic tie bar.

The shape of the female pelvis is different from that of the male. The iliac wings are more vertical and the symphysis is broader. The female's true pelvis is broader and more arcuate in contour than the male's. This broader, laterally curving pelvis makes surgical access to the true pelvis somewhat easier in the female than in the male.

Joints and Ligaments

The bones that form the pelvis are held together by a complex system of ligaments that span the symphysis pubis in front and the sacroiliac joints in back, as well as accessory ligaments attaching the ilium to the sacrum. The symphysis pubis joins the innominate bones anteriorly; the joint consists of a fibrocartilaginous interpubic disk spanned superiorly by pubic ligaments and inferiorly by an arcuate pubic ligament.

The sacroiliac joint has an anterior lip or shelf that protrudes from the iliac side of the joint and allows the sacrum to key into the ilium, adding stability. The sacroiliac joints are held together anteriorly by a ventral sacroiliac ligament that is broad but thin and separates the joint cavity from the pelvic cavity itself. The posterior sacroiliac capsule is formed by dorsal sacroiliac ligaments—the interosseous ligaments—which function to secure the ilium to the sacrum; these ligaments also function as a suspension bridge type mechanism for supporting the sacrum between the two innominate bones. The other two major ligaments of the pelvis that prevent forward rotation of the sacrum on the ilium are the sacrospinous and sacrotuberous ligaments. These ligaments limit the forward rotation of the sacrum on the pelvis.

Pelvic Trauma

Disruption of the pelvis requires considerable force. Injuries associated with fractures of the pelvis and acetabulum therefore can be severe and involve virtually all the major organ systems. The reported mortality rate for patients who have pelvic fractures is between 5% and 20%. More than 50% of patients with pelvic fractures have major additional injuries. Among patients who have open pelvic fractures and major vessel injury, the mortality rate is 50%. If there is disruption of the posterior pelvis and major head or abdominal injury, the mortality rate is greater than 50%. The treating physician is dealing with a total system of injuries and must approach the problem in a systematic and complete fashion. Despite what the prognosis might be, it is the surgeon's obligation to treat each system as if the patient will make a full recovery.

Neurologic Injury

The incidence of neurologic injuries associated with pelvic fractures has been reported to be between 1.2% and 12%. In patients who have bilateral vertical shear injuries, however, the incidence of neurologic injuries can be as high as 46%. These injuries commonly involve the obturator nerve, sciatic nerve, or nerve roots avulsed at the lumbosacral plexus. The nerve root avulsions can be intradural. Nerve lesions are usually peripheral and are more common if there is a sacral fracture or sacroiliac dislocation. Early electromyography as well as myelography are useful to identify the level of the lesion or to serve as a baseline for evaluation of possible return of function.

Gastrointestinal Injury

The incidence of gastrointestinal injuries is relatively low in pelvic fractures but, when bowel disruption does occur, it is potentially a very serious injury. Physical examination can be difficult to perform or its results may be misleading because retroperitoneal bleeding causes pressure on the abdominal contents through the peritoneum and simulates intra-abdominal injury. Diagnostic peritoneal lavage or "mini-laparotomy" may be required.

Genitourinary Injury

The overall incidence of bladder and urethral injuries in pelvic fractures is 13%. Most urethral injuries occur in males. The diagnosis of urethral injury is based on 1) inability to void, 2) blood at the urethral meatus spontaneously or after milking the urethra, or 3) mobile or high-riding prostate on rectal examination. An intravenous pyelogram can show an intact but elevated bladder that is compressed by a pelvic hematoma. The diagnosis is confirmed by dynamic retrograde urethrography with radiographs taken while the contrast material is being injected. All patients who have hematuria after acute pelvic trauma should undergo intravenous pyelography.

Vascular Injury

Open reduction of pelvic fractures within the first 72 hours results in a markedly increased blood loss compared to delayed operation. However, it may be important to stabilize the pelvis to decrease the amount of bleeding, especially in open-book type injuries. The external fixator is an effective means of maintaining stability of the pelvis, thereby controlling intrapelvic bleeding after pelvic and acetabular fractures.

Stabilizing a pelvic fracture by using an external fixator has been found to contribute to a low mortality rate. Firm interfragmentary compression of the pelvis with an external compression frame was reported to decrease bleeding. External fixators usually cannot control vertical displacement. However, the anterior half-frames can be used in cases of posterior disruption to achieve partial stabilization of an unstable vertical shear fracture. Stabilization of the pelvis or reduction of the volume of the pelvis by closing any anterior defects can decrease hemorrhage by a tamponade effect.

Retroperitoneal bleeding can lead to symptoms of an intraperitoneal hemorrhage because the blood surrounds the bladder and rectum and places pressure on the abdominal contents through the peritoneum. This can cause abdominal muscle spasm, abdominal wall rigidity and tenderness, and decreased bowel sounds. If bleeding cannot be controlled and the source is not known, angiography should be performed. Bleeding usually comes from the venous system, which makes radiographic diagnosis and treatment difficult. Bleeding due to severe pelvic injuries usually comes from branches of the hypogastric artery. A transfemoral catheter can be threaded into the aorta, and angiography can be performed to localize sites of arterial bleeding. Selective catheterization with infusion of autologous blood clot or Gelfoam or insertion of detachable balloons has been successful in controlling severe intrapelvic bleeding.

Open Fractures

Approximately 5% of pelvic fractures are open. These fractures carry higher morbidity and mortality rates than closed fractures do because they are caused by higher energy.

The most common causes of death are hemorrhage, sepsis, and head injury. The average blood replacement for patients with open fractures is 18 units; that for closed fractures is 6 units. Some patients may require in excess of 100 units of blood products.

The average incidence of associated injuries with open pelvic fractures is 2.7 per patient. These occur to the vascular system (20%), gastrointestinal system (45%, with as many as 39% of these patients requiring laparotomy), and genitourinary system (19% to 75%).

Small perineal or gluteal lacerations should always be considered to be a sign of open fracture until proved otherwise. Blood in the rectum or vagina is presumptive evidence of an open pelvic fracture. Pelvic fractures associated with bladder or gastrointestinal tract rupture should be treated as open fractures.

The steps that might be needed in managing a patient with an open pelvic fracture with active hemorrhage are: 1) wound packing, 2) MAST suit, 3) external fixation to stabilize the pelvis and decrease bleeding, 4) angiographic embolization, 5) ligation of hypogastric arteries, 6) exposure of the aorta and vena cava below the renal vessels with dissection and repair of the vascular tree, and 7) hemipelvectomy as a life-saving measure in extreme situations.

Irrigation and debridement should be carried out routinely. In the case of buttock or perineal lacerations, fecal diversion should be accomplished by means of a colostomy. A diverting colostomy should be created in all patients who have major open pelvic fractures. If there is a rectal tear, the retrorectal or presacral space should be drained to prevent abscess formation. After colostomy or presacral drainage is completed, rectal irrigation should be performed.

Vaginal lacerations smaller than 1 cm should be left open; if larger, they should be repaired. In either case, the vagina should be irrigated and the fracture sites should be irrigated and drained through the space of Retzius by approaching the site through a Pfannenstiel incision. Vaginal irrigation should be performed at the bedside twice a day with a dilute povidone-iodine (Betadine) solution or an antimicrobial agent solution.

The bladder should be drained by using a Foley catheter or suprapubic catheter, depending on the nature of the injury.

Open pelvic fractures should be stabilized—for example, with an external fixator—even if this achieves only posterior stability. Most Malgaigne-type fractures with posterior instability and many fractures with anterior ring disruption are best treated by internal fixation at the time of initial irrigation and debridement. Many of these fractures require little further dissection to expose the fracture sites and are readily stabilized by internal fixation. Open pelvic fractures have a high incidence of infection and, if stabilized, are easier to manage. The surgical wounds can be closed over the fixation device and drained. Traumatic wounds should be left open. The patient should be returned to the operating room at 48 hours for repeat debridement.

Pelvic Ring Injuries

Radiography

Initial radiographic examination of the pelvis should include an anteroposterior view as well as the 40° caudad and 40° cephalad projections described by Pennal and Tile. The oblique projections further delineate the fracture lines and also show the displacements that are present. The caudad projection ("inlet view") best defines posterior lesions and their displacement into the pelvic ring. This projection also shows sacroiliac dislocation and displacement of sacral fractures. It makes the pelvis appear as a ring and gives an end-on view of the sacrum. A cephalad projection ("outlet view") of the pelvis shows cephalad or caudad displacements of segments of the pelvis in both the anterior and posterior portions of the ring. It is projected in a line perpendicular to the plane of the sacrum (Fig. 1 *A-C*).

Additional radiographic views that often are very useful are 45° oblique views of the pelvis. Oblique views can disclose fractures of the acetabulum that are not visible on anteroposterior projections as well as provide a better view of the sacroiliac joint, iliac wing, and pubic ramus. If a fracture of the posterior pelvic rim is suspected but not visible on radiographs, computed tomography should be performed. These scans are particularly useful for delineating sacral fractures and diastasis pubis and also can reveal additional injuries previously unsuspected (Fig. 1 *D*).

Classification

Several classification systems for pelvic ring injuries have been described. Pennal and Tile classified these injuries according to the mechanism of the injury: anteroposterior compression, lateral compression, and vertical shear. A typical anteroposterior compression injury involves disruption of the symphysis pubis, causing widening of the

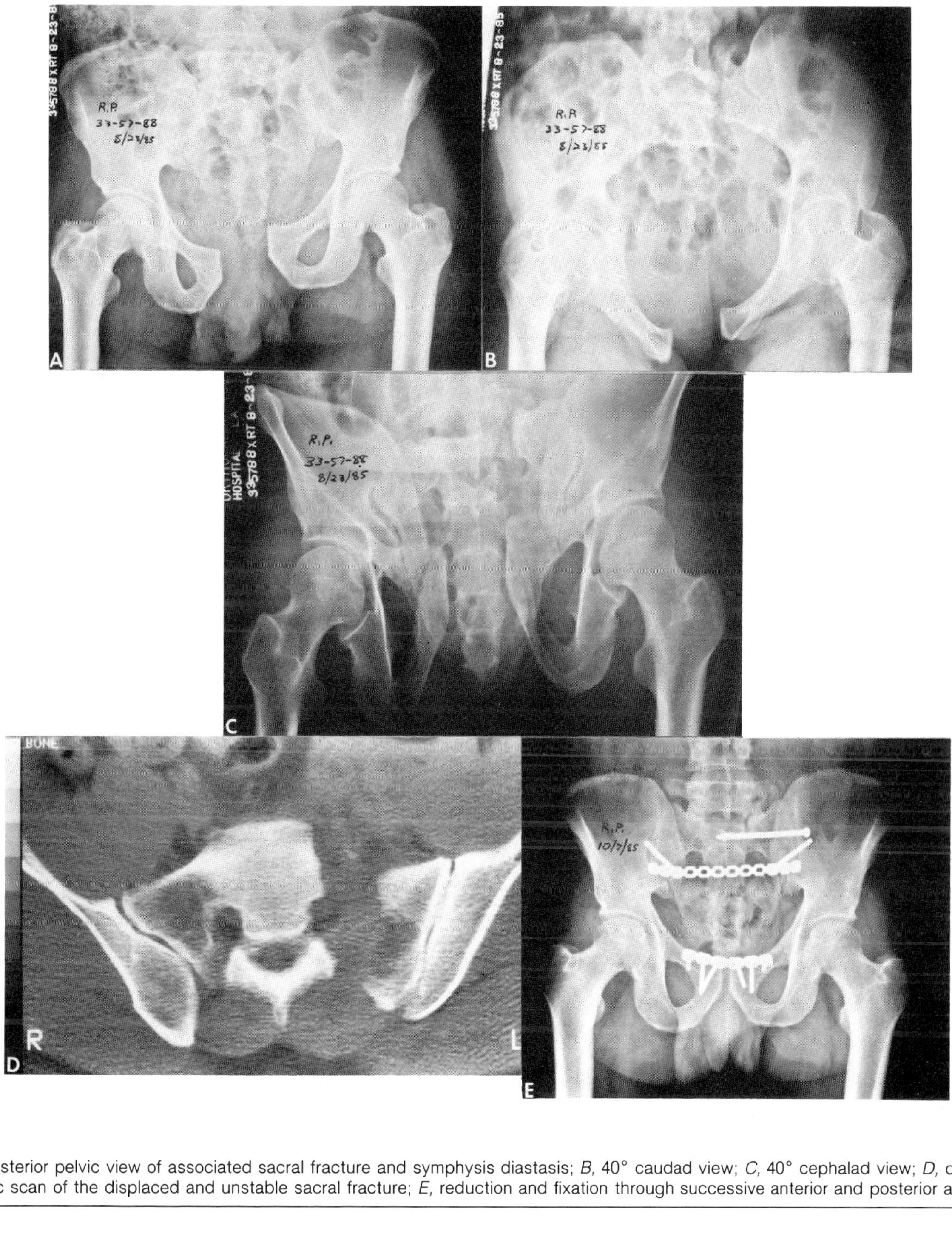

Figure 1

A, Anteroposterior pelvic view of associated sacral fracture and symphysis diastasis; *B,* 40° caudad view; *C,* 40° cephalad view; *D,* computed tomographic scan of the displaced and unstable sacral fracture; *E,* reduction and fixation through successive anterior and posterior approaches.

symphysis pubis and disruption of the anterior sacroiliac joint but no disruption of the posterior sacroiliac ligaments.

A typical lateral compression injury involves fracture of one or both anterior pubic rami. This injury results from a direct blow to the lateral pelvis, such as when a pedestrian is struck by an automobile. Posteriorly, there may be no radiographic evidence of injury or there may be an anterior impaction fracture of the sacrum or a minimally displaced fracture of the iliac wing.

A vertical shear type injury results from axial loading of the pelvis, usually to one side. However, both sides can be injured. This type of injury can occur if a patient falls from a height and lands on an outstretched leg or is in a motor vehicle accident such that force is transmitted through the lower limb to drive the hemipelvis proximally. Vertical shear injuries are typically fractures of the pubic rami or disruptions of the symphysis pubis anteriorly. Posteriorly, the disruption can occur through the iliac wing, the sacroiliac joint, or the sacrum. A characteristic feature is vertical translation of the hemipelvis. In addition, there often is considerable disruption of ligaments. If radiographs show an avulsion fracture of the ischial spine or a bony fragment fractured from the inferior border of the sacrum, these are signs of sacrospinal ligament avulsion. Fracture of the L-5 transverse process often is evidence of avulsion of the iliolumbar ligaments.

Another fracture classification is based on information gained from dissection of many cadavers with pelvic fractures (Fig. 2). The type I injury has good anterior and posterior stability with minimally displaced anterior fractures and a minimally displaced but stable posterior fracture or just posterior ligament stretching. Type II injuries include anterior pelvic ring disruption with partial posterior instability; an example is symphysis pubis diastasis with anterior opening of the sacroiliac joint. Type III injuries include unstable anterior and posterior pelvic ring disruptions.

A third classification of pelvic ring injuries simply names the disruption as either anterior or posterior. The types of anterior disruptions are disruption of the symphysis pubis, a double vertical fracture through the pubic rami, and a combination of these injuries. The types of posterior injury are iliac wing fracture, sacroiliac joint dislocation, fracture-dislocation of the sacroiliac joint, and pure sacral fracture.

All three classification systems are useful in the management of patients with pelvic ring injuries. They help in understanding the mechanism of injury, in assessing the stability of the pelvic ring, and in identifying the specific anatomic sites of injury.

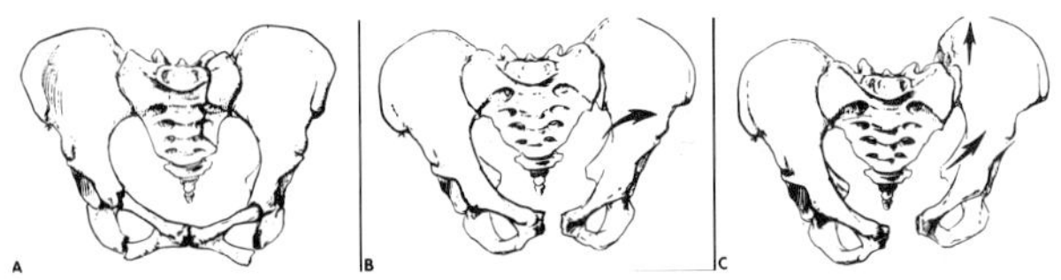

Figure 2

Pelvic ring fracture classification of Bucholz. *A*, Type I. Stable anterior and posterior injuries. *B*, Type II. Anterior instability with partial posterior instability. *C*, Type III. Complete anterior and posterior instability.

Assessment of Pelvic Ring Stability

The stability of a pelvic fracture is influenced not only by the bony configuration of the fracture but to a large extent also by the soft tissue or ligament injury associated with the fracture. The most reliable sign of pelvic instability is the amount of displacement of the posterior elements of the pelvic ring on the initial radiographs. Translational displacement of the sacroiliac joint is a sign of an unstable pelvis because this involves a purely ligamentous disruption of the very strong posterior sacroiliac ligaments. Fractures of the sacrum are probably stable if they are minimally displaced or impacted. However, sacral fractures are probably very unstable if significant displacement is seen or diastasis is present.

When fracture-dislocation of the sacroiliac joint with significant displacement is present, the pelvis almost always is unstable. Fractures of the iliac wing are unstable when displaced. Anterior diastasis of the symphysis pubis produces anterior instability of the pelvic ring because the anterior ligaments are disrupted. Fractures of the pubic rami can allow proximal or distal migration of the pelvic ring when combined with an unstable posterior lesion. Diastasis pubis usually does not occur when the rami are fractured. The anterior ligaments, including Poupart's and Cooper's ligaments, usually remain intact.

Treatment Principles

The goals of orthopaedic management are to achieve bony union in satisfactory position and to rehabilitate the patient as quickly as possible. Pelvic deformity can lead to leg length inequality, problems in sitting due to proximal displacement of one or both ischial tuberosities, and possible dyspareunia or difficulties with parturition in women. Nonunion or late sacroiliac joint instability can cause pain and limitation of function.

Most pelvic ring injuries are stable and can be treated by closed methods. If only the anterior pubic rami are fractured or if the injury is a combination of an anterior pubic ramus fracture plus a nondisplaced posterior ring fracture, the treatment can be bed rest until the patient is comfortable. The patient is then allowed to ambulate with crutches and progress to weight-bearing as tolerated. Serial radiographs should be taken to be sure that an apparently stable lesion does not displace.

Some minimally displaced fractures of the pelvic ring can appear to be stable but in fact can be potentially unstable. An example is a vertical fracture through the sacrum in which anteroposterior or caudad-cephalad migration of the hemipelvis is minimal. Computed tomography can reveal considerable diastasis pubis and comminution. In this case, there are two treatment choices: one is to perform initial surgical stabilization of the unstable posterior lesion; the other is to apply traction to the affected extremity and keep the patient at bed rest in traction for 8 to 12 weeks, until bone union has occurred. Serial radiographs should be taken.

Fractures that are known to be unstable or displaced initially are best treated by early open reduction and internal fixation. When treating unstable pelvic ring injuries nonoperatively with skeletal traction, several guidelines should be followed. After application of the skeletal traction, satisfactory reduction of the pelvic ring must be obtained. To obtain a satisfactory union of the pelvic disruption in traction there must be an unstable fracture anteriorly and posteriorly. If the anterior lesion is a disruption of the symphysis pubis or if the posterior lesion is a disruption of the sacroiliac joint, skeletal traction will not result in satisfactory union of the ligaments. Occasionally, a dislocated sacroiliac joint will heal by spontaneous fusion, but nonunion and malunion are common.

Nonunions through sacral or iliac wing fractures are not uncommon after closed treatment. If the fracture is treated by skeletal traction for the usual period of 8 to 12 weeks, a small loss of reduction typically occurs after discontinuation of the traction.

The Bucholz type II injuries that have diastasis of the symphysis pubis of more than 3 cm should be treated by open reduction. The Bucholz type III injuries should be treated by open reduction and internal fixation of the posterior pelvic disruption in all cases; internal fixation of the anterior disruption is required for diastasis of the symphysis pubis or severely displaced fractures of the pubic ramus. Open reduction and internal fixation of the pelvic ring should be performed when it is important to mobilize the patient because of other injuries, when an acetabular fracture is also present, or when there is cephalad displacement of the posterior pelvic ring greater than 1 cm.

Open Reduction/Internal Fixation

The disruptions of the posterior pelvic ring that may be treated by open reduction and internal fixation are fracture of the iliac wing, dislocation of the sacroiliac joint, fracture of the sacrum, and fracture-dislocation of either side of the sacroiliac joint. All posterior lesions, except for the iliac wing fracture, can be reached through a common posterior surgical approach. A vertical incision is made 2 cm lateral to the posterior superior iliac spine. The incision starts proximal to the iliac crest and proceeds over the buttock distal to the sciatic notch. The gluteal muscles are reflected from their origins on the iliac wing laterally. The gluteus maximus is partially mobilized from its sacral origin; the erector spinae as well as the multifidi overlying the sacrum are mobilized to variable degrees depending upon whether or not it is necessary to visualize the posterior sacral lamina.

To be able to assess reduction of sacral fractures or sacroiliac joint dislocations, the piriformis is mobilized at the greater sciatic notch so that a finger can be placed into the greater sciatic notch. It is thus possible to palpate anteriorly along the sacrum and sacroiliac joint (Fig. 3). Palpation through the greater sciatic notch also reveals the location of the sacral foramina and their accompanying sacral nerve roots. This posterior incision is normally performed with the patient in the prone position. Fractures of the iliac wing are usually approached through an incision paralleling the iliac crest. Exposure of the external or internal surface of the iliac wing can be accomplished as needed.

Posterior Lesions For open reduction and internal fixation of posterior lesions—such as fractures of the sacrum, dislocations of the sacroiliac joint, or fracture-dislocations of the sacroiliac joint—the patient should be prone on a radiolucent table to allow the use of an image intensifier during operation. Internal fixation of these posterior pelvic ring disruptions usually involves placement of screws from the ilium into the sacrum. Intraoperative monitoring with the image intensifier helps ensure proper placement of the screws, avoiding the sacral nerve roots and cauda equina.

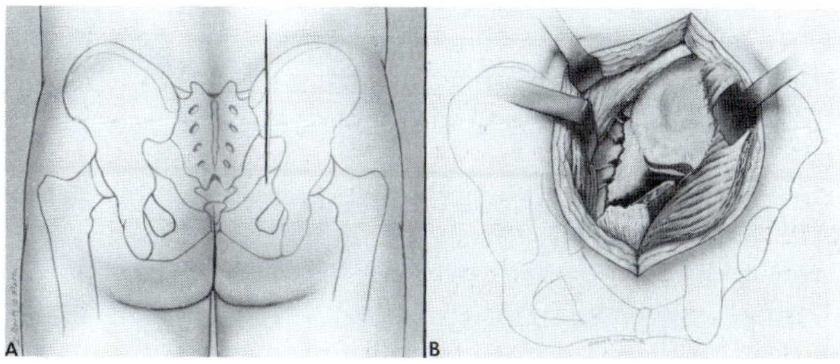

Figure 3

A, Posterior skin incision for exposure of the sacroiliac joint, fracture-dislocation of the sacroiliac joint, and fracture of the sacrum. *B,* Final exposure of the posterior iliac crest, sacroiliac joint, and sacral lamina. (By permission of J.M. Matta.)

The patient should be positioned so that an anteroposterior view can be taken as well as 40° cephalad and caudad projections to best show the adequacy of reduction as well as the location of internal fixation hardware.

When an entire hemipelvis is displaced, it usually moves in a proximal and posterior direction. There can be additional rotational components that also must be corrected. A good technique for internal fixation of sacroiliac joint dislocation is to place two screws perpendicular to the iliac wing directed toward the S-1 sacral ala (Fig. 4). Drill bit and screw position are checked during operation by using the three views on the image intensifier.

An alternative for fixing the sacroiliac joint is to approach the joint from the anterior aspect and place two-hole metal plates from the anterior sacral ala to the internal iliac fossa. This technique is most useful when an anterior approach to the acetabulum is necessary.

Sacrum Internal fixation of sacral fractures can be best achieved through the vertical posterior incision. If access is necessary for placement of fixation between the two iliac wings, an additional vertical incision is made. A sacral fracture is reduced by using pointed reduction forceps. Adequacy of the reduction can be seen on the posterior sacral lamina and palpated through the sciatic notch. Before the fracture is reduced, the fracture should be distracted to

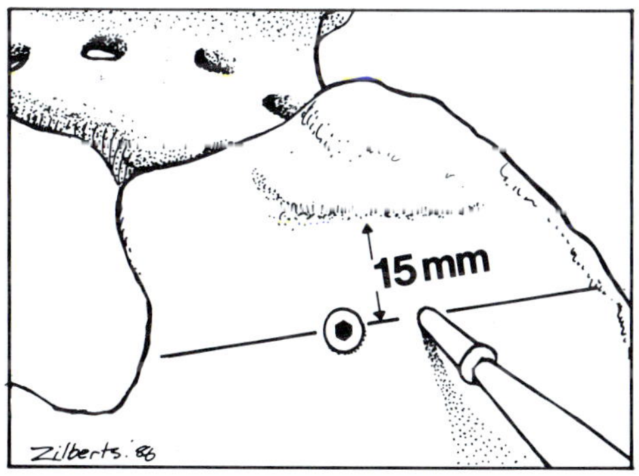

Figure 4

Screw insertion for sacroiliac joint and sacrum fracture fixation: 15 mm anterior to crista glutea, midway between iliac crest and sciatic notch, and directed perpendicularly to iliac wing.

permit visualization of the sacral nerve roots. Also, the nerve roots should be palpated through the sciatic notch during the reduction maneuver to ensure that they are not compressed by bony fragments.

One method of fixation is to place a single 6.5-mm screw into the lateral iliac wing and to advance this screw into the S-1 vertebral body. Multiple anteroposterior and oblique views taken with the image intensifier are used during drilling of the screw hole and placement of the screw to be sure of the exact location of the hardware (Fig. 5).

This screw fixation is augmented by use of a long flexible metal plate that is placed from one iliac wing to the other across the posterior sacrum just above the level of the greater sciatic notch. An osteotomy of the spinous process of the sacrum can be performed to allow placement of the plate under the multifidi of the sacrum and the osteotomized spinous process. With this fixation method, the screw in the S-1 vertebral body controls translational displacement and prevents diastasis of the superior portion of the sacrum while the plate prevents diastasis of the inferior portion of the sacrum (Fig. 1 *E*). Use of a transverse "double cobra plate" to fix complex or bilateral posterior pelvic ring disruptions has been recommended.

Fracture-dislocations of the sacroiliac joint and fractures of the ilium or iliac wing can be fixed internally by using long screws placed between the two tables of the ilium or by plates placed along the surface of the ilium. The reduction is usually achieved by using a two-screw technique in which reduction forceps grip a screw on each side of the fracture line.

Anterior Lesions Open reduction and internal fixation is sometimes indicated to treat separations of the symphysis pubis and fractures of the pubic rami. Disruption of the symphysis pubis commonly requires open reduction whereas fracture of the pubic rami does not. Internal fixation of the symphysis pubis is performed through an anterior incision, vertical midline or transverse, placed 2 cm proximal to the symphysis pubis. After the skin and subcutaneous tissue are retracted, the linea alba is split between the two heads of the rectus abdominis. One head of the rectus abdominis is often avulsed from the symphysis by the injury. If it is intact, the insertion of the rectus abdominis on the superior aspect of the pubis is elevated anteriorly to expose the superior aspect of the pubic rami without completely detaching the insertion. The dissection stays outside the peritoneum and anterior to the bladder and urethra (Fig. 6).

Fractures of the pubic ramus also can be approached through a transverse lower abdominal incision extended laterally as in the ilioinguinal approach. It is possible to reduce and plate the entire superior pubic ramus and to stay medial to the external iliac vessels; however, exposure of pubic ramus fracture usually requires identification and retraction of the spermatic cord.

Open reduction of an acute dislocation of the symphysis pubis usually can be accomplished without difficulty by placing the points of a pointed reduction forceps on each side of the symphysis and closing the diastasis. A six-hole 3.5-mm curved plate can be placed along the superior aspect of the pubic symphysis and pubic rami posterior to the insertion of the rectus abdominis. Use of a two-hole plate attached with a single 6.5-mm screw on either side of the symphysis has been recommended. This technique is adequate for a simple diastasis of the symphysis but should be used with caution if there is a tendency for one side of the symphysis to translate vertically in relation to the other. With the combination of a symphysis pubis diastasis and pubic ramus fracture, the symphysis alone can be fixed if the ramus fracture is displaced only slightly. Pubic ramus fractures with wide diastasis can be fixed internally with a curved plate and 3.5-mm screws.

The key to achieving stability of an unstable pelvic ring fracture is in the reduction and internal fixation of the posterior lesion. The posterior lesion is usually approached first with the patient in the prone position. If the anterior lesion consists of fractures of the rami that are widely displaced after the posterior fixation has been accomplished, internal fixation of the anterior lesion is not necessary. If the anterior lesion is pubis diastasis of the symphysis or a widely displaced fracture of the pubic ramus, internal fixation should be performed after completion of the posterior operation. It is not necessary to use an external fixator to stabilize moderately displaced anterior pelvic ring fractures if internal fixation of the posterior ring disruption has been accomplished.

If stable internal fixation of a pelvic ring disruption has been achieved, it is beneficial to mobilize the patient as quickly as possible. Gait training is usually begun at 5 to

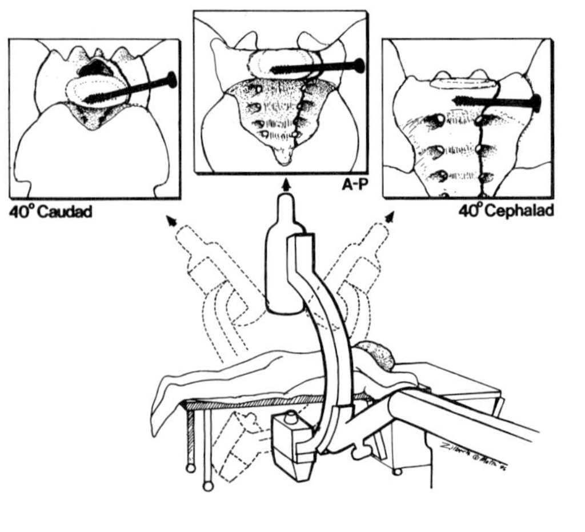

Figure 5

Positioning of the patient and use of the image intensifier for sacroiliac joint and sacrum fracture fixation, showing anteroposterior view of sacral fracture and proper drill bit position, 40° caudad view, and 40° cephalad view. (By permission of J.M. Matta.)

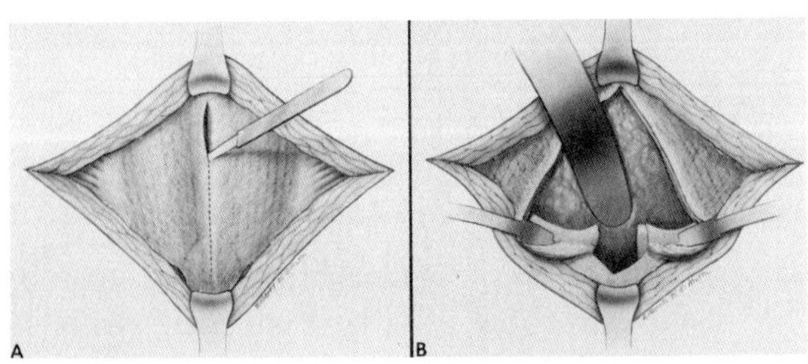

Figure 6

A, Skin incision for fixation of the symphysis pubis. *B*, Final exposure of the symphysis pubis. (By permission of J.M. Matta.)

7 days after operation. If the injury is unilateral, partial weight-bearing is allowed on the affected side. If injury is bilateral, the patient is usually permitted to do standing pivot transfers from bed to wheelchair, and gait training is not started until 6 weeks postoperatively. Full weight-bearing usually can be allowed at 6 to 8 weeks after operative stabilization.

External Fixation

External fixation is useful to stabilize an acute, displaced pelvic fracture in order to decrease the volume of the pelvis and help control blood loss. In most instances, however, the role of external fixation in pelvic fractures is limited. External fixation is best in treating a Bucholz type II injury of the pelvic ring with diastasis of the anterior ring and intact posterior sacroiliac ligaments. The anterior tension band element of the external fixator can maintain reduction of the pelvic ring. The method of applying an internal fixation plate on the symphysis pubis has the advantage of ensuring a better reduction and fixation and is better tolerated by the patient.

Nonunions and Malunions

Nonunion or malunion is not uncommon after a pelvic fracture that has a very unstable posterior ring disruption if primary stable internal fixation is not performed. The treatment of malunions and nonunions of the pelvic ring is much more difficult and dangerous to the patient than is the acute treatment of the injury. Surgical correction of nonunions and malunions is difficult and often must be done in several stages. The risk of neurologic injury is high when proximal migration of the hemipelvis and mobilization of nonunion sites are performed. Intraoperative monitoring of cortical evoked potentials assists in preventing sacral or other nerve root injury.

Pelvic Fractures in Children

Most pelvic ring injuries in children are stable. The radiographic evaluation should include anteroposterior, inlet, outlet, and oblique views. Computed tomography is useful for evaluating the posterior pelvic ring. Several authors have reported the possibility of late deformity that is not corrected with growth in the case of pelvic ring injuries in children. Among 154 cases reviewed, there were 15 with significant pelvic deformity at the time of injury; of these 15 patients, 4 healed with deformity that was symptomatic. All had unreduced sacroiliac dislocations. In 69 children who had sacroiliac joint injuries, results were good if diastasis of the joint was the only injury. Residual pain was frequent, however, in patients with persistent joint subluxation due to either ligament disruption or fracture. Reduction of pelvic ring fractures in children should be performed when significant displacement is present. This is particularly true when there is persistent sacroiliac joint dislocation.

Acetabular Fractures

Radiography

Routine radiographic views for diagnosis of acetabular fractures include anteroposterior views of the pelvis and hip and 45° oblique views of the pelvis (Fig. 7). Diagnosis

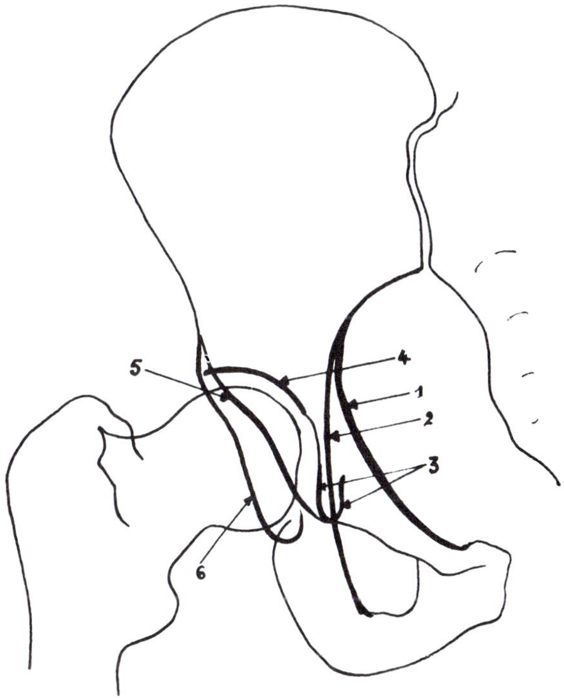

Figure 7

Anteroposterior view of the acetabulum. Lines: 1, iliopectineal line; 2, ilioischial line; 3, radiographic "U"; 4, roof; 5, anterior rim; 6, posterior rim.

of acetabular fractures is dependent on careful radiographic assessment (Table 1; Fig. 8). The purpose of the classification shown in Table 2 is to aid in the selection of treatment for the individual patient and allow comparison of treatment results.

On the anteroposterior view the anterior column is identified by the iliopectineal line or pelvic brim. The ilioischial line corresponds to the posterior column. The roof or dome of the acetabulum and posterior lip or wall of the acetabulum are well visualized on this view. A very important feature is the constant relationship of the radiographic teardrop sign to the ilioischial line.

The obturator oblique view demonstrates the superior pubic ramus and anterior column as well as the posterior wall of the acetabulum (Fig. 9). The iliac oblique view demonstrates the anterior wall of the acetabulum and clearly outlines the posterior column (Fig. 10).

Elementary acetabular fractures include fractures of the posterior wall, posterior column, anterior wall, anterior column, and transverse acetabulum. Wall fractures occur through portions of the acetabular rim and can be isolated or occur in association with column fractures. Isolated disruption of the ilioischial line is indicative of a posterior column fracture. Disruption of the iliopectineal line indicates an anterior column fracture. In a simple transverse fracture, the innominate bone is divided into two parts through a portion of the acetabulum. The distal portions of the anterior and posterior columns remain together and are usually displaced medially. No distortion of the teardrop and its relationship with the iliopectineal and ilioischial lines is noted.

Table 1. Radiographic Diagnosis of Acetabular Fractures*

Fracture	Posterior rim	Anterior rim	Ilioischial line	Iliopectineal line	Roof	Obturator foramen	Ilium
Posterior wall	+	−	−	−	−	−	−
Posterior column	+	−	+	−	−	±	−
Anterior wall	−	+	−	+	−	±	−
Anterior column	−	+	−	+	±	±	±
Transverse, with or without dissociated posterior wall	+	+	+	+	−	−	−
T-shaped	+	+	+	+	−	+	−
Associated anterior plus posterior hemitransverse	+	+	+	+	±	±	±
Both-column	+	+	+	+	+	±	+

*+, positive radiographic finding; −, negative; ±, present in some cases but not all.
From Letournel, E., and Judet, R.: Fractures of the Acetabulum. (Translated and edited by R.A. Elson.) New York, Springer-Verlag, 1981. By permission of the publisher.

Associated fractures are complex acetabular fractures which include combinations of elementary fractures. Both-column and T-shaped fractures are included in this category. A T-shaped fracture is a comminuted form of a transverse fracture with an additional fracture line extending through the obturator foramen, usually through the inferior pubic ramus. When both columns fracture, a fracture line divides the columns above the acetabulum through the iliac wing, with additional fracture lines running through the acetabulum and the obturator foramen. This is usually accompanied by central dislocation of the femoral head. All radiographic landmarks are disrupted.

A useful adjunct is the computed tomogram. This enables detection of occult fractures through the sacrum, minimally displaced and incomplete fractures through the iliac wing, fractures through the quadrilateral surface, incarcerated fragments within the joint, and rotational displacement of the anterior and posterior columns. However, this scan can be deceptive if interpreted without the anteroposterior and oblique radiographs of the pelvis. Loose fragments of bone within the hip joint can be erroneously diagnosed when one is simply seeing a cross section through the small end of a larger fracture fragment. Interpretation of the lower portion of the anterior column can be con-

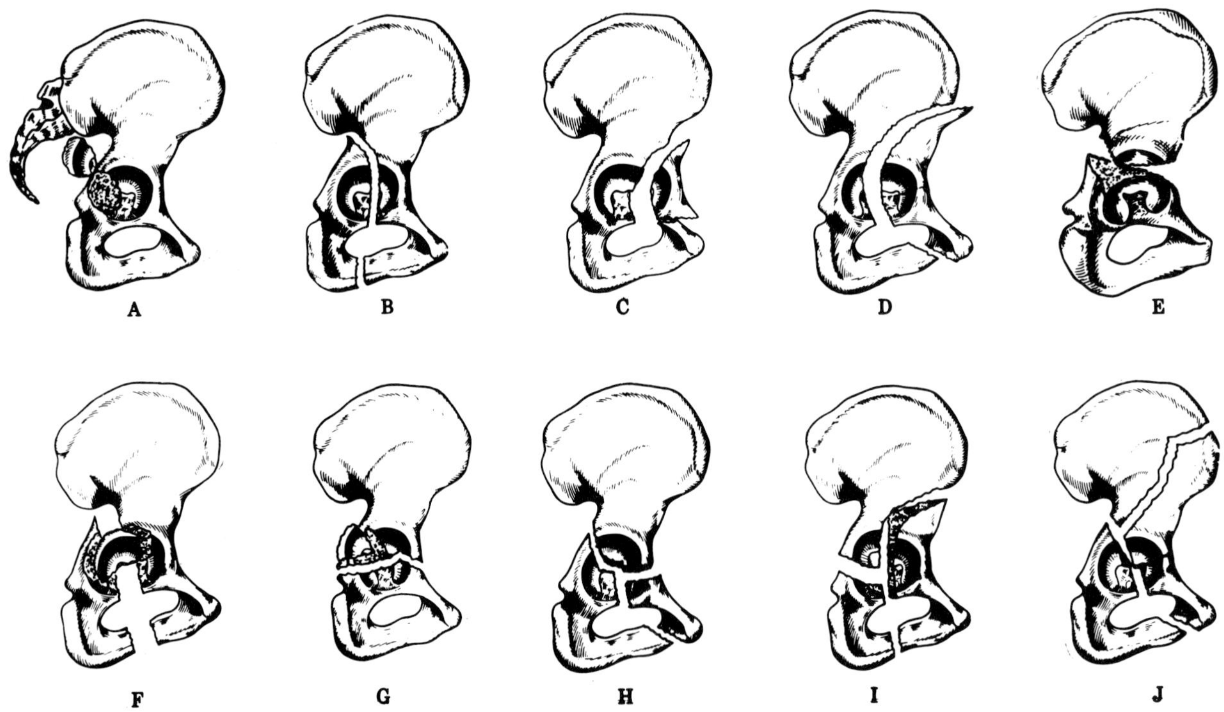

Figure 8

Classification of Letournel: *A*, posterior wall fracture; *B*, posterior column fracture; *C*, anterior wall fracture; *D*, anterior column fracture; *E*, transverse fracture; *F*, associated posterior column and posterior wall fracture; *G*, associated transverse and posterior wall fracture; *H*, T-shaped fracture; *I*, associated anterior column and posterior hemitransverse fracture; *J*, both-column fracture.

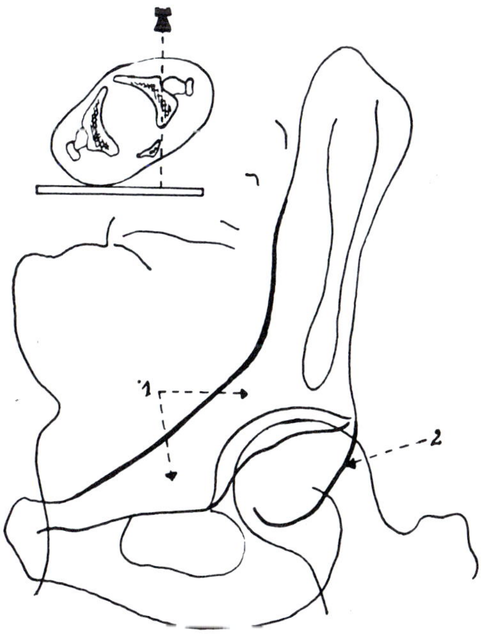

Figure 9
Obturator oblique view of the acetabulum. Lines: 1, anterior column; 2, posterior column.

fusing because the fracture appears more comminuted than it actually is. Three-dimensional computed tomography is a recent innovation that demonstrates the overall configuration and displacement of the fracture fragments. Fine details of bone, however, cannot be seen with existing techniques (Fig. 11).

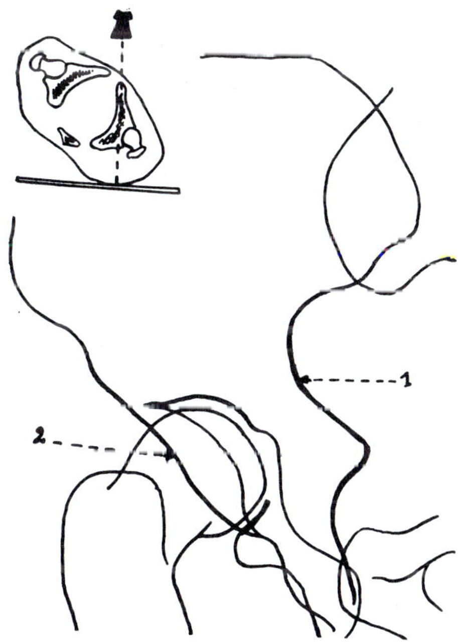

Figure 10
Iliac oblique view of the acetabulum. Lines: 1, posterior column; 2, anterior rim.

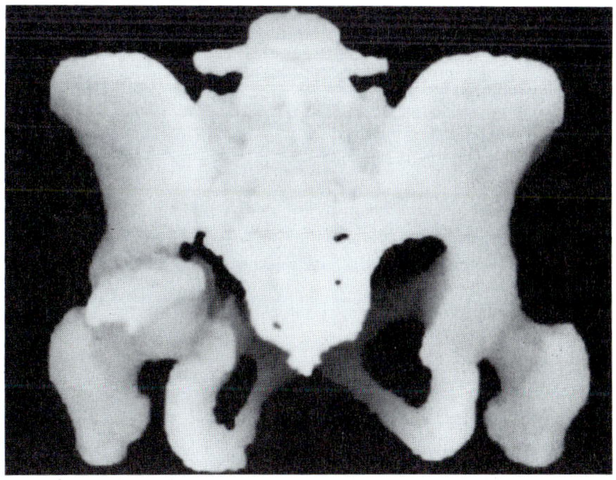

Figure 11
Three-dimensional computed tomogram of a displaced T-shaped fracture.

Treatment Principles

The goals of treatment are restoration of function and prevention of post-traumatic arthritis. Although articular cartilage can be damaged at the time of original injury or by unrecognized incarcerated osteochondral fragments, the most usual cause of post-traumatic arthritis is residual joint incongruity from an imperfect reduction. With intra-articular displacement greater than 1 to 2 mm, especially in the weight-bearing portion of the acetabulum, the articular cartilage cannot withstand the alteration in pressure distribution, and degenerative changes ensue.

Certain displaced intra-articular fractures can be treated successfully with skeletal traction. A both-column fracture without wide displacement and with apparent congruence on the three standard radiographic views can be treated in this manner (Fig. 12). Similarly, a low transverse fracture

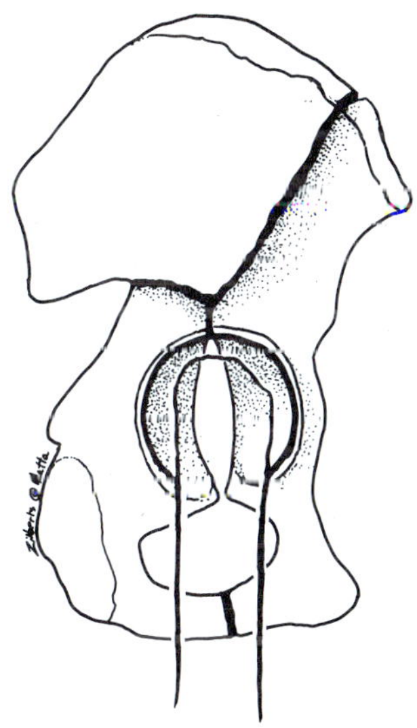

Figure 12
Typical rotational displacement of a both-column fracture with significant separation of fragments but minimal decrease in contact area. (By permission of J.M. Matta.)

not involving the weight-bearing dome usually can be reduced by using skeletal traction. Most displaced intra-articular fractures, however, require open reduction. The decision of whether or not to operate usually can be made on the basis of the initial radiographs and computed tomogram. Of additional help is the use of a system to estimate the amount of acetabular dome remaining intact after fracture. This system utilizes three measurements: the medial roof arc, the anterior roof arc, and the posterior roof arc.

These three measurements are made on the anteroposterior view, obturator oblique view, and iliac oblique view of the pelvis, respectively. Medial roof arc is measured by drawing a vertical line through the roof of the acetabulum to the geometric center of the acetabulum. A second line is then drawn from the point where the fracture line intersects the roof of the acetabulum to the geometric center of the acetabulum. The angle between these lines is the medial roof arc (Fig. 13). The anterior roof and posterior roof arcs are measured similarly. This measurement method is most useful in cases of posterior column fracture, anterior column fracture, transverse fracture, T-shaped fracture, and associated anterior column and posterior hemitransverse fractures. Roof arc measurements have limited usefulness for evaluating both-column fracture and fracture of the posterior wall.

The following criteria should be met for nonoperative treatment to be selected: 1) the femoral head should remain congruent with the roof of the acetabulum if the patient is taken out of traction; 2) the anterior roof arc, medial roof arc, and posterior roof arc all should be greater than 45°; 3) adequacy of the remaining acetabular rim in posterior wall fractures should be assessed by plain radiographs and computed tomography because roof arc measurements are unreliable.

Neufeld type roller traction is a useful form of nonoperative treatment because it allows active lower extremity exercises. Traction must be maintained for 4 to 8 weeks to achieve bony union.

Operative Treatment

Except with a coexisting anterior or posterior hip dislocation irreducible by closed means, open reduction and internal fixation of acetabular fractures is best undertaken no sooner than 2 to 3 days after injury, to allow the initial bleeding from the fracture site and pelvic vessels to subside. In the preoperative period, the patient is usually placed in skeletal traction through a distal femoral pin. This is particularly important in the case of a T-shaped or transverse fracture of the acetabular roof because the femoral head can be damaged by sharp fracture surfaces. Operation should not be delayed past 3 weeks because resorption of the fracture surfaces will have occurred and callus will have formed.

The most useful surgical approaches for open reduction and internal fixation of acetabular fractures are the Kocher-Langenbeck, ilioinguinal, and extended iliofemoral. The use of a triradiate incision that can be extended to give an exposure similar to the extended iliofemoral approach has been advocated (Fig. 14). With the exception of isolated anterior wall and posterior wall acetabular fractures, exposure of the innominate bone is required. Reduction of the innominate bone is usually necessary to achieve an accurate reduction of the acetabulum. No single surgical approach has been found to provide ideal exposure for all fracture types. Proper classification of the fracture configuration preoperatively is essential in the selection of the best approach in order to achieve an anatomic reduction of the fracture (Table 2).

The Kocher-Langenbeck approach is performed with the patient in the prone position on a fracture table. Access is obtained to the retroacetabular surface as far distally as the ischial tuberosity (Fig. 15). Only the most inferior portion of the iliac wing is accessible. Proximal access is limited by the superior gluteal vessels and nerve. The quadrilateral surface and pelvic rim are accessible by palpation through the greater sciatic notch. The greater and lesser sciatic notches are exposed by transecting the tendons of the piriformis and obturatorius internus in the trochanteric fossa. The inferior aspect of the iliac wing is exposed by osteotomy of the trochanter or transection of the gluteus medius tendon. Visualization of the interior of the joint can be obtained through a capsulotomy performed along the acetabular rim.

The ilioinguinal approach is performed with the patient supine on a fracture table (Fig. 16). This allows access to the internal aspect of the innominate bone and exposes the entire internal iliac fossa, anterior sacroiliac joint, pelvic rim, and quadrilateral surfaces. Limited access is possible to the anterior portion of the external iliac wing. The incision begins at a point two-thirds of the way posterior

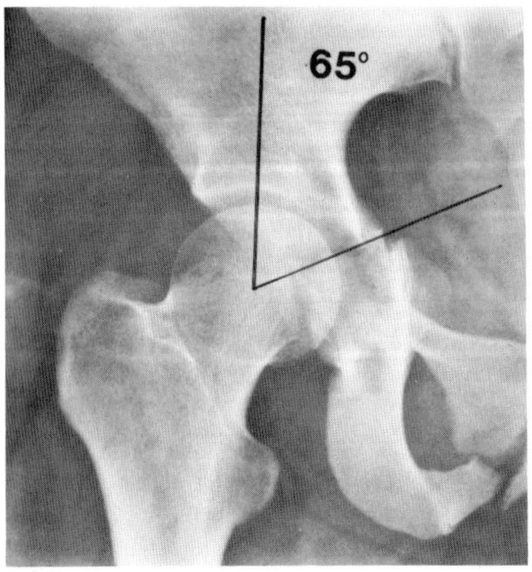

Figure 13

Measurement of the medial roof arc of a very low T-shaped fracture.

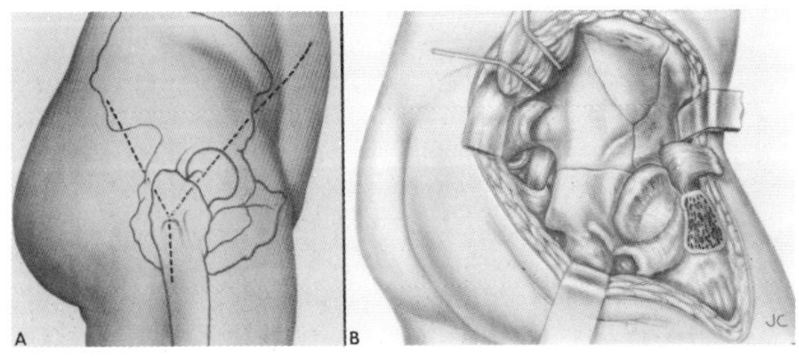

Figure 14

Triradiate approach. *A*, Skin incision. *B*, Exposure of the lateral ilium and the retroacetabular surface.

Table 2. Surgical Approaches in Acetabular Fractures, by Anatomic Diagnosis

Diagnosis	Approach		
	Kocher-Langenbeck	Ilioinguinal	Extended iliofemoral
Posterior wall	x		
Posterior column	x		
Transverse	x		
Associated transverse plus posterior wall	x		
Old associated transverse & posterior wall			x
T-shaped			x
Anterior column & anterior wall		x	
Associated anterior column & posterior hemitransverse		x	
Both-column			

From Letournel, E., and Judet, R.: Fractures of the Acetabulum. (Translated and edited by R.A. Elson.) New York, Springer-Verlag, 1981. By permission of the publisher.

along the iliac crest, proceeds forward to the anterior superior iliac spine, and then moves transversely along the lower abdomen to a point two fingerbreadths above the symphysis pubis. The abdominis and iliacus are mobilized from the crest and anterior iliac fossa. The inguinal canal is opened on both its roof and floor to mobilize the abdominis muscles and transversalis fascia from the inguinal ligament. The structures passing across the inguinal ligament—including the spermatic cord, external iliac vessels, iliopsoas muscle, and femoral nerve—are identified and retracted according to the segment of pelvis that is being reduced or internally fixed. This is primarily an approach to the anterior column; however, access to the posterior column can be gained by retracting the external iliac vessels medially and the iliopsoas and femoral nerve laterally. Open reduction and internal fixation at times can be difficult through this exposure. The advantages, however, include a cosmetically acceptable scar and a lower incidence of operative morbidity and postoperative heterotopic bone formation due to minimal muscle stripping from the innominate bone.

The extended iliofemoral approach is performed with the patient in the lateral position on the fracture table (Fig. 17). This approach gives wide access to the entire external aspect of the iliac wing and the retroacetabular surface distal to the ischial tuberosity and limited access to the anterior column as far distally as the pectineal eminence. The incision begins at the posterior superior iliac spine, proceeds anteriorly along the crest to the anterior superior iliac spine, and then gently curves toward the anterior aspect of the greater trochanter and extends distally along the proximal lateral border of the femur. The incision follows a plane between nerves, reflecting the muscles innervated by the superior and inferior gluteal nerves posteriorly and the muscles innervated by the femoral nerve medially. The gluteal muscles and tensor fascia lata are reflected from the external aspect of the iliac wing and their tendons are divided at their trochanteric insertions. The obturatorius internus and piriformis tendons are divided in the trochanteric fossa. Elevation of the iliacus from the internal iliac fossa and detachment of the rectus femoris origin from above the acetabulum and the anterior inferior iliac spine gives further access to the anterior column. Visualization of the internal aspect of the hip joint is possible by division of the hip capsule next to the acetabular rim. This exposure provides the most commanding access to the innominate bone. The amount of dissection required, however, leads to a longer period of postoperative rehabilitation.

The choice of surgical approach is made with the expectation that the entire operation can be performed through a single surgical incision. Intraoperative traction distracts the femoral head from its displaced position, allowing reduction of the acetabular fragments. The ASIF femoral distractor can be used as an alternative to the fracture table. When traction is utilized, it is important to flex the knee at least 60° in order to relax the sciatic nerve.

Various reduction forceps are available for use in the reduction of fragments (Fig. 18). Pointed reduction forceps can be directly applied to the bone to maintain reduction. Additional control can be achieved with the use of specialized reduction forceps attached by positional screws on both sides of the fracture line. It is important to correct all components of the deformity, including diastasis, translational displacement, and rotational displacement. Rotation of the posterior column along its longitudinal axis is best controlled by using a femoral head corkscrew type extractor inserted into the ischial tuberosity. Rotation of a high anterior column fracture can be controlled with a Farabeuf reduction forceps placed along the anterior border of the innominate bone at the level of the anterior inferior iliac spine. Fracture reduction usually cannot be achieved in a single step. It is often necessary to proceed by stepwise reduction of single fracture fragments to intact portions of the pelvis. In general, precise reduction of extra-articular fragments will aid in the final articular reduction. Incarcerated fragments and impacted articular surfaces must be recognized preoperatively to allow correction by manipulation.

Fracture fixation is achieved with a combination of interfragmentary screws and plates. Rarely is screw fixation alone satisfactory. Screws should be available in several diameters from 2.5 to 6.5 mm and in lengths up to 110 mm. Plates should be available in various lengths, and plate-bending devices are useful (Fig. 19). Provisional fixation is with screws alone. Lag screws are preferred to provide interfragmentary compression, enhancing fracture stability. Fixation is completed with the application of plates, usually along the pelvic brim or paralleling the rim of the acetabulum. Direct visualization and palpation of the articular surface is essential to recognize inadvertent penetration of the joint with screws.

Treatment of Specific Fractures

Posterior Wall Fractures Fixation is performed through a Kocher-Langenbeck approach. The first step is irrigation and debridement to be sure there are no loose osteocartilaginous fragments in the hip joint. It is important to recognize any marginal impaction of articular surface that can be corrected by elevation of the impacted segment. If

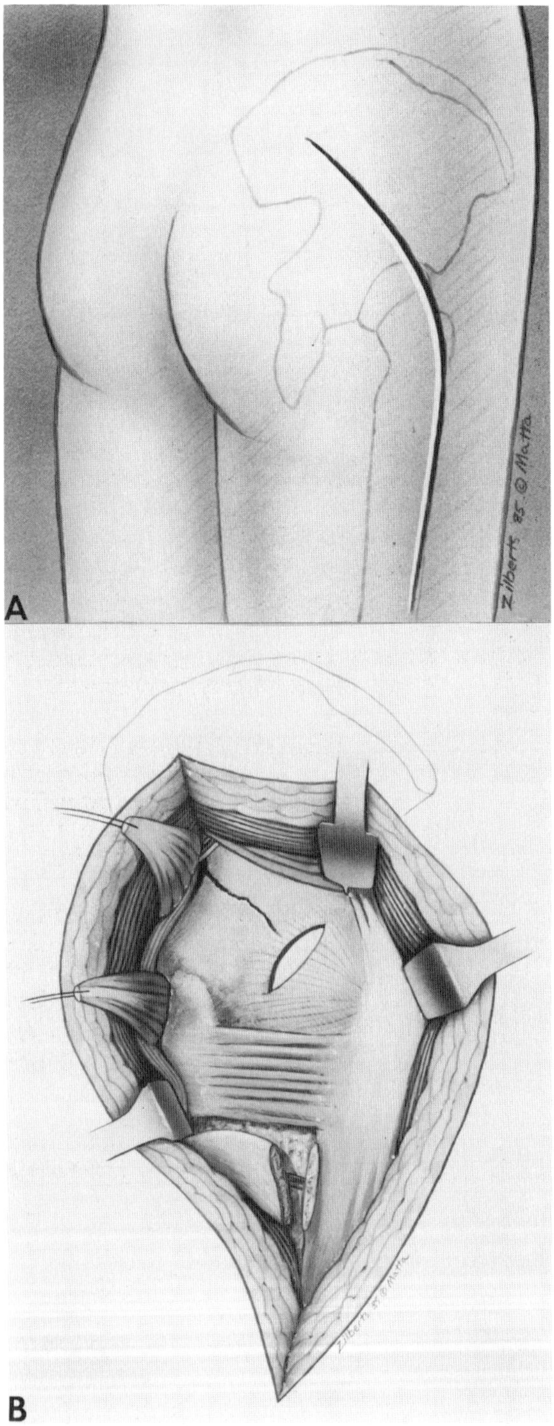

Figure 15

Kocher-Langenbeck approach. *A*, Skin incision. *B*, Exposure of the retroacetabular surface. (By permission of J.M. Matta.)

significant impaction is present, additional bone grafting may be necessary. Fixation should use lag screws traversing the fragments and a posterior buttressing plate paralleling the posterior rim of the acetabulum (Fig. 20).

Posterior Column Fractures Isolated fractures of this type are exposed through a Kocher-Langenbeck approach with

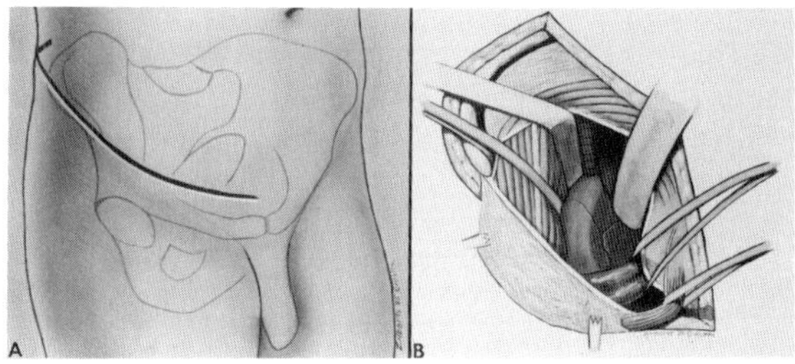

Figure 16

Ilioinguinal approach. *A*, Skin incision. *B*, Exposure of the pelvic brim and quadrilateral surface. (By permission of J.M. Matta.)

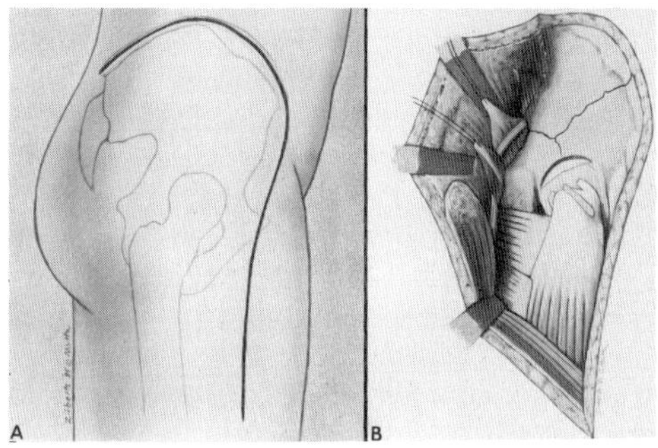

Figure 17

Extended iliofemoral approach. *A*, Skin incision. *B*, Exposure of the lateral ilium and retroacetabular surface. (By permission of J.M. Matta.)

the patient in the prone position. Reduction is performed and visually assessed on the retroacetabular surface. Fixation is obtained by using a small reconstruction or dynamic compression plate applied from the ischial tuberosity to the lateral ilium along the retroacetabular surface.

Transverse Fractures Exposure is usually through the Kocher-Langenbeck approach with the patient prone. Re-

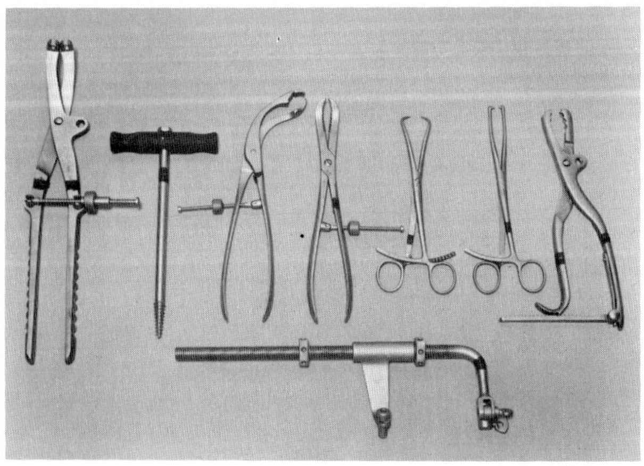

Figure 18

Instruments used for reduction of acetabulum fractures.

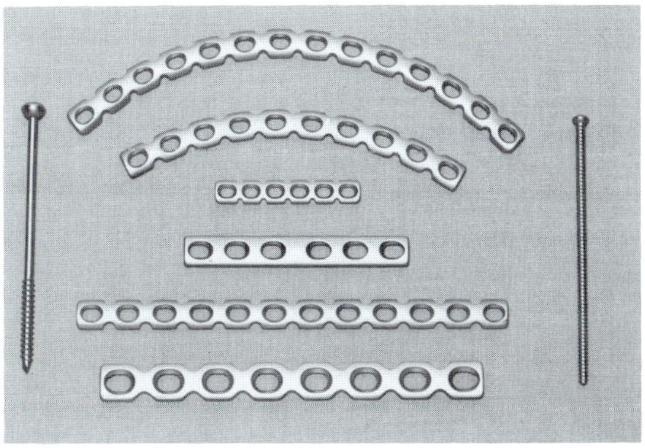

Figure 19
Screws and plates used for fixation of acetabulum fractures.

duction is carried out in a fashion similar to that for isolated posterior column fractures, and fixation of the posterior column is carried out with a buttress plate. A long 6.5-mm cancellous screw is inserted across the anterior portion of the fracture into the superior pubic ramus. If the anterior component of the transverse fracture is situated high, exposure is best obtained through the ilioinguinal approach.

Associated Transverse and Posterior Wall Fractures Most of these can be exposed through the Kocher-Langenbeck approach with the patient prone on the fracture table (Fig. 21). These fractures are often associated with posterior dislocation of the femoral head and incarceration of loose osteocartilaginous fragments. Distraction of the femoral head is necessary for thorough inspection of the interior of the joint and removal of these fragments. The transverse fracture is reduced and provisionally fixed, followed by reduction of the posterior wall fracture and application of a buttress plate. The extended iliofemoral approach may be necessary for a particularly difficult or old associated transverse and posterior wall fracture.

T-Shaped Fractures The majority can be reduced and fixed through the Kocher-Langenbeck approach by reducing the posterior column in the usual manner and manipulating

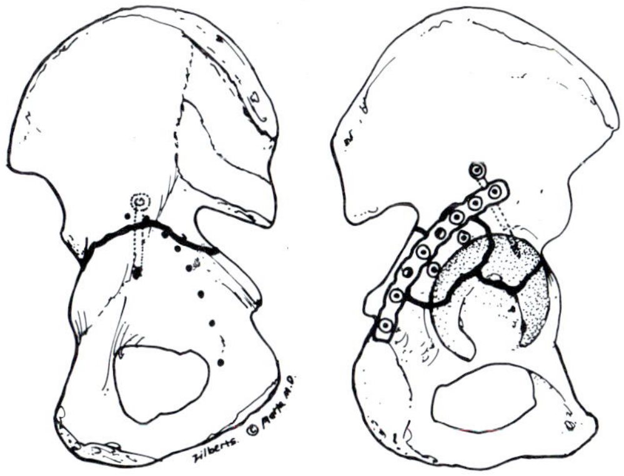

Figure 21
Fixation of an associated transverse and posterior wall fracture through the Kocher-Langenbeck approach. (By permission of J.M. Matta.)

the anterior column either through the sciatic notch or from an intra-articular approach. If anterior column reduction is not possible at operation, a subsequent ilioinguinal approach is required. Therefore, initial use of the extended iliofemoral approach may be preferred.

Anterior Column and Anterior Wall Fractures These are best exposed through the ilioinguinal approach which provides access to the entire length of the anterior column. Fixation is accomplished with lag screws initially and completed with application of a plate along the pelvic brim.

Associated Anterior Column and Posterior Hemitransverse Fractures The ilioinguinal approach with the patient supine on the fracture table is best. After anterior column reduction and fixation, the posterior column is reduced by manipulation of the quadrilateral surface and fixed by passing long lag screws from the pelvic brim to the posterior column near the ischial spine (Fig. 22).

Both-Column Fractures These are the most difficult acetabular fractures to reduce and fix satisfactorily. Best exposure

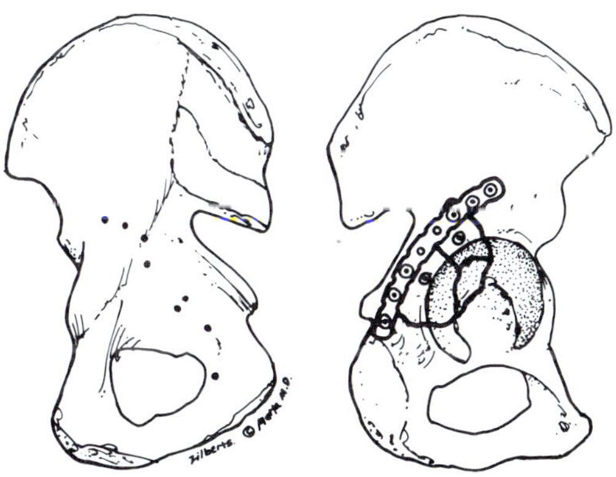

Figure 20
Fixation of a posterior wall fracture through the Kocher-Langenbeck approach. (By permission of J.M. Matta.)

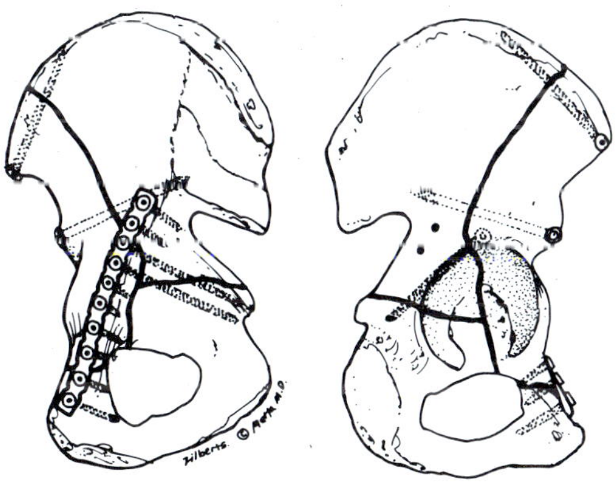

Figure 22
Fixation of an associated anterior column and posterior hemitransverse fracture through the ilioinguinal approach. (By permission of J.M. Matta.)

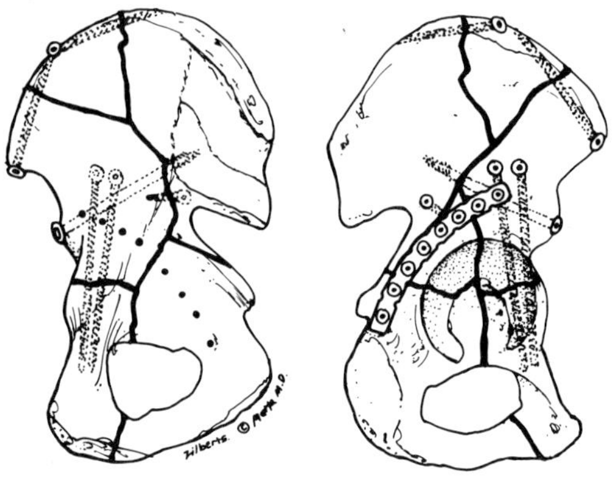

Figure 23

Fixation of a both-column fracture through the extended iliofemoral approach. (By permission of J.M. Matta.)

is obtained with the extended iliofemoral approach with the patient in a lateral position on the fracture table. The anterior column is reduced and fixed to the ilium (Fig. 23). The posterior column is then reduced; the reduction is judged by visualization of the quadrilateral surface. Fixation is performed with interfragmentary lag screws and supplementary reconstruction or buttress plate.

Postoperative Management

Closed suction drainage is continued postoperatively for 48 hours. Antimicrobial agents are used for 48 to 72 hours after operation. Passive motion of the hip is started at postoperative day 2 or 3. Crutch walking, allowing up to 14 kg of weight-bearing, is allowed at postoperative day 4 to 7, when pain permits. Weight-bearing is limited for the first 8 weeks and then progressively increased.

Complications include infection, nerve palsy, pulmonary embolism, and heterotopic bone formation which can markedly limit hip motion. Heterotopic bone formation occurs almost exclusively in approaches that strip the external aspect of the innominate bone. This includes the Kocher-Langenbeck, extended iliofemoral, and triradiate approaches. Unfortunately, the ilioinguinal approach, which has the advantage of a negligible incidence of ectopic bone formation, is useful in only approximately 30% of the acetabular fractures that require open reduction and internal fixation. Currently, there is no known treatment regimen that is both effective and safe for preventing ectopic bone formation.

Combined Acetabular and Pelvic Injuries

Occasionally, acetabular fractures are associated with significant injury to the posterior pelvic ring—that is, sacroiliac joint dislocation or sacral fracture. In these complex cases, reduction and stabilization of the posterior pelvic ring is required prior to attempts at reduction of the acetabular fracture. Precise reduction of a displaced acetabular fracture cannot be achieved when the pelvic ring is distorted. Fixation of the sacroiliac joint often can be done through a single surgical incision that also exposes the acetabulum. The sacroiliac joint can be exposed by either the Kocher-Langenbeck approach with a cephalad extension or an extended iliofemoral approach. The ilioinguinal approach can be used for access to both the anterior sacroiliac joint and the symphysis pubis.

Old Fractures

If operation is delayed beyond 3 weeks after injury, organized callus will be present about the fracture lines, impairing reduction. In younger patients with unacceptable displacement, and especially with an elementary fracture configuration, open reduction and internal fixation should be undertaken even if osteotomy of a partially or totally healed fracture is required. If the patient is older and has a complex fracture with minimal to moderate deformity, operation can be deferred. The extended iliofemoral approach provides maximal access to the innominate bone for the necessary removal of fracture callus or osteotomy.

Acetabular Fractures in Children

Acetabular fractures occur in approximately 2% of all pelvic fractures in children. Injury to the triradiate cartilage can result in growth arrest with subsequent acetabular deformity. The number of reported cases, however, is less than 10. Post-traumatic arthritis is the most common complication after acetabular fracture in children. In one series, 18 of 25 children with displaced acetabular fractures subsequently had arthritis; 2 patients had premature closure of the triradiate cartilage in this series. Displaced acetabular fractures in children require anatomic reduction, just as in adults, to prevent malunion and late traumatic arthritis. If closed methods are unsuccessful, open reduction and internal fixation is required.

Annotated Bibliography

Anatomy

Hollinshead, W.H.: Anatomy for Surgeons, pp. 635–647. Vol. 3. Second edition. New York, Harper & Row, Publishers, 1969.

Basic anatomy of the pelvis is reviewed with emphasis on soft tissue attachments. Joints of the pelvic girdle are described completely.

Tile, M.: Fractures of the Pelvis and Acetabulum. Baltimore, Williams & Wilkins, 1984.

This text details radiology, classification, and surgical and nonsurgical treatments of acetabulum and pelvic fractures.

Pelvic Trauma

Colapinto, V.: Trauma to the pelvis: Urethral injury. Clin. Orthop. 151:46–55, 1980.

Urethral injuries are reviewed with a classification outlined. Diagnostic as well as therapeutic regimens are discussed.

Naam, N.H.; Brown, W.M.; Hurd, R.; Burdge, R.E.; and Kaminski, D.L.: Major pelvic fractures. Arch. Surg. 118:610–616, 1983.

Pelvic fractures in 593 patients are reviewed. Mortality may be as high as 60%. Factors influencing morbidity and mortality are discussed. Advanced treatment methods are outlined.

Perry, J.F., Jr.: Pelvic open fractures. Clin. Orthop. 151:41–45, 1980.

A series of 738 patients included 31 open fractures. These are reviewed in terms of complications, associated injuries, and mortality.

Saibil, E.A.; Maggisano, R.; and Witchell, S.S.: Angiography in the diagnosis and treatment of trauma. J. Can. Assoc. Radiol. 34:218–227, 1983.

The role of angiography in the diagnostic work-up of the trauma patient is discussed. Transcatheter arterial embolization is described as possibly the definitive therapeutic procedure in pelvic bleeding.

Tile, M.: Fractures of the Pelvis and Acetabulum. Baltimore, Williams & Wilkins, 1984.

(For annotation, see entry under *Anatomy* above.)

Pelvic Ring Injuries

Alho, A., and Horn, A.: External fixation of pelvic fracture ex vivo. Ann. Chir. Gynaecol. 72:308–311, 1983.

Craniad dislocation of the fractured hemipelvis is the most difficult component to reduce and to control by external fixation. The stabilizing effect of several external frames was studied by using a cadaver pelvis. Single frames, double frames, trapezoid frames, and double trapezoid frames were mounted in three-pin units on each anterior iliac crest. Successively increasing the number of transverse connecting rods increased the stability of the construction. Wiring of the symphysis had the same effect when constructions with one or two transverse rods were used. Double fixation sites of the pin units in the anterior pelvis added only marginally to the stability. The highest rigidity was achieved by using a circumferential frame with pin units in both anterior and posterior iliac crests.

Bucholz, R.W.: The pathologic anatomy of Malgaigne fracture-dislocations of the pelvis. J. Bone Joint Surg. 63A:400–404, 1981.

Multiple fresh dissections of cadavers with pelvis fractures were performed to determine the nature of the injury and the stability. All pelvic ring fractures were found to have some degree of anterior as well as posterior injury. A classification of three types based on stability was formulated.

Gill, K., and Bucholz, R.W.: The role of computerized tomographic scanning in the evaluation of major pelvic fractures. J. Bone Joint Surg. 66A:34–39, 1984.

Twenty-five patients with double vertical fractures of the pelvic ring were evaluated by both plain radiography and computed tomography of the pelvis. In 8 of the 25 patients, the interpretation from the plain radiographs, based on the classification of Pennal et al., changed when additional anatomic information was provided by the computed tomogram. The authors recommend that computed tomography be used for: 1) double vertical fracture-dislocations of the pelvic ring in which plain radiographs are inadequate for judging pelvic stability, 2) fractures of the pelvic ring with extension into the acetabulum, and 3) major injuries to the hemipelvis that are to be treated by open reduction and internal fixation. However, due to the increased cost and radiation exposure, routine computed tomographic scanning is not justified for all injuries to the pelvic ring.

Klassen, R.A., and Hall, B.B.: Pelvic fractures in children: A long-term follow-up study (abstract). Orthop. Trans. 6:323, 1982.

The late results in 69 children with sacroiliac joint injury were examined. In patients who only had diastasis the long-term results were generally good; however, if initial subluxation of the joint was present, the majority had late pain.

Lange, R.H., and Hansen, S.T., Jr.: Pelvic ring disruptions with symphysis pubis diastasis: Indications, technique, and limitations of anterior internal fixation. Clin. Orthop. 201:130–137, 1985.

Twenty-four patients with symphysis diastasis were treated with a two-hole plate technique, with overall satisfactory results.

McDonald, G.A.: Pelvic disruptions in children. Clin. Orthop. 151:130–134, 1980.

One hundred fifty-four cases of pelvis fractures in children were examined, and 15 were found to have had significant initial deformity. Of these 15 patients, those who had unreduced sacroiliac dislocation had late symptomatic deformity.

Mears, D.C., and Rubash, H.: Pelvic and Acetabular Fractures. Thorofare, N.J., Slack, 1986.

An extensive exposure to the innominate bone is described. The approach proceeds through a triradiate incision and has a final exposure very similar to the extended iliofemoral approach. Satisfactory reductions with an acceptable complication rate were achieved through this approach. Other surgical techniques for acetabulum and pelvis fractures are detailed.

Rang, M.: Children's Fractures, pp. 150–154. Philadelphia, J.B. Lippincott Company, 1974.

The majority of pelvic ring injuries in children may be treated conservatively and a satisfactory result expected. If significant initial deformity of the pelvic ring is present, this deformity must be corrected because pelvic ring deformities are most likely not to correct with growth. Acetabulum fractures are a rare injury in children.

Semba, R.T.; Yasukawa, K.; and Gustilo, R.B.: Critical analysis of results of 53 Malgaigne fractures of the pelvis. J. Trauma 23:535–537, 1983.

Critical analysis of 53 Malgaigne fractures of the pelvis was undertaken at Hennepin County Medical Center, Minneapolis, over a 10-year period (1968–1978) with particular emphasis on immediate and late complications. Thirty patients were followed for 2 to 12 years after injury. Eleven patients were asymptomatic, 11 had paresthesias of the lower extremity on the same side as the fracture, 9 had gait disturbance, 8 had severe low back pain, 4 had groin pain, and 2 had fecal incontinence. Low back pain as a late sequela was related to sacral or sacroiliac injury. There appeared to be a correlation between the amount of displacement of the detached hemipelvis and the frequency of subsequent low back pain. Reduction of the upward displacement of the hemipelvis, by any means, to anatomic configuration can be of help in reducing late sequelae.

Tile, M.: Fractures of the Pelvis and Acetabulum. Baltimore, Williams & Wilkins, 1984.

(For annotation, see entry under *Anatomy* above.)

Acetabular Fractures

Burk, D.L., Jr.; Mears, D.C.; Kennedy, W.H.; Cooperstein, L.A.; and Herbert, D.L.: Three-dimensional computed tomography of acetabular fractures. Radiology 155:183–186, 1985.

Computer programs that produce three-dimensional surface reformations from sets of contiguous axial computed tomography scans were used in evaluating various acetabular fractures in 20 patients. The three-dimensional images were easily correlated with plain radiographs, and new views were produced that provided a unique perspective not obtainable by conventional radiography. The three-dimensional images were useful in complex displaced fractures in cases in which the interpretation of plain radiographs was difficult. Plain radiographs and conventional computed tomography scans were more sensitive than the three-dimensional images in detecting undisplaced fractures.

Epstein, H.C.: Traumatic Dislocation of the Hip. Baltimore, Williams & Wilkins Company, 1980.

Posterior dislocation of the hip combined with acetabulum fracture leads to a high incidence of post-traumatic arthritis. The long-term results were best in those patients who underwent primary open reduction of the dislocation with removal of intra-articular bone fragments and internal fixation of the fracture.

Hall, B.B., and Klassen, R.A.: Acetabular fractures in children: A long-term follow-up study (abstract). Orthop. Trans. 6:355, 1982.

As in adults, post-traumatic arthritis is the most common problem after acetabular fracture in children. Two of 25 children had premature triradiate cartilage closure.

Hallel, T., and Salvati, E.A.: Premature closure of the triradiate cartilage: A case report and animal experiment. Clin. Orthop. 124:278–281, 1977.

Documentation is provided for a limited number of case reports of premature closure of the triradiate cartilage after acetabulum fracture in children. This premature closure produces a very shallow acetabulum.

Harley, J.D.; Mack, L.A.; and Winquist, R.A.: CT of acetabular fractures: Comparison with conventional radiography. A.J.R. 138:413–417, 1982.

Computed tomography is recommended for routine evaluation of all acetabulum fractures. Efficacy is greatest in demonstrating fractures of the roof, quadrilateral surface, and posterior wall and in diagnosing intra-articular free bony fragments.

Judet, R.; Judet, J.; and Letournel, E.: Fractures of the acetabulum: Classification and surgical approaches for open reduction. J. Bone Joint Surg. 46A:1615–1646, 1964.

The initial findings and techniques in open reduction and internal fixation of acetabulum fractures are presented. A descriptive anatomic classification is provided that continues to be the most useful acetabulum fracture classification available.

Letournel, E., and Judet, R.: Fractures of the Acetabulum. (Translated and edited by R.A. Elson.) New York, Springer-Verlag, 1981.

A thorough anatomic and radiographic description of the 10 major acetabulum fracture types is given. After analysis of an acetabulum fracture and assignment of the classification, decision-making proceeds to selection of a surgical approach for open reduction and internal fixation. The long-term functional results have a high degree of correlation with the accuracy of surgical reduction.

Matta, J.; Anderson, L.; Epstein, H.; and Henricks, P.: Fractures of the acetabulum: A retrospective analysis. Clin. Orthop. 205:230–240, 1986.

A retrospective analysis was performed of 64 cases of major fractures of the acetabulum. A radiographic method of measuring the acetabular dome after fracture proved to have prognostic significance for those fractures that were treated nonoperatively or had inadequate surgical reductions. In fractures treated operatively, the accuracy of surgical reduction correlated significantly with the final clinical results.

Matta, J.M.; Mehne, D.K.; and Roffi, R.: Fractures of the acetabulum: Early results of a prospective study. Clin. Orthop. 205:241–250, 1986.

In a prospective series of major acetabulum fractures, open reduction and internal fixation was found to be necessary for the majority. Utilizing the techniques described by Letournel, accurate surgical reduction was possible in a large majority of the cases while maintaining an acceptable complication rate. The early clinical results were overall satisfactory.

Mays, J., and Neufeld, A.J.: Skeletal traction methods. Clin. Orthop. 102:144–151, 1974.

The technique of Neufeld roller traction is described. In this type of traction, the leg is suspended free while in traction and may be actively exercised in all directions while traction is maintained.

Mears, D.C., and Rubash, H.: Pelvic and Acetabular Fractures. Thorofare, N.J., Slack, 1986.

(For annotation, see entry under *Pelvic Ring Injuries* above.)

Müller, M.E.; Allgöwer, M.; Schneider, R.; and Willenegger, H.: Manual of Internal Fixation, pp. 28–41. Berlin, Springer-Verlag, 1979.

The principle as well as technical application of the lag screw for internal fixation of fractures is described. In this technique a screw glides freely through the first bone fragment and purchases only the distal fragment.

Rang, M.: Children's Fractures, pp. 150–154. Philadelphia, J.B. Lippincott Company, 1974.

(For annotation, see entry under *Pelvic Ring Injuries* above.)

31

Trauma: Hip

This chapter reviews current treatment of trauma in and about the hip. Simple dislocations without associated fractures are reduced as soon as possible, and graded weight-bearing is started after 6 to 10 days of bed rest. Hip dislocations associated with fractures are treated more aggressively—open reduction, removal of bone fragments from the joint, and stabilization of fractures as necessary to produce a stable, concentric hip joint. Femoral neck fractures are treated by anatomic reduction and stable fixation in the majority of cases. Completely displaced neck fractures in debilitated patients may require a hemiprosthesis. Femoral neck fractures in young patients are treated by anatomic reduction and multiple pin fixation. For intertrochanteric fractures, a collapsible nail or screw plate device is used that allows impaction of the fracture fragments to a stable configuration. Ender pins are not used in fixation of intertrochanteric fractures, except in selected cases. Subtrochanteric fractures are treated with intramedullary devices such as the Zickel nail or a strong nail or screw plate sliding device. The choice of fixation depends on the configuration of the fracture, and bone grafting of medial comminution is of value.

Hip Dislocations

Hip dislocations are the result of high-energy trauma and occur most commonly in the young. Osteonecrosis causes up to 15% of dislocations. The majority occur within 1 year after injury, but they can occur up to 3 years after injury. Degenerative osteoarthritis is a long-term complication; an incidence of up to 75% is noted in long-term follow-ups. Careful management of hip dislocations with removal of osteocartilaginous fragments from the joint decreases this complication. Because this is a high-energy injury, other associated musculoskeletal trauma occurs in 30% to 40% of the cases.

The recommended treatment is immediate reduction, closed or open if necessary, with evaluation of the hip joint to ensure that there are no osteocartilaginous fragments remaining. In uncomplicated hip dislocations without significant acetabular fracture, the hip may be reduced and tested for stability. If the hip is stable and a concentric reduction is obtained, the patient is treated symptomatically with bed rest for 6 to 10 days, and then ambulation is started with partial weight-bearing as tolerated. The patient remains on crutches with partial weight-bearing for 4 to 6 weeks (until soft tissue is healed) and then progresses to full weight-bearing. If there are osteocartilaginous fragments within the joint, surgical removal is necessary. The surgeon must evaluate the joint carefully for stability after reduction. Associated acetabular fractures, the most common of which is of the posterior lip, must be internally fixed to reconstruct a stable joint if instability is present.

The most useful classification of posterior fracture dislocations of the acetabulum is that developed by Epstein (Table 1).

Anterior Dislocations

Anterior dislocations occur in approximately 15% of all traumatic hip dislocations. Femoral head damage is common, occurring in up to 85% of patients, and is most commonly an indentation fracture. It has been documented that indentation fractures deeper than 4 mm have a poor prognosis. Osteonecrosis occurs in up to 15% of these dislocations, and the majority of anterior dislocations progress to degenerative arthritis. Closed reduction is accomplished by traction, extension, and internal rotation of the hip. Tomography is indicated if there is any question of osteocartilaginous fragments in the joint.

Posterior Dislocations

This is by far the most common hip dislocation and may be associated with a posterior acetabular defect. The straight posterior dislocation without acetabular injury can be reduced with adduction, flexion, traction, abduction, and external rotation under general anesthesia. If closed reduction under general anesthesia cannot be performed, then open reduction through a posterior approach should be used. The femoral head can be buttonholed through the capsule or interposed behind the piriformis, preventing reduction.

In fracture-dislocations involving portions of the acetabulum, it is recommended that open reduction be performed with irrigation of the joint to remove debris and fixation of the acetabular component as necessary to reconstruct a stable hip. If closed reduction is successful, computed tomography is helpful to detect the presence of an inverted labrum or osteocartilaginous loose bodies, particularly if a nonconcentric joint is noted on the radiographs.

Osteonecrosis of the femoral head may occur in up to 10% of cases after straight posterior dislocation. This complication must be watched for as long as 3 years after injury. Degenerative post-traumatic arthritis is dependent on the severity of the hip injury, contusion to the articular cartilage, and the presence of osteocartilaginous fragments remaining in the hip joint. The incidence is documented to

Table 1. Epstein's Classification of Posterior Hip Dislocations

Type	Description
I	No or only minor fracture
II	Large posterior acetabular rim fracture
III	Comminuted fracture of posterior rim, with or without major fragment
IV	Fracture of both acetabular rim and floor
V	Fracture of femoral head with or without other fragments

be 33% at 10 years and up to 75% after 30 years. Posterior dislocations may go unrecognized, particularly in the multiple trauma patients in whom there is an ipsilateral femoral shaft fracture. One must evaluate the pelvic radiograph carefully and be aware of the position of the hip if a femoral shaft fracture is present in a multiply injured patient. A radiograph with the hip in flexion and adduction may reveal a posterior dislocation when there is an ipsilateral femoral shaft fracture (Fig. 1).

In 242 posterior fracture-dislocations of the hip, long-term satisfactory results were obtained by primary open reduction, internal fixation of the fracture, and removal of loose fragments.

In dislocations that are 3 weeks or more old, the acetabulum is generally filled with fibrous tissue, and closed reduction is no longer possible. Open reduction must be performed at this time. Late reduction is associated with osteonecrosis in more than 50% of patients. In the young patient, attempted reduction and acetabular repair is indicated. In the elderly, primary arthroplasty is indicated.

Posterior Dislocations With Femoral Head Fractures

This rare injury is seen in only 7% of all hip dislocations. Pipkin's classification is the most useful in categorizing femoral head fractures (Fig. 2). This injury commonly occurs in vehicular accidents when the knee strikes the dashboard while the hip is adducted and flexed less than 50°. The femoral head is driven into the thick portion of the posterior rim of the acetabulum, and a fragment of the head is sheared off. Computed tomography is of great value in identifying the location and degree of the fracture. Careful attention should be paid to the femoral neck so that a nondisplaced femoral neck fracture is not missed (displacement of the fracture could occur during the attempt to reduce the hip). If a femoral neck fracture is associated with a hip dislocation, open reduction is mandatory. Closed reduction can be attempted in Pipkin's type I, II, and IV injuries. If concentric reduction is obtained by the closed technique, the extremity can be held in traction for 6 weeks; then, the patient is mobilized with graded weight-bearing. Open reduction is indicated if reduction cannot be obtained closed or if there are loose osteocartilaginous fragments that block a concentric reduction of the hip and fractured femoral head. Most authors recommend a surgical approach to the posterolateral aspect of the hip for open reduction and fixation so that the anterior femoral head vasculature can be preserved.

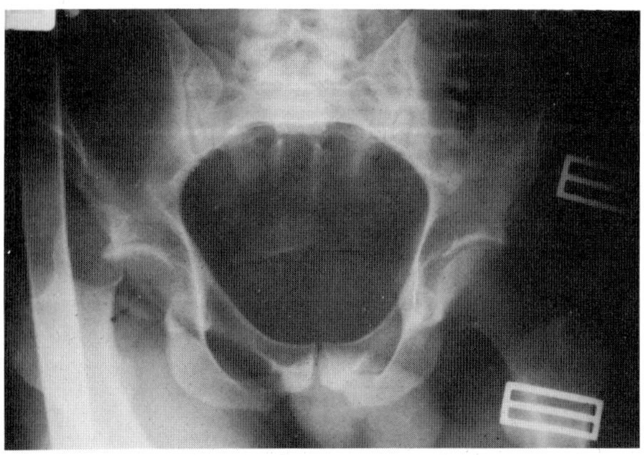

Figure 1

Multiply injured patient with ipsilateral shaft fracture and posterior hip dislocation. Note the flexed, adducted position of the hip.

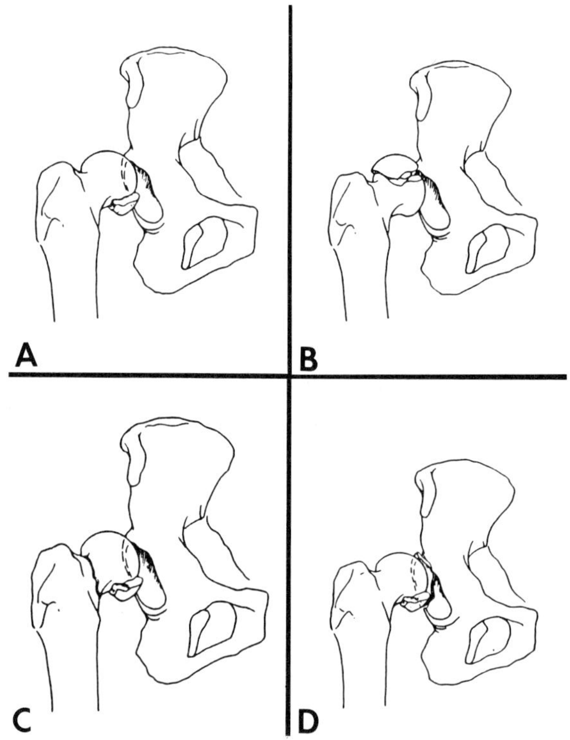

Figure 2

Pipkin's classification of femoral head fractures. *A*, Type I, fracture of femoral head caudad to fovea. *B*, Type II, fracture of femoral head cephalad to fovea. *C*, Type III, type I or II injury plus fracture of femoral neck. *D*, Type IV, type I or II injury plus fracture of acetabular rim.

Small femoral head fragments should be excised during open reduction. There is some controversy over large femoral head fragments, but most authors believe that fixation should be attempted to prevent later degenerative arthritis. In type III injuries, the femoral neck fracture should be stabilized with multiple pins, and other fragments should be either excised or fixed, depending on their size. In young patients, if a femoral neck fracture is missed and displacement results, open reduction with multiple internal pin fixation is necessary. After open reduction and internal fixation, limited weight-bearing is allowed for 6 to 8 weeks; then, the patient progresses to full weight-bearing as tolerated. In the elderly, this injury is quite rare, but arthroplasty is indicated if it occurs.

Summary

Hip dislocations generally occur secondary to high-energy trauma and, for this reason, are more frequent in the young. The incidence of osteonecrosis after dislocation ranges from 10% to 15%, and the long-term incidence of post-traumatic arthritis is extremely high. The rate of development of post-traumatic arthritis is increased if loose fragments remain within the joint. Therefore, open reduction is indicated for fractures of the acetabulum or femoral head in the majority of cases. It is mandatory if a concentric reduction is not obtained. In all injuries, the patient must be warned that the sequelae of osteonecrosis can occur several years after injury, and the patient should be followed for an extended period of time. The patient should also be warned about the possible development of posttraumatic arthritis.

Hip Fractures

Incidence and Mortality

The number and severity of hip fractures are increasing rapidly as the average age of our population increases. The number of hip fractures in the United States tripled between the years 1965 and 1981. Other studies have predicted that, over the next 2 decades, the number of hip fractures will again triple. This results, in part, from the advancing age of our population due to better medical care. At the present time, 250,000 hip fractures occur annually in the United States and result in health care costs of more than 1.25 billion dollars.

The mortality rates associated with hip fractures vary from 13% to 30% within the first year after injury. After that, the life expectancy of the patient returns to normal. In general, there is a slightly greater mortality rate with intertrochanteric fractures than with intracapsular fractures; this corresponds to the slightly more advanced age of patients who suffer the former. Patients living in nursing homes prior to fracture have the highest morbidity and mortality rates (30%) and are least likely to resume ambulation. In the socially independent population, the majority of patients recover to their previous levels of function if complications do not occur.

The average age of the population will be 40 years by 1990, with a large percentage of it in the age group in which hip fractures are common. For this reason it is absolutely essential that the orthopaedic surgeon understand the nature of hip fractures as well as their current treatment.

Etiology

Falls are the single largest cause of hip fractures in the United States. In the younger population, high-energy trauma from motor vehicle accidents is the leading cause of hip injuries.

Studies have shown no increased incidence of osteoporosis in patients with fracture compared with those without fracture. Muscular paresis, weakness, and instability from neurologic conditions are the main causes of falls. These problems are directly correlated with the incidence of hip fracture in the elderly. Because simple falls do not result in a fractured hip in the young, it is likely that osteoporosis in the elderly is a contributing factor in causing hip fractures, even though it is not the initiating event. The identification of factors leading to osteoporosis and their treatment are paramount in the prevention of this rapidly increasing problem.

Preoperative Evaluation

Recent studies have shown that improved rehabilitation postoperatively can be achieved by proper evaluation of the patient preoperatively.

The patient should be assessed in the emergency room for degree of blood loss, particularly with an intertrochanteric fracture. One in five elderly patients suffers from cardiac disease, senility, or neurologic impairment, and these must be evaluated and stabilized prior to surgical intervention. The timing of operation has been debated in many articles; the most recent recommend thorough medical evaluation and stabilization before operation. This must be carried out as rapidly as possible and usually can be accomplished within 12 to 24 hours. Several recent reports prove the value of prophylactic administration of antimicrobial agents started preoperatively. Infection rates have been decreased from 5% to less than 1% with the use of broad-spectrum agents before and for 1 day after operation. Prolonged use of prophylactic antimicrobial therapy has not been shown to be beneficial. The prevention of decubitus ulcers during recumbency before and after operation is also important because development of decubitus ulcers is associated with a 30% mortality rate and prolonged hospitalization.

Thromboembolic Disease

Low-dose heparin therapy has not been effective in preventing thromboembolic disease. Warfarin (Coumadin) has been found to be the most effective drug in preventing thromboembolic disease, but hematoma formation can complicate anticoagulant treatment if the prothrombin time is not kept within the recommended range (15–18 sec). Aspirin has been shown to be an effective prophylactic drug. Continuous passive motion and intermittent positive-pressure splints may be of value but require specialized apparatus and, in some cases, prolonged recumbency. Stable fixation of the fracture and rapid mobilization of the patient is the most effective method of preventing thromboembolic disease and, in conjunction with administration of either warfarin or aspirin, is the best way to prevent pulmonary embolism.

Preoperative Planning for Special Problems

Special problems can be encountered, depending on the age and the condition of the patient with the hip fracture.

Young Adults With Hip Fracture The lower extremities, upper extremities, chest, abdomen, head, and neck can be involved as a result of high-energy trauma. These multiply injured patients must be stabilized immediately by fixation of all long-bone fractures in the lower extremity; specific care must be paid to the hip fractures to save satisfactory hip function.

Senile Patients The senile patient who is combative and who will pose difficult postoperative management problems should be treated with the goal of obtaining a stable hip. This can require multiple pins, screw plate fixation, or hemiarthroplasty. Stable internal fixation of femoral neck fractures, whenever possible, is preferable to avoid the complications of prosthetic arthroplasty. If the patient has a completely displaced femoral neck fracture or has a painful fracture that is old, the use of an anterior approach for hemiarthroplasty has been found to decrease the incidence of hip dislocation. This is also true in the patient who is unable to walk preoperatively and the patient who has hip flexion contractures. If the senile, nonambulatory patient experiences little pain secondary to the hip fracture, a few days of traction followed by progression to a bed-chair status can be the treatment of choice.

Femoral Neck Fractures in the Elderly Undisplaced femoral neck fractures (Garden type I and II) in elderly patients are best treated with multiple pins or screw fixation and immediate weight-bearing. If a single telescoping hip screw or nail device is used for internal fixation, an additional stabilizing pin or screw above is recommended to achieve more torsional stability. Rigid nail plate devices (i.e., Smith-Peterson nail) must not be used for femoral neck fractures, irrespective of age of patient or type of fracture, because of the high rate of osteonecrosis and nonunion.

For displaced femoral neck fractures (type III and IV), closed reduction and fixation with multiple pins or screws is effective if anatomic reduction is obtained. The osteonecrosis and nonunion rates for Garden type I and type II femoral neck fracture are less than 10%; for Garden types III and IV femoral neck fractures, they are 15% to 20% and 15% to 30%, respectively.

Delay of operation (up to 3 days) and early weight-bearing do not appear to influence the incidence of osteonecrosis and nonunion. However, anatomic reduction and method and quality of fixation greatly influence the end result.

Early studies of hemiarthroplasty for femoral neck fractures showed higher morbidity and mortality rates compared to internal fixation with multiple pins or a collapsing device. However, excellent results with a low sepsis rate and infrequent dislocations have been reported recently with the use of cemented hemiarthroplasty or cemented bipolar prosthesis. This is attributed to good preoperative medical work-up, prophylactic antimicrobial therapy, and appropriate surgical approaches that consider the patient's mental and ambulatory status. An anterior approach is recommended for the senile patient who otherwise tends to dislocate his prosthesis in flexion, which is common in the posterior approach. Bipolar prostheses appear to lessen protrusio or central migration, compared with conventional hemiarthroplasty. Disassembly of a bipolar prosthesis after dislocation or in an attempt to reduce the dislocated prosthesis has not been a problem recently because the locking devices have been improved.

Mortality and morbidity are high in primary total hip replacement for femoral neck fractures. The only indication for primary total hip replacement in femoral neck fractures is evidence of severe osteoarthritis or rheumatoid arthritis.

Neurologically Impaired Patients Neurologically impaired patients have a poor prognosis, and mortality has been reported to be as high as 30% to 50% after treatment with an endoprosthesis. One study found a 100% mortality rate in patients who dislocated their prostheses. Internal fixation of these hip fractures is indicated when possible. Prosthetic replacement should be done through an anterolateral approach. In old patients who have displaced femoral neck fractures and are being treated with phenytoin (Dilantin), endoprosthetic replacement is indicated because of the decreased rate of fracture union.

Rheumatoid Arthritis Patients Mortality and morbidity rates are high in rheumatoid arthritis patients who sustain hip fractures. With intracapsular fractures, the incidences of nonunion and osteonecrosis are high compared to those in the general population. With intertrochanteric and intracapsular fractures, the rates of infection, overall morbidity, and failure of internal fixation devices are much higher than in the general population. For this reason, in this group of patients, arthroplasty is often the treatment of choice for femoral neck fractures.

Pathologic Fractures If the life expectancy of the patient who has a pathologic fracture is greater than 6 weeks, the fracture should be fixed internally or prosthetic replacement should be performed. An impending pathologic fracture should be fixed if it is painful, if the lytic lesion is more than 2.5 cm in diameter, or if the process has destroyed 50% or more of the cortex of a long bone. Internal fixation of an impending fracture is easier than treatment of a fracture and therefore is the treatment of choice if the lesion is discovered early enough. Preoperative evaluation and preparation of the patient for operation are the same as for other patients who have hip fractures. Special attention should be paid to serum calcium levels, both prior to and after internal fixation. With tumors that are sensitive to irradiation, treatment should begin prior to or immediately after internal fixation of the fracture. Effective doses of radiotherapy have not been shown to decrease soft tissue healing. However, radiotherapy does decrease incorporation of bone graft, and therefore methyl methacrylate is used to fill defects left after tumor removal. Abduction muscles can be sewn into the iliotibial band. Special care must be taken with these patients to prevent hip dislocation in the immediate postoperative period if the trochanteric area of the femur is removed.

In patients who have acetabular damage, a cemented acetabular prosthesis is used. Portions of the ilium are rebuilt with methyl methacrylate, wire mesh, and Steinmann pins or screws. Protrusio rings, expanded polyethylene components, and large bipolar prostheses also can be of benefit in these patients.

For subtrochanteric pathologic fractures without head or neck involvement, the Zickel nail with or without cement has been the fixation device of choice. Cerclage wiring is used if needed, and methyl methacrylate can be added after the fracture has been fixed.

Pain relief and early mobilization of patients with pathologic fractures have been shown to enhance the quality of life, even in a very short-term situation.

Intracapsular Fractures Intracapsular fractures of the hip are the result of high-energy trauma in healthy young persons and of simple falls in the majority of the elderly.

In the young, closed or open reduction with internal fixation is the accepted method of treatment. In the elderly, the undisplaced femoral neck fracture is treated with internal fixation, but there is controversy over treatment of the displaced femoral neck fracture. Both open reduction with internal fixation and prosthetic replacement including hemiarthroplasty and total hip arthroplasty have been advocated.

Femoral Neck Fractures

Young Patients

The majority of femoral neck fractures in young patients occur secondary to high-energy trauma from motor vehicle accidents or falls from heights; more than 50% of these victims also have other serious injuries to the skeletal system. The incidences of osteonecrosis and nonunion have been reported to be high in the past. More recent studies have shown the rates of osteonecrosis and nonunion to be quite acceptable and comparable to those associated with well-fixed femoral neck fracture in old patients.

Closed reduction with gentle traction and internal rotation is successful in most patients. If the fracture cannot be reduced by closed methods, it should be opened, anatomically reduced, and then fixed internally. Bone in young patients is hard, and so nails should not be used to fix these fractures because the blood supply to the femoral head can be damaged during the pounding process. The best results have been obtained with multiple pin fixation. The current recommended treatment in the young patient with femoral neck fracture is closed or open anatomic reduction with multiple pin fixation.

Advocates of posterior muscle pedicle and bone graft have shown that osteonecrosis and nonunion rates can be decreased by using these procedures. More recent studies have not confirmed their value, and a higher incidence of infection has been reported when they are used. There still remains controversy in this area of treatment of femoral neck fractures.

In the multiply injured young patient who has a femoral neck fracture, anatomic reduction of the hip fracture should be performed with multiple pin fixation of the hip, followed by fixation of the long bone fractures by other means of internal fixation, depending upon the type of fractures.

The usefulness of radionuclide scanning to predict the future development of osteonecrosis of the hip immediately after fracture fixation is controversial. There is probably some value in bone scans to compare the affected hip with the unaffected hip. Aspiration of the hip joint to relieve pressure has been shown to have little or no value because of the small amount of blood that is aspirated and the small pressure gradients that were found in the study evaluating this procedure. With proper treatment, the young patient who has a displaced femoral neck fracture should have a nonunion rate no greater than 15% and a necrosis rate no greater than 20% (Fig. 3).

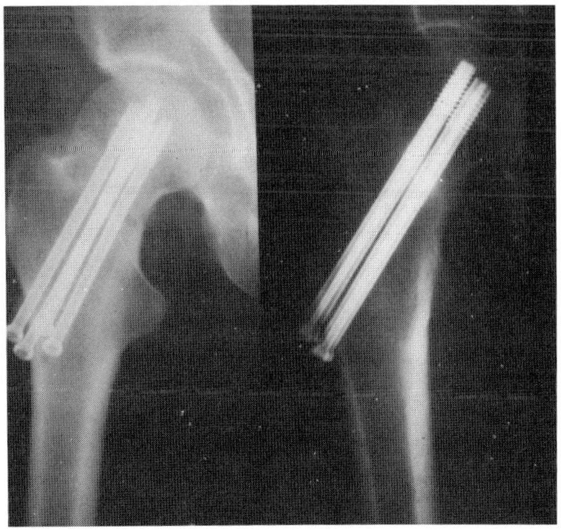

Figure 3

In young patients, femoral neck fracture fixed with multiple pins after anatomic reduction should have a nonunion rate of less than 15% and an osteonecrosis rate of less than 20%.

Elderly Patients

Femoral neck fractures usually are the result of simple falls. Concurrent medical problems are quite common, however, and these must be addressed prior to surgical intervention. A valgus angulation of up to 15° is acceptable. The final alignment of the femoral neck after reduction is less than 10° of either anterior or posterior angulation. Two-point fixation appears to offer better stability and long-term results than use of one large device. Excellent results have been obtained with multiple pins. Immediate weight-bearing after multiple pin fixation does not appear to increase the incidence of failure compared with limited weight-bearing. Excellent results also have been obtained by using a single impaction screw device with a stabilizing pin above it. Less satisfactory, and indeed unacceptable, results have been reported with rigid nail plate devices. Damage to the blood supply of the femoral head has been found when the flanged nail is driven into it.

For Garden types I and II (nondisplaced impacted femoral neck fractures in slight valgus), internal fixation and immediate mobilization is advocated. For Garden types III and IV (displaced femoral neck fractures), controversy exists. Most authors advocate open reduction and internal fixation of femoral neck fractures in young and active patients and primary hemiarthroplasty in older patients.

Osteonecrosis and nonunion rates should be less than 7% after undisplaced Garden type I or II fractures. Nonunion rates should range from 15% to 20% and osteonecrosis rates from 15% to 30% in displaced femoral neck fractures. These complications can be kept to a minimum by achieving anatomic reduction—closed if possible, open if necessary—and stable internal fixation. Fixation should not be done by using a nail in intracapsular fractures; if a large screw is used, optimal fixation can be obtained by inserting at least one additional smaller screw to prevent rotation.

Prosthetic Replacement

If the patient with a completely displaced femoral neck fracture has a physiologic age of 75 years or more, most authorities recommend a hemiarthroplasty. Different types of hemiarthroplasties have been used. Early studies showed that a cemented prosthesis gave better results than an uncemented prosthesis in terms of pain relief. The cemented bipolar component gave excellent pain relief, and at least one study found no evidence of acetabular erosion with the bipolar components. There is no definitive report, however, on the best hemiprosthesis to use in these instances. Early studies on hemiarthroplasty replacement showed a higher rate of morbidity and mortality with prosthetic replacement than with fracture fixation. However, recent studies show that, with new technologic advances and the prophylactic use of antimicrobial agents and anticoagulants, the morbidity and mortality rates with the two treatment approaches are equivalent. These studies also point out that, in the older studies, the patients receiving a prosthesis generally were the more debilitated ones. Modern prostheses also allow a better press fit compared to older prostheses. The question of whether it is better to use cement or a solid press-fit prosthesis has not been answered yet. Disassembly of bipolar prostheses in the postoperative period has been a problem in the past, but the current bipolar prostheses are locked together and disassembly in the patient is less of a problem. Dislocation rates of bipolar and solid hemiarthroplasty prostheses have not been shown to be different, but closed reduction of the bipolar prosthesis may be more difficult.

There are several reports on use of primary hip arthroplasty to treat femoral neck fractures, but other reports show excellent results when delayed arthroplasty was used to treat late complications of femoral neck fractures. The salvage procedure that can be used to treat the patient who has a poor result after femoral neck fracture is so good that primary total hip arthroplasty for this injury is rarely warranted. Primary total hip arthroplasty, however, is the method of choice in the patient who has a femoral neck fracture and also has advanced rheumatoid arthritis or osteoarthritis.

Summary

In the young patient who has a femoral neck fracture, anatomic closed or open reduction and internal fixation with multiple pins is recommended. The nonunion rates should not exceed 15% and the necrosis rate should not exceed 20%.

In the old but active patient, open reduction and internal fixation is recommended. In both young and old patients, acceptable reduction has limits of 15° of valgus angulation, no varus angulation, and no more than 10° of posterior or anterior angulation.

The Garden type I and II fractures heal with few problems compared to Garden type III and IV displaced fractures which have a higher morbidity. In debilitated patients or patients who have pathologic fractures, hemiarthroplasty is the treatment of choice.

Total hip replacement after femoral neck fracture should be considered in the patient who has rheumatoid arthritis, osteoarthritis, or tumor involving the acetabulum. It is not the recommended treatment for most femoral neck fractures.

Intertrochanteric Fractures

Incidence and Severity

The number and severity of intertrochanteric hip fractures are increasing as the average age of the population increases. Approximately 60% of intertrochanteric fractures are classified as stable and 40%, as unstable. In more recent studies, the percentage of unstable fractures has increased, and this trend is expected to continue due to the increasing age of the population.

Treatment

Intertrochanteric fractures cause considerable bleeding at the fracture site. Therefore, patients must be stabilized and monitored carefully prior to operation. In the early 1900s, before the advent of surgical intervention, use of conservative treatment and bed rest led to numerous complications and ultimate death in the majority of patients. Optimal results can be obtained with internal fixation of these fractures when the patient has been medically stabilized, ideally within the first 24 hours after injury. The best fixation device is a collapsible nail plate or screw plate device that allows bone impaction into a stable position. This allows early mobilization and rehabilitation of the patient. Mortality rates should not exceed 20% in the first year after injury.

Attempts, in the past, to fix these fractures with rigid nail plate devices led to complication rates ranging up to 40% for the difficult-to-reduce unstable fractures. In unstable fractures, the posteromedial buttress of the proximal femur is completely lost, and fixation with a rigid device leads to a high rate of nail penetration, breakage, or cut-out as the fracture impacts into a stable position (Fig. 4). Muscular forces across the hip can be 3 to 5 times body weight. If impaction is prevented by use of rigid nail plate devices, a large bending moment is transmitted to the nail plate junction, which may result in failure.

In the early 1960s, displacement osteotomies were used to create a stable fracture complex and eliminate collapse about a rigid nail plate. The Dimon and Hughston medial displacement osteotomy and the Sarmiento valgus osteotomy were popular. Subsequent studies have shown that, despite the use of osteotomies, impaction still occurred. An anatomic reduction and fixation in slight valgus with a sliding device allows spontaneous impaction and medial displacement, without the additional operation that is required to perform displacement osteotomy. Even fractures that appear to be stable by radiographic criteria may impact and displace medially. Therefore, a sliding device is better than a rigid fixation device.

In the early 1970s, sliding nail and screw devices were popularized. These devices allow solid fixation of the femoral head to the distal femoral shaft and impaction of the fracture fragments into a stable position (Fig. 5). They control bending and rotation while allowing impaction. This converts the hip fixation device into a load-sharing device rather than being a rigid load-sparing device.

Intramedullary devices were introduced in the middle to late 1970s in the form of the Ender nails and condylocephalic nails for fixation of intertrochanteric fractures. The mechanical advantage of these devices is their intramedullary position which places them closer to the resultant force across the hip, reducing the bending moment on the device. In addition, the use of distal sites of insertion was reported to decrease operative time and blood loss

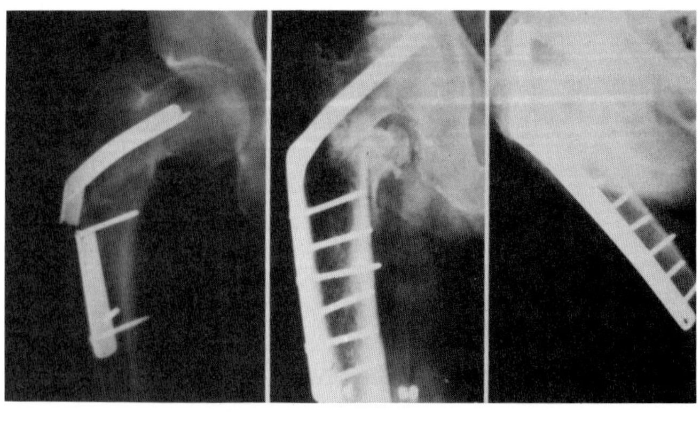

Figure 4

Fixation of unstable intertrochanteric fractures with rigid devices often results in nail plate failure, penetration, or cut-out of the device.

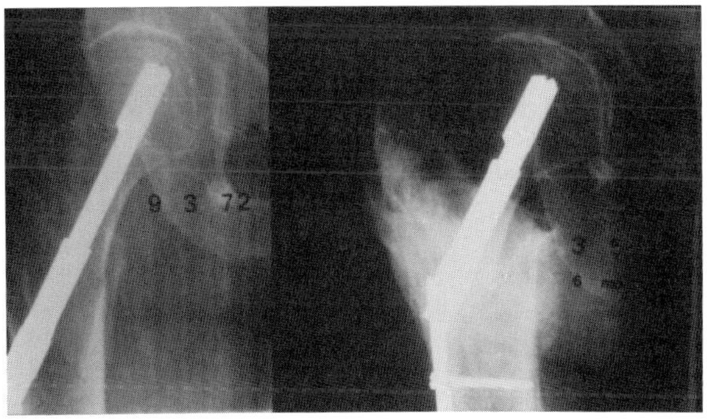

Figure 5

Fixation of unstable intertrochanteric fractures with a sliding device allows impaction and spontaneous medial displacement to a stable position.

compared to use of proximal sites. This surgical technique was made possible by the use of image intensification. The procedure was promoted as a closed method of fixation of intertrochanteric fractures.

Numerous recent reports have described a high incidence of varus deformity and knee pain caused by distal migration of the pins (Fig. 6). This leads to a high incidence of reoperation for pin extraction and correction of deformity. In the majority of these series the high failure rate resulted from loss of reduction, shortening, and external rotation. This has led most authorities to recommend complete abandonment of intramedullary devices as methods of fixation of intertrochanteric fractures.

Others believe that there is still a place for the intramedullary devices in elderly, debilitated patients who have a stable fracture and who can tolerate only minimal operative intervention. An adequate number of pins must be used, and they must be driven deeply into the femoral head to be successful. The poorest results with the Ender and condylocephalic nails have been in subtrochanteric fractures and in unstable intertrochanteric fractures.

The current recommended treatment of both stable and unstable intertrochanteric fractures of the femur in most cases is anatomic reduction and internal fixation of the fracture with a sliding nail or screw that allows spontaneous impaction of the fracture fragments into a stable position.

Surgical Technique The nail should be placed in the center of the femoral head within 1 cm of subchondral bone. This is best accomplished by accurate placement of a guide pin under image intensification and correct measurement to determine the length of the sliding device. Eccentric placement of the screw in the femoral head does not allow deep penetration into the central, dense cancellous bone that is resistant to cut-out. Eccentric placement, particularly in the superolateral aspect of the femoral head, results in a higher complication rate with loss of fixation and nail cut-out (Fig. 7).

There is debate as to the optimal nail plate angle to be used with collapsible hip fixation devices. The combined vector force across the hip acts at 159° to the horizontal. Theoretically, a sliding device that has a screw plate angle closest to this combined vector force allows optimal ease of sliding and impaction (Fig. 8). The larger the nail plate angle, the closer the angle is to the resultant force across the hip and the more the force available to assist impaction. Devices at a smaller angle decrease the available parallel force to the sliding axis of the device and increase the perpendicular or jamming force that acts on the device to prevent impaction. Technically, however, the surgeon is unable to place the sliding device at an angle greater than 150°. This is the optimal angle that is technically possible because it most closely approximates the combined vector force acting across the hip and on the sliding device. The need to position the nail at the ideal angle should not overshadow the need for secure purchase in the femoral head. If the surgeon cannot place a high-angle device deep into the center of the femoral head, a smaller-angle device should be used so that optimal placement can be obtained. This is determined by placing the guide pin under image intensification. The smaller-angle devices must be used in pa-

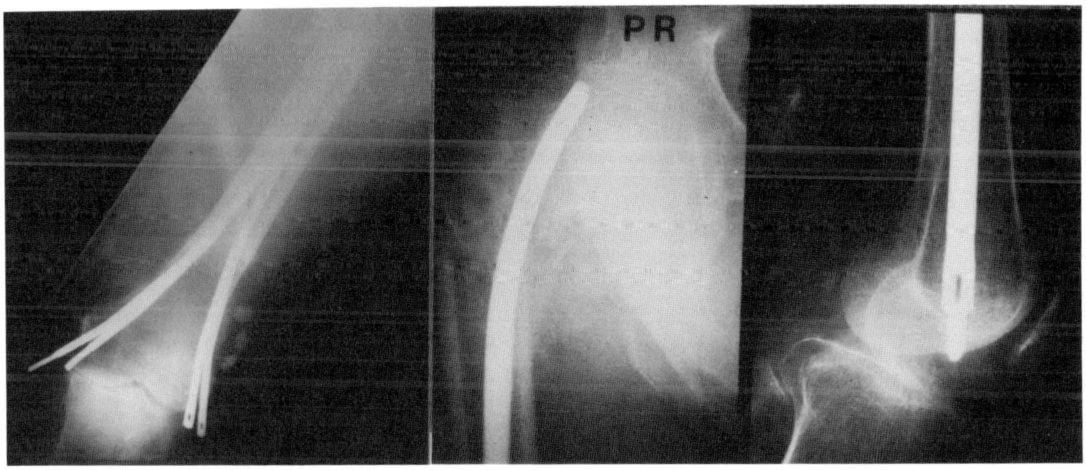

Figure 6

There is a high incidence of varus deformity and knee pain after the use of Ender and other intramedullary devices in fixation of unstable intertrochanteric fractures.

FAILURE RATE VERSUS NAIL POSITION IN TYPE-III FRACTURES

	Position	Incidence No.	Incidence Per cent	AP/Lat. Distance of Nail Tip from Subchondral Bone (mm)	Failures No.	Failures Per cent
2/2	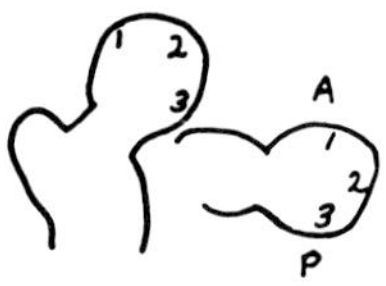	34	46	11/12	0	0
2/3		22	30	14/7	1	4.5
2/1		4	5	9/5	0	0
1/2		6	8	12/18	2	33
1/3		4	5	14/11	1	25
3/3		4	5	15/16	1	25

Figure 7

Device placement in the superolateral aspect of the femoral head results in a higher complication rate, loss of fixation, and nail cut-out.

tients who are small and have varus hips. Because most sliding devices now are available in 5° increments at the nail plate junction, the largest angle that allows proper placement can be selected in each instance. This optimizes both fixation of the fracture and ease of sliding of the device, allowing impaction of the fracture fragments. Mechanical testing has shown that, if fracture fragments are allowed to impact, they can carry a large portion of the load transmitted across the hip. Impaction is essential to reduce the stresses on the fixation device and prevent failure. Use of sliding devices, properly placed after anatomic reduction, allows spontaneous impaction and medial displacement of all intertrochanteric fractures into a stable configuration, permitting early mobilization and weight-bearing.

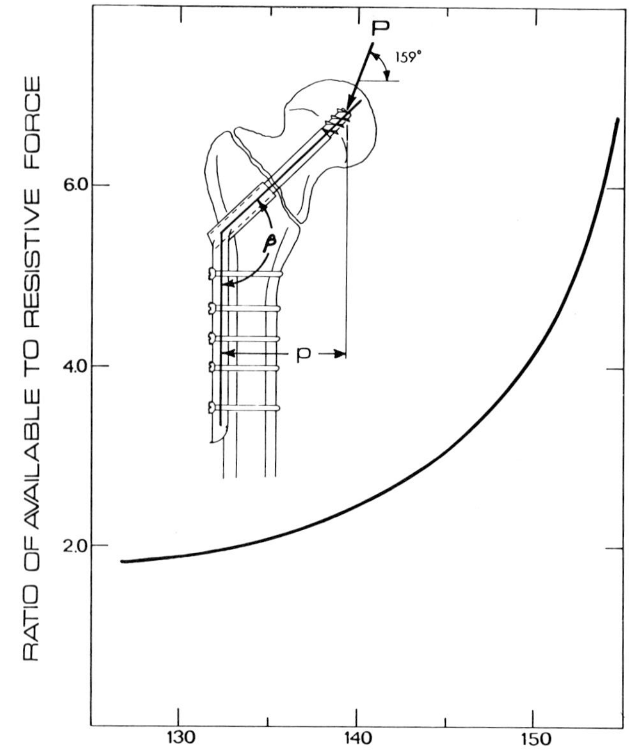

Figure 8

The larger the nail plate angle, the closer the angle is to the resultant force across the hip and the more force available to the sliding device.

Perioperative and Postoperative Care Postoperative care includes early mobilization of the patient; sitting is begun as soon as the patient is medically stable. Ambulation is begun as soon as the patient is strong enough to attempt to walk with assistance in parallel bars. The patient is usually able to sit on postoperative day 1 and able to start ambulation and physical therapy on postoperative day 3. When the fracture is adequately fixed with a collapsible device, weight-bearing can be instituted immediately. Studies have shown that anticoagulation, with either aspirin or warfarin (Coumadin), is effective in decreasing the incidence of thrombophlebitis and fatal pulmonary embolism.

Summary

Optimal care of the patient with intertrochanteric fracture requires medical stabilization, the prophylactic use of antimicrobial agents, and early surgical intervention. Operation should achieve anatomic or slight valgus reduction of the fracture with a device that allows impaction and load-sharing of the fracture fragments. Solid fixation requires penetration into the center of the femoral head to within 1 cm of subchondral bone and solid fixation to the shaft of the femur. Large-angle nailing is desirable without compromising fixation in the central portion of the femoral head. For this reason, a slight valgus reduction may be necessary. Postoperative anticoagulation, early mobilization, and ambulation with full weight-bearing can be allowed when adequate fixation has been obtained.

Subtrochanteric Fractures

Subtrochanteric fractures comprise approximately 15% of hip fractures. No one classification system has withstood the test of time. A subtrochanteric fracture is defined as a fracture of the proximal femur that starts at or below the lesser trochanter and involves the proximal femoral shaft.

With weight-bearing, stresses in the subtrochanteric region are among the highest in the body. Subtrochanteric fractures with significant comminution medially have been reported to have failure rates as high as 50% after nail plate fixation alone. The use of intramedullary devices has decreased this failure rate and is recommended to treat the true subtrochanteric fracture. The device that has given the highest percentage of successful results in numerous

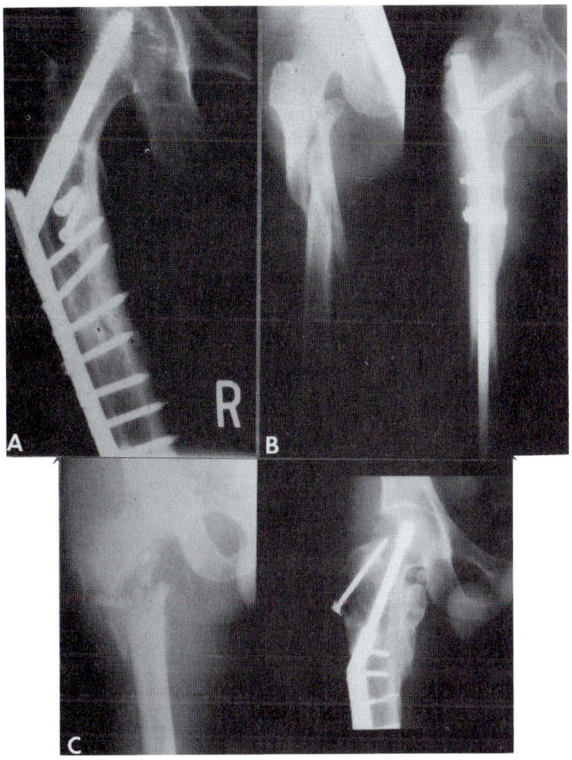

Figure 9

Success in the subtrochanteric fracture can be obtained with the use of the Zickel nail or a strong nail plate sliding device in the intertrochanteric/high subtrochanteric fracture.

studies is the Zickel nail. This requires open reduction and internal fixation of the fracture. Interfragmentary fixation or cerclage wiring is often needed to reconstitute stability and prevent shortening. If there is severe comminution medially, bone grafting of this area should be performed.

Results with use of Ender nails to treat fractures in the subtrochanteric region are variable. Some studies report high success rates and others report high failure rates. Interlocking nails have recently been used to treat subtrochanteric fractures when the lesser trochanter is intact and there is comminution of the proximal shaft in the subtrochanteric region. Reports of varus deformity and failure of this device in subtrochanteric fractures have been published. The safety and efficacy of interlocking nails in the treatment of subtrochanteric fractures have not been determined yet.

Recent reports describe a high success rate with new, strong, sliding nail plate devices in selected patients with subtrochanteric fractures. These collapsible nail plate devices are of particular value in the treatment of intertrochanteric/subtrochanteric fracture in which impaction of the intertrochanteric portion of the fracture is needed to achieve stability. Bone graft in fractures that are comminuted medially is of great value.

In high subtrochanteric fractures in which the collapsible device can act as an intramedullary device and allow impaction of the proximal fragment into the distal fragment, early weight-bearing is allowed. In the subtrochanteric fracture that has medial comminution that extends down the proximal shaft or that has lateral and medial comminution and loss of integrity of the shaft, weight-bearing is not allowed until callus formation is observed on radiographs (this generally occurs at 6 to 8 weeks).

With proper selection of a strong nail plate device that allows impaction of the intertrochanteric/subtrochanteric fracture and with use of the Zickel nail in the pure subtrochanteric fracture, a high success rate can be obtained in treating these difficult fractures (Fig. 9). The Zickel nail is of particular value in fixing the pathologic subtrochanteric fracture because it combines proximal fixation with a long intramedullary rod that can be used to bridge more distal lesions.

Annotated Bibliography

General Considerations

Aitken, J.M.: Relevance of osteoporosis in women with fracture of the femoral neck. Br. Med. J. [Clin. Res.] 288:597–601, 1984.

Osteoporotic individuals did not sustain fractures more frequently than the general population; however, history of a previous hip fracture did correlate with a high incidence of fracture of the opposite hip. Trochanteric fractures occurred more commonly in severely osteoporotic women, and postural instability was the major determinant for femoral neck fracture rather than generalized osteoporosis.

Alho, A.; Stangeland, L.; Røttingen, J.; and Wiig, J.N.: Prophylaxis of venous thromboembolism by aspirin, warfarin and heparin in patients with hip fracture: A prospective clinical study with cost-benefit analysis. Ann. Chir. Gynaecol. 73:225–228, 1984.

The authors recommend aspirin as a general prophylaxis against pulmonary embolism in orthopaedic patients and warfarin in patients with established risk of thromboembolic complications.

Cummings, S.R.: Are patients with hip fractures more osteoporotic? Review of the evidence. Am. J. Med. 78:487–494, 1985.

Patients with hip fractures do not appear to be distinctly more osteoporotic than other persons of similar age.

Farmer, M.E.; White, L.R.; Brody, J.A.; and Bailey, K.R.: Race and sex differences in hip fracture incidence. Am. J. Public Health 74:1374–1380, 1984.

White women are at the highest risk for hip fracture and are at twice the risk for hip fracture (controlled for age) compared with black women and 2.7 times the risk for hip fractures compared to white men.

Frandsen, P.A., and Kruse, T.: Hip fractures in the county of Funen, Denmark: Implications of demographic aging and changes in incidence rates. Acta Orthop. Scand. 54:681–686, 1983.

In 3,096 hip fractures in Funen, Denmark, studied, there was an exponential increase in hip fractures with age in both sexes. If the trend continues, there will be a 3-fold increase in the number of hip fractures over a 20-year period.

Kenzora, J.E.; McCarthy, R.E.; Lowell, J.D.; and Sledge, C.B.: Hip fracture mortality: Relation to age, treatment, preoperative illness, time of surgery, and complications. Clin. Orthop. 186:45–56, 1984.

A retrospective study of 406 fractures of the proximal femur identified preexisting medical conditions at the time of operation and after admission to be highly significant factors influencing patient mortality. Patients with subcapital fractures had a mortality rate of 13% and patients with intertrochanteric fractures had a mortality rate of 15%, with the expectant mortality rate of the normal population of a similar age being 9%. The recommendation was for serious medical conditions to be maximally stabilized for at least 24 hours preoperatively.

Lawton, J.O.; Baker, M.R.; and Dickson, R.A.: Femoral neck fractures—two populations. Lancet 2:70–72, 1983.

A survey of 128 patients with femoral neck fractures emphasized the difference in physical condition and clinical behavior between this group and those with trochanteric fractures. Patients with trochanteric fractures that manifested advanced biologic aging presented a greater health care problem.

Norden, C.W.: A critical review of antibiotic prophylaxis in orthopedic surgery. Rev. Infect. Dis. 5:928–932, 1983.

Two well-designed and well-documented studies support the efficacy of prophylactic use of antimicrobial agents in the prevention of wound infection in surgical treatment of hip fractures.

Strömqvist, B.: Hip fracture in rheumatoid arthritis. Acta Orthop. Scand. 55:624–628, 1984.

In persons with rheumatoid arthritis, hip fractures occur at a younger age. After femoral neck fractures and intertrochanteric fractures, failure rates are higher than in the general population. Serious complications such as septicemia and nonunion occur with increased frequency.

Hip Dislocations

Epstein, H.C.: Traumatic Dislocation of the Hip. Baltimore, Williams & Wilkins, 1980.

This book presents a long-term follow-up of a very large experience with various groups of fractures and fracture-dislocations of the hip. It presents Epstein's classification of traumatic hip dislocations.

Stein, H.: Computerized tomography for ascertaining osteocartilaginous intraarticular (slice) fractures of the femoral head. Isr. J. Med. Sci. 19:180–184, 1983.

Computed tomography is of value for diagnosis of slice fractures of the femoral head after posterior hip dislocation.

Upadhyay, S.S., and Moulton, A.: The long-term results of traumatic posterior dislocation of the hip. J. Bone Joint Surg. 63B:548–551, 1981.

Eighty-one patients are reviewed with a mean follow-up of 12.5 years. There was a direct correlation between the severity of the initial injury and the long-term results. The incidence of osteoarthritis was 33% at 10 years and 100% at 30 years.

Femoral Neck Fractures

Arnold, W.D.: The effect of early weight-bearing on the stability of femoral neck fractures treated with Knowles pins. J. Bone Joint Surg. 66A:847–852, 1984.

In a retrospective study, displaced femoral neck fractures that had been adequately fixed with Knowles pins and allowed to bear weight early were compared to a similar group not allowed to bear weight. No difference in complication rate, morbidity, or healing rate was noted in the early-weight-bearing group.

Devas, M., and Hinves, B.: Prevention of acetabular erosion after hemiarthroplasty for fractured neck of femur. J. Bone Joint Surg. 65B:548–551, 1983.

In 161 femoral neck fractures with a 4-year follow-up after treatment with a bipolar prosthesis, no acetabular erosion was seen.

Frandsen, P.A.; Andersen, P.E., Jr.; Christoffersen, H.; and Thomsen, P.B.: Osteosynthesis of femoral neck fracture: The sliding-screw-plate with or without compression. Acta Orthop. Scand. 55:620–623, 1984.

A prospective series of 220 displaced femoral neck fractures was treated with and without compression with a sliding screw plate device. Compression was not found to be beneficial in treatment of femoral neck fractures with this device.

Giliberty, R.P.: Hemiarthroplasty of the hip using a low-friction bipolar endoprosthesis. Clin. Orthop. 175:86–92, 1983.

In 75 patients with a bipolar type prosthesis, primarily for displaced femoral neck fractures, 92% had satisfactory results. The author recommends a bipolar prosthesis for hemiarthroplasty of the hip in femoral neck fractures.

Hägglund, G.; Nordstrom, B.; and Lidgren, L.: Total hip replacement after nailing failure in femoral neck fractures. Arch. Orthop. Trauma Surg. 103:125–127, 1984.

Forty patients were treated by means of total hip arthroplasty after failed femoral neck nailing. Excellent results were obtained, and this is considered to be the salvage operation of choice after failed femoral neck surgery.

Holmberg, S., and Thorngren, K.G.: Preoperative ^{99m}Tc-MDP scintimetry of femoral neck fractures. Acta Orthop. Scand. 55:430–435, 1984.

Preoperative ^{99m}Tc-MDP scintimetry in 117 patients proved to be of value in the choice of primary treatment of femoral neck fractures. A ratio of 0.90 correlated well with uneventful healing in both displaced and undisplaced femoral neck fractures.

Kofoed, H., and Kofod, J.: Moore prosthesis in the treatment of fresh femoral neck fractures: A critical review with special attention to secondary acetabular degeneration. Injury 14:531–540, 1982–1983.

A consecutive series of 106 patients with displaced femoral neck fractures was treated with Moore prostheses. Of the 71 patients followed 2 years, 37% required a total hip replacement secondary to hip pain. The authors concluded that active patients, regardless of age, should not be treated with a one-piece prosthesis and they preferred satisfactory reduction and pinning; hip replacement is performed only if the fracture cannot be reduced.

Maxted, M.J., and Denham, R.A.: Failure of hemiarthroplasty for fractures of the neck of the femur. Injury 15:224–226, 1983–1984.

A review of 92 patients 4 years after hemiarthroplasty for displaced subcapital fractures revealed that 19% required further operations. A separate review of 70 patients who had undergone a revision after hemiarthroplasty showed that over half needed the operation within 3 years. The authors recommend the hemiarthroplasty be reserved for patients over age 79 or for those over 65 who are medically unfit.

Strömqvist, B., and Hansson, L.I.: Femoral head vitality

in femoral neck fracture after hook-pin internal fixation. Clin. Orthop. 191:105–109, 1984.

A study of the vitality of the femoral head in 317 femoral neck fractures by tetracycline and ^{99m}Tc-MDP scintimetry revealed a rate of avascular healing complication in 7% of undisplaced and 32% of displaced femoral neck fractures treated with hook pins.

Strömqvist, B.; Hansson, L.I.; Nilsson, L.T.; and Thorngren, K.-G.: Two-year follow-up of femoral neck fractures: Comparison of osteosynthesis methods. Acta Orthop. Scand. 55:521–525, 1984.

In a prospective series of 152 femoral neck fractures, half fixed with hook pins and half fixed with four-flanged nail, the hook pins were far superior in both displaced and undisplaced fractures. Less than 1 patient in 12 needed reoperation with total hip replacement within 2 years after fixation with a hook pin, and therefore fixation was favored over primary arthroplasty.

Strömqvist, B.; Hansson, L.I.; Palmer, J.; Ceder, L.; and Thorngren, K.-G.: Scintimetric evaluation of nailed femoral neck fractures with special reference to type of osteosynthesis. Acta Orthop. Scand. 54:340–347, 1983.

Using ^{99m}Tc-MDP scintimetry prior to nailing and 1 to 2 weeks after nailing, the authors demonstrated that a four-flanged nail is harmful to the vascular supply of the femoral head, compared to a Hansson screw, and therefore a four-flanged nail is not recommended in femoral neck fractures.

Swiontkowski, M.F.; Hansen, S.T., Jr.; and Kellam, J.: Ipsilateral fractures of the femoral neck and shaft: A treatment protocol. J. Bone Joint Surg. 66A:260–268, 1984.

Eighty-three cases with ipsilateral femoral neck and shaft fractures reported in the literature were reviewed and the conclusion is that anatomic reduction of the femoral neck fracture should be achieved first and multiple pin fixation and the shaft addressed secondarily. One-third of femoral neck fractures were missed in this combined injury.

Swiontkowski, M.F.; Winquist, R.A.; and Hansen, S.T., Jr.: Fractures of the femoral neck in patients between the ages of twelve and forty-nine years. J. Bone Joint Surg. 66A:837–846, 1984.

A series of 27 consecutive patients younger than 50 years old with femoral neck fractures was reviewed; no nonunions and an aseptic necrosis rate of 20% were reported. Early fixation of femoral neck fractures with multiple pins after anatomic reduction was advocated for young patients.

Welch, R.B.: The rationale for primary hemiarthroplasty in the treatment of fractures of the femoral neck in elderly patients. Hip 11:42–50, 1983.

The author believes that hemiarthroplasty is the treatment of choice for displaced femoral neck fractures in the elderly and results in no greater morbidity or mortality than other forms of intervention. Mortality and morbidity may even decrease when modern technology is used.

Zindrick, M.R.; Daley, R.J.; Hollyfield, R.L.; Jobski, R.; Kinzler, G.M.; Schwartz, C.M.; and Wood, W.S.: Femoral neck fractures in the geriatric population: The influence of perioperative health upon the selection of surgical treatment. J. Am. Geriatr. Soc. 33:104–108, 1985.

Patients with femoral neck fractures fixed by internal fixation or hemiarthroplasty were reviewed retrospectively. The increased morbidity and mortality associated with arthroplasty compared with internal fixation may be a result of biased patient selection in that the more elderly, debilitated patients were given a hemiarthroplasty.

Intertrochanteric Fractures

Harper, M.C., and Walsh, T.: Ender nailing for peritrochanteric fractures of the femur: An analysis of indications, factors related to mechanical failure, and postoperative results. J. Bone Joint Surg. 67A:79–88, 1985.

Ender nails are advocated for both stable and unstable intertrochanteric fractures if a good reduction can be obtained, the canal can be filled, the surgeon is experienced with the technique, and the fracture is relatively stable. They are not recommended for use in subtrochanteric fractures.

Kyle, R.F.; Gustilo, R.B.; and Premer, R.F.: Analysis of six hundred and twenty-two intertrochanteric hip fractures. J. Bone Joint Surg. 61A:216–221, 1979.

A review of over 600 intertrochanteric fractures shows that a collapsible device is superior to a rigid device in successful fixation of intertrochanteric fractures and that central head placement with a collapsible device will give a 90% success rate even in unstable intertrochanteric fractures.

Kyle, R.F.; Wright, T.M.; and Burstein, A.H.: Biomechanical analysis of the sliding characteristics of compression hip screws. J. Bone Joint Surg. 62A:1308–1314, 1980.

The single most important factor in impaction of compression hip screws is the angle at which the screw is placed in fixation of fractures. The larger the angle, the greater the ease of sliding. This is an exponential phenomenon.

MacEachern, A.G., and Heyse-Moore, G.H.: Stable intertrochanteric femoral fractures: A misnomer? J. Bone Joint Surg. 65B:582–583, 1983.

Both stable and unstable intertrochanteric fractures impact to a stable position after anatomic reduction and fixation with a sliding device. Medial displacement is not needed. Failure is more likely to occur when a rigid Jewett nail is used.

Sherk, H.H., and Foster, M.D.: Hip fractures: Condylocephalic rod *versus* compression screw. Clin. Orthop. 192:255–259, 1985.

Seventy consecutive intertrochanteric fractures were fixed with a condylocephalic nail or a compression sliding screw. There was a significantly higher complication rate with the condylocephalic nail.

Strathy, G.M., and Johnson, E.W., Jr.: Ender's pinning for fractures about the hip. Mayo Clin. Proc. 59:411–414, 1984.

Four years of experience with Ender nails in intertrochanteric fractures revealed knee pain in 41% of the patients followed; 31% required additional surgical procedures secondary to migration of the pins. The authors recommend the use of Ender nails only in stable fractures in patients who cannot tolerate more extensive procedures.

Zain Elabdien, B.S.; Olerud, S.; and Karlström, G.: The influence of age on the morphology of trochanteric fracture. Arch. Orthop. Trauma Surg. 103:156–161, 1984.

In 127 trochanteric fractures it was found that there was a continuous decrease in the quality of bone with age as well as a direct relationship between bone quality and severity of the pattern of the trochanteric fracture. Skeletal aging starts before menopause in women; after age 85, the process is more rapid in men than in women. Because of the longevity of the patient population, the unstable trochanteric fracture has increased by a factor of 3 over the past 3 decades.

Subtrochanteric Fractures

Wile, P.B.; Panjabi, M.M.; and Southwick, W.O.: Treatment of subtrochanteric fractures with a high-angle compression hip screw. Clin. Orthop. 175:72–78, 1983.

Twenty-five subtrochanteric fractures were transfixed with a large-angle compression hip screw with excellent results. No mechanical failures, delayed unions, or nonunions were found. In certain subtrochanteric fractures, fixation with a large-angle compression hip screw is reliable and advantageous.

Zain Elabdien, B.S.; Olerud, S.; and Karlström, G.: Subtrochanteric fractures: Classification and results of Ender nailing. Arch. Orthop. Trauma Surg. 103:241–250, 1984.

Twenty-seven subtrochanteric fractures were fixed with Ender nails, with a 17% complication rate and a good or excellent result in 79% of patients.

Zickel, R.E.: Subtrochanteric femoral fractures. Orthop. Clin. North Am. 11:555–568, July 1980.

A review of the biomechanical stresses acting on subtrochanteric fractures emphasizes the desirable features in intramedullary fixation.

32 Trauma: Femur

This chapter will discuss classification and treatment of femoral shaft fractures. Use of interlocking nails and complications such as fat embolism, infection, nonunion, shortening, malrotation, and angulation will be discussed.

General Aspects

Multiple Trauma Patient

Treatment of the patient with multiple injuries has improved dramatically over the last decade. With the evolution of rapid transportation and early stabilization of the patient as well as aggressive management, the survival rate has increased. Early stabilization of the femoral fracture is an integral part of resuscitation. The incidences of acute respiratory distress syndrome and death are decreased by this early stabilization, and no study suggests that it increases morbidity or mortality. Furthermore, early stabilization allows mobilization of the patient to a sitting position.

Vascular Injuries

Vascular injuries are uncommon with femoral shaft fractures but can occur when there is marked displacement of transverse fractures of the distal fourth of the femur. The femoral artery can become entrapped as it enters the adductor canal, causing injury at this level. Intimal injuries to the arteries and arterial injuries caused by gunshot wounds to the distal femur are frequently difficult to diagnose. An arteriogram should be obtained if there is any question of vascular injury. The treatment of arterial injuries varies depending on the severity of vascular compromise and the time that has elapsed since the injury. If the arterial injury is minimal, the fracture should be stabilized first. Vascular flow should then be restored with an interpositional vein graft or a synthetic graft.

If the arterial injury is severe, such as with complete laceration, or if ischemia has been present for several hours, the first step is temporary shunting of the artery followed by fasciotomy. Next, the femoral fracture can be internally stabilized and then the artery is repaired, all in a single procedure. The femoral vein must be repaired as well. Associated sciatic nerve injuries are generally caused by contusions or stretch injuries and rarely need surgical repair.

Types of Injuries

Ipsilateral Fractures

Femoral Neck and Shaft Ipsilateral fracture of the femoral neck is seen in approximately 2.5% of patients with femoral shaft fractures. In most published reports, one-third of these femoral neck fractures are not diagnosed initially. This occurs for two reasons: radiographs of the femoral neck often are not taken as part of the standard diagnostic work-up, and the proximal femur rotates externally and the femoral neck in this position is not well visualized on radiography. Because it is difficult to rotate the femur internally, the entire patient must be rotated to obtain a better radiographic view of the femoral neck. Complications resulting from treating the femoral shaft are infrequent but include nonunion and malunion with shortening and malrotation.

Complications of treating the femoral neck can be severe and lead to osteonecrosis. In young patients there are no satisfactory options available for treating osteonecrosis. Therefore, proper initial treatment of the femoral neck fracture in young patients is extremely important. The ideal treatment of femoral neck fractures in children and young adults is early anatomic reduction and stable internal fixation. Treatment should be performed on an emergency basis, and open reduction of the femoral neck fracture via anterior capsulotomy is necessary if anatomic reduction cannot be achieved. The effect of anterior capsulotomy to release a hematoma is still in question. The best stabilization for the femoral neck in the young adult appears to be use of multiple lag screws.

After the femoral neck fracture has been reduced and fixed, the next step is stabilization of the femoral shaft fracture. In all major reported series of treatment of combined femoral neck and shaft fractures, the best results were achieved by stabilizing both fractures. After the femoral neck fracture has been stabilized with multiple screws, the femoral shaft fracture can be stabilized with a retrograde intramedullary nail, multiple Ender nails or Rush rods placed through the distal femoral condyles, or compression plating of the femoral shaft. The relative advantages and disadvantages of each of these treatment methods will be discussed in the section on treatment of fractures of the femoral shaft.

Several other methods have been recommended for treating ipsilateral fractures of the femoral neck and shaft. If an intramedullary nail has been used to fix the femoral shaft fracture before the femoral neck fracture has been diagnosed, multiple screws can be placed around the nail to stabilize the femoral neck fracture. Two other methods can be used to fix both fractures simultaneously: 1) Ender nails driven up from the medial femoral condyle, and 2) interlocking nails with the left nail inserted on the right side to allow placement of the proximal interlocking screw in the femoral neck. Neither of these methods gives adequate mechanical stability to the femoral neck fracture. The Ender nails do not provide stable anatomic reduction of the femoral shaft fracture. Therefore, neither is recommended as fixation for ipsilateral fractures of the femoral shaft and neck.

Femoral Shaft and Tibial Shaft ("Floating Knee") Ipsilateral fractures of the femoral shaft and tibial shaft are seen in approximately 10% of patients who have femoral shaft fractures. These are life-threatening injuries and are associated with a 13% incidence of fat embolism and a mortality rate ranging from 5% to 15%. Approximately 33% of patients have additional injuries such as to the head, chest, or abdomen. There is a high incidence of open fractures: 20% of the femoral fractures and over 50% of the tibial fractures are open. Treatment of such a multiply injured patient focuses on resuscitation and management of these major injuries. The key to treatment of the floating knee is early stabilization of the femoral fracture and early restoration of range of motion of the knee. The femoral shaft fracture usually requires internal fixation. The best results reportedly have been obtained by stabilizing both the femoral and the tibial fracture. With this form of treatment, 80% and 86% of patients achieved good or excellent results in two separate series. In comparisons of operative and nonoperative treatments of the tibia, the results are improved with stabilization of the tibia.

Internal fixation of tibial fractures carries a high risk. In a series of 222 patients, 26% had nonunion and 30% had osteomyelitis. Therefore, a more conservative approach should be considered. The ideal treatment for fracture of the femoral shaft appears to be intramedullary nailing with interlocking nails when necessary. The treatment of the tibial shaft fracture should be individualized. Immobilization of the knee for no more than 6 weeks gives a good result. If the tibial fracture is minimally displaced, is distal in location, and can be treated in a patellar tendon bearing cast, early knee motion can be allowed. For a closed fracture of the mid tibia, intramedullary nailing is a good method of treatment. With a comminuted, displaced fracture of the tibia, either an interlocking tibial nail or a compression plate and screw fixation is the method of choice. For open fractures, an external fixator offers the safest approach and still allows early motion of the knee. The treatment of choice for a supracondylar fracture of the femur or an intra-articular tibial plateau fracture should include primary anatomic reduction by stable internal fixation and early range of motion mobility of the knee.

Ipsilateral Injuries to Femoral Shaft and Knee

Coexisting femoral shaft fractures and ipsilateral knee ligament injuries are seen in approximately 5% of patients with femoral fractures and frequently are not diagnosed throughout the course of treatment. If ligament injury is suspected, physical examination should be performed after internal fixation of the femur. Arthroscopy can be performed at the same time if indicated.

Open Femoral Fractures

The nature of the injury that caused the open fracture is an important factor in the end result of treatment. Patients injured by shotgun blast tend to do extremely poorly. Farm injuries carry a high rate of severe infection. The standard treatment of open femoral fracture includes thorough debridement and irrigation. The wound is left open but the surgical extension of the wound can be closed.

The major question focuses on management of the fracture. The long-time standard of treatment has been debridement with delayed closure at 5 to 7 days, followed by stabilization of the fracture at 10 to 14 days. Recent reports have advocated primary internal fixation of the open femoral fracture. The rate of deep infection has not changed for grade I and grade II open fractures treated by internal fixation with intramedullary nails or interlocking femoral nails. In grade III fractures, internal fixation with nails or plates has led to high rates of infection. Therefore, external fixators can be used in these fractures.

Classification of Fractures of the Femoral Shaft

Fractures of the femoral shaft are classified by their location as well as by the fracture pattern and degree of comminution (Fig. 1). The classification discussed here includes fractures below the lesser trochanter and fractures that do not enter the knee joint. The use of interlocking nails has made it possible to stabilize fractures in the proximal and distal parts of the femoral shaft.

Proximal and distal femoral fractures may heal with shortening and malrotation. Spiral and long oblique fractures are rarely seen in young adults but are the most common femoral shaft fractures seen in the elderly. They can be located anywhere from the proximal to the distal shaft and generally are caused by low-velocity injuries in patients with large medullary canals and porotic bone. Comminuted fractures have been classified into types I through IV.

A type I fracture has a very small butterfly fragment (25% or less of the width of the bone).

In a type II comminuted fracture, the butterfly fragment is 50% or less of the width of the bone. If the fracture line in the opposite cortex at that level is transverse, adequate cortex remains to maintain length and rotation. If the component opposite the butterfly fragment is oblique or spiral, control of rotation and length may not be possible. With type II comminuted fracture locations more proximally or distally into the metaphyseal flares, the degree of instability increases.

The type III comminuted fracture consists of a very large butterfly segment (more than 50% of the width of the bone) with only a very small spike of bone remaining intact. Therefore, it is difficult to determine the length of the femur. These fractures are unstable and it is difficult to maintain position in regard to rotation and axial length. The instability increases as these fractures occur closer to the proximal and distal ends of the femoral shaft.

A type IV comminuted fracture has comminution of an entire segment of bone and can be a simple split segmental fracture or a fracture with multiple fragments. There is no inherent stability in terms of length or rotation.

An additional type of comminuted fracture is the segmental fracture with the segment intact. The treatment is determined by the pattern of fracture at each end of the segment. A central segment with transverse components at both ends has a stable fracture pattern. If the fracture is oblique or comminuted at either end of the segmental fracture, further treatment is necessary to control length and rotation.

A final fracture type (type V) is one with segmental bone loss.

Methods of Treatment

The ideal treatment for fractures of the femoral shaft should include early mobilization of the patient whenever possi-

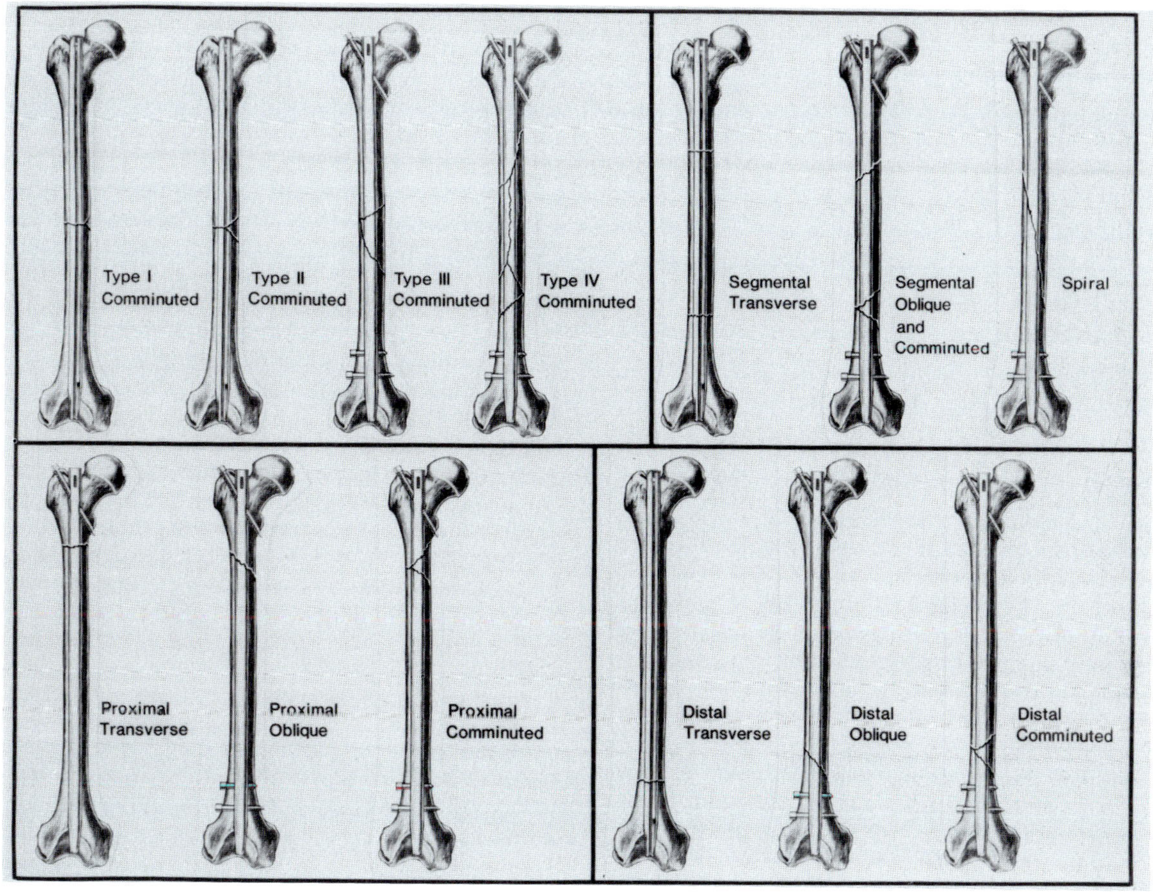

Figure 1

Classification of femoral shaft fractures and preferred methods of treatment.

ble. Early motion of the knee is desirable to prevent joint stiffness. Anatomic reduction and fixation will prevent deformities of angulation, rotation, and shortening.

Traction and Cast Brace

Through the years, traction and prolonged casting has been the standard method of treatment of fractures of the femur. Although this method carries a low risk of infection, the results are often unacceptable because of excessive knee stiffness and malunion. Use of the functional brace such as a cast brace allows early mobilization of the patient and early knee motion. With roller traction, the alert patient can even be mobilized well in bed. The time in traction varies from a few days to a few weeks, but the patient is generally out of traction and in a tight fitting cast brace by 4 weeks. Angulation has been a problem with proximal fractures which tend to drift into varus.

Good and excellent results from cast bracing have been reported in 43% to 86% of cases. Complications have been frequent. Knee motion is not as good as in patients treated by internal fixation. The major problems with the cast brace treatment method are nonunion and malunion. Mean shortening in most reports was more than 1 cm. The mean hospital time was more than 30 days and usually was twice as long as that required for a patient treated by internal fixation. Angulation of more than 10° was seen in as many as 62% of patients. Therefore, the use of cast braces in the treatment of femoral shaft fractures is limited. A comminuted fracture of the distal femur with minimal shortening on initial radiographs usually can be treated well with a cast brace.

External Fixation

External fixation of femoral shaft fractures has limited application. This treatment method allows early mobilization of the patient but frequently does not permit early motion of the knee. The operative risks are extremely low. This method achieves stabilization of a severely injured patient without additional blood loss. However, the late problems of knee stiffness, pin track infections, and delayed union and nonunion as well as problems with angulation detract from its value.

A Wagner apparatus can be used as a single frame on the lateral aspect of the femur. This apparatus does not impale the anterior quadriceps femoris and takes a very short time to apply. It is only partially adjustable, so it is essential that the overall alignment of the femur be quite good before application of the frame.

A more stable apparatus is the dihedral frame with pins placed laterally and anteriorly. It offers a great addition in strength but it impales the anterior quadriceps femoris and makes early motion of the knee more difficult.

Fifty percent of patients treated with external fixation lose knee motion. The use of external fixators for femoral shaft fractures therefore should be limited. The ideal application for an external fixator is with a grade III open femoral fracture when simultaneous debridement of the fracture is performed. The external fixator is applied and maintained until soft tissue healing occurs. The fixator is later removed with substitution of a cast brace or intramedullary fixation if the pin tracks have been cleaned.

Compression Plates

With the use of compression plates many of the goals of treatment of femoral fractures can be achieved. They allow early mobilization of the patient and motion of the knee. They provide anatomic reduction and stable internal fixation. Axial alignment as well as proper length can be maintained. Stress shielding of the bone is excessive if two plates are used. Therefore, a single plate is used on the lateral aspect of the femur with medial bone grafting added if there is any comminution. The operation is best performed with the patient in the lateral position on a standard fracture table. An intraoperative distraction device is frequently needed. Soft tissue stripping should be held to a minimum. Interfragmental lag screws should be used if there is comminution, and bone grafting should be added to fill defects. A wide compression plate should be used to fix femoral shaft fractures and it should be applied with screws that engage at least eight cortices proximally and distally to the fracture.

The use of compression plates has disadvantages. The infection rate is high. The rate of late complications—plate failure, fracture at the end of the plate, screw failure, loosening of the plate from nonunions, and delayed healing of the fracture—indicates that mechanically this method is less than ideal for treating fractures of the femur. Compression plate fixation, therefore, should be used when a fracture extends into the knee joint and requires intra-articular stabilization and neutralization with a plate. Compression plate fixation also can be used for midshaft fractures that are associated with injuries of either the proximal or distal femur, making intramedullary fixation difficult.

Intramedullary Nails

Intramedullary Nails in Unreamed Femur Intramedullary nails in the unreamed femur make it possible to achieve most of the goals of treatment of femoral fractures. They allow early mobilization of the patient. The final range of motion of the knee usually is excellent, and the rate of union is high. The major problems with the technique are malrotation and shortening of the fracture and angulation and failure of the implant. The instrumentation is simple and the cost of the equipment is low. The surgical technique is relatively simple, requiring a small incision if antegrade nailing is done or a large incision if open reduction of the fracture and retrograde nailing is performed. When the nails are used to fix transverse or short oblique fractures of the midshaft, the success rate is very high. When the nails are used to fix fractures of the proximal or distal femur or comminuted fractures, the incidence of shortening and external rotation is high. The method appears to be excellent for treating stable fractures. Union is slower with nails in the unreamed femur. The infection rate is higher if the fracture is opened to insert the nail. Although the results of intramedullary nailing of the unreamed femur are superior to those of functional brace treatment, they have not been as good as those with intramedullary nails in reamed femurs or with interlocking nails.

Intramedullary Nails With Cerclage Wires Comminuted fractures treated with conventional nails in reamed or unreamed femurs have had a high rate of failure because of shortening and malrotation. Additional fixation is necessary in these fractures. Intramedullary nailing with open reduction and cerclage wire has been offered as the solution. This technique requires opening the fracture. The length is restored by using a femoral distractor, and cerclage wires are placed at 1-cm intervals around the fracture fragments. The standard examination and insertion of an intramedullary nail are performed. Postoperative management includes early mobilization of the patient with postoperative support in traction or casts or no additional support.

Although the technique appears to be simple, reported results vary from excellent in two series to inferior in another because of a mean shortening of 1.3 cm and a 15% infection rate. Although this form of treatment appears to be excellent for comminuted fractures, it is a large, open procedure. Use of interlocking nails can be a better alternative.

Intramedullary Nails in Reamed Femur and Interlocking Femoral Nails These two methods are currently the best for treatment of most fractures of the femoral shaft. They allow early mobilization of the patient and of the joint. They achieve the highest rates of union and, when done by the closed method, result in the lowest rate of infection. They lead to the lowest rate of malunion and shortening when properly performed and give excellent results in approximately 95% of patients. The major disadvantage of these techniques is the cost of the special instruments that are required, such as the image intensifier and fracture table. The technique for inserting the nail, particularly the interlocking nail, requires special surgical training, a second assistant who does not scrub, and a radiology technician in the operating room.

Biomechanics of Intramedullary Fixation Small, straight intramedullary nails are weak and tend to undergo fatigue failure. Large intramedullary nails require intramedullary reaming for insertion because the femur is bowed in various patterns. The flexible nail that has an open slot anteriorly, a bullet tip, and a nail curvature radius of 137 cm solves many of these problems.

The intramedullary nail that has a longitudinal slot on its posterior aspect has increased bending strength but, unfortunately, less flexibility. This can cause additional comminution during insertion at an anterior fracture site or anterior shaft fractures in treating distal fractures. The newer nails have an anterior slot to improve flexibility. A conical bolt that is threaded into the proximal end of the nail aids in the insertion of the device. However, this is a stress riser and can cause fatigue of the nail at the proximal end of the slot, even after the fracture has healed. Unfortunately, some of these design features are being introduced into new interlocking nails. Over-reaming is essential for these stiff nails, and frequently the fracture should be over-reamed by a full 1 mm. Fatigue failure through screw holes also can develop. Unslotted nails with holes and completely circularized nails will require over-reaming (1 to 2 mm) to prevent further comminution during insertion. The bal-

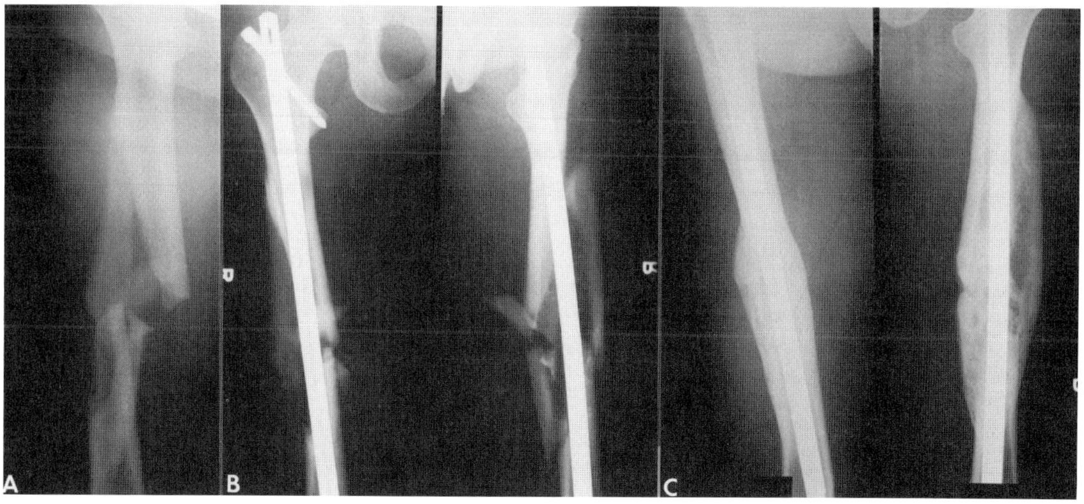

Figure 2
Type IV comminuted fracture of the femoral shaft in young girl. *A*, Preoperatively. *B*, Postoperative radiographs. *C*, Radiographs after healing.

ance between flexibility and strength is an important one and will require careful observation during development of new nails.

Preoperative Management If operative treatment of a femoral fracture will be performed after a delay, skeletal traction should be applied with a proximal tibial pin to prevent contamination of the femoral canal. Initial traction should use 11 to 16 kg for women and up to 20 kg for men. If femoral length is not maintained in the preoperative period, then closed reduction and closed intramedullary nailing can be exceedingly difficult. A lateral radiograph should be taken to be certain that femoral length is maintained during longitudinal traction in the preoperative period.

Prophylactic intravenous antimicrobial therapy is used during operation. It should be begun immediately prior to the procedure and continued for 12 to 24 hours afterward.

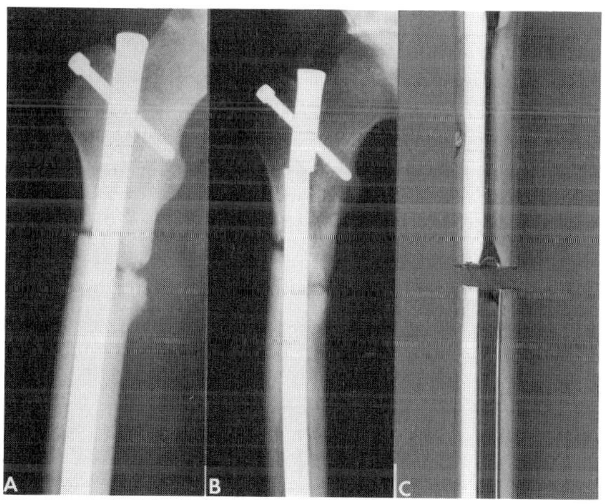

Figure 3
Short, oblique, proximal femoral fracture in a young man, fixed with proximal dynamic locking with a Grosse-Kempf nail. *A*, Postoperative radiograph. *B*, Radiograph at 5 months postoperatively, showing broken intramedullary nail at the top of the slot. *C*, Broken intramedullary nail.

The diameter of the femur can be measured on anteroposterior and lateral radiographs. The medullary canal appears to be 2 mm wider on the lateral radiograph than on the anteroposterior view in the midsection of the diaphysis. This lateral measurement generally is the proper nail size. The length of the nail is best selected by measuring the normal femur from the tip of the trochanter to the lateral joint line.

Although many reports have suggested a higher rate of healing when operation is delayed for 5 to 7 days after injury, the importance of early stabilization in the multiply injured patient outweighs this factor. In comparing patients treated with early internal fixation and those treated by delayed internal fixation, the healing rates are the same for simple fractures but for comminuted fractures the early internal fixation gives a slightly lower rate, particularly with interlocking nails.

Most children and adults who have a closed head injury in addition to a femoral fracture require internal fixation. The combative patient is difficult to manage in traction. The femoral fracture in a comatose patient should be treated with the expectation that the neurologic recovery will be complete. The age of the patient is a factor when intramedullary nailing is being considered. The ideal patient is an adult. Children under 10 years of age are best managed with initial spica cast application with traction first and then a spica cast. In patients between ages 10 and 15, intramedullary nailing can be done if the epiphyses are closed. If the epiphyses are open, treatment can be either traction and then use of a functional brace or intramedullary nailing.

Operative Technique The technique of fixation of comminuted femoral shaft fractures by using interlocking nails is similar to that for intramedullary nail fixation. However, interlocking screws must be added. An effort should be made to insert the nail in the correct rotation so that the screws will go directly through the lateral cortex of the femur. If the nail is externally rotated it is difficult to get the distal screws in through the lateral posterior border of

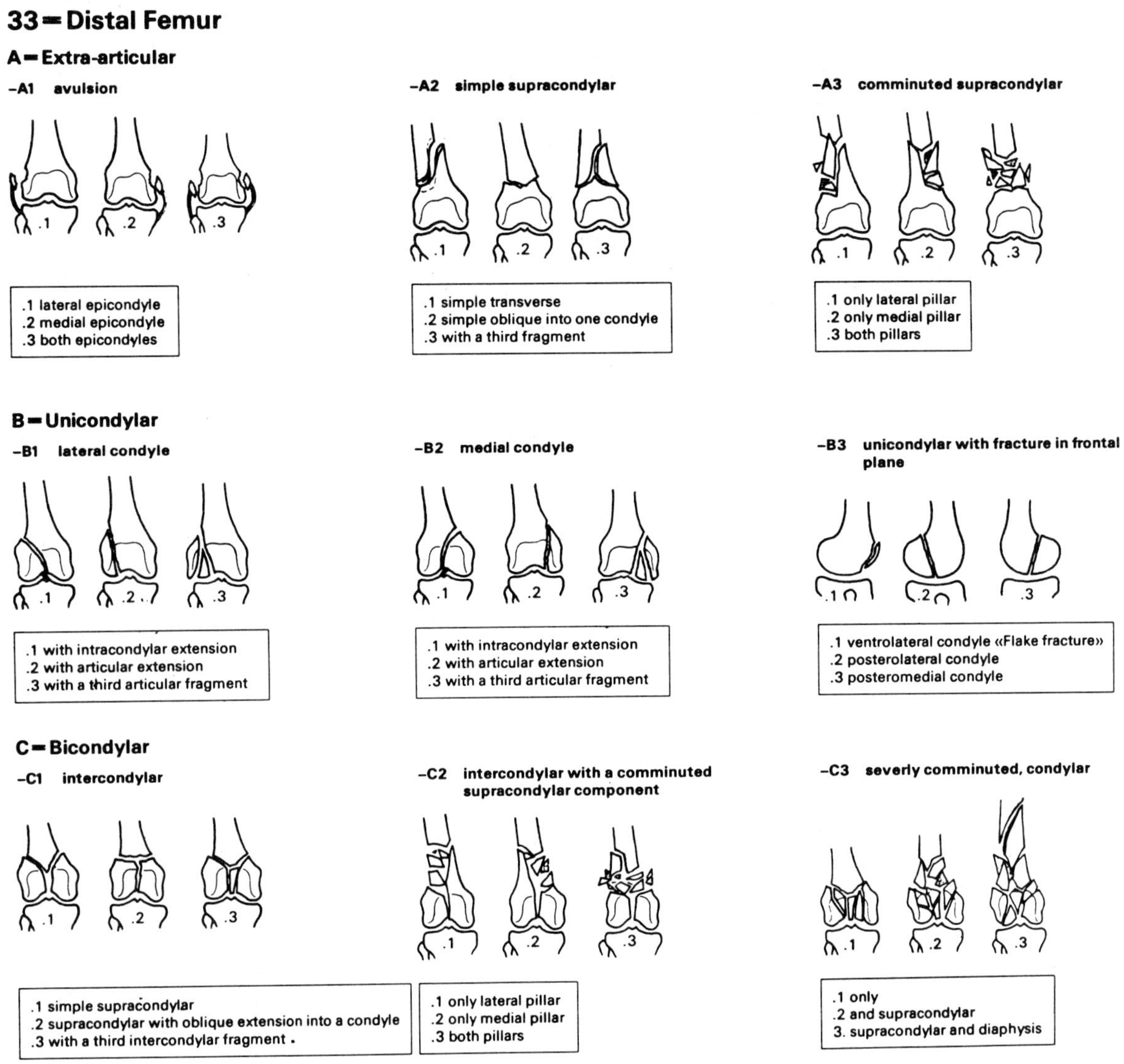

Figure 4
AO/ASIF classification of supracondylar femoral fractures.

the femur. The drills tend to slip off this area because it is extremely sclerotic. Placement of the proximal screw usually is not difficult. The aiming device for most interlocking nails works well proximally. A drill sleeve is used, and the proximal hole is observed during drilling. The hole is measured and the proper screws are selected. A second sleeve is available for placement of the screw. The final placement should be assessed in two planes to be certain the screw has not glanced off the anterior or posterior edge of the nail.

Placement of the distal screw is more difficult. Most of the targeting devices have not worked very well, including the devices attached to the proximal end of the nail, the hand-held targeting devices, and the targeting devices attached to the image intensifier. The image intensifier is rotated in two planes to ensure that the distal hole is perfectly round. A very sharp Steinmann pin or crow-tipped pin is then placed in the center of the circle on the cortex of the bone to start the near hole. After this hole is completed a drill bit is placed through the hole and through the nail. The far cortex is drilled. The femur is measured and a screw of the correct size is placed. Fully threaded screws are much easier to place than screws threaded only in the opposite cortex. The use of 4.5-mm screws in this area has made the job of insertion easier but has led to fatigue and breakage of the screws.

Postoperative Management In injuries close to the knee, early motion of the knee can be instituted with a continuous passive motion machine. One to 2 days postoperatively, quadriceps femoris exercises are started. Electrical stimulation can be helpful if the patient has difficulty contracting the quadriceps femoris. As soon as the patient has control of the quadriceps, ambulation is started. The patient is dismissed when he or she can use crutches safely; non-weight-bearing or toe-touch weight-bearing is maintained for 6 to 8 weeks.

Occasionally, excessive callus develops at the fracture site, limiting the range of motion of the knee. Such patients

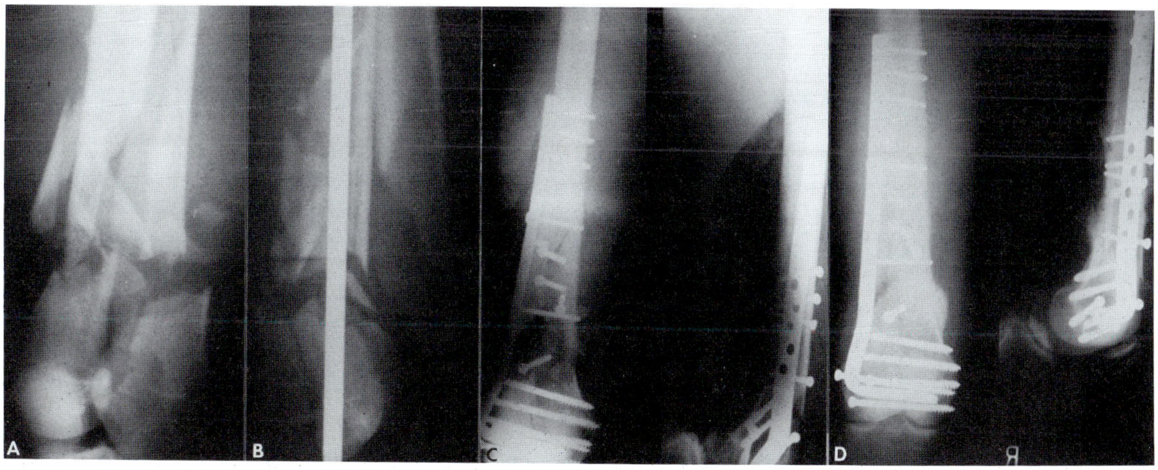

Figure 5

Comminuted intercondylar femoral fracture. *A*, Anteroposterior radiograph. *B*, Lateral radiograph. *C*, Postoperative radiograph, showing blade plate and lag screw fixation. *D*, At 1 year postoperatively, showing fracture healing. Patient has 125° of knee flexion.

should be managed very carefully over 4 to 5 months to restore knee range of motion gradually. Manipulations under anesthesia usually are not helpful. Once 90° of knee flexion is achieved, the patient can get into the crawling position on hands and knees and gently sit back on the heels to gain further flexion.

Results of Intramedullary Nailing Eighty-five percent of femoral fractures treated by intramedullary nailing heal within 3 months after injury. The mean range of motion of the knee is 125°, and full range of motion is attained by up to 97% of the patients. Seventy-eight percent of patients return to work within 6 months after injury, and 96% return to work within 12 months. Eighty-eight percent of patients have no subjective pain, and 91% are able to walk normally. Sixty-nine percent return to normal daily activities. Sixty-five percent of patients are able to return to previous sports.

Infection Infection rates after closed intramedullary nailing are reported to be 0% to 3%, usually 0.5% to 1%. The treatment of an acutely infected intramedullary nail site includes debridement of the fracture site with copious irrigation. The trochanteric area should be opened and a guide rod should be placed down to decompress the femoral canal. If the intramedullary nail is fitting properly, it should be left in place. The wounds are packed open and allowed to heal slowly. This treatment is adequate for the majority of acutely infected intramedullary nail sites. Only in rare circumstances is nail removal with a change to an external fixator indicated.

Nonunion Nonunions after closed intramedullary nailing of femoral fractures are reported to occur in 0% to 3% of cases. Nonunions can be treated by removal of the intramedullary nail, further intramedullary reaming, and placement of a larger nail.

Malunion The most frequent complications of intramedullary femoral nailing are shortening and rotary malunion. The incidences of malrotation and shortening increase as more comminuted fractures are included in the series. Malrotation of more than 20° is seen in 2% to 6% of patients. Shortening of more than 2 cm is seen in 0% to 2% of patients. Shortening of 1 to 2 cm is seen in as many as 18% of patients.

Rotational malunions occur for several reasons. One is malpositioning on the fracture table. Another is the patient's twisting in bed postoperatively or a fall within the first few weeks after operation. Fracture patterns that commonly lead to malrotation are type III and type IV comminuted fractures and fractures of the proximal femoral shaft.

Shortening is most commonly seen in comminuted fractures, with types III and IV shortening the most; type I and type II fractures in the proximal and distal shaft also tend to shorten. Spiral fractures can also shorten, but generally in the range of only 2 cm and most frequently in elderly patients.

Interlocking Nails

Interlocking nails are designed to allow intramedullary nailing of fractures near the lesser trochanter and the knee joint. Interlocking nails are very useful for treating comminuted fractures and should be used for type II proximal and distal comminuted fractures treated by intramedullary nailing. Type III and type IV comminuted fractures located anywhere in the femoral shaft also should be treated with interlocking nails (Fig. 2). Insertion of interlocking nails is more complex than insertion of standard nails; the major problem has been in placement of the distal interlocking screws.

Interlocking nails are useful to prevent shortening and rotation. Unfortunately, it has been difficult to judge both of these complications at the time of operation. A tendency has been to use interlocking nails that are too long in some patients. Up to 1 cm of femoral lengthening is not uncommon; this occurs because these fractures are extremely unstable, have lost their soft tissue envelope, and therefore can be over-distracted. An additional problem is judging the rotation correctly during positioning of the patient on the table, leading some surgeons to prefer using the supine position. In a large series in which interlocking nails were used, shortening occurred in 11% of patients; maximum shortening was 2.5 cm.

The biomechanics of interlocking nail systems are different from those of routine intramedullary nailing. Instead of a load-sharing device with the total load going through the bone, a partial-load-bearing device has been developed. The interlocking intramedullary nail is fixed by screws at each end of it. Theoretically a higher nonunion rate would be expected with this technique. Early removal of the screws or using them only at one end has been associated with excessive shortening. Most reports now describe leaving the screws in for at least 6 months. Weight-bearing begins 8 to 12 weeks after injury, when callus appears on radiographs. With the interlocking nail the nonunion rate is reported to be up to 7.6%; however, this is easier to treat than shortening of the femur.

If the nonunion persists, the nail may fail. With Grosse-Kempf nails, failure usually occurs at the proximal weld; other forms of interlocking nails most commonly break at the most proximal of the distal screw holes (Fig. 3). Screw breakage has been rare for 6-mm screws but is more common when 4.5-mm screws are used. Removal of broken screws and broken nails is not simple. The nonunion is treated by repeat intramedullary nailing. Unicortical failure is another problem. With comminuted fractures the butterfly fragments frequently are not reduced accurately and circumferential healing may not occur. Circumferential union occurs slowly and requires a long time. Some of the voids may never become filled with bone. Therefore, the period during which the nail is left in place is prolonged.

Supracondylar Fractures of the Femur

Supracondylar fractures usually are the result of high-energy trauma in young patients. They are also the result of low-velocity injuries in the elderly. Because these fractures are close to the knee joint and intra-articular extension is common, knee stiffness and degenerative joint disease are common sequelae.

Fracture Classification

Supracondylar fractures can be entirely extra-articular or intra-articular involving one or two condyles. The ASIF classification system divides fractures according to whether they are extra-articular (type A), unicondylar (type B), or bicondylar (type C) (Fig. 4).

Treatment

Functional Bracing Hinged cast application is an excellent method for treating nondisplaced extra-articular supracondylar fractures or comminuted extra-articular supracondylar fractures with minimal shortening and angulation. Traction can be used initially, before application of this cast. The functional bracing is continued for approximately 12 weeks, and motion of the knee is started early in the treatment. This treatment method is not suited for most comminuted fractures and intra-articular fractures.

Flexible Intramedullary Devices Flexible intramedullary devices are indicated primarily for elderly patients. These devices achieve good axial alignment and allow early mobilization of the patient but do not maintain accurate reduction or rigid stabilization of the fractures. Thus, some shortening usually occurs with this treatment method. It is ideal for the elderly patient who has a supracondylar fracture in which there is no significant comminution of the intra-articular component. Devices available include Rush rods, Ender nails, and Zickel supracondylar devices. The cross screws of the Zickel device allow both reduction and fixation of the intra-articular T component.

These devices frequently can be inserted without opening the fracture site. The two intramedullary devices must cross the fracture site simultaneously. The patient can be mobilized soon after fixation. Deep infections occur infrequently, and nonunion is rare. Good or excellent results are reported in 67% of the patients.

Blade Plate The condylar blade plate can provide the best fixation in most comminuted supracondylar fractures, particularly in young adults (Fig. 5). Simple lag screws can be adequate for avulsion fractures and unicondylar fractures, but comminuted fractures, particularly with intra-articular components, require additional internal fixation. The "Mercedes incision" has been associated with a high incidence of wound breakdown. Occasionally, a lateral incision with a separate medial incision is necessary. The initial step is open reduction of the condyles with lag screws used for fixation. It is important to place the lag screws so that they will not interfere with subsequent application of the plate. If a lag screw is inserted too far posteriorly, it will be in the intercondylar notch and overcompress the fracture.

Fixation with a properly applied blade plate produces good or excellent results in approximately 75% of patients. The most common technical complications are inadequate reduction of the articular surfaces, inaccurate positioning of the blade plate, and poor lag screw placement. The most common long-term complications are nonunions that eventually result in failure of the implant, knee joint stiffness, and degenerative joint disease if there has been joint injury. Infection is an uncommon but serious complication when it occurs.

Condylar Compression Screw The indications for using a condylar compression screw are similar to those for using a blade plate. The condylar compression screw is easier to insert and is put in over a guide wire. This technique allows compression across the intercondylar fracture. Rotation can be adjusted and therefore it is easier to line up the femoral shaft. Interfragment compression using lag screws must be performed accurately. The disadvantage of this technique is that it is difficult to achieve rigid stabilization distally. Stable fixation of the distal fragment(s) necessitates the insertion of a cancellous screw through the distal holes of the plate. Satisfactory results have been reported in 70% of cases.

Condylar Buttress Plate The condylar buttress plate is designed to fix fractures that have intra-articular comminution with involvement of the anterior or posterior condyles. A blade plate or compression screw would pass directly through these fracture planes and cannot be used unless stable lag screw fixation can first be achieved. The condylar buttress plate is easier to apply than a blade plate and is placed on the lateral cortex. Interfragmentary lag screw fixation is used for femoral condyle fractures or other large fragments. Anterior-to-posterior lag screws are needed to fix the fracture in the frontal plane. Unfortunately, the condylar buttress plate is not as strong as an angled blade plate and the distal fixation with the screws is not rigid, potentially allowing a varus deformity to develop. These patients should have more protection of the limb in the postoperative period. They should have early gentle motion but with careful monitoring to see if a varus deformity develops. The patients should remain non-weight-bearing until the fracture is healed. If there is severe comminution medially, a bone graft is necessary and occasionally an additional small medial T plate is required which is inserted through a medial approach.

Annotated Bibliography

Femoral Shaft Fractures

Classification of Fractures

Richards, R.R.; Waddell, J.P.; Sullivan, T.R.; Ashworth, M.A.; and Rorabeck, C.H.: Infra-isthmal fractures of the femur: A review of 82 cases. J. Trauma 24:735–741, 1984.

Intra-isthmal femoral fractures had a high complication rate when treated with plates or closed treatment. Intramedullary fixation is the treatment of choice for these fractures.

Winquist, R.A.; Hansen, S.T., Jr.; and Clawson, D.K.: Closed intramedullary nailing of femoral fractures: A report of five hundred and twenty cases. J. Bone Joint Surg. 66A:529–539, 1984.

A large series of femoral fractures was studied. A classification was developed for comminuted fractures. The union rate was 99.1% with a 0.9% infection rate. Shortening and malrotation were the most frequent complications.

Associated Injuries

Swiontkowski, M.F.; Hansen, S.T., Jr.; and Kellam, J.: Ipsilateral fractures of the femoral neck and shaft: A treatment protocol. J. Bone Joint Surg. 66A:260–268, 1984.

In ipsilateral fractures of the femoral neck and shaft, one-third of the neck fractures were missed initially. The treatment of choice is cancellous screws for the neck and a retrograde nail for the shaft.

Veith, R.G.; Winquist, R.A.; and Hansen, S.T., Jr.: Ipsilateral fractures of the femur and tibia: A report of fifty-seven consecutive cases. J. Bone Joint Surg. 66A:991–1002, 1984.

Patients with a "floating knee" had a high incidence of multiple system injury and fat embolism. The best results were obtained with early stabilization of the femur and tibia and motion of the knee.

Biomechanics

Cook, S.D.; Barrack, R.L.; Renz, E.; Anderson, R.C.; Harding, A.F.; Haddad, R.J., Jr.; and Milicic, M.: Retrieval and analysis of intramedullary rods: A follow-up study. Clin. Orthop. 191:269–273, 1984.

AO intramedullary nails were examined after removal. Twenty-five percent were cracked or fractured at the point of maximal stress, at the end of the slot.

Zimmerman, K.W., and Klasen, H.J.: Mechanical failure of intramedullary nails after fracture union. J. Bone Joint Surg. 65B:274–275, 1983.

Four AO nails were broken or cracked at the junction between the round cross section and the cloverleaf cross section.

Mechanism of Injury

Yvars, M.F., and Kanner, H.R.: Ski fractures of the femur. Am. J. Sports Med. 12:386–390, 1984.

An excellent review of femoral fractures resulting from skiing. There was a high incidence of collision injuries and high-speed accidents.

Fat Embolism

Talucci, R.C.; Manning, J.; Lampard, S.; Bach, A.; and Carrico, C.J.: Early intramedullary nailing of femoral shaft fractures: A cause of fat embolism syndrome. Am. J. Surg. 146:107–110, 1983.

Fat embolism was studied in immediate and delayed intramedullary nailing. The rate of fat embolism was higher with delayed nailing and, therefore, acute fixation of femoral fractures was advised.

Fractures in Children

Ziv, I.; Blackburn, N.; and Rang, M.: Femoral intramedullary nailing in the growing child. J. Trauma 24:432–434, 1984.

Femoral fractures in patients 5 to 12 years old were treated with intramedullary fixation. The authors concluded that retrograde Rush pins were safer than reamed Küntscher nails.

Ziv, I., and Rang, M.: Treatment of femoral fracture in the child with head injury. J. Bone Joint Surg. 65B:276–278, 1983.

Head-injured children with femoral fractures were studied. Eighty-four percent returned to ambulation without support. In older children, intramedullary nailing was the treatment of choice, and plates had a high infection rate.

Prophylactic Antibacterial Therapy

Jones, S.; DiPiro, J.T.; Nix, D.E.; and Bhatti, N.A.: Cephalosporins for prophylaxis in operative repair of femoral fractures: Levels in serum, muscle, and hematoma. J. Bone Joint Surg. 67A:921–924, 1985.

Prophylactic use of cefamandole, cefazolin, and cefoxitin was compared. Cefazolin produced significantly higher levels in the serum. Levels of cefazolin in the hematoma were twice as high as those of cefamandole or cefoxitin.

Anatomy

Kristiansen, T.; Seligson, D.; and Blakeslee, M.: Hip arthrograms following femoral intramedullary nailing. Unfallheilkunde 87:129–131, 1984.

Hip arthrograms were obtained of 24 femurs at the time of intramedullary nail removal. There was no communication with the nail despite a surgical starting point medial to the trochanter.

Methods of Treatment

Cast Brace

Breen, T.F., Jr.; Jones, G.S.; and Seligson, D.: Fractures of the femoral shaft in a regional hospital setting. J. Trauma 23:483–487, 1983.

One hundred fifty femoral fractures were treated by various methods. The results were very poor with traction and cast braces, and the authors favored the use of intramedullary nails.

Hardy, A.E.: The treatment of femoral fractures by cast-brace application and early ambulation: A prospective review of one hundred and six patients. J. Bone Joint Surg. 65A:56–65, 1983.

A multitude of problems were noted with cast brace treatment of femoral fractures. These included a mean shortening of 10.9 mm as well as angulation and knee stiffness. There was a high rate of knee instability and hyperextension.

Iwegbu, C.G.: Preliminary results of treatment of fractures of the femur by cast-bracing using the Zaria metal hinge. Injury 15:250–254, 1984.

Cast bracing is ideal in developing countries because it is effective, simple, and inexpensive. Among 27 patients, there was shortening of more than 2.5 cm in 3 patients and angulation of more than 10° in 6 patients.

McIvor, J.B.; Ross, P.; Landry, G.; and Davis, L.A.: Treatment of femoral fractures with the cast brace. Can. J. Surg. 27:592–594, 1984.

Traction and cast bracing was used to treat 82 patients with femoral fractures. Eighty-eight percent had satisfactory results, with a mean shortening of 1.4 cm and additional problems with ambulation and nonunion.

Suman, R.K.: Functional bracing in lower limb fractures. Ital. J. Orthop. Traumatol. 9:201–209, June 1983.

Functional bracing was used to treat femoral fractures, ipsilateral femoral neck fractures, and ipsilateral femoral shaft and tibial shaft fractures. The results were satisfactory in 96% of cases.

External Fixator

Coppola, A.J., Jr., and Anzel, S.H.: Use of the Hoffmann external fixator in the treatment of femoral fractures. Clin. Orthop. 180:78–82, 1983.

The Hoffmann external fixator was applied in a dihedral frame for open fractures, soft tissue wounds, infection, open physis, and extensive comminution. Pin track infections were common but did not alter the result. The nonunion rate was high in these difficult fractures.

Dabezies, E.J.; D'Ambrosia, R.; Shoji, H.; Norris, R.; and Murphy, G.: Fractures of the femoral shaft treated by external fixation with the Wagner device. J. Bone Joint Surg. 66A:360–364, 1984.

The Wagner external fixator was used in open and comminuted femoral fractures. There were no cases of osteomyelitis, but knee stiffness and shortening were problems.

Plates

Rinaldi, E., and Marenghi, P.: Plate and screw fixation by autogenous corticocancellous grafts in comminuted fractures of the femur. Ital. J. Orthop. Traumatol. 10:349–354, September 1984.

Femoral fractures were treated with single lateral plates with or without additional autogenous bone graft. The group of fractures with bone graft were more difficult but results were better and there were no complications.

Sprenger, T.R.: Fractures of the shaft of the femur treated with a single AO plate. South. Med. J. 76:471–474, 1983.

A single AO plate was used. There was a high rate of delayed union and nonunion. There were no nonunions in patients receiving primary bone grafts with the plating.

Ender Nails

Browner, B.D.; Burgess, A.R.; Robertson, R.J.; Baugher, W.H.; Freedman, M.T.; and Edwards, C.C.: Immediate closed antegrade Ender nailing of femoral fractures in polytrauma patients. J. Trauma 24:921–925, 1984.

Ender nailing of femoral shaft fractures was achieved through a proximal starting point in multiple trauma patients. Early stabilization improved the general patient management but the reoperation rate (28%) led the authors to the conclusion that other techniques were better.

Goldie, I.; Althoff, B.; and Hallström, E.: Ender's nailing of femoral shaft fractures. Injury 14:312–317, 1983.

Ender nails were used for traumatic femoral fractures, refractures, pathologic fractures, and nonunions. The complication rate was high, and the technique is advised only for the elderly.

Intramedullary Nails

Chan, K.M.; Tse, P.Y.T.; Chow, Y.Y.N.; and Leung, P.C.: Closed medullary nailing for fractured shaft of the femur—A comparison between the Küntscher and the AO techniques. Injury 15:381–387, 1984.

Small unreamed nails and larger reamed AO nails were compared. Ambulation, healing, and return to work were achieved sooner with AO nails, but the final outcome was similar in both groups.

Harper, M.C.: Fractures of the femur treated by open and closed intramedullary nailing using the fluted rod. J. Bone Joint Surg. 67A:699–708, 1985.

Femoral fractures were treated with the fluted rod inserted by the open or closed technique. Operative morbidity was greater with the open technique, and intraoperative complications were higher with the closed technique.

Høgh, J., and Mikkelsen, P.: Hansen-Street nailing of fractures of the femoral shaft: A study of 70 consecutive cases. Injury 14:440–446, 1983.

The Hansen-Street nail provides good results and does not require advanced technique skills or equipment.

Ker, N.B.; Maempel, F.Z.; and Paton, D.F.: Bone cement as an adjunct to medullary nailing in fractures of the distal third of the femur in elderly patients. Injury 16:102–107, 1984.

A combination of intramedullary nailing and bone cement was used in 14 elderly patients with acute or pathologic fractures. Fixation failed in one patient and there were no nonunions.

Murti, G.S., and Ring, P.A.: Closed medullary nailing of fractures of the femoral shaft using the AO method. Injury 14:318–323, 1983.

The AO closed intramedullary nail was used in 61 femoral fractures; there were 2 infections and otherwise results were excellent.

Interlocking Nails

Johnson, K.D.; Johnston, D.W.C.; and Parker, B.: Comminuted femoral-shaft fractures: Treatment by roller traction, cerclage wires and an intramedullary nail, or an interlocking intramedullary nail. J. Bone Joint Surg. 66A:1222–1235, 1984.

Seventy-nine type III and type IV comminuted fractures were treated with roller traction, cerclage wire, intramedullary nailing, and interlocking nails. The failure rates were: roller traction, 66%; intramedullary nail and cerclage wire, 39%; and interlocking nails, 4%.

Kempf, I.; Grosse, A.; and Beck, G.: Closed locked intramedullary nailing: Its application to comminuted fractures of the femur. J. Bone Joint Surg. 67A:709–720, 1985.

Locked nails expand the indications for closed nailing of the femur to fractures proximal, distal, spiral, comminuted, and with segmental bone loss.

Thoresen, B.O.; Alho, A.; Ekeland, A.; Strømsøe, K.; Follerås, G.; Haukebø, A.: Interlocking intramedullary nailing in femoral shaft fractures: A report of forty-eight cases. J. Bone Joint Surg. 67A:1313–1320, 1985.

Forty-seven patients with femoral fractures were treated with dynamic or static Grosse-Kempf interlocking nails. The results were better with static locking, and delayed union did not occur.

Supracondylar Femur Fractures

Halpenny, J., and Rorabeck, C.H.: Supracondylar fractures of the femur: Results of treatment of 61 patients. Can. J. Surg. 27:606–609, 1984.

Supracondylar and intercondylar fractures in patients less than 60 years old were treated and followed 1–9 years. Extra-articular and unicondylar fractures achieved better results with open reduction. Intra-articular T and Y fractures had unsatisfactory results in 45% with either operative or nonoperative treatment.

Healy, W.L., and Brooker, A.F., Jr.: Distal femoral fractures: Comparison of open and closed methods of treatment. Clin. Orthop. 174:166–171, 1983.

Supracondylar fractures of the femur were studied in groups treated by operative and nonoperative methods. Patients treated with open reductions had better functional results, less hospital time, earlier return to prefracture activity, and a lower incidence of nonunion and other complications compared to the patients treated with closed methods.

Kolmert, L.; Egund, N.; and Persson, B.M.: Internal fixation of supracondylar and bicondylar femoral fractures using a new semielastic device. Clin. Orthop. 181:204–219, 1983.

Flexible nails with distal screws were utilized in 34 elderly patients with supracondylar fractures. The semielastic character of the system prevented the failures usually seen when rigid internal fixation is used in osteoporotic bone.

Pritchett, J.W.: Supracondylar fractures of the femur. Clin. Orthop. 184:173–177, 1984.

A 90° supracondylar compression screw was used to fix 23 distal femur fractures. Most of these were extra-articular or had minimal joint displacement. The surgical technique is easier than that with an AO blade plate, and the results were 74% excellent or good.

Femoral Neck Fractures

Arnold, W.D.: The effect of early weight-bearing on the stability of femoral neck fractures treated with Knowles pins. J. Bone Joint Surg. 66A:847–852, 1984.

In a retrospective study, displaced femoral neck fractures that had been adequately fixed with Knowles pins and allowed to bear weight early were compared to a similar group not allowed to bear weight. No differences in complication rate, morbidity, or healing rate were noted.

Brümmer, R.: Natural course in nailed fractures of the femoral neck: A five-year prospective investigation. Arch. Orthop. Trauma Surg. 103:52–56, 1984.

Forty patients were followed for 5 years by ^{85}Sr scintimetry and radiography, and the test results were correlated with clinical examinations. After nailing, 13 fractures healed without complications, 20 had necrosis, and 5 showed nonunion. Not all osteonecrosis patients were symptomatic or required arthroplasty, and it was concluded that primary arthroplasty in fracture of the femoral neck should be avoided.

Brümmer, R.; Hansson, L.I.; and Mortensson, W.: A radiographic five-year follow-up of femoral neck fractures. Acta Orthop. Scand. 54:865–871, 1983.

Forty femoral neck fractures were followed for 5 years in a prospective clinical, radiographic, and scintimetric investigation. It was recommended that patients requiring arthroplasty after fractures should be identified on clinical grounds after early radionuclide scintimetry.

Devas, M., and Hinves, B.: Prevention of acetabular erosion after hemiarthroplasty for fractured neck of femur. J. Bone Joint Surg. 65B:548–551, 1983.

In 161 femoral neck fractures treated with a bipolar prosthesis, no acetabular erosion was seen at 4-year follow-up.

Giliberty, R.P.: Hemiarthroplasty of the hip using a low-friction bipolar endoprosthesis. Clin. Orthop. 175:86–92, 1983.

Of 75 patients with a bipolar type prosthesis, primarily for displaced femoral neck fractures, 92% had satisfactory results. The author recommends a bipolar prosthesis for hemiarthroplasty of the hip in femoral neck fractures.

Hägglund, G.; Nordström, B.; and Lidgren, L.: Total hip replacement after nailing failure in femoral neck fractures. Arch. Orthop. Trauma Surg. 103:125–127, 1984.

Forty patients were treated by total hip arthroplasty after failed femoral neck nailing. Excellent results were obtained, and this is considered to be the salvage operation of choice after failed femoral neck surgery.

Holmberg, S., and Thorngren, K.-G.: Preoperative ^{99m}Tc-MDP scintimetry of femoral neck fractures. Acta Orthop. Scand. 55:430–435, 1984.

Preoperative ^{99m}Tc-MDP scintimetry in 117 patients proved to be of value in the choice of primary treatment of femoral neck fractures. A ratio of 0.90 correlated well with uneventful healing in both displaced and undisplaced femoral neck fractures.

Kofoed, H., and Kofod, J.: Moore prosthesis in the treatment of fresh femoral neck fractures: A critical review with special attention to secondary acetabular degeneration. Injury 14:531–540, 1983.

One hundred six consecutive patients with displaced femoral neck fractures were treated with Moore prostheses. At 2-year follow-up of 71 patients, 37% required a total hip replacement because of hip pain. The authors concluded that active patients, regardless of age, should not be treated with a one-piece prosthesis, and they preferred satisfactory reduction and pin ning. Hip replacement is performed only if the fracture cannot be reduced.

Maxted, M.J., and Denham, R.A.: Failure of hemiarthroplasty for fractures of the neck of the femur. Injury 15:224–226, 1984.

A review of 92 patients 4 years after hemiarthroplasty for displaced subcapital fractures revealed that 19% required further operations; a separate review of 70 patients who had undergone a revision after hemiarthroplasty showed that over half needed the operation within 3 years. The authors recommend that hemiarthroplasty be reserved for patients over age 79 or those over 65 who are medically unfit.

Ort, P.J., and LaMont, J.: Treatment of femoral neck

fractures with a sliding compression screw and two Knowles pins. Clin. Orthop. 190:158–162, 1984.

Twenty-two patients over age 65 with displaced femoral neck fractures had fixation with sliding hip screw and two Knowles pins. The rate of union was 100%; osteonecrosis occurred in 24%.

Sim, F.H.: Displaced femoral neck fractures: The rationale for primary total hip replacement. Hip 11:51–61, 1983.

A series of femoral neck fractures treated with primary total hip arthroplasty is presented with adequate results.

Stewart, H.D.: Pugh's nail fixation versus Thompson's prosthesis for displaced subcapital fractures of the femur. Injury 15:227–231, 1984.

A retrospective study of 100 patients with displaced subcapital fractures fixed with either a Pugh nail or primary Thompson prosthesis revealed that, up to 3 months, the mortality rate was higher with the Thompson prosthesis; after 1 year the rates were comparable. Nail fixation resulted in higher failure rate and need for reoperation.

Strömqvist, B.; Brismar, J.; Hansson, L.I.; and Palmer, J.: Technetium-99m-methylenediphosphonate scintimetry after femoral neck fracture: A three-year follow-up study. Clin. Orthop. 182:177–189, 1984.

In 39 patients with femoral neck fractures followed by ^{99m}Tc-MDP scintimetry 1–3 weeks after operation, the fractured/intact side ratio of 1.0 corresponded to uneventful healing, and defective uptake (ratio <1.0) correlated with healing complications. At 4 months, the ratio was always <1.0. Early ^{99m}Tc-MDP scintimetry was of predictive value in this study.

Strömqvist, B., and Hansson, L.I.: Femoral head vitality after femoral neck fracture. Comparison between pre- and peroperative tetracycline labeling. Arch. Orthop. Trauma Surg. 101:251–257, 1983.

Labeling with tetracycline in 370 femoral neck fractures revealed that undisplaced fractures had a much higher uptake than displaced fractures; no difference was found between the degrees of displacement.

Strömqvist, B., and Hansson, L.I.: Femoral head vitality in femoral neck fracture after hook-pin internal fixation. Clin. Orthop. 191:105–109, 1984.

A study of the vitality of the femoral head in 317 femoral neck fractures by tetracycline labeling and ^{99m}Tc-MDP scintimetry revealed a rate of avascular healing complication of 7% in undisplaced and of 32% in displaced femoral neck fractures treated with hook pins.

Strömqvist, B.; Hansson, L.I.; Nilsson, L.T.; and Thorngren, K.-G.: Two-year follow-up of femoral neck fractures: Comparison of osteosynthesis methods. Acta Orthop. Scand. 55:521–525, 1984.

In a prospective series of 152 femoral neck fractures, half fixed with hook pins and half fixed with tri-flanged nail, the hook pins were far superior in both displaced and undisplaced fractures. Less than 1 patient in 12 needed reoperation with total hip replacement within 2 years after fixation with a hook pin, and therefore fixation was favored over primary arthroplasty.

Strömqvist, B.; Hansson, L.I.; Palmer, J.; Ceder, L.; and Thorngren, K.G.: Scintimetric evaluation of nailed femoral neck fractures with special reference to type of osteosynthesis. Acta Orthop. Scand. 54:340–347, 1983.

Using ^{99m}Tc-MDP scintimetry prior to nailing and 1–2 weeks after nailing, the authors demonstrated that a four-flanged nail is harmful to the vascular supply of the femoral head compared to a Hansson screw; therefore, a four-flanged nail is not recommended in femoral neck fractures.

Svenningsen, S.; Benum, P.; Nesse, O.; and Furset, O.I.: Internal fixation of femoral neck fractures: Compression screw compared with nail plate fixation. Acta Orthop. Scand. 55:423–429, 1984.

Fixation of femoral neck fractures by using a compression screw device gave fewer failures without disadvantages compared to nail plate fixation.

Swiontkowski, M.F.; Hansen, S.T., Jr.; and Kellam, J.: Ipsilateral fractures of the femoral neck and shaft: A treatment protocol. J. Bone Joint Surg. 66A:260–268, 1984.

Eighty-three cases of ipsilateral femoral neck and shaft fractures reported in the literature were reviewed and the conclusion is that anatomic reduction of the femoral neck fracture should be done first, followed by multiple pin fixation, and the shaft should be addressed secondarily. One-third of femoral neck fractures were missed in this combined injury.

Swiontkowski, M.F.; Winquist, R.A.; and Hansen, S.T., Jr.: Fractures of the femoral neck in patients between the ages of twelve and forty-nine years. J. Bone Joint Surg. 66A:837–846, 1984.

A series of 27 consecutive patients less than 50 years old with femoral neck fractures was reviewed; no nonunions and an aseptic necrosis rate of 20% were reported. Early fixation of femoral neck fractures with multiple pins after anatomic reduction was advocated for these younger patients.

Turner, A., and Wroblewski, B.M.: Charnley low-friction arthroplasty for the treatment of hips with late complications of femoral neck fractures. Clin. Orthop. 185:126–130, 1984.

Two hundred five Charnley low-friction arthroplasties were used in patients after complications from femoral neck fractures, with excellent results. The infection rate was high (3.9%) and was related to a high incidence of previous superficial wound infection.

Welch, R.B.: The rationale for primary hemiarthroplasty in the treatment of fractures of the femoral neck in elderly patients. Hip 11:42–50, 1983.

The author believes that hemiarthroplasty is the treatment of choice for displaced femoral neck fractures in the elderly and results in no greater morbidity or mortality than other forms of intervention. Mortality and morbidity may even decrease when modern technology is used.

Intertrochanteric Fractures

Harper, M.C., and Walsh, T.: Ender nailing for peritrochanteric fractures of the femur: An analysis of indications, factors related to mechanical failure, and postoperative results. J. Bone Joint Surg. 67A:79–88, 1985.

Ender nails are advocated for both stable and unstable intertrochanteric fractures if a good reduction can be obtained, the canal can be filled, the surgeon is experienced with the technique, and the fracture is relatively stable. They are not recommended in subtrochanteric fractures.

Hayse-Moore, G.H.; MacEachern, A.G.; and Evans, D.C.J.: Treatment of intertrochanteric fractures of the femur: A comparison of the Richards screw-plate with the Jewett nail-plate. J. Bone Joint Surg. 65B:262–267, 1983.

One hundred seven patients with intertrochanteric fractures of the femur treated with the Richards screw were compared with 103 similar patients treated with a Jewett nail. The former became mobile more quickly and left the hospital sooner, and more returned to their home.

Hayward, S.J.; Lowe, L.W.; and Tzevelekos, S.: Intertrochanteric fractures: A comparison between fixation with a two-piece nail plate and Ender's nails. Int. Orthop. 7:153–158, 1983.

One hundred eight-two patients with intertrochanteric fractures were treated with the McLaughlin nail plates and Ender intramedullary nails. The solid nail plate system failed in varus; the Ender nails failed by backing out with protrusion into the knee. Unstable intertrochanteric fractures occur more frequently in the elderly.

Kyle, R.F.; Gustilo, R.B.; and Premer, R.F.: Analysis of six hundred and twenty-two intertrochanteric hip fractures. J. Bone Joint Surg. 61A:216–221, 1979.

A review of over 600 intertrochanteric fractures shows that a collapsible device is superior to a rigid device in successful fixation of intertrochanteric fractures and that central head placement with a collapsible device will give a 90% success rate, even in unstable intertrochanteric fractures.

Kyle, R.F.; Wright, T.M.; and Burstein, A.H.: Biomechanical analysis of the sliding characteristics of compression hip screws. J. Bone Joint Surg. 62A:1308–1314, 1980.

The single most important factor in impaction of compression hip screws is the angle at which the screw is placed in fixation of fractures. The higher the angle, the greater the ease of sliding. This is an exponential phenomenon.

MacEachern, A.G., and Heyse-Moore, G.H.: Stable intertrochanteric femoral fractures: A misnomer? J. Bone Joint Surg. 65B:582–583, 1983.

Both stable and unstable intertrochanteric fractures impact to a stable position after anatomic reduction and fixation with a sliding device. Medial displacement is not needed. Failure is more likely to occur when a rigid Jewett nail is used.

Møller, B.N.; Lucht, U.; Grymer, F.; and Bartholdy, N.J.: Instability of trochanteric hip fractures following internal fixation: A radiographic comparison of the Richards sliding screw-plate and the McLaughlin nail-plate. Acta Orthop. Scand. 55:517–520, 1984.

In a comparative series of intertrochanteric hip fractures fixed with the McLaughlin nail plate and Richards sliding screw, a much higher complication and reoperation rate occurred with the McLaughlin nail plate. The compression screw is superior to the rigid nail plate device in both stable and unstable fractures.

Rao, J.P.; Banzon, M.T.; Weiss, A.B.; and Rayhack, J.: Treatment of unstable intertrochanteric fractures with anatomic reduction and compression hip screw fixation. Clin. Orthop. 175:65–71, 1983.

One hundred sixty-two cases of unstable intertrochanteric fractures treated by anatomic reduction and compression hip screw fixation showed that over 92% displaced medially and impacted to a more stable position. Displacement osteotomies had no advantage over anatomic reduction and fixation with a compression screw device.

Sherk, H.H., and Foster, M.D.: Hip fractures: Condylocephalic rod *versus* compression screw. Clin. Orthop. 192:255–259, 1985.

Seventy consecutive intertrochanteric fractures were fixed with a condylocephalic nail and a compression sliding screw. There was a significantly higher complication rate with the condylocephalic nail.

Strathy, G.M., and Johnson, E.W., Jr.: Ender's pinning for fractures about the hip. Mayo Clin. Proc. 59:411–414, 1984.

Four years of experience with Ender nails in intertrochanteric fractures revealed knee pain in 41% of the patients followed; 31% required additional surgical procedures secondary to migration of the pins. The authors recommend the use of Ender nails only in stable fractures in patients who cannot tolerate more extensive procedures.

Zain Elabdien, B.S.; Olerud, S.; and Karlström, G.: The influence of age on the morphology of trochanteric fracture. Arch. Orthop. Trauma Surg. 103:156–161, 1984.

One hundred twenty-seven trochanteric fractures were analyzed, and it was found that there was a continuous decrease in the quality of bone with age as well as a direct relationship to bone quality and severity of the pattern of the trochanteric fracture. Skeletal aging starts in premenopausal women; after age 85, the process is more rapid in men than in women. Because of the longevity of the patient population, the incidence of unstable trochanteric fracture has increased by a factor of 3 over the past 3 decades.

Subtrochanteric Fractures

Wile, P.B.; Panjabi, M.M.; and Southwick, W.O.: Treatment of subtrochanteric fractures with a high-angle compression hip screw. Clin. Orthop. 175:72–78, 1983.

Twenty-five subtrochanteric fractures were transfixed with a high-angle compression hip screw with excellent results. No mechanical failures, delayed unions, or nonunions occurred. In certain subtrochanteric fractures, fixation with a high-angle compression hip screw is reliable and advantageous.

Zain Elabdien, B.S.; Olerud, S.; and Karlström, G.: Subtrochanteric fractures: Classification and results of Ender nailing. Arch. Orthop. Trauma Surg. 103:241–250, 1984.

Twenty-seven subtrochanteric fractures were fixed with Ender nails with a 17% complication rate and a good or excellent result in 79% of patients.

Zickel, R.E.: Subtrochanteric femoral fractures. Orthop. Clin. North Am. 11:555–568, July 1980.

A review of the biomechanical stresses acting on subtrochanteric fractures, emphasizing the desirable features in intramedullary fixation.

33

Hip Reconstruction: Total Hip Replacement

The dramatic early results of total hip replacement led to approximately 100,000 hip replacements being done per year in the United States by the late 1970s. Longer-term results have included some disappointing failures which require major revision by complex and challenging hip surgery. These failures and the resultant difficult revisions have led, in the mid-1980s, to widespread enthusiasm for attempting to obtain the same relief from pain and improvement in hip function without using poly(methyl methacrylate). This chapter discusses cemented total hip replacement, revision total hip replacement, and uncemented total hip replacement.

Cemented Total Hip Replacement

Long-Term Follow-Up

Clinical studies show dramatic results in the first 2 years after total hip replacement, with very low incidences of death (0.1% to 0.5%), infection (0.5% to 4%), and mechanical problems necessitating reoperation on the hip (less than 5%). Studies at 5 years show an increased incidence of mechanical loosening, and at 10 to 15 years loosening has emerged as the most common complication. Two categories of loosening have been identified in these long-term studies: radiologic and clinical. Different authors have defined radiologic loosening in various ways and thus reported incidences of radiographic loosening have ranged from 10% to 40%.

All authors agree that change in position of a prosthesis (migration) represents radiologic loosening (Fig. 1). Most agree that 2 mm or more of circumferential lucency surrounding the acetabular cup or femoral component represents radiologic loosening. Fracture of the cement mantle or the appearance of radiolucency at the cement-prosthesis interface suggests radiologic loosening. The most definitive radiographic sign of actual loosening of prosthetic components is a progressively enlarging radiolucent line on serial radiographs. Many hips show obvious radiolucencies on radiographs but the patient has no onset or progression of clinical symptoms (Fig. 2).

The incidence of symptomatic loosening requiring revision ranges from 5% to 20% in long-term follow-ups. In the first 5 years postoperatively, most loosening problems that require revision involve the femoral component. When follow-up extends beyond 8 years, the incidence of loosening of the acetabular component appears to increase exponentially. Incidences of 14% for significant radiologic demarcation and 11% for acetabular component migration were reported in 112 hips followed for 12 to 15 years.

Long-term studies reported in the 1980s obviously reflect the outcome of the surgical techniques and experience and the prosthesis and patient selection decisions of the early 1970s. Clearly, the choice of prosthesis has significant bearing on long-term outcome. A 10-year follow-up of first-generation curved-stem Mueller prostheses revealed a revision rate of 20% and signs suggestive of radiologic loosening in 40%. In contrast, several follow-ups of series in which Charnley prostheses were used in the early 1970s found revision rates of only 5% to 10% and radiologic loosening rates below 20%.

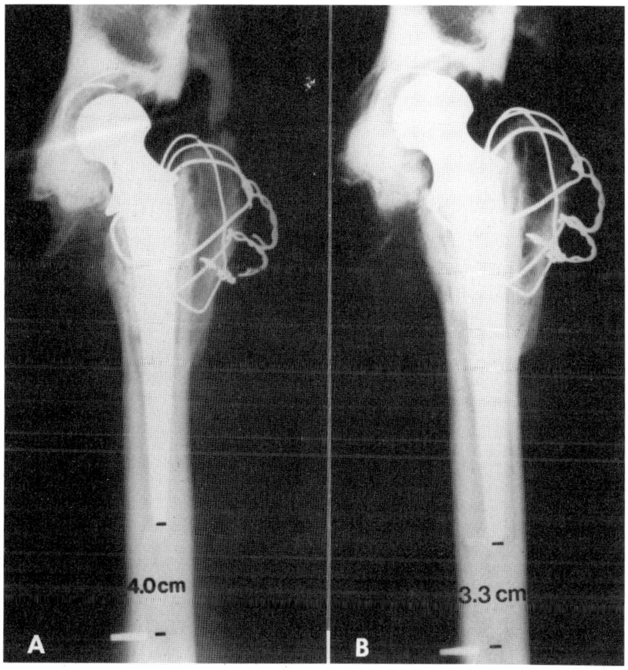

Figure 1

Migration of femoral component in 28-year-old woman, resulting in symptomatic loosening and requiring revision. *A,* At 4 years postoperatively; fragment of screw from childhood osteotomy for CDH provides landmark. *B,* At 6 years, easily measurable distal subsidence has occurred. (From Collis, D.K. Hip 10:1–26, 1982. By permission of C.V. Mosby Company.)

In patients under 30 years of age, one study of 33 total hip replacements found a 57% incidence of actual or potential loosening of one component within 5 years. A subsequent study confirmed a relationship between loosening and poor surgical technique. Another report indicated a 9% revision rate in 45 operations in patients under 50 years of age followed 7.3 years; 13% were thought to show progressive radiologic demarcation. It was strongly recommended that young patients be counseled emphatically to avoid running, jumping, and lifting. Cemented total hip

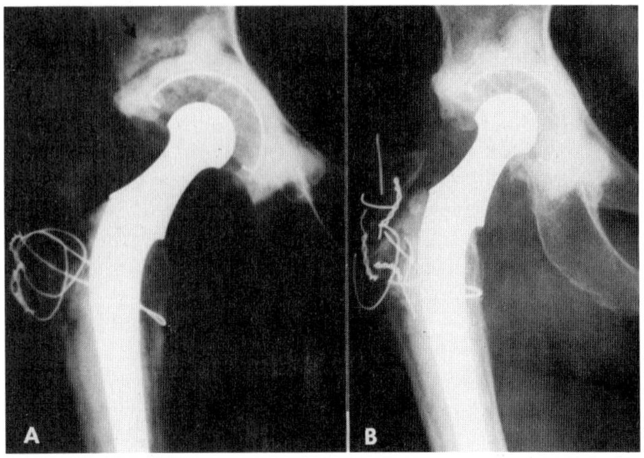

Figure 2

A, Wide radiolucencies superior to the acetabular cup in 61-year-old woman seen on postoperative radiograph. *B,* At 10 years later, no progression (and possible improvement) in the radiolucency and no clinical symptoms.

replacement in this age group should be performed only on patients who are willing to cooperate with this recommendation.

Rheumatoid arthritis often causes enough pain and disability from diminished hip function to necessitate reconstructive surgical procedures, even in very young patients. One follow-up found 96% good clinical results 7 years after operation. Multiple joint involvement and soft osteopenic bone can create special surgical challenges. Even in these patients with low functional requirements, mechanical loosening with clinical failure has been observed. When the acetabulum was not positioned anatomically—i.e., left in a position of protrusio or placed superior and lateral to the notch—higher failure rates were seen. A higher incidence of infection has been reported in patients with rheumatoid arthritis in most series of total hip replacements.

Results With Modern Surgical Techniques

Improvements in Femoral Prosthesis Numerous laboratory and clinical studies have addressed design and composition of the femoral prosthesis. Superalloys of forged cobalt/chromium and titanium have fatigue strengths several times greater than those of earlier stainless steel or other cast alloys. Only rare clinical case reports of stem breakage with these new metals have been published in the last few years, indicating that use of these stronger metals markedly decreased the problem of stem breakage. Geometric design recommendations from laboratory studies, including three-dimensional finite-element stress analysis, support eliminating sharp corners on the prostheses and broadening the femoral component in the anterior-posterior dimension to distribute stresses to the cement more broadly.

Controversy exists regarding the appropriate modulus of elasticity of the femoral component. A higher modulus (stiffer material, such as cobalt/chromium) will increase stresses in the stem and decrease stress in the cement. Such transfer of the stress into the stem distally potentially could stress-shield the proximal femur and lead to disuse bone resorption. Lower modulus (more flexible stems of titanium) stresses the bone but could increase the stress on, and thus fatigue, the proximal cement mantle, causing increased loosening. Prostheses with proximal collars theoretically stress the bone more proximally, but achieving contact between collar and bone at operation is difficult. Some reports suggest that absence of a collar may allow the femoral component to undergo favorable (painless) subsidence within the femoral canal. Clinical data to support selection of prostheses on the basis of modulus of elasticity or presence or absence of a collar are inconclusive so far. Therefore, surgeons must select these design parameters on the basis of laboratory data.

Improvements in Acetabular Component Several laboratory studies established that use of metal backing on polyethylene acetabular components reduces peak stresses in cement and trabecular bone. Use of thick polyethylene provides a similar but lesser improvement. One clinical study of 51 hips in which cemented metal-backed acetabular components were used in young people, all followed more than 5 years, found only three loose components, all in patients under age 25 at operation. Another clinical follow-up of patients with cemented metal-backed acetabular components found 3 aseptic loosenings in 40 hips followed 5 to 10 years.

Bone Preparation and Prosthesis Placement Loose bone should be removed from the canal with a curette or brush. The femoral cortex should not be perforated. The femoral stem should be placed in neutral or slight valgus.

The acetabular bone bed is best prepared by maintaining the subchondral cortex of the acetabular bone stock surrounding the acetabular component but still using numerous keying holes in it for cement fixation. Finite element analysis predicts that placement of the acetabulum in its anatomic position at the level of the true notch will decrease stresses and increase longevity of the component. Several clinical studies confirm this, reporting a higher acetabular component failure rate when the acetabular component is not positioned anatomically. Clinical studies in hips in which protrusio is present show that either bone graft or cement can be used to fill in the floor of the acetabular bed to facilitate such anatomic positioning.

Optimal Cement Technique Early reports suggest that slower mixing of the cement for a shorter time decreases the air voids within the cement and thus improves its strength characteristics. The physical characteristics of poly(methyl methacrylate) are markedly improved by centrifugation: one study found a 24% increase in mean ultimate tensile strength, 54% improvement in mean ultimate tensile strain, and 136% increase in mean fatigue life. Initial reports suggest that mixing the cement under reduced pressure may decrease retained air and increase cement strength. Introduction of cement into its bed at an earlier stage, when its viscosity is lower, improves its intrusion characteristics but requires special care and handling so that it can be pressurized effectively into the bone bed. Special low-viscosity cements have been developed to improve intrusion characteristics but these show decreased fracture toughness. Preparation of the bone bed for the cement requires removal of any loose cancellous bone debris, blood, or tissue. Cleansing the bed with water pick lavage is helpful. Routine mechanical drying of both acetabular and femoral surfaces is important. Some authors advocate utilizing hypotensive anesthesia to keep blood away from the bone-cement interface at the time of cementing.

Mechanical compression of the cement in order to facilitate intrusion into the bony bed is important and can be facilitated by delivering the cement with a syringe. In the acetabulum, the bony floor must be maintained intact or restored with bone graft, cement, or artificial materials to facilitate this pressurization. In the femoral canal, distal plugging with bone, cement, Silastic, or polyethylene allows retrograde filling of the canal and permits better pressurization. Several clinical follow-up studies demonstrate that 1 to 2 cm of poly(methyl methacrylate) distal to the tip of the femoral stem decreases the incidence of radiologic demarcation that often precedes clinical loosening. Several authors have suggested that the cement mantle should be 5 to 10 mm thick proximally and medially and an intact cement mantle of several millimeters should surround the entire stem. Laboratory data are available to support all of these surgical techniques and some follow-up clinical data are available. However, no double-blind studies have been done and, to date, clinical studies are of insufficient length to demonstrate the degree of improvement over earlier techniques.

Complications

Implant Interface There is increasing evidence that component loosening may be attributable in part to a biologic reaction to particulate debris. Polyethylene, metal, and poly(methyl methacrylate) particles stimulate the benign fibrous membrane to become a resorptive membrane by recruiting and stimulating macrophages. Membrane removed from the bone-cement interface during revision arthroplasty was found to be histologically and biochemically differentiated so that synovium-like cells were adjacent to the cement layer. Deep to them, the predominant cell type was macrophages. The membrane had the capacity to produce large amounts of prostaglandin E_2 and collagenase. It was postulated that aggressive lysis of bone might be explained by the biochemical activity of this reactive tissue, either through the direct activity of the macrophages or through their interaction with other cells.

More recently, a deleterious effect on DNA replication has been demonstrated in a mouse macrophage cell line in which phagocytized poly(methyl methacrylate) particles were present. In a rabbit wound model, the effect of particle size as well as particle composition was examined. Whereas polyethylene or poly(methyl methacrylate) in bulk form elicited a bland fibrous tissue response, the same materials in smaller particulate form initiated an inflammatory foreign cell reaction. These and other studies strongly suggest that loosening of cemented prostheses results not only from mechanical factors such as suboptimal implant design and inadequate cement technique but also from biologic factors as well. In particular, a factor of critical importance may be the ability of the host's immune system to accommodate to particulate debris at the host-implant interface.

Mechanical Loosening The most frequent cause of failure is mechanical loosening. The incidence of this after hip replacements done 10 to 15 years ago is discussed above. The improved surgical techniques outlined may decrease this complication, but several survivorship studies of earlier series show this to be occurring at rates of about 1% per year.

Material Failure Stem fracture rates as high as 33% have been reported in large active men after replacements by the earlier surgical techniques and with the earlier prosthesis designs. Use of the techniques, designs, and materials described above appears to have decreased this to rare cases. Initially, potential acetabular wear was of great concern but clinical studies document wear rates of less than 0.1 mm per year. Wear rates sometimes are larger with loose prostheses or when acrylic debris erodes the surface. The significance of the small fragments of abraded polyethylene seen in microscopic sections of soft tissues removed at the revision of failed total hip prostheses is unclear.

Methacrylate Failure The mechanical properties of methacrylate are inferior to those of metal and polyethylene. Use of the surgical techniques described above can dramatically improve the clinical properties of methyl methacrylate. Most cases of loose components are associated with some fracturing of the methacrylate mantle. Even when the mantle of cement remains intact but loose, studies of the soft tissue-bone-cement interface reveal histologic and histochemical characteristics of a synovium-like membrane with macrophages but no inflammatory cells. One study revealed that this tissue has the capacity to generate prostaglandin E_2 and collagenase and this could explain the progressive lysis of bone at the interface. Another study found no obvious signs of cytotoxicity and rare inflammatory cells. An electron microscopic study of three non-loose cemented femoral stems found viable bone alternating with areas of soft tissue containing macrophages (Fig. 3). These findings support the theory of mechanical instability as the prime cause of tissue reaction and bone loss, rather than a biologic intolerance to methyl methacrylate itself.

Infection. ***Prevention*** Deep infection is one of the most serious postoperative complications of total hip replacement, making prevention of such an infection critically important. Patients who have a systemic illness or rheumatoid arthritis or who are taking steroids have higher rates of infection. Any systemic infection should be eliminated prior to elective hip surgery. After all total hip replacements, antimicrobial agents should be given prophylactically when the patient has dental or urologic procedures or any other potential cause of bacteremia.

At operation, careful preparation and draping and minimizing traffic flow into and out of the operating room have been shown to decrease infection rates. Numerous studies have established that prophylactic systemic antimicrobial therapy significantly decreases infections after total hip replacement. In most cases the agent should be a broad-spectrum variety, given just before operation and continued only for 12 to 24 hours postoperatively. In many total hip replacement series in which prophylactic antimicrobial therapy was used, infection rates were less than 1%. In a large multicenter retrospective study of 8,000 joint replacements in England, use of ultraclean air and body exhaust systems decreased the infection rate to 0.14%. Use of ultraviolet light decreased the incidence of postoperative infection to 0.15% after 1,322 total hip replacements. In another study, a history of previous surgery on the hip, failure to use prophylactic antimicrobial therapy, failure of the surgical wound to heal within 3 to 4 weeks, and the presence of postoperative infections elsewhere in the body all

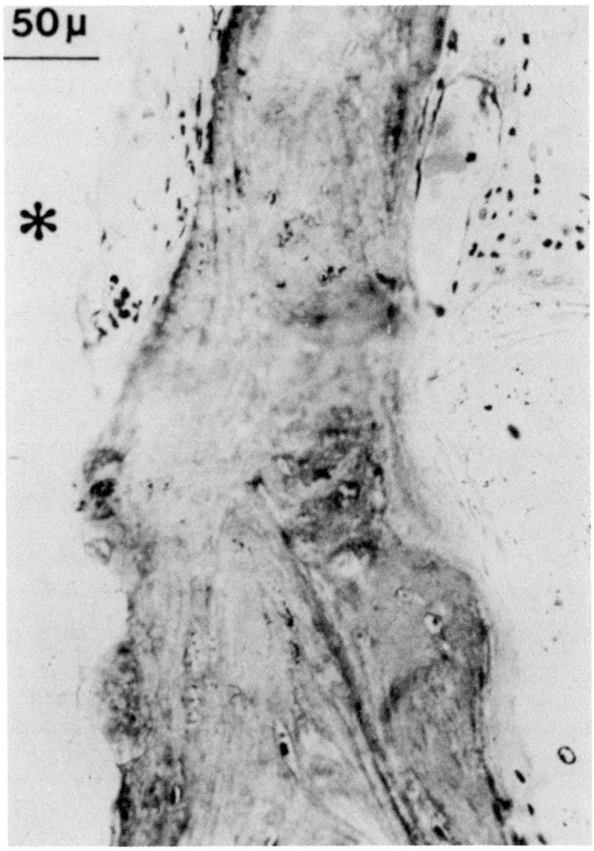

Figure 3

Bone-cement interface with a stem that was not loose, demonstrating viable bone next to methyl methacrylate. Cement dissolved during embedding process. (Methylene blue; scale = 50 μm.) (From Linder, L., and Hansson, H.A. J. Bone Joint Surg. 65B:646–649, 1983. By permission of the British Editorial Society of Bone and Joint Surgery.)

were related to an increased incidence of deep wound infection after total hip replacement. There is no current evidence to support the use of antimicrobial agents in the cement in uncomplicated primary total hip replacement.

Diagnosis Infections may occur at any time after a total hip replacement, from a few days to many years. Infections after the first few weeks usually do not present with the classic findings of wound drainage, fever, and changes in leukocyte count or sedimentation rate. Numerous authors have indicated that unexplained pain after total hip replacement must arouse suspicion of infection. Indium-111 has been reported by some as reliable for making a definitive diagnosis of infection. Aspiration of the joint itself, often under image intensification, remains the most definitive diagnostic test. However, even culture of material taken at operation and microscopically showing the presence of infected material has been shown to fail to grow microorganisms in up to 10% of cases.

Treatment No study has yet documented more than a rare successful treatment of deep infection after total hip replacement if antimicrobial agents alone are the treatment. Occasionally, when deep infection presents in the first few weeks postoperatively, immediate surgical drainage accompanied by immediate and long-term antimicrobial therapy appears to eradicate the infection permanently. Several authors condemn the use of closed irrigation-suction methods because of possible introduction of secondary infections. In most patients with chronic infection, surgeons advocate complete removal of the prosthesis and the cement. If gross purulence is present, delayed primary or secondary wound closure is appropriate. Primary closure over one or two closed suction drains has proved to be effective in the treatment of an infected total hip arthroplasty in which only granulation (without gross pus) is present. Parenteral antimicrobial therapy is recommended for several weeks, followed by oral therapy for 1 to several weeks. One study found such excisional arthroplasty effective in eradicating infections in 27 of 33 hips. A study with 6-year follow-up after resection arthroplasties found control of sepsis in 97% of the patients; the patients were left with shortened extremities and the need for external support in walking, but the results seemed to improve with time.

Numerous reports support the implantation of a new hip replacement at a later date, after adequate treatment of the infection. Recommendations for timing of the reimplantation vary from several weeks to several months, depending on the extent of the infection, the causal organism, and the surgeon's preference. In all series, gram-negative infections had a poorer prognosis for successful reimplantation (Table 1). In fact, reconstruction can be accomplished successfully earlier (3 months) with the less virulent microorganisms. When the causal organism is a gram-negative bacillus, reconstruction should be delayed for 12 months.

Primary exchange arthroplasty, consisting of treatment of an infected arthroplasty by removal of all implant materials and infection and reimplantation of a new implant with gentamicin-impregnated acrylic cement, has been recommended for many years by European authors. Recent follow-up of 825 such procedures found overall success rates of 70% at 6 years postoperatively and 50% at 11 years. In this country, gentamicin-impregnated acrylic cement has been available only under special FDA protocols. Surgeons in the United States have reported using tobramycin, erythromycin, colistin, and other heat-stable antimicrobial agents in a powdered form that can be mixed with the acrylic polymer powder in the operating room prior to

Table 1. Relationship of Delay in Reconstruction of Infected Total Hip Replacement and Causal Organism

- Earlier reconstruction (3 months):
  - Low-virulence microorganisms
    - Aerobic and anaerobic gram-positive cocci
      - *Staphylococcus epidermidis* (methicillin susceptible)
      - *Staphylococcus aureus* (methicillin susceptible)
      - Streptococci (except enterococci)
      - *Peptococcus* sp.
      - *Peptostreptococcus* sp.
      - *Propionibacterium acnes*
- Late reconstruction (≥12 months):
  - Virulent microorganisms
    - Aerobic and anaerobic gram-negative bacilli
      - *Pseudomonas* sp.
      - *Escherichia coli*
      - *Klebsiella* sp.
      - *Bacteroides* sp.
    - Aerobic gram-positive cocci
      - *Staphylococcus epidermidis* (methicillin resistant)
      - *Staphylococcus aureus* (methicillin resistant)

addition of the monomer. Other authors have reported treating the infection with antibiotic-impregnated methyl methacrylate beads as an interim procedure prior to reimplantation of new prosthetic components.

Thromboembolism Thrombophlebitis and pulmonary embolism are frequent complications after total hip replacement. Fortunately, the clinical presentation of either of these entities is almost always effectively treated by intravenous administration of heparin followed by oral warfarin (Coumadin) therapy with no eventual impairment of the outcome of the hip replacement. Numerous studies have shown clotting in the calf or thigh veins in up to 50% of patients after elective hip surgery. Most authors recommend early ambulation of the patient and use of graded pressure stockings, but the effectiveness of these measures is not well documented.

Various anticoagulants have been proposed for prophylactic use, including aspirin (1.2 g/day), low-dose heparin, mini-dose heparin, and low doses of warfarin. In one study, despite prophylactic warfarin therapy, routine lung scans showed an embolism incidence of 19%, and routine venography showed a 43% incidence of thrombosis in the deep veins. In this same study, obesity and operations exceeding 2½ hours in duration were associated with increased incidences of thromboembolism. Prophylaxis with aspirin is reported to be less effective in women than in men.

The use of compression devices that create intermittent pressure on the calf and thigh of the operated leg has been shown to decrease the incidence of thromboembolism. One recent report described an improved effect of this method when combined with low-molecular-weight dextran in small doses. Unfortunately, dextran and heparin have been associated with increased incidences of bleeding in the wound, as has been warfarin when prothrombin time is not kept at or below 1.5 times normal. Fortunately, almost all forms of prophylaxis have eliminated or drastically decreased the incidence of fatal pulmonary embolism compared with patients not given some form of prophylaxis.

Neurovascular The incidence of sciatic and femoral palsies after total hip replacement ranges from 1% to 3% in various series. Fortunately, the majority of these nerve deficits are partial, and the patients gain significant recovery. The specific cause is rarely identified, although case reports have implicated overlengthening of legs, major revision surgery, cement protrusion, and use of pointed retractors. Occasionally, a slowly developing palsy has been associated with a hematoma, especially in a patient on anticoagulation therapy; in these cases, relieving the pressure by draining the hematoma has led to dramatic recovery. Arterial injuries are even rarer than neurologic deficits and have been reported to occur in 0.1% to 0.2% of all total hip replacements. Surgical instruments have been identified as causes. Cement protrusion has been implicated as a cause of late-onset vascular compromise, and false aneurysms have been reported.

Dislocation Postoperative dislocation has been reported in 1% to 5% of total hip replacements in various studies. Two recent reports describe the posterior approach as having a higher dislocation rate than the anterolateral or transtrochanteric. Other causes identified include malposition of components, failure of the greater trochanter to unite after the transtrochanteric approach, and failure to attain adequate leg length. Most dislocations occur in the weeks immediately after operation and can be treated by simple reduction with the expectation of lasting stability. Casting or bracing has been reported to be effective, and these methods may allow the patient to regenerate a stabilizing hip capsule. If recurrent dislocations occur, surgical treatment may be necessary. When obvious correctable prosthetic malpositioning or anatomic deficiencies are not present, repeat persistent redislocations have been reported in up to a third of the patients. One recent study of 32 dislocations occurring for the first time 5 to 10 years after operation found that these patients had a greater range of motion than is usual after total hip replacement; these dislocations were attributed to gradual stretching of the pseudocapsule.

Trochanteric Osteotomy Because of problems in obtaining union of the greater trochanter after the transtrochanteric approach, more and more surgeons report using the trochanteric osteotomy approach only in the most complicated cases. Unfortunately, these are the very cases in which it is most difficult to obtain secure fixation and bony union. Trochanteric bursitis is the most common clinical problem and it often can be solved with a simple steroid injection. Surgical removal of fragmented or protruding trochanteric wires is simple and often pain relieving. When true trochanteric nonunion occurs with proximal displacement of the trochanter and weakness of abduction, surgical reapproximation of the trochanter may be warranted. This operation becomes more difficult as more time elapses between displacement and repair. Reattachment at the proper level is often difficult and requires significant soft tissue dissection and repair. On occasion, protection of the hip in abduction for several months postoperatively is required; sometimes, an above-the-knee spica cast must be used for a few weeks.

Heterotopic Bone The reported incidence of heterotopic bone formation after total hip replacement varies from 5% to 61%, depending upon the definition of how much bone constitutes heterotopic bone. Clinical problems related to heterotopic bone formation are infrequent, and even radiologically obvious heterotopic bone seems to cause little pain or to have little effect on hip mobility. Patients in high-risk diagnostic categories, such as men with hypertrophic osteoarthritis or patients with ankylosing spondylitis, are proposed by some to be candidates for prophylactic treatment with diphosphonates. This medication must be given for 1 month preoperatively and for 3 months postoperatively; it has been shown to prevent calcification of the osteoid matrix. After discontinuation of the medication, some calcification of this matrix often occurs. Most recent studies do not seem to be strongly in support of its effectiveness. Low-dose radiation, totaling 1,000 to 2,000 rads given in divided doses beginning immediately after operation and spread over 5 to 10 days, appears to be effective but has the obvious disadvantage of increased radiation burden.

Femur Fractures Fractures of the femur during total hip replacement can almost always be avoided by careful surgical technique, notably with good exposure, careful hip dislocation, careful utilization of power tools, and appropriate bone preparation to allow easy insertion of the prosthetic devices. Fractures occurring at operation usually should be treated by using a longer or larger prosthesis or some form of internal fixation or both.

Most postoperative femoral fractures can be prevented by avoiding injury to the bone during the hip replacement procedure. Fractures that do occur postoperatively usually can be treated by standard fracture principles. Fractures distal to the prosthesis often can be treated with traction or a cast brace if the fracture can be maintained in good alignment. If an open reduction is required, care must be taken to avoid damage to the cement or prosthesis by any internal fixation device used. One recent report described using plate fixation with screws distally and cerclage wires proximally in order to avoid damage to the existing prosthetic device. If the prosthetic device has been loose and painful prior to fracture or appears to be loose on radiographs after the fracture, clearly a new prosthetic device should be used, usually with a longer stem to facilitate fracture stabilization.

Special Problems

Congenital Hip Dislocations Hips that require total hip replacement because of secondary degenerative arthritis from congenital dislocation present special problems of distorted anatomy and small bones. Careful preoperative planning is necessary in order to have prosthetic devices of the appropriate size available. Computed tomographic scanning is helpful. Care must be taken to obtain a proper leg length in order to avoid nerve or vessel stretch. Appropriate positioning of the prosthetic device is critical in order to avoid postoperative dislocations. Superior lateral bone grafting may be necessary in order to stabilize the acetabulum, but some authors have recommended that these bone deficits be replaced with cement. All authors concur that the goal is anatomic positioning of the acetabulum.

Bone Grafts Bone defects such as those with congenital hip dislocation or after failed surgical treatment of the hip often require bone grafting. Autogenous bone from the iliac crest or from the removed femoral head is preferred. Numerous authors have reported the use of fresh-frozen allografts from femoral head material or other sources, and some reports document early success with this material which seems to act as a good scaffolding for new bone formation.

Failed Prosthesis and Fusions Although hemiarthroplasty or bipolar hemiarthroplasty appears to be quite successful in the treatment of fresh femoral neck fractures, for hip joint disease involving both the acetabular and femoral articular surfaces the results have been inferior compared with replacement of both acetabular and femoral sides. Failed hemiarthroplasties present special problems of preparation of the endosteal surface of the femur to allow good cement interdigitation. The entire membrane surrounding the previous loose hemiarthroplasty must be removed. Conversion of a fused hip to a total hip replacement certainly can be successful. This requires attention to bony landmarks. If care is taken and the entire hip is mobilized, an excellent range of motion and long-term good results can be obtained.

Blood Replacement Autogenous blood replacement can be provided by most blood banks. This requires the patients to donate up to 4 units of their own blood at weekly intervals in the month prior to operation. With oral iron therapy given during this period, few problems are encountered. The recent concern about AIDS has further popularized this technique. Use of a blood cell-recovery system during revision may be advantageous to avoid the need for homologous blood.

Revision Total Hip Replacement

Indications

Revision of infected or chronically dislocating total hips has been discussed above. The most common indication for revision of a total hip prosthesis is loosening of the prosthesis and resultant pain. These procedures are of significant magnitude, and the results rarely equal those of primary total hip replacement. Before revision is indicated, pain almost always reaches such a level that the patient's hip function is significantly limited. However, radiologic signs of loosening in hips with little pain should be watched carefully with serial films and, if major bone destruction progresses, revision should be considered even if the current pain is not too disabling. Revision certainly should be accomplished before there is bone destruction of such magnitude that successful revision is less likely to be successful (Fig. 4).

Surgical Techniques

These lengthy, complex procedures should be undertaken in settings where the entire surgical team's experience is significant and the hospital has available numerous specialized pieces of equipment for prosthesis and cement removal and a large inventory of revision prosthetic components. Some authors recommend routine trochanteric osteotomy, and all recommend wide exposure of the hip joint with removal of the pseudocapsule to expose the entire proximal end of the femur and the entire circumference of the acetabulum, permitting careful implant removal. The acetabular cup often can be removed intact with curved gouges, but sometimes it must be split into several segments and removed in pieces. The acetabular cement mass must be totally removed, including the cement plugs that often remain firmly fixed to bone. This must be accom-

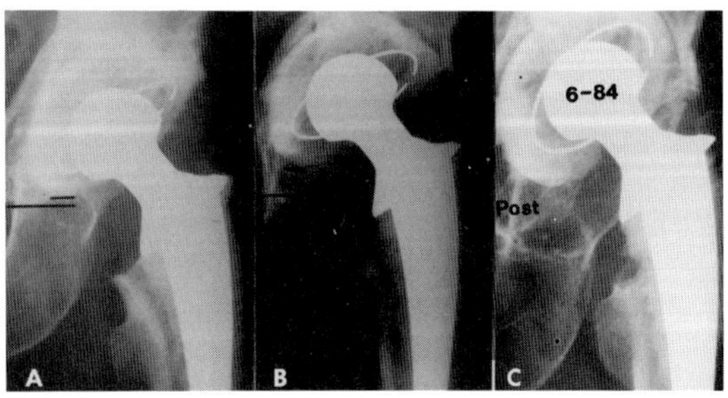

Figure 4

Progressive bone loss around a loose acetabular cup. *A,* At 6 weeks postoperatively. *B,* At 6½ years postoperatively, loose cup with superior migration apparent radiologically. *C,* At 10 years postoperatively, bone destruction is apparent superiorly to above the inferior sacroiliac joint. The surgical revision recommended at 6 years postoperatively was refused because pain was minimal. The amount of bone destruction complicated eventual revision.

plished while avoiding removal of remaining bone stock. If the acetabular floor is already penetrated, care must be taken to avoid the underlying vessels. Removal of a loose femoral component is usually accomplished quite readily. Some remaining cement mantle will usually be still tightly attached to the bone and must be removed with great care in order to prevent penetration of the femoral shaft. High-speed drills are available for cement removal; however, it has been pointed out by several authors that with these drills bone is removed more easily than the harder methacrylate. Numerous specially designed hand chisels are available for cement removal and are recommended by some authors as less damaging to the femoral shaft. Image intensification has been proposed as extremely useful in avoiding bone damage but introduces the risks of increased radiation and potential contamination. Light must be introduced into the internal surface of the femur, and fiberoptic, headlamp, and disposable thin battery-powered sources have been proposed.

Broken femoral stems pose a special problem during revision surgery because the remaining distal portion of the stem often is rigidly held in its cement bed. Early authors proposed creation of a window in the femur over the broken stem. These windows weaken the bone least if they are placed in the anterior portion of the retained femur. A method using high-speed drills to cut an offset hole in the fractured surface of the broken stem permits attachment of an extraction device and removal of the stem in this fashion. A recently proposed method uses a large circular trephine saw that drills over the entire stem length, dividing the surrounding cement by frictional sawing (Fig. 5). Once the prosthesis and cement have been removed, the entire endosteal surface of the femoral canal must be freed of any membrane or debris with brushes and curettes. Water pick lavage is helpful to clean the surfaces of both the acetabular and femoral bone.

Reimplantation

If reimplantation is to be accomplished with cement, all the techniques described in the preceding major section must be used (Fig. 6). The bone surfaces must be clean and dry. For these lengthy operations, hypotensive anesthesia can be helpful in decreasing blood loss and obtaining dry surfaces. If bone defects are present in either the acetabulum or the femur, they should be filled by bone grafting. The patient's own iliac crest bone is preferable but may not provide enough bone. Many hospitals now have allograft bone available, often in the form of frozen femoral heads taken from previous primary arthroplasty patients. Use of more massive allograft replacement of the proximal femur or pelvis with cadaver bone is being reported; however, these procedures have been done so far in large institutions on a very experimental basis under strict investigational protocols.

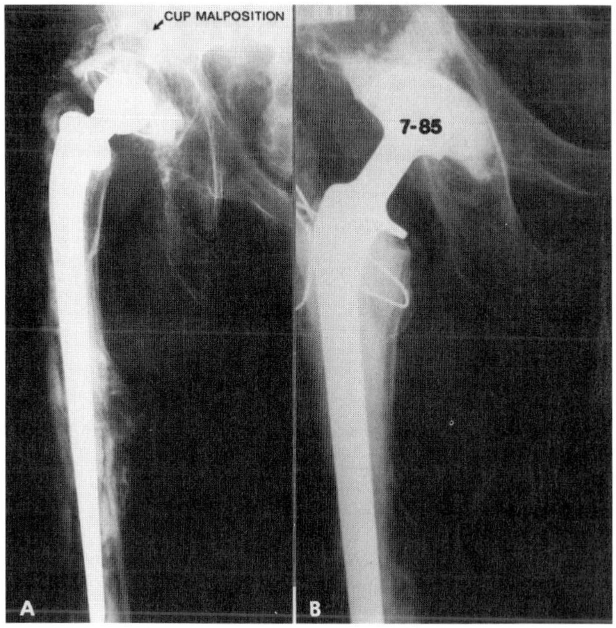

Figure 6

Initial revision of a failed total hip prosthesis was accomplished without revising a malpositioned cup and using only a 200 mm stem which inadequately spanned the midshaft fracture of the femur. This resulted in nonunion of the femur, a loose femoral component, and easily dislocatable hip (*A*). Patient is asymptomatic with good function of the hip at 2 years after the second revision with an appropriately positioned acetabular cup, a 300-mm prosthesis to span the fracture adequately (full length not shown), and good cementing techniques (*B*).

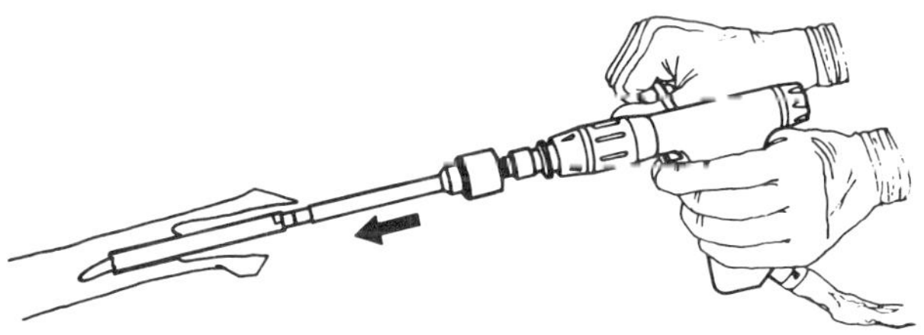

Figure 5

Large, circular, low-speed, power-driven saw cutting the cement surrounding a broken stem. (From Collis, D., and Dubrul, W.: The removal of fractured prosthetic components from medullary cavities: A new technique. Contemp. Orthop. 8:61–65, 1984. By permission of Bobit Publishing Company.)

Prosthesis Selection

Most hips can be revised with standard or factory-available "custom" prosthetic replacements for the type of hip system the surgeon uses. Usually, devices with longer stems are needed in the femur, and many authors have recommended that the stem length bypass any defect in the femur by 1 to 3 diameters of the femoral canal, depending on the size of the defect. Occasionally, special prostheses of specific dimensions are needed. A computed tomographic scan will help define the bone dimensions, and computer-assisted design and manufacturing techniques (CAD/CAM) can provide individualized and precisely shaped prostheses (these may be prohibitively expensive).

Complications

All of the complications seen in primary arthroplasty are even more likely after the extensive surgery required for revision. The likelihood of nerve, vessel, or bone injury is increased. The length of the procedure increases the need for more blood replacement and increases the possibilities of infection. Some authors have recommended routinely mixing antimicrobial agents with the cement in all revision procedures in the hope of decreasing the likelihood of infection.

Results

Initial reported clinical results after revision of cemented total hip arthroplasty with recemented implants were quite good, often approaching those of the initial replacements. If the initial procedure had failed because of some technical inadequacy, such as malposition of components or inadequate cement techniques, the result of the revision procedure can exceed that of the initial procedure. For the most part, as with any revision surgery, this is not the case. In one series of 166 revisions followed 2 or more years, there was clinical improvement in 90%, but radiologic evaluation found loosening of the acetabular components in 20% and loosening of the femoral components in 44%. Symptomatic clinical loosening was seen in 35 hips, and a second revision was required for 15 hips. Fifteen hips had had one or more episodes of dislocation, and seven of them had required a second revision for recurrent dislocations.

Another study with extended follow-up of revision total hip replacement was done at two separate teaching institutions; the previous 3.4-year mean follow-up of 110 revisions was extended for 99 of the revisions followed for a mean of 8.1 years. In the 5 years between the studies, the mechanical failure rate increased from 14% to 29%. Sixty-three percent of these hips had a good or excellent result at 8 years and 7% had a fair result. These authors concluded that, although initially an uncomplicated revision compares favorably with a primary total hip replacement in terms of quality, the durability of the result is substantially diminished. Comparison of revisions done after 1979 at one of these institutions, using some of the newer techniques described above, demonstrated modest improvement over the results of revisions done before 1979 but no change in the re-revision rate.

Uncemented Arthroplasty

The failures of cemented total hip arthroplasty and, more significantly, the results after the revisions of these failed cemented arthroplasties have led many surgeons to attempt total hip replacement without utilizing cement. Unfortunately, many of the developments in this area are just now being proposed, and published significant supporting clinical follow-up data are not yet available. Because of the timeliness of this subject, some of this section will be based on unpublished data given in lecture form by various proponents of uncemented arthroplasty.

There are two different types of prostheses available for uncemented joint replacement: press-fit prostheses, and interference fit devices which have some type of porous surface that permits fibrous or bony ingrowth into the surface of the prosthesis to enhance fixation. The initial uncemented arthroplasties used a press-fit femoral component (Austin Moore) with the acetabulum treated merely by reaming and without prosthetic replacement; these had only limited success. One recent clinical follow-up after use of a press-fit femoral prosthesis with a straight stem and no collar (but small amounts of cement were used) found good clinical results. Femoral cortex cracking was noted but subsidence, early loosening, and calcar resorption were not seen at early follow-up. These authors have now added a porous surface to the press-fit design and stopped using cement. Clinical follow-up is too short to be meaningful.

Macrointerlock

Much developmental work on cementless prostheses was done in Europe during the 1970s. Large irregular surfaces were used in the hope of obtaining some form of tissue prosthesis interlock. The isolastic macroporosity prosthesis, in use since 1973, introduced not only the macroporosity but also an increased flexibility of the femoral component stem. Several design changes have been implemented to solve early clinical problems.

Ceramic prosthetic components for total hip arthroplasty were introduced in North America in 1981. These systems use a ceramic cup with large peripheral threads for immediate rigid peripheral acetabulum rim fixation (Fig. 7). Although the system has been used by many surgeons in the United States, the change to new materials and fixation methods, even with short follow-up, has yet to show results surpassing, or even equalling, those after cemented arthroplasty.

Madreporic cementless hips use a screw-in cup and a

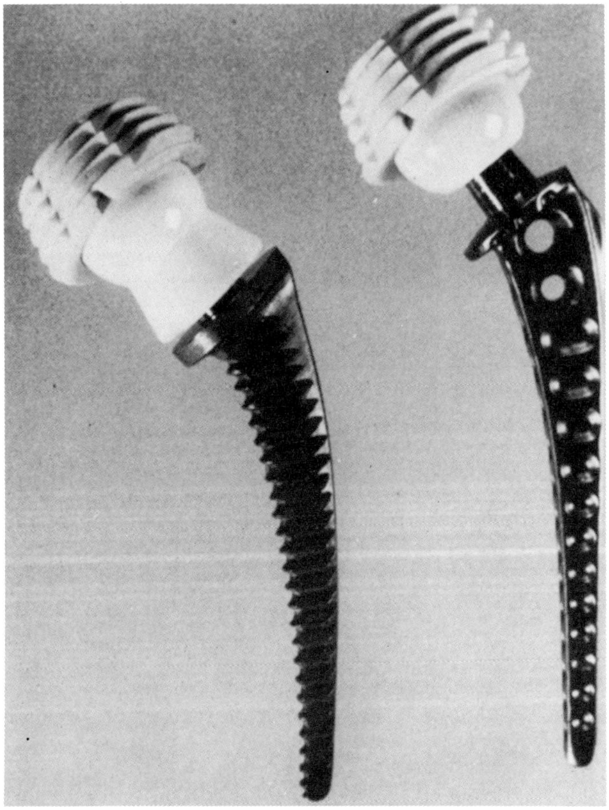

Figure 7

Autophor ceramic macrointerlock hip prosthesis. (From Mittelmeier, H.: Ceramic prosthetic devices. Hip 12:146–160, 1984. By permission of C.V. Mosby Company.)

rough-surfaced large-beaded femoral component. Good early results were reported in more than 1,500 arthroplasties done by 1982. Revision of these firmly fixed irregular-surfaced femoral prostheses produced significant bone destruction during extraction. Also, several authors warn of the rare but serious potential risk of significant proximal femoral cortical atrophy—presumably resulting from stress-shielding secondary to rigid fixation. This device in its original form has been abandoned by the inventor.

Microinterlock

In the United States there has been more interest in using microlock prostheses with a smaller pore size which theoretically allows true bony ingrowth and thus more lasting fixation. Early animal studies showed that bone will grow into such a porous surface (Fig. 8). One femoral implant using a porous coating of Proplast (80% porosity) had a high rate of failure in clinical use. This was attributed to the weakness of the material which failed by shear within its substance. The optimal pore size for bony ingrowth is 50 to 400 μm. The longest clinical application of such a microporous surface used a femoral prosthesis coated with porous material to the distal tip of its stem (Fig. 9). Some hips show stress-shielding of the proximal femur, possibly because of secure bony ingrowth and fixation distally. Clinical follow-up at 2 to 4 years has shown some bony ingrowth in specimens retrieved post mortem. Stems that fit the bony contours best appear to show the best results on clinical and radiologic follow-up.

At present, two metal surfaces are popular in the United States: one has cobalt/chromium beads on a cobalt/chromium prosthesis, and the other has pure titanium mesh implanted in pads on the titanium alloy stems. Most recent designs limit these porous surfaces to the proximal portion of the femoral stem to preclude the distal bony ingrowth that could complicate subsequent removal should it become necessary and may cause proximal stress-shielding. Unfortunately, engineering studies have shown that applying either titanium mesh or cobalt/chromium beads significantly weakens the structural strength of the femoral components. Compared with the recent so-called superalloys, the same size prosthesis fabricated with porous material is approximately one-third as strong. Fortunately, when the stem is not being cemented, relatively larger prostheses are often used in order to get good cortical bone contact.

Two forms of fitting the femoral prosthesis into the femur have evolved. Straight-stem devices require internal reshaping of the bone and depend on three-point fixation for rigid initial fixation. Curved or proximally anteverted

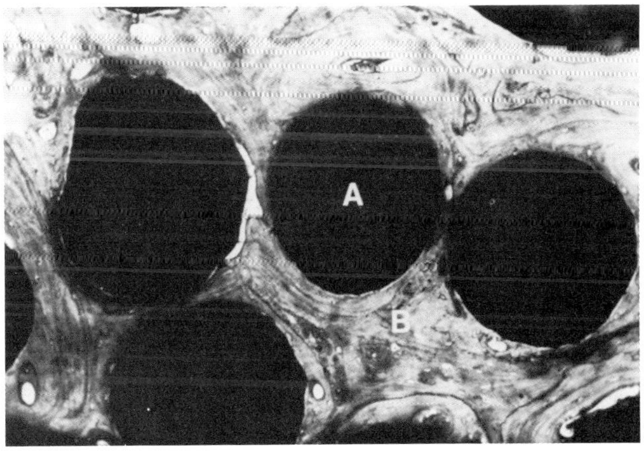

Figure 8

Bone (*B*) growing into appropriately sized openings in a metal surface. (From Galante, J.O.: Overview of current attempts to eliminate methylmethacrylate. Hip 11:181–189, 1983. By permission of C.V. Mosby Company.)

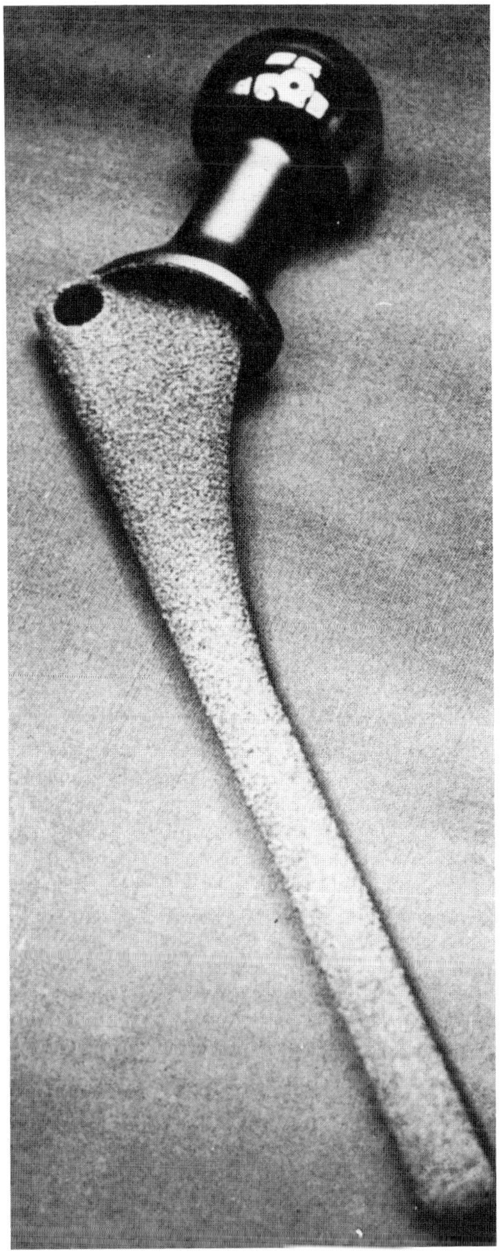

Figure 9

Femoral prosthesis stem fully coated with microporous surface, used in early clinical work. Subsequent prosthetic designs have limited the porous surface to the proximal stem. (From Engh, C.A.; Bobyn, J.D.; and Matthews, J.G., II: Biologic function of a modified Moore prosthesis. Part I. Evaluation of early clinical results. Hip 12:95–110, 1984. By permission of C.V. Mosby Company.)

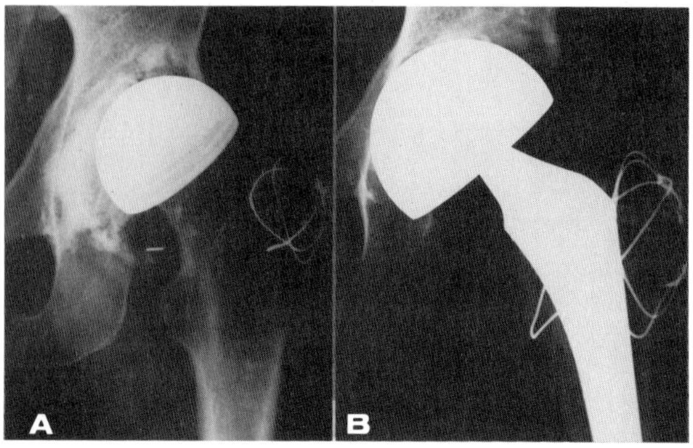

Figure 10

Failed resurface arthroplasty in 41-year-old man. *A*, Loose acetabular cup at 5 years postoperatively. *B*, After revision with an uncemented bipolar prosthesis. Note the grafting with morcellized, tightly packed bone in the ilium superior and lateral to the cup.

stems attain initial fixation by a more anatomic fit into the curved metaphyseal region. Of course, right and left stems are required.

Various geometric designs have been proposed for cementless acetabular components: cylindrical, square, ellipsoid, conical, and truncated cone. All of these require more bone removal than was needed with hemispherically shaped prostheses. In addition to the porous surface that eventually may anchor the prosthesis, spikes, screws, and pegs are used to obtain more immediate fixation. Large cups threaded on their outer surface require significant forces to insert and allow no alteration of orientation once the tapping of the large screw has begun. Nearly all of these components are metal-backed. In Europe, non-metal-backed polyethylene cups have been inserted without cement. In retrieved specimens, tiny particles of polyethylene have been found in the surrounding tissues, leading to the conclusion that the polyethylene surface needs to be coated.

Young Patients and Revisions

Because of the lack of satisfactorily high success rates after revision arthroplasty with cement and the higher failure rate in young patients with primary cemented total hip replacements, these two groups represent the most common diagnostic categories for which uncemented arthroplasty is proposed. Careful utilization of porous-coated devices in the young age group is under investigation. When such devices are implanted the porous coating should be limited to the proximal portion of the femoral component. In the late 1970s, resurface arthroplasty was proposed as a conservative answer, especially for hip problems in the young. Three- to 5-year clinical follow-ups established a 20% to 50% failure rate for resurface arthroplasty (Fig. 10 *A*). It is hoped that this will not be the case with uncemented arthroplasty. One of the unknowns of uncemented arthroplasty is the effect of devices with porous surfaces after long-term direct contact with the body. Loose rough-surface prostheses could well have a deleterious effect on the bone comparable to that of loose fragments of methyl methacrylate. In addition, these porous coatings expose the body to a much greater surface area of metal. The potential problems associated with the release of metal ions are under investigation.

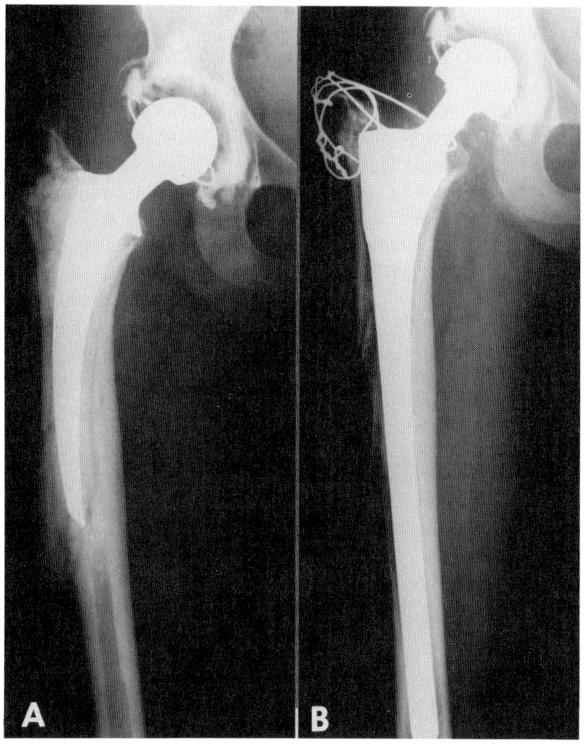

Figure 11

Revision with porous ingrowth femoral component. *A*, Two previous cemented femoral prostheses had failed in 27-year-old woman. Each was of inadequate stem length, and a large lateral femoral cortical defect had been created with extrusion of cement and prosthesis. *B*, Revision with uncemented femoral component and large autogenous bone graft laterally; also, small bone grafts were packed in the intramedullary canal to achieve more rigid initial fixation.

With regard to revision arthroplasty, some authors report that their results are so poor with cemented revisions that they do all revisions without cement, often with massive amounts of bone graft (Fig. 11). Autogenous or homologous grafts are used to pack the space between the prosthesis and the bone, to improve the fit of the prosthetic device on both the acetabulum and the femoral side. Not even short-term results are published on these procedures. One special form of uncemented revision for patients with extensive acetabular bone loss uses only a bipolar femoral component articulated against an acetabulum filled with a tightly packed morcellized bone graft (Fig. 10 *B*). The fate of these grafts has not yet been determined but the limited experience (2 years) is that they appear to be incorporating.

Follow-Up

Uncemented porous ingrowth prostheses have been in routine clinical use only since 1983. Early clinical data indicate that these patients seem to have more thigh discomfort. Even at 1-year follow-up, the incidences of pain and limp seem to be higher than in patients with a cemented arthroplasty. Because the clinical follow-up is short, data are insufficient for justification of routine use of uncemented total hip replacements.

Annotated Bibliography

Surgical Techniques

Burke, D.W.; Gates, E.I.; and Harris, W.H.: Centrifugation as a method of improving tensile and fatigue properties of acrylic bone cement. J. Bone Joint Surg. 66A:1265–1273, 1984.

Centrifugation of methyl methacrylate dramatically decreased the porosity and improved the ultimate tensile strength and fatigue life with no reported detrimental changes. A cement centrifugation system for use in the operating room was presented.

Crowninshield, R.D.; Brand, R.A.; and Pedersen, D.R.: A stress analysis of acetabular reconstruction in protrusio acetabuli. J. Bone Joint Surg. 65A:495–499, 1983.

Finite-element analysis of acetabular reconstruction in total hip replacement shows that normal anatomic placement of the component decreases stresses on the medial part of the pelvic wall. Metal backing of polyethylene acetabular components decreases the peak cement and trabecular bone stresses.

Harris, W.H., and White, R.E., Jr.: Advantages of metal-backed acetabular components for a total hip replacement: A clinical assessment with a minimum 5-year follow-up. Hip 11:240–246, 1983.

Metal-backed cups used in cemented arthroplasty in patients followed at least 5 years showed a very low incidence of loosening, even in relatively young patients.

Roberts, J.M.; Fu, F.H.; McClain, E.J.; and Ferguson, A.B., Jr.: A comparison of the posterolateral and anterolateral approaches to total hip arthroplasty. Clin. Orthop. 187:205–210, 1984.

The posterolateral approach was associated with shorter operating time and less blood loss, but the anterolateral approach produced fewer dislocations and loose components.

Vicar, A.J., and Coleman, C.R.: A comparison of the anterolateral, transtrochanteric, and posterior surgical approaches in primary total hip arthroplasty. Clin. Orthop. 188:152–159, 1984.

Dislocation rates were highest after the posterior approach, heterotopic bone formation was highest after the anterolateral and transtrochanteric approaches, and trochanteric bursitis was highest after the transtrochanteric approach. No differences were seen in the prosthesis positioning by the three approaches.

Infection

Bourne, R.B.; Hunter, G.A.; Rorabeck, C.H., and Macnab, J.J.: A six-year follow-up of infected total hip replacements managed by Girdlestone's arthroplasty. J. Bone Joint Surg. 66B:340–343, 1984.

Satisfactory pain relief was obtained in 91% of the patients and infection was controlled in 97%, but the patients were left with shortened extremities and the need for external support. However, the results seemed to improve with time.

Buchholz, H.W.; Elson, R.A.; and Heinert, K.: Antibiotic-loaded acrylic cement: Current concepts. Clin. Orthop. 190:96–108, 1984.

This report extends the follow-up of 825 previously reported one-stage reimplantations in which antibiotic-loaded acrylic was used for infected total hip replacements. *Pseudomonas* infections did poorly, but the overall success rate 5 years after operation was 77%.

Canner, G.C.; Steinberg, M.E.; Heppenstall, R.B.; and Balderston, R.: The infected hip after total hip arthroplasty. J. Bone Joint Surg. 66A:1393–1399, 1984.

Nearly half of the patients with infected hips had had an operation prior to the index arthroplasty. In nearly all, a single organism grew on culture, usually *Staphylococcus epidermidis, Staphylococcus aureus,* or *Escherichia coli.* Antibiotic therapy alone was not effective in eradicating infection, but excisional arthroplasty eradicated infection in 27 of 33 hips.

Lidwell, O.M.; Lowbury, E.J.; Whyte, W.; Blowers, R.; Stanley, S.J.; and Lowe, D.: Infection and sepsis after operations for total hip or knee-joint replacement: Influence of ultraclean air, prophylactic antibiotics and other factors. J. Hyg. (Lond.) 93:505–529, 1984.

A large multicenter retrospective study of 8,000 joint replacements found that the prophylactic use of antimicrobials decreased the incidence of joint sepsis from 3.4% to 0.85%. In addition, use of ultraclean air decreased it to 0.42% and the further addition of body exhaust systems further decreased the incidence to 0.14%.

Surin, V.V.; Sundholm, K.; and Bäckman, L.: Infection after total hip replacement: With special reference to a discharge from the wound. J. Bone Joint Surg. 65B:412–418, 1983.

Previous hip surgery, failure to use prophylactic antimicrobial therapy at the time of total hip replacement, failure of the surgical wound to heal within 3 to 4 weeks, and postoperative infections elsewhere in the body all were related to an increased incidence of a deep wound infection after total hip replacement.

Bone-Cement Interface

Goldring, S.R.; Schiller, A.L.; Roelke, M.; Rourke, C.M.; O'Neill, D.A.; and Harris, W.H.: The synovial-like membrane at the bone cement interface in loose total hip replacements and its proposed role in bone lysis. J. Bone Joint Surg. 65A:575–584, 1983.

The membrane present at the bone-cement interface was retrieved from 20 patients with loose, aseptic, failed total hip replacements. This membrane contained synovium-like cells and macrophages that could secrete enzymes capable of bone lysis.

Lewis, J.L., and Galante, J.O. (eds.): A Workshop on the Bone-Implant Interface. Proceedings of a Conference Held in Chicago, September 13–16, 1983. Chicago, American Academy of Orthopaedic Surgeons, 1985.

A collection of papers presented at a symposium on the prosthesis-bone interface in which mechanical and biologic factors that contribute to loosening were investigated.

Linder, L., and Hansson, H.A.: Ultrastructural aspects of the interface between bone and cement in man: Report of three cases. J. Bone Joint Surg. 65B:646–649, 1983.

Electron microscopic study of three nonloose cemented femoral stems found viable bone alternating with areas of soft tissue containing macrophages. Living bone may remain in contact with bone cement even after many years of service.

Linder, L.; Lindberg, L.; and Carlsson, Å.: Aseptic loosening of hip prostheses: A histologic and enzyme histochemical study. Clin. Orthop. 175:93–104, 1983.

Soft tissue membrane at the cement-bone interface was infiltrated with macrophages with a high acid phosphatase activity. Inflammatory cells were rare or absent. The role of the bone cement was obscure because there were no obvious local signs of cytotoxicity. The findings support the theory of mechanical instability as the prime cause of this tissue reaction.

Complications

Ling, R.S.M.: Complications of Total Hip Replacement. Edinburgh, Churchill Livingstone, 1984.

Excellent general discussions of complications of total hip arthroplasty, especially the editor's discussion of loosening.

Suomalainen, O.; Kettunen, K.; Rissanen, V.; Karjalainen, P.; Länsimies, E.; and Tanska, S.: Postoperative thromboembolism and risk factors in elective hip surgery. Ann. Chir. Gynaecol. 72:207–213, 1983.

In patients given prophylactic warfarin therapy, lung scans showed a 19% incidence of pulmonary embolism; venography showed a 43% incidence of deep vein thrombosis. Obesity and operations exceeding 2½ hours in duration increased the incidence of thromboembolism.

Follow-Up Assessment

Collis, D.K.: Cemented total hip replacement in patients who are less than fifty years old. J. Bone Joint Surg. 66A:353–359, 1984.

Good clinical and radiologic results were found in patients with an average age of 40 years followed 5 to 11 years postoperatively, with a revision rate of less than 10%. The need to advise against heavy strenuous activities in this age group was stressed.

Dorr, L.D.; Takei, G.K.; and Conaty, J.P.: Total hip arthroplasties in patients less than forty-five years old. J. Bone Joint Surg. 65A:474–479, 1983.

Patients under age 30 had poorer results. Good surgical technique with cementing and prosthetic positioning yielded satisfactory clinical results in 93%.

O'Neill, D.A., and Harris, W.H.: Failed total hip replacement: Assessment by plain radiographs, arthrograms, and aspiration of the hip joint. J. Bone Joint Surg. 66A:540–546, 1984.

Plain radiographs correctly showed the status of the prosthesis fixation in over 90% of the femoral components but in only 60% of the acetabular components. Arthrography helped in the diagnosis of loosening only of the acetabular component. Aspiration of the joint proved reliable in excluding the possibility of infection.

Poss, R.; Maloney, J.P.; Ewald, F.C.; Thomas, W.H.; Batte, N.J.; Hartness, C.; and Sledge, C.B.: Six- to 11-year results of total hip arthroplasty in rheumatoid arthritis. Clin. Orthop. 182:109–116, 1984.

Clinical improvement was maintained at follow-up in nearly all patients but radiologic analysis showed that, even in these patients with low functional requirements, mechanical loosening occurs and failures can be expected. High incidence of infection, osteopenic bone, and multiple joint involvement are special problems. Failure to restore the anatomic position of the acetabulum predisposes it to loosening and migration.

Ranawat, C.S.; Atkinson, R.E.; Salvati, E.A.; and Wilson, P.D., Jr.: Conventional total hip arthroplasty for degenerative joint disease in patients between the ages of forty and sixty years. J. Bone Joint Surg. 66A:745–752, 1984.

Clinical results were excellent in 90% of the patients at 5 to 10 years after operation. Ten of 103 hips required revision. Seventy percent of the femoral components and 80% of the acetabular components had no progressive radiologic evidence of loosening.

Radiologic Evaluation

Collis, D.K.: Long-term radiologic follow-up of total hip replacements. Hip 10:1–26, 1982.

Heterotopic bone formation, calcar resorption, and distal cortical hypertrophy were radiologic findings that had little effect on clinical results. Most incomplete lucent lines did not progress and did not correlate with clinical deficiencies. Progressive radiolucent lines were not seen frequently in 129 hips followed 8 to 10 years.

Green, D.L.; Bahniuk, E.; Liebelt, R.A.; Fender, E.; and Mirkov, P.: Biplane radiographic measurements of reversible displacement (including clinical loosening) and migration of total joint replacements. J. Bone Joint Surg. 65A:1134–1143, 1983.

By using metallic markers and biplane radiography, reversible displacement of the prostheses in weight-bearing and non-weight-bearing films could be measured in 75% of the cases. Radiolucent lines correlated with measured reversible displacement. The incidence of actual clinical loosening was less than 10%.

Revision Total Hip Replacement

Kavanagh, B.F.; Ilstrup, D.M.; and Fitzgerald, R.H.: Revision total hip arthroplasty. J. Bone Joint Surg. 67A:517–526, 1985.

One hundred forty-five of 166 hips were improved with revision. Radiographic analysis showed probable loosening in 20% of the acetabular components and 44% of the femoral components. Thirty-five hips had symptomatic loosening, and 15 hips required a second revision.

Pellicci, P.M.; Wilson, P.D., Jr.; Sledge, C.B.; Salvati, E.A.; Ranawat, C.S.; Poss, R.; and Callaghan, J.J.: Long-term results of revision total hip replacements: A follow-up report. J. Bone Joint Surg. 67A:513–516, 1985.

As the previously reported follow-up was extended from 3 years to 8 years, the failure rate increased to 29%. Most new failures occurred in hips that had shown progressive radiolucency at initial follow-up.

Uncemented Arthroplasty

Brown, I.W., and Ring, P.A.: Osteolytic changes in the upper femoral shaft following porous-coated hip replacement. J. Bone Joint Surg. 67B:218–221, 1985.

Ten uncemented porous-coated femoral components showed a high incidence of extensive stress-relieving changes with loss of medial femoral bone stalk and osteoporosis.

Engh, C.A.: Hip arthroplasty with a Moore prosthesis with porous coating: A five-year study. Clin. Orthop. 176:52–66, 1983.

One-third of 26 hips at 2 years showed radiopaque lines, suggesting that micromotion was present, but 4-year follow-up radiographs in 10 hips were interpreted as showing tissue ingrowth, providing uniform fixation and no bone resorption.

Lord, G., and Bancel, P.: The Madreporic cementless total hip arthroplasty: New experimental data and a seven-year clinical follow-up study. Clin. Orthop. 176:67–76, 1983.

Early good results of 1,509 cementless arthroplasties done between 1975 and 1982 are reported. The need for longer follow-up to confirm indications for this technique is stressed.

Morscher, E.: The Cementless Fixation of Hip Endoprostheses. Berlin, Springer-Verlag, 1984.

This extensive overview, by 73 authors, of the European experience with cementless fixation includes numerous brief presentations of techniques and short follow-ups of various prosthetic devices.

Pilliar, R.M.: Powder metal-made orthopedic implants with porous surface for fixation by tissue ingrowth. Clin. Orthop. 176:42–51, 1983.

In vivo tests demonstrated the need for initial implant stability in order to achieve bony ingrowth. Optimal pore size was 50 to 400 μm.

Swanson, R.L., and Evarts, C.M.: Dual-lock total hip arthroplasty: A preliminary experience. Clin. Orthop. 191:224–231, 1984.

This prosthesis has a femoral component design with a straight stem and no collar, to allow primary fixation by press-fit to the bone using only small amounts of surrounding cement. Femoral cracking was noted to be a problem, but subsidence, early loosening, and calcar changes were not seen in this early follow-up.

Tullos, H.S.; McCaskill, B.L.; Dickey, R.; and Davidson, J.: Total hip arthroplasty with a low-modulus porous-coated femoral component. J. Bone Joint Surg. 66A:888–898, 1984.

A 36% clinical failure rate was attributed to a porous coating (Proplast) that failed by shear within its substance and appeared to be too weak to withstand normal weight-bearing loads.

34
Hip Reconstruction: Non-Implant

Reconstructive hip surgery without implantation of a prosthetic device is still an important part of orthopaedic surgery. Arthrodesis should be the primary reconstructive procedure for unilateral destructive disease of the hip in adolescents and young adults. Osteotomy of the hip can provide effective pain relief for up to 10 years in carefully selected patients. Osteonecrosis of the hip remains a difficult problem. No surgical treatment regimen has been proved to be universally successful. Prevention of steroid-induced osteonecrosis may prove to be efficacious until an improved understanding of the pathophysiology permits development of better treatment modalities.

Arthrodesis

Arthrodesis should be considered for unilateral post-traumatic arthritis of the hip in young adults. The advantages include a return to nearly normal physical activity level (including manual labor) and excellent relief of pain. A solidly fused hip is uniformly painless but exposes the ipsilateral knee and the lower back to increased stresses. Therefore, a normal ipsilateral knee and a healthy low back are prerequisites in the preoperative screening. The patients must understand and accept the limitations of motion that result from the procedure and the compensatory maneuvers that will be necessary for the activities of daily living. A method that has proved to be useful is the application of a hip spica cast as a preoperative rehearsal.

Indications and Contraindications

Indications for arthrodesis include arthritis secondary to sepsis or osteomyelitis, failed osteotomy, arthritis secondary to slipped capital femoral epiphysis or Legg-Calvé-Perthes disease, and failed cup arthroplasty in the young patient. The presence of osteonecrosis poses a difficult challenge because loss of bone stock may result in a shorter leg or more difficulty in achieving union.

Contraindications include a noncooperative patient, poor general condition, and presence of low back or ipsilateral knee disorders.

Bilateral arthrodesis is contraindicated. However, fusion of one side with total hip replacement on the other is supported in the literature.

Surgical Technique

An important consideration is choosing a technique that preserves the hip abductors so that subsequent conversion to total hip arthroplasty will be possible. The technique should allow accurate positioning of the leg. A hip position of neutral rotation, neutral abduction/adduction, and 30° of flexion is recommended. Up to 5° of external rotation and 10° of adduction are well tolerated; abduction and internal rotation are to be avoided.

Two techniques for internal fixation are recommended.

Barr Bolts After hip dislocation and reaming of the acetabulum and femoral head, transarticular bolting is performed with Barr bolts. The bolts are inserted through the femoral head and neck and into the ilium. Nuts are fastened under direct vision on the inner surface of the wing of the ilium. Bolts can be passed above the level of the superior neck of the femur from the greater trochanter to the ilium as well. This procedure avoids any insult to the abductor musculature, does not require pelvic osteotomy, and does not prevent future reconstruction.

A hip spica cast is applied when the patient can stand comfortably for 20 to 30 minutes, usually on postoperative day 2 or 3. Ambulation with partial weight-bearing is permitted with crutches.

Cobra Plate Alternatively, the AO cobra plate has been used with success. This device provides rigid stabilization and eliminates the need for a brace or cast postoperatively. Exposure includes complete detachment of the gluteus medius and gluteus maximus from the greater trochanter and proximal reflection of the musculature.

A pelvic transverse osteotomy is performed 1 cm above the acetabular roof, and the distal fragment is displaced medially. The greater trochanter is osteotomized and may be used as a source of graft between the cobra plate and the femoral neck. The cobra plate is fixed to the ilium, and then the hip is placed under tension by using the AO compression device. The abductors are sutured to the vastus lateralis.

The enhanced stability afforded by the cobra plate must be weighed against the disturbance to the abductor musculature that is necessary. Respect for the anatomy is an important principle, particularly with regard to the abductor musculature, if later conversion to total hip arthroplasty may be contemplated.

Results

Complications of arthrodesis include malposition of the extremity, nonunion or delayed union, and excessive shortening of the leg. Long-term problems include ipsilateral knee instability or degenerative arthritis, lumbar spine degenerative changes, and contralateral hip problems.

Even with the use of the cobra plate, a pseudarthrosis rate of approximately 8% and a malposition rate of approximately 16% can be anticipated. Reoperation with bone grafting and corrective osteotomy results in satisfactory resolution of these difficulties in most instances. Shortening by 1 cm is desired. If shortening greater than this occurs, a lift is prescribed.

Long-term follow-up studies, one with a minimum follow-up of 20 years, demonstrated up to 80% patient satisfaction with arthrodesis. Of particular interest is the report that women were satisfied with their results. Arthrodesis was not incompatible with sexual function and normal childbirth; however, 38% of the women and 24% of the men reported moderate impairment of sexual function. Only one patient reported severe difficulties.

Results were better in patients who were young (age 18 years or younger) at the time of arthrodesis.

Back pain was absent in 16% and only mild after strenuous activity in an additional 27%. No patient had incapacitating back pain or radicular symptoms. None required back surgery.

Ipsilateral knee laxity was common and four operations had been required for knee arthritis in four patients (osteotomies in two and total knee replacement in two).

Fewer than 20% had problems with the contralateral hip.

Resection Arthroplasty

Only rarely is resection arthroplasty considered as a primary procedure. The indications include incurable infection, extensive post-irradiation bone necrosis, and developmental or congenital painful hip disease in patients whose medical status or condition precludes other reconstructive procedures. It is more commonly performed as a salvage procedure for failed arthroplasty. Resection arthroplasty of the femoral head and neck is successful in the relief of pain in 80% or more of patients.

Many modifications of the technique have been advocated, such as simultaneous or staged subtrochanteric osteotomy or resection of the acetabular rim. However, none of the modified procedures has resulted in outcomes superior to the results with simple resection of the femoral head and neck without interpositional arthroplasty. It is important to preserve muscle attachments and bone stock of the proximal femur and acetabulum as much as is consistent with the clinical condition of the patient so that later reconstruction is possible.

The results tend to be stable or even slowly improve with time. Shortening of 2 to 5 cm is to be expected, as well as a Trendelenburg gait pattern. Most patients will require a cane, crutches, or a walker for walking other than at home. Approximately 25% will be able to walk without any type of support.

Although the indications are few, this procedure has a useful role. Almost all patients retain or regain the ability to transfer and to walk independently. It can be performed bilaterally.

Trochanteric Advancement Osteotomy

Not uncommonly, a high-riding trochanter is found after disturbance of growth of the capital epiphysis. This condition often is associated with weak abductors, a Trendelenburg gait, and poor walking endurance. Clinically, it is encountered most commonly after osteonecrosis has complicated the treatment of congenital dislocation of the hip or as a residual of Legg-Calvé-Perthes disease. It is also seen in conjunction with congenital or developmental coxa vara and as a sequela of varus intertrochanteric osteotomy.

Treatment involves distal and lateral transfer of the greater trochanter. In order to avoid a symptomatic and unsightly lateral bulge of the upper thigh, a wedge of appropriate size is removed. It is important to avoid the superior neck of the femur in removing the wedge and performing the trochanteric osteotomy. A stress riser in this region can lead to a displaced intracapsular fracture of the femoral neck or an insult to the pericapsular retinacular vessels. In some patients it is necessary to combine the trochanteric advancement with intertrochanteric valgus osteotomy. Use of a fluoroscope intraoperatively is recommended to verify accuracy of the bony osteotomies and blade placement if an intertrochanteric osteotomy is performed.

Postoperative care does not require use of cast immobilization. Patients can begin touch-down weight-bearing with crutches as soon as their general condition permits. Sitting is discouraged for 3 weeks. It usually is possible to progress to a single crutch at 6 weeks and to independent walking at 3 months. Walking without a limp should be achieved before gait support is discontinued. Immobilization in abduction is an acceptable alternative.

Complications are uncommon.

Osteotomies About the Hip

General Considerations

Conceptually, it is important to segregate osteotomies into two basic categories: those done to correct structural deformities prior to the development of significant arthritis in young patients, and those done to intervene when advanced degenerative disease is present.

In the latter category, proximal femoral intertrochanteric osteotomies dominated as the procedure of choice for advanced osteoarthritis, particularly in Europe, prior to the widespread use of total hip arthroplasty. In the middle to late 1970s, the emerging problem of loosening of the femoral and acetabular components led to a resurgence of interest in osteotomy. The indications for this procedure were refined.

It is important to emphasize that total hip replacement remains the procedure of choice for most patients with advanced degenerative hip disease. Varus intertrochanteric osteotomy is rarely indicated in patients with advanced arthritis with obliteration of the joint space and osteophytes and cysts. In some patients with residual subluxation associated with coxa magna in which a mushroom-cap type of deformity is present in the femoral head, valgus and extension osteotomies have been shown to be effective in approximately 75% of the patients over a 10-year period. The effectiveness of osteotomy is generally limited to relief of pain, however. Any restriction of motion present preoperatively rarely improves after the operation.

Osteotomies are valuable in restoration of a more normal anatomy and mechanics in young patients with structural hip deformities. Frequently, the symptoms are minimal when the patient first seeks medical attention. It is difficult to justify major surgery, with its attendant potential complications, in these patients. They should be informed of the potential for deterioration of the hip joint and invited to return for follow-up at appropriate intervals.

Assessment of the Deformity

It is useful to approach the assessment of a structurally abnormal hip with independent review of the acetabular and femoral sides of the articulation. Some cases are well suited for a surgical solution on the femoral side alone; others are best approached from the acetabular side. Certain cases require surgical procedures on both the acetabular and the femoral side.

On the femoral side, factors that must be assessed include the position of the greater trochanter, the sphericity of the femoral head, the angle of the neck to the shaft, and the quality of the bone (i.e., osteoporosis, cysts).

On the acetabular side the inclination of the weight-bearing surface as reflected in the acetabular index in the frontal plane radiograph and the degree of coverage of the femoral head in both the mediolateral and anteroposterior views need to be assessed.

More than one surgical solution may be available for any one patient or category of deformity. For example, a young adult with a symptomatic dyplastic hip manifested by a valgus neck-shaft angle, mild to moderate lack of coverage, and a spherical femoral head with well-preserved joint space would be an ideal candidate for varus or varus/extension intertrochanteric osteotomy. For this patient, pelvic osteotomy also represents an excellent solution, particularly if the valgus angulation is not severe.

Surgical Technique

If excellent coverage of the femoral head can be demonstrated on preoperative anteroposterior radiographs in moderate abduction, intertrochanteric varus osteotomy is indicated. It can be combined with extension osteotomy and trochanteric advancement as staged procedures. In patients with deficient acetabular coverages, corrective pelvic osteotomy alone has been effective even with an uncorrected valgus deformity. The principal advantage of pelvic procedures is the avoidance of the distortion of the femoral anatomy that occurs with intertrochanteric osteotomy. Excessive fragment displacement significantly increases technical difficulty with subsequent total hip arthroplasty. Frequently there are structural deformities on both the femoral and pelvic sides of the hip, so procedures on both sides are required to achieve adequate coverage.

Intertrochanteric osteotomy is indicated when abnormality of the proximal femur is the dominant feature. When residual subluxation of the hip is associated with early symptoms in young or middle-aged adults, varus intertrochanteric osteotomy has been demonstrated to be effective in numerous published series. Good candidates are those with a spherical, nondeformed femoral head, well-preserved joint space, good mobility in the flexion arc (90° or more) and in rotation, a valgus neck shift angle of 140° or more, and no evidence of inflammatory arthritis or osteopenia.

Preoperatively, significant enhancement of femoral head coverage should be apparent in abduction radiographs in the anteroposterior plane. Clinically, passive abduction of at least 15° is considered mandatory because a varus osteotomy results in relative adduction of the limb. Marked impairment of abduction preoperatively will predispose to restricted abduction postoperatively, which is poorly accepted.

Most cases of dysplasia of the hip are associated with insufficient coverage of the femoral head anteriorly as well as laterally. To compensate for the anterior deficiency, a sagittal plane correction can be incorporated into the osteotomy, equivalent to taking a posteriorly based closing wedge. This has been referred to as an "extension osteotomy" in the European literature. It provides increased anterior coverage of the femoral head articular cartilage. The trochanter can be advanced to compensate for the weakening of the abductors that occurs with varus osteotomy. However, this is optional and can be done later if necessary. In one long-term study of osteotomy without simultaneous transfer of the trochanter, 70% of patients recovered normal walking patterns within 18 months; 30% had persistent Trendelenburg gait of varying severity. In the latter circumstance, a trochanteric advancement osteotomy can be combined with hardware removal in order to achieve a more normal gait pattern.

Complications unique to varus osteotomy include nonunion, delayed union, trochanteric bursitis (over the plate), and persistent limp. In general, complications are few. Consequences of the procedure include a fullness of the proximal thigh, a scar, shortening of the extremity, and a longer period of crutch dependency and muscle weakness compared to patients who have a cemented total hip arthroplasty.

Results

Long-term good and excellent results in more than 80% of patients have been reported with follow-ups of up to 10 years. Patients generally experience prompt and substantial relief of pain. This was noted even after medial displacement osteotomies in the past.

Pelvic Osteotomies

Pelvic or periacetabular osteotomies fall into two distinct categories: those that redirect or displace the articular cartilage-bearing bone of the acetabulum into a more favorable position, and those that use extra-articular periacetabular bone to augment the weight-bearing surface area of the acetabulum. The Steel triple innominate osteotomy, the Sutherland double osteotomy, the Salter innominate osteotomy, the Pemberton pericapsular osteotomy, and the Wagner dome osteotomy are examples of the articular cartilage redirection category of pelvic osteotomies. The Chiari osteotomy of the ilium and extra-articular shelf procedures are examples of the latter category.

A fundamental prerequisite common to all redirection osteotomies is the presence of a congruent joint space. This implies, of course, that these procedures are indicated only in cases of acetabular deficiency associated with arthrosis or arthritis in its earliest stages. Their goal is to postpone, if not arrest, the otherwise inevitable evolution of progressive arthritis secondary to the structural deformity.

On the other hand, the Chiari osteotomy is a salvage procedure. It is useful in patients with more advanced arthritis with deformity. The ilium is brought over the superolateral capsule of the hip joint to provide a bone buttress over uncovered portions of the femoral head. The capsule of the hip joint serves as an interpositional layer between the raw surface of the transiliac osteotomy and the articular cartilage of the femoral head. The shelf grafts or shelf arthroplasties are bone grafts of various types adjacent to the bony margins of the acetabulum that depend on the integrity of the capsule.

Salter Osteotomy

Open hinged innominate osteotomy with autogenous bone grafts from the iliac crest was first performed by Salter in 1957 to treat children with congenital subluxation of the hip. Gradually, the operation came to be performed on older children and adolescents. More recently it has been used in the treatment of hip problems in young adults.

The hip must be congruent and have at least 50% of the articular cartilage space well-preserved, articular acceptability, and mobility of at least 60% of normal.

The osteotomy is maintained open by placement of an iliac crest wedge graft, secured by two or three stout Steinmann pins. The pins are directed so as to enter the distal fragment in its posteromedial aspect, thereby avoiding the joint space. Placement of the pins is a critical point of the procedure. Intraoperative radiographs in two planes are not always reliable in demonstrating the extra-articular position of the pins or screws. If doubt exists as to the safety of the pin tracks, the pins and the graft can be removed. A K-wire can be placed into the track under direct vision. It is difficult to rotate the acetabulum in patients past adolescence. Thus, this procedure must be used judiciously for hip problems in adults.

If patients are selected according to the criteria outlined above, 90% can be expected to have no pain or only minimal discomfort, approximately 60% will walk without any limp, and most will experience no significant loss of mobility.

The complications unique to this operation include possible injury to the femoral or sciatic nerve and associated vessels, intra-articular placement of the pins, graft displacement, and postoperative stiffness. It is technically a demanding procedure.

Steel Osteotomy

This is designed to sever all three bony pillars of support for the acetabulum. Separate exposure of the ischium is accomplished by a transverse incision just distal to the palpable prominence of the ischial tuberosity with the hip in 90° flexion. The gluteus maximus is reflected to expose the ischial tuberosity. The conjoined tendon of the biceps femoris and semitendinosus is incised longitudinally, and the bone is exposed by reflection of the biceps off the ischial ramus laterally. Care must be taken to visualize and protect the sciatic nerve which lies lateral to the tendinous origin of the semimembranosus. An osteotome is used to divide the ischial ramus. This wound is closed and the remaining portions of the procedure are performed with a separate set of instruments after regowning and regloving of the surgical team.

In the second stage, an iliofemoral approach is used to expose the bone from the anterior-superior spine to just below the pectineal tubercle. The pubic ramus is divided about 1 cm medial to the pectineal tubercle. Care must be taken to protect the obturator artery, vein, and nerve which are located just medial to the osteotomy site. The triple bony division is completed by performing a Salter osteotomy of the innominate bone. To finish the liberation of the acetabular segment, the periosteum and fascia of the medial pelvic wall are cut.

At this point the capsule is opened and an open reduction of the hip joint is performed with resection of the redundant tissue medially. The acetabular segment is then rotated laterally and anteriorly until good coverage of the femoral head has been achieved. The displaced position is stabilized with an iliac crest autogenous graft and fixed with extra-articular pins. Cast immobilization is used postoperatively.

Good results, with residual subluxation, have been reported for approximately 80% of the patients.

The increase in redirectional capabilities must be weighed against the added complexity of the surgical procedure, the loss of inherent stability of the pelvis after redirection, and the need for postoperative cast immobilization.

Rotational Dome or Dial Osteotomies

These have also been used effectively. In this technique the cartilaginous acetabulum with 1 cm of subchondral bone is freed with a curved osteotome that conforms to the circumferential curvature of the acetabulum.

The indications for this procedure are quite strict. The articulation must be concentric with good preservation of articular cartilage. There must be a satisfactory thickness of the medial wall. The triradiate cartilage must be closed. It is not useful for severely dysplastic hips.

Technically the operation is quite demanding. Special curved osteotomes are required.

The complications include osteonecrosis of the acetabular segment and intra-articular penetration by the osteotome.

Osteonecrosis

Establishing the diagnosis of osteonecrosis in patients with unexplained hip pain can be just as difficult as the treatment once osteonecrosis is established. As a general principle, it is important to search for osteonecrosis in any patient who has unexplained hip pain.

Magnetic resonance imaging is emerging as a sensitive noninvasive diagnostic method for osteonecrosis, even when bone scan and plain radiographs are normal. Because of the high incidence of bilaterality, this method also is useful in the assessment of the contralateral hip. Bilateral hip involvement eventually will develop in up to 50% of patients with idiopathic osteonecrosis and 80% of patients with steroid-induced osteonecrosis. Intraosseous manometry might be a helpful method of identifying patients with either preclinical or early stages of the disease, but it is invasive. Magnetic resonance imaging appears to be superior to the manometry technique.

Staging of Osteonecrosis

Five stages of osteonecrosis have been described (Fig. 1).

Stage 0 This refers to a hip that is normal in every respect except for increased intraosseous pressure. Such hips have been found when a clinically normal contralateral hip has been studied during intraosseous pressure manometry. Approximately 60% of such hips eventually are affected by biopsy-proved osteonecrosis.

Stage I Early clinical symptoms are present. Subtle physical findings, such as limited internal rotation of the hip, also may be present. The bone scan may arouse suspicion but is nondiagnostic. Plain radiographs are normal. Magnetic resonance imaging has been useful in establishing the diagnosis at this stage of involvement.

Stage II Sclerosis of the necrotic segment, often in the form of a wedge, becomes apparent on plain radiographs but sphericity of the femoral head is unequivocally maintained. The subchondral bone plate remains intact.

Stages	Joint Line	Contour	Trabeculae	Schema	Diagnosis
0 and I	N	N	N	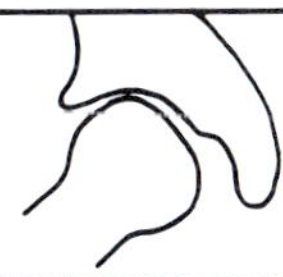	Impossible
II	N	N	Diffuse porosis or sclerosis cysts (mixed)	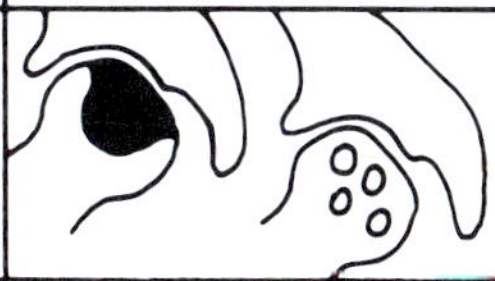	Probable
III	N	Broken	Sequestrum	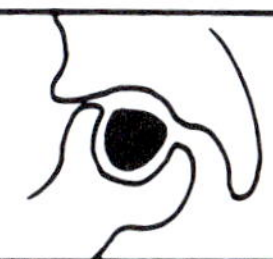	Certain
IV	Decreased	Flattened	Collapse	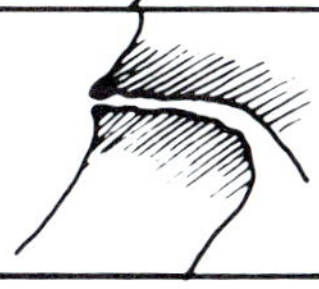	Arthrosis

Figure 1

Stages of osteonecrosis. (From Ficat, R.P.: Treatment of avascular necrosis of the femoral head. Hip 11:279–295, 1983. By permission of C.V. Mosby Company.)

Stage III Violation of the subchondral plate is manifested by flattening of the femoral head or subsidence of the necrotic wedge into the head. Clinically, arthritis symptoms intensify significantly.

Stage IV Full-scale joint arthritis is evident with unequivocal pathologic change on the acetabular side on plain radiographs.

Treatment

The treatment of osteonecrosis is complicated by the fact that the condition characteristically affects young adults. Surface replacement has been unacceptable in the treatment of this condition. The preliminary experience with implantation of a bipolar prosthesis in the treatment of osteonecrosis of the femoral head has been good. In a recent study of 28 patients with a mean age of 46 years, 17 (77%) had a good or excellent result at 1 to 4 years postoperatively. Among the eight patients with a poor result, two required total hip arthroplasty and three had significant hip pain.

In the early stages of osteonecrosis, revascularization and preservation of sphericity of the femoral head are the primary goals of treatment. Although the originators of core decompression remain enthusiastic, independent investigators have not been able to substantiate their results. Until controlled studies are reported, caution is advised.

Numerous osteotomies have been attempted in treatment of osteonecrosis, including intertrochanteric angular, rotational, and displacement osteotomies. These include the flexion osteotomy commonly performed in Europe and the rotational osteotomy of Sugioka. No general consensus exists with regard to the type or timing of intertrochanteric osteotomy for osteonecrosis. Furthermore, a complex intertrochanteric osteotomy may render subsequent insertion of a femoral component substantially more difficult if conversion to total hip arthroplasty becomes necessary in the immediate aftermath of a failed osteotomy.

Segmental fresh osteochondral allograft transplantation is currently in human trials. Also, direct intraosseous electrical stimulation as well as external pulse electromagnetic field stimulation are under clinical investigation.

Once stage III or stage IV involvement has been reached, treatment options are indeed limited. Stage III osteonecrosis can be best treated by insertion of a press-fit or porous ingrowth bipolar prosthesis. For stage IV osteonecrosis, it usually will be necessary to resort to a cementless total hip arthroplasty.

The management of osteonecrosis in the young adult is one of the most difficult problems facing an orthopaedic surgeon. Education of colleagues in other fields of medicine in regard to the musculoskeletal complications of use of steroids may prove to be one of the best methods of decreasing the numbers of these devastating problems.

Annotated Bibliography

Arthrodesis

Liechti, R.: Hip Arthrodesis and Associated Problems. Berlin, Springer-Verlag, 1978.

The technique for using the cobra plate and follow-up of a large number of patients are reviewed (more than 40% of the patients were female). No problems were encountered with hip arthrodesis contralateral to a total hip prosthesis. Conversion of failed arthrodeses to total hip arthroplasty was possible as long as the insertion of the abductors had been protected during the previous operation.

Sponseller, P.D.; McBeath, A.A.; and Perpich, M.: Hip arthrodesis in young patients. J. Bone Joint Surg. 66A:853–859, 1984.

At more than 20 years postoperatively (mean, 38 years), 80% of 53 patients were working and satisfied with their result; 34% of the patients could not think of any significant functional limitation when asked to do so. No patient had disabling back pain or radicular symptoms, and none had required lumbar surgery. Of the seven conversions to total hip arthroplasty, three were done for ipsilateral knee complaints and three for low back pain. This conversion was successful for relief of back pain, but two of the three patients with knee problems required subsequent total knee replacement.

Resection Arthroplasty

Haw, C.S., and Gray, D.H.: Excision arthroplasty of the hip. J. Bone Joint Surg. 58B:44–47, 1976.

A review of 40 hips at a mean follow-up of 10 years demonstrated 90% patient satisfaction with resection as a salvage procedure and 50% satisfaction when it was done as a primary procedure. Only one patient could not walk at follow-up.

Trochanteric Advancement Osteotomy

Kelikian, A.S.; Tachdjian, M.O.; Askew, M.J.; and Jasty, M.: Greater trochanteric advancement of the proximal femur: A clinical and biomechanical study. Hip 11:77–105, 1983.

Thirty-nine of 40 patients (ages 8–21 years; mean, 13 years) experienced complete correction of gluteus medius lurch and elimination of the Trendelenburg gait after greater trochanteric advancement. The excellent results could not be explained entirely on the basis of biomechanical calculations. Developmental muscle adaptation in the growing child was thought to play an important role in the observed increases in abductor muscle strength. The underlying diagnoses were osteonecrosis of the femoral head in 26 cases and residual deformity after Legg-Calvé-Perthes disease in 14.

Lloyd-Roberts, G.C.; Wetherill, M.H.; and Fraser, M.: Trochanteric advancement for premature arrest of the femoral capital growth plate. J. Bone Joint Surg. 67B:21–24, 1985.

Results of trochanteric advancement for growth arrest of the capital epiphysis associated with Legg-Calvé-Perthes disease were good in all nine hips studied. Good results were achieved in five of eight hips with a similar problem secondary to congenital dysplasia. These patients were children.

Quaglia, F.; Bertini, G.; Dettoni, A.; Peveraro, A.; and Rossi, P.: Transposition of the great trochanter in the treatment of congenital dysplasia of the hip and Perthes disease. Ital. J. Orthop. Traumatol. 10:67–74, 1984.

Marked improvement in muscle strength, gait, and motion in abduction (previously limited by impingement) was obtained by distal and lateral transfer of the greater trochanter in 14 of 17 cases (age at operation, 9–19 years; mean age, 13 years). Fifteen cases represented necrosis complicating treatment for congenital dysplasia of the hip and two were secondary to Legg-Calvé-Perthes disease.

Osteotomies

Benson, M.K.D., and Evans, D.C.J.: The pelvic osteotomy of Chiari: An anatomical study of the hazards and misleading radiographic appearances. J. Bone Joint Surg. 58B:164–168, 1976.

Anatomic demonstration of 1.5 cm of true lateral coverage with proper displacement of the pelvis was reported. Vulnerability of the sciatic nerve and inferior gluteal vessels was demonstrated, as well as the technical error of hinging on the sciatic notch.

Ninomiya, S., and Tagawa, H.: Rotational acetabular osteotomy for the dysplastic hip. J. Bone Joint Surg. 66A:430–436, 1984.

At follow-up of 3 years or more in 41 patients (45 hips), 35 had no pain and 6 had mild pain. One case of necrosis of the acetabular segment with subsequent healing and two cases of penetration of the joint by the osteotome were reported.

Poss, R.: The role of osteotomy in the treatment of osteoarthritis of the hip. J. Bone Joint Surg. 66A:144–151, 1984.

The evolution of modern osteotomy approaches is reviewed. This paper also addresses the questions of patient selection, choice of operative procedure, and meaning of reported results.

Salter, R.B.; Hansson, G.; and Thompson, G.H.: Innominate osteotomy in the management of residual congenital subluxation of the hip in young adults. Clin. Orthop. 182:53–68, 1984.

Mobility that was 60% of normal, articular cartilage space of at least 50% of normal for the age, good radiographic congruity of the hip joint, and residual subluxation all are required. One failure occurred among 55 hips followed 2 to 21 years; 91% had follow-up of 4 or more years postoperatively. Mobility was improved in only one patient; the others were the same as or stiffer than at the time of operation.

Santore, R.F., and Bombelli, R.: Long-term follow-up of the Bombelli experience with osteotomy for osteoarthritis: Results at 11 years in the hip. Proceedings of the Eleventh Open Scientific Meeting, pp. 106–128. C.V. Mosby, St. Louis and Toronto, 1983.

Of 45 patients followed for a minimum of 11 years after intertrochanteric osteotomy, 34 (76%) were rated excellent or good. No patient required conversion to total hip arthroplasty. Operations included 40 valgus osteotomies for advanced arthritis secondary to residual subluxation and 10 varus intertrochanteric osteotomies for less advanced arthritic changes.

Schatzker, J. (ed.): The Intertrochanteric Osteotomy. Berlin, Springer-Verlag, 1984.

Contributions by eminent European surgeons on patient selection, operative technique, and results of intertrochanteric osteotomy are presented.

Schreiber, A.: Long term results of Chiari pelvic osteotomies. Prog. Orthop. Surg. 4:31–37, 1980.

At follow-up (10–19 years), 80% of 51 adult patients showed radiographic evidence of arrest or regression of arthritis. A simplification of the surgical technique was developed—straight transverse iliac osteotomy with gentle cranial inclination. Valgus intertrochanteric osteotomy was done in nearly 50% of cases.

Steel, H.H.: Triple osteotomy of the innominate bone. J. Bone Joint Surg. 55A:343–350, 1973.

Ability to displace and rotate the acetabulum can be enhanced by osteotomy of the pubis and ischium in addition to the iliac osteotomy.

Wainwright, D.: The shelf operation for hip dysplasia in adolescence. J. Bone Joint Surg. 58B:159–163, 1976.

Results were excellent in 13 of 17 patients followed 5–20 years (mean, 9 years). With proper placement of graft adjacent to the capsule, resorption was not seen. Mobility was preserved consistently. Failures were attributed to high placement of graft in one and inadequate size in another.

Shelf Procedure

Judet, J., and Judet, H.: Long term results of acetabular shelf arthroplasty. Prog. Orthop. Surg. 4:45–55, 1980.

A follow-up of 10 years or more of 655 hips is presented. Of 168 hips with acetabular dysplasia without significant secondary arthritis at the time of operation, 86% were good at follow-up, compared with an overall good rating of 65% for the entire group. Results tended to deteriorate at 17–20 years postoperatively.

White, R.E., and Sherman, F.C.: The hip-shelf procedure: A long-term evaluation. J. Bone Joint Surg. 62A:928–932, 1980.

In 21 cases, follow-up of 10 years or more demonstrated 1 excellent, 8 satisfactory, and 12 poor results. More than half had pain and degenerative changes within 20 years after the operation. All procedures were done with open reduction of the hip; 85% were done with an iliac turn-down technique with cancellous graft. Mean age at operation was only 7 years.

Osteonecrosis

Genant, H.K.; Jergeson, H.E.; Heller, M.; Richardson, M.L.; Gillespy, T., III; Helmes, C.A.; Moore, S.G.; Bovill, E.G.; Maurer, R.; and Murray, W.R.: Magnetic resonance imaging of the hip. Hip 13:150–156, 1985.

Early detection of osteonecrosis by magnetic resonance imaging is possible on the basis of a homogeneous loss of normal high-density signal in the femoral head. Also, in known cases of osteonecrosis, this technique may be useful in clarifying the extent of involvement in segmental lesions.

Hungerford, D.S. (ed.): Avascular necrosis of the femoral head. Hip 11:247–330, 1983.

This collection of five papers reviews in detail the pathogenesis, diagnostic techniques, staging, and treatment alternatives for osteonecrotic femoral heads. Excellent descriptions of the technique for intraosseous pressure manometry and core decompression biopsy are given.

Weil, U.H. (ed.): Segmental idiopathic necrosis of the femoral head. Prog. Orthop. Surg. 5:1–116, 1981.

This is a compilation of eight articles that review in detail the pathogenesis, staging, and treatment of osteonecrosis. Vascular bundle transplantation, flexion osteotomy for segmental femoral head necrosis, modified cup arthroplasty, rotational intertrochanteric osteotomy, and surface replacement are discussed.

35

Knee and Leg: Pediatric Aspects

The topics considered in this section include congenital and developmental anomalies of the knee and leg, patellar problems, developmental angular deformity, inflammation and infection, trauma to the knee, and limb length inequality.

Congenital and Developmental Anomalies

Congenital Deficiencies

Congenital femoral deficiencies can vary from hypoplasia with a nearly normal hip and a normal knee to complete absence of the proximal femur. In simple hypoplasia, the major problem is limb length inequality. Lengthening can be considered if one is aware of the risk, if the hip joint is normal, and if the anticipated lengthening is 10% to 15% of the bone to be lengthened. Proximal femoral focal deficiency (PFFD) varies from a mild deformity of the proximal femur to complete absence of the proximal femur. In the unilateral variety, the major problems are the great discrepancy in the limb length and hip stability rotation. These are frequently managed by unilateral knee fusion, Syme amputation, and fitting with a prosthesis. The Van Nes rotation-plasty can be considered in some patients. Treatment of patients with bilateral PFFD must be individualized. Some are best left untreated; others can be fitted with custom prostheses.

Congenital deficiency of the fibula is often associated with other lower extremity anomalies including tarsal coalition and partial absence of the lateral rays of the foot. Patients with hypoplasia always have a limb length inequality. Particularly when associated with other foot anomalies, complete absence of the fibula usually requires Syme or Boyd amputation and prosthesis fitting. A fibrocartilaginous band nearly always is present in these patients. It probably represents a fibular *Anlage.* If the foot is to be preserved, this band should be resected because it can increase the equinovalgus deformity of the foot as the limb grows. If the foot is to be disarticulated, resection of this band as a separate procedure is not necessary because it causes no problems once the foot is removed.

Congenital absence of the tibia can result in a severe disability, depending on how much of the tibia is missing. When the proximal portion of the tibia is present, the usual treatment is to disarticulate the foot and perform a synostosis of the proximal tibia to the fibula which is usually normal. The heel pad is placed over the distal fibula and the weight is transmitted from the fibula to the proximal tibia by means of the synostosis. Attempts at substituting a totally intact fibula for a completely absent tibia have produced very poor and highly unpredictable results. In nearly all cases, disarticulation of the knee is a much more preferable procedure. With partial absence of the tibia, a Syme amputation may be performed or the fibula may be transferred and fused to the proximal tibial fragment, particularly if the knee is normal.

Congenital Angular Deformity

There are two types of congenital angular deformity of the tibia.

One is posteromedial bowing of the tibia. This deformity most likely is due to the influences of intrauterine posture. Because this deformity is self-correcting, neither bracing nor surgical treatment is indicated. There is no association with pseudarthrosis of the tibia. These patients must be followed until skeletal maturity because some will have a leg length discrepancy requiring a limb equalization procedure.

The other entity presents with an anterolateral bowing or with congenital pseudarthrosis of the tibia; it carries a less favorable prognosis. Neurofibromatosis is present in approximately 50% of the patients who have congenital pseudarthrosis (5% to 11% of patients with neurofibromatosis have congenital pseudarthrosis). The final answer for treatment is not available but the following guidelines should be followed.

If the patient does not have a fracture, the tibia should be protected with an orthosis. The parents should be advised at the outset of the possibility of repeated fractures, the need for repeated surgical procedures, the probability of limb length discrepancy, and the ultimate possibility of amputation. Autogenous bone grafting procedures are considered to be the best initial approach to gain union. Recent efforts have emphasized the use of intramedullary fixation of the tibia, internal fixation of the fibula (if fractured) when possible, and autogenous iliac bone grafting to both bones. More recently, microvascular fibular bone grafting has shown promise in that one of the proposed reasons for failure of union is considered to be the avascularity of the bone and soft tissues in the area of the pseudarthrosis (Fig. 1). The results, however, are preliminary, and there is concern about the fact that two abnormal legs are being created by removing a vascularized fibular graft from a normal growing limb as a donor site.

Pulsed electromagnetic fields have been used by several investigators, but the long-term results are preliminary and uncertain and this method has not achieved universal acceptance as treatment for this condition.

Amputation should be considered if the projected limb length discrepancy at maturity will be unacceptable or after multiple attempts to achieve union have failed or if the foot size and configuration are unacceptable. Disarticulation of the foot (Syme principle) is the procedure of choice. This technique not only provides a longer stump with good end-bearing skin but also obviates or reduces the likelihood of the need for repeat stump revisions during subsequent growth.

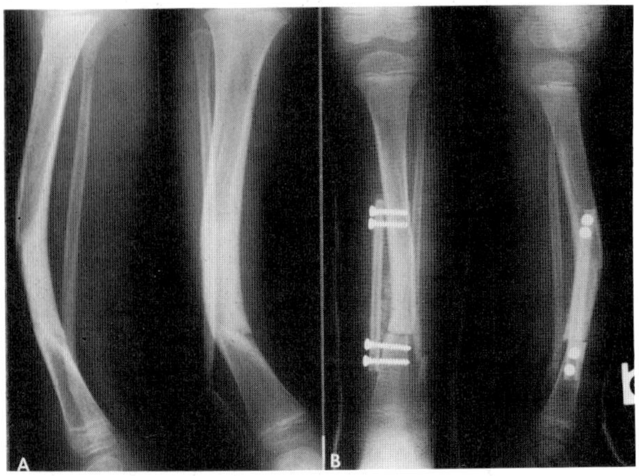

Figure 1

Treatment of congenital pseudarthrosis of the tibia with a free vascularized fibular transfer. *A*, Anteroposterior and lateral radiographs demonstrating recalcitrant pseudarthrosis with angulation deformity. *B*, Postoperative radiographs, showing free vascularized fibular flap bridging the site after osteotomy to improve the malalignment.

Abnormalities of the Knee

The knee is a frequent site of pain in the pediatric patient. There are several types of osteochondrosis and other pathologic conditions that can occur in this joint. In a patient presenting with knee pain, the hip must always be evaluated to rule out disorders such as Legg-Calvé-Perthes disease or slipped capital epiphysis.

Irregular centers of ossification in either the medial or lateral condyle of the femur may be discovered as an incidental radiographic finding. (That they cause pain is controversial.)

Typically, osteochondritis dissecans occurs in the lateral aspect of the medial femoral condyle. Trauma and circulatory disturbances have been postulated as the mechanism although the true cause is unknown. A history of pain, locking, and snapping and the presence of effusion are suggestive.

Osteochondritis dissecans usually is not a severe condition in children. Healing can be expected after rest with immobilization of the knee. Rarely, immobilization in a cylinder cast with 60° to 90° of flexion may be necessary for 6 to 10 weeks. In adolescents, this condition is more likely to cause effusion and synovitis. Arthrography or arthroscopy can be used to detect a loose fragment that should be removed. Drilling and pinning of the free osteochondral fragment and bone grafting with screw fixation have been used. Removal of the osteochondral flap and trephination of the remaining defect is sometimes needed.

Osgood-Schlatter disease—fatigue failure of the apophyseal cartilage of the tibial tubercle—is caused by excessive repeated tension of the knee extensor mechanism in a growing child. The radiographs can be normal or they can show irregularity and fragmentation of the tibial tubercle. This is a self-limiting condition that resolves when the tubercle apophysis fuses. Treatment is symptomatic and conservative. Occasionally, a separate ossicle remains in the patellar tendon at the tibial tubercle. It can be removed if it is causing symptoms. Often the tubercle remains enlarged as a consequence of prior Osgood-Schlatter disease.

In Sinding-Larsen-Johanson syndrome there is sclerosis, decalcification, and fragmentation of the distal pole of the patella. This is similar to patellar tendinitis ("jumper's knee"). These conditions are caused by excessive tensile stress at the junction of the inferior pole of the patella and the patellar ligament.

Patellar Problems

Patellar instability includes lateral patellar dislocation and subluxation. The first time that acute patellar dislocation occurs, it should be treated by immobilization for 3 to 6 weeks. Dislocation may not recur, particularly if the first dislocation was caused by significant trauma. Recurrent dislocation is often associated with bony anomalies such as genu valgum, external tibial torsion, high quadriceps angle, lateral tilt of the patella, patella alta, and hypoplasia of the lateral femoral condyle. Patients who have recurrent patellar instability tend to have soft tissue anomalies such as hypoplasia of the vastus medialis obliquis and medial capsular laxity. Patients with patellar malalignment form a very large group of pediatric patients who have knee pain. Operative correction should be attempted only if symptoms are severe. Soft tissue procedures involve lateral capsular release or lengthening and either repair or reefing of the medial capsular tissues. In patients who have severe deformities, operation on bone may be indicated to correct genu valgum or another alignment problem. If the patient is skeletally immature, operation involving the tibial tubercle must be avoided because of potential for genu recurvatum from arrest of the anterior portion of the growth plate.

Patellar subluxation is due to the same conditions that cause patellar dislocation. However, the diagnosis may be difficult. To be thorough, the examination should include assessment of knee and hip ranges of motion, quadriceps angle, patella alta, knee stability, muscle strength, and patellar stability to lateral pressure. After a site of malalignment is identified, a conservative program to correct or compensate for the underlying problem should be instituted.

If the conservative program fails and the symptoms become disabling, surgical correction should be considered. This could include proximal or distal realignment and can improve knee function in properly selected patients. Proximal realignment should lengthen, not just release, the lateral fascial and capsular layers and shorten (by reefing) the medial capsule and fascia. Arthroscopic lateral release has a lower success rate and a higher incidence of complications compared with open surgical procedures. For distal realignment, the Maquet type appears to be the best. The tibial tubercle should not be advanced distally.

"Chondromalacia patellae" refers to a pathologic condition in which there is fibrillation and softening of the articular cartilage on the undersurface of the patella. The term frequently is misused with pediatric patients. It should not be used to describe a clinical condition even though there may be pain and crepitation with direct compression of the patellofemoral joint and possibly an effusion. The diagnosis is best made by direct inspection (arthroscopy or arthrotomy). Any existing malalignment of the patella should be corrected.

Patellar tendinitis ("jumper's knee") is a common cause of knee pain in adolescents and young adults. It usually is overlooked or is misdiagnosed as chondromalacia patellae. The condition is characterized by point tenderness at the inferior pole of the patella and is a type of fatigue failure.

Developmental and Angular Deformity

Angular deviations about the knees are usually physiologic and do not require treatment. Knowledge of the natural history is necessary to rule out conditions that will not correct spontaneously and to counsel parents about the expected prognosis. Most children have a genu varum at birth that peaks at age 18 months. By age 3 years, most children will have genu valgum. The adult posture of approximately 6° genu valgum is achieved by age 5 to 8. Normal ranges that will correct spontaneously are approximately 30° of varus and 20° of valgus.

Blount's disease is the most common cause of nonphysiologic genu varum. This disturbance of the medial tibial physis is divided into infantile and adolescent varieties. The metaphyseal-diaphyseal angle of the tibia has been suggested as a means of differentiating infantile Blount's disease from physiologic bowing: less than 11° indicates a physiologic process, and values over 11° suggest Blount's disease (Fig. 2). In the early stages of Blount's disease a valgus-producing osteotomy may completely eradicate the process. In advanced stages, physeal bridge resection or repeat osteotomies may be necessary. The adolescent variety tends to be less severe. When associated with significant deformity or pain, an osteotomy may be indicated.

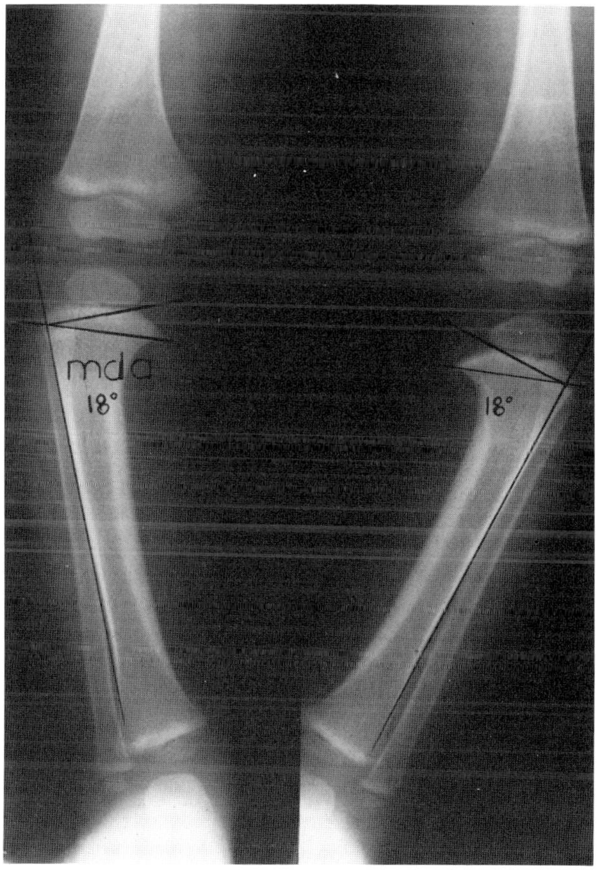

Figure 2

Anteroposterior radiograph, showing metaphyseal-diaphyseal angle of 18°, consistent with a diagnosis of infantile Blount's disease.

Persistent angular deformities that result from pathologic processes such as renal disease may require surgical management if improvement is not seen after appropriate medical management. This surgical treatment can be corrective osteotomy or selective stapling. Results from stapling are less predictable because resumption of growth cannot be guaranteed after removal of the staples.

Inflammation and Infection

Septic arthritis frequently involves the knee. Correct diagnosis depends on aspiration of joint fluid for analysis and culture. Cultures of blood and of specimens from any other site of potential seeding are mandatory. Because fluid is readily available for analysis in cases of septic arthritis, radionuclide scanning is rarely indicated or beneficial. If the infection is detected within 5 days, intravenous antimicrobial therapy, immobilization, and aspiration of the joint would be appropriate management. Surgical drainage of the joint should be considered if the diagnosis has been delayed or the organism is especially virulent (i.e., *Staphylococcus aureus*). The optimal duration of treatment with antimicrobial agents is uncertain but probably is 14 to 21 days. Oral therapy on an outpatient basis can be considered if the organism is sensitive to an appropriate agent, if satisfactory serum bactericidal levels can be obtained and monitored, and if compliance is ensured.

Acute hematogenous osteomyelitis frequently occurs in the distal femoral and proximal tibial metaphyses. Diagnosis can be suspected from the findings of fever, localized tenderness, and appropriate increases in the leukocyte count and erythrocyte sedimentation rate. Aspiration of pus from the metaphyseal area confirms the diagnosis. Failure to obtain pus by aspiration requires diagnostic investigations. Radiographic alterations are not seen until late in the process (7 to 14 days). Imaging with technetium-99m may reveal intense uptake, photopenic areas, or extended uptake. The last represents a reflex hyperemia of the affected limb in response to the infection. These variations represent the different complex pathologic processes that can occur within an infected osseous structure. Appropriate treatment is surgical drilling or windowing of the metaphyseal cortex and intravenous administration of antimicrobial agents. Oral antimicrobial therapy can be used after the initial clinical response if appropriate serum bactericidal activity can be obtained and monitored. (See Chapter 6, Infection.)

Hemophilia and juvenile rheumatoid arthritis, two conditions with very different causes, can both affect the knee joint. The principles of management are similar: rest, appropriate medical management, prevention of deformity, maintenance of motion, and, occasionally, surgical therapy. Patients with hemophilia eventually may require synovectomy to control bleeding and to prevent articular destruction. The synovectomy may be done by arthrotomy or arthroscopically. Postoperatively, constant passive motion is useful to maintain the range of motion. Synovectomy is rarely used in children but may be indicated in a patient with juvenile rheumatoid arthritis that does not respond to more conservative management. Soft tissue contractures can be prevented by appropriate physical therapy and use of casts.

Trauma

The physes are the weakest point in the bone-ligament complex, making physeal separations more common than ligamentous injuries about the knee. Ligamentous injuries can occur, however, and are usually associated with high-energy trauma. In some patients, both physeal injury and ligament injury occur at the same time. These must be accurately diagnosed by physical examination, stress radiographic evaluation, and arthroscopy (when indicated). Repair of ligamentous structures should be carried out if several ligaments are completely disrupted. Whenever instability to valgus or varus stress about the knee is detected by physical examination, stress radiographs should be obtained (Fig. 3).

Although Salter type II physeal fractures generally have a good prognosis, when they occur in the distal femur the prognosis is guarded. Malalignment and physeal arrest are more likely in this location than in other locations.

Physeal fracture or dislocation should be gently reduced, usually under general anesthesia. If the articular surface is disrupted, it must be anatomically reduced and held. With a Salter type II physeal fracture at the distal femur, maintenance of reduction can be difficult in a long leg or hip spica cast. Percutaneous pinning (with smooth pins) is necessary when anatomic reduction cannot be maintained with a cast (Fig. 4).

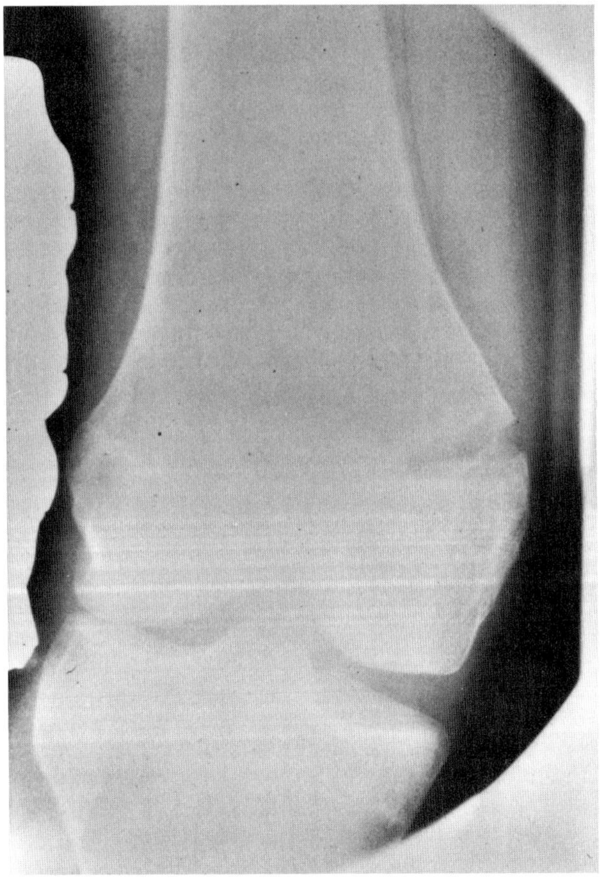

Figure 3

Lateral stress radiograph in an adolescent with knee injury. The stress view reveals a physeal fracture at the medial aspect of the distal femur.

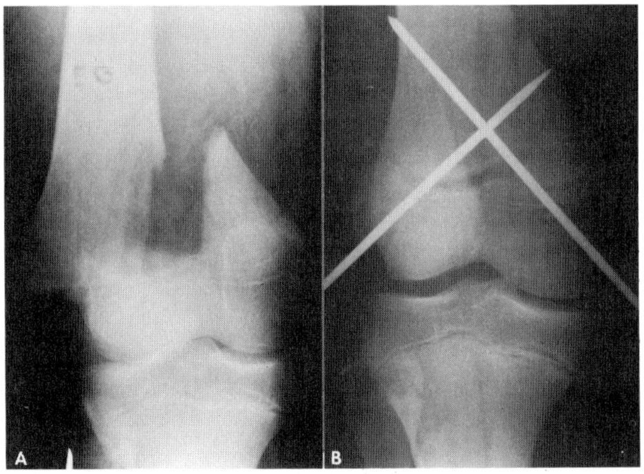

Figure 4

A, Anteroposterior radiograph, showing physeal fracture (Salter type II) of the distal femur. *B*, Fracture was unstable after closed reduction. Percutaneous smooth pins were used to maintain reduction.

The tibial spines (intercondylar eminences) are adjacent to the points of attachment of the cruciate ligaments and can be avulsed in injuries to the knee. These avulsions are graded 1, 2, or 3, depending on the amount of displacement. At times the fragment can be reduced by placing the knee in extension. Reduction should be confirmed by a lateral radiograph. If the fragment is unreduced, an arthrotomy should be performed and the reduction held with sutures brought out through drill holes that do not cross the physeal plate.

Osteochondral fractures of the knee at times are difficult to diagnose. Plain radiography, arthrography, and arthroscopy may be required to make the exact diagnosis. Fragments should be replaced whenever possible and held in place with smooth pins. Powerful contraction of the quadriceps can avulse the tibial tubercle. Watson Jones has graded these as grades I, II, and III. Grade I (a hinged fragment) usually can be managed by closed reduction; grade II, which has retraction of the fragment, and grade III, which has complete disruption of the articular surface, must be managed by open reduction and internal fixation. Fragments should be replaced anatomically and held with smooth pins or with a screw placed so as to avoid the physeal line.

Injuries to the knee may be associated with severe complications. Fracture separation of the proximal tibial epiphysis can damage the popliteal artery which is closely tethered to the bone by the geniculate branches and fascia. Arteriography is diagnostic. The complications of missing this diagnosis are disastrous. Proximal tibial metaphyseal fractures can result in progressive valgus deformity, particularly if the fibula is intact. This fracture occurs in children less than 5 years old. Bracing has not been successful. A high recurrence rate has been reported with surgical correction. The deformity seems to correct spontaneously.

Proximal tibial physeal damage can occur from tibial traction pins, even when the pin apparently does not violate the physis. Therefore, care should be exercised with proximal tibial traction. If at all possible, pins should be placed in the distal femur rather than in the proximal tibia because genu recurvatum can occur if the physis is damaged.

Stress fractures occur in the long bones in children as a result of repetitive microtrauma. The history usually suggests the diagnosis. Initial radiographs may be negative. A radionuclide bone scan may be diagnostic. The differential diagnosis includes infection, osteoid osteoma, shin splints, and malignant tumors. Stress fractures are treated symptomatically.

Meniscal tears are somewhat unusual in children but do occur. The diagnosis is made as in adults and is best confirmed arthroscopically. Meniscus repairs should be performed whenever possible in peripheral tears because meniscectomy is not a benign procedure in children. Partial meniscectomy for displaced bucket-handle tears usually is successful in children.

Discoid lateral meniscus is a condition in which the meniscus is discoid rather than elliptic. The usual symptom is a popping or snapping sensation. Unless symptoms are painful or interfere with function, nothing need be done. Tears tend to be of the vertical longitudinal variety and partial meniscectomy often is sufficient treatment.

Limb Length Inequality

The goal of treatment of limb length inequality is to achieve equality (within 2 cm) by maturity. This degree of inequality is compatible with normal function. Difficulty increases when the discrepancy exceeds 3 cm. Difference in limb lengths can result from trauma, infection, congenital anomalies, vascular abnormalities, or generalized systemic diseases.

The cause of the limb length inequality must be determined first and then its status as progressive or static must be documented by either of two methods. In both methods a scanogram and a radiograph must be obtained of a wrist at regular intervals for determining bone age. In the first, the tables of Green and Anderson are used. The growth inhibition of the involved extremity is calculated and, by using the growth-remaining table, the projected discrepancy is calculated. Whenever possible the patient should be followed over 2 to 3 years to obtain accurate information and establish a trend. In the other method, the Moseley line graph is used to obtain such longitudinal data and allows plotting and calculation of the growth inhibition of the involved extremity. Appropriate times for epiphyseodesis are displayed. Limb lengthenings also can be plotted on the Moseley graph.

The treatment selected for dealing with limb length inequality must be based on the underlying pathologic condition and the projected discrepancy at maturation. The patient and the family should participate in selecting the treatment modality, and consideration should be given to projected overall height, the level of the knees, and the risk-benefit ratio of the various methods.

For discrepancies up to 5 cm, selected epiphyseodesis is probably the treatment of choice.

A single-stage shortening on the longer side can be performed in a skeletally mature patient. Its main use is for discrepancies in the femur, and 3 to 5 cm can be corrected by this technique.

When the discrepancy exceeds 5 cm, one should consider limb lengthening. By using the Wagner technique, additional length of up to 15% of the original bone length can be obtained (approximately 6 cm in the femur and 5 cm in the tibia). The patient must understand at the outset that the treatment is prolonged and usually is associated with complications. The femur is osteotomized and then the Wagner apparatus is used to provide distraction at a rate of 1 mm per day. Throughout the entire procedure, careful attention must be paid to detail, and the protocol should be followed rigidly. Once the desired amount of length is obtained, open reduction with a specialized plate and bone grafting is performed. The patient is protected with a non-weight-bearing cast until solid union is achieved. The plate is removed once the medullary canal has been reestablished and the cortex has formed (approximately 1 year later). Because of the complication of late fracture, some surgeons are now advocating removing the original plate and replacing it with a smaller plate that subsequently is removed.

Function should never be sacrificed for length. Careful attention must be paid to maintaining 90° of motion at the knee and to meticulous pin track care. Because of the cooperation required from the patient, this procedure is mainly for patients who have at least a 5-cm projected discrepancy and preferably are in their teens. It is a demanding technique that should be utilized only by those familiar with it.

Recently described techniques use the apparatus of Ilizarov with K-wires run through the bone and then placed under tension, allowing use of a small-diameter pin placed percutaneously. In the first method, the lengthening occurs through the physis, but this method has been associated with a high incidence of physeal closure and should only be used in adolescents. The second method seems more promising because the lengthening occurs through a metaphyseal osteotomy. The procedures are complicated, and careful study of the original descriptions is necessary before one attempts them.

Annotated Bibliography

Developmental and Acquired Deformities

Balthazar, D.A., and Pappas, A.M.: Acquired valgus deformity of the tibia in children. J. Pediatr. Orthop. 4:538–541, 1984.

Tibial metaphyseal fractures in young children can result in a progressive valgus deformity during the first 2 years after injury; the deformity may then remain static or correct spontaneously. In those treated surgically, there has been an unacceptably high rate of recurrence, making nonoperative management the treatment of choice.

Hughston, J.C.; Hergenroeder, P.T.; and Courtenay, B.G.: Osteochondritis dissecans of the femoral condyles. J. Bone Joint Surg. 66A:1340–1348, 1984.

Patients treated either surgically or conservatively for osteochondritis dissecans were reviewed. Overall results in the two groups were similar, with conservative care working well before epiphyseal closure and surgical care working well afterward.

Jacobsen, S.T.; Crawford, A.H.; Millar, E.A.; and Steel, H.H.: The Syme amputation in patients with congenital pseudarthrosis of the tibia. J. Bone Joint Surg. 65A:533–537, 1983.

The most popular current surgical technique for amputation in congenital pseudarthrosis of the tibia is a Syme amputation. This operation provides a longer stump, better skin coverage, and more potential for future growth than other amputations do.

Kling, T.F., Jr., and Hensinger, R.N.: Angular and torsional deformities of the lower limbs in children. Clin. Orthop. 176:136–147, 1983.

The common torsional malalignments of the lower extremity, including calcaneal valgus foot, internal tibial torsion, genu varum, genu valgum, and femoral anteversion, usually become corrected with growth. It is important, however, to recognize those requiring further evaluation and treatment.

Pappas, A.M.: Congenital posteromedial bowing of the tibia and fibula. J. Pediatr. Orthop. 4:525–531, 1984.

Posteromedial bowing, which usually is associated with a calcaneovalgus foot, corrects with growth and is not related to congenital pseudarthrosis of the tibia. These patients must be followed until adult life; leg length discrepancy can vary to as much as 6.3 cm.

Schoenecker, P.L.; Meade, W.C.; Pierron, R.L.; Sheridan, J.J.; and Capelli, A.M.: Blount's disease: A retrospective review and recommendations for treatment. J. Pediatr. Orthop. 5:181–186, 1985.

Thirty-two patients treated over 30 years are reviewed for comparison of the results of surgical and conservative treatments. Patients with stage 1 or 2 Blount's disease responded to treatment. Those less than 5 years old and not responding to bracing or who had more severe disease responded to a proximal tibial osteotomy. After age 4 and with advanced stages of disease and increasing deformity, various other surgical procedures are necessary.

Sharrard, W.J.W.: Treatment of congenital and infantile pseudarthrosis of the tibia with pulsing electromagnetic fields. Orthop. Clin. North Am. 15:143–162, January 1984.

Proponents of therapeutic use of pulsed electromagnetic fields continue to report a success rate of 70% in patients with congenital pseudarthrosis of the tibia. These results are short term and will require further follow-up for validation.

Staheli, L.T.; Corbett, M.; Wyss, C.; and King, H.: Lower-extremity rotational problems in children: Normal values to guide management. J. Bone Joint Surg. 67A:39–47, 1985.

One thousand normal lower extremities of children and adults were studied to establish normal values for the rotational profile. These values allow quantitative clinical evaluation of lower extremity problems and provide a basis for counselling parents regarding the normal developmental pattern.

Limb Length Discrepancy

Grill, F.: Distraction of the epiphyseal cartilage as a method of limb lengthening. J. Pediatr. Orthop. 4:105–108, 1984.

This method, which has been used in Russia and in some parts of Europe and only recently in the United States, is reviewed. Its major disadvantage is frequent closure of the physis after lengthening, making it unacceptable for use in young children.

Mezhenina, E.P.; Roulla, E.A.; Pechersky, A.G.; Babich, V.D.; Shadrina, E.L.; and Mizhevich, T.V.: Methods of limb elongation with congenital inequality in children. J. Pediatr. Orthop. 4:201–207, 1984.

Seventy-eight children treated by epiphyseal distraction with an external fixator or with corticectomy and external fixation are reviewed. A general description of the technique and results are included but the data on the number of complications and on the fine points of the method are sparse.

Monticelli, G., and Spinelli, R.: Leg lengthening by closed metaphyseal corticotomy. Ital. J. Orthop. Traumatol. 9:139–150, 1983.

This new method of limb lengthening, which is gradually coming into use in the United States, is discussed. It involves a corticectomy in the metaphyseal area and gradual distraction by a special encircling external fixation device using crossed wires under tension. It is claimed to be more reliable and quicker and to have fewer complications than standard techniques.

Stephens, D.C.: Femoral and tibial lengthening. J. Pediatr. Orthop. 3:424–430, 1983.

The operative techniques, results, and complications of Wagner's technique of limb lengthening are discussed. The method is exacting, and complications, although remediable, should be expected frequently. The method remains a significant advance in the management of limb length inequality.

36

Knee and Leg: Soft Tissue Trauma

The recent advances in the management of knee injuries include further development of arthroscopic methods in the treatment of meniscus and ligament lesions and the demonstration of successful meniscus repair in properly selected patients. The importance of repair or reconstruction of the anterior cruciate ligament (ACL) in athletes and the need for early limited motion after ligament repair remain valid concepts. Also, advances have been made in the use of instruments to measure knee laxity, in procedures for ACL repair and reconstruction, and in understanding of the reverse pivot shift as a sign of posterolateral rotary instability. Complications associated with arthroscopic lateral parapatellar release, meniscus repairs, and operative procedures that combine open arthrotomy with arthroscopic techniques are now recognized.

Examination of the Knee

Physical examination for joint laxity should evaluate excessive joint motion in all directions. In assessing joint laxity in the anterior, posterior, medial, or lateral direction, the four primary restraints provided by the anterior cruciate, posterior cruciate, medial collateral, and fibular collateral ligaments are tested. The measurements obtained always should be compared to those from the normal knee. Differences are recorded as increased laxity. The degree to which these four ligaments restrain their respective motions depends upon the knee flexion angle. As the knee approaches extension, the participation of isolated ligaments lessens and the role of secondary restraints increases.

Rotation is an important but often disregarded normal motion of the knee. Attempts should be made to measure the degree of rotational laxity in knees. Anterior and posterior motions of the tibia (i.e., drawer signs) should be evaluated in varying degrees of rotation. However, the posteromedial and lateral capsules are relaxed at 90° of flexion and contribute little to stability in flexion.

The most sensitive test for determining the presence of a torn ACL is the anterior drawer performed at 25° of knee flexion (Lachman test). Posterior cruciate ligament (PCL) disruption is best measured by the posterior drawer test performed at 70° to 90° of flexion. Medial collateral ligament (MCL) laxity is best evaluated by the valgus stress test performed at 30° of flexion. Fibular collateral ligament and lateral capsule laxity are tested by the varus stress test at 30° of flexion. The pivot shift test is similar to the Lachman test—i.e., anterior subluxation or reduction of the tibia—but is performed under load and rotation. The reverse pivot shift test indicates excessive posterior subluxation of the lateral tibial condyle as the knee is moved from a flexed to an extended position accompanied by forced external rotation and valgus force (Fig. 1).

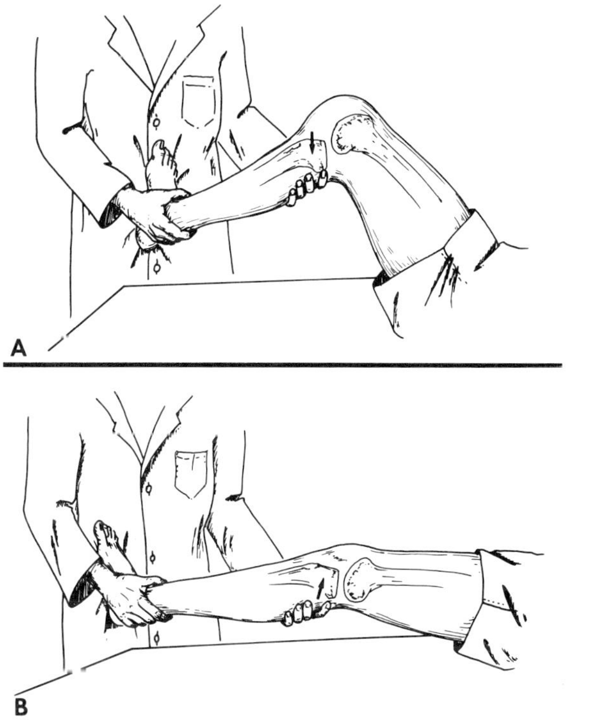

Figure 1

Reverse pivot shift test to detect posterolateral instability. *A*, Beginning at 80° of flexion, with the foot externally rotated and a slight valgus force applied, the leg is slowly brought into extension. *B*, At approximately 20° of flexion, the tibia reduces by sliding forward.

Anterior Cruciate Ligament

The ACL is the primary restraint to anterior tibial subluxation. In combination with the PCL, it is an important secondary restraint to varus and valgus forces.

Diagnosis

If the ACL is torn, the functional instability that results usually occurs during pivoting, jumping, or twisting maneuvers. The natural history of ACL deficiency is one of frequent episodes of knee instability and resultant injury to menisci and articular surfaces. Severe swelling within 2 to 6 hours after a sudden deceleration/valgus/rotational injury or a hyperextension injury is highly suggestive of a torn ACL. In the majority of cases, the diagnosis can be made by history and clinical examination alone. The value of arthroscopy to diagnose an acute tear of the ACL has been overemphasized, and it should be reserved for detecting associated joint damage. After an acute knee injury, the most reliable test for detecting a torn ACL is the Lachman test. Both the amount of anterior excursion and the quality of the end point must be determined. If there is little excursion but a soft end point, the test should be considered to be positive.

It is important to grade the amount of laxity in a knee that has a torn ACL. The amount of excess joint laxity correlates with subsequent functional instability and also is an indicator of additional joint pathology such as damage to the capsule or meniscus. In most clinical grading systems, grade I laxity represents up to 5 mm of motion, grade II means 6 to 10 mm, grade III means 11 to 15 mm, and grade IV means more than 15 mm. However, instrumented measurements are challenging these concepts, and more accurate classification systems are being adopted.

It is difficult to know which patients with acute ACL injury should be treated by primary surgical repair and which should be treated nonoperatively. Forty percent of patients who have a torn ACL reportedly can lead nearly normal but unathletic life-styles without surgical treatment. Another 40%, although unhappy with their disabled knee, will modify their life-styles by avoiding sports or decreasing their extent of activity. The remaining 20% continue athletic activity, experience multiple giving-way episodes, and subsequently require reconstructive surgery. Early surgical intervention in this third group of patients can prevent or forestall the associated morbidity that comes with repeated injury. Patients who are willing to modify their life-style should be educated regarding their knee problem and treated by rehabilitation and functional bracing.

When surgical treatment is recommended for a patient with a torn ACL, the amount of knee laxity that is present should be taken into consideration. Patients who have grade I or II knee laxity usually remain "functionally" stable after rehabilitation, bracing, and modification of their activity. Patients who have grade IV knee laxity usually have functional instability with daily activities even if they do not participate in sports. Therefore, they often require surgical stabilization whether they are athletic or not. In the gray zone are patients who have a grade III knee laxity. These patients usually can avoid surgical treatment if they reduce their sports activities, particularly events that require jumping, pivoting, and decelerating. Patients with a torn ACL and grade III knee laxity who wish to continue to participate in sports, especially if young, should have reconstructive surgery. Other factors that usually tip the balance toward need for reconstructing a torn ACL are: 1) complete tear of another primary restraint such as the MCL, 2) coexisting patellofemoral instability, and 3) a "repairable" meniscal tear.

Although one generally should operate for "functional instability" rather than for "knee laxity," the patient who fits into one or more of the high-risk categories noted above for developing problems should be identified soon after injury and offered surgical stabilization. As a general rule, whenever the physician or patient is in doubt as to the need for surgical intervention, the patient should be treated nonoperatively so that the functional instability can become apparent prior to operation. Whenever the decision to operate hinges on the amount of laxity or the presence of injury to secondary restraints in borderline cases, examination under anesthesia and diagnostic arthroscopy should be performed.

ACL Repair and Reconstruction

The operative methods designed to stabilize a knee with a torn ACL are intra-articular techniques, extra-articular techniques, and combinations of both. The principles that are important in obtaining good results from ACL reconstructive surgery are: 1) correction of all components of the instability (i.e., primary as well as secondary restraints); 2) use of strong tissue for grafts (the patellar tendon has been shown to be the strongest available tissue for intra-articular procedures and the iliotibial band, for extra-articular procedures); 3) use of secure fixation to allow early motion; 4) placement of the grafts in isometric positions; 5) use of static instead of "dynamic" repairs; 6) use of early limited motion; 7) delaying the patient's return to high-force activities for at least 1 year postoperatively; and 8) always protecting the knee with a brace for active sports.

Isometric placement of grafts is the only way to achieve a full range of knee motion without permanent ligament deformation. The use of strong tissues to replace the function of the ACL is essential to the success of either intra- or extra-articular methods. Any intra-articular procedure that does not attach the distal end of the graft at the anatomic attachment site of the ACL to the tibia or near the isometric position of the lateral femoral intercondylar wall (5 to 6 mm anterior to the over-the-top position) will probably stretch out when full range of motion is attained (Fig. 2 *Left*). Similarly, extra-articular procedures that do not attach the graft distally at Gerdy's tubercle and proximally at an isometric point just distal and posterior to the attachment of the lateral intermuscular septum to the femur should be questioned (Fig. 2 *Right*). Laxities of other restraints such as the MCL posteromedial capsule or lateral capsule should be corrected at the time of operation.

Isometric placement of strong tissues is the most important element in achieving successful repair after an ACL injury. Recently, arthroscopic methods have been used in trying to attain these goals. It is too early to assess the efficacy of these procedures. Synthetic, xenograft, and allograft ligaments have also been tried experimentally.

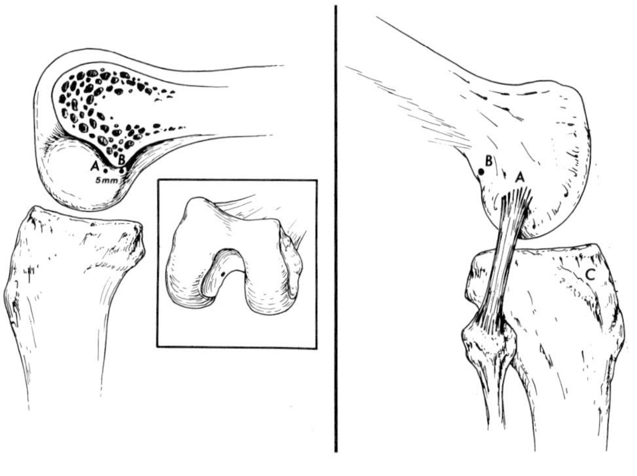

Figure 2

Left, Isometric ACL attachment point on the femur. This is located approximately 5 mm distal to the "over-the-top" position. *Inset,* Location on frontal view. *Right,* Point B is the optimal location for fixing an extra-articular tenodesis. A, Lateral femoral epicondyle; B, desired point of tenodesis of the iliotibial band distal to the attachment of the lateral intermuscular septum; C, Gerdy's tubercle.

However, none of the synthetic ligaments has been approved for general use at this time, and no long-term reports regarding their safety or efficacy are available.

Primary repair alone as a surgical technique for an acutely torn ACL is rarely successful. Intra-articular repair of the ACL by using staples has been attempted but violates biomechanical principles and is ineffective. Several reports of results after ACL repair alone show a progressive loss in joint stability over time. "Dynamic" muscle or tendon transfers—of structures such as the pes anserinus, semitendinosus tendon, and biceps femoris—are probably ineffective and should not be relied on to stabilize a joint.

Concepts regarding rehabilitation after ACL surgery have also changed. With the use of securely fixed, high-strength, isometric grafts, progressive rehabilitation protocols can now be prescribed that include early protected motion, neuromuscular rehabilitation, and patellofemoral joint mobilization. However, all rehabilitation programs must take into consideration that ligaments require a long time to heal. There is a 50% decrease in tissue strength of tissue grafts inside the joint after intra-articular transfer for ACL reconstruction, compared with their strength *in situ*. By extrapolation from animal studies, one would predict healing periods for human ligaments to be in excess of 12 months. Comparison of stresses on the ACL from daily living activities to the strength of the ACL graft at 1 year shows why some surgical procedures fail in the postoperative period and why muscle rehabilitation is so critical (Fig. 3).

In the knee flexion range of 0° to 40°, even low forces strain the ACL (Fig. 4). Therefore, early mobilization programs should restrict the knee from going into this range of knee extension until secure graft fixation has occurred. Progressive resistive exercises from 0° to 40° of knee flexion should be delayed until approximately 5 to 6 months postoperatively. A patient should not return to forceful athletic activities until at least 12 months postoperatively. This time period allows for collagen maturation and proper healing of the graft. The criteria for allowing an athlete to resume play are no pain or swelling, full range of motion, and strength at least 90% of normal. To judge strength, total quadriceps power of one knee should be compared with that of the opposite knee as well as with body weight (an estimate of the desired strength of the quadriceps upon isokinetic testing is that strength in foot pounds should be close to the patient's weight in pounds). Normal hamstring strength is approximately two-thirds of quadriceps strength. The hamstring muscles should be strengthened to achieve a quadriceps/hamstring ratio close to 1:1 after ACL surgery. Protective (functional) knee braces are prescribed if the patient is returning to active sports.

Instrumented knee testing devices permit objective measurement of knee laxity before and after operation. If knees are tested at low force (7 kg) and at a higher force (18 kg), ligament compliance can be estimated. Knees that have more laxity at high force compared to low are said to have an increased compliance factor. This suggests that at high force situations such as in athletics, the knee can be un-

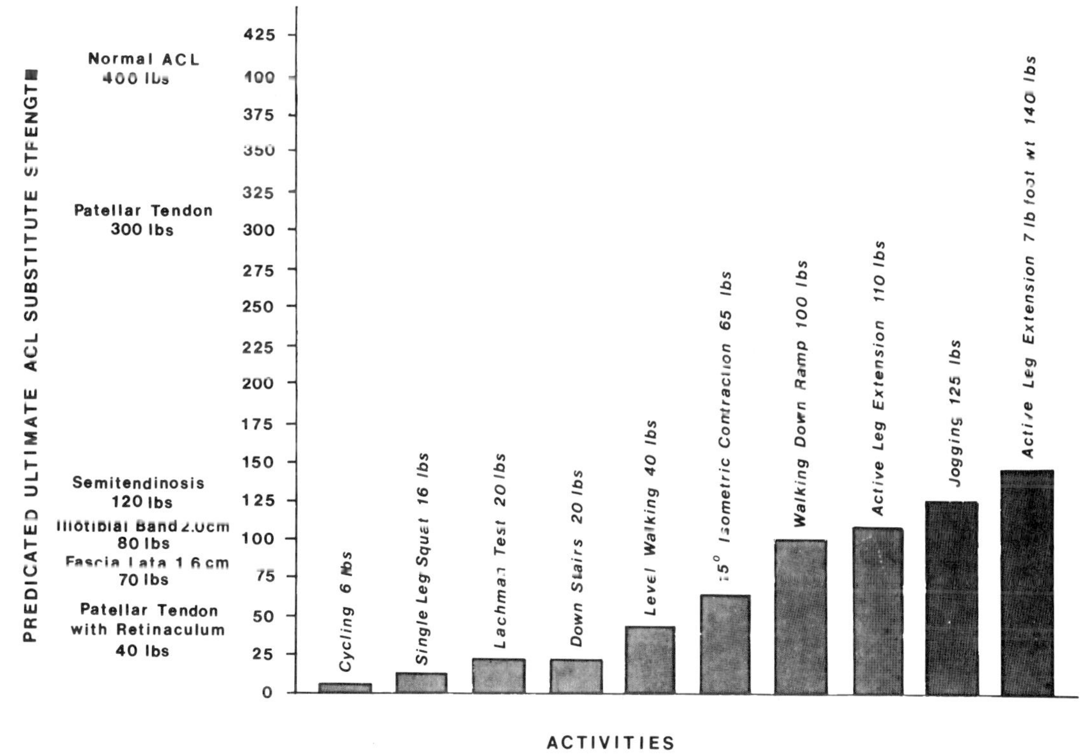

Figure 3

Ligament strength versus ACL forces. The *y* axis represents the predicted strengths, at 1 year postoperatively, of the various tissues used to reconstruct the ACL. The *x* axis represents calculated or measured strains on the ACL during various activities.

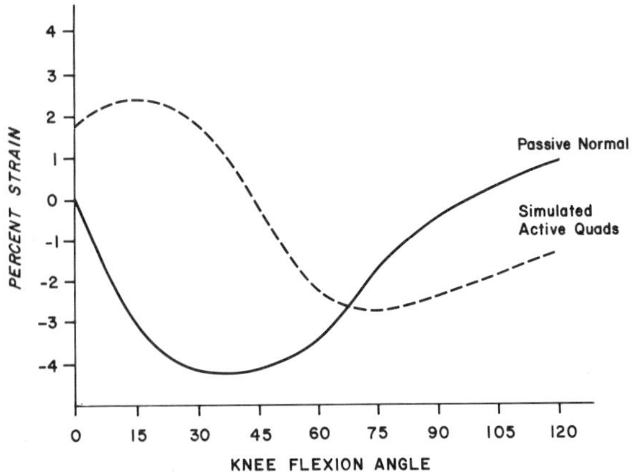

Figure 4

Strain on the ACL at different knee flexion angles at passive motion and simulated active quadriceps contraction.

stable or the graft can deform. Athletes who are found to have a high compliance ratio after ligament reconstruction should be encouraged to limit forceful sports activities and to wear functional braces for sports.

Posterior Cruciate Ligament

The PCL is the primary restraint to posterior subluxation of the tibia. The posterolateral complex is the most important secondary restraint. The tensile strength of the PCL is approximately the same as the strength of the ACL and the tibial MCL. Rupture of the PCL does not necessarily result in a poorly functioning knee. Knees with an "isolated" PCL disruption often have a good prognosis when treated nonoperatively. A poor functional outcome is often the result when the posterior instability is associated with other types of instability, additional intra-articular damage such as to meniscal and articular cartilage, poor quadriceps strength, or gross posterior laxity.

Diagnosis

Injury to the PCL generally is caused by violent trauma; therefore, serious injury to other structures is common. However, isolated PCL tears can occur from a blow to the anterior tibia when the knee is flexed 90°, such as in hitting the dashboard in an automobile accident or in a fall on a flexed knee. Hemarthrosis is not usually a characteristic feature. Whereas the knee with a torn ACL usually has "instability" symptoms, the knee with a torn PCL has "disability" symptoms. Patients who have posterior knee instability often have medial compartment arthritis (60%), patellofemoral arthritis (70%), and symptoms of swelling and pain related to activity (40%).

The posterior drawer test at 90° knee flexion is the best way to diagnose a torn PCL. However, the posterior drawer sign can be negative in some cases of acute tears of the PCL. In these cases, instability to valgus stress testing in full knee extension or hyperextension is a sign of PCL disruption. Palpating the anterior joint lines in a knee that has a posterior drawer sign at 90° flexion shows the absence of normal anterior tibial plateau protuberance (it should extend 10 mm beyond the femoral condyles). The posterior sag or gravity test (Godfrey test) and the 90° active drawer test also are informative. The latter test can detect mild to moderate instability and is performed with the patient lying supine, the knee flexed to 90°, and the examiner holding the foot against the examining table (Fig. 5). The patient is instructed to contract the quadriceps and to try to extend the knee by pushing the restricted foot down toward the end of the examining table. Normally, the tibia will either remain in the neutral position or move slightly posteriorly; when a knee has a torn PCL, the tibia will move forward because of the unbalanced force vectors of the quadriceps and patellar tendons.

Repair and Reconstruction

Whether or not to reconstruct a torn PCL surgically remains a controversial issue because poor results after surgical treatment have been reported. If an operation is to be performed, the procedures should be based on sound biomechanical principles: strong grafts attached anatomically on the tibia and at an isometric point on the femur. This isometric point is located approximately 10 mm proximal from the edge of the articular surface and in the anterior intercondylar notch at the 11 o'clock position for the left knee or 1 o'clock for the right knee (Fig. 6). When the graft is attached to other locations or muscle or tendon transfers are used, improvement is not likely when results are tested objectively.

For the acutely torn PCL, surgical repair with augmentation by tissues such as a portion of the patellar tendon or semitendinosus and gracilis tendons should be performed when there is gross posterior laxity. Acute repair with augmentation appears to have a better success rate than does delayed reconstruction.

To prevent posterior tibial subluxation in the postoperative period, transarticular fixation with Steinmann pins has been used. However, complications such as deep pin track infection, skin slough, and pin migration often offset the advantages of this method. Alternate methods to prevent the tibia from dropping posteriorly include immobilizing the knee in near extension and passing a Steinmann pin through the patella into the tibia.

Unless synthetic ligaments (which are still experimental) are used, early postoperative motion after PCL repair usually is not recommended. A period of 4 to 6 weeks of immobilization is recommended to allow healing of the

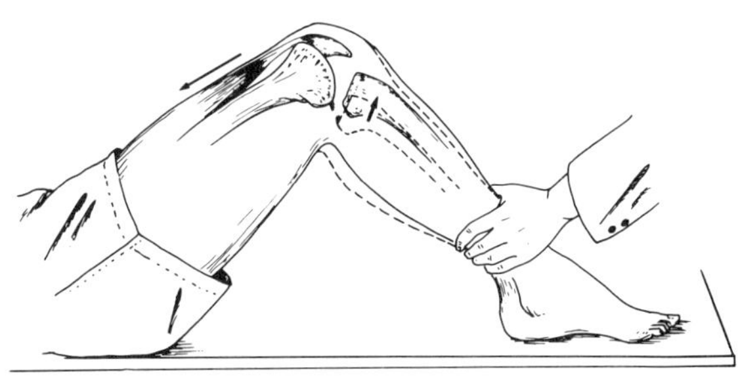

Figure 5

The 90° active drawer test for PCL disruption. With the patient supine and the knee flexed to 90°, the patient is asked to extend the leg against the examiner's hand. Anterior translation of the proximal tibia is seen if one PCL has been torn.

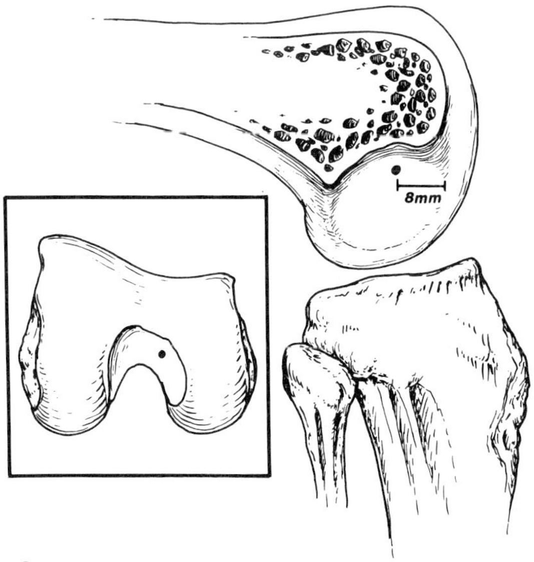

Figure 6

Isometric attachment point of the PCL to the femur. This point is approximately 10 mm proximal to the articular margin, in the anterior aspect of the intercondylar notch. When viewed from the front the PCL attachment point is at the 11 o'clock or 1 o'clock position, 10 mm from the articular surface (*Inset*).

grafts within the bone tunnels prior to initiating joint motion. Protected motion and exercises minimizing hamstring use and maximizing quadriceps use are stressed. Also, initiating exercises in the prone position minimizes posterior forces on the repair. Prolonged use of crutches is important, particularly if posterolateral rotary instability has also been corrected. If isokinetic exercise devices are used to rehabilitate the limb, the force pad should be placed near the ankle to minimize the posterior forces on the knee. Although several knee braces have been designed for the knee with a torn PCL, none adequately controls posterior tibial translation. For this reason, active quadriceps strengthening exercises should be begun early to help control the knee during the stance phase. The quadriceps must be strong enough to stabilize the knee before use of crutches is discontinued.

Posterolateral Rotary Instability

Pathologic joint laxity leading to posterior subluxation of the lateral tibial condyle in relation to the femur is caused by injury to the posterolateral corner of the knee—i.e., the fibular collateral ligament (FCL), the popliteus tendon, and the arcuate ligament complex. A common cause is a blow to the anteromedial portion of the tibia. This same trauma mechanism usually also ruptures the PCL. Posterior instability due to a torn PCL and posterolateral rotary instability frequently are present together.

Posterolateral rotary instability is diagnosed by the reverse pivot shift test. One confirmatory test is the gravity rotation test in which the tibia is suspended with the knee at 90° flexion and the tibia is externally rotated on the femur. Increased external rotation compared to the opposite side indicates increased laxity of the posterolateral structures. A posterolateral drawer test also can be performed with the knee flexed at 90° and the foot resting on the examining table. The amount of posterior dropback in external tibial rotation reflects the severity of the laxity. These tests for posterolateral instability are most sensitive when performed at 30° of knee flexion because at 90° the PCL helps to restrain this motion. By testing at 30° of flexion, the stabilizing effects of the PCL are minimized. Increased posterior tibial subluxation at both 30° and 90° of flexion indicates a combined PCL and posterior lateral complex injury. Increased posterolateral drawer at 30° of flexion compared to 90° usually indicates that the posterolateral complex has been injured and the PCL is intact. Thus, the posterolateral drawer test and straight posterior drawer test should be performed at both 30° and 90° of knee flexion.

Surgical procedures to correct posterolateral tibia subluxation have been described in which the arcuate ligament complex, popliteus tendon, and FCL are transferred anterosuperiorly on the lateral femoral condyle. This results in nonisometric placement of the restraints and a high percentage of poor results. Secure fixation at isometric points augmented by autogenous or allograft tissue appears to yield more satisfactory results.

Rehabilitation procedures after surgical repair of the posterolateral complex or FCL should be specific and should be selected according to the procedure that was performed. If ligaments are transferred anteriorly and superiorly on the femur (nonisometric), then prolonged protection with double-caliper braces and pelvic band is required. If the tissues have been fixed to isometric points on the femur, routine postoperative braces are sufficient. Regardless of the operative procedure, it must be combined with a prolonged period of crutch use. Upon weight-bearing, medial joint compression and lateral joint distraction occur. This tends to stretch the tissues on the lateral side of the joint. Tissue maturation and healing must be in advanced stages prior to weight-bearing. Because of the action of the biceps femoris, active knee flexion exercises should be minimized until late in the rehabilitation program. By contrast, quadriceps exercises should be encouraged early.

If genu varum or tibia vara is also present in the knee that has posterolateral instability, in addition to ligamentous repair on the lateral side of the joint, a valgus osteotomy might be required to reduce the distracting forces at the lateral compartment.

Fibular Collateral Ligament

The fibular collateral ligament (FCL) serves as the primary restraint to varus force at the knee in extension. If the FCL alone tears, little if any functional instability is produced in most cases. Therefore, an isolated FCL injury usually can be treated nonoperatively.

The lateral capsule is a very important secondary restraint to varus force and may be as important as the FCL. The cruciate ligaments, particularly the ACL, also act as important secondary restraints. If these secondary restraints are torn, functional instability is common. These lesions usually should be corrected surgically.

Procedures that transfer the iliotibial band from the lateral side of the knee to other sites place the knee at risk of increased varus laxity. The risk is even greater if the iliotibial band replacement fails in its new location.

Injuries that are likely to cause functional instability to varus stress are those in which the cruciate ligaments and the posterolateral capsule and FCL are disrupted. This varus instability should be recognized and corrected, especially when other instabilities are more obvious.

When an acutely torn FCL is repaired, often the repair is not strong enough to sustain the high forces on the lateral side of the joint. Therefore, augmentation with such tissues as fascia lata or biceps femoris tendon is advised. Rehabilitation after repair of the FCL should follow the guidelines outlined for the PCL and for posterolateral rotary instability.

Medial Collateral Ligament

Significant changes have occurred in concepts regarding treatment of MCL injuries. In the past, grade II or III MCL sprains usually were treated by casting or operation. Now, even complete tears of the MCL are usually treated nonoperatively except if the ACL or other major restraints are torn. It is now apparent that the major morbidity after disruption of both the ACL and MCL is from the ACL injury, not the MCL injury. Weight-bearing forces tend to compress the medial side of the joint, thus aiding stability. The MCL has excellent secondary supporting structures (i.e., the posterior oblique ligament and cruciate ligaments). Finally, the MCL injury can be protected adequately with bracing.

When an MCL disruption is combined with another major ligament injury, surgical treatment usually is indicated. The combination of torn ACL and MCL is most common although the PCL can also be torn in a knee that has a torn MCL. Findings suggesting injury to multiple ligaments are acute hemarthrosis, valgus instability in full extension, anterior subluxation of the medial tibia on the femur in external rotation at 90° of flexion, and tibial dropback as demonstrated by the gravity test. Disruption of the medial retinaculum and vastus medialis occurs in approximately 20% of the knees that have MCL injury. Associated patellar dislocation must always be suspected, especially in the female who has sustained an MCL injury. Recognition and correction of this associated injury should be carried out in addition to early surgical repair of an MCL tear. The incidence of medial meniscus tears with grade I or II MCL sprains is very low. Therefore, in the absence of joint swelling or hemarthrosis, arthroscopy usually is not indicated for a sprained MCL.

When the acutely torn MCL is repaired surgically so that tissues are repaired to their anatomic locations, long-term results usually are excellent. If the torn MCL cannot be repaired securely, it can be reinforced by using transfer of the tibial arm of the semimembranosus or part of the adductor magnus tendon. When the MCL and entire medial capsule are torn from the femur, the tissues are best repaired by using isometric techniques without advancing or transposing tissues (Fig. 7). When the MCL is disrupted from the tibia, fixation with sutures passed through drill holes in the bone is better than fixation with staples.

Rehabilitation after most MCL injuries can progress fairly rapidly. After nonoperative treatment or surgical repair of the medial ligament complex to isometric locations, early protected motion can be used with functional braces to prevent excess valgus motions.

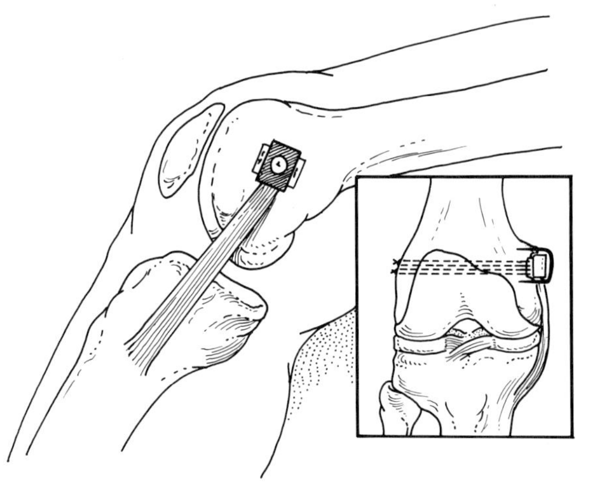

Figure 7

MCL recession. For medial side laxity secondary to MCL damage at the femur, the MCL can be recessed into a bony trough created at the distal femur with sutures brought through and tied over the lateral side. This re-creates the anatomic insertion site for the MCL and improves isometricity of the ligament repair.

Knee Dislocation

Multiple knee ligament disruptions and vascular injuries can occur with complete dislocation of the knee. Recognition and treatment of these injuries must be prompt because of the importance of the neurovascular structures. Anterior knee dislocation has a high frequency of vascular injury due to traction on the popliteal artery; this injury usually results in an intraluminal thrombus which can occur soon after injury or can be delayed for up to 2 weeks. Posterior knee dislocation can cause acute popliteal laceration. In all instances of knee dislocation, both cruciates and one or both collateral ligaments are disrupted. Popliteal artery injuries are reported in 10% to 50% of knee dislocations; peroneal nerve injury is seen in 20% to 40% of these cases. The vascular injury must be corrected within 6 to 8 hours after injury to decrease the need for limb amputation. Amputation is required in approximately 10% of knee dislocations. Early treatment should consist of closed reduction, arteriography, and immediate vascular repair if needed. Repair of torn ligaments should be performed only after the vascular supply has been restored, the overall status of the limb has stabilized, and artery or vein repairs have healed (usually 2 to 4 weeks).

The Menisci

The medial and lateral menisci play major roles in load transmission, joint stability, lubrication, and nutrition of articular cartilage. Long-term studies show progressive osteoarthritic changes in patients who have had either the medial or the lateral meniscus removed. In the knee that has a tear of the ACL, the loss of menisci is the prime factor causing long-term progressive disability.

The most frequent causes of meniscus tears are injuries that disrupt one or both cruciate ligaments. Noncontact is most common and usually involves knee flexion or rotation. When excess stress causes forward tibial motion, the ACL tears. The meniscus becomes trapped between the femoral condyle and the tibia and tears in a vertical-longitudinal (circumferential) direction.

Meniscus injuries can cause mechanical symptoms or pain. Displaceable tears cause sensations of catching, popping, or locking. The symptom of giving-way of the knee is due to instability because of loss of the ACL and not because of the meniscus tear. Degenerative tears, such as horizontal cleavage tears or flap tears, cause different types of symptoms which tend to be more subtle. Symptoms of dull aching and pain that gradually gets worse with use are due to degenerative joint changes and not to a torn meniscus.

The peripheral 10% to 30% of the meniscus and the anterior and posterior meniscus horns are well vascularized and have the potential for healing. The vascular supply originates from the geniculate arteries. These vessels give rise to the perimeniscal capillary plexus that supplies the peripheral border of the meniscus. There is also a layer of synovial tissue that covers the peripheral portion and anterior and posterior horns of both menisci. In the lateral meniscus, an avascular region exists in the posterolateral section adjacent to the popliteus tendon. There is evidence that meniscus tears in the vascular regions can heal when repaired.

In young patients who have vertical-longitudinal tears within the peripheral 3 mm of the meniscus or at the meniscocapsular junction, the meniscus usually should be repaired rather than removed. Healing of circumferential tears farther from the periphery and other tear patterns has not been established. When performing any meniscus repair, arthroscopically or via arthrotomy, the neurovascular structures must be protected. If arthroscopic repair is attempted, an incision is necessary so that the saphenous nerve can be identified medially and the peroneal nerve can be identified and protected laterally from injury.

Partial meniscectomy with removal of the unstable portion of the meniscus is preferred to complete meniscectomy. Removal of as little meniscal tissue as possible, so that a balanced, stable rim is created, is important.

Degenerative meniscus tears are best treated by partial meniscectomy if the patient has mechanical symptoms such as popping associated with pain. Weight-bearing radiographs of the knee flexed 30° to 45° help determine the degree of articular cartilage loss (Fig. 8). With significant joint space narrowing, partial meniscectomy can aggravate symptoms and hasten the progression of osteoarthritis.

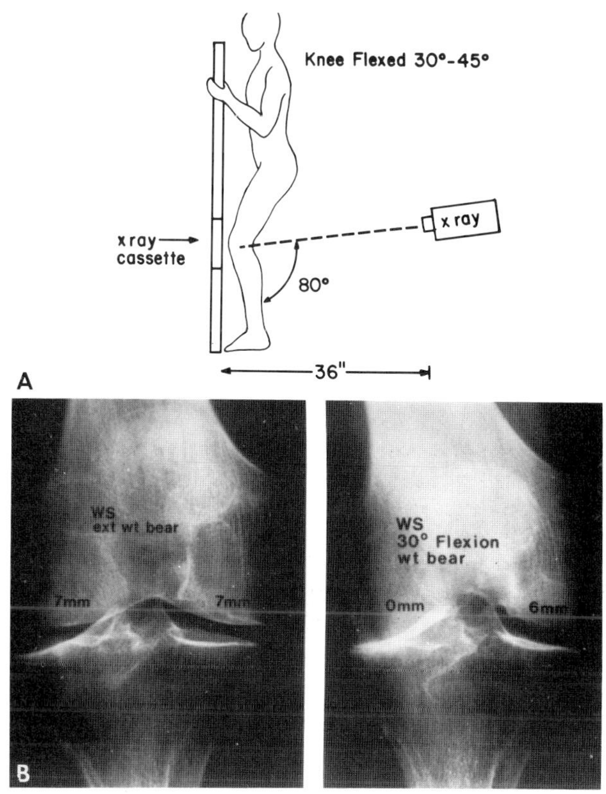

Figure 8

Weight-bearing with the knee flexed, showing bone-on-bone contact of the medial or lateral compartment. *A*, Technique for obtaining 30° to 45° flexion weight-bearing radiograph. *B*, Standing anteroposterior radiograph in extension (*Left*) and at 30° flexion (*Right*).

The Patella

Patellofemoral disorders are often difficult to diagnose and to treat. Patellofemoral alignment and stability can be evaluated by several tests. The passive patellar tilt test (Fig. 9 *A*) assesses patellar laxity when the lateral patellar edge is elevated from the femoral condyle. A 0° or a negative patellar tilt angle usually reflects excessive lateral retinacular tightness. The passive patellar glide test estimates lateral patellar excursion. The test can be performed with the knee in full extension and at varying degrees of flexion; this test helps determine the tightness of the medial patellar restraints. To estimate lateral patellar excursion, the width of the patella is divided into fourths longitudinally (Fig. 9 *B*); lateral overhang in excess of half the width of the patella usually indicates lax or torn medial patellofemoral restraints.

Although the quadriceps (Q) angle has not proved to be significant in many pathologic patellofemoral conditions, determination of the "functional" Q angle appears to be useful. The active lateral patellar glide test helps estimate the functional Q angle. With the knee flexed at 20°, the patient is asked to contract the quadriceps, and the amount of lateral patellar excursion is estimated. If lateral patellar excursion exceeds superior excursion, this reflects an increased functional Q angle, indicating an excessive lateral quadriceps vector (Fig. 9 *C*).

The integrity of patellar articular cartilage can be assessed by active knee extension starting with the hips and knees flexed to 90°. As the patient flexes and extends the knee, the amount of crepitus heard and felt correlates with the degree of chondrosis in the patellofemoral articulation.

Excessive compression of a lateral patellar facet has been implicated as a cause of patellofemoral pain. This is seen in patients who have lateral patellar tilt and tight lateral restraints. Radiography can show an increased lateral tilt on the tangential view taken with the knee between 20° and 40° of flexion (Fig. 10). Lateral patellar compression can often be reduced with a lateral release done either arthroscopically or as an open procedure. Hemarthrosis is the most common complication of lateral release and should be avoided by meticulous attention to hemostasis of the superior and inferior lateral geniculate vessels. Lateral release should not be performed indiscriminately for patients with patellofemoral pain. Lateral release for undiagnosed patellofemoral disorders or in knees with a gross patellar laxity or large Q angle is inappropriate. This conclusion is

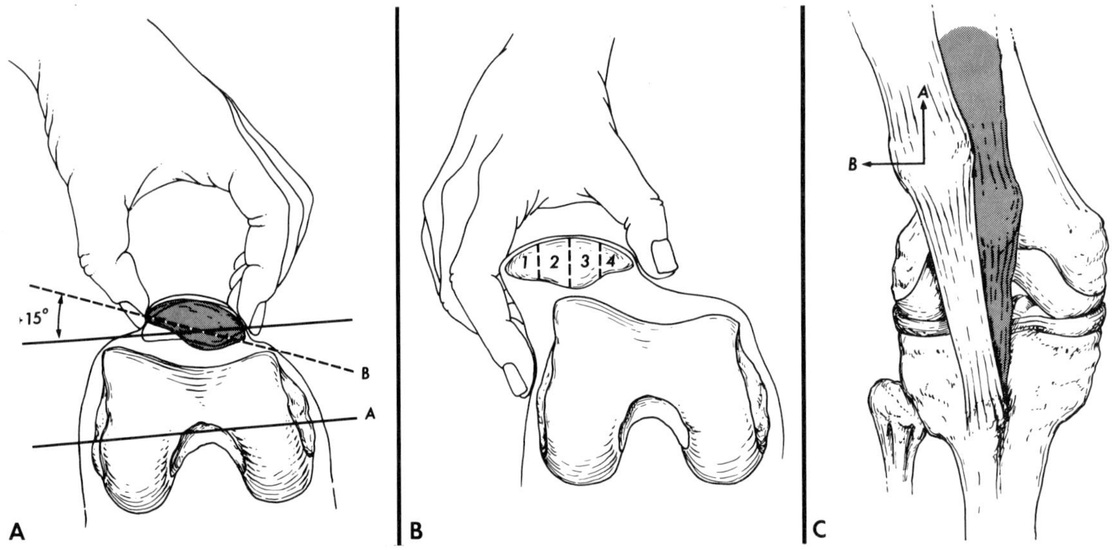

Figure 9

A, Passive patellar tilt of +15° is demonstrated. A tilt of 0° or less indicates tight lateral restraints. *B*, Passive lateral glide test, demonstrating a patella being subluxated laterally to half its width; subluxation beyond this point is a sign of excess laxity of the medial restraints. *C*, Active lateral glide test, demonstrating lateral excursion of the patella upon active quadriceps contraction. If lateral excursion (B) exceeds proximal excursion (A), an increased "functional" Q angle is present.

supported by long-term studies that show poor results in these problems.

Patients who have patellar subluxation or dislocation should be evaluated for: 1) lateral restraint tightness, 2) medial restraint laxity, and 3) functional Q angle. Patellar subluxation in the presence of tight lateral patellar restraints alone can be treated with lateral retinacular release only. A passive patellar glide test that reveals overhang greater than 75% of the width of the patella signifies laxity of the medial restraints. This type of knee problem should be treated with a medial reefing procedure and a lateral release. If the patella demonstrates excessive lateral excursion and if the Q angle is high, proximal and distal realignment should be performed. In patients who have

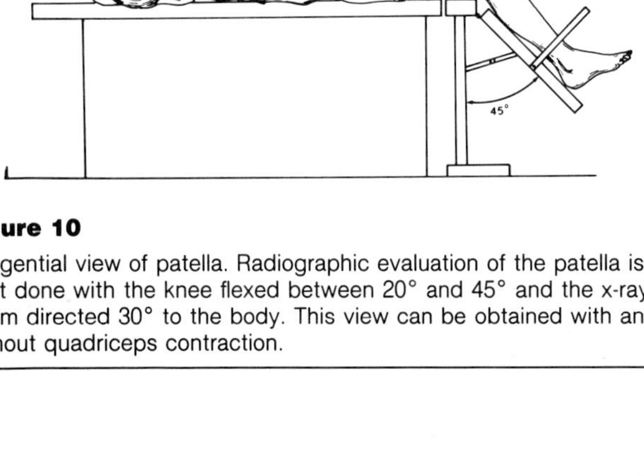

Figure 10

Tangential view of patella. Radiographic evaluation of the patella is best done with the knee flexed between 20° and 45° and the x-ray beam directed 30° to the body. This view can be obtained with and without quadriceps contraction.

long-standing patellar instability with severe chondrosis of the patellofemoral joint, realignment can be combined with a tibial tubercle elevation or patellectomy.

If a patient has an acute patellar dislocation and hemarthrosis, arthroscopy can be useful. An osteochondral fracture of the medial patellar facet or lateral femoral condyle is common in these patients.

If the patient has patellofemoral arthrosis due to long-standing malalignment or trauma, anterior transposition of the tibial tubercle (Maquet procedure) can relieve the symptoms in some patients. The goal of this procedure is to decrease the patellofemoral compression force. Anterior transposition can be combined with other realignment procedures. Biomechanical studies show that this procedure decreases the contact force on the patellofemoral articular cartilage. Long-term clinical studies have shown satisfactory results in properly selected patients. Patellectomy is an effective procedure to decrease severe pain due to patellofemoral arthrosis. Although patellectomy weakens quadriceps strength, it can produce functional increases in strength and satisfactory long-term results.

A common diagnosis is chondromalacia patellae. This is a pathologic diagnosis, not a clinical term. Causes of anterior knee pain such as patellar tendinitis must also be considered. Chondromalacia patellae is usually a result of repetitive overload of the articular surface that results in articular cartilage breakdown. It usually is a self-limited condition that is best treated nonoperatively. Lateral release is seldom successful in chondromalacia patellae that is not associated with excessive lateral patellar compression. In patients who have severe pain, swelling, and crepitus due to chondromalacia patellae, arthroscopic debridement can relieve symptoms, at least for the short term.

The Proximal Tibiofibular Joint

The proximal articulation of the tibia and fibula, with its own synovial cavity, is separate from the tibial-femoral joint. Its stability is provided by bony geometry: The head of the fibula rests in a sulcus provided by the lateral aspect of the proximal tibia. Anterior and posterior tibiofibular ligaments help to stabilize the joint. Dislocation of the proximal tibiofibular joint can occur in three directions. Posterior-medial dislocation is rare and is usually the result of direct trauma to the head of the fibula. Posterior dislocation, equally rare, is usually associated with proximal tibial fracture. Anterior-lateral dislocation is most common and usually is the result of a fall on an inverted foot with the knee flexed as the leg is adducted (this is a common skating injury).

Dislocation or subluxation of the tibiofibular joint should be suspected if there is obvious prominence of the head of the fibula or a history of recurrent locking or catching at the lateral aspect of the knee joint. Radiographs demonstrate lateral displacement of the fibula on the anteroposterior view if the fibula is displaced. Radiographs are usually normal if the joint subluxates. Physical examination demonstrates increased anteroposterior laxity of the fibular head in relation to the tibia, compared with the contralateral knee. In acute dislocations, peroneal nerve injury can be present. Closed reduction followed by 6 weeks of immobilization is recommended. In the knee that has a chronic unreduced dislocation or a recurrent subluxation, fibular head resection or soft tissue reconstruction is usually effective.

Knee Arthroscopy

The usefulness of arthroscopy and arthroscopic surgery has increased dramatically in the past several years. In the acutely injured knee, arthroscopy combined with examination under anesthesia can give information needed to make appropriate decisions regarding treatment.

The standard arthroscope (4 or 5 mm in diameter; 25° oblique view) is used for most procedures. A 70° oblique arthroscope can be used to obtain better visualization of the posterior compartments. The 70° arthroscope is passed into the posterior compartments between the femoral condyle and cruciate ligament. The standard portals used in arthroscopy are the anterolateral portal located 2 cm above the joint line close to the patellar tendon and the anteromedial portal also located 2 cm proximal to the joint line but 1 cm medial to the patellar tendon (Fig. 11). Other portals can be placed posteromedially and posterolaterally to remove loose bodies, to perform synovectomy posteriorly, or for access to the meniscus. Superolateral and superomedial portals give good access to the patellofemoral joint and the suprapatellar pouch. The transpatellar tendon or central portal is utilized less often than the others but is useful as a third portal for meniscus surgery, especially for access to the posteromedial compartment. Triangulation, the method used for performing most arthroscopic surgical procedures, is performed by inserting an instrument through one portal while viewing through another. Video arthroscopy has the advantages of direct viewing on the video monitor, video recording, and sterility but can be difficult to learn.

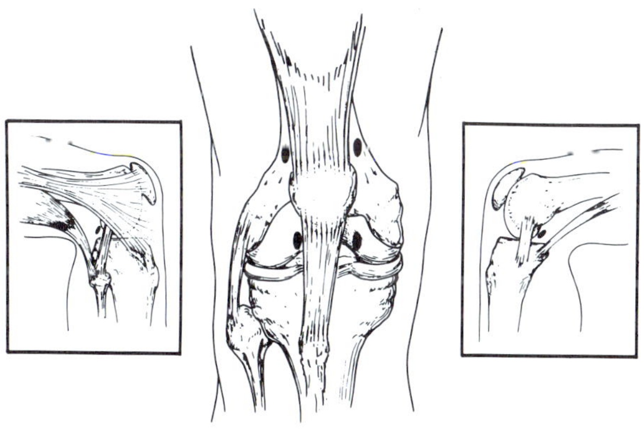

Figure 11

The six portals most commonly used for arthroscopic surgery.

Loose bodies can be located in the anterior intercondylar area, in the suprapatellar pouch, posteriorly in the intercondylar notch region, or in the lateral gutter. Occasionally, loose bodies are in the popliteus tendon sheath or near the tibial attachment of the PCL. The arthroscope should be inserted into the posterior compartments either through the notch or posteromedial and posterolateral portals if a loose body is suspected but not found.

The medial synovial plica or shelf is a synovial fold found in 60% of normal knees. Rarely, this plica becomes thickened and fibrotic, causing anteromedial joint pain and snapping. In these cases, arthroscopic excision of the plica results in relief of symptoms. However, most plicae are asymptomatic and should be left undisturbed.

Many synovial disorders can be treated with the aid of arthroscopy. Synovectomy to treat rheumatoid arthritis or pigmented villonodular synovitis can be performed by using a six-portal technique. This gives access to the posterior compartments. Arthroscopic synovectomy is a difficult and time-consuming procedure. However, postoperative rehabilitation is easier for the patient.

Arthroscopy is not without complications, however. A recent national survey found an overall complication rate of at least 0.8%. Complications include infection, hemarthrosis, instrument breakage within the joint, thrombophlebitis, and neurovascular complications. The most common complication is damage to the articular surfaces from the arthroscopic instruments, especially when complicated procedures are performed and high-energy mechanical instruments are used.

Rehabilitation

Recent changes in surgical techniques for knee ligament repair and reconstruction have resulted in significant changes in the rehabilitation protocol. Ligament repair using strong grafts, isometric or anatomic placement, and secure fixation has allowed important modifications in rehabilitation to help prevent the undesirable consequences of immobility. Early, limited joint motion but avoiding excessive stresses on healing ligament tissue is a well-established principle. Proper postoperative rehabilitation and bracing are essential to ensure a consistent outcome after operation.

Patients should be encouraged to perform voluntary isometric muscle contractions after operation. Galvanic neuromuscular stimulators also can be used. Isometric exercise does not prevent disuse atrophy but helps to maintain neuromuscular coordination so that atrophy can be reversed more easily when immobility is discontinued. Recently developed high-frequency muscle stimulators can provide more intense stimulation than earlier units. These are less painful and can give better strength gains. The muscles should be stimulated early in the postoperative period and frequently. Specific muscle groups should be stimulated, depending upon the nature of the injury or the operation. For example, the hamstrings should be stimulated after ACL surgery and the quadriceps, after PCL surgery.

Continuous passive motion has been used experimentally after certain knee ligament reconstructive operations; the ligament fixation must be extremely secure and the motion should be restricted and passive. Knee motion to the extremes of flexion and extension increases strain on repaired ligaments and attachment sites, and ligament failure can occur, especially if active motion is too early.

Active range of motion effort usually is delayed for 4 to 6 weeks after ligament repair, but this depends on the procedure that was performed. Full extension is blocked to prevent the quadriceps from straining the repair in the range 0° to 40° of flexion. Gradually increasing the range is then allowed until full range of motion is obtained. If the patient fails to gain an increase in range of motion by 3 or 4 months after operation, closed manipulation or arthroscopic release should be considered.

The mainstay of muscle rehabilitation is progressive resistance exercise. This approach, popularized in the 1940s, uses isotonic exercises in gradually increasing amounts. Because the resistance is constant in isotonic exercise, the muscles are not loaded to maximal capacity at all joint positions. Variable resistance exercise devices have been developed that use cams to provide high resistance throughout the full range of joint motion. Although there is some question about whether these devices actually achieve this goal, they are widely used.

Isokinetic exercises that limit the rate at which the joint can move allow variable resistance at a constant velocity. This can develop strength at varying joint speeds. Isokinetic devices have the disadvantages of variable resistance that is patient-controlled and unpredictable vector forces at the knee. This is particularly true for the patellofemoral joint which is extremely vulnerable to excess force in the range of 30° to 60° of flexion.

Recently, attention has been directed toward rehabilitating muscles both concentrically (resistance with muscle shortening) and eccentrically (resistance with muscle lengthening). Computer-assisted exercise machines have been developed that control exercise rate (isokinetic devices) and also provide resistance in concentric and eccentric modes. Extreme caution must be used with these types of machines because muscle or tendon overload is possible in the eccentric phase.

Despite the various types of exercise devices and regimens that are available, the underlying exercise principle is the same: a muscle responds to an applied force with hypertrophy. If the physician selectively controls the demands that are placed on the muscles about the knee, he can protect healing tissues and yet develop muscle power and coordination with the simplest of devices. Isometric, isotonic, and isokinetic exercises all can be part of a rehabilitation protocol. Nevertheless, prescriptions should be individualized rather than applied to all patients indiscriminately. Factors that influence which exercises can be safely prescribed postoperatively are 1) whether the surgical procedure was intra- or extra-articular; 2) whether or not the repair was isometric; 3) whether other procedures, in addition to the ligament repair, were performed (i.e., patellofemoral realignment or meniscus repair); 4) individual patient characteristics that affect injury and healing (such as generalized hypermobility of joints); and 5) level of athletic activity or expected demands on the joint.

Knee Bracing

Knee braces are designed to control instability, limit motion, and allow controlled range of motion. They can be classified as *rehabilitative braces, "prophylactic" braces,* and *functional braces.*

Rehabilitative braces protect injured knees and limit their motion. They are used after injury or postoperatively. These braces have replaced casts and hinged casts in many instances. Their advantages include light weight, ease of application and removal, and ability to regulate motion. Their disadvantages include lack of ability to control rotation and, in some instances, translation. Braces are easily removed but can shift on the leg, thus changing the hinge position. When maximal control of motion and position are critical, they should not be used.

"Prophylactic" knee braces, such as the lateral knee braces used in football, are becoming increasingly popular although there has been no clinical or laboratory proof to substantiate the claim that they prevent valgus injuries. In fact, several studies have shown either no change or a slight increase in knee injuries with use of these braces. Most currently available models are structurally too weak to prevent medial joint opening with valgus forces. There is a need to develop stronger braces with better hinge designs and to perform additional prospective studies to determine the efficacy of braces in preventing knee injury.

Functional knee braces are used in athletics by patients who have chronic knee instability or to protect the knee after ligament repair. Beginning with "derotation" braces in the 1970s, their number has expanded rapidly. Functional braces are designed to prevent excess joint motion during work or sports. Functional knee braces do not effectively control gross laxity or rotation. Functional braces that prevent anterior tibial subluxation due to a torn ACL are most effective if hyperextension is prevented. Braces that have thigh and calf shells and are designed to have a four-point restraining system appear to be most effective.

Running Injuries

Soft tissue injuries about the knee and leg secondary to long-distance running have increased dramatically with the increased number of runners. Running injuries usually result from overuse secondary to stress failure of collagen tissue. In these instances, the rate of breakdown exceeds the rate of the reparative process.

Anterior Knee Pain

This is the most common knee complaint of runners and is due to excessive repetitive stress on the patellofemoral joint and extensor mechanism. A common pathologic condition causing anterior knee pain is chronic patellar tendinitis or "jumper's knee." This often occurs in patients who have patellofemoral malalignment or tight hamstrings. It also occurs if the runner lands too hard on the forefoot repetitively during running. Excessive foot pronation can contribute to patellofemoral malalignment and should be corrected by using orthotics if present. Running on level surfaces and avoiding hills and stairs should be stressed to the patient.

Iliotibial Band Friction Syndrome ("Runner's Knee")

This is characterized by pain in the region of the lateral epicondyle of the femur. The underlying pathologic condition can be popliteus tendinitis in some instances. This syndrome generally results from excessive hill running, particularly downhill. Tenderness at the lateral femoral epicondyle, full range of motion, and absence of effusion or joint line tenderness are typical physical findings. Treatment consists of rest, anti-inflammatory medication, and not running on hills until the symptoms have abated.

Pes Anserinus Bursitis

The characteristic is pain in the region of the medial tibia 6 cm below the joint line. Visible swelling and tenderness at the pes anserinus insertion usually are found. As with all "overuse syndromes," anti-inflammatory medication, application of cold, rest, stretching, and strengthening exercises are important in treatment. Pain at the medial proximal tibia also can be caused by a stress fracture. A radionuclide scan is useful in making the distinction if radiographs are negative for fracture.

Chondral Stress Fracture

A common but often misdiagnosed condition, this usually involves the medial femoral condyle. The patient complains of medial compartment pain aggravated by walking and running. Occasionally, medial compartment catching and crepitation are also noted. Medial joint pain can lead to an erroneous diagnosis of a peripheral meniscal tear. A technetium radionuclide scan can demonstrate increased uptake in the medial femoral condyle suggestive of subchondral bone microfracture. At arthroscopy, chondral blistering, fragmentation, or fibrillation is seen. Arthroscopic chondral debridement, abrasion, and drilling of the condylar defect as in the treatment of osteochondritis dissecans has had success in relieving symptoms but not in returning patients to running.

Medial-Tibial Stress Syndrome ("Shin Splints")

This occurs in athletes and causes exercise-induced pain along the posterior-medial aspect of the tibia at the junction of the middle and distal thirds. Intramuscular and intracompartmental pressures in these patients generally are normal or return quickly to normal after exercise. "Periostitis" can be the underlying condition. This condition usually heals with rest. Good results have been obtained after release of the fascial insertion at the posterior-medial aspect of the tibia in the patient who has chronic pain. The medial stress syndrome can be differentiated from chronic compartment syndrome of the deep posterior compartment by comparing compartment pressures at rest and after exercise. It is possible that "shin splints" is a precursor of stress fracture.

Stress Fracture

These fractures of the tibia or fibula secondary to excessive running are not uncommon. The most accurate way of diagnosing a stress fracture is the technetium radionuclide scan. Diffuse uptake along the tibial periosteum is suggestive of periostitis whereas discrete uptake at one or several areas along the tibia or fibula indicates a stress fracture. The treatment for stress fractures requires the avoidance of running and jumping for an extended period (6 to 12 weeks). After point tenderness has subsided from the area of the stress fracture, active rehabilitation exercises that include muscle stretching and strengthening are instituted. Malalignment should be corrected if possible. When the patient resumes running, it should be on soft surfaces on alternate days and the increase in mileage run should be no more than 10% per week until well into the training program.

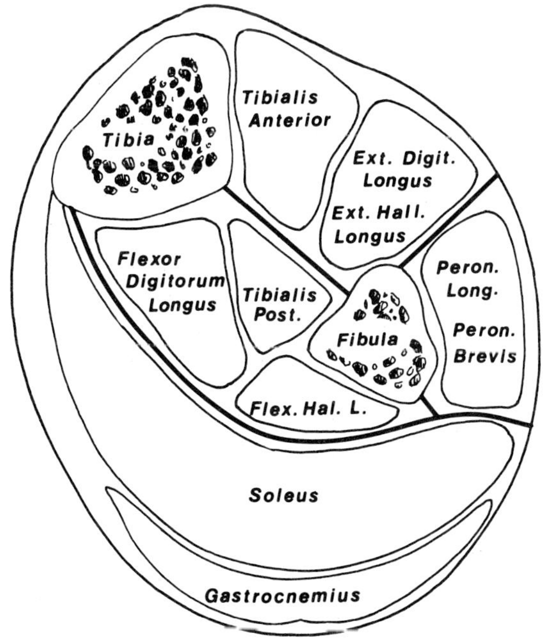

Figure 12

Compartments of the leg at the level of the soleus bridge. Chronic exertional compartment syndrome can affect any compartment but frequently affects the deep posterior compartment or individual muscles within that compartment.

Compartment Syndrome

In this condition, excess pressure occurs within a confined space. It can be acute or chronic. An acute compartment syndrome usually occurs after major trauma to the extremity, although it sometimes can occur after a single major overuse event. Intracompartment pressure above 30 mm Hg for 6 or more hours is sufficient to cause muscle necrosis. A chronic compartment syndrome is an exercise-induced condition in which an excessive increase of intracompartment pressure causes pain shortly after exercise is begun. The pain from increased tissue pressure can be brought on by a 20% increase in muscle mass in the limited space of the compartment. In a patient with a chronic compartment syndrome, compartment pressure is more than 10 mm Hg (normal, −4 to +4 mm Hg). Intracompartment pressure increases to more than 100 mm Hg during exercise and fails to return to less than 15 mm Hg after 30 minutes of rest. Release of the fascia that envelopes the involved compartment usually is curative. Release of individual myofascial compartments is required for the relief of symptoms (Fig. 12).

Annotated Bibliography

Anterior Cruciate Ligament

Natural History

McDaniel, W.J., Jr., and Dameron, T.B., Jr.: The untreated anterior cruciate ligament rupture. Clin. Orthop. 172:158–163, 1983.

Forty-nine patients (52 knees) with untreated ACL ruptures were evaluated a mean of 14 years after injury. The results were compared with those of a 10-year follow-up study in the same patients. Eighty-six percent of the knees had one or both menisci removed. There had been little change in symptoms since the 10-year study except that the incidence of giving-way had decreased. The incidence of degenerative changes on the radiographs had increased, with one-third of the knees demonstrating joint space narrowing or unequivocal evidence of osteoarthritis. Development of degenerative changes was associated with varus deformity, meniscectomy, and relatively heavy body weight.

Diagnosis

Donaldson, W.F., III; Warren, R.F.; and Wickiewicz, T.: A comparison of acute anterior cruciate ligament examinations: Initial versus examination under anesthesia. Am. J. Sports Med. 13:5–10, 1985.

Results of the preoperative examination, findings under anesthesia, and findings at operation were compared for acutely injured knees with a documented ACL tear. The Lachman test was positive initially in 99% and under anesthesia in 100%. The pivot shift was positive in 35% initially and improved to 98% under anesthesia. The anterior drawer test was positive initially in 70% and increased to 91% under anesthesia. The Lachman test was unaffected by associated ligamentous injuries and was very reliable, having an absence of end point in all complete ACL tears.

Markolf, K.L.; Kochan, A.; and Amstutz, H.C.: Measurement of knee stiffness and laxity in patients with documented absence of anterior cruciate ligament. J. Bone Joint Surg. 66A:242–253, 1984.

Thirty-five patients with documented absence of their ACL were tested on an instrumented clinical knee-testing apparatus, and the response curves for the following test modes were measured: anteroposterior (AP) force versus displacement at 0°, 20°, and 90° of flexion; varus-valgus moment versus angulation at 0° and 20°; tibial torque versus rotation at 20°. The AP laxity was greatest at 20° of flexion with a mean increase of 5.5 mm at 200 N of applied AP force (compared to 3.1 mm and 2.5 mm at 0° and 90°). At 20° and 90°, the AP laxity was greatest with 15° of external rotation of the foot. Varus-valgus laxity was moderately increased, pointing out the secondary restraint function of the ACL.

Intra-articular

Bartlett, E.C.: Arthroscopic repair and augmentation of the anterior cruciate ligament in cadaver knees. Clin. Orthop. 172:107–111, 1983.

An experimental method for arthroscopic repair and augmentation of the ACL was designed in cadaver specimens. The manner of arthroscopic repair is described; it avoids the adverse effects of arthrotomy and patellar dislocation. A specially designed drill guide as well as a braided internal suture and fascia lata graft are used. The principles of treatment of ACL injury, isometric placement, preservation of vascularity, and preservation of normal structures are followed.

Clancy, W.G., Jr.: Anterior cruciate ligament functional instability. A static intra-articular and dynamic extra-articular procedure. Clin. Orthop. 172:102–106, 1983.

Fifty patients were evaluated at a minimum of 2 years after intra- and extra-articular ligament reconstruction for chronic ACL instability. The central one-third of the patellar tendon with its attached patella and tibial bone was used. A biceps transfer and pes transfer was done extra-articularly. The results were encouraging, with a return to sports reported in 46 of 49, and 47 of 49 had good to excellent results.

Jensen, J.E.; Slocum, D.B.; Larson, R.L.; James, S.L.; and Singer, K.M.: Reconstruction procedures for anterior cruciate ligament insufficiency: A computer analysis of clinical results. Am. J. Sports Med. 11:240–248, 1983.

A preoperative and postoperative study of 205 patients who had surgical reconstruction of the ACL of the knee was evaluated with a prototype computer program. At mean follow-up of 4.1 years, there was a 27% decrease in subjective complaints and an 8% improvement in objective findings. The anterior drawer was improved in 25%, and subluxation of the lateral tibial plateau was improved in 58%, correlating highly with a good result. Seventy-four percent of patients had undergone medial meniscectomy, 58% had lateral meniscectomy, and 41% had both menisci removed at follow-up after reconstruction.

Kochan, A.; Markolf, K.L.; and More, R.C.: Anterior-posterior stiffness and laxity of the knee after major ligament reconstruction. J. Bone Joint Surg. 66A:1460–1465, 1984.

Eighteen patients with chronic ACL instability were evaluated for stiffness and laxity, both preoperatively and postoperatively at 3 years. Patients who received only an extracapsular stabilization procedure showed no change in the injured knee in either laxity or stiffness at 20° and 90°. Those who underwent intra-articular repair (using one-third of the patellar tendon) and extracapsular repair showed a significant decrease in anterior laxity with an increase in anterior stiffness at 20° of flexion. These improvements in stability were not seen at 90°. Six patients with intra- and extra-articular reconstruction tested at both 1 and 3 years postoperatively showed no changes, indicating that their graft had not stretched.

Odensten, M.; Lysholm, J.; and Gillquist, J.: Suture of fresh ruptures of the anterior cruciate ligament: A 5-year follow-up. Acta Orthop. Scand. 55:270–272, 1984.

Thirty-five of 41 consecutive patients were followed for 5 years after early primary suture of the acutely torn ACL and repair of all other injured structures. The ACL repair was not augmented. Twenty-three patients were evaluated early (at 2 years postoperatively). From the early to the late follow-up, the function of the knees operated on decreased significantly.

Paulos, L.E.; Butler, D.L.; Noyes, F.R.; and Grood, E.S.: Intra-articular cruciate reconstruction. II: Replacement with vascularized patellar tendon. Clin. Orthop. 172:78–84, 1983.

The patellar tendon offers a number of advantages (strength, location, bone-to-bone fixation, vascularity) as a tissue for intra-articular ACL reconstruction. The authors present a new technique using the medial one-third of the patellar tendon and its contiguous neurovascular supply. This procedure was used in 100 patients over a 3-year period with encouraging results.

Extra-articular

Krackow, K.A., and Brooks, R.L.: Optimization of knee ligament position for lateral extraarticular reconstruction. Am. J. Sports Med. 11:293–302, 1983.

A kinematic study of cadaver knees was undertaken, using

multiple pairs of markers on the lateral aspect of the distal femur and proximal tibia and measuring their separation distances as the knee was taken through full range of motion. The optimal tibial attachment site appears to be anterior to Gerdy's tubercle. This would be paired with a femoral attachment proximal and posterior to the natural lateral collateral ligament origin. Reduction of the variance of separation distances may reduce the "stretching out" seen with many extra-articular procedures.

Odensten, M.; Lysholm, J.; and Gillquist, J.: Long-term follow-up study of a distal iliotibial band transfer (DIT) for anterolateral knee instability. Clin. Orthop. 176:129–135, 1983.

A prospective study of 60 consecutive patients who underwent distal iliotibial band transfer for anterolateral knee instability. A knee function score was obtained preoperatively and at 17 and 40 months postoperatively. Although improved at 17 months, the knee score decreased significantly at 40 months. Stability tests revealed 80% stable at 17 months but only 42% stable at 40 months.

Synthetic Replacement

Bolton, C.W., and Bruchman, W.C.: The GORE-TEX™ expanded polytetrafluoroethylene prosthetic ligament: An *in vitro* and *in vivo* evaluation. Clin. Orthop. 196:202–213, 1985.

An *in vitro* and *in vivo* analysis of the Gore-Tex ACL prosthesis is presented. Tensile strength is 3 times that of the normal ACL. *In vivo* tests using sheep showed good stability and fixation strength. Early results of clinical evaluation at 15 different centers are encouraging.

Roth, J.H.; Kennedy, J.C.; Lockstadt, H.; McCallum, C.L.; and Cunning, L.A.: Polypropylene braid augmented and nonaugmented intraarticular anterior cruciate ligament reconstruction. Am. J. Sports Med. 13:321–326, 1985.

A restorative study of the efficacy of a polypropylene braid (PB) used to augment an intra-articular ACL autograft (central one-third patellar tendon and quadriceps tendon). Two consecutive series, 38 nonaugmented and 45 augmented, are compared. On objective laxity and function testing, the PB-augmented had better results. On subjective questioning, physician's examination, and radiography, the PB-augmented did better.

Posterior Cruciate Ligament

Baker, C.L., Jr.; Norwood, L.A.; and Hughston, J.C.: Acute combined posterior cruciate and posterolateral instability of the knee. Am. J. Sports Med. 12:204–208, 1984.

Thirteen patients are reviewed who underwent operative treatment for acute combined posterior cruciate and posterolateral instability. The diagnosis can be made with a combined positive response to the posterior drawer test, the anterior drawer test with tibia internally rotated, adduction and abduction stress with knee fully extended, posterolateral drawer test, and external rotation-recurvatum test. This combination occurs more often than appreciated and, when all structures are repaired, functional and subjective results will be good.

Clancy, W.G., Jr.; Shelbourne, K.D.; Zoellner, G.B.; Keene, J.S.; Reider, B.; and Rosenberg, T.D.: Treatment of knee joint instability secondary to rupture of the posterior cruciate ligament. J. Bone Joint Surg. 65A:310–322, 1983.

Both chronic and acute PCL injuries were repaired with a free graft of one-third of the patella tendon with its tibial and patellar attachments. Articular damage to the medial femoral condyle showed a high correlation to interval of instability in the chronic cases. The procedure had good overall functional and static results in both acute and chronic cases.

Cross, M.J., and Powell, J.F.: Long-term followup of posterior cruciate ligament rupture: A study of 116 cases. Am. J. Sports Med. 12:292–297, 1984.

A retrospective review of 116 cases of PCL instability showed the benefit of conservative treatment. Quadriceps tone correlated well with eventual results: increased tone and strength was associated with better results. Posterior drawer sign had poor correlation with eventual results. Patients with sport-related injuries did much better than those with traffic accident injuries.

Hughston, J.C., and Jacobson, K.E.: Chronic posterolateral rotatory instability of the knee. J. Bone Joint Surg. 67A:351–359, 1985.

Ninety-five patients with a 2- to 13-year follow-up are reviewed after reconstruction for chronic posterolateral rotary instability. The diagnosis was dependent on the posterolateral drawer chest and external rotation-recurvatum tests. The procedure consisted of advancement of the arcuate ligament complex with its osseous attachment. Results were good in approximately 80%.

Posterolateral Laxity

Jakob, R.P.; Hassler, H.; and Staeubli, H.-U.: Observations on rotatory instability in the lateral compartment of the knee. Acta Orthop. Scand. [Suppl.] 191:1–32, 1981.

The reversed pivot shift sign is a constant finding in acute or chronic posterolateral instability. It represents the posterior subluxation of the lateral tibial plateau and its jerk-like reduction. It is tested by holding the tibia externally rotated with a slight valgus stress and bringing the knee from 70° of flexion to extension. Reduction occurs at approximately 20°.

Lateral Collateral Ligament

DeLee, J.C.; Riley, M.B.; and Rockwood, C.A., Jr.: Acute straight lateral instability of the knee. Am. J. Sports Med. 11:404–411, 1983.

Ten patients are reviewed who underwent repair for acute straight lateral instability. In all knees, the ACL, PCL, and arcuate complex were severely disrupted. Direct repair of all ligament tears resulted in good functional results.

Medial Collateral Ligament

Hunter, S.C.; Marascalco, R.; and Hughston, J.C.: Disruption of the vastus medialis obliquus with medial knee ligament injuries. Am. J. Sports Med. 11:427–431, 1983.

A retrospective review of 189 consecutive MCL injuries surgically repaired was undertaken to determine the frequency of vastus medialis disruption concurrent with MCL tears. Forty disruptions were observed, of which 31 were avulsions from the adductor tubercle. Recognizing and treating disruptions of the vastus medialis can prevent chronic disorders of the extensor mechanisms.

Indelicato, P.A.: Non-operative treatment of complete tears of the medial collateral ligament of the knee. J. Bone Joint Surg. 65A:323–329, 1983.

This prospective study compared the results of operative and nonoperative treatment for isolated grade III MCL tears. All patients underwent arthroscopy to rule out associated damage. The results showed no advantage with surgical repair; rehabilitation was expedited in the patients treated with cast-bracing only.

Multiple Ligament and Neuromuscular Injuries

Sisto, D.J., and Warren, R.F.: Complete knee dislocation: A follow-up study of operative treatment. Clin. Orthop. 198:94–101, 1985.

Twenty knee dislocations occurring over a period of 20 years are reviewed. Sixteen knees underwent ligamentous reconstruction, of which 13 were acute. Vascular injury occurred in 10% and peroneal nerve injury, in 40%. Early operative repair followed by cast-bracing and manipulation at 3 months (if flexion is less than 90°) is recommended in young, active adults.

Meniscus Symptoms

Hamberg, P.; Gillquist, J.; and Lysholm, J.: Suture of new and old peripheral meniscus tears. J. Bone Joint Surg. 65A:193–197, 1983.

Fifty-one patients underwent open meniscal repair for peripheral tears, of which 35 were chronic. At 18-month follow-up, 84% had healed clinically. Repeat arthroscopy in 27 patients showed that all had healed. There were eight second tears after the initial repair.

Northmore-Ball, M.D.; Dandy, D.J.; and Jackson, R.W.: Arthroscopic, open partial, and total meniscectomy: A comparative study. J. Bone Joint Surg. 65B:400–404, 1983.

The results of three different types of meniscectomy are compared in 219 knees: arthroscopic partial meniscectomy in 71, open partial meniscectomy in 45, and open total meniscectomy in 103. Mean follow-up was 4.3 years. Knees treated by arthroscopic partial meniscectomy did considerably better by all criteria. Partial meniscectomy did better than total.

Patellofemoral Symptoms and Diagnosis

Jensen, C.M., and Roosen, J.U.: Acute traumatic dislocations of the patella. J. Trauma 25:160–162, 1985.

Twenty-three consecutive patients with acute traumatic patellar dislocations were followed for a mean of 39 months. All had a medial capsulorrhaphy and 8 had a lateral release. There were two dislocations, one in a lateral release patient. The patients in the lateral release group had a high incidence of chondromalacia at follow-up.

Ogilvie-Harris, D.J., and Jackson, R.W.: The arthroscopic treatment of chondromalacia patellae. J. Bone Joint Surg. 66B:660–665, 1984.

Three hundred nineteen patients who had chondromalacia patellae and persistent patellofemoral pain after 6 months of conservative management underwent arthroscopic surgery. Shaving was effective in relieving symptoms in the post-traumatic group. Lateral release and shaving were effective in the malalignment group. In the unstable patella, only one in four was aided by lateral release.

Simpson, L.A., and Barrett, J.P., Jr.: Factors associated with poor results following arthroscopic subcutaneous lateral retinacular release. Clin. Orthop. 186:165–171, 1984.

Forty-eight patients (55 knees) who underwent arthroscopic subcutaneous lateral retinacular release were followed for an average of 15 months. Factors contributing to a poor result include advancing age, postoperative hemarthrosis, incomplete release, incomplete quadriceps rehabilitation, and severe ligamentous laxity. During operation, release of the tight lateral tether is essential to produce a positive "tilt" sign, signifying complete release.

Tibia and Fibula

Turco, V.J., and Spinella, A.J.: Anterolateral dislocation of the head of the fibula in sports. Am. J. Sports Med. 13:209–215, 1985.

Seventeen cases of traumatic anterolateral dislocation of the head of the fibula are presented; 7 were acute and 10 were chronic. The mechanism of injury was a fall on the affected flexed knee with the leg adducted under the body and the ankle inverted. Physical examination and radiographic findings need to be carefully evaluated to make the diagnosis. Treatment options are closed or open reduction acutely and local strapping or fibular head resection in the chronic cases.

Rehabilitation

Knee

Hungerford, D.S., and Lennox, D.W.: Rehabilitation of the knee in disorders of the patellofemoral joint: Relevant biomechanics. Orthop. Clin. North Am. 14:397–402, April 1983.

Rehabilitation regimens for patellofemoral disorders should be based on sound biomechanical principles. Using free ankle weights for knee extension exercises will produce patellofemoral joint reactive forces above the physiologic range from 30° to 60°. Rehabilitation instead should include isometric exercises, terminal extension exercises, and minimal impact loading such as cycling and swimming.

Anterior Cruciate Ligament

Arms, S.W.; Pope, M.H.; Johnson, R.J.; Fischer, R.A.; Arvidsson, I.; and Eriksson, E.: The biomechanics of anterior cruciate ligament rehabilitation and reconstruction. Am. J. Sports Med. 12:8–18, 1984.

Strain analysis on cadaver knee ACLs showed that strain was significantly different depending on whether the knee angle changed passively or via simulated quadriceps contraction. Simulated isometric contraction of the quadriceps significantly increased anteromedial ACL strain in the range of 0° to 45° of knee flexion. The anteromedial capsule is an important aspect of strain protection for the ACL.

Henning, C.E.; Lynch, M.A.; and Glick, K.R., Jr.: An in vivo strain gage study of elongation of the anterior cruciate ligament. Am. J. Sports Med. 13:22–26, 1985.

The load-elongation characteristics of a grade II ACL sprain were studied at the time of local anesthesia. The results indicate that the proper order for a rehabilitation program should be crutch-walking, cycling, walking, and slow running. Knee extension exercises less than 45° of flexion caused high strain in the ACL and should be avoided during the first year after ACL injury or reconstruction.

Bracing

American Academy of Orthopaedic Surgeons: Knee Braces: Seminar Report. Chicago, 1985.

A knee brace seminar was held in August 1984 in Chicago to evaluate the various knee braces available to orthopaedists. Braces were divided into three groups: prophylactic knee braces, rehabilitative knee braces, and functional knee braces. The discussion of biomechanical testing and clinical studies showed a need for further delineation of the efficacy of all three types of braces.

Bassett, G.S., and Fleming, B.W.: The Lennox Hill brace in anterolateral rotatory instability. Am. J. Sports Med. 11:345–348, 1983.

Thirty-six patients with anterolateral rotary instability previously fitted with Lennox Hill braces were examined and graded with and without the brace. Patients with grade I instability alone were generally improved. Patients with grade II or combined anterolateral and anteromedial rotary instability had minimal improvement in stability (less than 50%) with use of the brace.

Running Injuries

Li, G.P.; Zhang, S.D.; Chen, G.; Chen, H.; and Wang, A.M.: Radiographic and histologic analyses of stress fracture in rabbit tibias. Am. J. Sports Med. 13:285–294, 1985.

Twenty rabbits were studied for the effects of controlled, excessive running and jumping on the internal structure of the tibia. Periosteal new bone formation was seen 12 days after the initial vascular changes and osteoclastic resorption. Cracks in the cement line were observed as well as incomplete stress fractures in two rabbits and complete fracture in one.

Compartment Syndrome

Davey, J.R.; Rorabeck, C.H.; and Fowler, P.J.: The tibialis posterior muscle compartment. An unrecognized cause of exertional compartment syndrome. Am. J. Sports Med. 12:391–397, 1984.

Cadaver studies revealed that the tibialis posterior is contained in its own osseofascial compartment. A compartment syndrome created in cadaver tibialis posterior specimens was not decompressed by opening the deep posterior fascia. In some cases of exertional compartment syndrome, separate decompression of the tibialis posterior fascia may be required.

37

Knee and Leg: Bone Trauma

Topics covered in this section are fractures of the patella, tibial plateau, and tibial shaft and nonunion of tibial shaft fractures. Compartment syndromes associated with tibial fractures are also discussed.

Patellar Fractures

The functions of the patella are 1) to increase the mechanical advantage of the quadriceps, 2) to aid in the nourishment of the articular surface of the femur, and 3) to protect the femoral condyle from injury. Fractures of the patella constitute approximately 1% of all skeletal injuries, occur more frequently in males (2:1), and can occur at all ages but are most common in persons 40 to 50 years old.

Fractures of the patella with 2 mm of distraction or less and an intact quadriceps mechanism are best managed by early weight-bearing in a cylinder cast for 3 to 6 weeks followed by progressively increasing range of motion exercises. Transverse fractures with more than 2 mm of distraction and disruption of the lateral and medial quadriceps expansions are best treated by anatomic reduction and internal fixation. Tension band wiring consisting of two Kirschner wires introduced vertically across the fracture and a wire loop passed behind the tips of the wires and over the anterior surface of the patella has been demonstrated to provide the strongest internal fixation in most instances. This method of tension band wiring allows early motion of the knee. Accurate repair of the patellar retinaculum must be undertaken at the time of open reduction. The goal of surgical treatment is anatomic reduction and early postoperative motion. This demands stable internal fixation.

Comminuted displaced fractures of the patella are best treated surgically. Partial excision of the patella with repair of the patella tendon or quadriceps tendon is generally successful as long as half of the gliding surface of the patella remains intact. Although total patellectomy may be required when there is extensive comminution and displacement of the fracture fragments, partial patellectomy usually produces better results than total patellectomy. In the elderly patient, especially if there is some preexisting arthritic change in the knee, strong consideration should be given to stable internal fixation, even of comminuted patellar fractures, in an effort to maintain patellar bone stock for possible later total knee arthroplasty. When total patellectomy is performed, one should ensure that the extensor mechanism is stable tracking within the intracondylar notch.

Tibial Plateau Fractures

Tibial plateau fractures usually result from vehicular accidents or falls. The normal knee has a slight valgus alignment and, therefore, the lateral tibial plateau is split or crushed by the lateral femoral condyle upon impact from a fall. Fractures of the medial femoral condyle are much less common. The lateral tibial plateau usually fails before excessive stress is placed on the medial ligament in adults over age 40, but concomitant injuries to medial knee ligaments are estimated to occur in 10% to 30% of the patients with tibial plateau fractures. Arterial and nerve complications are rare but might be overlooked unless evaluation is careful.

To visualize the extent of comminution and displacement, anteroposterior, lateral, and oblique radiographs are necessary. Computed tomography has been reported to provide better visualization of tibial plateau fractures than conventional tomography. Stress films under anesthesia can be useful to diagnose associated injury to the medial collateral ligament or capsule. However, such stress films can also cause increased displacement of the tibial plateau fracture.

If operative repair of a tibial plateau fracture is undertaken, careful planning of the surgical approach is essential. Because of the frequent need for later reconstructive surgery, such as total knee arthroplasty, surgical incisions for open reduction and internal fixation should be longitudinally oriented where possible. Knee stiffness can develop after operation, and prolonged rehabilitation often is necessary. Late traumatic and arthritic changes can occur.

Classification and Treatment

Type I This is a pure cleavage fracture. The lateral femoral condyle is driven into the articular surface of the tibia, creating a wedge-shaped fragment that is split off and displaced outward and downward. If the displacement can be reduced, these fractures can be treated with either hinged-cast immobilization or open reduction and internal fixation with equally good results. Early motion is a key factor in obtaining a satisfactory end result.

Type II This is a cleavage combined with depression. A lateral wedge is split off as in type I but also varying portions of the remaining lateral tibial plateau and articular surface are comminuted and depressed downward into the metaphysis. If there is less than 0.5 cm of depression (especially if the posterior aspect of the tibial plateau is all that is involved), these fractures can be treated with closed reduction with the knee manipulated into varus and held in a hinged cast for 4 to 6 weeks. If the depression is greater than 1 cm, the procedure of choice, particularly in a young patient, is open reduction and internal fixation using a buttress plate and cancellous screw. The depressed fragment should be elevated to its normal position and supported with supplementary bone graft. Early motion in a hinged cast is a critical feature in postoperative care, and prolonged non-weight-bearing must be maintained.

Type III This is a pure central depression fracture. The articular surface of the lateral tibial plateau is depressed and driven into the lateral tibial condyle. There is no lateral wedge, and the lateral cortex is intact. This fracture tends to occur in osteoporotic patients and is commonly due to simple falls with pure axial loading of the tibial plateau. If the depression is less than 1 cm and the knee is stable on examination under anesthesia, these injuries can be treated by hinged-cast immobilization. If the depression is greater than 1 cm, especially in young patients, or if significant valgus instability is found on examination, surgical treatment is recommended. Elevation and packing of bone graft beneath the elevated fragments should be done. Fixation with lag screws or buttress plate is advocated. Postoperative early motion in a cast brace and prolonged non-weight-bearing improves the end results.

Type IV This is a fracture of the medial tibial plateau. There are two distinct kinds. A pure cleavage fracture of the medial tibial plateau occurs in young patients who have sustained severe trauma. If these fractures are undisplaced they can be treated with a long-leg hinged cast for 4 to 6 weeks. If they are displaced more than 2 mm they should be reduced and internally fixed with cancellous screws. This can be accomplished by either closed manipulation and percutaneous insertion of the screws or by open reduction, depending upon the amount of instability and displacement of the fracture.

The other kind are depression fractures of the medial tibial plateau. These usually occur in older patients as a result of minor trauma and, in general, carry a poor prognosis. The anterior cruciate ligament also can be torn. Treatment is by open reduction and elevation of the tibial plateau with bone grafting and internal fixation with a buttress plate. If the anterior cruciate ligament is torn, the decision to repair or to reconstruct the ligament must be made on an individual basis.

Type V This is a pure bicondylar or inverted Y fracture. It is a rare fracture pattern. Although closed reduction and traction through a distal tibial pin have been recommended, results of use of this method have been reported to be less than satisfactory. However, this fracture often occurs in elderly patients who have osteopenic bone that will not hold stable internal fixation screws. In these instances, closed reduction and percutaneous pinning of the condylar fragments followed by treatment of the metaphyseal/diaphyseal fracture component in traction is satisfactory. Additionally, this method does not risk infection or failure of internal fixation, either of which might complicate later total knee arthroplasty. If open reduction is performed, use of medial and lateral buttress plates after accurate open reduction and supplemental bone grafting often is indicated.

The choice between open and closed treatment is most difficult to make with this type of tibial plateau fracture. These bicondylar fractures indeed may represent fracture-dislocations of the knee and can occur in young patients as the result of high-energy trauma. The long-term results may be poor, regardless of the method of treatment, because of injury to articular cartilage, difficulty in restoring anatomic position, and scarring.

Type VI This is a tibial plateau fracture in which there is disassociation of the metaphysis and diaphysis. The characteristic feature is the oblique fracture of the proximal tibia. Despite marked displacement and instability, surgical elevation of the tibial plateau fracture with the addition of a supportive bone graft and normal fixation with a long buttress plate for the metaphyseal/diaphyseal fracture can produce good results.

Tibial Shaft Fractures

The tibia is the long bone that is fractured most frequently. Significant complications can occur after treatment, including delayed union, malunion, nonunion, and infection. The single most important factor that delays healing is the extent of the initial fracture displacement. When the initial displacement of a fractured tibia is greater than the diameter of its shaft, the incidence of delayed union (defined as absence of healing after 20 weeks) is 50%. The energy expended in causing a fracture to undergo this much displacement also causes major soft tissue and bone damage. Tibial fractures that have little displacement usually result from indirect or low-energy trauma, and they heal more rapidly. The fracture sites that tend to heal most slowly are the middle third and the junction of the middle and proximal thirds. This is because direct trauma is most often the cause of fractures at these levels. The widely held belief that fractures in the distal third heal more slowly has not been substantiated. However, healing with malalignment is more common in this distal location.

Classification

Open fractures are classified into three categories according to the extent of associated soft tissue damage. Grade I fractures have skin perforation from the inside (usually caused by indirect trauma). Grade II includes fractures with skin contusion or perforation from the outside (usually caused by direct trauma). Grade III fractures have laceration of the skin and soft tissues with or without damage to blood vessels or nerves (caused by direct high-energy trauma).

Treatment

Most stable, closed, low-energy tibial fractures can be treated successfully by closed reduction and plaster immobilization with or without early weight-bearing. A long-leg plaster cast, a below-the-knee functional cast, or a functional brace can be used. In a recent review of the use of prefabricated functional braces in the treatment of tibial shaft fractures, the nonunion rate was only 2.5%. However, complications included a 7% rate of initial treatment failure requiring a change to other methods of fracture stabilization and a 9% rate of malunion (shortening, varus-valgus deformity, anterior-posterior angulation). Recent studies also show that loss of bone mineral from the upper ends of the tibia and fibula does not differ between patients with tibial shaft fractures who were allowed weight-bearing in a functional below-the-knee brace and those treated with a long-leg brace without weight-bearing.

Several well-controlled randomized studies have compared internal plate fixation with closed reduction and plaster immobilization as treatment of stable, closed, tibial shaft fractures. One study found that open reduction and internal fixation resulted in faster healing, less ankle joint stiffness, and earlier return to normal activity. This was true despite the disability that accompanied later removal of the implant. On the other hand, the factors of operating time and duration of hospitalization favor the nonsurgical method. The most important difference between the two treatment methods was infection rate: virtually nil in the nonsurgical group, and between 0% and 15% in patients treated by open reduction and plate fixation. Another study found that with closed functional bracing the nonunion rate was less than 1% and that 92% of fractures healed with less than 1 cm of shortening and 96% healed with an angular deformity of less than 10°.

Closed intramedullary nailing with a Lottes nail has been advocated for fractures of the tibia between 10 cm below the knee and 5 cm above the ankle. Postoperatively, the patients were allowed to walk in a patellar tendon-bearing brace. With this method of treatment, all fractures united within 7 to 8 weeks. An advantage of reamed intramedullary nailing is that it may not require postoperative cast immobilization because it provides rigid fixation. The union rate is reported to be as high as 96%.

The management of open (grades II and III) tibial fractures can be difficult. The extent of soft tissue damage is far more important than the fracture. Anatomic reduction and external stabilization is an excellent way to treat these injuries. This method allows access to the site of the soft tissue damage for dressing changes, local debridement, and soft tissue coverage procedures. Significant advances have been made in the treatment of major soft tissue defects after severe trauma. Muscle and musculocutaneous flaps can be used to cover large defects.

Open tibial fractures also have a high incidence of infection. In three prospective 1-year studies, the infection rate was found to be highest (24%) in patients with open fractures and not receiving antimicrobial agents and lowest (4.5%) in patients who received a combination of cephalosporin and aminoglycosides. These studies emphasize the importance of antimicrobial therapy at the time of initial treatment and subsequent debridement of open fractures. Rates of delayed union or nonunion are increased with open tibia fractures. Early cancellous bone grafting, if the wound is clean, should be considered for severe fracture comminution, segmental fractures, fractures with bone loss, and fractures with extensive periosteal stripping. This can be accomplished during wound coverage or 6 weeks after local or free flap transfer.

When an external fixator is used, excellent rigidity can be achieved when compression can be applied across the fracture site. The bone-pin interface is the least rigid link in the entire structure, particularly in the anteroposterior bending mode. The rigidity provided by the external fixator can be improved substantially by increasing the number of pins, by using fully threaded pins of large diameter, by decreasing the distances connecting the side rods, and by increasing the distance separating the pins in each pin group. Although stability of the fracture is increased by the use of the standard Hoffmann-Vidal frame, there are some disadvantages of bilateral external fixation frames when applied to the tibia. These include the possibility of injury to neurovascular structures and the transfixation of the tibialis anterior or peroneal muscles by the pins. Unilateral frames also provide better wound access than bilateral frames and allow for partial or full weight-bearing.

To prevent the transfixation of musculotendinous structures and to decrease the risk of neurovascular injury, two one-plate unilateral frames have been designed. These half-frames can be modified by the addition of pins and rods to provide improved two-plane rigidity and to accommodate unusual mechanical and clinical requirements.

In most reports, open fractures treated by plate fixation have been associated with a higher incidence of deep sepsis and delayed wound healing than those managed by closed reduction and external fixation. Plate fixation in open fractures should be limited to articular and metaphyseal fractures for which external fixation is not suitable to achieve fracture stability.

The use of intramedullary fixation without reaming the intramedullary canal is an alternative treatment method for unstable, open tibial fractures. However, obtaining good stability with nailing often requires reaming of the medullary canal to insert a nail large enough to obtain torsional bending stability. This reaming can adversely affect the healing potential of the endosteum in an open fracture in which periosteal circulation has been compromised by trauma.

Nonunion The four major treatment methods for delayed union or nonunion of the tibia are resection of the fibula and casting, posterolateral bone grafting, internal fixation (plates or nails with or without bone grafting), and electrical stimulation and casting (Table 1).

Resection of the Fibula When the fibula remains intact or heals before the tibia does, effective compression at the fracture site is prevented. Partial fibulectomy (removal of 1 cm) and controlled weight-bearing with a plaster cast has been reported to have a success rate of 77%. This approach is particularly effective in delayed union within 6 to 9 months after injury. An oblique osteotomy may heal before the tibia does and is not recommended.

Posterolateral Bone Grafting In tibial delayed union or nonunion with extensive soft tissue damage anteriorly, segmental bone defect, and indolent infection anteriorly, use of cancellous posterolateral bone grafting (Harmon approach) is effective treatment; the success rate is 92%. Fracture stability can be achieved by creating a tibiofibular synostosis. In most patients, once a stable tibiofibular synostosis is created above and below the fracture site and the fracture unites, wound drainage diminishes or ceases.

Internal Fixation With or Without Bone Grafting Hypertrophic, reactive nonunion often unites once stabilized by closed intramedullary nailing, with or without reaming, or by compression plating without bone grafting and excision of interposed pseudarthrosis tissue. Early mobilization can be started without external support. Closed intramedullary nailing with reaming is reported to be successful in 96% and plating in 93% to 94%. For atrophic or nonhypertrophic nonunion, bone grafting should be used in addition to plating.

Table 1 Methods for Treating Nonunion

Treatment	Subsequent union, %
Fibular resection	77
Electrical stimulation	81
Rigid internal fixation with or without bone grafting	96
Operation without internal fixation (posterolateral bone grafting)	92

Annotated Bibliography

Patellar Fractures

Böstman, O.; Kiviluoto, O.; and Nirhamo, J.: Comminuted displaced fractures of the patella. Injury 13:196–202, 1981.

In this retrospective analysis of 64 comminuted displaced fractures of the patella, the results of anterior tension band wire fixation were acceptable even in severe comminuted fractures. Partial excision produced satisfactory results provided that at least 60% of the patella could be preserved.

Böstman, O.; Kiviluoto, O.; Santavirta, S.; Nirhamo, J.; and Wilppula, E.: Fractures of the patella treated by operation. Arch. Orthop. Trauma Surg. 102:78–81, 1983.

Ninety-three fractures of the patella treated operatively are presented. Tension band fixation gave results superior to those of screw fixation. Patients under 30 years of age had better results than older patients. Partial patellectomy produced better results than total patellectomy. Tension band fixation and partial patellectomy are the methods of choice for patellar fractures that require operative treatment.

Haajanen, J., and Karaharju, E.: Fractures of the patella: One hundred consecutive cases. Ann. Chir. Gynaecol. 70:32–35, 1981.

Based on the results of treatment of 100 consecutive patellar fractures, partial excision of the patella was the best procedure for comminuted fractures in which at least half of the patella's gliding surface was intact. Tension band wiring fixation was effective in dealing with transverse fractures but not with comminuted fractures.

Weber, M.J.; Janecki, C.J.; McLeod, P.; Nelson, C.L.; and Thompson, J.A.: Efficacy of various forms of fixation of transverse fractures of the patella. J. Bone Joint Surg. 62A:215–220, 1980.

The patellae of 25 fresh cadaver knees were fractured transversely after the knees were mounted in machines capable of measuring quadriceps force, flexion angle, and fracture separation simultaneously. The fractures were fixed by using circumferential wiring, tension band wiring, and a modification of tension band wiring. Fracture separation was less in those patellae fixed with modified tension band wiring (a wire loop passed behind two Kirschner wires that had been introduced vertically across the fracture).

Fractures of the Tibial Plateau

Blokker, C.P.; Rorabeck, C.H.; and Bourne, R.B.: Tibial plateau fractures: An analysis of the results of treatment in 60 patients. Clin. Orthop. 182:193–199, 1984.

Sixty patients with fractures of the tibial plateau were evaluated in terms of fracture type, treatment method, adequacy of reduction, immobilization time, and associated ligamentous injury to identify factors important in determining outcome. Adequacy of reduction is the *single* most important factor influencing outcome. The method of achieving reduction and the duration of immobilization are not as critical. A residual step-off at the fracture site of greater than 5 mm was always associated with an unsatisfactory result.

Burri, C.; Bartzke, G.; Coldewey, J.; and Muggler, E.: Fractures of the tibial plateau. Clin. Orthop. 138:84–93, 1979.

In a collective review of the German study group of 342 patients with displaced tibial plateau fractures treated surgically, 278 were available for evaluation at a mean of 32 months postoperatively. Good results were obtained when accurate reduction and internal fixation with a buttress plate were accomplished and supplemental bone grafting was used.

Perry, C.R.; Evans, L.G.; Rice, S.; Fogarty, J.; and Burdge, R.E.: A new surgical approach to fractures of the lateral tibial plateau. J. Bone Joint Surg. 66A:1236–1240, 1984.

A new surgical approach is presented, consisting of incising and detaching only a segment of the anterior horn of the lateral meniscus so the split fragment can be opened like a book. The approach minimizes the need to detach a large portion of the lateral meniscus from its tibial attachment. Excellent results are reported.

Rafii, M.; Firooznia, H.; Golimbu, C.; and Bonamo, J.: Computed tomography of tibial plateau fractures. A.J.R. 142:1181–1186, 1984.

Computed tomography (CT) was compared to conventional tomography in 20 patients with tibial plateau fractures. CT resulted in less discomfort to the patient and produced optimal visualization of the plateau defect and split fragments. CT was more accurate than conventional tomography in assessing split fractures of the anterior and posterior borders of the plateau and in demonstrating fracture comminution.

Waddell, J.P.; Johnston, D.W.C.; and Neidre, A.: Fractures of the tibial plateau: A review of ninety-five patients and comparison of treatment methods. J. Trauma 21:376–381, 1981.

In 95 patients with tibial plateau fractures, adequacy of reduction was as important as early motion in obtaining a satisfactory result, regardless of the type of fracture treated. Tibial plateau fractures with depressions or widening of less than 1 cm did well when treated nonoperatively. If open reduction was undertaken, both internal fixation and bone grafting were required to obtain optimal results.

Compartment Syndromes Associated With Tibial Fractures

DeLee, J.C., and Stiehl, J.B.: Open tibia fracture with compartment syndrome. Clin. Orthop. 160:175–184, 1981.

Among 104 open tibial fractures, compartment syndromes, involving all four compartments of the lower leg, developed in 6. All six underwent four-compartment fasciotomies performed within 8 to 17 hours of the onset of symptoms. All had some residual footdrop as well as sensory deficits.

Halpern, A.A., and Nagel, D.A.: Anterior compartment pressures in patients with tibial fractures. J. Trauma 20:786–790, 1980.

In 20 patients with tibial fractures, tissue pressure in the anterior compartment was measured (with a mercury manometer) acutely and for the first 72 hours after injury. In normotensive patients in this series, fasciotomy was not necessary for tissue pressure less than 50 mm Hg in the absence of any sensory or motor compromise.

Matsen, F.A., III; Winquist, R.A.; and Krugmire, R.B., Jr.: Diagnosis and management of compartmental syndromes. J. Bone Joint Surg. 62A:286–291, 1980.

The 31 compartments at risk for compartmental syndrome were in patients who varied in their tolerance for increased tissue pressure. Thus, there was a range of intracompartmental pressures, of which some were associated with neurovascular deficits.

Rorabeck, C.H.: The treatment of compartment syndromes of the leg. J. Bone Joint Surg. 66B:93–97, 1984.

Eighteen patients with compartment syndromes below the

knee were treated with four-compartment fasciotomies by the double revision technique. Associated tibial fractures should be treated by some form of stabilization at the time of fasciotomy.

Nonunion of Tibial Diaphyseal Fractures

Ahl, T.; Andersson, G.; Herberts, P.; and Kalén, R.: Electrical treatment of non-united fractures. Acta Orthop. Scand. 55:585–588, 1984.

The semi-invasive technique of electrical stimulation of bone was used in 23 patients with nonunion. Solid union developed in 10. The results do not compare well with those of bone grafting.

Barker, A.T.; Dixon, R.A.; Sharrard, W.J.W.; and Sutcliffe, M.L.: Pulsed magnetic field therapy for tibial non-union: Interim results of a double-blind trial. Lancet 1:994–996, 1984.

Patients with nonunited tibial fractures for at least 52 weeks were randomly allocated to either active or dummy pulsed magnetic field stimulators and treated in full leg casts for 24 weeks. Union occurred in five of nine patients treated with active stimulators, and in five of seven treated with dummy stimulators. The high proportion of fractures uniting in the control group suggests that conservative treatment may explain some of the success attributed to pulsed magnetic field therapy.

Brighton, C.T.; Black, J.; Friedenberg, Z.B.; Esterhai, J.L.; Day, L.J.; and Connolly, J.F.: A multicenter study of the treatment of non-union with constant direct current. J. Bone Joint Surg. 63A:2–13, 1981.

Of 136 established nonunions of the tibia, 109 (80%) were successfully treated with semi-invasive constant direct current. The failures were believed to be due to inadequate electricity, the presence of synovial pseudarthrosis, infection, or dislodgement of the electrodes.

DeLee, J.C.; Heckman, J.D.; and Lewis, A.G.: Partial fibulectomy for ununited fractures of the tibia. J. Bone Joint Surg. 63A:1390–1395, 1981.

Partial fibulectomy proved to be a relatively effective and simple method of achieving union in 37 of 48 patients with established tibial nonunions. Failure of union after fibulectomy was associated with failure of the patient to bear weight postoperatively, the presence of pseudarthrosis at the fracture site, or previous prolonged treatment of the initial fracture with external fixation.

Heppenstall, R.B.: Constant direct-current treatment for established nonunion of the tibia. Clin. Orthop. 178:179–184, 1983.

Forty patients treated by constant direct current were evaluated in a prospective survey. Eighty-five percent of the fractures healed. When undetected synovial pseudarthroses are eliminated, the success rate increases to 93%.

Reckling, F.W., and Waters, C.H., III: Treatment of non-unions of fractures of the tibial diaphysis by posterolateral cortical cancellous bone-grafting. J. Bone Joint Surg. 62A:936–941, 1980.

Union was obtained in 43 of 44 tibial nonunions after cancellous bone grafts were inserted from the posterolateral approach. Three fractures required a second bone grafting. The majority of the fractures had been complicated by severe soft tissue damage, segmental bone loss, or infection, and multiple attempts had been made to obtain union prior to the posterolateral bone grafting procedure.

Tibial Shaft Fractures

Allum, R.L., and Mowbray, M.A.S.: A retrospective review of the healing of fractures of the shaft of the tibia with special reference to the mechanism of injury. Injury 11:304–308, 1979–1980.

A retrospective study of 500 fractures of the tibia confirmed Nicoll's cause of poor bone healing. If the fracture is open or comminuted, this has a similar but less pronounced effect on bone healing.

Behrens, F.; Comfort, T.H.; Searls, K.; Denis, F.; and Young, J.T.: Unilateral external fixation for severe open tibial fractures: Preliminary report of a prospective study. Clin. Orthop. 178:111–120, 1983.

Serious complications after severe open tibial fractures were considerably fewer after the use of relatively rigid one- or two-plane unilateral fixator frames than after internal fixation by plates and screws. Unilateral frames provide better wound access than bilateral frames and allow partial or full weight-bearing. This can have a positive effect on fracture healing.

Briggs, B.T., and Chao, E.Y.: The mechanical performance of the standard Hoffmann-Vidal external fixation apparatus. J. Bone Joint Surg. 64A:566–573, 1982.

A standard Hoffmann-Vidal quadrilateral fixation system for tibial fractures was analyzed by using different geometric and material variations of the basic configuration. The results show that the bone-pin interface is the least stiff link in the entire structure, particularly in the anteroposterior bending mode. Under both bending and torsional loads, the stiffness values are greatly increased when compression occurs at the fracture site. Rigidity of the device can be substantially improved by increasing the number of pins, using fully threaded pins with a large diameter, decreasing the distance connecting the side rod, and increasing the distance separating the pins in each group.

Patzakis, M.J.; Wilkins, J.; and Moore, T.M.: Use of antibiotics in open tibial fractures. Clin. Orthop. 178:31–35, 1983.

Three hundred sixty-three open tibial fractures were treated in three prospective 1-year studies. The infection rate was highest (24%) in patients with open fractures who received no antimicrobial agents and lowest (4.5%) in patients with fractures who received a combination of cephalosporin and aminoglycosides. The authors now use a combination of an aminoglycoside and a cephalosporin for all open fractures.

Sarmiento, A.; Sobol, P.A.; Sew Hoy, A.L.; Ross, S.D.K.; Racette, W.L.; and Tarr, R.R.: Prefabricated functional braces for the treatment of fractures of the tibial diaphysis. J. Bone Joint Surg. 66A:1328–1339, 1984.

Prefabricated functional braces were used in the treatment of 625 tibial diaphyseal fractures. Nonunion occurred in 2.5%. Ninety-one percent healed with 10 mm of shortening or less. Prefabricated functional braces are useful in most tibial diaphyseal fractures.

Sedlin, E.D., and Zitner, D.T.: The Lottes nail in the closed treatment of tibia fractures. Clin. Orthop. 192:185–192, 1985.

The Lottes nail was used in 63 consecutive cases of tibial fractures treated by closed intramedullary fixation. Only type III open wounds and fractures between 10 cm below the knee and 5 cm above the ankle were included. After the tibia was nailed, the patients were allowed to bear weight in a patellar tendon brace. All fractures united with a bridging callus in 7 to 8 weeks. Only one fracture became infected. The authors recommend Lottes nail as the preferred treatment for diaphyseal fractures of the tibia in adults.

Van Der Linden, W., and Larsson, K.: Plate fixation versus conservative treatment of tibial shaft fractures. J. Bone Joint Surg. 61A:873–878, 1979.

One hundred consecutive patients with displaced fractures of the tibial shaft were randomly assigned to two groups. One was treated with ASIF plate fixation and the other, with nonoperative methods. Duration of hospital stay was longer in the ASIF plate group, and there were more complications in that group. However, the median healing time was shorter and the anatomic end results were better than in patients treated nonoperatively. Closed longitudinal fractures were found to be suitable for ASIF plate fixation, but open fractures were not. In the group treated nonsurgically, most fractures that healed in malalignment were located in the distal third of the tibial shaft.

Velazco, A., and Fleming, L.L.: Open fractures of the tibia treated by the Hoffmann external fixator. Clin. Orthop. 180:125–132, 1983.

Forty consecutive open tibial fractures were treated with a Hoffmann external fixator, irrigation, and debridement, and all wounds were left open to be closed secondarily with skin grafts or muscle flaps. All wounds were classified as Gustilo's type II or III. At 18-month follow-up, there were five nonunions that healed after bone grafting and five amputations. Pin-site drainage was the most common complication; ring sequestrae that developed in five patients cleared after removal of the fixator and curettage.

38

Knee and Leg: Reconstruction

Various surgical options are available for the treatment of the arthritic patient after medical treatment has proved to be inadequate. This medical management includes anti-inflammatory medication and the appropriate use of analgesics. It includes a complete evaluation of the patient to identify associated knee pain referred from the hip or other sites. It includes the insistence that the patient make a concerted effort to lose weight when he or she is obese—the force transmitted across the knee during walking on level ground is as much as triple the patient's body weight. Periodic injections of steroid into the knee may be appropriate for some patients and give adequate temporary relief. The judicious use of a cane can relieve weight-bearing pain and increase a patient's walking and standing tolerance.

When all these measures fail to provide adequate relief of pain and reversal of disability, surgical options to be considered include synovectomy, debridement, osteotomy, hemiarthroplasty, unicompartmental total knee replacement, bicompartmental total knee replacement, tricompartmental total knee replacement, and arthrodesis.

Treatments

Synovectomy

The indications for knee synovectomy continue to be chronic synovitis (for at least 6 months) that does not respond to appropriate medical management. The standing radiographs should show preservation of articular cartilage space. Open surgical synovectomy probably should be performed through a single midline vertical skin incision and a parapatellar capsular incision. Such an approach provides the same exposure as would be necessary for total knee replacement and has the least chance of compromising subsequent arthrotomy for this purpose. If two incisions are used, wound healing problems may be encountered after future operations. In properly selected patients, the incidence of relief of swelling and pain 2 years postoperatively is about 80%.

Some centers are performing synovectomy through the arthroscope, but this technique has met with limited success. More encouraging is early experience with radiation synovectomy in which a radioactive substance with a short half-life and little tissue penetrability is injected into the affected joint. Short-term beneficial results have been seen in 60% to 70% of properly selected patients. The technique may have limited applicability in other joints such as the wrist or ankle.

Debridement Procedures

Open surgical debridement is of limited use today. Its best application is in patients with osteoarthritis, some preservation of joint space, no angular deformity, and significant intercondylar osteophytic formation with impingement. The intercondylar disease is best seen on a tunnel view of the knee.

Arthroscopic debridement may have some value in the treatment of degenerative arthritis, but its exact role has yet to be established. Most surgeons agree that, if significant angular deformity is present, abrasion arthroplasty will give only transient relief or may aggravate the condition. Patients with crystalline synovitis may benefit from repeated copious irrigation with simultaneous anti-inflammatory therapy. The patient with a degenerated meniscus may benefit temporarily from debridement of the torn fragments.

Valgus Osteotomy of the Proximal Tibia

The ideal candidate for a valgus osteotomy of the proximal tibia is an active patient who is heavy and has mild to moderate medial compartment osteoarthritis: deformity less than 10°, range of motion greater than 90°, a flexion contracture less than 15°, weight-bearing pain localized at the medial joint line, minimal synovitis, no rest pain, no internal derangement, and no subluxation. A good to excellent initial result can be anticipated in 80% to 85% of broadly selected patients. Appropriate preoperative planning requires standing, full-length radiographs. Early failures are usually characterized by persistent pain that is the result of inadequate correction of the deformity. The ideal postoperative alignment is such that a straight line drawn from the center of rotation of the hip to the center of the ankle passes through the lateral compartment of the knee (7° to 10° of valgus). The cosmetic problem associated with overcorrection to excessive valgus can be significant; therefore, careful attention to the resultant angle is required. However, a good result can be expected to last 10 years in only about 40% of the patients. Late failures are often caused by recurrence of the deformity in slightly undercorrected knees or by lateral compartment degeneration in subluxed or overcorrected knees.

Varus Osteotomy of the Distal Femur

The ideal candidate for a distal femoral osteotomy is a young, active patient who is heavy and has mild to moderate lateral compartment osteoarthritis: range of motion greater than 90°, deformity less than 10°, a flexion contracture less than 15°, pain localized to the lateral joint line, minimal synovitis, no rest pain, no internal derangement, and no subluxation. The ideal postoperative alignment of the knee is such that a straight line drawn from the center of rotation of the hip to the center of the ankle passes through the medial compartment of the knee. Distal femoral osteotomy is preferable to proximal tibial osteotomy in lateral compartment disease because a femoral osteotomy will shift the joint line closer to the horizontal whereas a tibial osteotomy for a valgus deformity will increase joint obliquity and predispose the knee to medial-lateral subluxation.

No large series of supracondylar osteotomies for arthritis have been reported with long-term results. There does not appear to be a consensus regarding surgical technique. Most agree on use of a medial closing wedge. Some recommend staple fixation while others use plate and screws. Supracondylar osteotomy appears to be technically more difficult than distal tibial osteotomy, and the success rate is not as high. Because the osteotomy crosses the quadriceps mechanism, there is more chance for quadriceps binding or contracture with subsequent loss of motion.

Arthrodesis

This operation now is rarely indicated as a primary procedure for treatment of arthritis. It usually is reserved as an end-stage procedure for salvage of a failed arthroplasty, especially when infection is present. Arthrodesis may be considered as a primary procedure for a young patient with advanced post-traumatic or septic arthritis or for a young, heavy laborer who has unilateral disease and cannot learn a sedentary occupation.

Conversion of arthrodesis to a total knee replacement is usually unsatisfactory and rarely is indicated. Range of motion is poor after arthroplasty, and these knees often are unstable unless a constrained prosthesis is used. Conversion may be indicated and beneficial for the patient who has knee fusion in marked flexion or has multiple joint involvement.

Total Knee Replacement

Unicompartmental Unicompartmental prosthetic total knee replacement appears to be an attractive alternative to high tibial osteotomy for the treatment of unicompartmental osteoarthritis in an elderly patient. It has been shown to have a higher initial success rate and fewer early complications than osteotomy. The procedure allows thorough examination of the joint and debridement of impinging osteophytes. No cast immobilization is required. Range of motion (both flexion and extension) can be improved by the procedure. In patients requiring bilateral operations, both can be performed during the same hospitalization, whereas bilateral osteotomies probably should be done 3 to 6 months apart.

Unicompartmental replacement has potential advantages over tricompartmental replacement in selected patients because it preserves both the anterior and posterior cruciate ligaments along with bone stock in the opposite compartment and patellofemoral joint. In the experience of one institution, patients with bilateral total knee replacement who had a tricompartmental replacement on one side and a unicompartmental replacement on the other usually preferred the unicompartmental knee because it felt more like a normal knee and had better function.

With proper selection of patients and surgical techniques, after unicompartmental replacement 90% of the patients can be expected to have good to excellent results at 10 years postoperatively. Knees with extreme deformity (more than 15° valgus or 10° varus) are not amenable to correction with this procedure. Undercorrection overloads the prosthetic compartment and will often lead to component subsidence or loosening. Overcorrection can lead to secondary degeneration of the opposite component. Care must be taken to avoid subluxation of the tibia on the femur and to achieve good congruency between the articulating surfaces of the femoral and tibial components to minimize the chance of excessive prosthesis wear. Metal-backed tibial components show less radiolucency at 2- to 4-year follow-up than do the all-plastic components.

Bicondylar Most bicondylar total knee replacement prosthetic devices now in use have evolved into a common design. The femoral component consists of condylar resurfacing and trochlear flange to resurface the femoral side of the patellofemoral joint. The shape of the prosthesis mimics the normal shape of the distal femur. Most systems are available in at least three or four anterior-posterior and medial-lateral dimensions to allow the surgeon to reproduce the dimensions of the specific femur as closely as possible. Right and left prostheses are usually available to allow capping of the cut bone surfaces without overhang of the metallic trochlear flange on the medial side. Most prostheses have condylar lugs to enhance fixation; some substitute an intramedullary femoral stem for these lugs.

Tibial components have evolved from modular two-piece prostheses to one-piece plateaus with some form of fixation extending into the tibial plateau. Some systems have spikes or lugs for this purpose and others make use of a central stem. *In vitro* testing indicates that the central stem might be the best method for buffering medial-lateral compression/distraction forces, rotational forces, and anterior-posterior rocking forces. Central stems as long as 70 mm have been found to share approximately 30% of the axial weight-bearing forces, thus unloading the tibial plateau. This may not be beneficial for the routine knee replacement but can be helpful when one or both plateaus are deficient in bone.

The evolution of tibial component designs has also included the use of metal backing to reinforce the high-density polyethylene. Although this provides more uniform distribution of the weight-bearing forces, the metal backing seems to be related to complications such as fracture of the metallic tray. These have usually resulted from the combination of malalignment with asymmetric weight-bearing forces, excessive patient weight and activity, and a tray design with a stress-riser that allows propagation of a fracture.

So far, symptomatic femoral component loosening has been a relatively rare complication after bicondylar total knee replacement. In one large series of knees it was seen in only 1% of patients after more than 3 years of follow-up. When femoral component loosening did occur, it was usually associated with loss of contact between the posterior condyle of the metal prosthesis and the posterior condylar bone. This gap allowed the femoral component to rock into flexion when it was loaded while the knee was flexed.

Patellofemoral Joint

Isolated patellofemoral arthritis still is a difficult entity to treat. Reports of tibial tubercle elevation procedures, such as the Maquet operation, still appear but this is not without significant potential morbidity including wound-healing problems, tibial fractures, compartment syndrome, and unacceptable cosmetic results. Patellectomy may be the procedure of choice for the younger patient and can yield satisfactory results when combined with a tubing of the quadriceps mechanism. It may result in quadriceps weakness and an extensor lag. It does not preclude excellent pain relief if total knee replacement is performed at some future date. Many patients with patellofemoral osteoarthritis can tolerate their condition by avoiding stairs and using arm support to rise from a chair. When their condition does deteriorate it often is because of secondary damage in the tibiofemoral joint, and total knee replacement is indicated.

Prostheses for replacement of the patellofemoral joint are available in the form of a metallic hemiarthroplasty or a metal-to-plastic resurfacing. The results of independent resurfacing have been inconsistent and the procedure has been associated with a high complication rate. Prosthetic replacement should be avoided in the younger patient.

Most total knee systems now have a polyethylene resurfacing that mates with the trochlear flange of the femoral component. It is still controversial as to whether the patella should always be resurfaced during total knee replacement. There is good evidence to suggest that all patients with inflammatory arthritis (especially rheumatoid) should undergo patellar resurfacing. This is to avoid eventual secondary degeneration of the patella and to prevent the possible return of active rheumatoid synovitis to the prosthetic joint. There is both laboratory and clinical evidence that leaving cartilage behind on the unresurfaced patella in the patient with rheumatoid arthritis permits interaction with regenerated rheumatoid synovium with the potential for symptomatic effusions and possible subsequent erosion of the bone-cement interface.

In the osteoarthritic patient, patellar resurfacing might not always be necessary. Follow-up of a large series of osteoarthritic patients showed that they did well without patellar resurfacing if they had no eburnated bone on the patella and had a normal anatomic shape and good tracking at the end of the procedure. The morbidity of patellar resurfacing includes stress fractures and long-term potential for wear and loosening.

Lateral retinacular release is performed much more routinely now to aid patellar tracking. Most surgeons perform the vertical release from inside the joint, isolating and preserving the lateral superior genicular artery for its blood supply to the patella and the lateral skin flap. Sacrifice of this artery has been associated with osteonecrosis of the patellar bone and subsequent stress fracture.

Posterior Cruciate Ligament Retention

At present, routine sacrifice of an intact posterior cruciate ligament during total knee replacement arthroplasty is controversial. Advocates of retaining the ligament claim that, after operation, the knee has more normal kinematics, greater potential range of motion, and greater anterior-posterior stability. In addition, less shear stress is imparted to the prosthesis and the bone-cement interface because of the less constrained prosthesis design. Advocates of routine sacrifice of the ligament claim that the operation is easier to perform, especially in a knee with severe angular deformity. Wider exposure of the tibia is possible, facilitating cementing technique.

Many different prosthesis designs are available for use with ligament sacrifice and preservation. Comparisons of short-term results with these prostheses do not yet show significant differences. At follow-up of at least 2 years, patients with the ligament-sparing condylar prosthesis had an 18% incidence of radiolucent lines at the bone-cement interface, compared with 19% in patients with a ligament-sacrificing device. The decision to save or sacrifice the posterior cruciate ligament, therefore, remains a matter of the individual surgeon's preference.

Continuous Passive Motion in Postoperative Care

Postoperative rehabilitation of the patient with a total knee replacement may be enhanced by use of the continuous passive motion machine but firm data are not available. These machines are now used immediately after operation to mobilize the knee. The range of motion is increased daily depending on the tolerance of the patient; in most instances, more than 90° of knee flexion is achieved several days earlier than if the machine had not been used. Results of retrospective studies suggest that less pain medication is required when the machine is used rather than conventional physical therapy methods. Other retrospective studies show a decreased incidence of thrombophlebitis.

Results

With the prostheses and cementing techniques currently available, good to excellent results can be anticipated in well over 90% of the patients in the first several years after operation. The first relatively long studies with condylar femoral components and one-piece central-stem tibial components have shown that results deteriorate at a rate of approximately 1% per year of follow-up. In a 5- to 9-year follow-up of the total condylar prosthesis, the reoperation rate was 7%.

Complications

Thrombophlebitis Preoperative and postoperative venography has shown that the incidence of clots in the calf can be as high as 40%. These findings do not correlate with the percentage of patients who develop thrombophlebitis or pulmonary embolism. This raises the question of how aggressively calf clots need to be treated with anticoagulation therapy. Most surgeons use some sort of prophylactic anticoagulation therapy regimen; aspirin and low-dose warfarin (Coumadin) are used the most frequently.

Infection This is the most catastrophic complication after total knee replacement. Fortunately, infection rates have been minimized by the prophylactic use of antimicrobial agents, provision of ultraclean operating rooms or ultraviolet lights, and careful attention to the handling of the soft tissues. Primary infection rates for condylar knee replacement should be less than 1%. Late infection can occur at about the same rate but is more common in patients with rheumatoid arthritis. Staphylococci are the most common causal organisms. Successful salvage of infected total knee replacements is being reported from many centers. Infections that occur in the immediate postoperative period can be treated by appropriate surgical intervention and administration of specific antimicrobial agents. For delayed infections, removal of the prosthesis components will be necessary. Most advocate delaying insertion of the new prosthesis for 4 and 6 weeks after removal if the infection is controlled. Some recommend using a temporary spacer block of antibiotic-impregnated bone cement. Some use cast immobilization and others recommend using the continuous passive motion machine between the removal and the reimplantation to mobilize the soft tissues. Removal of prosthesis components and arthrodesis is indicated for certain patients—e.g., those with loss of soft tissue or interruption of the quadriceps mechanism.

Loosening Loosening is occurring less frequently after total knee replacement with prostheses that are well aligned, less constrained, and implanted with modern cementing techniques. Increased prosthetic constraint results in increased stresses at the bone-cement interface. Malalignment causes weight-bearing forces to be transmitted asymmetrically across the knee and concentrated in the compartment on the concave side of the deformity. Several studies have correlated varus malalignment with an increased incidence of bone-cement demarcation under the medial tibial plateau. In order to minimize problems with postoperative malalignment, many new instrumentation systems have been devised to guide the surgeon. Those systems with intramedullary devices seem to give the most reproducible results.

Prostheses and Techniques for Revisions

Prostheses and techniques for revision total knee replacement are still evolving. Most surgeons adhere to the general principle that, for revision, the least-constrained prosthesis that will afford adequate stability to the knee should be utilized. This is to minimize stresses at the bone-cement interface that would be transmitted through the constraint of the prosthesis. Techniques have been described to aid in the exposure of the knee at operation for revision. These usually involve an inverted "V" incision proximally in the quadriceps tendon to allow for easier eversion of the patella and quadriceps mechanism without jeopardizing the patellar tendon insertion. This technique can be further developed into a "V-Y" quadriceps-plasty at the end of the procedure if necessary to gain motion in the ankylosed knee. The vast majority of revision total knee operations can be performed through the usual medioparapatellar incision.

Instruments have been developed to assist in extraction of both femoral and tibial components. These are indispensable if the surgeon is to minimize destruction of femoral and tibial bone stock during removal of failed components. Revision femoral and tibial components should be available with extended stems in order to enhance fixation when bone stock is deficient.

Methods available to restore deficient stock on both the femoral and tibial sides include the use of bone grafts, the use of cement alone, and the use of cement supplemented by screws or mesh, augmented components, custom components, or components that can be augmented at operation, depending on the defect, by spacers or wedges applied to the prosthesis. Use of autogenous bone (if available) or allograft bone is the most attractive method for restoration of bone stock. This appears to be uniformly successful for contained defects. The use of bone graft for peripheral defects has met with early success. Any resorption of the peripheral grafts, however, could lead to component subsidence and loosening. Of the other methods available, laboratory tests show that custom components and augmented components give better fixation than does filling the defects with cement alone or cement reinforced by screws. As yet, not much clinical data are available to support these observations.

Cementless Total Knee Replacement

In contrast to the situation with the hip, there seems to be no urgency to abandon the use of bone cement for prosthesis fixation in all but the most elderly patients. On the other hand, it would seem most appropriate to pursue cementless fixation for knee prostheses on an investigational basis in selected patients. Cementless prostheses are less forgiving than cemented components and require greater accuracy in the execution of bone cuts and in the restoration of neutral mechanical alignment. Although some early results seem promising, long-term results are unknown. There are concerns to be resolved about the potential for long-term stress shielding and metal toxicity.

Annotated Bibliography

Osteotomy

Coventry, M.B.: Upper tibial osteotomy. Clin. Orthop. 182:46–52, 1984.

A study of 213 knees with a 16-year follow-up showed 61% of the knees were satisfactory after 10 years. Mechanical axis valgus angulation of 3° to 5° is preferred. Joint replacement is recommended for inactive patients over 65 years of age.

Insall, J.N.; Joseph, D.M.; and Msika, C.: High tibial osteotomy for varus gonarthrosis: A long-term follow-up study. J. Bone Joint Surg. 66A:1040–1048, 1984.

At 2 years, 97% of the knees were good or excellent but of those knees followed more than 9 years, only 37% were painfree. Total knee arthroplasty is preferred over tibial osteotomy for elderly patients with a sedentary life-style.

Johnson, E.W., Jr., and Bodell, L.S.: Corrective supracondylar osteotomy for painful genu valgum. Mayo Clin. Proc. 56:87–92, 1981.

Fifty-three osteotomies were reviewed; 30% had poor results. Correction to a neutral anatomic axis is recommended. The best technique was use of an incomplete medially based closing wedge with staple fixation.

Keene, J.S., and Dyreby, J.R., Jr.: High tibial osteotomy in the treatment of osteoarthritis of the knee: The role of preoperative arthroscopy. J. Bone Joint Surg. 65A:36–42, 1983.

Arthroscopic findings prior to osteotomy appeared to have little, if any, predictive value in evaluating patients for high tibial osteotomy. Results were based on follow-up of the osteotomy for 2 to 3 years.

Synovectomy

Sledge, C.B.; Atcher, R.E.; Shortkroff, S.; Anderson, R.J.; Bloomer, W.D.; and Hurson, B.J.: Intra-articular radiation synovectomy. Clin. Orthop. 182:37–40, 1984.

Synovectomy by the instillation of an appropriate radionuclide shows promising early results in patients with rheumatoid disease in the knee.

Hemiarthroplasty

Scott, R.D.; Joyce, M.J.; Ewald, F.C.; and Thomas, W.H.: McKeever metallic hemiarthroplasty of the knee in unicompartmental degenerative arthritis. J. Bone Joint Surg. 67A:203–207, 1985.

Unicompartmental metallic hemiarthroplasty can be an attractive alternative in the treatment of unicompartmental degenerative arthritis when osteotomy is contraindicated and the patient is too young, heavy, or active to permit total knee replacement.

Total Knee Replacement

Results

Bae, D.K.; Guhl, J.F.; and Keane, S.P.: Unicompartmental knee arthroplasty for single compartment disease: Clinical experience with an average four-year follow-up study. Clin. Orthop. 176:233–238, 1983.

Seventy-two knees were followed for a mean of 4 years (minimum, 2 years). Pain relief was rated as excellent in 90% of the knees. One revision was performed for patellofemoral disease.

Ewald, F.C.; Jacobs, M.A.; Miegel, R.E.; Walker, P.S.; Poss, R.; and Sledge, C.B.: Kinematic total knee replacement. J. Bone Joint Surg. 66A:1032–1040, 1984.

One hundred twenty-four knees were followed for 2 to 4 years after insertion of a prosthesis with metal backing of the tibial component and retention of the posterior cruciate ligament. Ninety percent of the results were rated good or excellent. Tibial radiolucent lines were seen in 18% of the knees.

Insall, J.N.; Hood, R.W.; Flawn, L.B.; and Sullivan, D.J.: The total condylar knee prosthesis in gonarthrosis. A five to nine-year follow-up of the first one hundred consecutive replacements. J. Bone Joint Surg. 65A:619–628, 1983.

At follow-up, 91% of knees were good or excellent; 7% of the knees had been revised. Forty-one percent of the tibial components had evidence of radiolucent lines, of which 19% showed some progression.

Mallory, T.H., and Danyi, J.: Unicompartmental total knee arthroplasty: A five- to nine-year follow-up study of 42 procedures. Clin. Orthop. 175:135–138, 1983.

Forty-two knees were followed for 5 to 8 years. Thirteen failures occurred, usually because of tibial component loosening related to surgical technique and prosthesis design.

Rand, J.A.; Stauffer, R.N.; and Chao, E.Y.S.: Kinematic rotating hinge total knee arthroplasty (abstract). Orthop. Trans. 9:424, 1985.

Fifty knees were reviewed. Satisfactory results were achieved in only 80% of the primary cases and 56% of the revision cases. The complication rate was high.

Ritter, M.A.; Gioe, T.J.; Stringer, E.A.; and Littrell, D.: The posterior cruciate condylar total knee prosthesis: A five-year follow-up study. Clin. Orthop. 184:264–269, 1984.

Ninety-four knees were followed for a minimum of 5 years after a total condylar type of prosthesis with retention of the posterior cruciate ligament. Ninety percent of the knees were rated as good or excellent.

Sarokhan, A.J.; Scott, R.D.; Thomas, W.H.; Sledge, C.B.; Ewald, F.C.; and Cloos, D.W.: Total knee arthroplasty in juvenile rheumatoid arthritis. J. Bone Joint Surg. 65A:1071–1080, 1983.

The primary reason for operation often was to improve function rather than to relieve severe pain. The mean arc of motion improved from 45° preoperatively to 79° postoperatively. Failure to resurface the patella was the most common reason for reoperation.

Sledge, C.B., and Walker, P.S.: Total knee arthroplasty in rheumatoid arthritis. Clin. Orthop. 182:127–136, 1984.

Seven hundred ninety-eight arthroplasties in rheumatoid patients in which the posterior cruciate ligament was preserved were reviewed. The incidence of good and excellent results increased from 67% to 92% as prosthesis design changes evolved. Failures most often were due to loosening (1.3%), patellofemoral pain (1.8%), or infection (0.4%).

Complications

Inman, R.D.; Gallegos, K.B.; Brause, B.D.; Redecha, P.B.; and Christian, C.L.: Clinical and microbial features of prosthetic joint infection. Am. J. Med. 77:47–53, 1984.

Sixty-three prosthetic joint infections were studied. Half occurred more than 1 year after implantation. Staphylococci were the predominant organisms, and *Staphylococcus epidermidis* was the most common species in both early and late infections.

Lotke, P.A.; Ecker, M.L.; Alavi, A.; and Berkowitz, H.: Indications for the treatment of deep venous thrombosis following total knee replacement. J. Bone Joint Surg. 66A:202–208, 1984.

Postoperative venography revealed that 41% of patients had small thrombi in the calf and 31% had large thrombi. These findings do not correlate with those in patients who went on to develop pulmonary emboli. It is suggested that calf clots may not require aggressive anticoagulation therapy.

Pritsch, M.; Fitzgerald, R.H., Jr.; and Bryan, R.S.: Surgical treatment of ligamentous instability after total knee arthroplasty. Arch. Orthop. Trauma Surg. 102:154–158, 1984.

Ligamentous reconstruction failed to restore stability to the knee in any of the seven patients studied. Component revision is the appropriate treatment of the unstable knee after total knee arthroplasty.

Sisto, D.J.; Lachiewicz, P.F.; and Insall, J.N.: Treatment of supracondylar fractures following prosthetic arthroplasty of the knee. Clin. Orthop. 196:265–272, 1985.

Closed reduction and skeletal traction are recommended for the initial treatment.

Walker, R.H., and Schurman, D.J.: Management of infected total knee arthroplasties. Clin. Orthop. 186:81–89, 1984.

Delayed exchange total knee arthroplasty is a reasonable alternative to arthrodesis after resection of an infected total knee arthroplasty.

Patellofemoral Joint

Bayne, O., and Cameron, H.U.: Total knee arthroplasty following patellectomy. Clin. Orthop. 186:112–114, 1984.

Pain and instability may occur after total knee arthroplasty when patellectomy is performed. The posterior cruciate ligament should be retained or should be replaced by a prosthesis with inherent anteroposterior stability.

Ranawat, C.S.; Rose, H.A.; and Bryan, W.J.: Replacement of the patello-femoral joint with the total condylar knee arthroplasty. Int. Orthop. 8:61–65, 1984.

Complications associated with replacement of the patello-femoral joint in the total condylar knee arthroplasty have been seen in less than 5% of knees after 2 years. No subluxations or fractures were seen. Loosening was noted in only 1 of 206 knees. Discomfort was noted with eccentric placement of the prosthesis when bone was left uncovered.

Scott, R.D.; Ewald, F.C.; and Walker, P.S.: Stress fracture of the patella following duopatellar total knee arthroplasty. Clin. Orthop.

Stress fracture of the patella was initially seen in 3.5% of the osteoarthritic patients undergoing duopatellar total knee arthroplasty with patellar resurfacing. Predisposing factors include lateral release (leading to osteonecrosis of the patella), excessive bone resection, a large central fixation hole, and range of motion greater than 100° of flexion.

Techniques

Brooks, P.J.; Walker, P.S.; and Scott, R.D.: Tibial component fixation in deficient tibial bone stock. Clin. Orthop. 184:302–308, 1984.

Various nonbiologic methods to fill wedge-shaped medial plateau defects were tested in cadaver bone. The performance of cement alone was poor compared to integral custom-made tibial components. A metal wedge was considered an acceptable alternative to a custom-made component if securely fixed to the bottom of the tibial tray.

Ewald, F.C.; Jacobs, M.A.; Walker, P.S.; Thomas, W.H.; Scott, R.D.; and Sledge, C.B.: Accuracy of total knee replacement component position and relation to bone-cement interface reaction. *In* The Knee (First Scientific Meeting of the Knee Society), edited by L.D. Dorr, pp. 117–120. Baltimore, University Park Press, 1985.

Medial tibial bone-cement interface radiolucencies were associated with postoperative varus knees and varus tibial tray placement.

Hvid, I., and Nielsen, S.: Total condylar arthroplasty: Prosthetic component positioning and radiolucent lines. Acta Orthop. Scand. 55:160–165, 1984.

Radiolucent lines at the tibial component bone-cement interface were associated with a tilt of more than 4° of neutral alignment. The highest incidence was seen in rheumatoid patients with postoperative varus alignment.

Knutson, K.; Hovelius, L.; Lindstrand, A.; and Lidgren, L.: Arthrodesis after failed knee arthroplasty: A nationwide multicenter investigation of 91 cases. Clin. Orthop. 191:202–211, 1984.

Fusion was achieved in only 50% of attempts. Fusion rate was highest after unicompartmental replacement and in the absence of active infection. Infected knees may require a two-stage procedure, and rigid fixation is mandatory.

Scott, R.D., and Siliski, J.M.: The use of a modified V-Y quadricepsplasty during total knee replacement to gain exposure and improve flexion in the ankylosed knee. Orthopedics 8:45–48, 1985.

A modified "V-Y" quadriceps-plasty is an effective technique to aid in exposure of the ankylosed knee and in gaining postoperative range of motion. The initial extensor lag becomes sufficiently corrected in several months.

Cementless Arthroplasty

Freeman, M.A.R.; McCleod, H.C.; and Levai, J.-P.: Cementless fixation of prosthetic components in total arthroplasty of the knee and hip. Clin. Orthop. 176:88–94, 1983.

Cementless fixation without ingrowth can be successful in the short term. Factors leading to success include good initial primary fixation, low shear stresses at the prosthesis-bone interface, accurately cut bone surfaces, and accurate restoration of neutral mechanical alignment.

Hungerford, D.S.; Krackow, K.A.; and Kenna, R.V.: Clinical experience with the PCA prosthesis without cement (abstract). Orthop. Trans. 9:424–425, 1985.

A 2- to 5-year follow-up of the first 164 PCA prostheses implanted without bone cement showed 92% good or excellent results in rheumatoid patients and 96% good or excellent results in osteoarthritic patients. The reoperation rate was 8.5%, mainly for patellar loosening.

39

Ankle and Foot: Pediatric Aspects

Congenital and Developmental Problems

Idiopathic Equinovarus (Clubfoot)

The cause of congenital equinovarus has yet to be determined. It is thought to be a result of polygenic inheritance modified by environmental influences. The incidence among whites is 1.2/1,000 live births and increases to 2.1% for first-degree relatives.

During embryonic development, the foot assumes three different positions. At the 15-mm embryonic stage, the foot is in a straight line with the leg. By the time the embryo has grown to 30 mm, the foot passes into a marked equinovarus adducted position (embryonic position). Finally, at the 50-mm stage, the foot changes to a slight equinovarus adducted position (fetal position). The morphologic and structural changes of the foot from the initial to the embryonic position result from the rapid growth of the end of the fibula. The changes from the embryonic to the fetal position are due to growth of the distal end of the tibia and the skeletal rays of the medial foot during the tibial phase of rapid growth.

Environmental factors may interfere with the rapid growth phase of the fibula or tibia and may be of varying degrees of severity. If the interference occurs at the end of the fibular phase and during the first half of the tibial phase, the foot will remain in the marked equinovarus adducted position and a severe clubfoot will result. If it acts only during the last half of the tibial phase, a mild flexible clubfoot will result because by this stage most parts of the embryonic components have been corrected. If it occurs at the end of the tibial phase, a simple metatarsus adductus deformity will persist.

The pathologic changes involve the posterior and medial ligaments, muscles, tendons, and tendon sheaths and the tarsal bones. Histologic study of the short, thick ligaments reveals myoblastic and mass cells similar to the findings in Dupuytren's contracture. There is increased fibrous connective tissue in the sheaths of the short, thick Achilles tendon and the posterior tibial tendons. The os calcis is rotated from the subtalar joint posteriorly toward the fibula and anteriorly toward the tibia, and it simultaneously tilts into varus. In addition, there is ankle equinus, hindfoot varus, and midfoot and forefoot adduction but almost never internal tibial torsion.

The severity of the deformity is difficult to assess by clinical evaluation. Normal ligamentous laxity in young children allows apparent passive correction of the deformity without producing a rotation of the os calcis at the subtalar joint or reduction of the talonavicular joint. Assessment of the joint deformity is best confirmed and quantitated by standing or simulated standing lateral and anteroposterior radiographs. Ankle equinus is demonstrated by the calcaneal tibial angle. Subtalar varus, which includes inversion and adduction, is best inferred from the lateral talocalcaneal angle. The anterior-posterior talocalcaneal angle is helpful but is less accurate. Adduction occurs at the talonavicular joint and is demonstrable by the medial displacement of the navicular. Prior to ossification of the navicular bone at ages 1 to 5 years, adduction is best quantitated by the talar first metatarsal angle which normally should approximate 0°.

Corrective manipulation and serial cast application beginning in the immediate postnatal period remains the treatment of choice. This is effective in approximately half of the patients, which reflects the variable severity of the deformity. Often, there is initial partial correction and then an impasse is reached and further casting does not appear to gain any further correction. If this is documented by clinical and radiographic evaluation, surgical correction is necessary.

Over the last 20 years there has been an evolution in the surgical treatment for clubfoot. Although limited soft tissue releases or tendon lengthenings occasionally will produce satisfactory correction in mild deformities, the one-stage posteromedial release is the most effective surgical procedure and produces a higher percentage of satisfactory results. The experimental serial release of soft tissues in clubfeet of stillborn fetuses showed that release of all contracted tissues is necessary to correct the essential abnormality of dislocation of the talocalcaneal navicular joint. Release of the Achilles tendon and tibialis posterior produced very slight correction of varus. The addition of posterior ankle capsulotomy and posterior subtalar capsulotomy allowed full correction of equinus but did not correct the varus. The addition of plantar fasciotomy and deltoid ligament release increased the improvement of equinus and varus. Further addition of division of the talonavicular ligaments and the calcaneonavicular (spring ligament) produced further correction of the varus; however, the navicular hinged at the cuboid, opening the talonavicular joint. With the addition of anterior ankle capsulotomy, division of the anterior subtalar ligaments, calcaneocuboid ligaments, and lateral ankle ligament produced full correction of the deformity; however, there was some valgus instability unless the lateral calcaneocuboid and anterior talofibular ligaments were preserved.

The one stage posteromedial release is a difficult operation. It includes the following: 1) Achilles tendon Z-lengthening with secure reconstruction; 2) posterior release of the ankle and subtalar joint including the calcaneofibular and posterior talofibular ligaments; 3) Z-lengthening of the posterior tibial tendon; 4) medial release of the subtalar joint and the superficial deltoid which includes the calcaneotibial and tibionavicular ligaments; and 5) release of the calcaneal ligament. To achieve full correction of the deformity, the following releases are needed: calcaneonavicular ligament, talonavicular ligament, talonavicular ligament dorsally, bifurcate ligament, anterior calcaneal capsule, enough of the talocalcaneal interosseous ligament to allow rotation of the os calcis on the talus, and plantar release including the abductor hallucis, plantar fascia, short toe flexors, and abductor digiti minimi. The results of one-stage posteromedial release correlate best with correction of the lateral talocalcaneal and calcaneotibial angles to normal. The correction should be confirmed by postoperative radiographs. Unsatisfactory results commonly are associated with persistent medial subluxation of the navicular bone or with overcorrection of the navicular laterally, resulting in a planovalgus deformity. Positioning of the navicular on the talar head with a smooth Kirschner wire is recommended. Postoperative maintenance of the foot in the corrected position with plaster casts for 4 months or longer is important to prevent recurrent deformity. Nighttime splinting is recommended until normal functioning of the foot is achieved.

The most opportune time for performing the one-stage posteromedial release is controversial. Surgical correction in the neonatal period has been reported recently with excellent results; however, an adequate trial of serial casting is needed. The operation appears to be more difficult in the neonate, and delay of the procedure to age 1 year may be prudent.

Salvage of the foot overcorrected into planovalgus is very difficult. If the subtalar joint can be reduced adequately, extra-articular subtalar arthrodesis may be helpful. For the occasional young adolescent with unacceptable residual deformity, triple arthrodesis remains the treatment of choice.

Tarsal Coalition

Tarsal coalition appears to result from failure of segmentation of the primitive mesenchyme; it has an autosomal dominant inheritance pattern. Calcaneonavicular and talocalcaneal middle facet coalitions are the most common, but the coalition also may occur in the anterior or posterior facet. The calcaneonavicular coalition is best demonstrated by an oblique foot radiograph. The talocalcaneal coalitions are more difficult to demonstrate by radiographs. Middle facet coalition can be demonstrated in the Harris view, a 45° posterior plantar view. Lateral tomography may be necessary to confirm the diagnosis.

Symptoms usually appear in the second decade and consist of pain, limited subtalar motion, and occasional spasm of the peroneal muscles. These patients appear to have a greater risk of ankle sprain than seen in the normal population; however, most patients with tarsal coalition do not become symptomatic and do not require treatment.

In symptomatic patients, the symptoms sometimes are permanently relieved by temporary cast immobilization; however, manipulation is not helpful. For patients who remain symptomatic, surgical treatment is indicated. Triple arthrodesis has been the standard surgical procedure; however, in the young patient without degenerative changes in the talonavicular joint, resection of the coalition with interposition of either fat or muscle has relieved symptoms and restored subtalar motion. The talar beak as viewed on the lateral radiograph has been used as an indication of degeneration of the talonavicular joint and for performing a triple arthrodesis; however, a recent study has shown that the talar beak is not necessarily related to degenerative changes, and satisfactory excision of the coalition can be achieved in the presence of the talar beak. In these patients, the talonavicular joint is explored to determine degenerative changes before proceeding with excision of the tarsal coalition. If joint degeneration is found, a triple arthrodesis is performed.

Accessory Navicular

The accessory navicular is a normal anatomic and radiographic variant. It appears in approximately 12% of the population. There are two distinct patterns: 1) a sesamoid bone within the posterior tibial tendon, anatomically separated from the navicular and usually asymptomatic; and 2) an accessory ossification center which is closely associated with the navicular and is triangular in shape. It may be associated with painful foot, particularly in the athletic adolescent (Fig. 1). It is not a cause of hypermobile flatfoot but, because both are common, they may be present together. In the symptomatic patient, simple excision appears to be effective. When the patient has a hypermobile flatfoot, the Kidner procedure (excision of the accessory navicular and transfer of the posterior tibial tendon beneath the navicular) is preferred, although it may not produce a correction of the hypermobile flatfoot.

Hypermobile Flatfoot (Pes Planus)

The human foot is a well-developed biconcave structure by the end of the first trimester of gestation. At birth, the foot is in a position of equinus, adduction, and inversion as a result of the position *in utero.* Neonatal feet exhibit this appearance for several months. The plantar surface of the foot appears flat as a result of the thick fat pad, and this may persist for years. As children begin to stand and

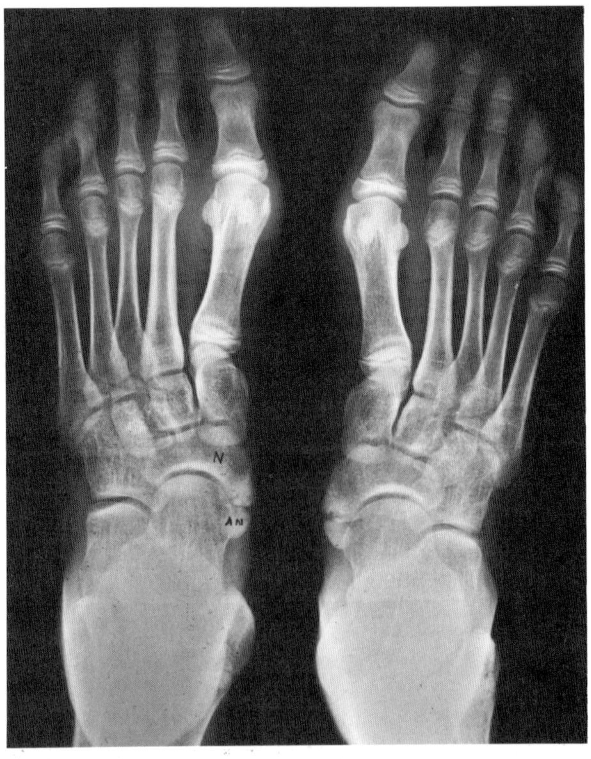

Figure 1

Type 2 accessory navicular (*AN*) adjacent to the medial and posterior margin of the navicular (*N*).

walk, they use a wide-based stance in which the weight is borne on a line passing medial to the foot, causing the flexible foot to assume a position of eversion and forefoot abduction. Normal medial rotation of the hip and knee tend to accentuate the pronation by coupled talar medial rotation and plantar flexion. The normal joint hypermobility peaks in children at 2 to 3 years of age and then gradually begins to decrease. At age 2, almost 97% of normal children will have some degree of flatfoot. By age 10, this has decreased to 4%. The effect of shoes on the development of the foot is questionable because examination of large primitive populations with comparison of shod and unshod portions of the population showed nearly equal incidences of flatfoot.

The diagnosis of a foot that appears flat should be based on physical and radiographic examinations. The foot should be assessed for forefoot and hindfoot mobility and for heel cord contracture. Presence or absence of generalized connective tissue laxity and neuromuscular abnormalities should also be assessed.

Radiographic examination is necessary to determine cause. The angles given are only approximate because they may vary depending on the position of the foot and the x-ray beam, even when the examination is performed in the standing position. The following are the key views for evaluation of the tarsal and arch alignments: 1) standing dorsoplanar view which shows the coverage of the talar head at the joint (the talocalcaneal angle should be 15° to 35°); 2) standing lateral view which shows the degree of equinus of the talus and the calcaneus and the amount of plantar displacement of the navicular (lateral talocalcaneal angle should be less than 35° and the talometatarsal angle should be approximately 0°); 3) inversion stress dorsiflexion view or special views to look for tarsal coalition if indicated (Fig. 2).

The diagnosis of flexible flatfoot is one of exclusion. Because of variations in ligamentous laxity, neuromuscular development, and structure of the foot, a small percentage of feet will remain in varying degrees of pronation into adulthood. Rarely will these feet become symptomatic.

The treatment of an asymptomatic flexible flatfoot in an otherwise normal child is observation. Early prophylactic treatment of asymptomatic feet is unwarranted. Use of corrective shoes, custom-molded orthotic devices, and exercises may ease parental anxiety but probably will not alter the natural formation of the arch based on hereditary and connective tissue laxity. Symptoms caused by flatfoot often will be relieved by an orthotic device that helps to support the longitudinal arch. Many surgical procedures have been tried for correction of the flexible flatfoot but few have stood the test of long-term review. Surgical procedures fall into three categories: 1) tendon transfer or lengthening; 2) arthrodesis; and 3) osteotomy.

Of the tendon procedures, Achilles tendon lengthening has been the most successful in patients with persistently tight heel cords that have not responded to stretching or serial casting. Generally, this is the only procedure that should be performed before skeletal maturity.

The majority of operations performed for flatfoot have been arthrodesis procedures. This procedure should never be performed for cosmetic reasons but should be reserved for the relief of disabling pain that has been refractory to every means of conservative therapy. The surgeon, the patient, and the parents must be willing to exchange a significant loss of inversion and eversion for the relief of pain and disability. The most successful arthrodesing procedures in the treatment of painful flatfoot in children are those that include the subtalar joint, such as a subtalar arthrodesis in a child or a triple arthrodesis in an adolescent.

Osteotomy procedures for painful flatfoot offer an advantage in that they do not create an iatrogenic tarsal coalition or ankylosis of the foot. Osteotomy of the os calcis realigns the weight-bearing line through the talocalcaneal axis of the hindfoot.

Congenital Vertical Talus

Congenital vertical talus is commonly associated with other abnormalities including: 1) neural tube defects; 2) neuromuscular disorders; 3) malformation syndromes; and 4) chromosomal aberrations. It may also occur as an isolated deformity. There is a high familial incidence in the idiopathic group. The deformity is characterized by fixed lateral and superior displacement of the talocalcaneal navicular complex. The peroneals, ankle extensors, and Achilles tendon as well as the superior talonavicular and the posterior tibiotalar capsules are shortened. The plantar calcaneonavicular ligament is elongated. The deformity is fixed and usually cannot be reduced by manipulation. A stress lateral radiograph of the foot often will give an indication of the correctability by manipulation and casting. If the angle between the talar axis and the first metatarsal base is less than 60° or that between the calcaneal axis and the first metatarsal base is less than 20°, then conservative treatment should be tried. Surgical correction should be considered if corrective casting in the extreme equinovarus position for 3 months fails to reduce the talar axis-first metatarsal base angle to 50° or less.

Surgical treatment is best performed between ages 6 and 12 months and is less successful after age 3 years. The deformity is best corrected in a one-stage procedure that includes anterolateral and posterior release with medial reefing and fixation of the reduced talonavicular joint with a Kirschner wire. Excision of the navicular is not advocated. Release of the subtalar joint medially, posteriorly, and laterally is needed in order to allow the os calcis to rotate under the navicular, reducing the anterior facet and providing support to the talar neck. Neurologic imbalance should be corrected by appropriate transfer or release of the muscles such as transfer of the tibialis anterior tendon to the neck of the talus or the peroneus longus or brevis to the posterior tibial tendon.

Persistent Medial Deviation of the Neck of the Talus

Children who walk with a toed-in gait may have many different abnormalities of their lower extremity, including excessive femoral anteversion, metatarsus adductus, and internal tibial-fibular torsion. In a recent study of children with toed-in gait, almost 18% were found to have external tibial-fibular torsion and internal axis deviation of the foot from the midsagittal plane. Anteroposterior radiographs showed that the major cause of toeing-in in this group was persistence of the fetal medial deviation of the talar neck, not internal tibial torsion. Spontaneous correction could be anticipated in children up to 3 years of age if the internal axis rotation was less than 10°. If it was greater than 10°, prognosis for correction appeared to be age-related, and in children more than 6 years of age little correction seemed possible. There is no evidence that treatment alters the natural history of this deformity. There also are no long-

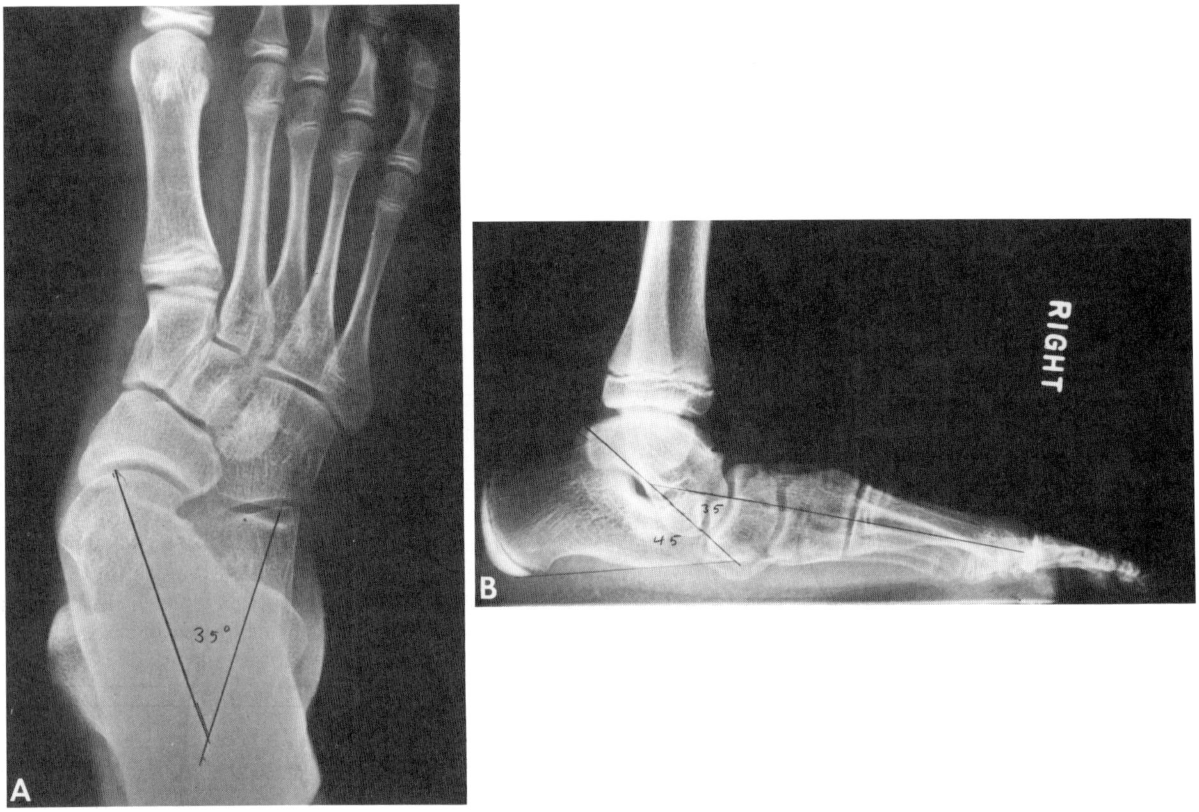

Figure 2

Radiographs of child with pes planus. *A*, Standing dorsoplanar view, showing uncoverage of the medial talar head and a late calcaneal angle of 35° (extreme of normal). *B*, Standing lateral view, showing talocalcaneal angle of 45° and talometatarsal angle of −25°.

term studies indicating if it causes disability in the adult. However, this deformity should be considered when evaluating a child with toed-in gait, to prevent making errors in diagnosis and treatment recommendations.

Hallux Valgus

Hallux valgus and bunion formation is a developmental deformity that has a familial predisposition. Modern shoes also may contribute somewhat to the development of the deformity. Metatarsus primus varus may or may not be present. Examination reveals valgus of the first metatarsal-phalangeal joint, pronation of the large toe, and varying degrees of varus alignment of the first metatarsal. There also may be varying degrees of loss of transverse arch with widening of the forefoot. Quantitation of the deformity is best performed on a standing anteroposterior radiograph taken 15° to the perpendicular.

Nonoperative treatment is usually unsuccessful but may decrease the discomfort. Operative treatment has been the mainstay for correction, and over 130 operative procedures have been described for this deformity. Operative treatment has been followed by a higher recurrence rate in adolescents than in adults. Therefore, if possible, it seems best to delay operative treatment until the child becomes an adult. Failure of conservative treatment to relieve pain and to permit proper shoe fitting are indications for operation. Surgical procedures at the distal end of the first metatarsal with internal fixation to prevent migration of the osteotomy fragments can give excellent results. Surgical procedures that center on the proximal end of the first metatarsal or muscle-balancing procedures have a much higher recurrence rate. The recurrence rate was 56% in children with hypermobile flatfoot and 50% in those who had a long first ray. From these reports, it would appear that a modified Mitchell operation is the preferred procedure in the adolescent.

Acquired Problems

Infection

Foot infections may result from hematogenous seeding or from puncture wounds. These infections are unusual, and the local signs of infections with absence of early systemic symptoms are often absent. The sedimentation rate may be increased, however. Diagnosis usually is delayed. Osteomyelitis of the metatarsals usually is due to puncture wounds, but acute hematogenous osteomyelitis of an isolated metatarsal may occur. The organisms usually are either

Staphylococcus aureus or *Streptococcus pyogenes*. Disturbance of growth of the metatarsal is common but usually does not cause disability.

Primary subacute osteomyelitis of the talus needs to be considered in patients who limp and complain of persistent pain in the foot. The radiographic findings are slow to appear and there is an absence of systemic reaction to the infection. Diagnosis is often delayed by 5 or 6 months before the lytic lesion becomes evident radiographically. Treatment by curettage, antimicrobials, and cast immobilization provides satisfactory results without growth disturbance or abnormalities of adjacent joints.

Trauma

In children under 10 years of age, rotational trauma of the lower leg usually results in fractures of the tibia and fibula whereas in older children, ankle fractures are more frequent. The most common ankle fractures are either supination-adduction or supination-eversion injuries. There are four stages of a supination-eversion injury. In stage I, there is a fracture of the anterolateral corner of the distal tibial epiphysis (Tillaux fragment) at the site of the insertion of the anterior tibiofibular ligament. Stage II includes periosteal detachment of the distal tibia superior to the anterior tibiofibular ligament and may include physeal fracture of the distal fibula. In stage III, the so-called triplane fracture, there may be two to four fragments. In stage IV, the distal fibular metaphysis is fractured.

Prediction of growth abnormalities after ankle fractures is often very difficult but is an important part in the management of this injury. Predictors for growth abnormalities include sex, skeletal maturity, type of trauma, anatomic classification, displacement, treatment, and associated tibial shaft fracture. When these factors are considered individually, treatment, displacement, and skeletal maturity are important, whereas the Salter-Harris classification system could not predict the growth pattern. Ankle fractures that involve both the distal tibia and fibula and require open reduction because of displacement are likely to undergo progressive growth retardation or growth arrest. Large displacement (greater than 2 mm) is common in supination-adduction and pronation-abduction stage II, supination-eversion stage IV-B, and pronation-eversion stages III and IV. These fractures can also appear when the remaining growth is considerable and, when displaced, represent high-risk injury. Special attention should be paid to injuries in girls up to 12 years old and boys up to 13 years old because they have 1 cm or more of growth remaining.

Soft Tissue Injuries

Soft tissue injuries are more difficult to diagnose in children. Ankle sprains are often thought to be minor injuries, although permanent instability may result. Despite the rapid healing in children, tears of the anterior talofibular ligament are surprisingly common in children and lead to permanent instability in up to 20% of the cases. Surgical repair of the ligament prevents the occurrence of chronic instability. It should be considered if a major tear of this ligament is present.

Neuromuscular Disease

Cerebral Palsy

Ankle equinus and foot varus or valgus are common major problems for cerebral palsy patients. Because of difficulties in assessment, surgical treatment generally is not recommended until the patient has established a gait pattern. Selection of surgical management and postoperative care remains controversial. The choices involve lengthening, and thereby weakening, a muscle, splitting a tendon of a muscle with a transfer of half of the tendon to the other side of the foot to distribute its force, or transferring a muscle to a different portion of the foot.

To clarify the pathomechanics of altered gait, dynamic electromyography has been performed. Four basic types of abnormal muscle activities have been identified. In the first, the phasing of the tibialis anterior and the tibialis posterior was thought to be essentially normal but a premature or continuous electromyographic signal was recorded from the soleus and gastrocnemius. Heel cord lengthening alone is suggested for these patients.

The second type of pattern was characterized by continuous firing of the tibialis anterior in combination with premature activation of the gastrocnemius and soleus. For these patients, the tibialis posterior was considered to be either normal or minimally premature in its phasic activity. Split anterior tibialis transfer combined with heel cord lengthening is suggested.

In the third type the tibialis posterior was either markedly premature or continuous in its myoelectric activity. In addition, there was abnormal activity in the gastrocnemius and soleus. Lengthening or release of the tibialis posterior combined with heel cord lengthening is suggested for these patients.

The fourth type of pattern is characterized by a tibialis posterior activity that is out of phase with the predominant myoelectric signal recorded during the swing phase of the gait cycle. There also is premature activity of the gastrocnemius and soleus. Transfer of the tibialis posterior to the dorsum of the foot and heel cord lengthening is suggested for this group.

Complications are frequent and include recurrence which seems to depend more on the pathophysiology of the muscle than on the type of lengthening procedure performed. Another complication is overlengthening which results in calcaneal deformity. The ankle should only be placed in 5° to 10° of dorsiflexion postoperatively, and a long-leg cast is applied with the knee in extension.

Valgus deformity of the foot can decrease the stability of the foot and make it difficult to wear shoes. In mild degrees of deformity, intramuscular lengthening of the peroneus brevis will decrease the power of the evertors by one muscle grade and correct the hindfoot valgus by one grade of severity. In more severe deformities, extra-articular arthrodesis with internal fixation has been successful in controlling the deformity.

The forefoot deformities include cavus, metatarsus adductus, hallux valgus, bunion, dorsal bunion, and toe flexion contractures. Prevention or correction of these deformities requires operation. Dynamic deformities caused by spastic muscles respond to tenotomy or lengthening of the tendons. Fixed deformities require osteotomies and arthrodesis of joints in addition to removing the deforming forces. In children 4 to 12 years of age, cavus deformity can be improved by soft tissue release of the plantar structures. In adolescents, triple arthrodesis usually is necessary.

Myelomeningocele

The most common deformity is equinovarus in the newborn and high-level paraplegics. Calcaneovalgus deformity of the foot and ankle valgus deformities are common in ambulatory children.

Nonoperative techniques rarely provide lasting correction of the paralytic equinovarus deformity, and surgical treatment usually is indicated. One-stage posteromedial release has been successful, with failures related primarily to technical problems or inability to provide follow-up splinting to the foot. It is important that the deformity be totally corrected at the time of operation and that follow-up splinting and bracing is used until maturity.

Progressive subtalar valgus may be associated with growth and ambulation. The deformity occurs both in the subtalar joint and in the ankle joint. In young children, if the fibular shortening is less than 10 mm, tenodesis of the Achilles tendon to the fibula may provide the desired correction. In older children, or if the deformity is more severe, supramalleolar osteotomy or epiphyseal stapling of the medial tibial epiphysis will provide satisfactory correction. In the adolescent, a combination of distal tibial osteotomy and triple arthrodesis often is required.

It is important to restore the muscle balance around the ankle joint to prevent recurrence of the valgus deformity. The simplest procedure is to release or tenotomize the peroneal and anterior compartment muscles if present. There is a temptation to perform transfers such as the posterior tibial tendon posteriorly to the calcaneus. This procedure does eliminate the calcaneal varus deformity, but significant equinus may occur. Dynamic electromyographic studies indicated that the transferred muscle did not develop the desired phasic contraction during the stance phase of walking. Bracing requirements are unaffected by this procedure.

Except for low-level sacral paraplegics, these patients perform best with an ankle-foot orthosis. This provides alignment control and stability in joints without sensation. The floor reaction force is transferred to the anterior shin with partial relief of pressure on the foot and increased sensory feedback to sensory-intact skin below the knee.

Arthrogryposis

Arthrogryposis multiplex congenita, a syndrome present at birth, may affect all four limbs and sometimes the spine. It is associated with muscular and ligamentous abnormalities that produce rigid contractures of joints. The foot and the ankle are most commonly affected, and rigid equinovarus is the most common foot deformity. Treatment by manipulation and serial plaster casts and soft tissue surgery alone have proved to be unsuccessful. Surgical treatment is therefore indicated. In mild cases, a complete posteromedial release may provide the desired correction. For severe deformities, talectomy or subchondral excision of the talus and cuboid (Verebelyi-Ogston procedure) provides satisfactory results; however, long-term orthotic management is necessary to prevent recurrence.

Muscular Dystrophy

Equinus deformity of the ankle is one of the serious orthopaedic problems associated with muscular dystrophy. Although it helps to stabilize the knee in the early stages of the disease, it eventually prevents use of an orthosis and prevents walking. Conservative treatment with orthotics only minimizes the progression of the deformity but does not appear to prolong the ability to walk. Surgical correction of the equinus has prolonged walking for several years, although the deformity and the progressive muscle weakness eventually confine the child to a wheelchair.

Radiologic evaluation of children with neuromuscular disease has shown many features in common with juvenile rheumatoid arthritis and hemophilia. These findings include apparent overgrowth of the epiphysis, periarticular osteoporosis, and joint space narrowing. There is accentuation of the trabecular pattern of the bone and evidence of soft tissue wasting. Tibiotalar slant and premature epiphyseal closure also are occasionally seen.

Muscle biopsies of the intrinsic musculature of the foot and the vastus lateralis in congenital myotonic dystrophy show structural changes that contribute to the force imbalance of the foot and result in clubfoot deformity.

Annotated Bibliography

Congenital and Developmental Problems

Idiopathic Equinovarus (Clubfoot)

Porat, S.; Milgrom, C.; and Bentley, G.: The history of treatment of congenital club foot at the Royal Liverpool Children's Hospital: Improvement of results by early posteromedial release. J. Pediatr. Orthop. 4:331–338, 1984.

The use of early Turco posteromedial release can offer excellent results in treating severe resistant clubfoot.

Victoria-Diaz, A., and Victoria-Diaz, J.: Pathogenesis of idiopathic club foot. Clin. Orthop. 185:14–24, 1984.

During embryonic development, the foot passes consecutively into three different positions. The clinical findings correspond to the stage at which development was interrupted.

Tarsal Coalition

Swiontkowski, M.F.; Scranton, P.E.; and Hansen, S.: Tarsal coalitions: Long-term results of surgical treatment. J. Pediatr. Orthop. 3:287–292, 1983.

Resection of the bar was successful if degenerative arthritis was not present. The talar "beak" is not necessarily a degenerative spur.

Accessory Navicular

Lawson, J.P.; Ogden, J.A.; Sella, E.; and Barwick, K.W.: The painful accessory navicular. Skeletal Radiol. 12:250–262, 1984.

The accessory navicular is a normal anatomic and radiographic variant. There are two distinct patterns: a sesamoid bone may be present within the posterior tibial tendon; and an accessory ossification center that may be associated with a painful foot, particularly in an athletic adolescent.

Hypermobile Flatfoot

Bordelon, R.L.: Hypermobile flatfoot in children: Comprehension, evaluation, and treatment. Clin. Orthop. 181:7–14, 1983.

The hypermobile flatfoot deformity depends on three structural deformities of the foot: 1) abduction of the forefoot relative to the weight-bearing line; 2) supination of the forefoot; and 3) heel valgus.

Congenital Vertical Talus

Hamanishi, C.: Congenital vertical talus: Classification with 69 cases and new measurement system. J. Pediatr. Orthop. 4:318–326, 1984.

Congenital vertical talus is classified into five groups according to association: 1) neural tube defects, 2) neuromuscular disorders, 3) malformation syndromes, 4) chromosomal aberrations, and 5) idiopathic.

Persistent Medial Deviation of the Neck of the Talus

Bleck, E.E., and Minaire, P.: Persistent medial deviation of the neck of the talus: A common cause of in-toeing in children. J. Pediatr. Orthop. 3:149–159, 1983.

Toeing-in children were found to have external tibial-fibular torsion and internal axial deviations of the foot from the midsagittal plane. From studies of newborn infants, radiographs, and anatomic specimens, the authors concluded that persistence of the fetal medial deviation of the talar neck was the major cause of toed-in gait.

Acquired Problems

Bunions

Luba, R., and Rosman, M.: Bunions in children: Treatment with a modified Mitchell osteotomy. J. Pediatr. Orthop. 4:44–47, 1984.

Modification of the original Mitchell osteotomy of the first metatarsal produced excellent results in growing children.

Scranton, P.E., Jr., and Zuckerman, J.O.: Bunion surgery in adolescents: Results of surgical treatment. J. Pediatr. Orthop. 4:39–43, 1984.

The failure rate was 36%. In children with hypermobile flatfoot or long first ray, the recurrence rate was 56% or 50%, respectively.

Osteomyelitis

Robb, J.E.: Primary acute haematogenous osteomyelitis of an isolated metatarsal in children. Acta Orthop. Scand. 55:334–338, 1984.

Acute hematogenous osteomyelitis is a rare condition in childhood. Organisms were either *Staphylococcus aureus* or *Streptococcus pyogenes.* Growth disturbances of the metatarsal were common but without disability.

Skevis, X.A.: Primary subacute osteomyelitis of the talus. J. Bone Joint Surg. 66B:101–103, 1984.

The only constant complaint was pain and limp. Treatment by curettage, antimicrobial agents, and plaster immobilization provided satisfactory results without growth disturbance or abnormalities of adjacent joints.

Trauma

Kärrholm, J.; Hansson, L.I.; and Svensson, K.: Prediction of growth pattern after ankle fractures in children. J. Pediatr. Orthop. 3:319–325, 1983.

The predictors of post-traumatic growth patterns included sex, skeletal maturity, traumatologic and anatomic classifications, displacement, treatment, and associated tibial shaft fracture. Displaced physeal injuries treated by reduction showed the highest risk of deformity.

Vahvanen, V.; Westerlund, M.; and Kajanti, M.: Sprained ankle in children: A clinical follow-up study of 90 children treated conservatively and by surgery. Ann. Chir. Gynaecol. 72:71–75, 1983.

Eighteen months after injury, 42% of children treated nonoperatively had symptoms of disability. All ankles treated operatively healed well, and the patients were symptom-free at follow-up. Lesions of the anterior tibofibular ligament are surprisingly common in children.

Neuromuscular Disease

Cerebral Palsy

Banks, H.H.: Equinus and cerebral palsy—its management. Foot Ankle 4:149–159, 1983.

Sliding lengthening of the heel cord gives excellent correction of fixed equinus deformity. However, postoperative management and long-term orthotic support during the growing period are necessary to prevent recurrent equinus. An exercise regimen to develop balanced muscle function is essential.

Barrasso, J.A.; Wile, P.B.; and Gage, J.R.: Extraarticular subtalar arthrodesis with internal fixation. J. Pediatr. Orthop. 4:555–559, 1984.

Extra-articular subtalar arthrodesis with internal fixation in children with mobile paralytic planovalgus deformity had good or excellent results in 95%.

Barto, P.S.; Supinski, R.S.; and Skinner, S.R.: Dynamic EMG findings in varus hindfoot deformity and spastic cerebral palsy. Dev. Med. Child. Neurol. 26:88–93, 1984.

Four different patterns of inappropriate muscle activity involving the tibialis anterior, tibialis posterior, gastrocnemius, and soleus were seen during walking.

Bleck, E.E.: Forefoot problems in cerebral palsy—diagnosis and management. Foot Ankle 4:188–194, 1984.

Forefoot deformities include cavus, metatarsus adductus, hallux valgus and bunion, dorsal bunion, and toe flexion contractures. Both prevention and correction of these deformities are surgical. Fixed deformities need osteotomies and arthrodesis of joints in addition to removing the face of the deforming muscle.

Eilert, R.E.: Cavus foot in cerebral palsy. Foot Ankle 4:185–187, 1984.

In children between 4 and 12 years of age, cavus deformity may be improved by soft tissue release of plantar structures, appropriate tendon lengthenings, and cast correction. In the adolescent, triple arthrodesis is often necessary.

Nather, A.; Fulford, G.E.; and Stewart, K.: Treatment of valgus hindfoot in cerebral palsy by peroneus brevis lengthening. Dev. Med. Child. Neurol. 26:335–340, 1984.

Mild hindfoot valgus deformity can be treated by intramuscular lengthening of the peroneus brevis. This method reduces the power of the muscle by one grade and corrects the hindfoot valgus by one grade of severity.

Root, L.: Varus and valgus foot in cerebral palsy and its management. Foot Ankle 4:174–179, 1984.

Although varus and valgus foot deformities are caused by muscle imbalance, the alignment of the hip and knee plays an important role in the production of the deformity. Once bone deformities are established, they must be corrected either prior to or simultaneously with muscle procedures.

Myelomeningocele

Burkus, J.K.; Moore, D.W.; and Raycroft, J.F.: Valgus deformity of the ankle in myelodysplastic patients: Correction by stapling of the medial part of the distal tibial physis. J. Bone Joint Surg. 65A:1157–1162, 1983.

Stapling of the medial part of the distal tibial physis bar proved to be a safe and simple procedure for correction of valgus deformities of the ankle. It was useful after failed previous muscle and bone surgery. There were no complications from this procedure.

Janda, J.P.S.; Skinner, S.R.; and Barto, P.S.: Posterior transfer of tibialis anterior in low-level myelodysplasia. Dev. Med. Child. Neurol. 26:100–103, 1984.

A clinical and electromyographic evaluation was performed on children who had undergone bilateral transfer of the tibialis anterior to the heel cord. The procedure eliminated the calcaneovarus deformity, but significant new deformity often occurred. Dynamic electromyographic studies indicated that the transferred muscle did not develop the desired phasic contraction during the stance phase of walking. Bracing requirements were unaffected by the procedure.

Malhotra, D.; Puri, R.; and Owen, R.: Valgus deformity of the ankle in children with spina bifida aperta. J. Bone Joint Surg. 66B:381–385, 1984.

In children suffering from spina bifida aperta, valgus deformity usually occurs in the ankle. Operations performed below the ankle (subtalar fusion or triple arthrodesis) are unlikely to succeed.

Nicol, R.O., and Menelaus, M.B.: Correction of combined tibial torsion and valgus deformity of the foot. J. Bone Joint Surg. 65B:641–645, 1983.

The combined deformity of ankle valgus and tibial torsion can be corrected by a single procedure: supramalleolar tibial osteotomy with a lateral inlay triple arthrodesis of the foot.

Arthrogryposis

Green, A.D.L.; Fixsen, J.A.; and Lloyd-Roberts, G.C.: Talectomy for arthrogryposis multiplex congenita. J. Bone Joint Surg. 66B:697–699, 1984.

Seventy-one percent satisfactory results were obtained in severe, rigid equinovarus deformity.

Spires, T.D.; Gross, R.H.; Low, W.; and Barringer, W.: Management of the resistant myelodysplastic or arthrogrypotic clubfoot with the Verebelyi-Ogston procedure. J. Pediatr. Orthop. 4:705–710, 1984.

Subchondral excision of the talus and cuboid achieved satisfactory correction in approximately half of the patients with rigid neuropathic clubfoot.

Muscular Dystrophy

Richardson, M.L.; Helms, C.A.; Vogler, J.B., III; and Genant, H.G.: Skeletal changes in neuromuscular disorders mimicking juvenile rheumatoid arthritis and hemophilia. A.J.R. 143:893–897, 1984.

Radiographic evaluation of children with neuromuscular disease showed many features in common with juvenile rheumatoid arthritis and hemophilia. These findings include apparent overgrowth of the epiphysis, periarticular osteoporosis and joint space narrowing, accentuation of the trabecular pattern, gracile bones and soft tissue wasting, tibiotalar slant, and premature epiphyseal closure.

Siegel, I.M.; Eisenberg, B.R.; and Glantz, R.H.: Contributory etiologic factor for talipes equinovarus in congenital myotonic dystrophy: Comparative biopsy study of intrinsic foot musculature and vastus lateralis in two cases. J. Pediatr. Orthop. 4:327–330, 1984.

Structural change in intrinsic foot muscles can contribute to the phase imbalance of the foot and produces clubfoot in this disease.

Williams, E.A.; Read, L.; Ellis, A.; Morris, P.; and Galasko, C.S.B.: The management of equinus deformity in Duchenne muscular dystrophy. J. Bone Joint Surg. 66B:546–550, 1984.

Conservative treatment could, at best, only minimize progression of the deformity. Surgical correction of equinus deformity benefits the patients for several years although the deformity may recur.

40

Ankle and Foot: Trauma

The first part of this section will cover soft tissue injuries of the ankle and foot: Achilles tendon injury, peroneal tendon dislocation, tibialis posterior rupture, tendon laceration, tibiofibular syndesmosis injury, ligament injury, dislocation, puncture wound, and reflex sympathetic dystrophy. The second section deals with bone injuries: fractures of the ankle, talus, calcaneus, and metatarsals.

Soft Tissue Injuries

Achilles Tendon Injury

Pathologic processes that can affect the Achilles tendon include tendinitis, peritendinitis, partial or complete ruptures, and achillobursitis. These conditions usually occur in patients in their fourth decade or older. The onset of symptoms can be insidious (such as from overuse in athletes) or sudden (such as in acute tendon rupture). Patients who have posterior calf and heel pain must be examined carefully to ensure that the Achilles tendon is intact and that there is no pathologic condition present to cause weakness of the tendon.

Achilles tendinitis is characterized by diffuse pain along the course of the tendon. It must be differentiated from a localized swollen tender area characteristic of a partial tear of the tendon, peritendinitis, and retrocalcaneal bursitis. The most common cause is overuse, such as a substantial increase in running mileage over a short period of time. The examination must distinguish among swelling or thickening of the peritendinous sheath, of the tendon itself, of the retrocalcaneal bursa, and of the insertion of the tendon into the os calcis. Radiographs should be examined for calcification in the tendon or a protruding bony prominence of the posterior superior calcaneus.

Nonsurgical treatment such as rest, nonsteroidal anti-inflammatory medications, and use of a heel lift usually relieves the symptoms. "Rest" can mean altering training habits, decreasing running mileage, or temporarily switching athletic workouts to activities that minimize tension on the Achilles tendon, such as swimming. Stretching, friction massage, and ultrasound may be of use. Steroids should not be injected into the Achilles tendon or its sheath because this can weaken the tendon.

Partial rupture of the Achilles tendon can be difficult to diagnose and may be the real cause of symptoms in many cases of "tendinitis."

Avulsion of the insertion of the medial head of the gastrocnemius ("tennis leg") should be differentiated from Achilles tendon injury. Rupture of the plantaris tendon probably does not exist as a clinical entity.

A partial Achilles tendon tear that causes persistent disabling symptoms should be repaired surgically. If the partial tear is located near the posterior superior prominence of the os calcis, this bone prominence and the adjacent bursa should be resected at the time the tendon is repaired.

Complete rupture of the Achilles tendon can occur with or without prior symptoms. When this occurs a defect in the tendon can be palpated and Thompson's test is positive. The patient will still be able to plantar flex the foot weakly by using the intact tibialis posterior and toe flexor muscles.

Both operative and nonoperative methods are effective in treating Achilles tendon disruptions, so treatment must be individualized. Elderly or sedentary patients can be treated with a below-the-knee non-weight-bearing cast in plantar flexion for 4 weeks followed by a below-the-knee walking cast for 4 weeks. A heel lift is used in the shoe until the ankle can dorsiflex past neutral.

For the professional or serious amateur athlete, operative repair usually can attain a better functional result than can be had from cast immobilization. The incision should be placed posteromedially to avoid the sural nerve laterally. The skin should not be incised directly posterior because there is a greater likelihood of skin slough in this location and because the scar can later create friction problems with a shoe's heel counter. The tendon should be repaired with nonabsorbable or slowly absorbable sutures, preferably by using several Dunnell-type "deep" sutures and superficial oversewing with 2-0 and 0 absorbable sutures. A below-the-knee non-weight-bearing cast is applied for 3 weeks. This is followed by a below-the-knee walking cast for an additional 3 weeks. In a secure repair, motion is possible even earlier but not weight-bearing.

A method for percutaneous pin fixation of the proximal end of the retracted Achilles tendon has been described (Fig. 1). This percutaneous suture technique offers the advantage of keeping the torn edges of the tendon apposed to enhance healing without the risks of a large open wound. After-care is similar to that for patients treated with open repair.

The incidence of re-rupture after Achilles tendon repair has been reported to be approximately half that after nonoperative treatment. Push-off strength is diminished in both groups.

Chronic ruptures (untreated for greater than 1 month) require special consideration. The proximal end has usually retracted, and a large gap exists that is filled with fibrous tissue. This tissue should be resected; then, the tendon ends are mobilized and repaired end to end. However, the repair should be reinforced by using additional tissue. A flap of proximal tendon can be turned down. The flexor digitorum longus tendon can be used for reinforcement by weaving it through the repaired tendon and inserting it into the calcaneus. The distal stump of the flexor digitorum longus tendon is sutured to the flexor hallucis longus tendon. The peroneus brevis tendon can also be used by di-

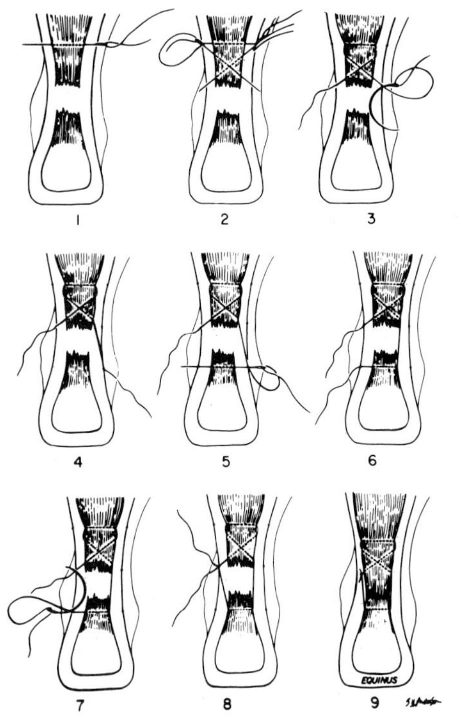

Figure 1

Closed suture technique for Achilles tendon repair. (From Ma, G.W.C., and Griffith, T.G. Clin. Orthop. 128:247–255, 1977. By permission of J.B. Lippincott Company.)

viding the insertion and transferring the tendon to the distal stump of the Achilles tendon and then proximally to reinforce the repair.

Other Tendon Injuries

Peroneal Tendon Dislocations Traumatic dislocation of the peroneal tendons most frequently occurs during snow skiing. Forced dorsiflexion or inversion can tear the peroneus brevis tendon from the peroneal retinacular sheath, causing the tendon to dislocate anteriorly. Reduction usually occurs spontaneously. The injury is frequently misdiagnosed as an ankle sprain and, in fact, a sprain may also occur at the time of the tendon dislocation.

Examination of the area behind the lateral malleolus reveals swelling and point tenderness. The swelling may extend down the peroneal tendon sheath. A diagnostic radiographic sign is a thin cortical fracture of the posterior lateral malleolus.

Acute injury can be treated with a below-the-knee walking cast for 3 weeks. To treat recurrent tendon subluxation, surgical reconstruction can be performed. The repair can be reinforced anteriorly by transposing the calcaneofibular ligament over the peroneal tendon. An alternative procedure is to transfer one-third of the lateral Achilles tendon to the lateral malleolus over the peroneal tendons. Fibular osteotomy to "deepen the groove" is technically difficult and it may result in painful peroneal tenosynovitis.

Posterior Tibialis Tendon Rupture Rupture of the posterior tibial tendon can be difficult to diagnose. It typically occurs in women in their fifth decade or older. The symptoms are similar to those of a "sprained ankle" at the time of rupture but there is no definite injury. The patient may have had pain in the tibialis tendon area prior to tendon rupture.

Examination frequently reveals medial ankle and midfoot swelling and asymmetric pes valgus. When viewed from behind, "too many toes" are seen on the involved side because the midfoot throws the forefoot into abduction. When the patient is standing on the toes, the involved side has less hindfoot inversion than the normal side. Tibialis posterior strength is best tested in plantar flexion. If inversion is tested in dorsiflexion, weakness will not be apparent. The exact site of rupture can be located by palpation. Lateral standing radiographs reveal asymmetric "sagging" of the talonavicular cuneiform arch (Fig. 2).

Complete ruptures are treated by open repair of the tendon and augmentation using flexor digitorum longus tendon transfer. An old rupture of the tibialis posterior can be repaired and augmented with tibialis anterior tendon transfer and naviculocuneiform arthrodesis. A chronic, painful rupture in a foot that has midtarsal joint degeneration is best treated by talonavicular arthrodesis or triple arthrodesis (in severe cases).

Ligament Injuries

Tibiofibular Syndesmosis Injury Disruption of the syndesmosis between the distal tibia and fibula is caused by external rotation or forced dorsiflexion. Four types of tibiofibular syndesmosis injuries have been described. Treatment is chosen on the basis of the severity of the diastasis and the type of ligament injury.

Pure rotational force can tear the anterior inferior tibiofibular ligament without disrupting the tibiofibular syndesmosis or posterior inferior tibiofibular ligament. Point tenderness at the anterior syndesmosis is the diagnostic physical finding. Stress films and arthrograms are normal. Treatment is symptomatic, and a cast usually is not required.

If the injury to the distal tibiofibular joint appears to be severe, an arthrogram or stress film can be helpful. If the syndesmosis has been disrupted and is wide, it should be reduced. A lag screw is passed through the distal fibula into the tibia and tightened while the foot is held in maximum dorsiflexion. Standard treatment has been to remove this screw. In a recent study it was found that removal of the screw was not necessary.

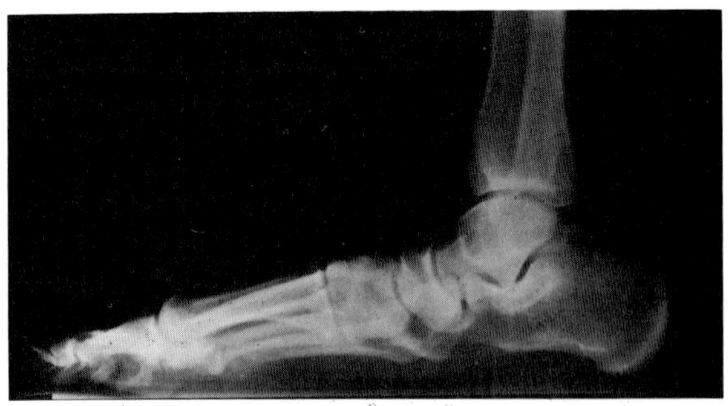

Figure 2

Talonavicular cuneiform "sagging" of the arch on a lateral standing radiograph after tibialis posterior rupture.

Deltoid Ligament Injury The anterior ankle capsule or the anterior deltoid ligament can be injured if the ankle is subjected to excessive plantar flexion. If an anterior drawer sign is present, the ankle is unstable and should be treated with a below-the-knee cast for 3 weeks.

Pure eversion injuries of the ankle are uncommon but can result in avulsion of the deltoid ligament. When the ankle reduces spontaneously, the deltoid ligament can remain interposed in the mortise. Radiographs reveal a wide ankle mortise and increased space between the medial malleolus and talus. Open reduction and deltoid ligament repair should be performed.

Lateral Ankle Ligament Injury Continued controversy exists regarding the diagnosis and treatment of lateral ankle sprains. Most lateral ligament injuries involve supination or adduction. The foot usually is plantar flexed at the time of injury and the anterior talofibular ligament usually is sprained. Supination of the foot in neutral flexion usually injures the calcaneofibular ligament. Supination and adduction injuries tear both the anterior tibiofibular and calcaneofibular ligaments. The posterior talofibular ligament is rarely injured.

The ankle must be examined in dorsiflexion and plantar flexion and tested for anterior drawer sign.

Ankle arthrography is rarely indicated in patients with acute ligament injuries. The radiographs are difficult to interpret and are unreliable in determining the degree of damage. The technique is expensive and can add to the morbidity of the injury. Stress radiographs likewise are rarely useful.

Primary repair of torn lateral ankle ligaments is rarely indicated. Open repair seems to offer no advantage over closed treatment.

Patients who have chronic ankle instability should be examined for excessive anteroposterior medial-lateral laxity as well as inversion-eversion laxity. Stress radiographs can be helpful. The Chrisman-Snook procedure has been reported to give good results in cases of chronic lateral ankle instability.

Dislocation of the Tarsal and Tarsometatarsal Joints Subtalar dislocations are uncommon. The mechanisms of injury described are forced inversion with forefoot plantar flexion or forced pronation. The incidence of osteonecrosis of the talus is related to the severity of the injury. An open subtalar dislocation with fracture of the neck of the talus has the highest risk of osteonecrosis. Open dislocations without talar neck fracture have a low incidence of osteonecrosis but a high incidence of subtalar stiffness. Closed dislocations are followed by a low incidence of osteonecrosis; the likelihood of subtalar arthritis or stiffness developing is proportional to the degree of soft tissue trauma at the initial injury.

Immediate open or closed reduction of subtalar dislocation is mandatory. If the talar neck is fractured, open reduction and internal fixation usually is required. Approaching the ankle through osteotomy of the medial malleolus can be helpful in providing the exposure needed for internal fixation. This method also preserves the blood supply to the medial talar body via the deltoid ligament. A compression splint and non-weight-bearing should be maintained until lucency becomes apparent under the subchondral talar bone on an anteroposterior radiograph. This finding indicates that talar vascularity is intact. If osteonecrosis occurs, non-weight-bearing or protection in a patellar tendon bearing foot-ankle orthosis should be continued. Protection for 2 years may be necessary for revascularization. If avascular collapse occurs, ankle arthrodesis is necessary.

Tarsometatarsal dislocations are frequently undiagnosed. Dislocations are usually caused by pronation or supination. Fracture dislocations are caused by excessive adduction, abduction, or dorsiflexion. Patients often report a snapping or "clunking" sensation in the foot. Forefoot swelling usually is excessive. Routine radiographs can be normal (Fig. 3). Comparison films or stress films under regional or general anesthesia can be essential in diagnosing the instability.

Simple tarsometatarsal dislocations that have reduced spontaneously require below-the-knee cast immobilization and non-weight-bearing for 6 weeks followed by use of a walking cast for 6 more weeks. A custom-made, rigid arch support is then worn in a lace-up shoe. Closed dislocations that require manual reduction should be transfixed with percutaneous Steinmann pins for 6 weeks, during which time a non-weight-bearing below-the-knee cast is worn. The pins are then removed and a below-the-knee walking cast is applied for 6 weeks. Lisfranc fracture-dislocations or tarsal or tarsometatarsal disruptions require open reduc-

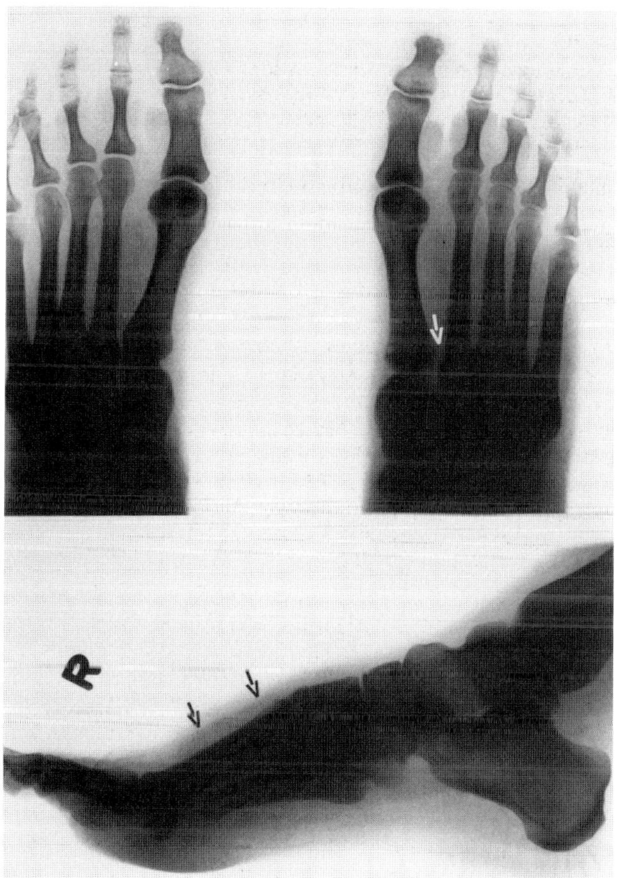

Figure 3

Lateral and anteroposterior radiographs of a patient with a spontaneously reduced metatarsocuneiform dislocation. Note the inordinate dorsal swelling (*arrows*) and the increased gap between the proximal first and second metatarsals.

tion with transfixing 6.5-mm cancellous bone screws. Severe intra-articular tarsal and tarsometatarsal fractures eventually may require an arthrodesis.

Isolated dislocations of tarsal bones are rare. Dislocations of the navicular, cuboid, or cuneiform bones have been reported, as have midtarsal dislocations. These injuries require closed or open reduction maintained by percutaneous pin fixation. Later, arthrodesis may be necessary, depending on the degree of joint instability, stiffness, pain, or arthritis.

Reflex Sympathetic Dystrophy

The clinical features of reflex sympathetic dystrophy, also known as causalgia or Sudeck's atrophy, are unusual pain and swelling; atrophic skin changes including atrophy, pigment changes, hypertrichosis, hyperhidrosis, and nail changes; vasomotor instability; and osteoporosis. The incidence is believed to be approximately 1 per 2,000 injuries.

In the lower extremity, reflex sympathetic dystrophy most frequently is a sequela of tarsometatarsal dislocation or supination-ankle sprain. This might be related to stretching of the superficial peroneal nerves. Some patients with severe symptoms have bilateral involvement, suggesting a central neural mechanism for the syndrome. A technetium-99m bone scan reveals diffuse increased uptake throughout the entire foot and ankle, with occasional increased uptake in the contralateral limb as well. This appearance on the bone scan occurs before the bone changes of patchy osteoporosis become visible on radiographs (Fig. 4).

The treatment of reflex sympathetic dystrophy is often delayed because it is difficult to recognize the syndrome in its early stages. Proper treatment of the initial injury and early mobilization are important in preventing its occurrence. The patient with reflex sympathetic dystrophy often has shown excessive anxiety regarding the injury and its treatment and apprehension in attempting mobilization and rehabilitation. A sympathetic block coordinated with physical therapy and gait training frequently can alleviate this syndrome.

When the patient has the full syndrome of reflex sympathetic dystrophy, including a swollen, discolored foot and ankle, diffuse osteoporosis, and a positive bone scan, further treatment is indicated. Various surgical procedures have been advocated in the past, but most of these have had limited or no success. These procedures include periarterial sympathectomy, stripping of the adventitia of major blood vessels, reserpine blocks, and repeated injections of anesthetic.

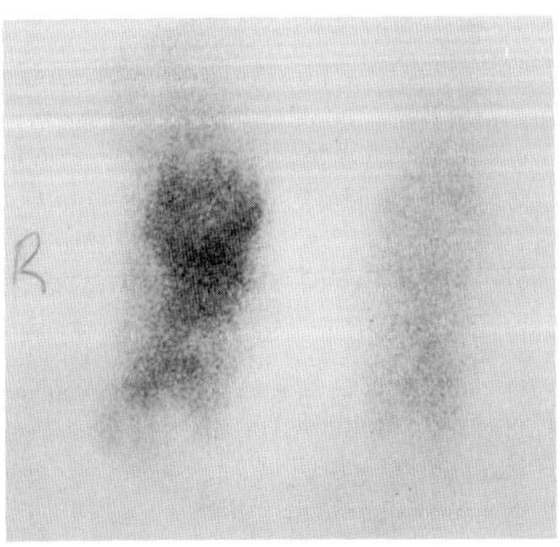

Figure 4

Diffuse increased radionuclide uptake in the foot and ankle of a patient with early causalgia, 3 months after ankle sprain.

Corticosteroid therapy has been recommended for treating patients who have reflex sympathetic dystrophy. Prednisone at 60 mg daily in divided doses is given for 1 week and then tapered to 5 mg daily over 2 weeks. Physical therapy and analgesics supplement the corticosteroid therapy, but the response to prednisone is reported to be immediate and dramatic.

Fractures of the Ankle and Foot

Fractures of the Ankle Joint

The ASIF classification system has three categories and is designed to be applied to operative treatment (Fig. 5). In this system, type A injuries occur below the tibiofibular syndesmosis. Ankle mortise instability is not common, and the result after anatomic closed reduction is likely to be satisfactory. In types B and C injuries, the incidence of injury to the tibiofibular syndesmosis and fracture of the posterior malleolus is 50% or greater. These fractures require anatomic open reduction, tibiofibular syndesmosis reduction and stabilization, and early joint mobilization for best results.

If anatomic reduction and stable internal fixation can be achieved, joint motion can begin early during hospitalization but not weight-bearing. Prior to dismissal, the ankle is immobilized in a cast that is worn for 3 weeks. Rigid internal fixation is not always achieved at operation. For these patients it is best to protect the ankle with a non-weight-bearing cast and to treat the injury as if no internal fixation had been used.

Pure axial force transmitted through the talus to the tibial plafond produces a so-called pilon fracture. These are divided into grades I through IV depending on the severity of injury. The objectives of treatment of pilon fractures are: 1) restoration of fibular length, 2) reduction of the articular surface of the tibia, 3) filling the tibial metaphyseal defect with cancellous bone graft, and 4) internal fixation of the medial aspect of the tibia by using a plate. Pilon and trimalleolar fractures usually extend into the articular weight-bearing surfaces. Despite anatomic rigid fixation and early joint mobilization, post-traumatic arthritis often develops (Fig. 6). It is important to document the degree of articular damage and to inform the patient of the prognosis at the time of the initial injury. Nonsteroidal anti-inflammatory agents and an ankle-foot orthosis with a shoe having a SACH heel and rocker bottom sole are helpful in conservative management. When pain due to post-traumatic arthritis can no longer be controlled by conservative means, ankle arthrodesis should be recommended (Fig. 6 *B*). The use of internal fixation and bone grafting appears to improve the rate of solid ankle fusion.

Fractures of the Talus

Osteochondral fractures of the dome of the talus can occur at the time of ankle ligament sprain or other injury. These injuries have been erroneously regarded as osteochondritis in the past.

The diagnosis can be difficult to confirm but it should be suspected in the patient who has persistent ankle pain.

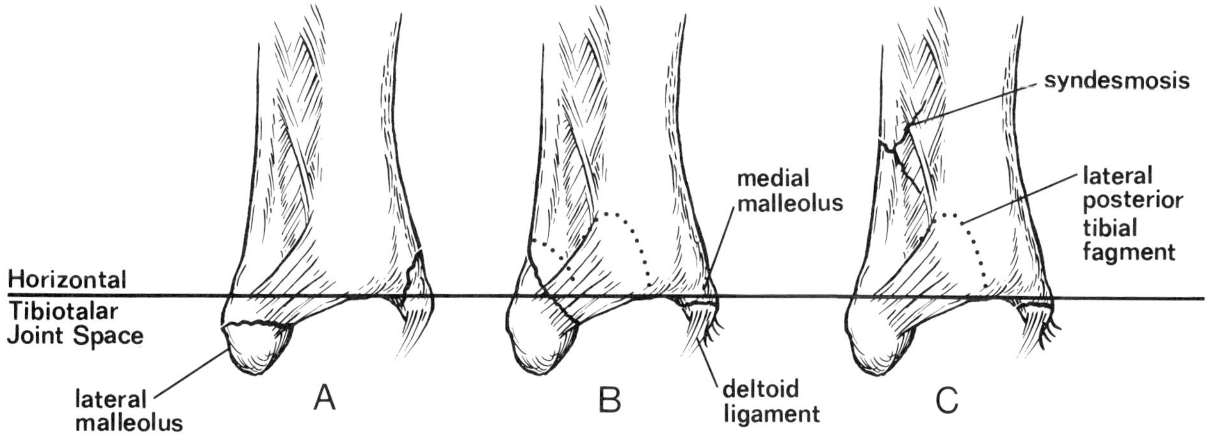

Figure 5

Diagram of classification system for ankle fractures.

Anteroposterior radiographs in maximum dorsiflexion and plantar flexion and an ankle arthrotomogram or a bone scan are useful diagnostic aids.

Surgical excision of the osteochondral fragment, drilling of the talar defect, and early motion, but without weight-bearing for up to 6 weeks, usually is recommended. The fragment can be removed either by arthroscopic methods or by arthrotomy, depending on the size and location of the lesion and the experience of the surgeon. Flexion-extension radiographs or tomograms assist in localizing the lesion so that an anterior or posterior approach can be chosen. A medial malleolar osteotomy approach usually is not required unless the fragment is very large and will be replaced and fixed. Drilling the medial malleolar screw hole before performing the osteotomy is helpful.

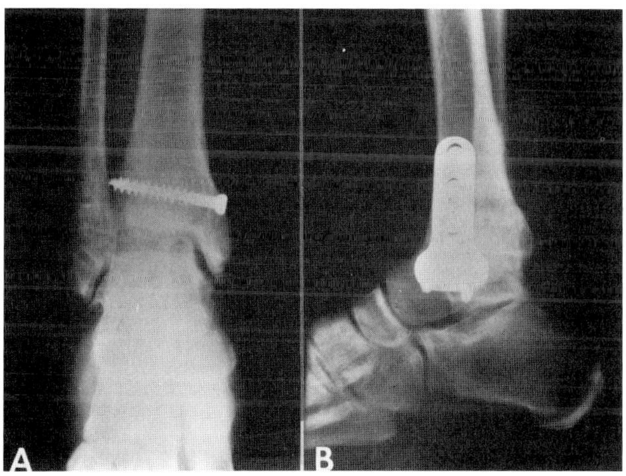

Figure 6

A, Anteroposterior radiograph of degenerative ankle 3 years after open reduction, internal fixation, and lateral plate removal. *B*, Lateral radiograph of same patient 1 year after arthrodesis.

The diagnosis, classification, and treatment of fractures of the talus were best described by Hawkins in 1970. The most common mechanism of injury is a fall from a height. Upon impact, the ankle is forced into dorsiflexion and the neck of the talus may fracture when it impacts against the anterior tibia. Undisplaced fractures of the talar neck require closed treatment only. Talar neck fractures displaced more than 1 mm require open reduction and internal fixation with anteroposterior cancellous compression screws. Surgical approaches vary depending on the location of the fracture. These approaches are designed to preserve the talar blood supply. A posterior approach to talar neck fractures preserves the dorsal blood supply. A medial malleolar osteotomy approach preserves the deltoid branch which supplies the medial talus. Weight-bearing should be prohibited until vascular integrity is ensured.

Fractures of the Calcaneus

The common cause of calcaneal fractures is a fall. An unexpected drop onto the heels from a height as low as 1 m has produced severe, bilateral, comminuted calcaneal fractures. Depending on the angle and degree of force, various fracture patterns may be seen. The classification of Essex-Lopresti is helpful in determining the type of fracture, however, it is not sufficiently appreciated that intra-articular fractures of the joint depression or the tongue type are preceded by fractures of the medial and lateral cortices.

The contouring of the calcaneus on the medial side to allow room for the tendon and neurovascular structures places the center of the talus slightly medial to the center of the tuberosity of the calcaneus. A downward force on the talus, as occurs in a fall onto the heel, therefore produces a shear stress along an oblique line through the body of the calcaneus, fracturing it along that line to produce two fragments—the sustentacular fragment anteromedially,

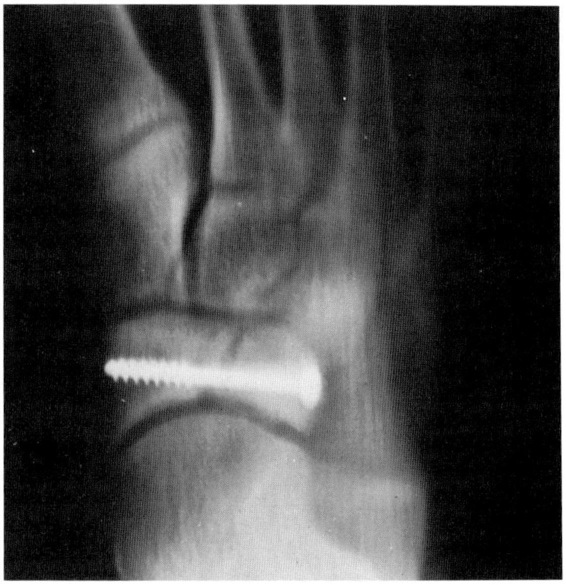

Figure 7

Tomogram of tarsal navicular bone treated by drilling and screw (2.7 mm) fixation for chronic stress fracture.

and the tuberosity fragment posterolaterally, with eventual overriding and displacement of the fragments on the medial side. The joint depression and tongue type fractures are additional components.

Although controversy still exists regarding the management of displaced intra-articular fractures, it is now increasingly accepted that an anatomically restored joint and calcaneus results in better function and that adequate reduction most often can be achieved only by operative methods.

A medial approach is now used more often in preference to the lateral approach or a combination of both surgical approaches is used to restore joint congruency. The medial approach appears to be logical in view of the fact that the sustentacular spike (of the anteromedial sustentacular fragment) is the key to reduction. Prior to the reduction of the tuberosity fragment in relation to the stable sustentacular fragment, the lateral bulge of the tuberosity is reduced as well as the joint depression or tongue type fragments through the medial approach. Occasionally, an additional lateral approach may be necessary.

Radiographic criteria that have been found to be useful in prediction of the final result are Bohler's angle, width of the calcaneus, and integrity of the medial arch. The quality of the result is in direct proportion to the degree to which these features are restored to normal by either conservative or operative treatment.

The markedly comminuted fracture in which an adequate reduction is not possible should be treated by nonsurgical means, preferably by compressive dressings, non-weight-bearing, and early joint mobilization.

Associated problems that might compromise the end results are injured calcaneal fat pad, traumatized posterior tibial nerve, and severe posterior articular facet damage despite relatively normal restored calcaneal anatomy. These residual problems need to be addressed separately.

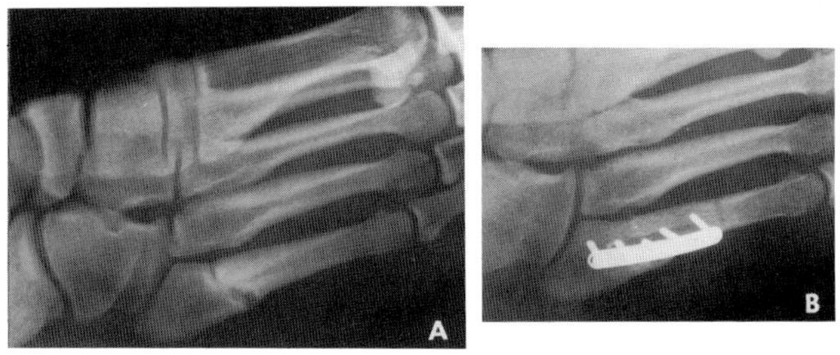

Figure 8

Jones fracture. *A*, Oblique radiograph, showing nonunion in recreational athlete. *B*, Healing after application of small plate and autogenous bone graft.

Fibular impingement or subtalar arthritis developing as a late complication after the fracture has healed can be treated by secondary reconstruction or a Grice-type extra-articular arthrodesis. Rarely, a triple arthrodesis is required.

Fractures of the anterior process of the calcaneus are caused by forced plantar flexion of the foot. They are best detected on oblique radiographs but commonly this diagnosis is missed. Treatment is a non-weight-bearing cast for 3 weeks followed by partial weight-bearing for an additional 3 weeks. Late excision of a painful nonunion of the anterior process results in satisfactory relief of symptoms.

Fractures of the Midtarsal and Metatarsal Bones

Fractures in the midtarsal region are usually associated with dislocations at Chopart's or Lisfranc's joint.

Stress fracture of the navicular bone can occur. It is characterized by insidious onset of vague medial midfoot pain. The fracture usually lies in the sagittal plane and is difficult to visualize on standard radiographs. A radionuclide scan should be performed if this fracture is suspected. Tomograms aid in localization of the fracture (Fig. 7).

If a navicular fracture is not diagnosed and treated early, there is a high incidence of osteonecrosis. This fracture should be treated by limiting weight-bearing to minimize fragmentation and collapse. An acute fracture is best treated by non-weight-bearing in a below-the-knee cast for 6 weeks followed by a walking cast for 6 weeks. Repeat tomograms are necessary to confirm healing. For chronic untreated fractures that have sclerotic borders, open reduction and internal fixation should be performed. A lateral approach

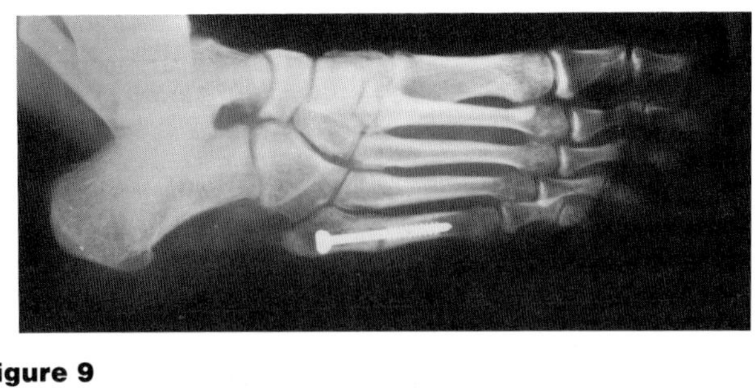

Figure 9

Lateral radiograph, showing Jones fracture at 6 months after it was treated by bone grafting and screw fixation.

preserves the dorsal blood supply to the navicular bone. Two 2.7-mm cancellous screws provide satisfactory fixation; drilling additional holes across the fracture site may promote fracture healing. A non-weight-bearing cast is worn for 6 weeks followed by use of a walking cast for 6 weeks.

Unstable metatarsal fractures can be fixed by using percutaneous Kirschner wires. If two or more metatarsals are fractured, it is best to keep the patient non-weight-bearing for 3 weeks and then remove the pins and apply a walking cast for 3 weeks.

Fractures of the base of the fifth metatarsal require special consideration. Supination injuries frequently cause avulsion fractures at the base (tuberosity) of the fifth metatarsal. These fractures are usually stable and should be treated as sprains. This type of fracture should be distinguished from the fracture that occurs distal to the tuberosity of the fifth metatarsal. The mechanism of injury and the healing characteristics are different.

These stress fractures carry the eponym "Jones fractures" (Fig. 8). Fractures at the base of the fifth metatarsal heal slowly and delayed union, nonunion, and refracture are common. Patients with an acute fracture of the proximal diaphysis of the fifth metatarsal should be placed in a non-weight-bearing cast for 4 weeks followed by a walking cast for 4 additional weeks. Because the incidence of nonunion can be high (67%) in young athletes with this fracture, some surgeons have advocated internal fixation with a malleolar screw. Stress fracture can also occur in this location and should be differentiated from these other injuries.

Stress fractures have been classified into three categories: 1) acute fractures with a narrow fracture line and no intramedullary sclerosis; 2) delayed union fractures with widening of the fracture line and evidence of intramedullary sclerosis, and 3) nonunion with complete sclerotic obliteration of the intramedullary canal. An acute fracture (category 1) can be treated by non-weight-bearing cast for 4 weeks followed by a walking cast for 4 more. Fractures in categories 2 and 3 are unlikely to heal, even with prolonged immobilization. Bone grafting and an intramedullary compression screw fixation at the time of injury seems to be the best form of treatment (Fig. 9). This is followed by non-weight-bearing for 6 weeks and then use of a walking cast for 6 weeks.

Annotated Bibliography

Syndesmotic Screw

de Souza, L.J.; Gustilo, R.B.; and Meyer, T.J.: Results of operative treatment of displaced external rotation-abduction fracture of the ankle. J. Bone Joint Surg. 67A:1066–1074, 1985.

In this review of 150 patients with displaced ankle fractures, it was found that the 30 patients treated with a suprasyndesmotic screw were able to walk without difficulty. In 18 of these 30, the screws were removed a mean of 1 year after insertion; in the 12 other patients the screws remained *in situ* without causing symptoms, from 2½ to 3½ years after insertion.

Tendon Injuries

Arrowsmith, S.R.; Fleming, L.L.; and Allman, F.L.: Traumatic dislocations of the peroneal tendons. Am. J. Sports Med. 11:142–146, 1983.

Violent inversion stress or dorsiflexion is the common mechanism of peroneal tendon dislocation. Conservative treatment for an initial injury is preferred, but operative repair or reconstruction is indicated in chronic cases.

Ma, G.W.C., and Griffith, T.G.: Percutaneous repair of acute closed ruptured Achilles tendon: A new technique. Clin. Orthop. 128:247–255, 1977.

The authors present a useful technique of percutaneous Achilles tendon repair that eliminates extensive surgical exposure and its attendant morbidity.

Mann, R.A., and Thompson, F.M.: Rupture of the posterior tibial tendon causing flat foot. J. Bone Joint Surg. 67A:556–561, 1985.

Rupture of the posterior tibial tendon results in a progressive painful flatfoot deformity. Surgical transfer of the flexor digitorum longus tendon into the navicular bone was a satisfactory salvage procedure.

Nistor, L.: Surgical and non-surgical treatment of Achilles tendon rupture: A prospective randomized study. J. Bone Joint Surg. 63A:394–399, 1981.

Forty-five patients were treated surgically and 60, by cast immobilization. Both treatment groups demonstrated loss of plantar flexion power, but no statistically significant difference existed. The group not treated surgically had a slightly higher rerupture rate, 8% compared with 4%.

Ankle Sprains

Broström, L.: Sprained ankles. VI. Surgical treatment of "chronic" ligament ruptures. Acta Chir. Scand. 132:551–565, 1966.

Various ligament reconstructions are reviewed, and the Broström-type repair is presented.

Edwards, G.S., and DeLee, J.C.: Ankle diastasis without fracture. Foot Ankle 4:305–312, 1984.

Four types of ankle diastasis are identified. Treatment is based on the type of diastasis as determined from stress radiographs.

Grace, D.L.: Lateral ankle ligament injuries: Inversion and anterior stress radiography. Clin. Orthop. 183:153–159, 1984.

Significant anterior talar subluxation will occur with stress when the anterior talofibular is incompetent. Significant lateral tilt occurs only when more than one component of the lateral ligament is incompetent.

Katznelson, A.; Lin, E.; and Militiano, J.: Ruptures of the ligaments about the tibio-fibular syndesmosis. Injury 15:170–172, 1983.

The history and clinical examination are key in making the diagnosis of diastasis. Arthrography can be helpful if necessary.

Niedermann, B.; Andersen, A.; Andersen, S.B.; Funder,

V.; Jørgensen, J.P.; Lindholmer, E.; and Vuust, M.: Rupture of the lateral ligaments of the ankle: Operation or plaster cast? A prospective study. Acta Orthop. Scand. 52:579–587, 1981.

Two hundred nine patients were treated randomly with either a cast for 5 weeks or surgical repair followed by non-weight-bearing in a cast for 5 weeks. Good results were obtained in 76% of the nonoperative group and 81% of the operative group. This is not a statistically significant difference.

Rasmussen, O.: Stability of the ankle joint: Analysis of the function and traumatology of the ankle ligaments. Acta Orthop. Scand. [Suppl.] 211:1–75, 1985.

The author correlates injuries to the lateral collateral ligaments with internal rotatory stability, talar tilt, and the anterior drawer sign.

Snook, G.A.; Chrisman, O.D.; and Wilson, T.C.: Long-term results of the Chrisman-Snook operation for reconstruction of the lateral ligaments of the ankle. J. Bone Joint Surg. 67A:1–7, 1985.

Mean follow-up of 10 years revealed good or excellent results in 45 of 48 ankles.

Midfoot Dislocations

Goossens, M., and De Stoop, N.: Lisfranc's fracture-dislocations: Etiology, radiology, and results of treatment; A review of 20 cases. Clin. Orthop. 176:154–162, 1983.

Fracture-dislocation at Lisfranc's joint is often missed because of spontaneous reduction. Anatomic reduction and transfixion with Kirschner wires is the treatment of choice.

Pediatric Ankle Fractures

Von Laer, L.: Classification, diagnosis, and treatment of transitional fractures of the distal part of the tibia. J. Bone Joint Surg. 67A:687–698, 1985.

Analysis of 32 transitional fractures of the distal tibia revealed three different configurations of fractures. Computed tomography will assist in determining whether fracture displacement of the weight-bearing epiphysis is greater than 2 mm and thus requires open reduction.

Adult Ankle Fractures

Alexander, A.H., and Lichtman, D.M.: Surgical treatment of transchondral talar-dome fractures (osteochondritis dissecans). J. Bone Joint Surg. 62A:646–652, 1980.

Transchondral fractures of the talar dome are associated with severe ankle sprains. Surgical excision of the fragment, followed by drilling, curettage, and non-weight-bearing motion, appears to be the best form of treatment.

Pettrone, F.A.; Gail, M.; Pee, D.; Fitzpatrick, T.; and Van Herpe, L.B.: Quantitative criteria for prediction of the results after displaced fracture of the ankle. J. Bone Joint Surg. 65A:66–77, 1983.

Open and closed treatments of ankle fractures are compared, and the influence of age, sex, side of injury, mechanism of injury, and severity of injury are evaluated. Open reduction was superior to closed treatment, and the outcome could be predicted on the basis of the accuracy of reduction and the severity of fracture.

Roberts, R.S.: Surgical treatment of displaced ankle fractures. Clin. Orthop. 172:164–170, 1983.

Pronation-eversion injuries had the poorest prognosis among ankle fractures. The best results occurred with the best anatomic reduction.

Ankle Salvage

Mazur, J.M.; Schwartz, E.; and Simon, S.: Ankle arthrodesis. Long-term follow-up with gait analysis. J. Bone Joint Surg. 61A:964–975, 1979.

Ankle arthrodesis patients are seen to have minimal disability at long-term follow-up after fusion. An ankle grading system provides an objective means to determine the quality of the functional result.

Morgan, C.D.; Henke, J.A.; Bailey, R.W.; and Kaufer, H.: Long-term results of tibiotalar arthrodesis. J. Bone Joint Surg. 67A:546–550, 1985.

One hundred one ankle arthrodeses had a union rate of 95%. Postoperative tarsal motion increased an average of 85%.

Scranton, P.: Use of internal compression in arthrodesis of the ankle. J. Bone Joint Surg. 67A:550–555, 1985.

A specially designed T-plate is used to provide stability and compression across the arthrodesis site. The medial approach provides excellent surgical exposure and permits supplementary bone graft.

Fractures of the Talus

Canale, S.T., and Kelly, F.B.: Fractures of the neck of the talus. J. Bone Joint Surg. 60A:143–156, 1978.

A detailed review of 71 fractures of the neck of the talus revealed that the incidence of osteonecrosis appeared to be related to the classification of the fracture. In a high percentage of patients, surgical treatment was regarded as the best form of treatment.

Fractures of the Calcaneus

Burdeaux, B.D.: Reduction of calcaneal fractures by the McReynolds medial approach technique and its experimental basis. Clin. Orthop. 177:87–103, 1983.

Hammesfahr, R., and Fleming, L.L.: Calcaneal fractures: A good prognosis. Foot Ankle 2:161–170, 1981.

Hunter, G.A., and James, E.T.R.: Amputation following os calcis fractures: A rare complication not previously emphasized (abstract). Orthop. Trans. 6:480–481, 1982.

41

Ankle and Foot: Reconstruction

Adaptation of the biomechanical principles of the human gait has led to a refinement in the treatment of forefoot and hindfoot disorders. A functional ankle arthrodesis requires the neutral position in the lateral plane and hindfoot valgus of 5°. Careful management of both the osseous and soft tissues is necessary in the surgical treatment of hallux valgus deformities. Most plantar keratoses can be treated nonoperatively. Management of heel pain from various causes, tendon injuries, and rheumatoid disease of the foot is detailed.

Biomechanical Considerations

When any type of fusion in the hindfoot region decreases the mobility of the joints, the degree of force dissipation is significantly altered. The greater the loss of mobility of the foot, the greater the stresses applied to the body; in fact, the level of activity of the patient can be diminished. Therefore, subtalar fusion is preferable to full triple arthrodesis because fewer joints are involved and greater mobility is maintained within the foot.

When ankle joint fusion is contemplated, the ankle position should be neutral insofar as dorsiflexion and plantar flexion are concerned. This creates a sort of "rocker bottom" effect which would enable the body to roll over the fused ankle joint rather than having to vault over it as would be required if it were in plantar flexion. Plantar flexion occasionally is required if there is loss of motor function about the knee joint. The degree of varus and valgus also needs to be considered carefully because, if the hindfoot is positioned so that the weight-bearing line of the lower extremity passes lateral to the heel, an unstable subtalar joint is created and the patient walks on the lateral aspect of the foot. Therefore, the alignment of the ankle fusion needs to be such that the calcaneus is placed in approximately 5° of valgus to prevent instability at the subtalar joint. The same considerations apply to a subtalar arthrodesis. The subtalar joint should be placed in approximately 5° of valgus to provide stability to the ankle joint. If it is placed in varus, the weight-bearing line will pass lateral to the heel and cause lateral ankle instability and foot pain.

The transverse tarsal joint, which consists of the talonavicular and calcaneocuboid joints, also plays a significant role in forefoot stability. When the calcaneus is in an inverted (varus) position, there is increased stability at the transverse tarsal joint; conversely, with the heel in an everted (valgus) position, there is decreased stability at this joint. Therefore, when the calcaneus is in a position of varus there is increased stability in the transverse tarsal joint and the body would tend to vault over the foot; in order to compensate for this, the foot is placed into an externally rotated position, thereby possibly placing strain along the medial side of the knee joint. For this reason, the positioning of the hindfoot affects not only the lateral stability of the foot and ankle but also the stability of the foot itself. Isolated fusion of the subtalar joint permits motion in the transverse tarsal joint, but fusion of the talonavicular joint essentially eliminates all of the motion in the subtalar and transverse tarsal joints. Therefore, when carrying out a talonavicular fusion, it is important that the hindfoot be positioned properly to provide the patient with a plantigrade foot.

Hallux Valgus

The hallux valgus deformity consists of lateral deviation of the proximal phalanx on the metatarsal head which results in a contracture of the lateral joint capsule, stretching, and some attenuation, depending upon the degree of deformity, of the medial joint capsule and the formation of a medial eminence of varying degree (the bunion). The first metatarsal head is pushed medially as the proximal phalanx drifts laterally, resulting in displacement of the metatarsal head off of the sesamoid sling. The sesamoids are anchored by the transverse metatarsal ligament which attaches to the lateral aspect of the fibular sesamoid and adductor hallucis. Depending upon the degree of deformity, the great toe no longer carries its share of the weight. As a result, weight is transferred onto the second metatarsal head, not infrequently resulting in metatarsalgia.

The pressure of the great toe against the second toe often causes a deformity of the second toe, which may take the form of either minor subluxation of the joint or a frank dislocation associated with a severe hammertoe. As a general rule, in severe deformities the second toe rests on top of the great toe, although occasionally it will be beneath it.

Treatment

The treatment of a hallux valgus deformity usually should be conservative. Use of a broad-toed, soft-soled shoe often produces a satisfactory clinical response. However, surgical intervention is indicated in some cases.

In surgical correction of severe hallux valgus deformity, the basic correction is release of the contracture along the lateral side of the metatarsophalangeal joint, which includes release of the lateral joint capsule, adductor hallucis, and transverse metatarsal ligament. This frees the lateral joint capsule and sesamoid sling of their contractures. On the medial aspect the medial eminence is removed 1 mm medial to the sagittal sulcus in line with the medial aspect of the metatarsal shaft, and the medial joint capsule is plicated.

The abnormal intermetatarsal angle also must be corrected. It is in this regard that most of the controversy regarding correction of a bunion exists. If needed, the correction can be made distally by carrying out a Mitchell or a chevron type of osteotomy or proximally by carrying out a crescentic, opening, or closing wedge osteotomy. The distal metatarsal osteotomies correct the intermetatarsal angle to varying degrees but can result in osteonecrosis of the metatarsal head or loss of position due to the difficulty in obtaining adequate fixation of the osteotomy site. The proximal osteotomies do not lead to an avascular change but, if done improperly, can result in shortening of the metatarsal or, not infrequently, dorsiflexion of the metatarsal or in loss of position if the osteotomy site is inadequately fixed.

Another method of treatment of severe hallux valgus deformity or hallux valgus deformity as a recurrence secondary to excessive excision of a portion of the medial eminence or due to degenerative arthritis is arthrodesis of the first metatarsophalangeal joint. This procedure is excellent for realignment of the metatarsophalangeal joint. The ideal position for an arthrodesed first metatarsophalangeal joint is approximately 15° of valgus and 25° of dorsiflexion in relation to the first metatarsal shaft. This alignment is important because, if the toe lacks valgus, the increased stress on the interphalangeal joint of the great toe may cause deterioration of the joint at an increased rate. Lack of adequate dorsiflexion would result in difficulty in passing over the foot, so that the patient would tend to rotate the lower extremity externally to avoid excessive stress on the interphalangeal joint. Excessive dorsiflexion should be avoided, to prevent the toe from striking the top of the shoe.

Use of a single-stem prosthesis in the base of the proximal phalanx does not seem to be indicated for primary hallux valgus deformity without significant degenerative arthritis. If such arthritis is present (which is uncommon), consideration should be given to use of a double-stem type of silicone prosthesis or possibly to arthrodesis.

Complications

The complications usually associated with release of the lateral joint capsule and excision of the medial eminence with plication of the medial joint capsule are recurrence of the deformity and possibly hallux varus. The recurrence usually is due to inadequate release of the lateral joint capsule and sesamoid sling along with failure to correct the metatarsus primus varus. If the metatarsus primus varus is not corrected, a soft tissue procedure *per se* cannot produce a satisfactory long-term result (a soft tissue procedure will not overcome a fixed contracture). Correction of recurrence is best achieved by revising the initial soft tissue procedure and adding to it a proximal metatarsal osteotomy.

Hallux varus is particularly likely if the lateral sesamoid is excised. It also can occur after excessive excision of the medial aspect of the metatarsal head or overplication of the medial capsular tissues. If the medial eminence is not excised in line with the medial aspect of the metatarsal, the medial buttress to a varus deformity is lost and this, along with some progressive soft tissue contracture, may result in a hallux varus deformity. This deformity can vary in degree from mild (1° to 7°) and only visible radiographically to severe associated with a cock-up deformity from loss of function of the flexor digitorum brevis through its insertion into the sesamoids and then into the base of the proximal phalanx. As a result of loss of flexor power of the proximal phalanx, the metatarsophalangeal joint hyperextends along with medial deviation; flexion of the interphalangeal joint may occur secondarily.

Hallux varus can be corrected in two ways: soft tissue reconstruction, and arthrodesis of the metatarsophalangeal joint. The soft tissue reconstruction can be achieved if the articular surface still present is adequate for the proximal phalanx (an excessive amount of medial eminence was not excised) and the interphalangeal joint of the great toe can be straightened passively. If the remaining metatarsal head is inadequate in amount or has undergone severe degenerative changes, arthrodesis of the joint would be the treatment of choice. A prosthesis would rarely be indicated for severe hallux varus deformity.

The soft tissue procedure, which is about 80% successful, consists of rerouting of the extensor hallucis longus tendon beneath the transverse metatarsal ligament and securing it into the base of the proximal phalanx of the great toe. Along with this, complete release of the contracted tissues on the medial aspect of the metatarsophalangeal joint along with repositioning of the sesamoid(s) must be achieved. If a fixed deformity of the interphalangeal joint of the great toe is present, arthrodesis is needed. This soft tissue correction provides a plantar lateral pull on the proximal phalanx, which usually brings it back into satisfactory alignment. The cause of failure of this procedure usually is inadequate medial soft tissue release. This procedure will result in satisfactory function of the metatarsophalangeal joint, although approximately 30% to 50% of the motion of the joint will be lost due to adhesions resulting from the initial operation and the reconstructive operation.

Salvage of the first metatarsophalangeal joint by arthrodesis for hallux varus usually produces a most satisfactory result. If a severe flexion contracture of the interphalangeal joint is present, it should be released at the time of operation to prevent a pressure problem on the tip of the great toe.

The incidence of osteonecrosis of the metatarsal head after Mitchell or chevron osteotomy is difficult to determine. If stripping of the lateral metatarsal head capsule is avoided, it usually will not occur.

Salvage is extremely difficult for complications after use of a prosthesis, particularly the single-stem variety. These complications consist of collapse of the prosthesis, silicone-induced synovitis, settling of the prosthesis into the proximal phalanx, and generalized stiffness of the metatarsophalangeal joint. Generally, for salvage the prosthesis must be removed and an arthrodesis of the metatarsophalangeal joint carried out. The arthrodesis can be carried out by bringing the base of the proximal phalanx and the metatarsal head together, which gives a satisfactory result although with a somewhat shortened toe, or by placing a bone graft across the joint to provide adequate length from a cosmetic standpoint. In either case, although a satisfactory plantigrade foot is achieved, the ability of the patient to participate in sports activities other than walking, swimming, and bicycle riding is significantly impaired. The conversion of a single-stem prosthesis to a double-stem prosthesis usually will not give a satisfactory result because the fibrosis present about the joint would preclude satisfactory motion even with a double-ended prosthesis. If a double-ended prosthesis fails, the salvage procedure of choice is an arthrodesis of the joint.

Deformities of Second Metatarsophalangeal Joint

As a rule, deformities of the second metatarsophalangeal joint are associated with a progressive hallux valgus deformity that causes pressure against the second toe, which may result in dorsal subluxation or frank dislocation of the joint and, not infrequently, a rather severe fixed hammertoe deformity. However, sometimes a spontaneous deformity develops in the second metatarsophalangeal joint. This may result in a cocking up of the second toe with a medial, but sometimes a lateral, deviation as well as a hammertoe deformity. In some patients, subluxation of the second metatarsophalangeal joint may occur as an isolated entity with no specific cause. The patient usually presents with pain in the forefoot; examination reveals thickening of the entire second metatarsophalangeal joint and, not infrequently, increased warmth.

Treatment

With Hallux Valgus When a deformity of the second toe is associated with a hallux valgus deformity, the principle of treatment is correction of the hallux valgus deformity to create a space in which the second toe can be placed. If there is a significant deformity of the second toe but no space between the great toe and the third toe, any type of surgical procedure carried out only on the second toe will fail.

Once the great toe is corrected, if the second metatarsophalangeal joint has only a mild cock-up deformity, release or lengthening of the extensor tendon and dorsal capsulotomy, along with postoperative splinting in a slightly plantar flexed position for 4 to 6 weeks, may result in satisfactory alignment. If there is dorsal subluxation of the joint that can be corrected passively but does not have adequate flexor power, complete medial and lateral capsulotomy also must be performed, followed by a Girdlestone flexor tendon transfer into the extensor mechanism (a tail of the flexor digitorum longus tendon is brought up on each side of the extensor hood and sutured into the extensor digitorum longus while the toe is held in approximately 20° of plantar flexion). This tendon transfer restores some plantar flexion function to the metatarsophalangeal joint.

Dislocation For complete dislocation of the metatarsophalangeal joint the treatment is somewhat more controversial. The base of the proximal phalanx should be saved because it provides insertion for the plantar aponeurosis and some of the intrinsic muscles of the foot. If the base of the proximal phalanx is resected, the toe may drift up into dorsiflexion, creating a significant problem for the patient. If the entire proximal phalanx is removed, a floppy, shortened toe results. If a syndactyly is carried out after these procedures, not infrequently the adjacent toe will also be drawn upward or become medially deviated as the second toe contracts after removal of the proximal phalanx. Arthroplasty at the level of the metatarsophalangeal joint is preferred for complete dislocation of the metatarsophalangeal joint.

The arthroplasty involves extensor tenotomy, dorsal capsulotomy, and release of the medial and lateral collateral ligaments. Then, not infrequently, synovectomy will be needed because of chronic synovitis. The toe is now pulled distally and the level at which the base of the proximal phalanx touches the metatarsal head is the site of resection of the distal portion of the metatarsal head.

Resection of the metatarsal head alone for the treatment of isolated dislocated metatarsophalangeal joint should not be carried out because it results in shortening of the involved toe as well as a transfer type of metatarsalgia which becomes refractory to conservative or operative management.

Swelling and Pain The patient with synovitis who presents with nonspecific swelling and pain in the second metatarsophalangeal joint initially should be treated conservatively with anti-inflammatory medications, a shoe of adequate size, and a soft metatarsal support. If the process fails to subside, synovectomy of the joint may produce a satisfactory result. However, in this type of condition the intrinsic muscles about the toe undergo some changes, and a hammertoe deformity often develops over a period of time. After synovectomy, the possibility of a hammertoe developing is diminished but not completely eliminated.

Lesser Toe Problems

The fixed hammertoe (a flexion deformity of the proximal interphalangeal joint) and the fixed mallet toe (a flexion deformity of the distal interphalangeal joint) can produce significant discomfort for the patient. At times these deformities may be associated with varying degrees of dorsiflexion at the metatarsophalangeal joint. (If a significant dorsiflexion contracture is present at the metatarsophalangeal joint, the condition is called a "claw toe deformity.") Generally speaking, hammertoe can be considered to be either a fixed or a dynamic deformity. With a fixed deformity, some type of bone procedure is needed; if it is a dynamic deformity, a tendon transfer may provide satisfactory correction of the problem.

Treatment

Conservative management of a lesser toe deformity involves the use of an adequate shoe, usually an extra-depth shoe with, at times, a Plastizote liner. Various types of felt supports are available to place underneath the toe to prevent the tip of the toe from striking the ground (this can produce a painful callus on the tip of the toe). If conservative management fails, surgical correction usually will produce a satisfactory result.

The mallet toe deformity can be treated by resection arthroplasty or arthrodesis. Resection arthroplasty involves resection of an ellipse of skin over the dorsal aspect of the distal interphalangeal joint, exposing the head of the middle phalanx, and removing the condylar portion of the middle phalanx. The articular surface of the base of the distal phalanx is left intact. With either a 0.045-inch Kirschner wire or Telfa bolsters, the deformity is corrected and held corrected for 6 weeks. A satisfactory long-term result can be expected. However, if the joint is not adequately decompressed or if the flexor tendon appears to be excessively tight, a long-term satisfactory result will not be achieved.

The fixed hammertoe deformity is corrected in a similar manner except that the skin incision is made over the dorsal aspect of the proximal interphalangeal joint. The distal portion of the proximal phalanx is exposed and the condyles are resected generously. The articular surface at the base of the middle phalanx is left intact. Fixation is with a 0.45-inch Kirschner wire or Telfa bolsters. If Telfa bolsters are used, they are left in place for only 1 week; then the toe is held in place with adhesive tape for the remainder of the 6 weeks of immobilization. If a Kirschner wire is used, it is left in place for approximately 3 weeks, and the remainder of the immobilization is with adhesive tape.

If a mild dorsiflexion contracture is present at the metatarsophalangeal joint, an extensor tenotomy and dorsal capsulotomy can be added to the mallet toe, the hammertoe, or the flexor tendon transfer in order to correct it. When releasing this contracture, it is important that the metatarsophalangeal joint be kept down in a corrected position for a total of 6 weeks to ensure that the contracture will be completely stretched out. At times, this may result in slight drooping of the toe, but this is more desirable than early recurrence of the deformity.

Intractable Plantar Keratoses

An intractable plantar keratosis, or plantar callus, is one of the causes of metatarsalgia. Other causes are interdigital neuroma, plantar wart, synovitis of a metatarsophalangeal joint, rheumatoid arthritis, stress fracture, and atrophy of the plantar fat pad. This discussion will be confined to the localized intractable plantar keratosis beneath a single metatarsal head.

These keratoses are divided into two types: well-localized discrete lesion with a central core, and diffuse. The causes of the two types differ in that the former may be due to a prominence of a condyle or a sesamoid and the latter is due to depression or excessive length of a metatarsal. To identify which is the cause, the lesion should be trimmed with a sharp scalpel to determine whether the lesion is a well-localized keratosis with a deep keratotic center or is a diffuse type of keratosis with no discrete central area. The trimming also enables one to differentiate the callus from a plantar wart which bleeds vigorously from end arteries when the superficial keratinized layer is removed.

Treatment

The conservative management of intractable plantar keratosis is based on managing the lesion itself with adequate debridement followed by selection of footwear that allows the foot to spread out and also increases the cushioning between the plantar aspect of the foot and the ground. A soft metatarsal support can be added, to relieve the involved area. Most intractable plantar keratoses can be managed in this manner, with debridement every 6 to 8 weeks. If the lesion remains significantly disabling, surgical intervention may give a satisfactory clinical result.

If operation is necessary, a DuVries type of condylectomy can be used in which the plantar half of the metatarsal head is removed. Additionally, arthroplasty of the metatarsophalangeal joint is carried out to round off the metatarsal head. If a transfer lesion occurs in the adjacent metatarsal, it is treated by a basilar metatarsal osteotomy.

A large, diffuse callus beneath the first metatarsal head presents an entirely different type of clinical problem. It is due to plantar flexion of the first metatarsal and can be corrected by a dorsiflexion osteotomy of the first metatarsal. This can be accomplished by a closing dorsal wedge osteotomy at the base of the first metatarsal to allow the metatarsal to rise.

Another plantar site where a diffuse callus occasionally arises is beneath the fifth metatarsal. Generally, this is associated with a tailor's bunion. However, not all tailor's bunions are associated with a plantar lesion. This problem can be treated by making an oblique osteotomy in the fifth metatarsal shaft in such a way that the deviation of the fifth metatarsal shaft—namely, the plantar flexion and lateral deviation—is corrected. The oblique osteotomy is made so that the metatarsal head moves both dorsally and medially. Once the metatarsal shaft is exposed, a long oblique osteotomy is produced and the osteotomy site is permitted to deviate dorsally and medially. It is then fixed with a small fragment screw or cerclage wire.

Much has been written about various types of metatarsal osteotomies for intractable plantar keratoses. As a general rule the osteotomy site should be fixed rather than permitting the metatarsal head to "float" to its new level. The cuts should be as accurate as possible and then the metatarsal should be fixed in position to keep the possibility of transfer lesions to a minimum. At times the healing of a metatarsal osteotomy seems to be progressing very slowly and no complete union is apparent radiographically, but usually after 8 to 10 weeks the osteotomy site is sufficiently healed by clinical examination that the immobilization can be discontinued. It is rare for a nonunion to occur although any time an osteotomy is produced the possibility of a nonunion is present.

Sesamoids

Pain about the sesamoids is not a common cause of metatarsalgia, although it does occur. The sesamoids are contained within the flexor hallucis brevis and insert, via a heavy ligamentous structure, into the base of the proximal phalanx of the great toe. This structure provides a fulcrum for the function of the plantar aponeurosis and flexor hallucis brevis. Because the sesamoids are intimately connected to the base of the proximal phalanx, any shift in the position of the sesamoids in relation to the first metatarsal brings about a change in the alignment of the great toe—i.e., pronation associated with hallux valgus. If the function of both sesamoids is disrupted, either through trauma or surgery, plantar flexion of the proximal phalanx is lost and the proximal phalanx will assume a dorsiflexed position on the metatarsal head. Therefore, only one sesamoid should be removed at a time.

The tibial sesamoid is bipartite in approximately 20% of cases, although this usually occurs bilaterally. Evaluation of sesamoid problems may be difficult because radiography may not reveal the cause of the chronic pain. Bone scanning with a pinhead collimator may demonstrate increased activity in a sesamoid with either a fracture or a collapse secondary to avascular change. If the scan is normal, stress fracture or avascular change of the sesamoid as a cause of pain is unlikely. Sesamoiditis is a common cause of pain. Other possible causes include synovitis, osteonecrosis, and stress fracture.

Treatment

Sesamoid pain should be treated conservatively by the use of anti-inflammatory medications and a low-heeled soft-soled shoe with a metatarsal support to relieve the force on the sesamoid area.

If fracture or collapse of the sesamoid occurs, a single sesamoid may be removed. The tibial sesamoid is easily removed through a medial plantar incision which is made on the non-weight-bearing surface. Great caution needs to be exercised to avoid damage to the plantar medial cutaneous nerve which runs along the medial aspect of the tibial sesamoid.

The fibular sesamoid should be removed through a dorsal approach in the first web space. The scar is on the dorsal side, away from the weight-bearing surface.

In the patient who has had a previous sesamoidectomy and now has pain in the remaining sesamoid, conservative management should be undertaken. If the pain persists and excision of the sesamoid is necessary, the possibility of a cock-up deformity developing because of lack of adequate reformation of the ligamentous tissue between the sesamoids and the base of the proximal phalanx may be a problem and should be carefully explained to the patient prior to operation.

Rheumatoid Arthritis

A major problem for patients with advanced rheumatoid arthritis involving the forefoot is metatarsalgia. As the metatarsophalangeal joints dislocate, the plantar fat pad is displaced distally, resulting in severe callus formation beneath the metatarsal heads. A severe hallux valgus deformity develops along with hammertoes.

Treatment

Conservative management of this problem, using the extra-depth shoe with a Plastizote liner, provides some patients with relief but, as the condition progresses, their level of pain becomes such that their ability to walk is severely impaired.

The goal of surgical treatment is to provide comfort during walking. This can be accomplished by resection of an appropriate amount of lesser toe metatarsal heads and arthrodesis of the first metatarsophalangeal joint. The hammering can be corrected by manipulation.

Use of a double-ended prosthesis for the first metatarsophalangeal joint may have a place in the treatment of the rheumatoid foot, but this would be mainly with the milder deformities in which adequate capsular tissue is present to hold the great toe in satisfactory realignment. The stability of the prosthesis is based not on the prosthesis itself but on the ability of the surgeon to reconstruct the surrounding soft tissues.

The management of the hindfoot in rheumatoid arthritis should be somewhat aggressive. Once it begins to show significant deterioration and loss of weight-bearing alignment, arthrodesis of the involved joint or joints is desirable before the foot becomes severely deformed. This is particularly useful at the talonavicular joint where early fusion will produce stabilization of the longitudinal arch of the foot and thus prevent further collapse of the midfoot region.

Heel Pain

Various causes have been proposed for pain about the heel.

1. Pain proximal to the tubercle of the calcaneus may be secondary to atrophy of the plantar fat pad or, possibly, a stress fracture. Treatment should be directed toward adequate padding for the former and immobilization for the latter. Bone scanning is helpful in the diagnosis.

2. Pain over the tubercle of the calcaneus may be secondary to a plantar fasciitis or, possibly, a tear at the origin of the plantar fascia. Treatment for this condition should be conservative, consisting of anti-inflammation medications, strapping, occasionally casting, and possibly shoe modification. Very rarely is a surgical procedure of any significant benefit to these patients.

3. Pain may be referred to the heel area secondary to an entrapment, possibly of the lateral plantar nerve or one of its terminal branches as it passes beneath the abductor hallucis origin, along its course adjacent to the medial edge of the plantar aponeurosis, or in the space on the plantar aspect of the foot between the plantar aponeurosis and the calcaneus. In these cases the diagnosis is often made when palpation at the origin of the abductor hallucis reproduces the pain on the plantar aspect of the foot. These patients usually respond to anti-inflammation medications, immobilization, or local steroid injections. On occasion, surgical release of the origin of the abductor hallucis or the plantar fascia, to decompress the lateral plantar nerve and its terminal branches, may result in a satisfactory clinical response, but this type of operation is rarely indicated except in extremely refractory cases. Medial calcaneal neurectomy is not a recommended procedure because it may result in a numb heel and painful neuroma.

4. Refractory pain in spite of previous surgical treatment frequently is due to disruption of one of the medial calcaneal branches or to partial disruption of the lateral plantar nerve. Clinically, these patients have exquisite tenderness in the area of the surgically induced neuroma. Anti-inflammation medications, adequate immobilization, local injections of a steroid in the area of the neuroma, use of a transcutaneous nerve stimulator, and, on occasion, use of a polypropylene ankle-foot orthosis may be tried. If all conservative management fails, surgical exploration of the area may be of benefit.

5. Other reported causes of heel pain include lumbar disk disease, peripheral neuritis secondary to diabetes mellitus, gout (rare), and Reiter's syndrome. In these refractory cases, a bone scan may aid in the diagnosis.

Tendons About the Foot and Ankle

The tendons about the foot and ankle are balanced to produce a plantigrade foot. Dysfunction of one of these tendons, as a consequence of trauma, attrition, or stroke, may disrupt this balance. Although the overall strength of the plantar flexors is approximately 6 times that of the dorsiflexors and that of the evertors is greater than that of the invertors, a balanced foot is maintained. Neurologic function is important in this balancing. If a tendon is lost secondary to a degenerative process, an imbalance is created.

Tendon Dysfunction

Posterior tibial tendon dysfunction occasionally occurs after nonspecific trauma and can cause a progressive flatfoot deformity. The patient notes progressive loss of height of the arch and medial pain. As the deformity increases, subfibular impingement can occur. On examination the arch of the involved foot is flatter and, when viewed from the rear, more toes are exposed on the lateral aspect of the involved foot than on the uninvolved foot. Patients may or may not be able to perform a single leg heel raise but, once on their tiptoes, may be able to maintain this position. Thickening of the tendon may be noted. A defect in the tendon is occasionally palpable when the patient is asked to invert the hindfoot.

Because the excursion of the posterior tibial tendon is about 2 cm, an intratendinous tear resulting in lengthening by 1 cm or more may produce a significant degree of weakness.

Conservative management consists of use of a supportive orthosis. If the deformity is fixed, an orthosis is less helpful except to cushion the prominent talonavicular joint.

If symptoms are severe, several surgical options are available. Synovitis about the tibialis posterior tendon that does not respond to nonoperative measures may be treated by synovectomy. For complete rupture of the tibialis posterior tendon, several options are available: reconstruction of the tibialis posterior using either the flexor digitorum longus or the flexor hallucis longus; bony stabilization by subtalar arthrodesis; talonavicular arthrodesis; or triple arthrodesis. Although satisfactory in terms of pain relief, reconstruction of the tendon does not correct the deformity. The site of the arthrodesis is determined by the site of the maximum deformity. If severe valgus of the hindfoot is present, subtalar arthrodesis may be satisfactory. If the talonavicular joint appears to be significantly subluxed, isolated fusion of the talonavicular joint would be of benefit. However, if the entire foot is involved, triple arthrodesis would be the treatment of choice.

Tendon Lacerations

There is general agreement that lacerations of the tendons about the ankle should be repaired surgically. Repair of lacerations within the plantar aspect of the foot or the dorsum of the foot is controversial.

On the dorsum of the foot the extensor hallucis longus tendon probably should be repaired surgically. Lesser toe extensors probably can be treated with a course of immobilization for 6 weeks with the foot in dorsiflexion. A laceration of the flexor hallucis longus probably should be repaired surgically. Loss of flexor function of the lesser toes can be treated conservatively because attempts at repair may result in a painful scar and possible neuroma formation in the plantar nerves.

Ankle Ligaments

During the clinical evaluation, it is important to learn how the injury happened because from this information the ligament(s) that has been disrupted may be identified. Most commonly the anterior talofibular ligament is injured. With further deformity, tears of the calcaneofibular ligament occur. In rare cases, the entire ligamentous complex is ruptured.

The vast majority of these injuries can be treated nonoperatively, but the presence of associated injuries must be ruled out carefully. Primary repair is necessary infrequently. There are many reconstruction options for patients with definite recurrent instability. However, accurate assessment preoperatively is mandatory because "weak ankle" is not always due to lateral instability.

Ankle Arthrodesis

Many techniques are available for ankle arthrodesis. Rates of complications and nonunion vary greatly. Regardless of type of fixation, smooth broad surfaces of raw bone must be created and apposed.

Positioning of an arthrodesed ankle should be optimal in neutral dorsiflexion and in plantar flexion and in 5° of heel valgus. The feet should be symmetric in terms of external and internal rotation.

Degenerative Arthritis of the Subtalar Joint

Arthritis of the subtalar joint usually occurs after trauma. Spontaneous arthrosis is rare. If the degenerative process is limited to the subtalar joint, subtalar arthrodesis will produce a satisfactory result. After subtalar arthrodesis, degenerative changes at the calcaneocuboid or talonavicular joint are unusual. Some lipping may develop on the dorsal aspect of the talus but it is thought to be a result of traction on the joint capsule by the increased stress after a subtalar arthrodesis, not degenerative lipping.

The subtalar fusion should be positioned so that approximately 5° to 7° of valgus is achieved.

Tarsal Coalitions

Although tarsal coalitions usually are looked on as a problem of adolescents, adults also are affected. The incidence of tarsal coalition in the general population is not known with certainty, but several studies have indicated that the incidence of asymptomatic tarsal coalition is high in relatives of patients with a symptomatic coalition. Computed tomographic scanning has been helpful in diagnosis.

If the patient has an isolated coalition involving the middle or posterior facet that is not resectable, a subtalar fusion alone is adequate. The presence of talar beaking which may represent a traction spur does not preclude the use of an isolated fusion. For the patient who has a calcaneonavicular bar but the remainder of the subtalar joint appears to be uninvolved, resection of the bar, even in the adult, may give a satisfactory clinical result.

Charcot-Marie-Tooth Disease

Charcot-Marie-Tooth disease, a hereditary condition of variable penetrance, may cause significant deformities of the foot. Although the more severe cases are treated in childhood and late adolescence, some patients do not become symptomatic until adulthood. Variable combinations of hindfoot varus, adduction of the forefoot, plantar flexion of the first, second, and sometimes third metatarsals, and contracture of the plantar aponeurosis (forefoot equinus) occur as a result of muscle imbalance and secondary contracture.

Treatment

Because the severity of deformity and combinations of deformities are variable, care must be individualized.

For the severe deformity, corrective triple arthrodesis is necessary. The "beak" type is successful because it will lower the longitudinal arch by placing the navicular bone under a notch in the talus. This also corrects the forefoot equinus.

If the deformity is less severe, a Dwyer osteotomy of the calcaneus to correct the heel varus, release of the plantar fascia, and dorsal flexion osteotomy of the first and possibly the second and third metatarsals to correct the forefoot equinus can be performed.

In the forefoot, the hammer great toe can be corrected by arthrodesis of its interphalangeal joint with transfer of the extensor hallucis longus into the neck of the first metatarsal. The profound clawing of the lesser toes can be treated by release of the dorsal capsule and extensor tendons and of the flexor digitorum longus and flexor digitorum brevis. Arthrodesis or resection arthroplasty of the interphalangeal joint allows correction of more severe deformities.

Accessory Navicular Bone

The accessory navicular bone varies in size but is in intimate contact with the tibialis posterior tendon at its insertion into the tarsal navicular. After significant trauma to the foot, such as from tripping or twisting, pain may begin. Initial treatment by immobilization and anti-inflammatory medication is appropriate. If the pain persists and is well localized to the area of the accessory navicular bone, it can be excised and the posterior tibial tendon plicated.

Annotated Bibliography

Biomechanics

Perry, J.: Anatomy and biomechanics of the hindfoot. Clin. Orthop. 177:9-15, 1983.

This summary of the biomechanics of the hindfoot during foot support points out that the subtalar joint experiences rapid eversion at heel strike and inversion at terminal stance. Although being one of energy absorption, this action places stress on the local soft tissues and controlling muscles. This stress is accentuated by increased activities such as running, and this can lead to clinical problems.

Acquired Disorders

Ankle

Ankle Fusion

Morgan, C.D.; Henke, J.A.; Bailey, R.W.; and Kaufer, H.: Long-term results of tibiotalar arthrodesis. J. Bone Joint Surg. 67A:546-550, 1985.

A review of 101 ankle fusions with a mean follow-up of 10 years. Use of cancellous compression screws gave a 95% fusion rate. An average increase in tarsal motion postoperatively of 11° was found.

Scranton, P.E., Jr.: Use of internal compression in arthrodesis of the ankle. J. Bone Joint Surg. 67A:550-555, 1985.

A series of 25 patients underwent ankle arthrodesis with a T compression plate mortised into the anteromedial aspect of the tibia; two screws fixed the talus. The fusion rate was 100%.

Stewart, M.J.; Beeler, T.C.; and McConnell, J.C.: Compression arthrodesis of the ankle: Evaluation of a cosmetic modification. J. Bone Joint Surg. 65A:219-225, 1983.

Twenty-eight patients underwent an ankle arthrodesis in which a portion of the medial and lateral sides of the ankle was removed through anteromedial and anterolateral incisions, thereby narrowing the ankle joint. The articular surfaces were likewise removed, and a compression device was used to hold the position. A 93% fusion rate was achieved but, more importantly, the ankle joint was narrowed, thereby eliminating irritation and abrasion of the soft tissues beneath the malleoli against the top of the shoe.

Chronic Ankle Instability

Anderson, M.E.: Reconstruction of the lateral ligaments of the ankle using the plantaris tendon. J. Bone Joint Surg. 67A:930-934, 1985.

Nine patients underwent reconstruction of the lateral collateral ligaments with the plantaris tendon. All patients had good results and there was no significant loss of the ankle or subtalar joint.

Evans, G.A.; Hardcastle, P.; and Frenyo, A.D.: Acute rupture of the lateral ligament of the ankle: To suture or not to suture? J. Bone Joint Surg. 66B:209-212, 1984.

One hundred patients with acute ruptures of the lateral ankle ligaments randomly underwent conservative treatment (plaster cast) or operative repair. In each group there were 30 patients with isolated anterior talofibular ruptures and 20 with additional calcaneofibular ruptures. The operative repair was associated with a higher incidence of complications in the first week and a slight delay in the patient's return to work. Two years later there was no evidence that the operative repair offered improved symptomatic or functional benefit.

Orava, S.; Jaroma, H.; Weitz, H.; Loikkanen, T.; and Suvela, M.: Radiographic instability of the ankle joint after Evan's repair. Acta Orthop. Scand. 54:734-738, 1983.

Forty-two unstable ankle joints were treated surgically by Evan's operation. At 6-month follow-up, clinical and radiologic examinations demonstrated that 18 patients had an anterior drawer sign radiologically, but this correlated poorly with the subjective end result. Clinically, only four patients were noted to have persistent instability.

Snook, G.A., Chrisman, O.D.; and Wilson, T.C.: Long term results of the Chrisman-Snook operation for reconstruction of the lateral ligaments of the ankle. J. Bone Joint Surg. 67A:1-7, 1985.

A long-term evaluation of 57 patients with a follow-up of 10 years demonstrated good lateral ankle stability, but about half the patients had some loss of inversion of the subtalar joint.

St. Pierre, R.K.; Andrews, L.; Allman, F.; and Fleming, L.L.: The Cybex II evaluation of lateral ankle ligamentous reconstructions. Am. J. Sports Med. 12:52-56, 1984.

The eversion strength at approximately 4 years after Chrisman-Snook reconstructions in 10 patients and Evan's lateral ligamentous reconstructions in 10 patients was evaluated compared to the uninvolved side. At slow speeds the strengths were 7% and 4% weaker, respectively. At higher speeds they were 9% and 8% weaker, respectively.

Van Der Rijt, A.J., and Evans, G.A.: The long-term results of Watson-Jones tenodesis. J. Bone Joint Surg. 66B:371-375, 1984.

Of nine patients with a mean follow-up of 22 years after the Watson-Jones tenodesis, only three had complete relief of symptoms. Two initial good results deteriorated by 7 and 10 years after the operation. Radiographic examination demonstrated persistent laxity in seven of the nine.

Foot

Gould, N.: Surgery in advanced Charcot-Marie-Tooth disease. Foot Ankle 4:267-273, 1984.

In a study of 10 cases (18 feet) with a 5-year follow-up, the mobility of the foot was maintained by carrying out plantar fasciotomy, Dwyer calcaneal osteotomy, dorsiflexion metatarsal osteotomy, and first toe Jones procedure rather than a triple arthrodesis.

Jahss, M.H.: Evaluation of the cavus foot for orthopedic treatment. Clin. Orthop. 181:52-63, 1983.

The article stresses careful evaluation of the cavus foot and maintaining flexibility when possible rather than sacrificing joint motion by carrying out an arthrodesis. Tendon transfers are often necessary to help balance muscle power in flexible joints.

Samilson, R.L., and Dillin, W.: Cavus, cavovarus and calcaneocavus: An update. Clin. Orthop. 177:125-132, 1983.

The article emphasizes the need for careful search for the cause, particularly intraspinal and especially in children. Surgical correction should be by soft tissue procedures when possible, particularly in the young patient, and by bony procedures in the older patient. Triple arthrodesis is a salvage operation for correcting cavus.

Siffert, R.S., and del Torto, U.: "Beak" triple arthrodesis for severe cavus deformity. Clin. Orthop. 181:64-67, 1983.

The article describes a 20-year experience with the "beak" type of triple arthrodesis for correction of the cavus deformity—depressing the anterior aspect of the foot by placing the navicular bone beneath the head of the talus.

Hallux Valgus

Clinical Assessment

Smith, R.W.; Reynolds, J.C.; and Stewart, M.J.: Hallux valgus assessment: Report of research committee of American Orthopaedic Foot and Ankle Society. Foot Ankle 5:92-103, 1984.

A literature review pertaining to the clinical and radiographic assessment of hallux valgus in an attempt to standardize the reporting of series with hallux valgus deformities.

Postoperative Complications

Johnson, K.A., and Spiegl, P.V.: Extensor hallucis longus transfer for hallux varus deformity. J. Bone Joint Surg. 66A:681-686, 1984.

Hallux varus results from a dynamic imbalance and most frequently occurs after McBride type procedures. The authors corrected the imbalance by transferring the extensor hallucis longus beneath the first intermetatarsal ligament into the base of the proximal phalanx, along with arthrodesis of the interphalangeal joint.

Kinnard, P., and Gordon, D.: A comparison between chevron and Mitchell osteotomies for hallux valgus. Foot Ankle 4:241-243, 1984.

Review of 15 Mitchell and 15 chevron osteotomies demonstrated satisfactory clinical results although there was a 40% incidence of lateral metatarsalgia secondary to altered weightbearing after the operation.

Lemon, R.A.; Engber, W.D.; and McBeath, A.A.: A complication of Silastic hemiarthroplasty in bunion surgery. Foot Ankle 4:262-266, 1984.

Seven cases of reactive synovitis after Silastic hemiarthroplasty are described. Abrasion of the Silastic implant creates floating silicone elastomer particles that may precipitate a reactive synovitis.

Meier, P.J., and Kenzora, J.E.: The risks and benefits of distal first metatarsal osteotomies. Foot Ankle 6:7-17, 1985.

After chevron osteotomy, 12 of 60 patients had varying degrees of osteonecrosis; after Mitchell bunionectomy 1 of 12 had osteonecrosis of the metatarsal head. There was a 30% incidence of damage to the proper digital nerve of the great toe.

Fusion

Chana, G.S.; Andrew, T.A.; and Cotterill, C.P.: A simple method of arthrodesis of the first metatarsophalangeal joint. J. Bone Joint Surg. 66B:703-705, 1984.

Eighty-seven first metatarsophalangeal joint arthrodeses were carried out with a 90% union rate and 94% rate of good and excellent subjective results. Fixation of the arthrodesis site was by chromic catgut.

Riggs, S.A., Jr., and Johnson, E.W., Jr.: McKeever arthrodesis for the painful hallux. Foot Ankle 3:248-253, 1983.

In 206 patients who had arthrodesis, with a mean follow-up of 15 years, 92% were without pain, 98% were wearing dress shoes of choice, and 86% were satisfied. The complication rate was 8%.

Arthritis

Beauchamp, C.G.; Kirby, T.; Rudge, S.R.; Worthington, B.S.; and Nelson, J.: Fusion of the first metatarsophalangeal joint in forefoot arthroplasty. Clin. Orthop. 190:249-253, 1984.

The results of 64 arthroplasties in 37 patients demonstrated that fusion produced a better cosmetic appearance and improved overall balance. Pedobarography demonstrated that relatively more weight was transmitted through the first ray after a fusion than after a resection.

Kampner, S.L.: Total joint prosthetic arthoplasty of the great toe—A 12-year experience. Foot Ankle 4:249-261, 1984.

The experience in 103 cases in which double-stem, flexible, hinged, silicone implants were used as a total joint replacement for the first metatarsophalangeal joint is reported. The mean follow-up was 7.4 years. The indications were osteoarthritis and rheumatoid arthritis. Overall results were good.

Mann, R.A., and Thompson, F.M.: Arthrodesis of the first metatarsophalangeal joint for hallux valgus in rheumatoid arthritis. J. Bone Joint Surg. 66A:687-692, 1984.

Eighteen fusions were carried out for rheumatoid arthritis, with a mean follow-up of 4.1 years. The fusion rate was 94%. The arthrodesis provided stability of the first metatarsophalangeal joint and, in combination with arthroplasties of the lesser metatarsophalangeal joints, relieved the patients' metatarsalgia.

Heel Pain

Baxter, D.E., and Thigpen, C.M.: Heel pain—Operative results. Foot Ankle 5:16-25, 1984.

An operative procedure was described involving neurolysis of a mixed nerve supplying the abductor digiti minimi pedis as it passes beneath the abductor hallucis and beneath the medial ridge of the calcaneus. The deep fascia of the abductor hallucis is released routinely, and any impinging heel spur or tight plantar fascia is partially removed or released if it is contributing to the nerve entrapment. Of the 34 patients, 32 had good results and 2 had poor results.

Bordelon, R.L.: Subcalcaneal pain: A method of evaluation and plan for treatment. Clin. Orthop. 177:49-53, 1983.

The author stresses that evaluation of subcalcaneal pain should be based on anatomic factors that produce the abnormality. If patients fail to respond to conservative management, a surgical procedure that includes release of the nerve entrapment, release of the plantar fascia, and excision of the bone spur is advocated.

Graham, C.E.: Painful heel syndrome: Rationale of diagnosis and treatment. Foot Ankle 3:261-267, 1983.

In 97.7% of cases of heel pain, the bone scan was positive on the side of the pain. Radiographs at a 45° angle on the medial side demonstrated bony condensation which was interpreted as a fatigue fracture.

Henricson, A.S., and Westlin, N.E.: Chronic calcaneal pain in athletes: Entrapment of the calcaneal nerve? Am. J. Sports Med. 12:152-154, 1984.

A surgical release is described for entrapment of the calcaneal branches of the tibial nerve. A satisfactory result was achieved in 10 of 11 heels.

Lesser Toe Deformities

Barbari, S.G., and Brevig, K.: Correction of clawtoes by the Girdlestone-Taylor flexor-extensor transfer procedure. Foot Ankle 5:67-73, 1984.

Evaluation of 39 feet in 31 patients with a mean follow-up of 38 months is presented. The procedure resulted in reduction of metatarsalgia and callosities and improved shape of the toes. The authors believe that more radical procedures are rarely acceptable, for cosmetic as well as functional reasons.

Tendons

Degeneration

Johnson, K.A.: Tibialis posterior tendon rupture. Clin. Orthop. 177:140-147, 1983.

Rupture of the posterior tibial tendon occurs most commonly in adult women. It causes insidious, painful, and progressive flatfoot deformity. Treatment selection depends on the site and extent of the tendon disruption. Early treatment was advised to prevent long-term functional impairment.

Mann, R.A., and Thompson, F.M.: Rupture of the posterior tibial tendon causing flat foot. J. Bone Joint Surg. 67A:556-561, 1985.

In 19 adults with progressive flatfoot due to rupture of the posterior tibial tendon secondary to degenerative changes, reconstruction was carried out by using the flexor digitorum longus.

Lacerations

Floyd, D.W.; Heckman, J.D.; and Rockwood, C.A., Jr.: Tendon lacerations in the foot. Foot Ankle 4:8-14, 1983.

From retrospective review of 46 patients with various tendon lacerations about the foot and ankle, it was concluded that, when feasible, the flexor hallucis longus and extensor hallucis longus should be repaired, whereas the lesser extensor and flexor tendons probably do not require surgical repair.

Accessory Navicular Bone

Lawson, J.P.; Ogden, J.A.; Sella, E.; and Barwick, K.W.: The painful accessory navicular. Skeletal Radiol. 12:250-262, 1984.

Two types of accessory navicular bones are noted: 1) sesamoid bone within the posterior tibial tendon, which is anatomically separate from the navicular; and 2) accessory ossification center medial to the navicular. The latter may be associated with a painful foot after trauma. Histologic examination of the surgically excised specimen revealed inflammatory chondro-osseous changes.

MacNicol, M.F., and Voutsinas, S.: Surgical treatment of the symptomatic accessory navicular. J. Bone Joint Surg. 66B:218-226, 1984.

Treatments of 62 symptomatic accessory navicular bones by the Kidner operation with rerouting of the posterior tibial tendon insertion and by excision of the ossicle were compared. Excision was as effective as the Kidner technique. They proposed that correction of the associated flatfoot was secondary to growth and maturation of the foot rather than to the operation.

Ray, S., and Goldberg, V.M.: Surgical treatment of the accessory navicular. Clin. Orthop. 177:61-66, 1983.

The authors report on the treatment of 29 symptomatic accessory navicular bones treated surgically; good or excellent results were obtained in 26. The treatment consisted of excision of the accessory navicular and suturing of the fibers of the posterior tibial tendon to the inferior surface of the navicular.

Tarsal Coalitions

Mosier, K.M., and Asher, M.: Tarsal coalitions and peroneal spastic flatfoot. J. Bone Joint Surg. 66A:976-984, 1984.

A review of all aspects of tarsal coalitions is presented. The talocalcaneal joint is involved slightly more often than the calcaneonavicular joint. Radiographic diagnosis and treatment are discussed in detail.

Storemont, D.M., and Peterson, H.A.: The relative incidence of tarsal coalition. Clin. Orthop. 181:28-36, 1983.

The overall incidence is far less than 1% in the general population. Calcaneonavicular coalition is the most common, at 53%; talocalcaneal coalitions are seen in 37%.

Swiontkowski, M.F.; Scranton, P.E.; and Hansen, S.: Tarsal coalitions: Long-term results of surgical treatment. J. Pediatr. Orthop. 3:287-292, 1983.

Ten patients underwent talocalcaneal coalitions with four successful resections; the remainder underwent arthrodeses. Among 39 patients with calcaneonavicular coalitions treated with calcaneonavicular resections and 5 treated with primary triple arthrodesis, results were satisfactory in all but 2. The authors point out that the talar "beak" is not necessarily a degenerative spur but rather a traction process secondary to increased motion.

Index

Page numbers in italics indicate illustrations.